Simon's Emergency Orthopedics

Simon's Emergency Orthopedics

Eighth Edition

Editor

Scott C. Sherman, MD
Associate Professor of Emergency Medicine
Rush Medical College
Associate Residency Director
Department of Emergency Medicine
Cook County (Stroger) Hospital
Chicago, Illinois

With illustrations by Susan Gilbert and Catherine Delphia

Mc
Graw
Hill
Education

New York Chicago San Francisco Lisbon London Madrid Mexico City
Milan New Delhi San Juan Seoul Singapore Sydney Toronto

This book was set in Adobe Garamond by Aptara, Inc.
The editors were Amanda Fielding and Christie Naglieri.
The production supervisor was Richard Ruzycka.
Project management was provided by Dinesh Pokhriyal, Aptara, Inc.
The cover designer was Randomatrix.

Library of Congress Cataloging-in-Publication Data

Names: Sherman, Scott C., editor.
Title: Simon's emergency orthopedics / editor, Scott C. Sherman.
Other titles: Emergency orthopedics (Simon)
Description: Eighth edition. | New York : McGraw-Hill, 2019. | Includes
  bibliographical references and index.
Identifiers: LCCN 2017058973 (print) | LCCN 2017060216 (ebook) | ISBN
  9781259860836 ISBN 9781259860829 (adhesive - hard)
Subjects: | MESH: Extremities—injuries | Spinal Injuries—therapy | Wounds
  and Injuries—therapy | Orthopedic Procedures—methods | Emergency
  Medicine—methods
Classification: LCC RD750 (ebook) | LCC RD750 (print) | NLM WE 800 | DDC
  617.5/8044—dc23
LC record available at https://na01.safelinks.protection.outlook.com/?url=https%3A%2F%2Flccn.loc.
gov%2F2017058973&data=01%7C01%7Cleah.carton%40mheducation.com%7Cecbd6d03919142
1fbdad08d548683acd%7Cf919b1efc0c347358fca0928ec39d8d5%7C0&sdata=xVQM0lQVufg%
2FR0VGZuno8FERHZWWtMRjsTvPimjjCXc%3D&reserved=0

To Dad, his greatest joy was spending time with his family.
— S.C. Sherman —

CONTENTS

PREFACE

A multitude of texts and publications currently exist directed at the "ER doc." The "ER doc" has rapidly been replaced by a new physician who practices only emergency medicine. No current orthopedics text is directed at this physician. As emergency medicine has developed, there must evolve a cooperative relationship between the orthopedic surgeon and the "emergentologist" based on acknowledging the experience and expertise of one another to make prudent decisions and to recognize areas beyond the limitations of each practitioner. It is this spirit that permeates this text.

Currently available publications can be divided into two groups: those that are directed to the orthopedic surgeon and those that, although supposedly directed toward a more advanced audience, are in reality directed to the junior medical student. When one considers that disorders and injuries to the extremities compose more than 50% of what the emergency physician will see and that, initially, he or she will see more acute injuries than will the orthopedic surgeon, can it be acceptable to give only bits of information rather than the full range of mechanism of injury, treatment, associated injuries, and complications of a particular fracture or injury?

—Orthopedics in Emergency Medicine, 1982

More than 35 years later, this quote makes me marvel at the accomplishments of our specialty, and at the same time, believe that there is work left to be done. This eighth edition represents the second opportunity for individual authors to contribute to each and every chapter. Their insights have added significantly to the quality of the material within these pages. Other additions include new clinical photos, radiographs, and videos. As in previous editions, a fracture index is presented at the front of the book and continues to be a unique feature. The emergency clinician can look at figures of a fractured bone, select which one the patient has, and refer directly to the page where all pertinent information about that particular fracture is provided.

The body of the text is divided into four parts: Part I. Orthopedic Principles and Management; Part II. Spine; Part III. Upper Extremities; and Part IV. Lower Extremities. Part I includes chapters on general principles, including emergency splinting, the selection of definitive treatment, and indications for operative treatment. In addition, anesthesia and analgesia, rheumatology, complications, special imaging techniques, and pediatrics are discussed. Chapter 5, Special Imaging Techniques, has been significantly revised to include much more data on musculoskeletal ultrasound, a growing area of practice. Part II includes four chapters on the spine. Part III on the upper extremities includes six chapters, one each on the hand, wrist, forearm, elbow, upper arm, and shoulder. Part IV on the lower extremities includes chapters on the pelvis, hip, thigh, knee, leg, ankle, and foot. Each chapter is organized so fractures are covered first, followed by a discussion of soft-tissue injuries. We present a detailed discussion of each type of fracture, including, where appropriate, essential anatomy, mechanism of injury, examination, imaging, associated injuries, and treatment.

The Appendix describes and illustrates the steps involved in placing a particular type of splint. References to the Appendix are made throughout the text.

For all videos referenced in the book, please visit www.accessemergencymedicine.com/SimonsVideos.

ACKNOWLEDGMENTS

This edition, the eighth, is the second edition of the text retitled as *Simon's Emergency Orthopedics*, acknowledging the major contributions of the book's founding author and editor, Robert R. Simon, MD. I met Dr. Simon when I was a resident in emergency medicine at Cook County Hospital in 1999. Unlike some department chairs, Dr. Simon always preferred bedside teaching to any important meeting. And his bedside teaching in emergency orthopedics was the best I have ever experienced. His 2-day emergency orthopedics course was a highlight of the residency, and we are fortunate to have him continue to volunteer his time for this course annually so present and future residents in our program are not cheated of the same experience. When I was a young faculty member, Dr. Simon was always available to provide advice and counsel. In addition to career advice, he reminded me to reserve time for my family and, in particular, my wife. Dr. Simon is a true emergency medicine pioneer and leader in our field. It has been an honor to know him. No one is more loyal or hard working. As a mentor and friend, he has taught me more than I could ever repay.

Jeff Schaider, MD, our current chairman, has been supportive of me and this book from the beginning. Jeff is the consummate multitasker with the most positive attitude of anyone I know. It is a joy to be around him. He serves as my role model even though I know I will never match his abilities. Steve Bowman, MD, our residency program director, is the ultimate professional—a perfect example for our young resident physicians. He has carried the heavy load of the residency and allowed his assistants to explore their academic interests. In addition, the current and former residents in Emergency Medicine at Cook County deserve special mention. Their contributions and efforts do not go unnoticed. It is their drive to learn and serve their patients that pushes me to do better.

I want to further thank my colleagues/teachers/friends in Emergency Medicine. This includes members of the 2002 Cook County EM residency: Joseph Weber, Dan Belmont, Carolyn Clayton, Marc Doucette, Stuart Feldman, Danish Haque, Craig Huston, Tom Kirages, Anita Kulkarni, Ann Nguyen, Rahul Patwari, Martin Pitts, Yanina Purim-Shem-Tov, Andy Skoubis, Courtney Wilemon, and Daniel Wu. Also, I would like to thank Connie Greene, Lauren Grossman, Shari Schabowski, Erik Nordquist, Shayle Miller, Ardena Flippin, Eric Reichman, Tricia Lanter, Chris Ross, Sharon Southe, Dave Levine, Dave Harter, Mark Kling, Mike McDermitt, Moses Lee, Leon Gussow, Isam Nasr, Kevin Kern, Steve Aks, Sean Bryant, Mark Mycyk, Jenny Lu, Mike Schindlbeck, Tarlan Hedayati, Dhara Amin, Rosi Fernandez, Sean Dyer, Patrick Hoffman, Trevor Lewis, Rob Feldman, Rashid Kysia, Neeraj Chhabra, Mike Nelson, Rebecca Roberts, John Bailitz, Michelle Sergel, Helen Straus, Joanne Routsolias, Kip Adrian, Dave Anthony, John Mulligan, Lucy Hammerberg, Roy Horras, Jennifer Rodgers, Karen Cosby, Lauren Smith, Pilar Guerrero, Austen Chai, Lisa Palivos, Jordan Moskoff, Joe Palter, Linda Kampe, Velma Richmond, Judy Williams, Mishele Taylor, Patricia Taylor, Estella Bravo, Hilda Nino, Lolita Adams, and Ethel Lee.

I would also like to acknowledge several others who brought this project to fruition. First, our authors, practicing across the United States, provided their unique perspectives in each chapter. You did an outstanding job, and I cannot thank you enough for your efforts. I also appreciate the work of Jessica Gonzalez and Christie Naglieri, who reliably assisted in the early stages of author communications and editorial support, and Brian Belval, who was always available with sound and professional advice. I would not want to leave out Dinesh Pokhriyal whose attention to detail and timely responses put these pages together and kept the project on time. I also want to thank our artist, Jason McAlexander, for this edition of the book.

Lastly, and most importantly, I would like to say thank you to my wife, Michelle, for all of her love and support during this latest edition of the text. My two boys, Mason and Colin, setting a good example for you is my most important priority. I'm very proud of you both and love you with all my heart. And to my biggest fan, Mom, for always believing in me.

—**Scott C. Sherman, MD**

CONTRIBUTORS

Kim L. Askew, MD
Associate Professor and Associate Dean of Clinical Education
Emergency Medicine
Wake Forest School of Medicine
Salem, North Carolina

Hany Y. Atallah, MD
Associate Professor
Department of Emergency Medicine
Emory University
Chief and Medical Director
Emergency Medicine
Grady Health System
Atlanta, Georgia

Rachel R. Bengtzen, MD
Assistant Professor
Department of Emergency Medicine
Department of Family Medicine (Sports Medicine)
Oregon Health & Science University
Portland, Oregon

Andrea L. Blome, MD
Department of Emergency Medicine
Temple University Hospital
Philadelphia, Pennsylvania

Michael C. Bond, MD
Associate Professor
Residency Program Director
Department of Emergency Medicine
University of Maryland School of Medicine
Associate Designated Institutional Official and Vice Chair of
   the Graduate Education Committee
University of Maryland Medical Center
Baltimore, Maryland

George T. Chiampas, DO
Assistant Professor
Department of Emergency Medicine and Orthopedic Surgery
Northwestern University, Feinberg School of Medicine
Medical Director, Northwestern Medicine Community and
   Sports Even Preparedness Management
Director, Northwestern Medicine CCARES
Chicago, Illinois

Moira Davenport, MD
Associate Residency Director
Department of Emergency Medicine
Allegheny General Hospital/Temple University School
   of Medicine
Pittsburgh, Pennsylvania

Sean Dyer, MD
Instructor
Department of Emergency Medicine
Rush Medical College
Attending Physician/Faculty
Department of Emergency Medicine
Cook County Health and Hospital System
Chicago, Illinois

Joy L. English, MD
Assistant Professor
Department of Orthopaedics
University of Utah
Salt Lake City, Utah

Madison M. Galasso, MD
Allegheny General Hospital
Pittsburgh, Pennsylvania

Carl A. Germann, MD
Associate Professor
Tufts University School of Medicine
Assistant Residency Program Director
Department of Emergency Medicine
Maine Medical Center
Portland, Maine

Casey Glass, MD
Assistant Professor of Emergency Medicine
Department of Emergency Medicine
Wake Forest School of Medicine
Wake Forest Baptist Hospital
Winston Salem, North Carolina

Brook M. Goddard, MD
Department of Emergency Medicine
Maine Medical Center
Portland, Maine

Jonah C. Gunalda, MD
Assistant Professor
Emergency Medicine
Clerkship Co-director
University of Mississippi Medical Center
Jackson, Mississippi

Dennis Hanlon, MD
Associate Professor of Emergency Medicine
Drexel School of Medicine
Clinical Associate Professor of Emergency Medicine
Temple University School of Medicine
Quality Director of Emergency Medicine
Department of Emergency Medicine
Allegheny General Hospital
Pittsburgh, Pennsylvania

Megan E. Healy, MD
Assistant Professor
Department of Emergency Medicine
Lewis Katz School of Medicine at Temple University
Department of Emergency Medicine, Temple University
    Hospital
Philadelphia, Pennsylvania

Tarlan Hedayati, MD
Assistant Professor
Associate Program Director
Department of Emergency Medicine
Cook County Health & Hospitals System
Chicago, Illinois

Gregory W. Hendey, MD
Professor and Chair of Emergency Medicine
David Geffen School of Medicine at UCLA
Ronald Reagan-UCLA Medical Center
Los Angeles, California

Adnan Hussain, MD
Clinical Faculty
Resurrection Emergency Medicine Residency
Assistant Medical Director
Director of Quality and Patient Experience
Northwest Community Hospital
Chicago, Illinois

Usama Khalid, MD
Assistant Professor
Ultrasound Faculty, Department of Emergency Medicine
Emory University School of Medicine
Emory University Hospital Midtown
Atlanta VA Medical Center
Atlanta, Georgia

Zheng Ben Ma, MD
Department of Emergency Medicine
Harvard Medical School
Massachusetts General Hospital and Brigham and
    Women's Hospital
Boston, Massachusetts

Sanjeev Malik, MD
CAQ in Primary Care Sports Medicine
Assistant Professor
Department of Emergency Medicine
Feinberg School of Medicine
Northwestern University
Medical Director
Department of Emergency Medicine
Northwestern Memorial Hospital
Chicago, Illinois

David E. Manthey, MD
Professor
Emergency Medicine
Wake Forest School of Medicine
Salem, North Carolina

Jehangir Meer, MD
Assistant Professor
Emory University School of Medicine
Director of Ultrasound
Department of Emergency Medicine
Grady Memorial Hospital
Atlanta, Georgia

Emily Senecal Miller, MD
Assistant Professor
Department of Emergency Medicine
Harvard Medical School
Department of Emergency Medicine
Massachusetts General Hospital
Boston, Massachusetts

Christopher Morris, DO
Department of Emergency Medicine
Allegheny General Hospital
Pittsburgh, Pennsylvania

R. Darrell Nelson, MD
Associate Professor, Emergency Medicine
Program Director EMS and Disaster Fellowship Wake
    Forest University Health Sciences
Winston-Salem, North Carolina

Michael E. Nelson, MD
Clinical Assistant Professor
Department of Emergency Medicine
University of Chicago
Chicago, Illinois
Attending Physician
Emergency Medicine, Medical Toxicology and Addiction
    Medicine
NorthShore University Health System
Evanston, Illinois
Clinical Assistant Professor
Department of Emergency Medicine
Rush University
Chicago, Illinois
Attending Physician
Emergency Medicine and Medical Toxicology
Cook County Health and Hospital System
John H. Stroger Jr. Hospital
Chicago, Illinois

Erik K. Nordquist, MD
Assistant Professor
Department of Emergency Medicine
Texas Tech University Health Sciences Center El Paso /
    Paul L. Foster School of Medicine
El Paso, Texas

Adriana Segura Olson, MD
Assistant Professor
Department of Emergency Medicine
University of Texas Health San Antonio
San Antonio, Texas

Andrew D. Perron, MD
Professor and Residency Program Director
Department of Emergency Medicine
Maine Medical Center
Portland, Maine

Ghazala Q. Sharieff, MD
Clinical Professor
University of California
Corporate Vice President, Chief Experience Officer
Scripps Health
San Diego, California

Alexander P. Skog, MD
Department of Emergency Medicine
Oregon Health & Science University
Portland, Oregon

Jacob Stelter, MD
McGaw Medical Center of Northwestern University
Chicago, Illinois

Todd Taylor, MD
Assistant Professor, Emergency Medicine
    Emory School of Medicine
Emory University
Grady Memorial Hospital
Atlanta, Georgia

Eric Toth, DO
Department of Emergency Medicine
Michigan State University College of Osteopathic Medicine
McLaren Oakland Hospital
Pontiac, Michigan

James Webley, MD
Clinical Assistant Professor
Michigan State University
McLaren Oakland Hospital
Pontiac, Michigan

Fracture Index

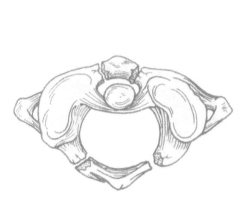

Figure 9–8. Jefferson fracture. **See page 161**.

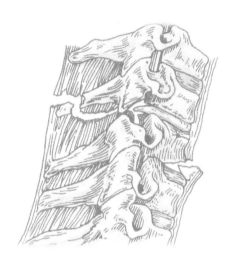

Figure 9–14. Flexion teardrop fracture. **See page 163**.

Type I   Type II   Type III

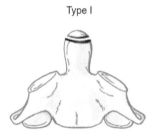 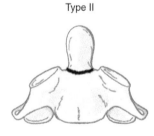 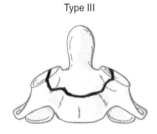

Figure 9–11. Odontoid fractures. **See page 162**.

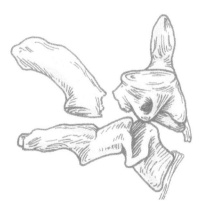

Figure 9–13. Hangman's fracture. **See page162**.

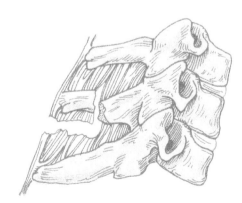

Figure 9–15. Clay shoveler's fracture. **See page 163**.

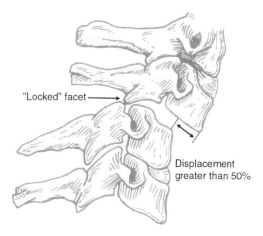

Figure 9–16. Bilateral facet dislocation. **See page 164**.

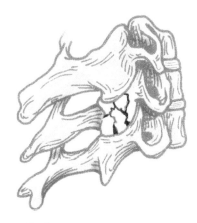

Figure 9–21. Pillar fracture. **See page 166**.

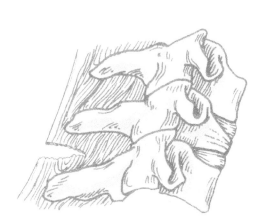

Figure 9–17. Wedge compression fracture. **See page 164**.

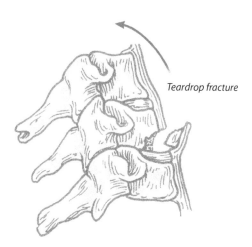

Figure 9–24. Extension teardrop fracture. **See page 167**.

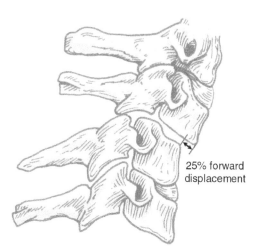

Figure 9–20. Unilateral facet dislocation. **See page 165**.

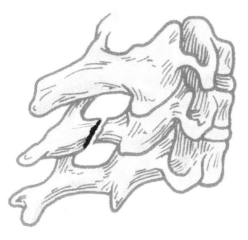

Figure 9–25. Laminar fracture. **See page 167**.

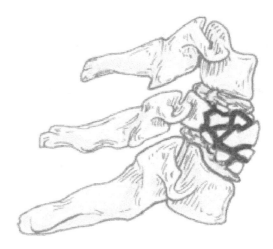

Figure 9–26. Burst fracture. **See page 168**.

CHAPTER 10 THORACOLUMBAR SPINE TRAUMA

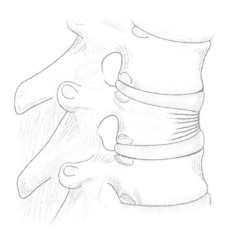

Figure 10–2. An anterior wedge compression fracture. **See page 171**.

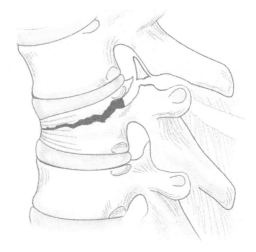

Figure 10–6. Chance fracture. **See page 172**.

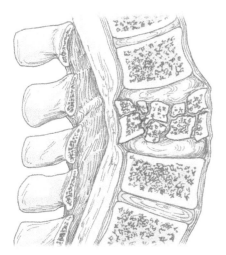

Figure 10–4. A burst fracture. **See page 171**.

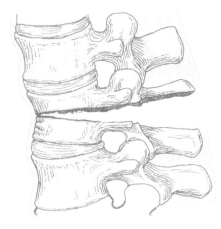

Figure 10–7. Flexion-distraction injury. **See page 173**.

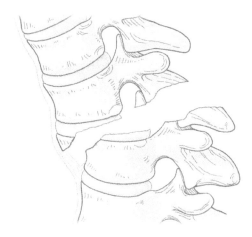

Figure 10–8. Fracture-dislocation (translational) injury due to a shearing force. **See page 173**.

CHAPTER 11 HAND

Longitudinal

Transverse

Comminuted

Transverse
with displacement

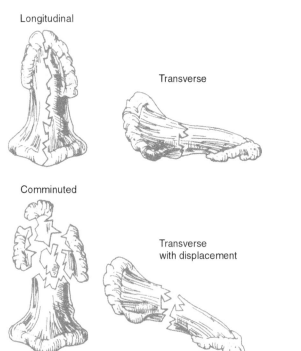

Figure 11–18. Extra-articular phalanx fractures. **See page 189**.

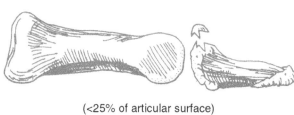

(<25% of articular surface)

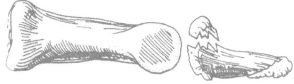

(>25% of articular surface)

Figure 11–24. Intra-articular distal phalanx avulsion fractures—dorsal surface. **See page 191**.

Volar avulsion fracture

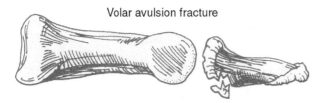

Figure 11–29. Intra-articular distal avulsion fracture—volar surface. **See page 192**.

Nondisplaced transverse

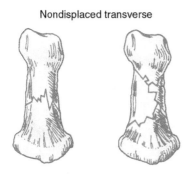

Displaced or angulated

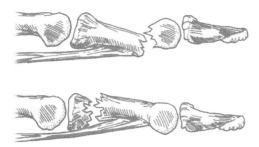

Spiral

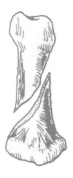

Figure 11–33. Middle phalanx fractures—extra-articular. **See page 194**.

Nondisplaced condylar	Displaced condylar	Comminuted basilar

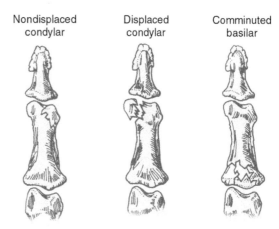

Figure 11–34. Middle phalanx fractures—intra-articular. **See page 195**.

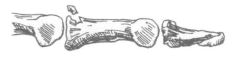

Avulsion fracture extensor surface

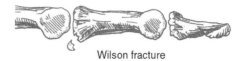

Wilson fracture

Collateral ligament avulsion fracture

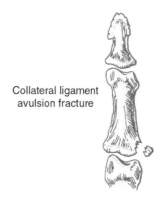

Figure 11–36. Middle phalanx fractures—avulsion. **See page 195**.

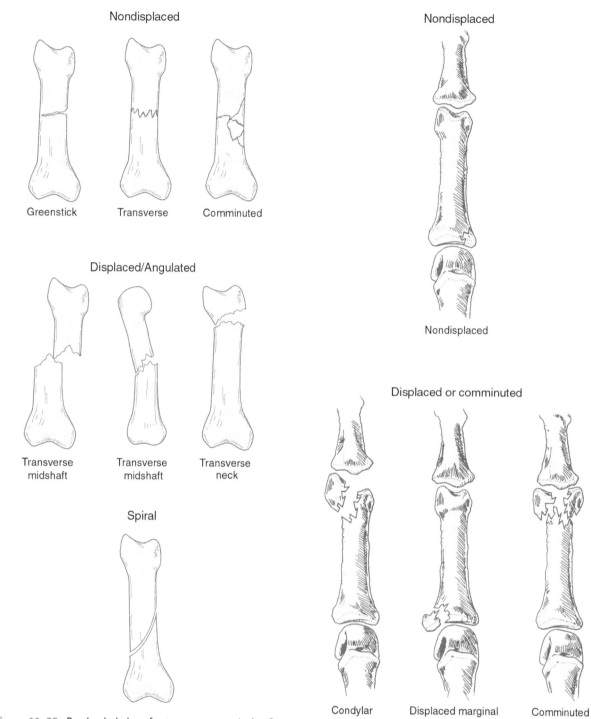

Nondisplaced

Greenstick   Transverse   Comminuted

Displaced/Angulated

Transverse   Transverse   Transverse
midshaft   midshaft   neck

Spiral

Figure 11–38. Proximal phalanx fractures—extra-articular. **See page 197.**

Nondisplaced

Nondisplaced

Displaced or comminuted

Condylar   Displaced marginal   Comminuted

Figure 11–40. Proximal phalanx fractures—intra-articular. **See page 198.**

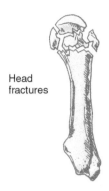

Head
fractures

Figure 11–43. Metacarpal fractures—head (2 through 5). **See page 199.**

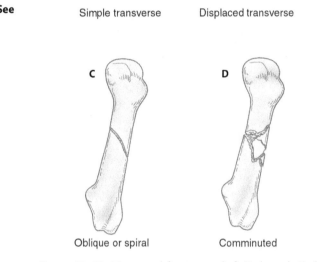

Simple transverse   Displaced transverse

Oblique or spiral   Comminuted

Figure 11–48. Metacarpal fractures—shaft (2 through 5). **See page 202.**

Neck fractures

Nondisplaced   Displaced or angulated

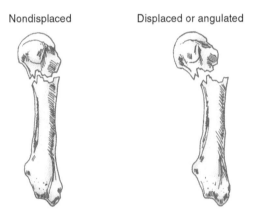

Figure 11–45. Metacarpal fractures—neck (2 through 5). **See page 200.**

Base fractures

Transverse   Comminuted   Avulsion

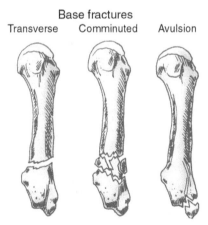

Figure 11–50. Metacarpal fractures—base (2 through 5). **See page 204.**

Transverse base fracture

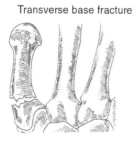

Transverse shaft fracture   Epiphyseal plate fracture
(in children)

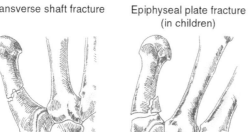

Figure 11–52. First metacarpal fractures—extra-articular. **See page 205**.

Intra-articular base fractures
Bennett fracture—dislocation

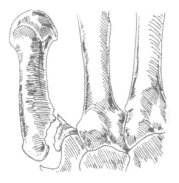

Rolando fracture

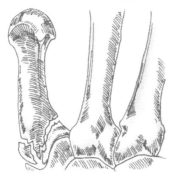

Figure 11–53. First metacarpal fractures—intra-articular. **See page 206**.

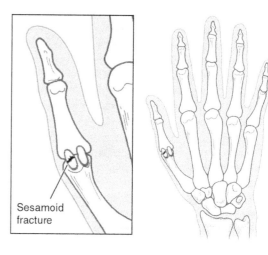

Figure 11–55. Thumb sesamoid fracture. **See page 207**.

CHAPTER 12 WRIST

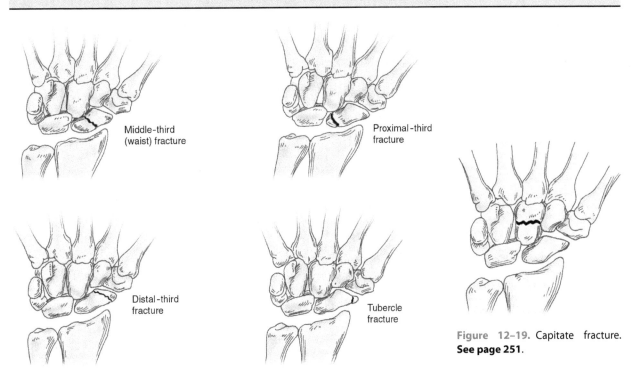

Middle-third
(waist) fracture

Proximal-third
fracture

Distal-third
fracture

Tubercle
fracture

Figure 12–19. Capitate fracture. **See page 251**.

Figure 12–12. Scaphoid fractures. **See page 247.**

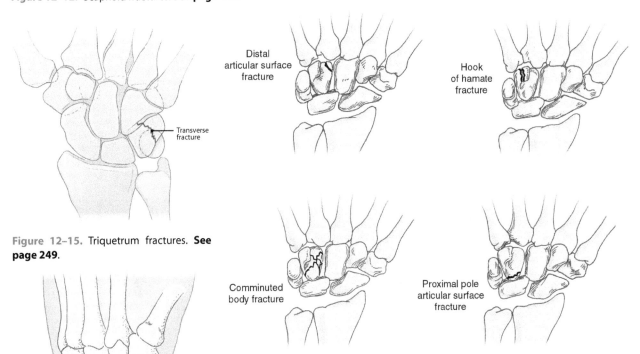

Transverse
fracture

Distal
articular surface
fracture

Hook
of hamate
fracture

Figure 12–15. Triquetrum fractures. **See page 249**.

Comminuted
body fracture

Proximal pole
articular surface
fracture

Figure 12–20. Hamate fractures. **See page 252.**

Figure 12–17. Lunate fracture. **See page 250.**

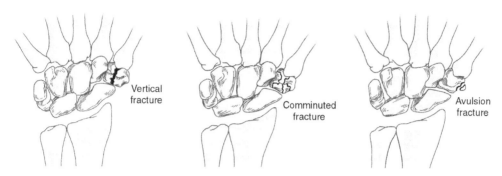

Figure 12–23. Trapezium fractures. **See page 254**.

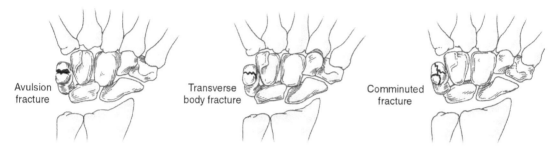

Figure 12–25. Pisiform fractures. **See page 255**.

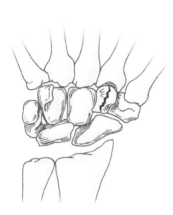

Figure 12–26. Trapezoid fracture. **See page 256**.

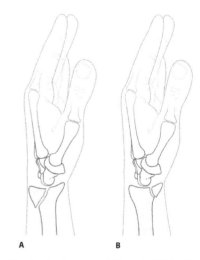

Figure 12–36. Barton fracture. **A.** Dorsal. **B.** Volar. **See page 264**.

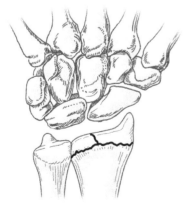

Figure 12–28. Distal radius fracture with intra-articular involvement. **See page 258**.

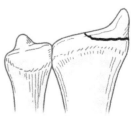

Figure 12–38. Radial styloid fracture (Hutchinson fracture). **See page 265**.

CHAPTER 13 FOREARM

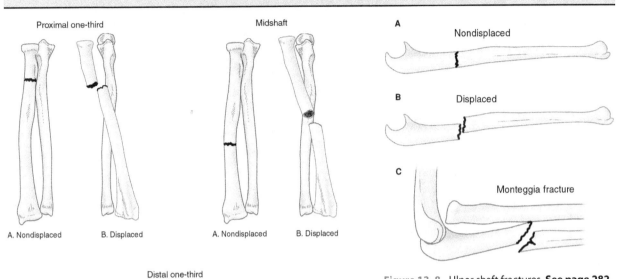

Proximal one-third

A. Nondisplaced   B. Displaced

Midshaft

A. Nondisplaced   B. Displaced

A Nondisplaced

B Displaced

C Monteggia fracture

Figure 13–8. Ulnar shaft fractures. **See page 282.**

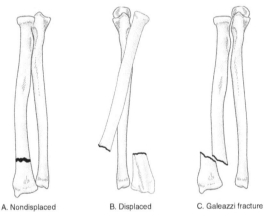

Distal one-third

A. Nondisplaced   B. Displaced   C. Galeazzi fracture

Figure 13–5. Radial shaft fractures. **See page 280.**

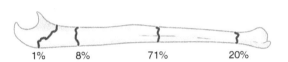

1%   8%   71%   20%

Figure 13–9. The midshaft of the ulna is the most common site for a fracture, often occurring due to a "nightstick"-type injury mechanism. **See page 283.**

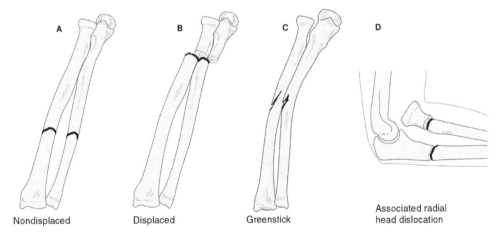

A   **B**   **C**   **D**

Nondisplaced   Displaced   Greenstick   Associated radial head dislocation

Figure 13–12. Classification of combination fractures of the shafts of the radius and ulna. **See page 285.**

CHAPTER 14 ELBOW

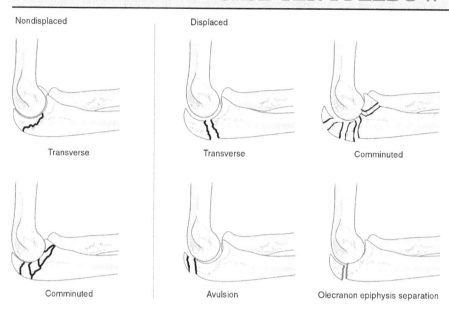

Nondisplaced

Displaced

Transverse

Transverse

Comminuted

Comminuted

Avulsion

Olecranon epiphysis separation

Figure 14–12. Olecranon fractures. **See page 297.**

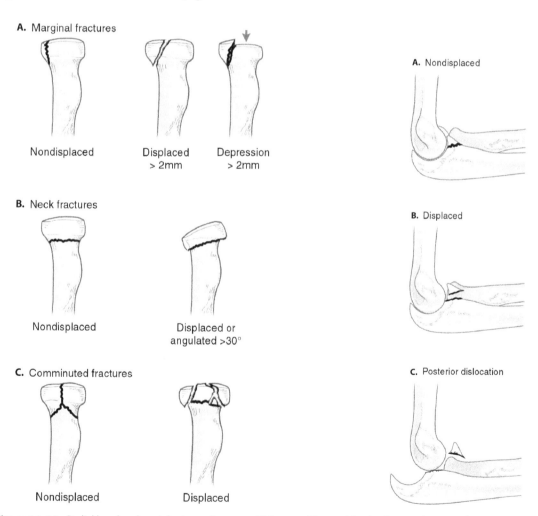

A. Marginal fractures

Nondisplaced

Displaced > 2mm

Depression > 2mm

B. Neck fractures

Nondisplaced

Displaced or angulated >30°

C. Comminuted fractures

Nondisplaced

Displaced

Figure 14–14. Radial head and neck fractures. **See page 298.**

A. Nondisplaced

B. Displaced

C. Posterior dislocation

Figure 14–19. Coronoid process fractures. **See page 301.**

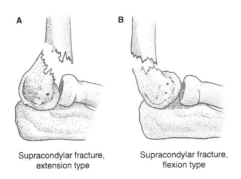

Supracondylar fracture, extension type

Supracondylar fracture, flexion type

Figure 14–20. Supracondylar fractures. **See page 302.**

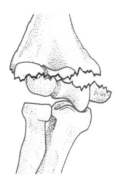

Figure 14–26. Transcondylar fracture. **See page 306.**

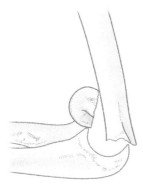

Figure 14–27. Posadas fracture. **See page 306.**

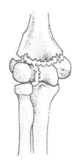

Nondisplaced

Figure 14–28. Intercondylar fractures. **See page 306.**

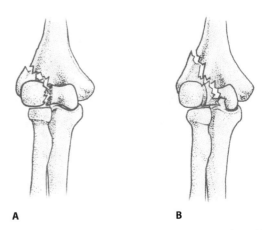

A

B

Figure 14–29. Lateral condylar fractures. **A.** Lateral trochlear ridge not included. **B.** Lateral trochlear ridge included. **See page 307.**

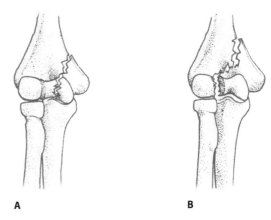

A

B

Figure 14–30. Medial condylar fractures. **A.** Lateral trochlear ridge not included. **B.** Lateral trochlear ridge included. **See page 308.**

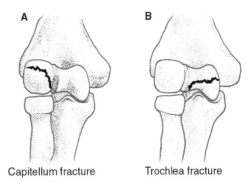

A

B

Capitellum fracture

Trochlea fracture

Figure 14–31. Articular surface fractures. **See page 309.**

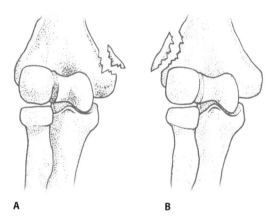

A   **B**

Figure 14–32. Epicondylar fractures. **A.** Medial epicondyle. **B.** Lateral epicondyle. **See page 309**.

CHAPTER 15 UPPER ARM

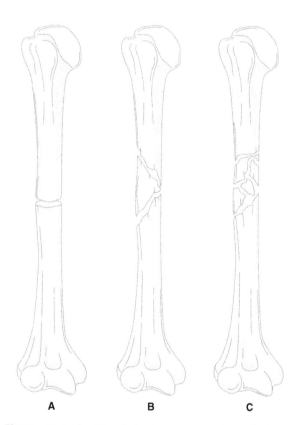

A   **B**   **C**

Figure 15–1. **A.** Type A fractures are simple and do not have an associated fracture fragment. They can be transverse, oblique, or spiral. **B.** Type B fractures have a free wedge-shaped fragment. The humeral shaft ends remain in close proximity. **C.** Type C fractures are complex (comminuted) fractures, where there is increased distance between the fractured ends of the humerus with interposed fracture fragments. **See page 323**.

CHAPTER 16 SHOULDER

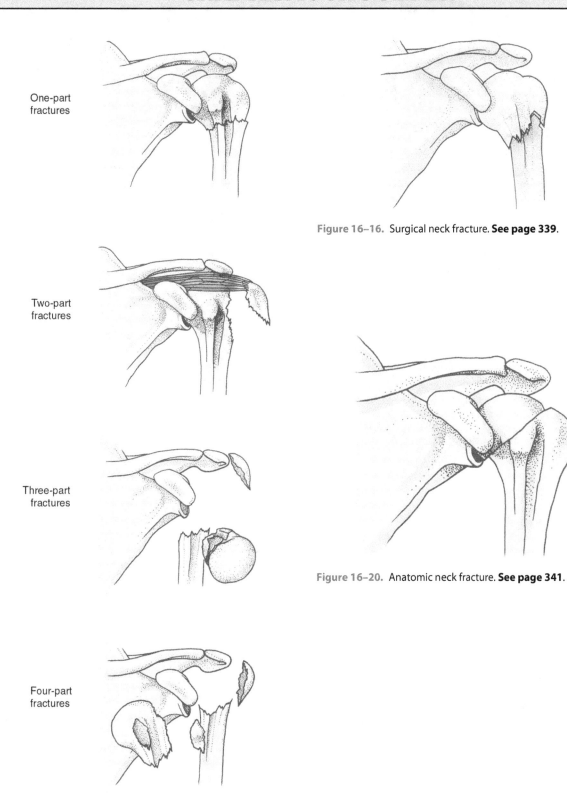

One-part
fractures

Figure 16–16. Surgical neck fracture. **See page 339**.

Two-part
fractures

Three-part
fractures

Figure 16–20. Anatomic neck fracture. **See page 341**.

Four-part
fractures

Figure 16–13. Examples of one-, two-, three-, and four-part
fractures as described by Neer. **See page 328**.

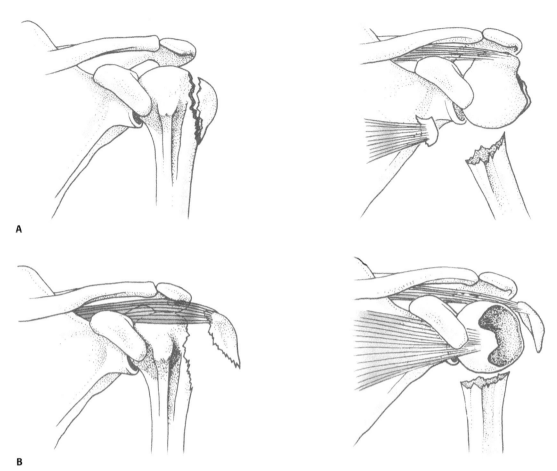

Figure 16–21. Greater tuberosity fractures. **A.** Nondisplaced. **B.** Displaced (>5 mm). **See page 341.**

Figure 16–24. Combination fractures—three-part fracture. **See page 343.**

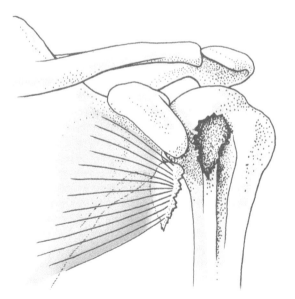

Figure 16–23. Lesser tuberosity fracture. **See page 342.**

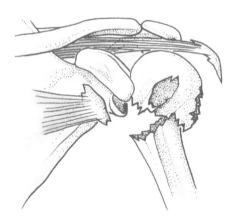

Figure 16–25. Combination fractures—four-part fracture. **See page 343.**

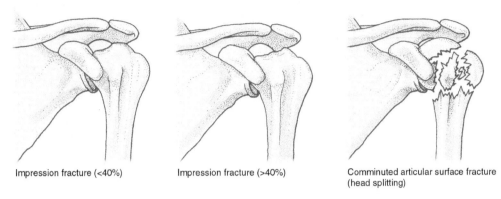

Impression fracture (<40%)   Impression fracture (>40%)   Comminuted articular surface fracture
                                                                        (head splitting)

Figure 16–27. Articular surface fractures. **See page 344.**

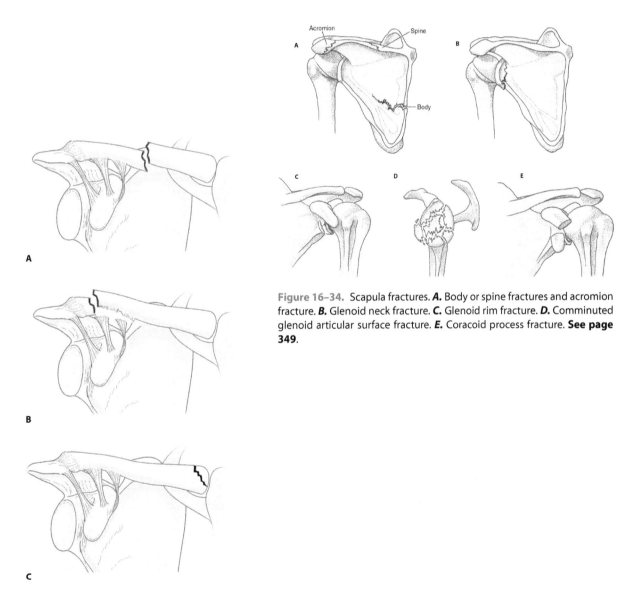

Figure 16–34. Scapula fractures. **A.** Body or spine fractures and acromion fracture. **B.** Glenoid neck fracture. **C.** Glenoid rim fracture. **D.** Comminuted glenoid articular surface fracture. **E.** Coracoid process fracture. **See page 349.**

Figure 16–29. Clavicle fractures. **A.** Middle third. **B.** Lateral third. **C.** Medial third (involving the sternoclavicular joint). **See page 345.**

CHAPTER 17 PELVIS

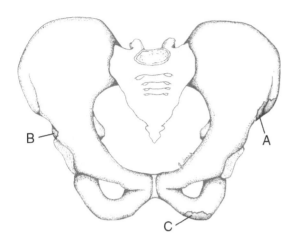

A = Avulsion of the anterior superior iliac spine
B = Avulsion of the anterior inferior iliac spine
C = Avulsion of the ischial tuberosity

Figure 17–8. Avulsion fractures. **See page 393.**

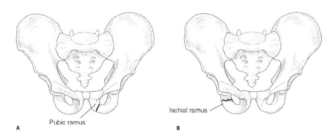

Figure 17–10. ***A.*** Single pubic ramus fracture. ***B.*** Ischial ramus fracture. **See page 394.**

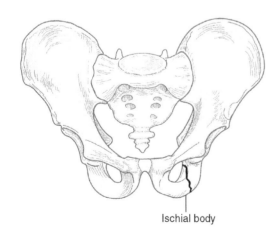

Figure 17–11. Ischial body fracture. **See page 395.**

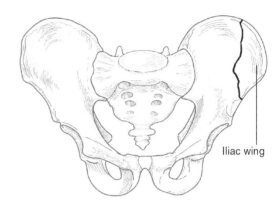

Figure 17–12. Iliac wing fracture (Duverney fracture). **See page 395.**

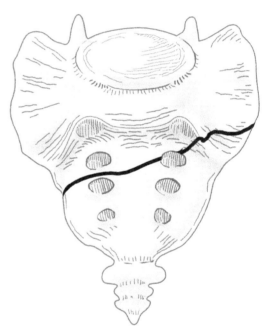

Figure 17–14. Horizontal sacral fracture. **See page 396.**

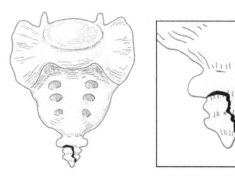

Figure 17–15. Coccyx fracture. **See page 397.**

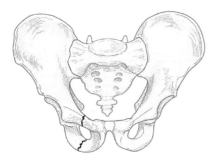

Figure 17–16. Superior and inferior pubic rami fractures (non-displaced). **See page 397.**

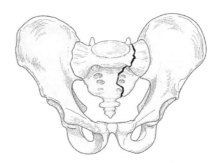

Figure 17–19. Vertical sacral fracture (nondisplaced). **See page 399.**

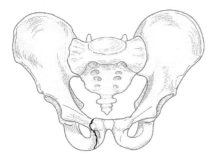

Figure 17–17. Pubic bone fracture (nondisplaced). **See page 398.**

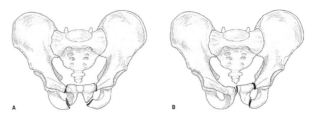

Figure 17–21. Straddle injuries. *A.* Bilateral pubic rami fractures. *B.* Pubic rami fractures and symphysis pubis disruption. **See page 400.**

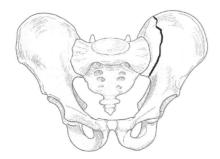

Figure 17–18. Ilium body fracture (nondisplaced). **See page 398.**

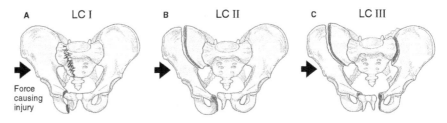

Figure 17–23. Lateral compression injuries. **See page 401.**

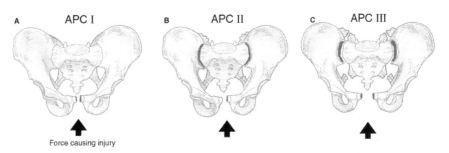

Figure 17–27. Anteroposterior compression injuries. **See page 403.**

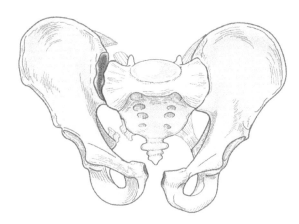

Figure 17–29. Vertical shear injury pattern. **See page 404**.

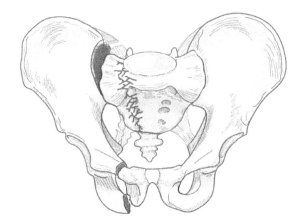

Figure 17–30. Combined mechanisms. **See page 405**.

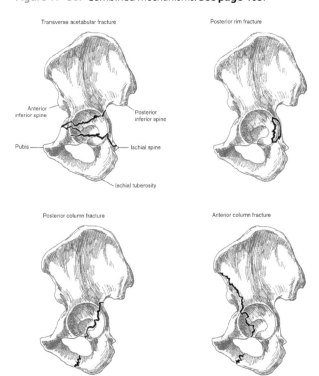

Figure 17–36. Nondisplaced acetabular fractures. Many variant types exist. **See page 410**.

Acetabular fractures

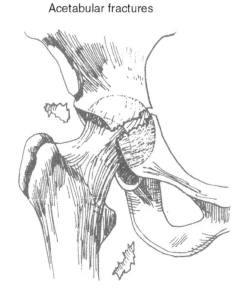

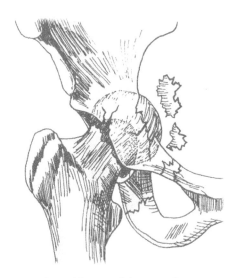

Figure 17–37. Central fracture dislocation. **See page 411**.

CHAPTER 18 HIP

Single fragment

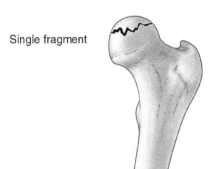

Comminuted

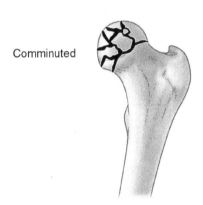

Figure 18–7. Femoral head fractures. **See page 422**.

A   Nondisplaced

Type I   Type II

B   Displaced

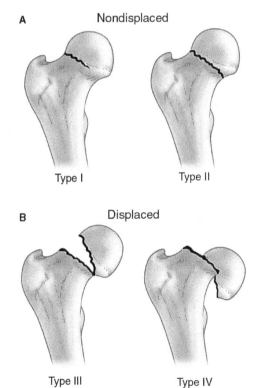

Type III   Type IV

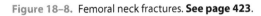

Figure 18–8. Femoral neck fractures. **See page 423**.

Stable   Unstable

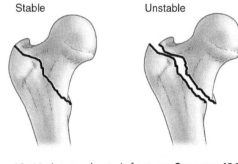

Figure 18–11. Intertrochanteric fractures. **See page 424**.

Greater
trochanteric
fracture

Lesser
trochanteric
fracture

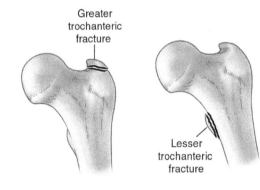

Figure 18–14. Trochanteric fractures. **See page 426**.

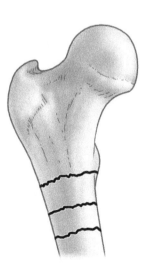

Figure 18–16. Subtrochanteric fractures. **See page 427**.

CHAPTER 19 THIGH

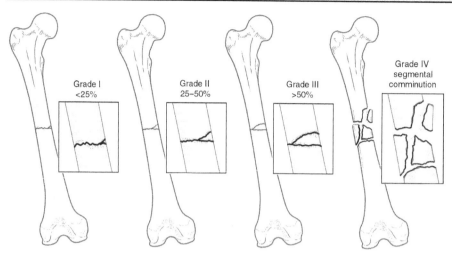

Figure 19–2. Winquist grading of femoral shaft fractures. **See page 446**.

CHAPTER 20 KNEE

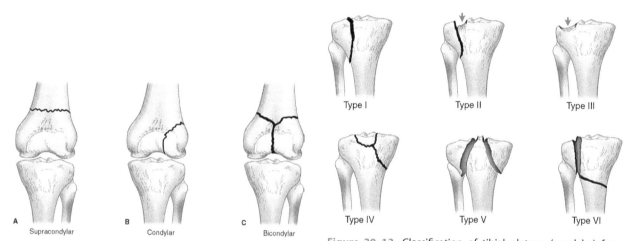

Figure 20–9. Distal femur fractures. **See page 463**.

Figure 20–13. Classification of tibial plateau (condylar) fractures. **See page 465**.

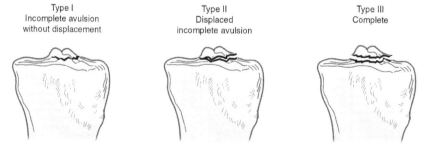

Figure 20–18. Tibial spine fractures. **See page 469**.

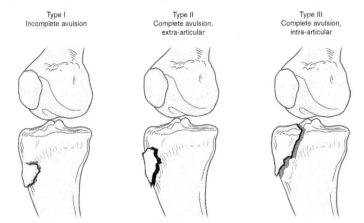

Figure 20–20. Tibial tuberosity fractures. **See page 470**.

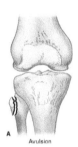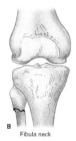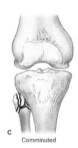

Figure 20–23. Proximal fibula fractures. **See page 472**.

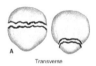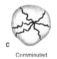

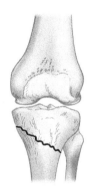

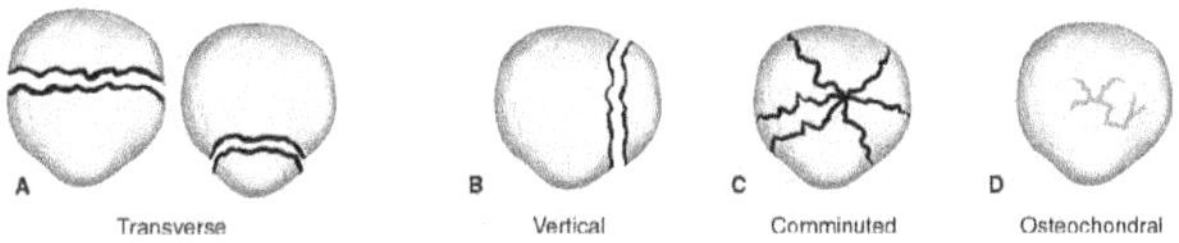

Figure 20–22. Proximal tibia fractures—subcondylar fractures.
See page 471.

Figure 20–25. Patella fractures. **See page 473**.

CHAPTER 21 LEG

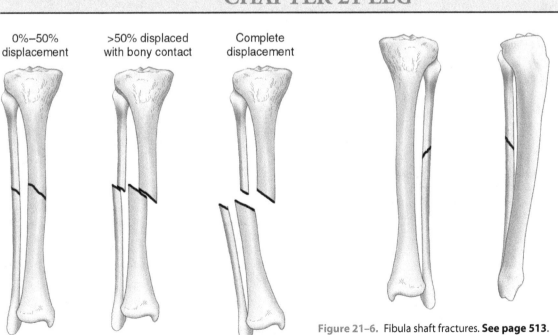

Figure 21–6. Fibula shaft fractures. **See page 513**.

Figure 21–1. Fractures of the tibia and fibula shaft. **See page 510**.

CHAPTER 22 ANKLE

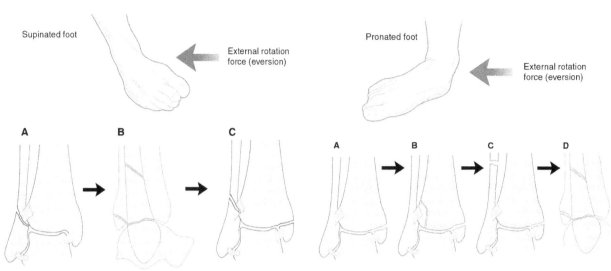

Figure 22–9. Schematic representing the progression of injury following forced eversion of the supinated foot. **A.** Distal oblique fibula fracture. **B.** With increasing force, the posterior malleolus avulses. **C.** Finally, the medial malleolus fractures, creating a trimalleolar fracture. **See page 524**.

Figure 22–11. Schematic representing the progression of injury following forced eversion of the pronated foot. **A.** Isolated medial malleolus fracture. **B.** With increasing force, the anterior tibiofibular ligament avulses a portion of the distal tibia. **C.** High fibula fracture. **D.** Posterior malleolus fracture. **See page 525**.

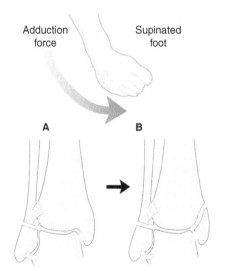

Figure 22–10. Schematic representing the progression of injury following forced adduction of the supinated foot. **A.** Distal transverse fibula fracture. **B.** With increasing force, the medial malleolus fractures, creating a bimalleolar fracture. **See page 524**.

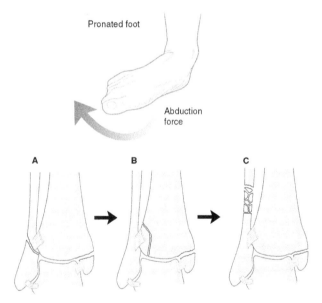

Figure 22–12. Schematic representing the progression of injury following forced abduction of the pronated foot. **A.** Isolated medial malleolus fracture. **B.** With increasing force, the anterior tibiofibular ligament avulses a portion of the distal tibia. **C.** Finally, a transverse or comminuted fibula fracture occurs. **See page 525**.

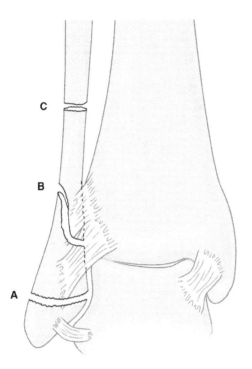

Figure 22–13. Weber classification system of ankle fractures. **See page 525**.

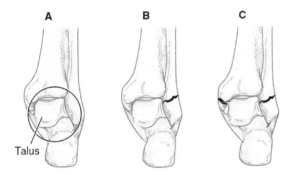

Figure 22–14. Closed ring classification system. **A.** The ankle is conceptualized as a closed ring surrounding the talus. **B.** A stable fracture is a single fracture without displacement. **C.** An unstable fracture involves a single fracture with a ligamentous disruption or two fractures in the ring. **See page 526**.

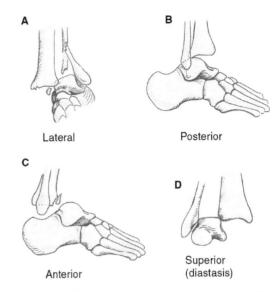

Figure 22–25. Ankle fracture—dislocations. **See page 531**.

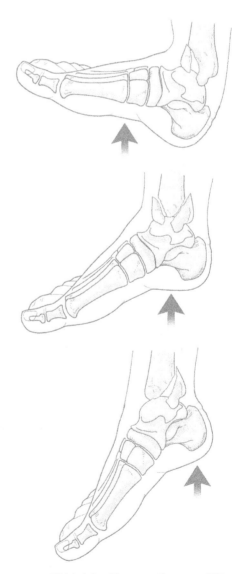

Figure 22–33. Tibial plafond fractures. **See page 535**.

CHAPTER 23 FOOT

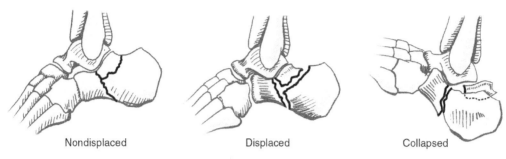

Nondisplaced   Displaced   Collapsed

Figure 23–5. Calcaneal body fractures—intra-articular. **See page 550**.

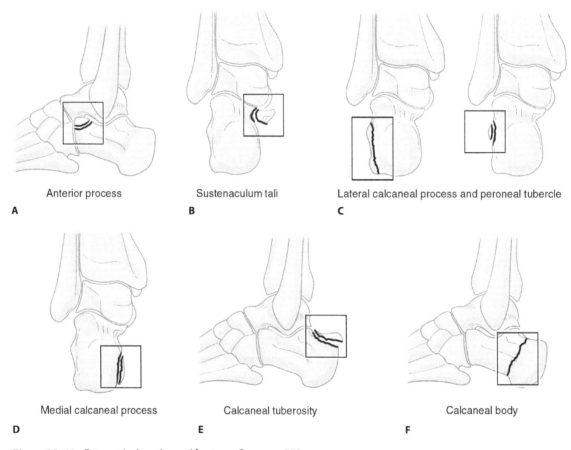

Anterior process   Sustenaculum tali   Lateral calcaneal process and peroneal tubercle

A   B   C

Medial calcaneal process   Calcaneal tuberosity   Calcaneal body

D   E   F

Figure 23–12. Extra-articular calcaneal fractures. **See page 553**.

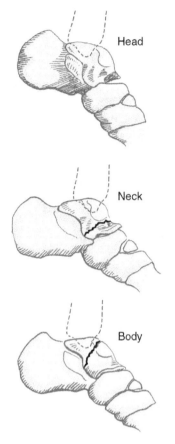

Head

Neck

Body

Figure 23–15. Talus fractures—major. **See page 556**.

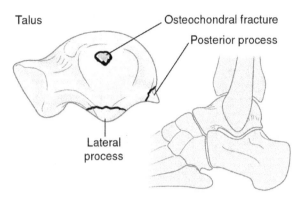

Talus

Osteochondral fracture

Posterior process

Lateral process

Figure 23–17. Talus fractures—minor. **See page 557**.

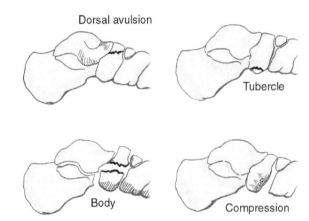

Dorsal avulsion

Tubercle

Body

Compression

Figure 23–18. Navicular fractures. **See page 558**.

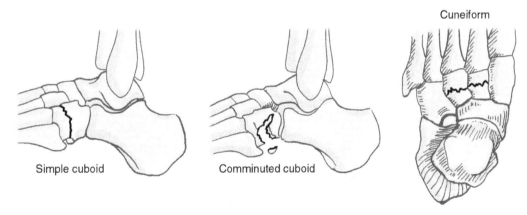

Cuneiform

Simple cuboid

Comminuted cuboid

Figure 23–21. Cuboid and cuneiform fractures. **See page 559**.

Homolateral   Divergent

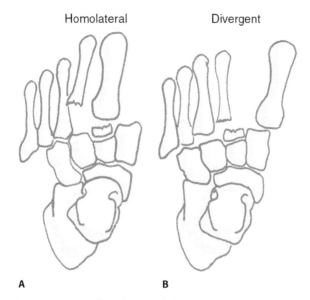

A   B

Figure 23-26. Lisfranc fracture dislocations. **See page 562**.

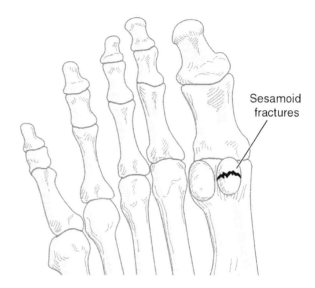

Sesamoid fractures

Figure 23-41. Sesamoid fractures. **See page 571**.

Comminuted distal phalangeal fracture

Proximal phalangeal fracture

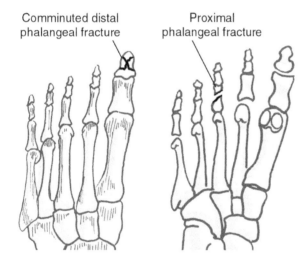

Figure 23-36. Toe fractures. **See page 569**.

PART I

Orthopedic Principles and Management

CHAPTER 1
General Principles

R. Darrell Nelson, MD and Jonah C. Gunalda, MD

FRACTURE PRINCIPLES

Biomechanics

An orthopedic fracture occurs when the stress applied to a bone exceeds the plastic strain beyond its yield point. A number of factors influence fracture patterns. These include the magnitude of force, its duration and direction, and the rate at which it acts. When a bone is subjected to repeated stresses, the bone may ultimately fracture even though the magnitude of any one individual stress is much lower than the ultimate tensile strength of the bone. The strength of a bone is related directly to its density, which is reduced by any condition, such as osteoporosis, where the osseous structure is changed, thus lowering its resistance to the stress.

Terminology

Fractures can be described in a number of ways. No one system of classification is all-encompassing, so physicians dealing with fractures on a day-to-day basis must be aware of the terminology to better understand and convey information to their colleagues. It should be noted that to adequately describe a fracture, at least two perpendicular radiographic views should be obtained.

Direction of Fracture Lines
* *Transverse:* A transverse fracture runs perpendicular to the bone (Fig. 1–1A).
* *Oblique:* An oblique fracture runs across the bone at an angle of 45 to 60 degrees (Fig. 1–1B). These fractures are due to compression and flexure at the fracture site.
* *Spiral:* A spiral fracture may be misdiagnosed as an oblique fracture; however, on closer study, a "corkscrew" appearance of the fracture is noted (Fig. 1–1C). It is a highly unstable fracture that is prone to poor healing. Spiral fractures are due to a torsional force. In pediatrics, a spiral fracture of the femur in a nonambulatory child is suspicious for nonaccidental trauma. However, a spiral fracture of the distal tibia in an ambulatory child is common and referred to as a "toddler's fracture".[1]
* *Comminuted:* A comminuted fracture is any fracture where there are more than two fragments (Fig. 1–1D). Other examples of comminuted fractures are the segmental and butterfly fractures (Fig. 1–1E and 1–1F).
* *Compression:* A compression fracture is one where the fractured ends are compressed together. These fractures are usually very stable (Fig. 1–1G). Compression fractures, also referred to as impacted fractures, are common in the vertebral bodies and lower extremities (e.g., calcaneus, femoral neck, and tibial plateau). When compression is significant, the fracture may become "depressed," or pushed in, and is referred to as a depression fracture (e.g., depressed calcaneus fracture).

Anatomic Location
* In a long bone, fractures are categorized as being in the proximal, middle, or distal portions of the bone.
* If the fracture extends into the joint space, it is described as intra-articular. Fractures that do not involve the joint are extra-articular.
* Other anatomic terms used to describe the location of a fracture are the head, neck, shaft, and base (e.g., metacarpal and metatarsal fractures).
* In pediatrics, fractures are described in relation to the growth plate (physis). Fractures that occur between the joint and the growth plate are epiphyseal fractures. Fractures of the diaphysis refer to the shaft of the bone. The metaphysis is the zone of growth of a bone between the epiphysis and the diaphysis.

Displacement
Displacement is used to describe the movement of fracture fragments from their usual position. Other terms that further describe fracture movements include:

* *Alignment* is the relationship between the axes of the bone fragments. To measure alignment, draw an imaginary line through the normal axis of the fractured proximal segment and then another line through the axis of the fractured distal segment, measuring the angle produced by the two lines. Alignment is described in degrees of angulation of the distal fragment in relation to the proximal fragment (Fig. 1–2). Lateral angulation of the distal fragment is also known as *valgus* deformity, whereas medial angulation is *varus* deformity. Angulation in the anteroposterior (AP) plane is referred to as volar and dorsal. Volar angulation of a distal fragment would be termed "volar angulation." Some orthopedists describe angulation based on the apex of a fracture. Therefore, "volar angulation" could also be described as "apex dorsal angulation."
* *Apposition* describes the amount of end-to-end contact between the fracture surfaces (Fig. 1–3). Apposition may be complete, partial, or absent (no contact).

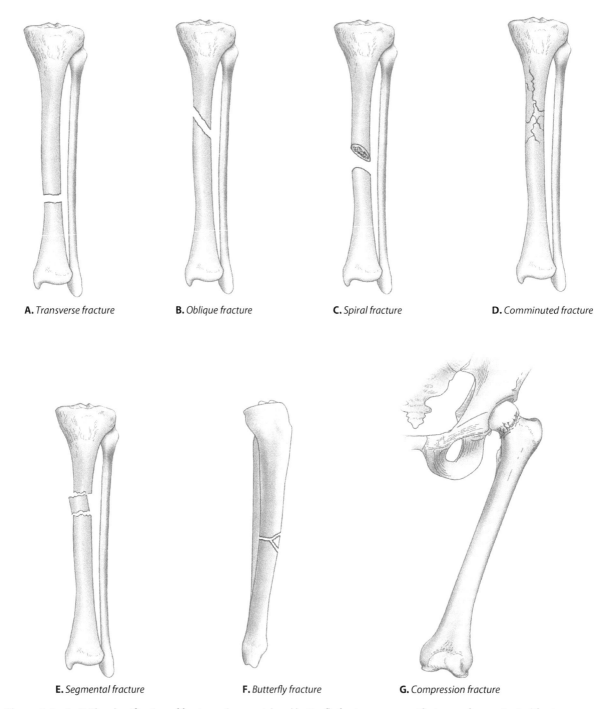

A. *Transverse fracture*   **B.** *Oblique fracture*   **C.** *Spiral fracture*   **D.** *Comminuted fracture*

E. *Segmental fracture*   **F.** *Butterfly fracture*   **G.** *Compression fracture*

Figure 1–1. ***A–G.*** The classification of fractures. Segmental and butterfly fractures are specific types of comminuted fractures.

- *Translation* is used to describe movement of fracture fragments from their usual position in a direction perpendicular to the long axes of the bone. Translation is described as a percentage of the bone's width. The direction of translation is described on the basis of the movement of the *distal* fragment in relation to the *proximal* fragment. In clinical practice, however, it is more common to use the more general term "displacement" to describe translation. For example, the fracture shown in Figure 1–3A

would be described as being 50% displaced in a lateral direction.

- *Bayonet apposition* is present when the fragments are not only 100% displaced but also overlapping (Fig. 1–3B). This is frequently seen in femoral and humeral shaft fractures.
- *Distraction* is the term used when the displacement is in the longitudinal axis of the bone (i.e., the bone fragments are "pulled apart") (Fig. 1–3C).

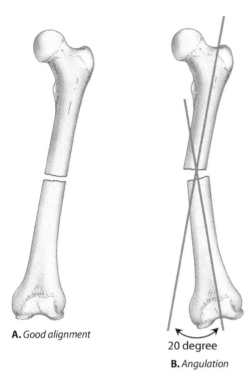

A. *Good alignment*

20 degree

B. *Angulation*

Figure 1–2. The description of fractures is according to the relationship between the distal segment and the proximal segment. **A.** There is no angulation, and this is referred to as good alignment of the fractured ends. **B.** There is lateral angulation of the distal segment of 20 degrees.

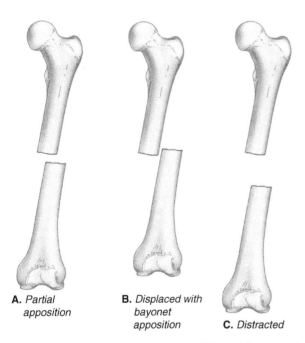

A. *Partial apposition*   **B.** *Displaced with bayonet apposition*   **C.** *Distracted*

Figure 1–3. Displacement or apposition. **A.** This partially apposed fracture can also be described as 50% laterally displaced. **B.** Bayonet apposition is when the two ends are no longer apposed and overlap with shortening of the normal length of the bone. **C.** Distraction occurs when the fracture ends are no longer apposed due to longitudinal separation rather than being separated in a side-to-side fashion.

- *Rotational deformity* can occur in any fracture, although it is common after spiral fractures. It can be detected clinically when radiographs reveal a nondisplaced fracture, yet the extremity appears abnormal, such as a finger pointing in the wrong direction. Subtle rotational deformity is detected by noting that the diameter of the bone on either side of the fracture line is different.

Soft-Tissue Injury

- *Closed:* A fracture in which the overlying skin remains intact.
- *Open:* A fracture in which the overlying skin is disrupted.
- *Complicated:* A fracture associated with neurovascular, visceral, ligamentous, or muscular damage. Intra-articular fractures are also considered complicated.
- *Uncomplicated (simple):* A fracture that has only a minimal amount of soft-tissue injury.

Stability

- *Stable fracture:* A fracture that does not tend to displace after reduction. Transverse fractures are frequently stable fractures.
- *Unstable fracture:* A fracture that tends to displace after reduction. Comminuted, oblique, and spiral fractures are more commonly unstable.

Mechanism of Injury

- *Direct* forces typically cause transverse, oblique, or comminuted fractures. An example of a direct force causing a fracture is the nightstick fracture via direct blow to the ulna. A comminuted fracture following a crush injury and a fracture due to a high-velocity bullet are also caused by direct impact.
- *Indirect* forces may also induce a fracture by transmitting energy to the bone. An example is the avulsion fracture due to ligamentous traction (Fig. 1–4A). A force, such as valgus stress at the knee, can result in a compression or depression fracture of the tibial condyle (Fig. 1–4B). A rotational or torsional force applied along the long axis of a bone results in a spiral fracture. A stress fracture, sometimes referred to as a fatigue fracture, results from repeated indirect stress applied to a bone. Some stress fractures are caused by repeated direct trauma.

Joint Injury

- *Dislocation:* Total disruption of the joint surface with loss of normal contact between the ends of two bones (Fig. 1–5A).
- *Subluxation:* Disruption of a joint with partial contact remaining between the two bones that make up the joint (Fig. 1–5B).
- *Diastasis:* Certain bones come together in a syndesmotic articulation in which there is little motion. An interosseous membrane that traverses the area between the two bones interconnects these joints. Two syndesmotic joints occur in

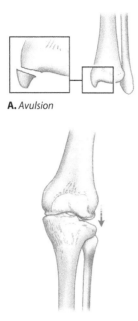

A. *Avulsion*

B. *Compression*

Figure 1–4. The mechanism of injury can frequently be deduced by the appearance of the fracture. **A.** Avulsion fracture due to the deltoid ligament pulling the medial malleolus from an eversion stress. **B.** Compression fracture caused by the femoral condyle contacting the tibial condyle following a valgus stress on the lower leg.

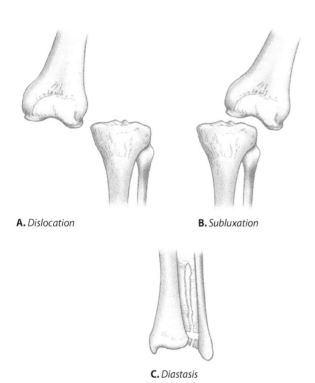

A. *Dislocation*   **B.** *Subluxation*

C. *Diastasis*

Figure 1–5. Joint injuries. **A.** A dislocation is complete separation of the two bones that make up the joint. **B.** Subluxation indicates partial displacement of the bone ends. **C.** Diastasis is separation at a syndesmotic joint.

humans between the radius and ulna and between the fibula and tibia. A disruption of the interosseous membrane connecting these two joints is called a diastasis (Fig. 1–5C).

Communication

The proper use of the terms provided to communicate with the orthopedic specialist is one of the most important aspects of orthopedic care performed by the emergency physician. In addition to fracture description, indicate the mechanism of injury, contamination of the injury, and overall patient status. A simple mnemonic to describe the fracture itself is NOLARD:

Neurovascular status

Open versus closed

Location

Angulation–Alignment–Articular involvement

Rotation

Displacement

Fracture Healing

Fracture healing can be divided into three phases—inflammatory, reparative, and remodeling (Fig. 1–6). The process is influenced by both fracture fixation or stability and the blood supply to the fracture site. Initially, after a fracture occurs, a hematoma forms at the site between the fracture ends and rapidly organizes to form a clot. This clot serves as a scaffold on which new fibrous tissue and bone is formed. Damage to the blood vessels of the bone deprives the osteocytes at the fracture site of their nutrition and they die. With this necrotic tissue, the *inflammatory phase* of fracture healing begins, accompanied by vasodilatation, edema formation, and the release of inflammatory mediators. In addition, polymorphonuclear leukocytes, macrophages, and osteoclasts migrate to the area to resorb the necrotic tissue.

The *reparative phase* begins with the migration of mesenchymal cells from the periosteum. These cells function to form the earliest bone. Osteoblasts from the endosteal surface also form a bone. Granulation tissue invades from surrounding vessels and replaces the hematoma. Most healing occurs around the capillary buds that invade the fracture site. Healing with new bone formation occurs primarily at the subperiosteal region; cartilage formation occurs in most other areas. Two types of bone healing occur: primary and secondary. Primary bone healing occurs when the fracture fragments are tightly affixed under compression without the formation of a callus. This occurs from osteoblast and osteoclast activity. Secondary bone healing is more common and occurs when interfragmentary motion occurs, creating a soft callus at the fracture site. This leads to a hard callus and then secondary bone formation through ossification of the callus. Osteoblasts are responsible for collagen formation, which is then followed by mineral deposition of calcium hydroxyapatite crystals. A callus forms, and the first signs of clinical union are noted.

During the *remodeling phase*, the healing fracture gains strength. As the process of healing continues, the bone

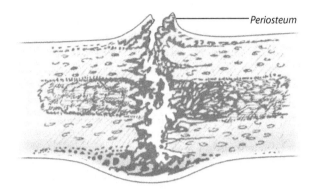

A. *Inflammatory phase*

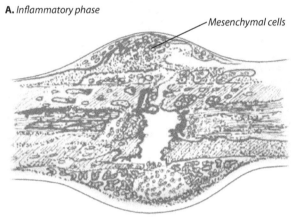

B. *Reparative phase*

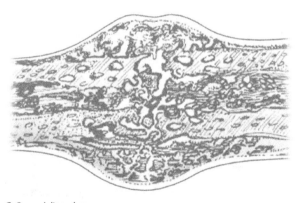

C. *Remodeling phase*

Figure 1–6. Phases of fracture healing.

organizes into trabeculae. Osteoclastic activity is first seen resorbing poorly formed trabeculae. New bone is then formed corresponding to the lines of force or stress.

An important concept to optimal fracture healing is strain. Insufficient strain or load may cause removal of the callus with delayed union (healing of a fracture that takes longer than expected) or nonunion (a fracture that does not heal). Excessive strain (e.g., weight bearing too early) can endanger the fracture healing process by causing fracture of callus formation. Several mechanisms influence healing, including the fracture geometry as well as the type and degree of fragment movement. These factors

influence the mechanical and biological signals for fracture repair.[5]

Many terms are used to describe fracture healing. *Union* refers to the healing of a fracture. Clinical union permits the resumption of motion of a limb and occurs earlier than radiographic union. Radiographic evidence of union is present when bone bridging of the fracture is seen on at least three cortices on orthogonal projections. Exercise increases the rate of repair and should be encouraged, particularly isometric exercise around an immobilized joint.

Malunion is the healing of a fracture with an unacceptable residual deformity such that angulation, rotation, or overriding fragments result in shortening of the limb. Shortening is better tolerated in the upper extremities (humerus) than lower extremities (femur or tibia). Generally, shortening greater than 1 inch is poorly tolerated in the lower extremity.

Delayed union is healing that takes a longer time than is usual. Delayed union is evident when periosteal new bone formation stops before union is achieved. In a long bone, delayed union is present if it has not fully united within 6 months.

Nonunion is defined as failure of the fracture to unite. The two most common reasons for fracture nonunion are an inadequate blood supply and poor fracture stabilization. Inadequate blood supply may be due to damaged nutrient vessels, stripping or injury to the periosteum and muscle, severe comminution with free fragments (butterfly and segmental fractures), or avascularity due to internal fixation devices. The amount of contact between the bone ends (apposition and distraction) and associated soft-tissue injuries adversely affect the rate of healing because the framework for bone repair is damaged.

The location of the fracture may impact the likelihood of nonunion. Cortical bone found in tubular bone diaphyses heals at a slower rate than does the cancellous bone in the epiphyses and metaphyses due to the differences in vascular supply and cellularity. Bones that have a higher incidence of nonunion include the distal tibia diaphysis, scaphoid, and proximal diaphysis of the fifth metatarsal.

Other causes of nonunion include soft-tissue interposition, bony distraction from traction or internal fixation, infection, age, fractures through pathologic bone, and medications. Patient age is a factor as children experience a higher affinity for rapid bone remodeling. The healing of intra-articular fractures is inhibited by exposure to the synovial fluid. The synovial fluid contains fibrinolysins that retard the initial stage of fracture healing, causing lysis of the clot. Certain drugs, such as corticosteroids, excessive thyroid hormone, and nicotine from cigarette smoke inhibit the rate of healing.[6] Chronic hypoxia and other comorbidities have been shown to inhibit bone healing in animal studies. The impact of nonsteroidal anti-inflammatory drugs (NSAIDs) on bone healing remains controversial, with many studies concluding conflicting results.[7]

Pseudoarthrosis results from an untreated and grossly mobile nonunion. In pseudoarthrosis, a false joint with a synovial-lined capsule appears that envelops the fracture ends.

Clinical Features

Assessment of fractures should begin with a thorough history, including the mechanism of injury, events since the injury, weight-bearing status, improvement or worsening symptoms, as well as medical and social history such as tobacco abuse and handedness. Examination of fractures should include visual inspection, palpation, movement of the affected area, and a neurovascular assessment.

Pain and tenderness are the most common presenting complaints associated with a fracture. Symptoms are usually well localized to the fracture site, but can be more diffuse if there is significant associated soft-tissue injury. Loss of normal function may be noted, but in patients with incomplete fractures (e.g., stress fracture) the functional impairment may be minimal. When the fractured ends are in poor apposition, abnormal mobility and crepitation may be elicited. These findings should not be sought on examination as they increase the chance of further soft-tissue damage. Patients with gross deformity or crepitation should be splinted immediately before they are moved or any radiographs are performed.

Point tenderness should be noted whenever it is elicited. A stress fracture may be tentatively diagnosed or suspected on the basis of bony tenderness even though a fracture might not be seen on radiographs for 10 to 14 days. In a similar manner, when evaluating a patient with an injury to a joint, consider an osteochondral fracture as the cause of pain.

No examination of a patient with a suspected fracture is complete without a neurovascular assessment. Injury to nerves and vessels should be documented and addressed where appropriate before and after any attempts at reduction. Furthermore, signs of compartment syndrome should be elicited such as spontaneous, intense pain or pain "out of proportion" to examination findings; enlarged or tense compartments; or pain on passive stretching of the muscles within the compartment. Paresthesias, poikilothermia, pulselessness, and/or paralysis may also be present, but are late findings.

Close visual inspection of the skin is necessary to exclude an open fracture. The injury to the skin may seem innocuous, but when present near the site of a fracture and the base of the wound cannot be identified, the injury should be considered an open fracture until proven otherwise (Fig. 1-7).

Evidence of blisters over a fracture site may occur when swelling is severe, often following high shear forces. Fracture blisters may appear as early as 6 hours after a fracture and as late as 3 weeks, but more commonly present in 24 to 48 hours after injury. Fracture blisters may also occur following a joint dislocation without fracture and following elective orthopedic surgical procedures. They may be clear or hemorrhagic. Hemorrhagic blisters indicate detachment between the dermal and epidermal layers and an associated worse prognosis (Fig. 1-8). Fracture blisters are most common in areas with bony prominences such as the elbow, foot, and distal tibia. Early reduction and stabilization of fractures decreases the incidence of blister formation, although blisters may form even when care has been optimal. Edema control with compression, elevation, and cryotherapy is also useful. The treatments for fracture

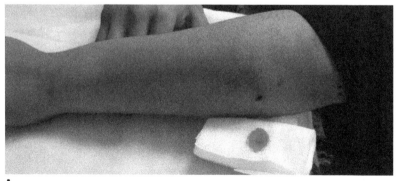

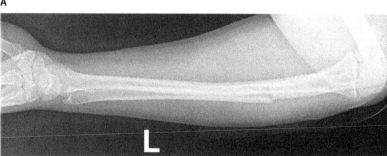

Figure 1–7. Open fracture. **A.** A small wound without an identifiable base is noted on the proximal forearm. **B.** The radiographs of the same patient demonstrate an ulna fracture in the proximity of the wound.

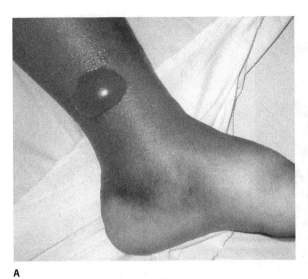
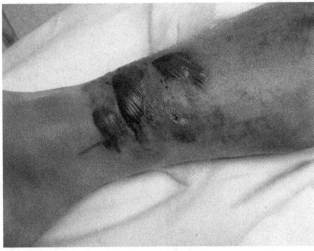

A **B**

Figure 1–8. Fracture blisters. **A.** Clear fracture blister in a patient following a bimalleolar ankle fracture. **B.** Hemorrhagic fracture blisters in a patient with a distal tibia fracture.

blisters are controversial, although most authorities leave them intact and cover them with povidone-iodine, antibiotic ointment or silver sulfadiazine dressing. Their presence frequently delays operative repair because they double the rate of infection and wound dehiscence.[10]

Bleeding is another potential problem following fractures, especially in long bones (e.g., femur) and the pelvis. A significant amount of blood loss can occur after a closed fracture, and the amount of bleeding is often not appreciated (Table 1–1). A patient with a significant pelvic fracture can experience hypovolemic shock from blood loss. This is especially true in the elderly, who are less able to vasoconstrict to support their blood pressure.

Radiographs

Plain radiographs are usually sufficient for fracture diagnosis. They not only allow identification of the fracture site, but they also provide information pertaining to the physiologic condition surrounding the injury (e.g., bone density; presence of infection, malignancy, or necrosis; joint space width; soft-tissue changes).[11] Fractures appear as a disruption of the smooth cortex of the bone with a radiolucent line delineating the fragments (Fig. 1–9). Acute fractures are usually linear

with irregular borders. Compression fractures are more difficult to detect and are noted when there is a loss of the normal trabecular pattern within the bone and when the bone appears more radiodense (Fig. 1–10).

Avoid treating accessory ossicles (i.e., sesamoid bones) as avulsion fractures by looking for their smooth border. When doubt exists, a comparison view of the opposite extremity can be obtained, although it should be noted that sesamoid bones are not always symmetric. The fabella of the knee, for instance, is bilateral in only 63% of people.

Two orthogonal views (e.g., AP and lateral) are obtained at a minimum. This serves to improve the rate of fracture diagnosis and to give the clinician a full understanding of the displacement of a fracture (Figs. 1–11 and 1–12). Additional views should be requested in select situations. Oblique views, for instance, are particularly helpful when imaging the distal extremities (e.g., hand, wrist, foot) and increase the sensitivity of fracture detection.

Radiographs may require the joint above and below the fracture, as this may be useful to detect distant fractures less symptomatic than the primary injury. For example, a medial malleolus fracture is commonly associated with a proximal fibula fracture in the Maisonneuve fracture pattern. Additionally, rotational deformities can be detected when joints are present in the radiographs of a long bone fracture. An AP view of one joint and a lateral view of the other joint suggest a significant rotational deformity (Fig. 1–13). Finally, shortening of one of the bones of the forearm or leg because of angulation or bayonet apposition suggests that another fracture is present in the other bone (e.g., tibia–fibula fracture) or that there is a joint dislocation (e.g., Monteggia fracture). These concomitant injuries will be diagnosed when the entire length of the long bone(s) and their proximal and distal joints are seen on radiographs. However, the routine acquisition of radiographs above and

▶ **TABLE 1–1. AVERAGE BLOOD LOSS WITH A CLOSED FRACTURE**

Fracture Site	Amount (mL)
Radius and ulna	150–250
Humerus	250
Pelvis	1500–3000
Femur	1000
Tibia and fibula	500

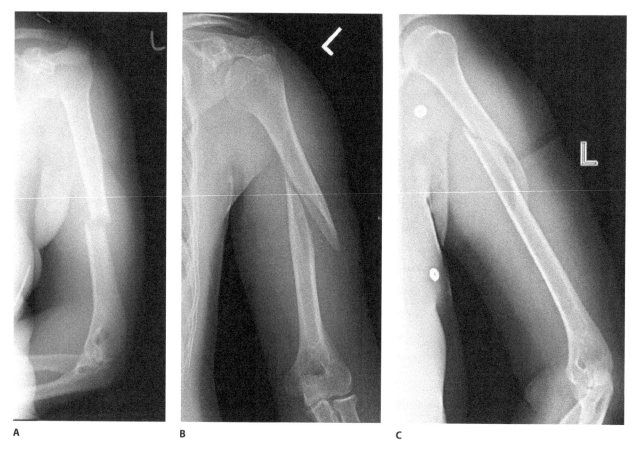

Figure 1–9. *A.* Transverse. *B.* Oblique. *C.* Spiral fractures of the humeral shaft.

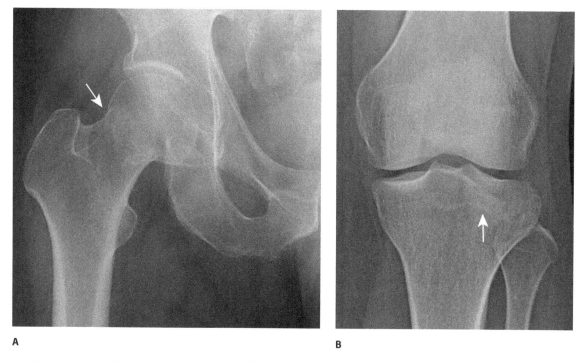

Figure 1–10. Compression fractures are present when an increased bone density is noted. They are frequently more difficult to appreciate (*arrows*). *A.* Femoral neck. *B.* Tibial plateau.

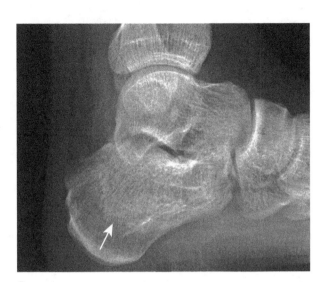

C

Figure 1–10. *(Continued)* **C.** Calcaneus.

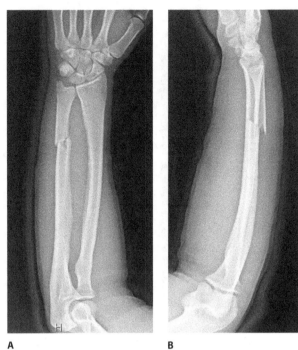

A   B

Figure 1–12. **A.** Anteroposterior (AP) view of the forearm demonstrates an ulna fracture. **B.** On the lateral view, displacement is seen that was not otherwise evident on the AP.

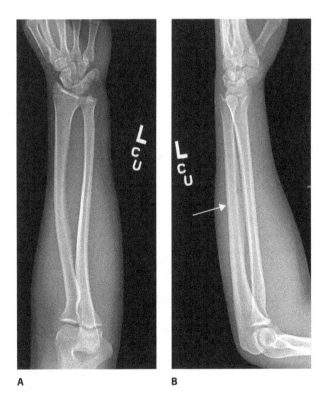

A   B

Figure 1–11. Two radiographs obtained at 90-degree angles aid in fracture detection and a fuller understanding of fracture displacement. **A.** Anteroposterior view of the forearm appears normal. **B.** On the lateral view, a more obvious nondisplaced fracture is seen in the shaft of the ulna *(arrow).*

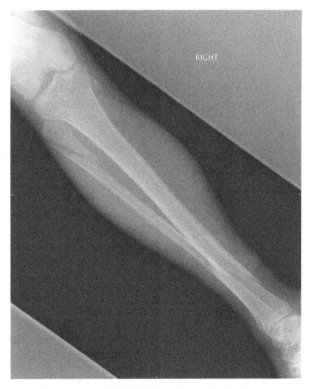

Figure 1–13. Including the joint above and below a long bone fracture will allow detection of rotational deformity as seen in this leg radiograph, where an anteroposterior view of the knee is seen with a lateral view of the ankle.

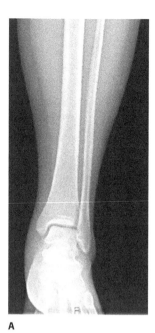 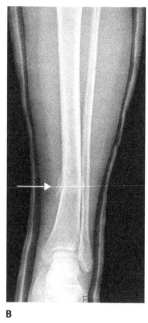

A   **B**

Figure 1–14. Occult fracture of the distal tibia. **A.** On the initial radiograph, no fracture is noted. **B.** One month later, a transverse fracture of the tibia with surrounding callus formation is seen (*arrow*).

below the suspected fracture as a rule has been shown to be of low yield in suspected ankle fractures. In patients who are able to participate in their exam, patient history, physical examination, and clinical suspicion should be used in decision making for additional radiographs.

A fracture may occur but may not be radiographically evident for as many as 10 to 14 days postinjury (Fig. 1–14). For this reason, the emergency physician should practice with the guideline that if there is significant trauma and focal bony tenderness suspicious of a fracture, it should be treated as such. This is especially true in the pediatric patient with pain over a growth plate.

There are some regions where occult fractures occur quite commonly and are frequently missed on initial evaluation. The scaphoid bone, for instance, is notorious for occult fractures (16%–27%) that are not radiographically visible for several weeks after injury. Occult fractures of the hip occur in close to 10% of elderly patients who present with trauma, hip pain, and negative initial radiographs.

When an occult fracture is suspected, the clinician should consider other diagnostic studies such as magnetic resonance imaging (MRI) and computed tomography (CT) scan. These imaging techniques have a much higher sensitivity for fracture detection. MRI has been shown to be close to 100% sensitive for diagnosing occult fractures of the scaphoid or hip. When further imaging is not obtained in the emergency department, splint the patient for the mere suspicion of such a fracture, even though it

is not radiographically visible, and arrange orthopedic follow-up.

Treatment

Prehospital Splinting

An unstable fracture must be stabilized by some form of external splinting or traction before movement of the patient. Proper splinting in the prehospital setting reduces pain and prevents further soft-tissue injury by the fracture fragments. A neurovascular examination should be performed both prior to splinting and immediately afterward.

A traction splint for a femur fracture is one of the most important splints to be placed in the prehospital setting. After a femur fracture, the overriding bone results in loss of soft-tissue tension in the thigh and an increased potential space for hemorrhage. Up to 1 L of blood can distend the soft tissues of the thigh. A traction splint maintains tension on the soft tissues, decreases the amount of hemorrhage, and subsequently improves outcome.

Perhaps the oldest known lower-extremity traction splint is the *Thomas splint*. This splint has been used since the late 1800s and became famous during World War I, when mortality was reduced by 50% after its introduction into battle. A modification of this splint is the *Hare traction splint*, in which a half-ring makes up the most proximal portion (Fig. 1–15). These splints provide traction of the fracture fragments, but cause a great deal of discomfort during transport. The splint should not be removed before radiographic evaluation.

The *Sager traction splint* (Minto Research and Development, Inc.) is our preference for emergency splinting of all proximal femur and femoral shaft fractures in both the pediatric and adult age groups (Fig. 1–16). The Sager splint has a single shaft that is placed on the inner aspect of the leg, but can be applied to the outer side of the leg if a pelvic fracture is present. The splint does not have a half-ring posteriorly, which has two important advantages: (1) it relieves any pressure on the sciatic nerve; and (2) it reduces hip flexion (which occurs up to 30 degrees in the Hare splint), thereby eliminating angulation of the fracture site.

Several other traction splints are available in prehospital, tactical, and military venues such as the *Faretec CT-6 Military Leg Traction Splint* (Faretec, Inc.), the *Slishman Traction Splint* (Rescue Essentials), and the *Tactical Traction Splint* (North American Rescue). Following similar principles to the previously mentioned splints, these offer lightweight options in tactical or military operations as well as in austere environments.

Other commercially available extremity splints include the SAM splint (SAM Medical Products, Inc.), *Fox splint* (Compliance Medical, Inc.), wire ladder splints, and inflatable splints. The SAM splint, made of malleable foam-covered aluminum, is lightweight, easy to use, and conforms well to the extremity. The Fox splint consists of cardboard

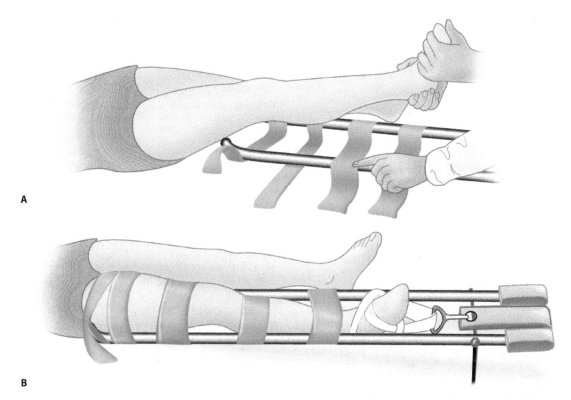

Figure 1–15. *A.* Hare traction comprises applying traction to the lower limb and elevating it with the knee held in extension. ***B.*** The splint is then inserted under the limb and the foot secured in the traction apparatus.

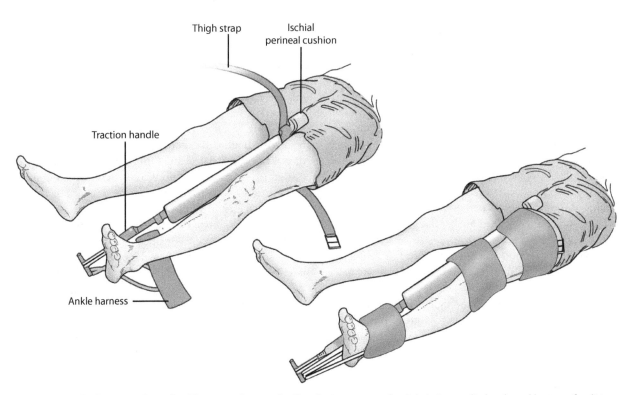

Figure 1–16. The Sager traction splint. The gauged meter distally tells the amount of weight being applied to the ankle straps for distraction. The splint can be applied to the outer side of the leg in patients with groin injuries or pelvic fractures who also have a femoral fracture.

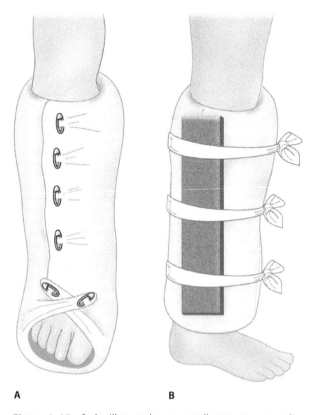

A   **B**

Figure 1–17. **A.** A pillow makes an excellent temporary splint for the prehospital management of a fracture to the ankle, foot, and distal tibia. **B.** A fracture of the lower leg can be stabilized by wrapping towels securely around the limb and then applying two splints of wood on either side and securing them to the extremity.

and foam rubber, therefore lacking malleability. Inflatable splints made of a double-walled polyvinyl jacket and ladder splints made of a moldable wire are also used, but they are not our preferred choice. Inflatable splints have the potential disadvantage of overinflation (limb ischemia) or underinflation (ineffective immobilization) and will change volume during air medical transport operations. These splints should not be applied over clothing as this can cause skin injury.

If medical attention has not yet arrived, a splint can be fashioned out of materials commonly found in most homes. An example is the *pillow splint* (Fig. 1–17A) formed by wrapping an ordinary pillow tightly around a lower-extremity fracture and securing it with safety pins. Alternatively, a splint can be made from towels wrapped around the limb and supported on either side by wood boards (Fig. 1–17B). The same type of splint can be used in the upper extremity with the addition of a sling to support the forearm.

Patients who present with open fractures should be splinted in a similar manner; however, the site of skin injury should be covered with a sterile dressing. One should

▶ TABLE 1–2. **JOINT POSITION FOR IMMOBILIZATION**

Joint	Position
Distal interphalangeal	0–10 degree flexion
Proximal interphalangeal	0–10 degree flexion
Metacarpophalangeal	60–90 degree flexion
Wrist	20–30 degree extension
Elbow	90 degree flexion
Shoulder	Adducted/internally rotated
Knee	20–30 degree flexion
Ankle	Neutral (avoid plantar flexion)
Toes	Neutral

be careful not to replace any exposed bone fragment back into the wound to avoid further contamination.

Emergency Department Immobilization

A fracture is immobilized in the emergency department to stabilize unstable fractures, relieve pain, and permit healing. The presence of a fracture, however, should not be automatically equated with the need for immobilization (e.g., clavicle fracture). The fundamental rules of splints and casts are identical. Ideally, at least one joint above and below the fracture should be immobilized. In general, the extremity should be placed in the position of function before it is immobilized, although there are exceptions to this rule depending on the injury (Table 1–2).

Splints

Splints differ from casts in that they are not circumferential and allow swelling of the extremity without a significant increase in tissue pressure. Ice packs can be applied closer to the skin in patients immobilized in a splint, thereby maximizing its effect. For these reasons, splints are more frequently used as the initial means of immobilization in the emergency department. Once swelling has decreased, casting is performed because splints permit more motion and provide less stability for a reduced fracture that needs to be maintained in a fixed position.

Splints and casts are strengthened by one of two different materials—plaster or fiberglass. The plaster rolls or slabs used in casting are stiffened by dextrose or starch and impregnated with a hemihydrate of calcium sulfate. When water is added to the calcium sulfate, a reaction occurs that liberates heat, which is noted by both the patient and the physician applying the cast.

$$CaSO_4 + H_2O \rightarrow H_2O \, CaSO_4 \cdot H_2O + Heat$$

Accelerator substances are added to the bandages that allow them to set at differing rates. Common table salt can be used to retard the setting of the plaster, if this is desired, by simply adding salt to the water. Acceleration of the setting occurs by increasing the temperature of the water. The

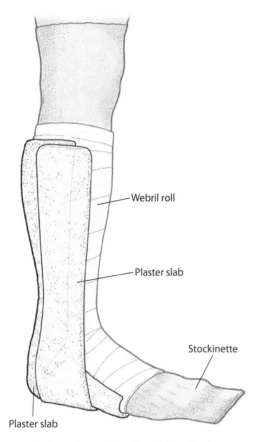

Webril roll

Plaster slab

Stockinette

Plaster slab

Figure 1–18. Posterior ankle splint. This splint is constructed by application of stockinette followed by padding (e.g., Webril). Finally, a posterior slab of plaster is applied. For additional stability, a "U"-shaped stirrup slab is used. An elastic bandage (not pictured) to secure the splint to the limb is the final step.

colder the water temperature, the longer the plaster takes to set.

For plaster splints, a stockinette is placed on the extremity with a generous amount allowed at the distal and proximal ends where the splint is to be applied (Fig. 1–18). Next, a soft layer of padding (e.g., Webril) is circumferentially placed around the extremity with special care to provide extra padding to areas where bony protuberances are most prominent (i.e., malleoli, heel). The plaster is measured and cut or torn to the appropriate length. For maximal strength, 8 to 10 layers should be used. The plaster layers are then immersed in warm water, smoothed for additional strength, and applied to the extremity. A strip of cast padding can be applied over the outer surface of the plaster so that the elastic bandage does not adhere. This will aid in the removal of the splint. Finally, an elastic bandage is applied to secure the splint to the limb. It is important to wrap the elastic bandage snugly, but not tightly enough to cause limb ischemia or a compartment syndrome.

Commercially available fiberglass splint materials, which incorporate the padding and fiberglass in one piece, are readily available. These splints are quick, clean, and easy to use for immobilizing joints following soft-tissue

injuries and most stable fractures. The fiberglass is activated with a small amount of water, and it dries quickly. Care should be taken to stretch the padding over the cut end of this splint material so contact with the skin is avoided. Dried fiberglass is sharp and will cause skin irritation and pain. For unstable fractures that require reduction, we recommend plaster splinting because it molds better to the limb.

Casts

Casts are applied in a similar manner to splints. First, stockinette is placed on the extremity so that extra is available on either side of where the cast will be placed. Next, cast padding is applied from the distal to the proximal end of the limb (Fig. 1–19A and B). The cast padding interposed between the skin and the plaster provides elastic pressure and enhances the fixation of the limb by compensating for slight shrinkage of the tissues after application of the cast. Too much padding reduces the efficacy of the cast and permits excessive motion. Generally, the more padding used, the more plaster needed (Video 1–1).

After placing a plaster roll in water, squeeze the ends together to eliminate excess water while retaining the plaster in the roll. The plaster bandage should be rolled in the same direction as the padding, and each turn should overlap the preceding one by 50%. The plaster should always be laid on transversely with the roll of bandage in contact with the surface of the limb almost continuously. The roll should be lightly guided around the limb, and pressure should be applied by the thenar eminence to mold the plaster. Each turn should be smoothed with the thenar eminence of the right hand as the left hand guides the roll around the limb. As the limb tapers, the casting material is made to lie evenly by small tucks made using the index finger and thumb of the right hand before each turn is smoothed into position (Fig. 1–19C). The palms and thenar eminences of the hands smooth the bandage when it is applied. Remember that the durability and strength of the cast depends on welding together each individual layer by the smoothing movements of both hands (Fig. 1–19D). Finally, the stockinette is folded back and the last roll of plaster is applied (Fig. 1–19E).

Some common casting mistakes include the following:

1. Making the center of the cast too thick. One should concentrate on making the two ends of the cast of adequate thickness because it is easy to make the center too thick. This provides no additional support at the fracture site (Fig. 1–20).
2. Using too many narrow bandages, rather than fewer wider rolls, creating a lumpy appearance to the cast. Bandages of widths of 4, 6, and 8 inches are most commonly used for casting.
3. Applying the plaster too loosely, especially over the proximal fleshy portion of the limb. A better fit is needed here than at the distal bony parts.

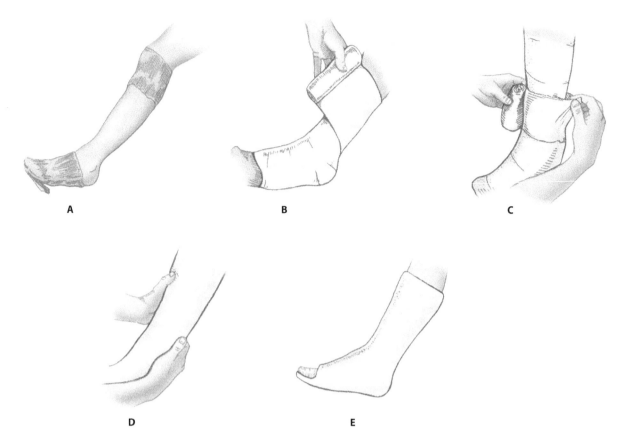

Figure 1–19. Applying a cast. **A.** Stockinette is used to cover the proximal and distal ends of the area to be casted. **B.** A soft padding material is used under the plaster roll. **C.** The plaster is applied with the roll held against the limb by the left hand. The right hand is used to smooth out the plaster and to pull and fold back the top corners, which are produced by the changing circumference of the limb. **D.** The plaster roll, once applied, is smoothed with the thenar eminence and palms of both hands to seal the interstices and to give additional support. **E.** The final step is to fold back the stockinette and apply the last roll of the plaster.

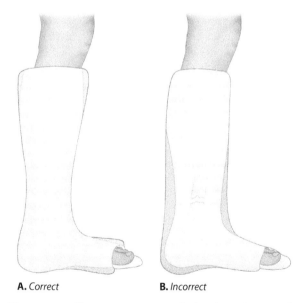

A. *Correct*   **B.** *Incorrect*

Figure 1–20. The correct way to apply the plaster is to use the same thickness throughout. **A.** For additional support, you may add extra thickness at the proximal and distal ends. **B.** A common mistake is for physicians to believe that one gains strength by adding thickness at the fracture site.

The application of a walking heel should be under the center of the foot (Fig. 1–21). The heel should be centered midway between the posterior tip of the calcaneus and the distal end of the "ball" of the foot. If one needs to reinforce the cast, as in an obese patient with a walking cast, this should be done by adding a fin to the front, *not* by adding excessive posterior splints to the back, as this only adds weight to the cast and does not make it stronger.

When applying a cast to the upper extremity, the hand should be left free by stopping the cast at the metacarpal heads dorsally and the proximal flexor crease of the palm volarly to permit normal finger motion (Fig. 1–22).

A window may be placed in a cast when a laceration or any skin lesion needs care while treating the fracture. To make a window, cover the wound with a bulky piece of sterile gauze and apply the cast over the dressing in the normal manner. Once the cast is complete, cut out the "bulge" created by the gauze dressing (Fig. 1–23). The cast defect should always be covered with a bulky dressing and held firmly in place with an elastic bandage to avoid herniation of the soft tissue and subsequent swelling and skin ulceration.

As mentioned previously, casts are not used as frequently in the emergency department as splints. Applying a

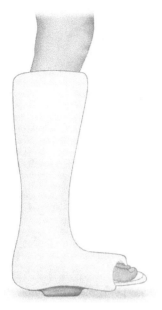

Figure 1–21. A walking cast.

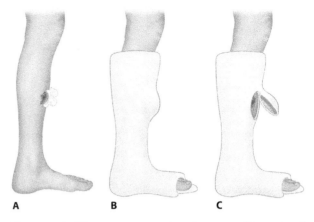

Figure 1–23. When an open wound requires care and is associated with a fracture to the extremity that must be casted, the following is a good technique for knowing where to cut a window in the cast for wound care and observation. **A.** The wound is covered with sterile dressings, which are wadded up in a ball over the wound. **B.** The cast is then applied in the routine fashion over the dressed wound. **C.** A window is cut out over the "bulge" produced in the cast.

circumferential cast in the acute setting can be problematic due to swelling and may result in a compartment syndrome. If a cast is placed in the emergency department and additional swelling is anticipated, the cast is cut on both sides and wrapped with an elastic bandage to hold it together. This process is known as "bivalving" the cast.

Fiberglass cast material is also used, as it is lightweight, strong, and radiolucent. Fiberglass casts can become wet without being softened or damaged. Fiberglass casts have limited applications to fresh fractures because fiberglass cannot be molded to the limb as well as the plaster. Another disadvantage is that the polyurethane resin within the fiberglass adheres to unprotected skin. Therefore, fiberglass casts are best used as a second or subsequent cast.

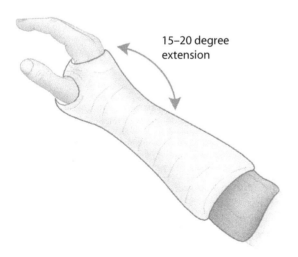

15–20 degree extension

Figure 1–22. A short arm cast with the wrist in 15 to 20 degree of extension and the fingers free at the metacarpophalangeal joint.

Checking Casts

Any patient with a circumferential cast should receive written instructions describing the symptoms of compartment syndrome from a tight cast. Increasing pain, swelling, coolness, or change in skin color of the distal portions of the extremity are signs that a cast is too tight, and the patient should be instructed to return immediately. As a general rule, we recommend that any circumferential cast be checked the following day for signs of circulatory compromise. The patient must be instructed to elevate the limb to avoid problems.

If a patient complains of discomfort at any point after cast application, it is best to remove the cast to check for compartment syndrome, pressure sores, or peripheral nerve injury. Alternatively, the cast can be split on both sides (i.e., bivalved) to decrease pressure. If the patient's complaints persist, the cast should be removed.

Figure 1–24 demonstrates the proper technique for removing or splitting a cast. The oscillating cast saw used to split plaster is generally safe, but can cut skin if not used carefully. One must remember to split not only the plaster casting but also the inner padding to significantly reduce the pressure. This was well demonstrated in a study that showed that no significant reduction in pressure occurred when only the plaster was opened. Splitting the plaster and the padding did result in a significant reduction in the soft-tissue pressure. Cast padding also affects pressure within the case. Evidence suggests that cotton-type padding offers the lowest pressure readings compared to synthetic and waterproof material.[17]

Closed Fracture Reduction

Fracture reduction is performed either open via surgery or closed. Closed reduction is carried out in the emergency department or operating room, depending on the circumstances.

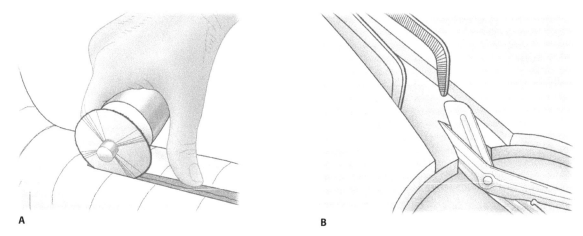

Figure 1–24. Cast removal using (*A*) cast saw and (*B*) cast spreader and safety bandage scissors.

Successful closed reduction is more likely if it is carried out as close to the time of injury as possible. Delaying reduction by several days will make the reduction more difficult.

Closed reduction should occur on an emergent basis when perfusion to the extremity is absent, especially in the setting of limited availability of orthopedic consultation. Because vascular injury can occur after any displaced fracture or dislocation, the clinician should note the presence of an expanding hematoma, absent distal pulses, or delayed capillary refill. An unperfused extremity has a finite period of time before nerve and muscle death occurs. For this reason, reduction should occur as soon as possible. The earlier the perfusion is regained, the better the chance of avoiding tissue necrosis.

Reduction in the emergency department is contraindicated in several instances:

1. The extremity is perfused and the patient will require immediate operative treatment. An open fracture in a perfused extremity, for example, should be reduced in the operating room, where an appropriate surgical washout can occur.
2. Remodeling is anticipated or the fracture will heal adequately without reduction. Remodeling, especially in children, may correct deformities gradually with healing and make the need for a painful reduction or the risk of procedural sedation unnecessary. In the adult skeleton, humeral shaft fractures and fifth metacarpal neck fractures are examples of bones in which some degree of residual angulation will not impact function, making reduction unnecessary.
3. Procedural sedation is inadequate or high risk. If adequate analgesia cannot be provided due to the patient's medical condition or the inability to appropriately monitor the patient, emergency department reduction should not be performed.
4. Vascular injury may be worsened by closed reduction. When vascular injury is suspected in a patient with a posterior sternoclavicular joint dislocation, for example,

reduction is best performed in the operating room with a cardiothoracic surgeon available because the distal clavicle may be tamponading a lacerated subclavian vessel. In a similar manner, supracondylar fractures require immediate reduction only when the extremity is pulseless and perfusion is absent.

The preparation of a patient for fracture reduction is dependent on the type of injury and the clinical setting. Explain the procedure to the patient and obtain consent. In performing the reduction, the patient should be supine whenever possible. The involved extremity should be fully exposed and any constricting pieces of clothing or jewelry both proximal and distal to the injury should be removed. If fluoroscopy is used, it should be moved into position. Frequently, splint material is set up prior to the start of the procedure so that it may be immediately applied to the extremity following reduction. This is especially helpful in the setting of an unstable fracture.

The basic principles to reduce fractures are similar and can be divided into four steps:

1. Distraction
2. Disengagement
3. Reapposition
4. Release

Distraction involves creating a longitudinal force to pull the bony fragments apart. This step is performed gradually and may require time to be effective in overcoming muscle spasm. Distraction is also important when the fractured ends of the bone are overriding. Distraction can be applied manually with the help of an assistant or by using weights.

Disengagement of the bony ends of the fracture allows for further disimpaction of the bone than does distraction alone. Disengagement can be achieved by rotating the distal fragment or by "re-creating the fracture deformity." It relieves tension on the soft tissues to allow interlocking fracture fragments to reposition.

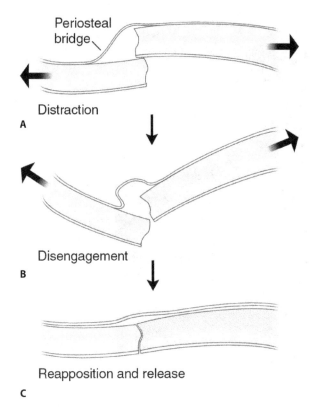

Periosteal
bridge

Distraction

A

Disengagement

B

Reapposition and release

C

Figure 1–25. Fracture reduction involves. **A.** Distraction. **B.** Disengagement. **C.** Reapposition and release. An intact periosteal bridge acts as a support to internally stabilize the fracture after reduction.

Reapposition is achieved by reversing the forces that caused the injury to bring the bone fragments back into alignment. A displaced fracture usually leaves the periosteum intact on one side. Without this intact periosteal bridge, reduction would be difficult to maintain (Fig. 1–25). An intact periosteal bridge will assist in the reduction and the maintenance of the reduction. Although this step seems simple conceptually, it may not be so easy in clinical practice. One important pitfall to avoid is ignoring a rotational deformity that might create functional problems if the bone went on to heal in this manner.

Release refers to the removal of the initial distracting force with the intent that alignment will be maintained. At this point, forces such as muscle contraction and gravity act on the fracture fragments, putting them at risk for becoming misaligned again. A properly applied splint or cast can protect from loss of fracture alignment. The patient should undergo repeat plain radiography or fluoroscopy in most cases to document the success of the reduction. Following reduction, the neurovascular status of the extremity should be reassessed to ensure pulses are present, the extremity is well perfused, and nerve function has not been compromised.

The astute clinician should also be aware of the limitations of the closed reduction technique. If soft tissue is interposed, for example, the fracture may be irreducible,

and no amount of distraction or alternative technique will obviate the situation. Additionally, fractures that are more than a week old are more difficult to reduce.

When performed properly, complications of fracture reduction are uncommon. However, even when techniques are properly adhered to, a complication may occur. These complications include converting a closed fracture to an open fracture, soft-tissue trauma during reduction that produces fracture instability or compartment syndrome, or neurovascular injury due to bony laceration or compression.

Definitive Treatment

The selection of definitive fracture treatment is a combined decision between the emergency physician and the referral physician. Some fractures can be treated safely with immobilization alone despite some angulation (e.g., humeral shaft, fifth metacarpal neck fracture). Others require closed reduction when displaced or angulated (e.g., Colles fracture). And still others require consultation for operative intervention (e.g., open fracture, femur fracture).

The management of individual fractures is discussed further in the remainder of the book. The emergency physician must be aware of the indications for operative intervention in managing fractures. Some general indications for operative management include the following:

- Displaced intra-articular fractures
- Associated arterial injury
- Experience shows that open treatment yields better results
- Closed methods fail to achieve or maintain acceptable alignment
- Fracture is through a metastatic lesion
- Early mobilization is desirable

Skeletal Traction

Traction can be applied to the skin (*skin traction*) or bone (*skeletal traction*) to align fractures. Skin traction has been used since popularized by Buck in the U.S. Civil War (Fig. 1–26). It was used as a temporary means to stabilize

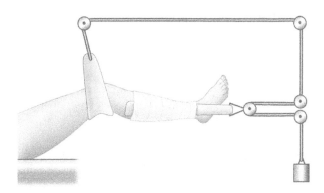

Figure 1–26. Skin traction can be used to temporarily distract a displaced fracture of the femur until the patient can be definitively managed the following day.

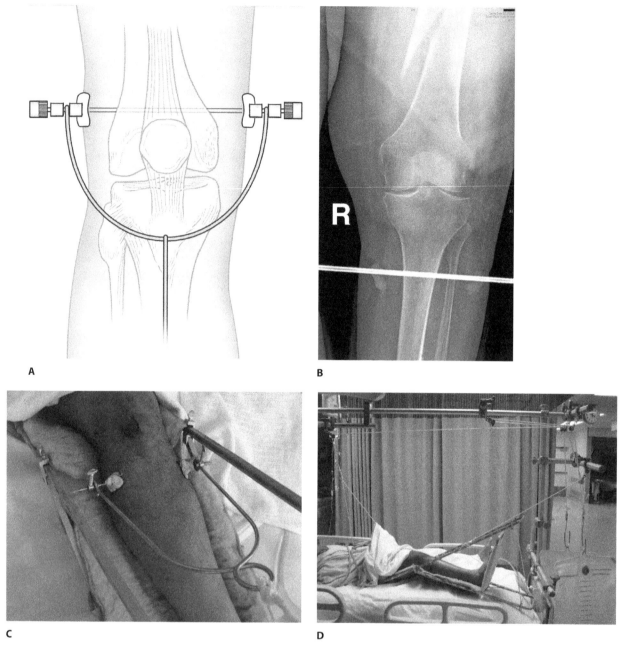

Figure 1–27. Skeletal traction. **A.** Schematic representation of a traction pin through the distal femur. **B.** Radiograph of a patient with a proximal tibia traction pin and a distal femur fracture. **C.** Clinical photograph of patient's leg. **D.** The entire apparatus with bags of water used as weights.

fractures of the hip; however, it is rarely used today. The use of adhesive tape and weights greater than 6 to 8 lb should be avoided as they may cause an avulsion of the superficial skin layers.

Skeletal traction, applied by an orthopedic consultant, is the preferred form of traction (Fig. 1–27). A pin (e.g., Steinmann pin) is passed through a bony prominence distal to the fracture site and weights are used to pull the fracture fragments into better alignment. This method is especially useful for comminuted fractures that cannot be held by plaster fixation. Skeletal traction may be used

as the sole treatment method when surgery is contraindicated, but it is more commonly used today as a temporary measure before a more definitive operative repair (i.e., intramedullary rod).

Skeletal traction is used most frequently in fractures of the femur and also in some tibia fractures, although it can be employed in the upper extremity to align humerus fractures. Common sites for pin placement in the lower extremity include the distal femur, proximal tibia, lower tibia, and calcaneus (Video 1–2). Complications include pin tract infections and overdistraction of the fracture.

Orthopedic Devices

A variety of devices are used to surgically stabilize an unstable fracture (Fig. 1–28). It is important for the emergency physician to have some familiarity with these devices and recognize their potential complications. The most common complications include implant failure (i.e., breakage), loss of fixation, and infections.

Plate and screws place the fracture ends in acceptable alignment to allow healing. If the fracture does not heal spontaneously, the plate will eventually break or the screws will come out. Healing occurs without the callus formation seen with casting. Screws may also be used independent of a plate. Examples include stabilization of a slipped capital femoral epiphysis and a displaced scaphoid fracture. The

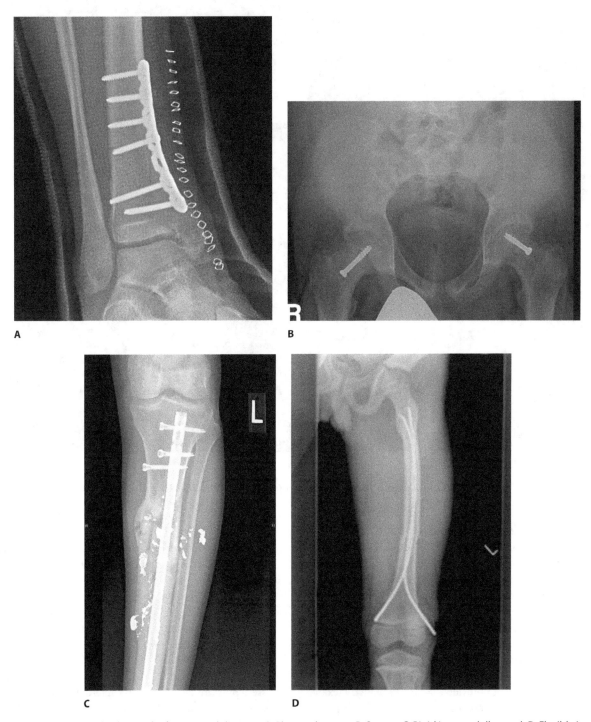

Figure 1–28. Orthopedic devices for fracture stabilization. *A.* Plate and screws. *B.* Screws. *C.* Rigid intramedullary rod. *D.* Flexible intramedullary rods. *(continued)*

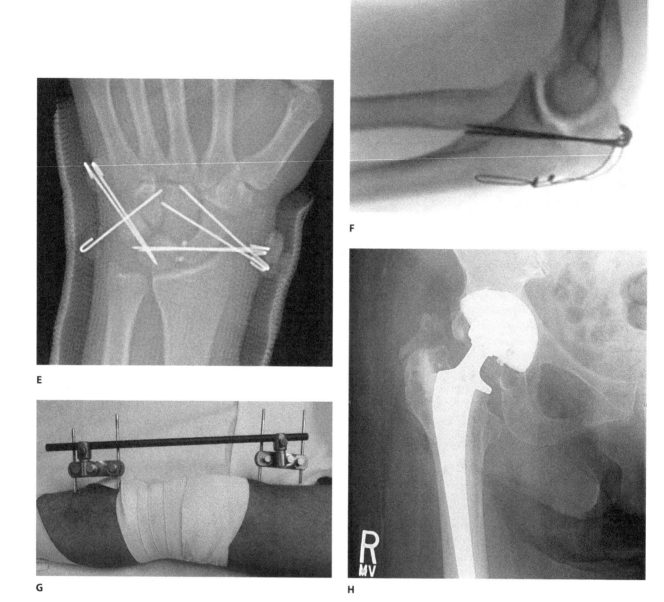

Figure 1–28. *(Continued)* **E.** Percutaneous pins. **F.** Tension band wires. **G.** External fixator. **H.** Total hip replacement.

most common complication of this type of internal fixation is wound infection.

Intramedullary rods (nails) are either rigid or flexible. Rigid intramedullary rods are used to treat long bone fractures. Because the fracture is not held in as much rigid alignment as a plate and screws, callus formation at the fracture site is more pronounced. Fracture healing is usually excellent because the periosteum and fracture hematoma are not disturbed when the rod is placed. Once the rod is placed, interlocking screws are frequently added to provide rotational stability. Flexible intramedullary rods are most common in the pediatric population because they can be inserted through the metaphyseal portion of the bone and avoid injury to the growth plate.

Rods are mechanically stronger than a plate and screws, but can break if the fracture does not unite. Infection is less common than with plate and screws. Flexible and unlocked rigid intramedullary rods can migrate out of the bone and into the soft tissues.

Percutaneous pins are used for fractures of the small bones of the hand and foot. As the name implies, the pin is inserted directly through the skin and then can be cut so that only a small portion of the pin is exposed. These stainless steel pins are also frequently referred to as Kirschner wires or K wires after Martin Kirschner who introduced them in 1909. Complications of these devices include pin tract infections, migration, or breakage.

Tension band wires are used to realign fractures that undergo distracting forces because of muscles. Examples include olecranon, greater tuberosity proximal humerus, and patella fractures. In this technique, the fracture fragments are aligned by percutaneous pins that also function as an anchor for a loop of flexible wire that serves to hold the fragments together. Complications of these devices include breakage, bursitis, and wire perforation through the skin.

External fixation has a frame that is supported by pins placed through the proximal and distal fracture fragments. These devices are used preferentially in the setting of open fractures as they allow for monitoring of soft tissues and the reduction of infection. They are also used to temporarily stabilize pelvis fractures and occasionally for the treatment of distal radius fractures. Pin tract infections and loosening of the device are the most common complications.

Prosthetic joints are available for almost every joint in the body. They are considered a total (complete) arthroplasty if both sides of the joint are replaced and a hemiarthroplasty (partial) if only one side of the joint is prosthetic. In the hip, total joint arthroplasty is used more commonly for arthritis, whereas hemiarthroplasty may be all that is required for a displaced femoral neck fracture. The most common type of total hip replacement uses a metal femoral prosthesis that articulates with a plastic acetabular cup. The plastic cup is secured to the acetabulum via a metal backing. The term "constrained" is used when the two portions of the prosthetic joint are locked together instead of being stabilized by the patient's intrinsic ligaments and tendons. Constrained devices are more likely to loosen. Another complication is dislocation, which can occur with both constrained and nonconstrained prosthetic joints. Reduction of a dislocated constrained device is rarely successful in the emergency department and may cause damage to the device if attempted. The other catastrophic complication of a prosthetic joint is infection. Consultation is advised in all cases of a suspected prosthetic joint infection.

Open Fractures

An open fracture occurs when a break in the skin and soft tissue directly communicates with a fracture and its hematoma. Although the diagnosis is straightforward in most cases, it can be difficult when there is a distance between the fracture fragments and the open wound.

A history should be obtained regarding the mechanism and location of injury. A high-energy farm injury, for example, would suggest a worse prognosis with higher rates of contamination than a low-energy fall on a sidewalk. The clinician must perform a neurovascular examination and immediately reduce the fracture only when associated with absent perfusion to the distal extremity.

Examination of the tissue within and around the wound should be performed, noting any contaminants. Lipid, in the form of fat globules, noted floating in the blood coming from a wound is evidence of an underlying open fracture.[18]

There should be no attempt to explore the wound digitally in the emergency department as little information will be provided and an increased risk of infection will result. If a question arises when a small wound is noted on the skin that overlies a fracture, one can safely check the wound with a sterile blunt probe to see whether the bone is touched.

Radiographs may aid in the diagnosis if air is seen within the soft tissues in patients who have suffered a recent injury. If it is still unclear whether the fracture is open, the prudent management would dictate to simply treat it as if it were open and obtain orthopedic consultation.

Gustilo and Anderson have classified open long bone fractures by the severity of associated soft-tissue damage and degree of wound contamination. This classification system is used widely and will allow the emergency physician to effectively communicate with an orthopedic consultant (Fig. 1–29). However, the interobserver reliability of the system is shown to be of poor to moderate agreement.[19]

- *Grade I* describes an open wound due to a low-energy injury. The wound is <1 cm in length and shows no evidence of contamination.[19] The fractures in grade I wounds are usually simple, transverse, or short oblique with minimal comminution. A fracture fragment piercing the skin from the inside usually causes these wounds.
- *Grade II* wounds involve a moderate amount of soft-tissue injury. Some comminution of the fracture and a moderate degree of contamination may be present. Grade II open fractures are characterized by a wound that is >1 cm in length. No soft tissue is stripped from the bone.
- *Grade IIIA* is a large wound (usually >10 cm). The degree of contamination is high, and the amount of soft-tissue injury is severe; however, there is adequate soft-tissue coverage of the bone. Comminution of the associated fracture is usually present.
- *Grade IIIB* is a large wound (usually >10 cm) with periosteal stripping and exposed bone. In this subclass, the degree of soft-tissue injury is such that reconstructive surgery is often necessary to cover the wound. Massive contamination and a severely comminuted fracture are noted in this subclass.[19]
- *Grade IIIC* is similar to the IIIB injury, but is associated with the additional finding of significant arterial injury that requires repair for salvage of the extremity.

Treatment in the prehospital setting consists of covering the wound with a sterile dressing and splinting the extremity. In the emergency department, foreign bodies or obvious debris should be removed sterilely either manually or with forceps. Tetanus prophylaxis is administered when indicated. Tdap (tetanus, diphtheria, and pertussis) should be administered to adults older than 19 once in their lifetime and to pregnant patients during each pregnancy regardless of Tdap interval.[20] The wound can be swabbed for a culture at the request of the orthopedic surgeon; however, there is evidence that predebridement cultures are of little value.

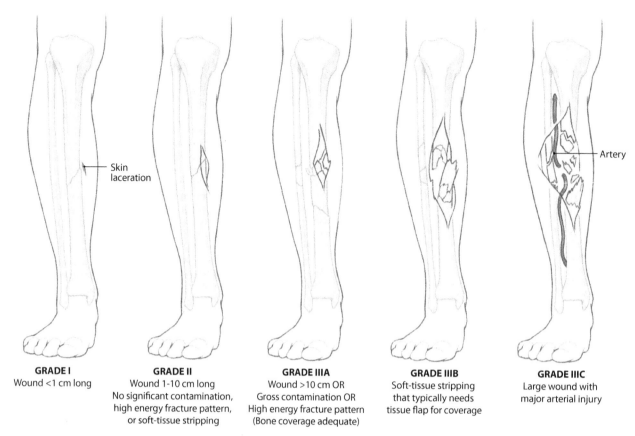

GRADE I
Wound <1 cm long

GRADE II
Wound 1-10 cm long
No significant contamination,
high energy fracture pattern,
or soft-tissue stripping

GRADE IIIA
Wound >10 cm OR
Gross contamination OR
High energy fracture pattern
(Bone coverage adequate)

GRADE IIIB
Soft-tissue stripping
that typically needs
tissue flap for coverage

GRADE IIIC
Large wound with
major arterial injury

Figure 1–29. Gustilo-Anderson classification of open long bone fractures.

Broad-spectrum antibiotics against both gram-positive and gram-negative organisms are recommended for use in open fractures. Antibiotics should be started as soon as possible after the injury. Antibiotics given within 3 hours have been shown to reduce infection rates from 7.4% to 4.7%. The most common organism producing infection is *Staphylococcus aureus*. The open fracture wound most susceptible to secondary infection is the close-range shotgun wound.

Following consultation with the orthopedic surgeon, a decision will be made regarding irrigation (wash-out) and debridement. Patients with open fractures have debridement performed in the operating room in most cases. One possible exception includes open hand (metacarpal and phalange) fractures, where studies have shown that small (<1 cm), clean injuries, without significant soft-tissue injury or fracture comminution have a low infection rate (1.5%).

If the patient is to be taken to the operating room for formal irrigation and debridement within 1 to 2 hours of injury, the sterile dressing and splint should be reapplied after obvious debris is removed. If there is a delay in taking the patient to the operating room beyond 2 hours, then the wound should be irrigated with 1 to 2 L of normal saline before the sterile dressing is reapplied. Recent evidence questions the optimal timing of debridement, with evidence now suggesting that debridement completed 6 to 24 hours post injury does not increase infection rates.

Note that keeping an open wound moist will increase the surface humidity, which is an important factor in healing. In addition, occlusive dressings will facilitate local healing by raising the wound temperature.

Gunshot Wounds

Gunshot wounds are commonplace in our society with as many as 500,000 occurring annually in the United States and 33,736 deaths reported in 2014. Many patients with these injuries present to the emergency department with associated fractures. Weapons are divided into two types— low velocity (<2000 ft/s) and high velocity (>2000 ft/s). Wounds inflicted by low-velocity weapons (e.g., handguns and shotguns) are still the most commonly seen; however, wounds from higher-velocity weapons (e.g., M-16, AK-47) are becoming more common.

Shotguns are low-velocity guns that are different from handguns because they propel hundreds of lead pellets (Fig. 1–30). Because the shotgun has a high efficacy of energy transfer at close range, it causes significant soft-tissue damage and bone injury leading to the highest risk of infection and compartment syndrome. Close-range shotgun blasts can be determined by measuring the diameter of the pellet spread on the patient. A wound with a diameter of <7 cm suggests a close-range shotgun injury.

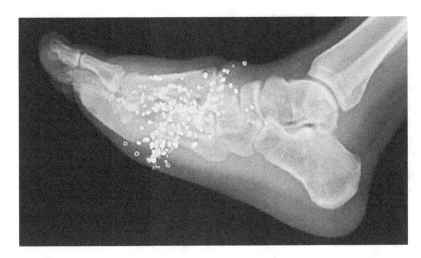

Figure 1–30. Multiple shotgun pellets in the foot.

When evaluating a patient with a gunshot wound to the extremity, the clinician must first address the ABCs of trauma care with a thorough primary survey. With regard to the injured extremity, the initial priority is the neurovascular status of the extremity. In patients with signs of vascular injury, angiography, and/or intraoperative exploration are warranted.

Most low-velocity gunshot wounds without evidence of vascular injury can be treated safely with local wound care, tetanus prophylaxis, and outpatient management. Antibiotics are controversial, but if used for routine prophylaxis, a short 3-day course of oral antibiotics (ciprofloxacin, cephalexin, or dicloxacillin) is likely sufficient. A recent review article did not find a significant difference in nonoperatively managed, low-velocity gunshot wound infection rates.[25] Associated fractures are treated according to accepted protocols for similar fractures in patients who were not shot. These injuries are treated as if they were "closed" fractures. Irrigation of the wound is followed by the application of a sterile dressing. The wound is left open and the fracture immobilized appropriately. Patients presenting more than 8 hours after injury may benefit from operative debridement because local wound care is less efficacious.

High-velocity injuries, close-range gunshot injuries, and grossly contaminated wounds require operative irrigation and debridement. These wounds are treated as open fractures. Intravenous antibiotics are indicated and should be started prior to surgery.[26]

Gunshot wounds that penetrate a joint generally require arthrotomy or arthroscopy for adequate debridement (Fig. 1–31). The presence of retained bullet fragments within the joint is an absolute indication for operative intervention. These wounds are associated with a high likelihood of injury to the soft tissues of the joint. Low-velocity injuries that penetrated the knee joint had a 42% incidence of meniscal injury and 15% incidence of chondral injury. These patients should receive at least 24 to 48 hours of intravenous antibiotics.

An important, yet often omitted, responsibility is careful documentation of the gunshot wound. A simple approach is to record the location of the wound, size or diameter, shape, and characteristics of the wound. Due to the difficulty in accurately determining whether the wound is an entrance or an exit wound do not attempt to describe the wound in these terms.

Another type of injury occurs after the accidental discharge of a nail gun with approximately 25,000 injuries occurring annually in the United States[27] (Fig. 1–32). The majority of injuries occur to the hand. High-velocity nail guns are capable of firing projectiles up to 10 cm into fully stressed concrete, and when discharged accidentally, have

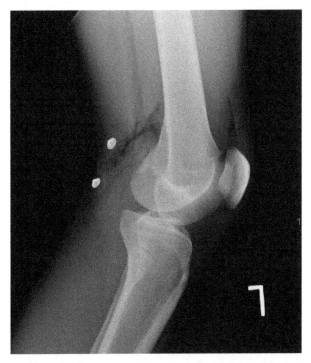

Figure 1–31. Gunshot wound causing traumatic arthrotomy of the knee joint. Note the presence of air within the joint.

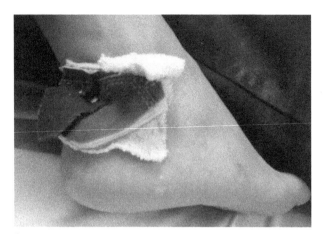
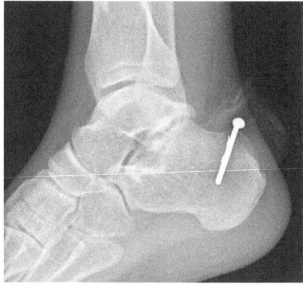

A   **B**

Figure 1–32. Nail gun injury. **A.** This construction worker accidentally discharged his nail gun through his heavy-duty construction boot and into his foot. **B.** Radiographs revealed that the nail was within the calcaneus. Note the barb present on the nail.

caused fatal injuries. If important vascular structures are not in proximity and the nail did not enter a joint space, it is safe to remove the nail in the emergency department.

Before removal, however, a radiograph should be obtained. The nails are held together within the gun by copper wires. This is significant because the copper may remain on the nail and create a barb that would make retrograde removal difficult. If such a barb is noted and the nail has pierced through the extremity, the head of the nail should be cut off and the nail pulled the remainder of the way through.

Following removal, the wound is thoroughly irrigated and debrided, and the patient is given tetanus prophylaxis as needed (with pertussis if indicated). Most authors recommend a dose of intravenous antibiotics followed by a short course of oral antibiotics.

Stress Fractures

A stress (fatigue) fracture is a common injury seen by health care professionals, particularly those who treat athletes. Under normal conditions of strain, bone hypertrophies. A stress fracture results when repetitive loading of the bone overwhelms the reparative ability of the skeletal system. People in poor physical condition who begin a strenuous fitness program are at a greater risk for developing a stress fracture. Alternatively, a conditioned athlete can develop a stress fracture after a recent increase in activity level. The diagnosis requires a thorough clinical examination with a high index of suspicion.

A number of possible factors may predispose a person to stress fractures. The type of surface (i.e., hard surface) may cause a stress fracture, as could a change in the intensity, speed, or distance at which a patient is doing exercise. Inappropriate shoes can result in stress fractures. Other factors include mechanical problems such as a leg length discrepancy, increased knee valgus, foot disorders, and decreased tibia bone width.

The most common sites for stress fractures are listed in Figure 1–33.[38] Stress fractures can occur in the upper extremities, but are much less common. Stress fractures are more common in women. Other conditions that should be considered in the differential of stress fractures include periostitis, infection, muscle strain, bursitis, exertional compartment syndrome, and nerve entrapment.

The patient presents with a complaint of pain and discomfort, describing an initial aching after exercise that progresses to pain localized to the site of the fracture. In general, the pain starts 4 weeks after the increase in physical activity. Pain progresses in severity during the activity until the exercise is discontinued. The time to diagnosis is variable and may be several weeks to months in some cases.

The physical examination will vary depending on the location of the stress fracture. A stress fracture of the proximal femur will reveal minimal clinical findings. Pain is usually present in the anterior groin. Hip motion, especially the extremes of internal and external rotation, exacerbates the pain. In addition, pain is produced when the patient is asked to hop on the affected extremity (hop test).

The initial plain films reveal a fracture in only 10% of cases.[39] A bone scan is more sensitive in detecting new stress fractures. It should be noted, however, that a positive bone scan is a nonspecific finding and can occur in other conditions. Other options to confirm the diagnosis when the initial plain films are negative include repeating the plain radiographs, MRI, or CT.

The treatment for stress fractures is conservative unless the location is considered high risk for a completed fracture that may be complicated by nonunion or avascular necrosis. The most common high-risk stress fracture is of the femoral neck. These patients should be treated as if they have an acute fracture and should not bear weight. Operative intervention is often required. Other high-risk stress fractures are the anterior cortex of the tibia, talus, medial malleolus, tarsal navicular, and the fifth metatarsal.

If the stress fracture is not high risk, conservative treatment involves a decrease in activity to the point that the pain is no longer present. It is rarely necessary to eliminate activities of daily living, but if pain is persistent, the patient is kept no weight bearing. Some authors recommend immediate cross training, such as bicycling, rollerblading, and pool running. Cessation of the precipitating activity for a minimum period of 4 weeks is required. After this period, the patient can gradually resume previous activities. NSAIDs are avoided due to their potential negative effects on bone healing.

Pathologic Fractures

A pathologic fracture occurs in bone that is abnormally weakened by a preexisting condition. Osteoporosis is the most common cause of a pathologic fracture, followed by metastatic lesions (Fig. 1–34). Table 1–3 lists other causes of pathologic fractures. Bony metastases represent the third most common location for metastasis after lung and liver. The most common sites for bony metastasis occur in the axial skeleton (e.g., spine, ribs, pelvis). However, most pathologic fractures from metastatic lesions occur

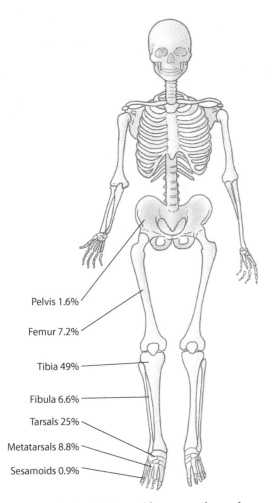

Pelvis 1.6%

Femur 7.2%

Tibia 49%

Fibula 6.6%

Tarsals 25%

Metatarsals 8.8%

Sesamoids 0.9%

Figure 1–33. The distribution and frequency of stress fractures.

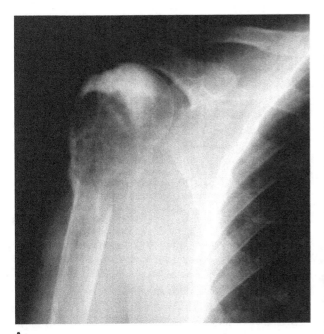

A

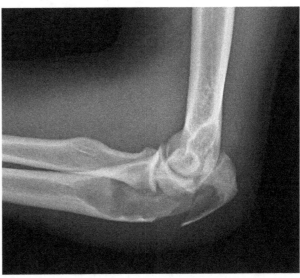

B

Figure 1–34. *A.* Lytic lesion of the humerus with pathologic fracture. *(Used with permission from J. Wanggaard, NP.)* ***B.*** Olecranon fracture in a patient with a prior benign bone cyst.

▶ TABLE 1-3. **CAUSES OF PATHOLOGIC FRACTURES**

Systemic Conditions
Osteoporosis
Paget disease
Osteogenesis imperfect
Osteopetrosis
Osteomalacia
Hyperparathyroid.ism
Vitamin D deficiency (Rickets)
Local Lesions
Metastatic lesions
  Breast, prostate, lung, kidney, thyroid
Osteomyelitis
Primary benign diseases
  Enchondroma
  Unicameral bone cysts
  Chondroblastoma
  Chondromyxofibroma
  Giant cell tumors
  Non-ossifying fibroma
Primary malignant diseases
  Multiple myeloma
  Ewing sarcoma
  Chondrosarcoma
  Fibrosarcoma
  Malignant fibrous histiocytoma

in the axial skeleton (e.g., femur, humerus). Metastatic pathologic fractures rarely occur distal to the knee and elbow. Enchondromas are benign tumors that commonly occur in the metacarpals and phalanges and may lead to fractures.

Any fracture that occurs from trivial trauma must be considered a pathologic fracture. Patients may note generalized bone pain or even painless swelling over the site of the pathologic fracture. Benign lesions are usually asymptomatic prior to the fracture. Bony pain prior to the fracture suggests that the lesion is more likely malignant.

The threshold to obtain plain films should be lower in patients with any of the systemic conditions listed in Table 1–3. On the radiograph, look for generalized osteopenia, periosteal reaction, thinning of the cortices, and changes in the trabecular pattern around the fracture site. The more severe the periosteal lesion, the more likely it is associated with a malignancy. Ultimately, the fracture should be splinted, and, depending on the suspicion for malignancy, the patient should be admitted for further diagnostic testing.

SOFT-TISSUE PRINCIPLES

Ligamentous Injury

Ligamentous injuries are divided into first-, second-, and third-degree sprains. A *first-degree* sprain is a tear of only a few fibers and is characterized by minimal swelling, no functional disability, and normal joint motion.

A *second-degree* sprain is a partial tear of the ligament. Second-degree sprains present with swelling, tenderness, and functional disability; however, there is generally no abnormal motion noted of the joint. Subsequent healing occurs in second-degree sprains, provided the joint is immobilized initially and protected from further mechanical stresses for approximately 6 weeks.

Third-degree sprains are characterized by complete disruption of the ligament and abnormal motion of the joint. Significant swelling occurs shortly after injury, and functional disability is readily apparent. Stress tests perpendicular to the normal plane of joint motion distinguishes second- from third-degree injuries. In patients with third-degree sprains, gross instability without pain is often demonstrated. In contrast, severe pain is caused when a partially damaged ligament is stretched, and the degree of opening of the joint is limited.

In third-degree sprains, direct apposition of the two severed ends of a ligament will result in a better outcome with minimal scar tissue than if the ligament ends have not been sutured. Apposition of the ligament ends hastens collagenization and restores normal ligament tissue. Ligaments divided and not immobilized heal with a gap. Sutured ligaments tested under tension compared to those not sutured showed the sutured ligaments to be stronger. The nonsutured ligaments failed at the scar. For these reasons, the authors would advocate repair of most third-degree (complete) disruptions of major supporting ligaments around weight-bearing joints within the first week after injury.

Bursitis and Tendonitis

Bursae are flattened sacs lined with a synovial membrane and filled with a thin layer of synovial fluid. They function to limit friction created by the movements of tendon and muscle over bony prominences. There are approximately 160 bursae throughout the body. Excessive frictional forces, trauma, or systemic diseases such as rheumatoid arthritis or gout may cause inflammation within a bursa and result in bursitis. The most common form of bursitis is subacromial (subdeltoid) bursitis. Other commonly encountered forms of bursitis include trochanteric, olecranon, calcaneal, anserine, and prepatellar bursitis. Treatment for bursitis consists of avoidance of the aggravating activity, rest of the involved extremity, an NSAID, and local steroid injection.

Tendonitis is an inflammatory process of the tendon involving its insertion into the bone. Tendonitis can result from chronic overuse or a single episode of strenuous activity. Chronic tendonitis results in atrophy of the tendon fibers. Clinically, tendonitis presents with pain during active range of motion and point tenderness near its bony insertion. Forced contraction of the muscle with pressure over the insertion of the tendon exacerbates the pain. Calcific tendonitis is associated with chronic inflammation and

▶ TABLE 1–4. **CORTICOSTEROID PREPARATIONS AVAILABLE FOR INJECTION**

Generic Name	Trade Name	Strength (mg/mL)	Relative Potency	Dose Range (mg)	Biological Half-Life (h)
Hydrocortisone acetate	Cortef Solu-Cortef	25	1	12.5–100	8–12
Triamcinolone acetonide	Kenalog-10	10	2.5	4.0–40	18–36
	Kenalog-40	40	10		
Triamcinolone hexacetonide	Aristospan	20	8	4.0–25	18–36
Dexamethasone acetate	Decadron, Hexadrol, Dexone	4, 8	20–30	0.8–4.0	36–54
Betamethasone sodium phosphate	Celestone	6	20–30	1.5–6.0	36–54
Methylprednisolone acetate	Medrol, Depo-Medrol, Solu-Medrol	20, 40, 80	5, 10, 20	4.0–30	18–36

Reproduced with permission from Reichman EF: *Emergency Medicine Procedures*, 2nd ed. New York: McGraw-Hill; 2013.

calcium deposition within the tendon that can be detected on plain radiographs. Common forms of tendonitis include patellar, quadriceps, rotator cuff, Achilles, lateral epicondylitis (tennis elbow), and de Quervain tenosynovitis. Like bursitis, treatment consists of rest, NSAIDs, and local steroid injection.

Local steroid injection for bursitis and tendonitis requires the physician to be familiar with the anatomy of the affected extremity. If used properly, corticosteroids serve to decrease inflammation, decrease pain, and promote healing. Contraindications to local steroid injection include an overlying cellulitis, suspicion of septic arthritis, coagulopathy, and more than three injections in 1 year.

Corticosteroid preparations available for injection are listed in Table 1–4. Triamcinolone hexacetonide (Aristospan) and triamcinolone acetonide (Kenalog) are preferred as they are potent preparations with long duration of action. The local effects of these agents may last for months. The amount of steroid to be injected depends on the indication. For large spaces such as the subacromial, olecranon, and trochanteric bursae, a dose of 20 to 30 mg of methylprednisolone acetate or its equivalent is appropriate, while tendon sheaths, such as de Quervain tenosynovitis, require a smaller dose of 5 to 15 mg of methylprednisolone acetate or its equivalent.

The addition of a local anesthetic to the steroid preparation provides two useful purposes. The patient is afforded immediate pain relief and the physician is comfortable that the location of the injection is anatomically correct. Lidocaine, bupivacaine, and mepivacaine are the most commonly used anesthetic agents.

Tendon Rupture

Tendons may be injured by either an avulsion or a laceration. Lacerations occur more commonly than tendon avulsion. Tendon avulsion occurs at the site of bony insertion or the muscle–tendon junction. The four most common avulsed tendons include the Achilles, quadriceps, biceps, and rotator cuff tendons (Fig. 1–35). The peroneal and patellar tendon also commonly rupture. Rupture of the extensor tendons of the hands occurs in patients with rheumatoid arthritis. Medications such as steroids and fluoroquinolones have also been associated with a higher incidence of tendon rupture. Achilles tendonitis and rupture are significantly associated with fluoroquinolone use. Age of 60 years or older, female gender, and body mass index less than 30 kg/m^2, concomitant use of steroids, diabetes, renal failure, or renal replacement therapy all increase risk associated with this class of antibiotics.

Tendon avulsions at bony attachments involve a fracture fragment or tendon that can be surgically reattached. Partial tendon ruptures usually heal well if further injury is prevented. Because gaps between the muscle–tendon junctions decrease the strength of the tendon after healing, complete tendon ruptures are repaired surgically. Rupture at the muscle–tendon junction is more difficult to repair surgically than rupture at the site of bony attachment due to the unpredictable nature of suturing tendon to muscle.

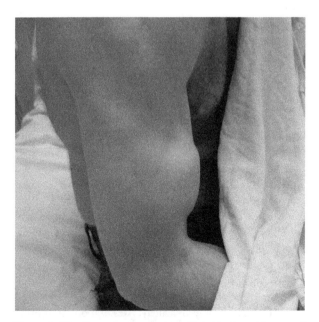

Figure 1–35. Biceps tendon rupture. Note the bunching up of the biceps muscle in the arm.

The flexor tendons of the hand are the most common tendons to be lacerated. These lacerations pose a unique challenge because the tendons pass through synovial-lined sheaths and fibrous pulleys. Adhesions to these structures, even when the tendon is surgically repaired, limit tendon function and restrict motion. If sutures are too taut, they can constrict the microcirculation of the tendon and impair healing. The commonly used Bunnell crisscross suture technique is particularly invasive. Controlled mobilization after tendon repair reduces adhesions and promotes healing, but excessive loading can result in reinjury.

Nerve Injury

Three types of nerve injuries can occur. A simple contusion of a nerve is called a *neurapraxia* and is treated by observation alone; a return to normal function is noted over the ensuing weeks or months. An *axonotmesis* is a more significant disruption that is followed by degeneration. The healing time is prolonged. Complete division of a nerve is called a *neurotmesis*, which typically requires surgical repair.

Muscle Disorders

Muscles are injured by direct and indirect trauma. A forceful blow can cause a localized contusion, hematoma, or laceration of the overlying fascia resulting in herniation. Indirect mechanisms of muscle injury are due to overstretching and result in tearing of the muscle fibers with ensuing hemorrhage and a partial loss of function—muscle strain. Complications of severe muscle injury are seen early in rhabdomyolysis and late in traumatic myositis ossificans. Muscle injury may also result from a systemic inflammatory response in the form of myositis.

Muscle Contusion

The wounding capacity of an object striking a muscle is directly proportional to its mass and the square of its velocity. Direct blunt trauma to a muscle results in partial disruption of the muscle fibers and capillary rupture. Ecchymosis is seen externally, while internally an inflammatory response and edema formation are noted.

Contusions are classified as mild, moderate, and severe. A mild contusion retains normal range of motion, and when it occurs in the lower extremity, it does not affect the gait. Localized tenderness is present, but there is no apparent swelling. Moderate contusions are characterized by reduction in range of motion, obvious swelling, and gait disturbance. Severe muscle contusions result in significant reduction in range of motion. Severe tenderness, edema, and an obvious limp are present. If bleeding is severe, a muscular hematoma forms.

Treatment involves restricting range of motion to minimize the risk of hemorrhage. Ice, elevation, and compression are also employed acutely. Restoration of motion occurs gradually as return to activity too early may result in reinjury and a significantly prolonged disability.

Muscle Herniation

Muscle herniates through a defect in the overlying fascia. A soft "tumor" may be palpated through the defect, which is not tethered to the overlying skin. The patient may complain of a swelling or bulge of the muscle when contracted and weakness may be noted. An audible snap associated with severe pain during a strong contraction may be noted. The mass is reduced by compression when the muscle is at rest. The muscles most commonly involved with this condition are the biceps, rectus femoris, and gastrocnemius. The treatment is contingent on the symptoms. If there are significant symptoms, the patient should be referred for repair of the defect.

Muscle Strain

Muscle strain occur secondary to excessive use (chronic strain) or excessive stress (acute strain). Although a strain can occur at any point within the muscle, the most common location is the distal muscle–tendon junction. Muscles that cross two joints and consist of more fast-twitch fibers (e.g., gastrocnemius, quadriceps, and hamstring) are more susceptible to strains. Strains are divided into first (mild), second (moderate), and third (severe) degree based on the amount of pain, spasm, and disability.

First-Degree Strain. The patient complains of mild localized pain, cramping, or tightness with movement or muscle tension. Pain is frequently not present until after the activity is over. Mild spasm and localized tenderness may be present. Routine function of the muscle is usually preserved with mild limitation. For instance, in the lower extremity, the patient is able to ambulate.

The patient is advised to place ice packs over the injured muscle and to rest for a few days. Mobilization may safely be started as tolerated. The use of an NSAID is indicated in the acute setting.

Second-Degree Strain. More forceful muscle contraction or stretch results in a greater disruption of muscle fibers. Swelling and ecchymosis are frequently present, in addition to tenderness and muscle spasm (Fig. 1–36). Pain is immediate in onset in relation to the activity. When the injury is in the lower extremity, it significantly limits ambulation.

In patients with second-degree strains, the injured muscle must be immobilized, the limb elevated, and ice packs applied for the first 3 to 7 days. While conclusive evidence is lacking for cryotherapy, recommended regimens range with cold application for 15 to 20 minutes every 30 minutes to 2 hours. After this, the muscle should be *"placed at rest"* using crutches for ambulation (lower extremity) or a sling (upper extremity) until the swelling and tenderness subsides, usually a period of 3 to 7 days. Passive stretching should be discouraged when there is significant hemorrhage and swelling as this may result in increased fibrosis, resulting in calcium deposition and a delay in healing. Ambulation (lower

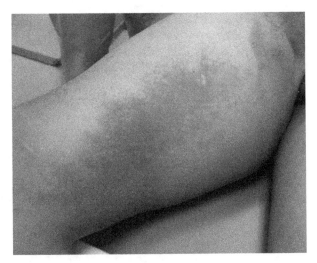

Figure 1–36. Second-degree adductor muscle strain. This patient had significant pain with thigh adduction. Note the ecchymosis from muscle fiber disruption.

extremity) or use of the injured muscle (upper extremity) should not be initiated until the pain has resolved.

After a brief period of immobilization, usually lasting no longer than a week, progressive active exercises can be started to the limit of pain. This stage of treatment should be accompanied by heat application. One of the more common complications is injury recurrence due to early return to normal activity, particularly in the athlete. Calcium deposition in the muscle, leading to prolonged disability, is another common complication, and is also a result of premature return to activity.[34]

Third-Degree Strain. There is complete disruption of the muscle, and the overlying fascia may be ruptured. The patient experiences severe pain and muscle spasm accompanied by swelling and ecchymosis. A large hematoma, localized tenderness, and loss of muscle function are noted, as well as bulging or bunching up of the muscle, particularly if the injury involves the musculotendinous junction.

Third-degree strains should be immobilized in a splint with ice packs applied, and the limb should be elevated. The patient should be referred for consultation as surgical repair may be indicated depending on age, the location of the tear, and which muscle is involved.

Rhabdomyolysis

This condition occurs when a large enough muscular injury results in the disruption of the integrity of the cell membrane with release of the cellular contents, including myoglobin. Rhabdomyolysis may be a result of a crush injury, prolonged immobility, hyperthermia, muscle ischemia, drugs or toxins, infection, or exertion. Muscle pain is present in only 50% of cases. Treatment is supportive and consists of fluid hydration and alkalinization of the urine to prevent myoglobin deposition within the kidney and subsequent renal failure.

Traumatic Myositis Ossificans

Myositis ossificans is a benign, solitary, self-limiting, localized muscular ossification that is due to skeletal muscle injury in 75% of cases and usually involves young male athletes. The formation of bone in muscle can follow a single blow or a series of repeated minor traumas to the muscle. The remainder of cases are seen in paraplegics or burn victims, or they may be congenital or idiopathic. The definition is complicated by historical controversies in that myositis ossificans definitions have ranged from benign to oncologic, are difficult to diagnosis, and usually require a multidisciplinary team approach. The incidence of traumatic myositis ossificans is reported with frequencies of 9% to 17% following muscle contusions. The most common muscles affected are the quadriceps and brachialis anticus.[35]

The mechanism is not completely understood, but a hematoma is usually a necessary prerequisite for the process to occur, and this condition is rarely seen after muscle strains. Extraskeletal bone formation may depend on endothelial-mesenchymal transition, where injury induces a local inflammatory cascade. This leads to cytokine release whereby the cytokine act on vascular endothelial cells and cause the endothelial-mesenchymal transition. The mesenchymal cells may then differentiate into chondrocytes or osteoblasts, with chondrocytes undergoing bone formation.[35]

The site having the highest predilection for myositis ossificans is the brachialis anticus muscle anterior to the elbow joint. Injury usually occurs after a posterior dislocation of the elbow. When a mass of bone forms, active and passive motion is restricted. Later, pain and swelling are reduced and a hard, tumor-like mass is palpable over the anterior aspect of the elbow. Active extension of the joint is limited by "inelasticity" of the muscle. Flexion is also prevented by obstruction from the mass. In some cases, a complete ossifying bridge may form at the joint.

Radiographs show the calcified mass beginning to form by the third to fourth week post injury, and definite radiographic evidence should be present by four weeks (Fig. 1–37). These lesions must be differentiated from the expanding heterotopic bone formation of an osteosarcoma. Bone scintigraphy, CT, and MRI are also useful aids in diagnosing, with MRI being the single best modality.[35]

The mass of bone may be connected to the shaft of a long bone by a pedicle or may be completely separate. Spontaneous repair may occur with complete disappearance of the osseous mass. The process usually ceases spontaneously in 3 to 6 months.

The osseous growth should not be disturbed in its early stage. Rest is indicated with the extremity immobilized by a splint or lightweight cast for 3 to 7 days. When the elbow is involved, the proper position of immobilization is with the forearm in a neutral position and the elbow flexed to 90 degrees. No surgery is indicated for 6 to 18 months because spontaneous resorption can occur with complete disappearance of the mass.[32] Some studies suggest that intravenous bisphosphonate therapy (e.g., pamidronate)

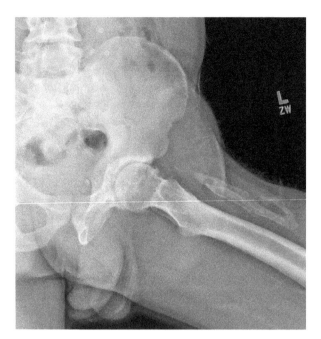

Figure 1–37. Traumatic myositis ossificans of the quadriceps muscle. Note the heterotopic ossification above the femur.

may have potential treatment benefits. Early surgical intervention may result in recurrence of the calcification and is usually indicated only for intractable pain from mechanical irritation of tendons, bursa, joints, or compression of neurovascular structures.

Myositis

Myositis is an inflammation of a muscle that may be due to an infectious agent, such as bacteria, or an autoimmune disorder. For a further discussion of necrotizing soft-tissue infections, the reader is referred to Chapter 4.

Infectious Myositis. Infectious agents that cause myositis include bacteria, mycobacteria, fungi, viruses, and parasitic agents. Bacteria invade muscle by contiguous extension more frequently than hematogenous spread. Acute suppurative myositis with abscess formation in the muscle, *pyomyositis*, is an unusual but important condition to consider because it is easily missed. Pyomyositis often presents following muscle trauma (20%–50% of cases), and due to the intramuscular nature of the abscess, many of the superficial findings associated with a soft-tissue infection are absent. Fever, chills, or an unexplained leukocytosis should help differentiate this condition from other causes of muscle pain. CT scanning may be very useful for detection. Systemic manifestations of sepsis may also occur, but this is usually a later finding.

Pyomyositis was initially believed to predominate in tropical climates but has, more recently, had increasing prevalence in more temperate climates. It occurs with greater frequency in patients with certain immunocompromised conditions (e.g., diabetes, malignancy, alcoholism, HIV).

Pyomyositis is usually secondary to spread of infection from an adjacent focus such as osteomyelitis or a puncture wound. The majority of cases occur in a single muscle or muscle group (e.g., quadriceps, gluteus). The most common causative agents are *Staphylococcus* (75%–95%) and *Streptococcus* organisms. The treatment includes immediate drainage of the abscess either percutaneously or in the operating room. Intravenous antibiotics should be administered early. Hot, moist compresses with elevation of the limb and splinting of the involved extremity are useful adjuncts.

Autoimmune Inflammatory Myositis. Three major types of autoimmune inflammatory myositis have been identified: polymyositis, dermatomyositis, and inclusion-body myositis. Newer entities, such as statin-induced necrotizing autoimmune myositis, are currently being identified and are under investigation. Patients present with varying degrees of muscle weakness that develop slowly over weeks to months. Weakness is most severe in the proximal muscles, and patients complain of difficulty getting out of a chair, getting into or out of a car, climbing stairs, and combing their hair. Distal muscles and fine motor movements are more commonly affected in inclusion-body myositis. Myalgias are not a common complaint and are present in less than 30% of patients. In patients with dermatomyositis, a rash precedes the onset of muscle weakness. The rash can be either a purplish color around the eyes (heliotrope rash) or an erythematous, a raised rash on the face, neck, chest, back, or joints, and may be a marker of skin malignancies. Polymyositis and dermatomyositis are associated with other malignancies such as breast, lung, nasopharyngeal, colorectal, and lymphoma.

Diagnostic features include an increase in creatine kinase levels that is seen in more than 95% of cases. In active disease, the creatine kinase level can be elevated to 50 times normal. Antibody testing may be helpful, with anti-Jo-1 conferring the greatest specificity. Muscle biopsy is the most important confirmatory test. Treatment includes administration of corticosteroids and immunosuppressive agents. Intravenous and subcutaneous immunoglobulin are effective in improving muscle strength and resolving the underlying immunopathology.

REFERENCES

1. Maguire S, Cowley L, Mann M. What does the recent literature add to the identification and investigation of fractures in child abuse: an overview of review updates 2005–2013. *Evid Based Child Health.* 2013;8(5):2044–2057.
2. Oakes R, Urban A, Levy P. The mangled extremity. *J Emerg Med.* 2008;35(4):437–444.
3. Claes L, Recknagael S, Ignatius A. Fracture healing under healthy and inflammatory conditions. *Nat Rev Rheumatol.* 2012;8(3):133–143.

4. Ghiasi MS, Chen J, Vaziri A, Rodriguez EK, Nazarian A. Bone fracture healing in mechano-biological modeling: a review of principles and methods. *Bone Rep.* 2017;6:87–100.

5. Mavčič B, Antolič V. Optimal mechanical environment of the healing bone fracture/osteotomy. *Int Orthop.* 2012;36:689–695.

6. Patel RA, Wilson RF, Palmer RM. The effect of smoking on bone healing. *Bone Joint Res.* 2013;2(6):102–111.

7. Pountos I, Georgouli T, Calori GM, et al. Do nonsteroidal anti-inflammatory drugs affect bone healing? A critical analysis. *Sci World J.* 2012. doi:10.1100/2012/606404.

8. White TO, Mackenzie SP, Gray AJ. Fractures and fracture management. *McRae's Orthopedic Trauma and Emergency Fracture Management*, 3rd ed. Edinburgh: Elsevier; 2016.

9. Falcon-Chevere MD, Jorge L. Critical trauma skills and procedures in the emergency department. *Emerg Med Clin North Am.* 2013;31:291–334.

10. Tolpinrud WL, Rebolledo BJ, Lorich DG. A case of extensive fracture bullae: a multidisciplinary approach for acute management. *JAAD Case Rep.* 2015;1(3):132–135.

11. Nelson FRT, Blauvelt CT. Imaging techniques. In: Nelson FRT, Blauvelt CT, eds. *A Manual of Orthopaedic Terminology*. 8th ed. Philadelphia, PA: Elsevier; 2015.

12. Antoci V, Patel SP, Weaver MJ, et al. Relevance of adjacent joint imaging in the evaluation of ankle fractures. *Injury.* 2016;47(10):2366–2369.

13. Mallee WH, Henny EP, van Dijk CN, Kamminga SP, van Enst WA, Kloen P. Clinical diagnostic evaluation for scaphoid fractures: a systematic review and meta-analysis. *J Hand Surg Am.* 2014;39(9):1683–1691.

14. Medero CR, Chilstrom ML. Diagnosis of an occult hip fracture by point-of-care ultrasound. *J Emerg Med.* 2015;49(6):916–919.

15. Henry BJ, Vrahas MS. The Thomas splint. Questionable boast of an indispensable tool. *Am J Orthop.* 1996;25(9):602–604.

16. Rowlands TK, Clasper J. The Thomas splint—a necessary tool in the management of battlefield injuries. *J R Army Med Corps.* 2003;149(4):291–293.

17. Roberts A, Shaw KA, Boomsma SE, et al. Effect of casting material on the cast pressure after sequential cast splitting. *J Pediatr Orthop.* 2017;37(1):74–77.

18. Emet M, Atac K, Aydin A, et al. Spotted lipid sign floating on the blood to differentiate obscured open fractures from simple wound lacerations. *Am J Emerg Med.* 2015;33(2):312.e1–312.e2.

19. Kim PH, Leopold SS. Gustilo-Anderson classification. *Clin Orthop Relat Res.* 2012;470(11):3270–3274.

20. Centers for Disease Control and Prevention (CDC). Advisory Committee on Immunization Practices (ACIP) recommended immunization schedules for persons aged 0 through 18 years and adults aged 19 years and older—United States, 2013. *MMWR Surveill Summ.* 2013;62(suppl 1):1.

21. Rodriguez L, Jung HS, Goulet JA. Evidence-based protocol for prophylactic antibiotics in open fractures: improved antibiotic stewardship with no increase in infection rates. *J Trauma Acute Care Surg.* 2014;77(3):400–408.

22. Swanson TV, Szabo RM, Anderson DD. Open hand fractures: prognosis and classification. *J Hand Surg Am.* 1991;16(1):101–107.

23. McLain RF, Steyers C, Stoddard M. Infections in open fractures of the hand. *J Hand Surg Am.* 1991;16(1):108–112.

24. Mauffrey C, Bailey JR, Bowles RJ, et al. Acute management of open fractures: proposal of a new multidisciplinary algorithm. *Orthopedics.* 2012;35(10):877–881.

25. Centers for Disease Control and Prevention (CDC). *FastStats All Firearm Deaths 2014*. Hyattsville, MD: Author; 2014. http://www.cdc.gov/nchs/fastats/injury.htm. Accessed May 24, 2017.

26. Papasoulis E, Patzakis MJ, Zalavras CG. Antibiotics in the treatment of low-velocity gunshot-induced fractures: a systemic literature review. *Clin Orthop Relat Res.* 2013;471(12):3937–3944.

27. Seng VS, Masquelet AC. Management of civilian ballistic fractures. *Orthop Traumatol Surg Res.* 2013;99(8):953–958.

28. Lipscomb HJ, Schoenfisch AL. Nail gun injuries treated in US emergency departments, 2006–2011: not just a worker safety issue. *Am J Ind Med.* 2015;58(8):880–885.

29. Matheson GO, Clement DB, McKenzie DC, Taunton JE, Lloyd-Smith DR, MacIntyre JG. Stress fractures in athletes. A study of 320 cases. *Am J Sports Med.* 1987;15(1):46–58.

30. Bryson DJ, Wicks L, Ashford RU. The investigation and management of suspected malignant pathologic fractures: a review for the general orthopaedic surgeon. *Injury.* 2015;46(10):1891–1899.

31. Wise BL, Peloquin C, Choi H, et al. Impact of age, sex, obesity, and steroid use on quinolone-associated tendon disorders. *Am J Med.* 2012;125(12):1223–1228.

32. Stephenson AL, Wu W, Cortes D, et al. Tendon injury and fluoroquinolone use: a systematic review. *Drug Safety.* 2013;36(9):709–721.

33. Wise BL, Peloquin C, Choi H, Lane NE, Zhang Y. Impact of age, sex, obesity and steroid use on quinolone-associated tendon disorders. *Am J Med.* 2012;125:1228.

34. Baoge L, Van Den Steen E, Rimbaut S, et al. Treatment of skeletal muscle injury: a review. *ISRN Orthop.* 2012. doi: 10.5402/2012/689012.

35. Walczak B, Johnson CN, Howe BM. Myositis ossificans. *J Am Acad Orthop Surg.* 2015;23(10):612–622.

36. Mani-Babu S, Wolman R, Keen R. Quadriceps traumatic myositis ossificans in a football player: management with intravenous pamidronate. *Clin J Sport Med.* 2014;24(5):e56–e58.

37. Crum NF. Bacterial pyomyositis in the United States. *Am J Med.* 2004;117(6):420–428.

38. Comegna L, Guidone PI, Prezioso G, et al. Pyomyositis is not only a tropical pathology: a case series. *J Med Case Rep.* 2016;10(1):372.

39. Dalakas MC, Hohlfeld R. Polymyositis and dermatomyositis. *Lancet.* 2003;362(9388):971–982.

40. Troyanov Y, Landon-Cardinal O, Fritzler MJ, et al. Atorvastatin-induced necrotizing autoimmune myositis: an emerging dominant entity in patients with autoimmune myositis presenting with pure polymyositis phenotype. *Medicine (Balt).* 2017;96(3):e5694.

41. Antiochos BB, Brown LA, Li Z, Tosteson TD, Wortmann RL, Rigby WF. Malignancy is associated with dermatomyositis but not polymyositis in Northern New England, USA. *J Rheumatol.* 2009;36(12):2704–2710.

42. Fang YF, Wu YJ, Kuo CF, Luo SF, Yu KH. Malignancy in dermatomyositis and polymyositis: analysis of 192 patients. *Clin Rheumatol.* 2016;35(8):1977–1984.

43. Cherin P, Belizna C, Cartry O, et al. Long-term subcutaneous immunoglobulin use in inflammatory myopathies: a retrospective review of 19 cases. *Autoimmun Rev.* 2016;15(3):281–286.

CHAPTER 2
Anesthesia and Analgesia

Tarlan Hedayati, MD

The relief of pain and suffering is one of the most important acts that a physician undertakes. Pain relief following orthopedic injuries should be provided universally and promptly, with rare exception. In addition, throughout this book, there are descriptions of fracture and dislocation reductions as well as soft-tissue repairs that will require significant anesthesia to perform successfully and compassionately. As such, this chapter serves as a reference for the safe and effective use of pain medications, procedural sedation, local anesthesia, and regional anesthesia used in emergency orthopedics. Finally, the clinical use of heat and cold is reviewed in patients with orthopedic injuries.

PAIN MANAGEMENT

The largest study to date of patients with closed fractures of the extremities or clavicle revealed that one-third of these patients did not receive pain medications while in the emergency department (ED). Underuse of analgesics after orthopedic injuries is well documented in the literature. Groups at risk for "oligoanesthesia" include pediatric patients, minority ethnic groups, and women. Children younger than 2 years seem to be at higher risk than school-age children.

Despite the frequent underuse of analgesics by physicians, there is evidence that practice habits can change. One study documented that physicians prescribed pain medications following orthopedic injuries with a 95% compliance rate when an aggressive educational program was instituted.

Once the decision has been made to give an analgesic agent, the next question is which analgesic to provide. Nonsteroidal anti-inflammatory drugs (NSAIDs) should be avoided in patients with healing fractures, as these agents have been shown to diminish bone formation, healing, and remodeling.

The evidence for the use of nonsteroidal agents in patients with soft-tissue injuries is not as clear. NSAID use in blunt muscle trauma (especially the quadriceps) will decrease the incidence of heterotopic ossification. The majority of randomized controlled studies have shown a benefit for the use of an NSAID after various sprains and strains, although the positive effect is not universally noted. The use of an NSAID after exercise-induced muscle injury may also be beneficial for short-term recovery of muscle function. In general, the use of an NSAID in soft-tissue injury is recommended

for its potential to stimulate collagen synthesis and the early phases of skin and ligament repair.

Of the opioid analgesics, codeine is the weakest agent, and in one study, it was no better than a placebo. Other oral narcotic medications include hydromorphone (Dilaudid), hydrocodone (Vicodin, Lorcet), and oxycodone (Percodan, Percocet). Complications include constipation, nausea, and vomiting. Patients should be instructed not to drive while taking these medications, although up to 7% of patients admit to doing just the same, despite warnings.

PROCEDURAL SEDATION AND ANALGESIA

The physician treating emergent orthopedic injuries will use procedural sedation and analgesia (PSA) frequently. It is not without significant complications, especially when it is performed hastily or without understanding the pharmacology of the medications involved. However, a substantial body of literature supports the safe use of PSA by emergency physicians.

The goal of PSA is to induce a state of tolerance to emergency procedures while preserving airway reflexes. This is usually accomplished by administering a sedative or dissociative agent, as well as an analgesic agent. However, certain fundamental principles must be adhered to well before the first agent is used. Requirements include appropriate personnel, thorough patient assessment and consent, adequate equipment, patient monitoring, and documentation. It is only after these requirements are satisfied that the physician can begin to consider drug administration.

PSA should only be performed by an individual who possesses an understanding of the medications used, an ability to monitor the patient's response, and the skills necessary to address any airway or cardiovascular complications that may occur. In general, this requires a second clinician, other than the physician performing the procedure.

Patient assessment should begin with a past medical history, including anesthetic history, medications, and allergies. PSA in individuals with an American Society of Anesthesiology Physical Status Class III (severe systemic disease with definite functional limitation) or higher should be avoided. Specific fasting periods before procedural sedation are not supported by the available medical literature, and the traditional guideline of 2 hours after clear liquids and 6 hours after solids and other liquids is not always practical in the ED, as often the procedure in question cannot be delayed.

▶ TABLE 2-1. **PROCEDURAL SEDATION MEDICATIONS AND REVERSAL AGENTS**

Agent	Initial IV Dose	Duration (min)	Important Complications
Midazolam (Versed)	0.05 mg/kg every 3–5 min	30–60	Respiratory depression, hypotension
Fentanyl (Sublimaze)	0.5–1.0 µg/kg every 3–5 min	20–30	Respiratory depression, hypotension, rigid chest syndrome
Ketamine (Ketalar)	0.5–1.0 mg/kg	45	Increased secretions, emergence reactions, laryngospasm, elevated ICP
Etomidate (Amidate)	0.1 mg/kg	20	Myoclonus (up to 20%), respiratory depression, vomiting
Methohexital (Brevital)	1–1.5 mg/kg	5–7	Respiratory depression, fasciculations, burning at IV site
Propofol (Diprivan)	1.0 mg/kg[a]	3–5	Respiratory depression, hypotension
Naloxone (Narcan)	0.1 mg/kg	20–40	Resedation, agitation
Flumazenil (Romazicon)	0.02 mg/kg	20–40	Resedation, seizures

ICP, intracranial pressure.
[a]Some recommend initial doses of 10 to 20 mg (adult) administered every 30 s until adequate sedation is achieved.

A prospective, observational study of 1014 children identified no difference in airway complications, emesis, or other adverse events between patients who met and did not meet the fasting guidelines. Moreover, no aspiration events were noted in either group. However, the authors did note that the study was underpowered to fully detect differences in rates of emesis due to the extremely rare nature of such events.[20] Therefore, although recent food intake is not a contraindication to administering procedural sedation, it should be considered in targeting the depth of sedation.[16]

Necessary equipment includes oxygen, suction, advanced life support equipment, and appropriate reversal agents (when applicable). Intravenous access should be established, and the patient should be placed on a monitor with continuous pulse oximetry and capnometry, if available. Supplemental oxygen via a nasal cannula, although controversial in the literature, is generally recommended. A departmentally developed checklist will help ensure compliance and improve documentation.[21]

There are a numerous options for PSA in the ED, which include midazolam, fentanyl, ketamine, etomidate, propofol, and various combinations of these medications. The ideal agent varies depending on the clinical circumstances. Whichever agents are used, a key to safe administration involves slow titration of the drug until the desired effect is achieved.[16,22] Rapid administration may lead to a higher rate of complications, including hypotension and respiratory depression. A review of the most commonly used agents as well as reversal agents is provided in Table 2–1.

Commonly Used Agents
Midazolam (Versed)
This agent should be dosed in increments of 0.05 mg/kg (up to 1–2 mg increments in adults) every 3 to 5 minutes to get the desired effect. A dose of 0.1 mg/kg will usually produce sedation within 2 to 3 minutes. This agent is the ideal benzodiazepine for procedural sedation due to its amnestic properties, as well as its short duration of action (30–60 minutes). The most important complication from midazolam use is respiratory depression. This effect appears to be augmented in patients receiving concomitant opioids or who have underlying pulmonary disease. Other adverse reactions include hypotension, vomiting, hallucinations, and hiccups. Of note, 1% of children under the age of 5 years may experience paradoxical excitation, which can be reversed with flumazenil.[23]

Fentanyl (Sublimaze)
This agent is the preferred opioid for procedural sedation due to its rapid onset and short duration of action. Peak analgesia is accomplished in 2 to 3 minutes, and the duration of action is only 20 to 30 minutes. It is recommended to use incremental doses of 1 µg/kg IV in adults and children, given slowly to a total dose of 2 to 3 µg/kg. Fentanyl is contraindicated in children younger than 6 months because of the risk of severe laryngospasm. In addition to respiratory depression and hypotension, fentanyl is also associated with chest wall rigidity. Rigid chest syndrome appears to occur at very high doses (>15 µg/kg) when the drug is administered rapidly.

Ketamine (Ketalar)
This agent has dissociative properties and is one of the most commonly used anesthetic agents for procedural sedation. Patients who have been administered this drug have blunted sensory perceptions and no memory of the events. Ketamine is advantageous for procedural sedation because it is not associated with a loss of protective airway reflexes and is the only sedative that also has analgesic properties. The recommended dose is 1 to 2 mg/kg intravenously. The onset of action is 1 minute with duration of 45 minutes.

Contraindications include age younger than 3 months, increased intraocular pressure, cardiovascular disease, or active respiratory infections. Adverse reactions include increased respiratory secretions, emergence reactions, and laryngospasm. Administering atropine or glycopyrrolate at 0.01 mg/kg 10 minutes before giving ketamine can decrease the respiratory secretions. Emergence reactions are hallucinations that occur during the recovery period. They are seen in up to 50% of adults and 10% of children. They are rare in children younger than 10 years. Concurrent administration of midazolam is sometimes given with the hope of decreasing the frequency of emergence reactions, although one randomized controlled trial refuted its effectiveness. Laryngospasm is a rare complication of ketamine administration that can often be treated with positive pressure ventilation. Rarely, succinylcholine is required for adequate ventilation if laryngospasm is severe or persists. Postrecovery nausea and vomiting may occur and can generally be treated with antiemetics, such as ondansetron.

Etomidate (Amidate)

This agent is a nonbarbiturate, imidazole hypnotic that has been gaining popularity for procedural sedation in the ED due to its rapid onset (30–60 seconds), short duration, and low side-effect profile. A dose of 0.1 mg/kg is given slowly, with additional doses of 0.05 mg/kg given every 3 to 5 minutes until appropriate sedation is achieved. Ninety-five percent of patients obtain full recovery within 30 minutes of administration. Side effects include respiratory depression, myoclonus, vomiting, and pain with injection. Myoclonus occurs in up to 20% of patients and is usually mild and self-limited, but occasionally may interfere with the procedure. Etomidate has not been shown to produce seizure activity when observed by an electroencephalogram. Respiratory depression, as represented by an oxygen saturation of <94%, occurs in 3% to 8% of patients. Adrenocortical dysfunction is transient, and the clinical significance of this finding is unclear. Some authors recommend caution when using this agent in patients with septic shock, but it is unlikely to be clinically significant in the ED PSA setting.

Methohexital (Brevital)

Methohexital is an ultrashort-acting barbiturate. One of the advantages of methohexital is that it has a rapid onset with maximal sedation in less than 1 minute in most cases. The initial dose is 1 to 1.5 mg/kg, followed by repeat doses of 0.5 mg/kg every 3 to 5 minutes as needed for further sedation. Alteration in hemodynamics is unusual, but respiratory depression is not uncommon. In one study of 76 adult patients, methohexital caused apnea in eight patients (10.5%) for an average duration of 64 seconds. Bag-valve mask ventilation was required in these patients, but none needed intubation. In another study, 4 of 52 patients (8%) receiving methohexital required bag-valve mask ventilation.

Propofol (Diprivan)

Propofol is a nonopioid, nonbarbiturate, sedative-hypnotic agent that can be administered at an initial dose of 0.5 to 1.0 mg/kg. Others prefer to give smaller initial amounts (10–20 mg intravenous push every 30 seconds until adequate sedation is achieved). This avoids overshooting with your initial bolus. Subsequent maintenance dosing can be as a continuous infusion or with 0.25 to 0.5 mg/kg boluses every 3 minutes as needed. Propofol is remarkable because it produces a very rapid onset (approximately 45 seconds) of a deep and effective sedation with a short duration (3–5 minutes). When compared with midazolam and fentanyl, both onset and duration are significantly shorter. Additional benefits are its potent antiemetic properties and its ability to reduce intracranial pressure. This must be balanced against the propensity of propofol to cause transient decreases in blood pressure, although the significance in otherwise healthy patients is debatable.

The depth of sedation provided by propofol requires extra vigilance in the observation of the patient to detect early complications, respiratory compromise, and hypotension. In one study, the rate of oxygen desaturation was 8% and assisted ventilation with bag-valve mask was 4%. In the only study to compare propofol with etomidate, rates of bag-valve mask use, airway repositioning, and stimulation to induce breathing were the same. Intravenous fluids should be available to administer if the patient becomes hypotensive during the use of propofol. Despite these potential problems, multiple studies looking at the use of propofol in the ED have shown it to be safe and cost effective for both adults and children when compared with other agents.

Propofol is a potent amnestic agent that lacks intrinsic analgesic properties. For this reason, it is frequently used with fentanyl, although a lower dose of ketamine (0.3 mg/kg) appears to reduce the rate of adverse events fivefold. Other authors have noted that because patients who receive only propofol without an analgesic generally have no recollection of the procedure and high satisfaction scores, an accompanying analgesic may not be necessary.

Ketofol

Ketofol is a newer procedural agent composed of equal amounts of ketamine and propofol. The initial dose ranges from 0.375 to 0.7 mg/kg each of ketamine and propofol, which can either be given individually or mixed together in the same syringe. The concept behind this mixture was to balance the hypotensive, respiratory depressant, and antiemetic components of propofol with the hypertensive, respiratory drive preserving, emetogenic, and analgesic components of ketamine. When compared with ketamine, there were decreased episodes of vomiting, decreased emergence reactions, greater patient satisfaction, and decreased sedation and recovery times. However, when compared with propofol, there appeared to be little difference in respiratory events or patient satisfaction. At this time, further studies are needed, but this combination may be used more frequently in the future.

Reversal Agents

Naloxone (Narcan)

This agent will reverse the effects of opioids. An intravenous dose of 1 to 2 mg (0.1 mg/kg in children) will reverse respiratory depression in most situations. Onset is rapid, but duration of action is relatively short (20–40 minutes), so resedation may occur if longer-acting opioids were used.

Flumazenil (Romazicon)

This agent will reverse the effects of benzodiazepine administration. The intravenous dose in an adult is 0.2 mg over 15 seconds (0.02 mg/kg in a child) that can be repeated at 1-minute intervals until the desired effect is achieved. In a manner similar to naloxone, resedation may occur if the effects of the benzodiazepine outlast the 20- to 40-minute duration of action of flumazenil. It is recommended to use this agent with caution, as it is known to lower the seizure threshold and can produce refractory seizures in chronic benzodiazepine users.

Postprocedure Monitoring

Monitoring in the postprocedure period is still important, as complications may occur following the removal of noxious stimuli. In children, the risk for adverse events is greatest within the first 10 minutes after the administration of a medication and in the immediate postrecovery phase.[52] Discharge criteria should include a patient who is conscious and responding appropriately, has normal vital signs, has normal respiratory status, and is able to tolerate oral liquids.[16]

LOCAL ANESTHESIA

Local anesthetic agents are used for abscess drainage, acute wounds, and regional anesthesia. The advantages of using local anesthesia are that it is often quicker, safer, and provides better hemostasis (via direct distension of tissue and concurrent use of epinephrine) than regional or general anesthesia. The disadvantages include the relatively larger amount of anesthetic required and the potential tissue distortion.

These agents are classified as esters or amides on the basis of their intermediate chain. Lidocaine, mepivacaine, and bupivacaine are amide anesthetics, whereas procaine is the prototypical ester local anesthetic agent. Their mechanism of action is based on blockage of sodium channels, thus inhibiting nerve cell depolarization. Longer-acting agents bind to sodium channels for prolonged periods of time. The addition of epinephrine increases the duration of action by causing vasoconstriction and a subsequent decrease in the absorption of the agent into the systemic circulation. To reduce the pain associated with anesthetic infiltration, it has been recommended to buffer the solution with 8.4% sodium bicarbonate, warm the solution to room temperature, inject slowly with a small-gauge needle, and infiltrate through wound edges.[53]

Contraindications to the use of a local anesthetic include an allergy to the agent. A true IgE-mediated allergy to a local anesthetic is rare, and there is no cross-reactivity between esters and amides, although the reaction may be due to a preservative in the vial. In such cases, avoid using multidose vials. In patients with a history of an allergic reaction to an unknown local anesthetic, 1% diphenhydramine solution can be used as a substitute agent. To create this, dilute 1 mL of the standard 5% parenteral solution into 4 mL of normal saline.

Systemic toxicity can be avoided by being aware of maximal recommended doses of local anesthetic agents. Maximum doses and other properties of the most commonly used local anesthetic agents are listed in Table 2–2. When calculating the maximum dose, it is important remember that 1% lidocaine contains 10 mg/mL and 2% lidocaine contains 20 mg/mL. Therefore, in a 100 kg individual, for example, the maximum dose of 1% lidocaine without epinephrine is 450 mg or 45 mL.

REGIONAL ANESTHESIA

Regional anesthesia offers many advantages over procedural sedation for fracture and dislocation reduction. In general, a successful block will provide complete anesthesia within the desired nerve distribution without the potential complications of procedural sedation. In addition, regional anesthesia does not require a prolonged postprocedural observation

▶ TABLE 2–2. **PROPERTIES OF COMMONLY USED LOCAL ANESTHETIC AGENTS**

Anesthetic Agent	Onset of Action (min)	Duration of Action (min)	Maximum Dose (mg/kg)	Maximum Dose with Epidural (mg/kg)
Lidocaine (Xylocaine)	2–5	30–60	4.5	7.0
Mepivacaine (Carbocaine)	2–5	120–240	8.0	7.0[a]
Bupivacaine (Marcaine)	3–7	90–360	2.0	3.0
Procaine[b] (Novocaine)	10–20	60–90	7.0	9.0

[a]Epinephrine adds to the potential cardiac toxicity of mepivacaine, and therefore, a lower maximum dose is recommended.
[b]Procaine is an ester; the other agents listed in the table are amides.

period following reduction, thus shortening ED length of stays and decreasing the requirement for nursing care.

The supplies needed for regional anesthesia include a local anesthetic agent, a syringe, a 25- or 27-gauge needle, an alcohol swab, a sterile drape, and a healthy knowledge of anatomy. Ultrasound is currently used for a variety of applications, including nerve blocks, and is briefly discussed in this chapter where applicable. Please refer to an ultrasound textbook for further discussion of ultrasound-guided nerve blocks.

Epinephrine can be added to the local anesthetic for most blocks to increase their duration of action. Epinephrine injection is classically avoided in the hand and digit due to the potential fear of digital ischemia, although the concentrations used with local anesthetic agents are low and unlikely to cause ischemia. In fact, no long-term complications or necrosis have been reported after injection of as much as 0.3 mg of epinephrine into a digit. Obvious contraindications to regional anesthesia include a bleeding disorder or the need to traverse infected tissue. Nerve function should be properly tested and documented before and after the procedure.

Anatomic landmarks should be identified, and sterile procedure should be maintained. The needle is inserted with care to watch for the presence of paresthesias. If paresthesias are noted, the tip of the needle is likely within the fibrous outer sheath of the nerve. Injection at this point may result in permanent nerve damage; therefore, the needle should be withdrawn until paresthesias dissipate. Then, the anesthetic can be injected. Depending on the agent used and the accuracy of the injection, anesthesia will be complete within 10 to 15 minutes. The closer the needle is to the nerve, the faster the onset of anesthesia. When in doubt about the proximity of the needle to the nerve, err on the side of injecting more anesthetic. A comprehensive discussion of regional anesthesia is beyond the scope of this text; however, the most commonly used extremity blocks are described subsequently.

Digital Blocks

Ring and Half-Ring Blocks

These are commonly used blocks to provide anesthesia to fingers or toes. The digits possess two dorsal and two palmar nerves that run along the phalanges in the 2, 4, 8, and 10 o'clock positions. The ring block is successfully performed by blocking these nerves in a circumferential pattern around the base of the digit. The half-ring block is an alternative method with similar success in which anesthetic is injected on either side of the base of the digit. To perform the half-ring block, insert the needle through the dorsal aspect of the hand into the web space just lateral to the corresponding metacarpophalangeal joint. One milliliter of anesthetic is injected in the subdermal area. The needle is advanced until it reaches an equivalent depth on the volar side, and then another 1 mL is injected. This is repeated on the medial side (Fig. 2–1 and Video 2–1). For blocking the great toe, a circumferential ring of anesthetic is recommended due to the greater distance between the nerves.

Metacarpal Block

Alternatively, the digit can be anesthetized by blocking the common digital nerves before they divide to innervate the digits. With this block, the needle is inserted on the dorsal

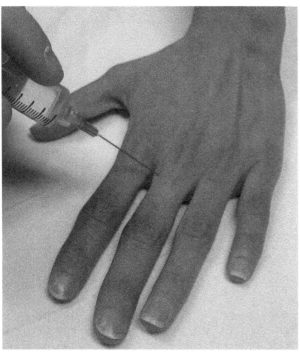
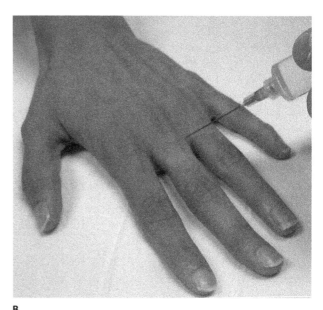

A   **B**

Figure 2–1. Digital half-ring block of the third digit. **A.** Radial injection site. **B.** Ulnar injection site.

aspect of the hand in the web space between the digits. The needle is directed toward the metacarpal heads and the palm of the hand (Video 2–2). For this block to be successful, anesthetic agent should be injected all the way to the palmar aspect of the hand to anesthetize the palmar branches of the nerve. Swelling should be noted on the palm between the metacarpal heads after infiltration. The opposite side of the metacarpal should be injected to anesthetize the entire digit. This method, although favored by some, has some disadvantages. In one study, the digital half-ring block outperformed the metacarpal block in terms of pain scores, failure rate, and time to complete the procedure.[54]

Transthecal Block

An advantage of the transthecal block is that it requires only one injection at a site that avoids proximity to the neurovascular bundle of the digit.[55] Anesthetic is injected directly into the flexor tendon sheath. In the initial description, the anesthetic was injected into the distal palmar crease of the hand.[56] This technique was shown to be similar to the digital half-ring block in both pain score and time to anesthesia.[57] A simpler, but equally efficacious, modified approach has been described that uses the center of the proximal digital crease on the volar surface of the digit as the site of needle insertion (Fig. 2–2).[58] A 25-gauge needle is inserted to the bone and then withdrawn slowly while applying pressure to the syringe plunger (Video 2–3). The resistance to anesthetic flow decreases when the needle tip is resting within the tendon sheath. At this point, approximately 2 mL of anesthetic agent is injected while proximal pressure is applied to the volar surface to aid distal diffusion.

Wrist Block

The wrist block provides anesthesia to the entire hand and is useful for many soft-tissue procedures and reductions of

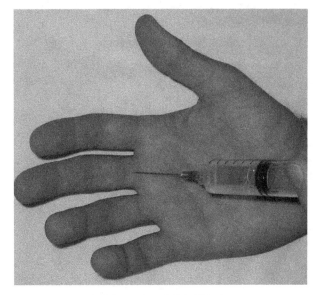

Figure 2–2. Modified transthecal digital block.

the bones in the hand. Proper technique requires the deposition of local anesthetic to block the radial, median, and ulnar nerves at the wrist.

Radial Nerve

The radial nerve is blocked at the wrist using two injections. The initial injection is made at the proximal wrist crease just lateral to the radial artery. Three milliliters of anesthetic are injected at a depth of approximately 0.5 cm. Because dorsal branches of the radial nerve arise more proximally, a second injection is required. A superficial skin wheal is created on the dorsum of the hand extending from the lateral aspect of the wrist at the dorsal wrist crease to the base of the fourth metacarpal bone. An additional 5 mL of local anesthetic is injected here (Fig. 2–3 and Video 2–4).[59]

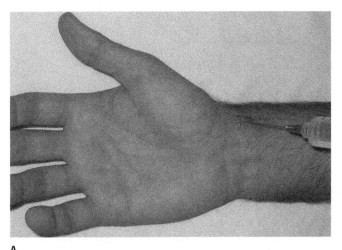

A

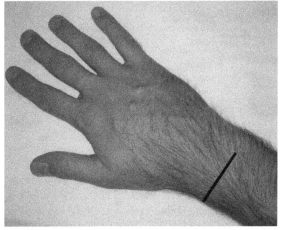

B

Figure 2–3. Radial nerve block at the wrist. **A.** Initial injection to block the main branch of the nerve. **B.** A second superficial injection along the dorsal surface of the wrist is used to block branches that arise more proximally.

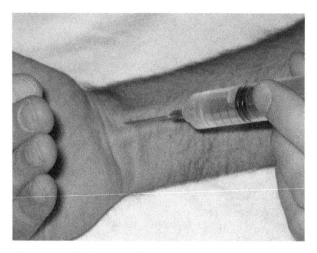

Figure 2–4. Median nerve block at the wrist.

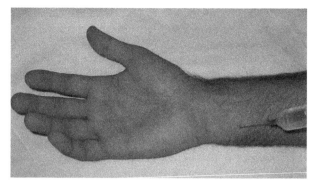

Figure 2–5. Ulnar nerve block at the wrist.

Median Nerve

The median nerve is located directly below or slightly lateral to the palmaris longus tendon. The palmaris longus tendon is absent in 10% to 20% of individuals, but if present, it can be palpated by having the patient flex the wrist against resistance. To block this nerve, insert the needle perpendicular to the skin and along the radial border of the palmaris longus tendon (or 1 cm medial to the flexor carpi radialis tendon if this is not present) to a depth of 1 cm. A "pop" should be felt when the needle penetrates the flexor retinaculum, and the presence of paresthesias signifies that the nerve is located. Withdraw slightly and inject 3 to 5 mL of local anesthetic. If no paresthesias are elicited, redirect slightly in an ulnar direction and inject the full 5 mL (Fig. 2–4 and Video 2–5).

Ulnar Nerve

The ulnar nerve is located between the flexor carpi ulnaris and the ulnar artery in the volar aspect of the wrist. It can be blocked by injecting 3 to 5 mL of local anesthetic agent just lateral to the flexor carpi ulnaris tendon, while remaining medial to the ulnar artery. This block is performed 2 cm proximal to the wrist crease to block the dorsal branch before its takeoff. A depth of 0.5 cm is sufficient for the ulnar nerve block (Fig. 2–5 and Video 2–6).

Femoral Nerve Block

This block is useful for relieving pain due to femoral neck fractures, intertrochanteric femur fractures, and femoral shaft fractures.[60-62] The femoral nerve also supplies innervation to the anterior and medial aspects of the thigh and leg. The femoral nerve is located just lateral to the femoral artery and can be blocked using either the landmark-based or ultrasound-guided approach.

Using the landmark-based approach, locate the femoral artery and insert the needle approximately 1 to 1.5 cm lateral to the artery and 1 to 2 cm distal to the inguinal crease at a 45-degree angle to a depth of about 3 to 4 cm. Two distinct "pops" should be felt as the needle crosses the fascia lata and fascia iliaca. This block usually requires 15 to 25 mL of local anesthetic.

The ultrasound-guided approach is an increasingly popular alternative, wherein a 6 to 18 MHz linear probe is placed in the inguinal crease and slid transversely until the vessels and nerve are located. The needle is inserted in-plane from the lateral aspect of the probe and advanced until the fascia lata and fascia iliaca are punctured. Small, 1-mL boluses are injected to surround the nerve, confirming proper placement under ultrasound visualization. As noted in the preceding paragraph, a total of 15 to 25 mL of anesthetic is usually required.

Ankle Block

The ankle block is the most challenging of the regional blocks. To provide complete anesthesia to the foot, a total of five nerves must be blocked—the saphenous nerve, the sural nerve, the posterior tibial nerve, the superficial peroneal nerve, and the deep peroneal nerve. To anesthetize the sole of the foot only, the posterior tibial nerve and sural nerve must be blocked. The patient should be positioned prone on the stretcher with the foot dangling off the edge. These blocks are performed at a level just superior to the malleoli.

Saphenous Nerve

The saphenous nerve is blocked at the anterior border of the medial malleolus just posterior to the greater saphenous vein. The needle is inserted approximately 1 to 2 cm above the superior aspect of the medial malleolus, and 3 to 5 mL of anesthetic solution is injected.

Sural Nerve

The sural nerve is blocked by raising a wheal using 3 to 5 mL of local anesthetic from the lateral border of the Achilles tendon to the fibula at the level of the superior malleoli. Anesthetizing this nerve and the posterior tibial nerve will provide anesthesia to the plantar aspect of the foot (Fig. 2–6 and Video 2–7).

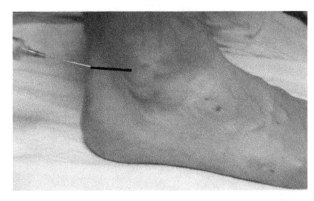

Figure 2–6. Sural nerve block.

Posterior Tibial Nerve

The posterior tibial nerve is located on the posteromedial ankle between the medial malleolus and the Achilles tendon. Palpate the posterior tibial artery and insert the needle 0.5 to 1 cm posterolateral to a depth of 0.5 to 1 cm. Paresthesias should be elicited during this block. At that time, withdraw the needle approximately 1 mm and inject 3 to 5 mL of anesthetic solution (Fig. 2–7 and Video 2–8).

Superficial Peroneal Nerve

The superficial peroneal nerve is blocked 1 to 2 cm above the malleoli by raising a wheal using 6 to 10 mL of anesthetic from the anterior edge of the tibia to the anterior edge of the fibula. This nerve provides sensory innervation to the dorsum of the foot and toes.

Deep Peroneal Nerve

The deep peroneal nerve is located on the anterior and dorsal aspect of the foot, just deep to the extensor hallucis

longus tendon. After anesthetizing the superficial peroneal nerve, insert the needle just medial to the extensor hallucis longus 30 degrees laterally until the tibia is encountered. Withdraw 1 mm and inject 1 mL of anesthetic. This nerve provides sensory innervation to the web space between the first and second toe.

HEMATOMA BLOCK

This technique is frequently employed for anesthesia during reduction of distal radius (Colles) fractures, but the principles apply to any type of fracture. The infiltration of local anesthetic agent within a fracture serves to block the nerve fibers of the surrounding soft tissues and periosteum (Fig. 2–8). To perform this procedure, a large bore needle is used to withdraw blood from the fracture and replace it with local anesthetic agent. For a distal radius fracture, a total of 10 to 15 mL of 1% lidocaine is injected directly into the fracture site (Video 2–9). Following the injection, place an elastic bandage around the wrist and allow 10 minutes for proper anesthesia.[63] Multiple studies have shown that hematoma blocks result in decreased pain scores when compared with procedural sedation.[64,65] Of note, this technique is only effective during acute management, when the hematoma has not yet become coagulated.

USE OF THERAPEUTIC HEAT AND COLD

There are identifiable and measurable physiologic effects produced by heat and cold that are therapeutically desirable. Although both heat and cold are known to reduce muscle spasm and decrease the pain associated with injuries, the mechanisms and indications for each are different.[66]

Superficial application of heat relieves pain through three primary mechanisms. Heat-induced vasodilation increases blood flow, thereby "washing out" the inflammatory cytokines. In addition, heat will relax muscle fibers, thereby relieving muscle spasm. Finally, heat decreases synovial fluid viscosity,

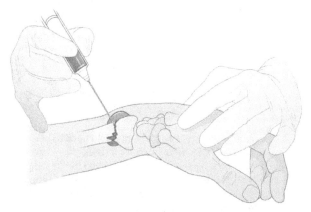

Figure 2–8. Hematoma block to provide anesthesia in a patient who will undergo reduction of a distal radius fracture.

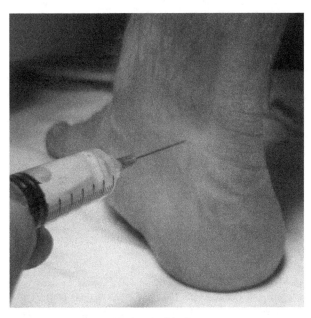

Figure 2–7. Posterior tibial nerve block.

which allows for better joint mobility. However, because of the aforementioned vasodilation, heat can also increase initial bleeding and edema in acute injuries. Therefore, heat is predominately used for subacute and chronic injuries.

Cold therapy will decrease the metabolic rate, as well as slow nerve conduction, with a combined effect of decreasing the amount of pain experienced. Moreover, cold therapy will decrease blood flow, thereby decreasing bleeding and edema after acute injuries. This is further supplemented with the use of compression and elevation—hence, the popular RICE (Rest, Ice, Compression, Elevation) therapy commonly recommended after acute orthopedic injuries. Some studies have also shown that cold can decrease muscle spasm, although the mechanism of this is unclear. Consequently, cold therapy may be used for acute, subacute, and chronic injuries.   In general, during the acute phase after injury, pain relief is best obtained with cold.   Despite this almost universal recommendation, there is little evidence-based medicine beyond observational studies and animal studies to support the use of cold. Even less evidence exists regarding the ideal duration of treatment, frequency, and mode of application.

Nonetheless, enough of a consensus exists to allow for some recommendations. The goal of therapy is a reduction in tissue temperature of 10°C to 15°C while avoiding injury to the superficial layers and skin. This is best performed by using melting iced water applied through a wet towel for a period of 10 to 15 minutes.   Longer application is appropriate in areas with more subcutaneous fat (20–30 minutes if >2 cm of fat). Using repeated, rather than continuous applications will help sustain reduced muscle temperatures without causing cold-induced tissue injury to the superficial layers (Fig. 2-9). Treatment should continue

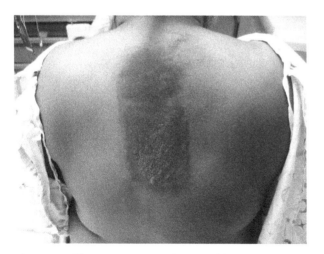

Figure 2-9. This woman was applying a cold pack to her back following epidural injections for chronic back pain. She had removed the protective covering and alternated the frozen pack with another that she kept in her freezer. Whenever cold application for soft-tissue injury is prescribed by the emergency physician, patients should be instructed about its proper usage—10 to 15 minutes every 2 to 3 hours with a protective barrier in the form of a wet towel between the tissue and ice.

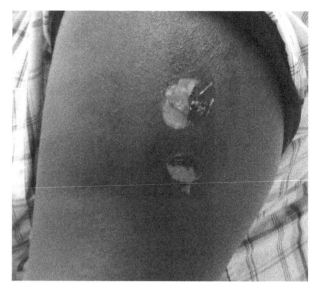

Figure 2-10. This patient sustained burns to the skin after using a topical anesthetic followed by a heating pad.

every 1 to 2 hours initially and continue for a period of 48 to 72 hours.

In the subacute stage, mild superficial heat with hot packs is preferable, but ice may also be used.   As with cold therapy, heat should be applied intermittently for 10 to 30 minutes with care to avoid skin injury, although there is very limited literature to support this. The combined application of heat and passive range of motion may significantly improve the range of motion of patients with hip and shoulder problems.

Of note, neither cold nor heat should be used in combination with topical methyl salicylate/menthol (Bengay or Icy Hot) or other related products. Topical anesthesia to the skin and superficial layers will blunt the ability of the patient to sense any damaging effects of temperature change (hot or cold) and may produce burns (Fig. 2-10).

REFERENCES

1. Brown JC, Klein EJ, Lewis CW, Johnston BD, Cummings P. Emergency department analgesia for fracture pain. *Ann Emerg Med.* 2003;42(2):197–205.
2. McIntosh SE, Leffler S. Pain management after discharge from the ED. *Am J Emerg Med.* 2004;22(2):98–100.
3. Petrack EM, Christopher NC, Kriwinsky J. Pain management in the emergency department: patterns of analgesic utilization. *Pediatrics.* 1997;99(5):711–714.
4. Alexander J, Manno M. Underuse of analgesia in very young pediatric patients with isolated painful injuries. *Ann Emerg Med.* 2003;41(5):617–622.
5. Todd KH, Deaton C, D'Adamo AP, Goe L. Ethnicity and analgesic practice. *Ann Emerg Med.* 2000;35(1):11–16.
6. Lewis LM, Lasater LC, Brooks CB. Are emergency physicians too stingy with analgesics? *South Med J.* 1994;87(1):7–9.

7. Holdgate A, Shepherd SA, Huckson S. Patterns of analgesia for fractured neck of femur in Australian emergency departments. *Emerg Med Australas.* 2010;22(1):3–8.

8. Chen EH, Shofer FS, Dean AJ, et al. Gender disparity in analgesic treatment of emergency department patients with acute abdominal pain. *Acad Emerg Med.* 2008;15(5):414–418.

9. Chan L, Verdile VP. Do patients receive adequate pain control after discharge from the ED? *Am J Emerg Med.* 1998;16(7):705–707.

10. Dahners LE, Mullis BH. Effects of nonsteroidal anti-inflammatory drugs on bone formation and soft-tissue healing. *J Am Acad Orthop Surg.* 2004;12(3):139–143.

11. Baldwin LA. Use of nonsteroidal anti-inflammatory drugs following exercise-induced muscle injury. *Sports Med.* 2003;33(3):177–185.

12. Bloomfield SS, Barden TP, Mitchell J. Naproxen, aspirin, and codeine in postpartum uterine pain. *Clin Pharmacol Ther.* 1977;21(4):414–421.

13. Skokan EG, Pribble C, Bassett KE, Nelson DS. Use of propofol sedation in a pediatric emergency department: a prospective study. *Clin Pediatr (Phila).* 2001;40(12):663–671.

14. Burton JH, Bock AJ, Strout TD, Marcolini EG. Etomidate and midazolam for reduction of anterior shoulder dislocation: a randomized, controlled trial. *Ann Emerg Med.* 2002;40(5):496–504.

15. Guenther E, Pribble CG, Junkins EP Jr, Kadish HA, Bassett KE, Nelson DS. Propofol sedation by emergency physicians for elective pediatric outpatient procedures. *Ann Emerg Med.* 2003;42(6):783–791.

16. Godwin SA, Caro DA, Wolf SJ, et al. Clinical policy: procedural sedation and analgesia in the emergency department. *Ann Emerg Med.* 2005;45(2):177–196.

17. Roback MG, Bajaj L, Wathen JE, Bothner J. Preprocedural fasting and adverse events in procedural sedation and analgesia in a pediatric emergency department: are they related? *Ann Emerg Med.* 2004;44(5):454–459.

18. Green SM, Krauss B. Pulmonary aspiration risk during emergency department procedural sedation—an examination of the role of fasting and sedation depth. *Acad Emerg Med.* 2002;9(1):35–42.

19. Treston G. Prolonged pre-procedure fasting time is unnecessary when using titrated intravenous ketamine for paediatric procedural sedation. *Emerg Med Australas.* 2004;16(2):145–150.

20. Agrawal D, Manzi SF, Gupta R, Krauss B. Preprocedural fasting state and adverse events in children undergoing procedural sedation and analgesia in a pediatric emergency department. *Ann Emerg Med.* 2003;42(5):636–646.

21. Reichman EF, Simon RR. *Emergency Medicine Procedures.* New York, NY: McGraw-Hill; 2004.

22. Innes G, Murphy M, Nijssen-Jordan C, Ducharme J, Drummond A. Procedural sedation and analgesia in the emergency department. Canadian Consensus Guidelines. *J Emerg Med.* 1999;17(1):145–156.

23. Sanders JC. Flumazenil reverses a paradoxical reaction to intravenous midazolam in a child with uneventful prior exposure to midazolam. *Paediatr Anaesth.* 2003;13(4):369–370.

24. Sherwin TS, Green SM, Khan A, Chapman DS, Dannenberg B. Does adjunctive midazolam reduce recovery agitation after ketamine sedation for pediatric procedures? A randomized, double-blind, placebo-controlled trial. *Ann Emerg Med.* 2000;35(3):229–238.

25. Vinson DR, Bradbury DR. Etomidate for procedural sedation in emergency medicine. *Ann Emerg Med.* 2002;39(6):592–598.

26. Van Keulen SG, Burton JH. Myoclonus associated with etomidate for ED procedural sedation and analgesia. *Am J Emerg Med.* 2003;21(7):556–558.

27. Ruth WJ, Burton JH, Bock AJ. Intravenous etomidate for procedural sedation in emergency department patients. *Acad Emerg Med.* 2001;8(1):13–18.

28. Hunt GS, Spencer MT, Hays DP. Etomidate and midazolam for procedural sedation: prospective, randomized trial. *Am J Emerg Med.* 2005;23(3):299–303.

29. Doenicke AW, Roizen MF, Kugler J, Kroll H, Foss J, Ostwald P. Reducing myoclonus after etomidate. *Anesthesiology.* 1999;90(1):113–119.

30. Schenarts CL, Burton JH, Riker RR. Adrenocortical dysfunction following etomidate induction in emergency department patients. *Acad Emerg Med.* 2001;8(1):1–7.

31. Jackson WL Jr. Should we use etomidate as an induction agent for endotracheal intubation in patients with septic shock?: a critical appraisal. *Chest.* 2005;127(3):1031–1038.

32. Lerman B, Yoshida D, Levitt MA. A prospective evaluation of the safety and efficacy of methohexital in the emergency department. *Am J Emerg Med.* 1996;14(4):351–354.

33. Miner JR, Biros M, Krieg S, Johnson C, Heegaard W, Plummer D. Randomized clinical trial of propofol versus methohexital for procedural sedation during fracture and dislocation reduction in the emergency department. *Acad Emerg Med.* 2003;10(9):931–937.

34. Frank LR, Strote J, Hauff SR, Bigelow SK, Fay K. Propofol by infusion protocol for ED procedural sedation. *Am J Emerg Med.* 2006;24(5):599–602.

35. Taylor DM, O'Brien D, Ritchie P, Pasco J, Cameron PA. Propofol versus midazolam/fentanyl for reduction of anterior shoulder dislocation. *Acad Emerg Med.* 2005;12(1):13–19.

36. Bahn EL, Holt KR. Procedural sedation and analgesia: a review and new concepts. *Emerg Med Clin North Am.* 2005;23(2):503–517.

37. Burton JH, Miner JR, Shipley ER, Strout TD, Becker C, Thode HC Jr. Propofol for emergency department procedural sedation and analgesia: a tale of three centers. *Acad Emerg Med.* 2006;13(1):24–30.

38. Hohl CM, Sadatsafavi M, Nosyk B, Strout TD, Becker C, Thode HC Jr. Safety and clinical effectiveness of midazolam versus propofol for procedural sedation in the emergency department: a systematic review. *Acad Emerg Med.* 2008;15(1):1–8.

39. Hohl CM, Nosyk B, Sadatsafavi M, Anis AH. A cost-effectiveness analysis of propofol versus midazolam for procedural sedation in the emergency department. *Acad Emerg Med.* 2008;15(1):32–39.

40. Zed PJ, Abu-Laban RB, Chan WW, Harrison DW. Efficacy, safety and patient satisfaction of propofol for procedural sedation and analgesia in the emergency department: a prospective study. *CJEM.* 2007;9(6):421–427.

41. Weaver CS, Hauter WE, Brizendine EJ, Harrison DW. Emergency department procedural sedation with propofol: is it safe? *J Emerg Med.* 2007;33(4):355–361.

42. Pershad J, Godambe SA. Propofol for procedural sedation in the pediatric emergency department. *J Emerg Med.* 2004;27(1):11–14.

43. Holger JS, Satterlee PA, Haugen S. Nursing use between 2 methods of procedural sedation: midazolam versus propofol. *Am J Emerg Med.* 2005;23(3):248–252.

44. Miner JR, Danahy M, Moch A, Biros M. Randomized clinical trial of etomidate versus propofol for procedural sedation in the emergency department. *Ann Emerg Med.* 2007; 49(1):15–22.

45. Symington L, Thakore S. A review of the use of propofol for procedural sedation in the emergency department. *Emerg Med J.* 2006;23(2):89–93.

46. Messenger DW, Murray HE, Dungey PE, van Vlymen J, Sivilotti ML. Subdissociative-dose ketamine versus fentanyl for analgesia during propofol procedural sedation: a randomized clinical trial. *Acad Emerg Med.* 2008;15(10):877–886.

47. Frazee BW, Park RS, Lowery D, Baire M. Propofol for deep procedural sedation in the ED. *Am J Emerg Med.* 2005;23(2):190–195.

48. Shah A, Mosdossy G, McLeod S, Lehnhardt K, Peddle M, Rieder M. A blinded, randomized controlled trial to evaluate ketamine/propofol versus ketamine alone for procedural sedation in children. *Ann Emerg Med.* 2011;57(5):425–433.

49. Nejati A, Moharari RS, Ashraf H, Labaf A, Golshani K. Ketamine/propofol versus midazolam/fentanyl for procedural sedation and analgesia in the emergency department: a randomized, prospective, double-blind trial. *Acad Emerg Med.* 2011;18(8):800–806.

50. Andolfatto G, Abu-Laban RB, Zed PJ, et al. Ketamine-propofol combination (ketofol) versus propofol alone for emergency department procedural sedation and analgesia: a randomized double-blind trial. *Ann Emerg Med.* 2012;59(6):504–512.

51. Donelly R, Willman E, Andolfatto G. Stability of ketamine-propofol mixtures for procedural sedation and analgesia in the emergency department. *Can J Hosp Pharm.* 2008;61(6): 426–430.

52. Flood RG, Krauss B. Procedural sedation and analgesia for children in the emergency department. *Emerg Med Clin North Am.* 2003;21(1):121–139.

53. Colaric KB, Overton DT, Moore K. Pain reduction in lidocaine administration through buffering and warming. *Am J Emerg Med.* 1998;16(4):353–356.

54. Knoop K, Trott A, Syverud S. Comparison of digital versus metacarpal blocks for repair of finger injuries. *Ann Emerg Med.* 1994;23(6):1296–1300.

55. Hart RG, Fernandas FA, Kutz JE. Transthecal digital block: an underutilized technique in the ED. *Am J Emerg Med.* 2005;23(3):340–342.

56. Chiu DT. Transthecal digital block: flexor tendon sheath used for anesthetic infusion. *J Hand Surg [Am].* 1990;15(3): 471–477.

57. Hill RG Jr, Patterson JW, Parker JC, Bauer J, Wright E, Heller MB. Comparison of transthecal digital block and traditional digital block for anesthesia of the finger. *Ann Emerg Med.* 1995;25(5):604–607.

58. Cummings AJ, Tisol WB, Meyer LE. Modified transthecal digital block versus traditional digital block for anesthesia of the finger. *J Hand Surg [Am].* 2004;29(1):44–48.

59. McCahon RA, Bedforth NM. Peripheral nerve block at the elbow and wrist. *Contin Educ Anaesth Crit Care Pain.* 2007;7(2):42–44.

60. Haddad FS, Williams RL. Femoral nerve block in extracapsular femoral neck fractures. *J Bone Joint Surg Br.* 1995; 77(6):922–923.

61. Finlayson BJ, Underhill TJ. Femoral nerve block for analgesia in fractures of the femoral neck. *Arch Emerg Med.* 1988;5(3):173–176.

62. Fletcher AK, Rigby AS, Heyes FL. Three-in-one femoral nerve block as analgesia for fractured neck of femur in the emergency department: a randomized, controlled trial. *Ann Emerg Med.* 2003;41(2):227–233.

63. Perry C, Elstrom JA, Pankovich AM. *Handbook of Fractures.* New York, NY: McGraw-Hill; 1995.

64. Furia JP, Alioto RJ, Marquardt JD. The efficacy and safety of the hematoma block for fracture reduction in closed, isolated fractures. *Orthopedics.* 1997;20(5):423–426.

65. Singh GK, Manglik RK, Lakhtakia PK, Singh A. Analgesia for the reduction of Colles fracture. A comparison of hematoma block and intravenous sedation. *Online J Curr Clin Trials.* 1992; Doc No 23.

66. Lehmann JF, Warren CG, Scham SM. Therapeutic heat and cold. *Clin Orthop.* 1974;99:207–245.

67. Lane E, Latham T. Managing pain using heat and cold therapy. *Paediatr Nurs.* 2009;21(6):14–18.

68. Deal DN, Tipton J, Rosencrance E, Curl WW, Smith TL. Ice reduces edema. A study of microvascular permeability in rats. *J Bone Joint Surg Am.* 2002;84-A(9):1573–1578.

69. Mac Auley DC. Ice therapy: how good is the evidence? *Int J Sports Med.* 2001;22(5):379–384.

70. MacAuley D. Do textbooks agree on their advice on ice? *Clin J Sport Med.* 2001;11(2):67–72.

71. Bleakley C, McDonough S, MacAuley D. The use of ice in the treatment of acute soft-tissue injury: a systematic review of randomized controlled trials. *Am J Sports Med.* 2004; 32(1):251–261.

CHAPTER 3

Rheumatology

Todd Taylor, MD, Usama Khalid, MD, and Jehangir Meer, MD

GENERAL PRINCIPLES

Although more than 100 different causes of arthritis exist, none is more important to the emergency physician than the diagnosis of septic (bacterial) arthritis. Mortality from untreated septic arthritis can be as high as 11%.[1] The rapid destruction of articular tissue is inevitable and can occur in as little as 2 to 3 days. Most of the following diagnoses in this chapter are not made primarily in the emergency department (ED); instead, patients will come in for symptom control due to acute exacerbations. There are many overlapping themes found here, but most importantly, the emergency physician must be cautious as many of the following types of arthritis can mimic septic arthritis.

Like everything else in medicine, the evaluation begins with a thorough history. The physician should first determine when the pain started and if there have been similar attacks in the past. An acute onset without previous similar presentations suggests trauma or infection. A history of similar attacks may support the diagnosis of crystal-induced arthritis or other noninfectious causes, although this cannot completely rule out an infectious etiology. Chronic joint pain usually suggests a chronic problem, but the clinician should be careful to note any new features that are unusual to the patient's previous presentations and might signify a concomitant condition (i.e., a septic joint in a patient with gout or rheumatoid arthritis).

The distribution of affected joints will also narrow down the differential. Monoarthritis involves one joint, oligoarthritis involves two to three joints, and polyarthritis occurs in more than three joints.[2] For example, symmetric involvement that is additive and initially involves the small joints is indicative of rheumatoid arthritis, whereas an arthritis that has a migratory pattern, especially if it occurs in conjunction with fevers, is more consistent with gonococcal arthritis. Infectious arthritis is typically monoarticular, but in 10% to 20% of cases, more than one joint is affected.[3-6] Further discussion of the differential diagnoses of monoarthritis and polyarthritis are provided later in this chapter.

Next, the patients should be questioned about constitutional symptoms (e.g., fever) and trauma. Fever and weight loss are important signs because they signify systemic illness. If a patient states that he/she has had fevers, the physician should think of septic arthritis first and foremost. Patients who have a history of trauma should be thought of as possibly having a fracture, which may not be seen on the initial x-ray, particularly in the lower extremity where

fractures may be occult. Diarrhea, urethritis, or uveitis suggests a reactive type of arthritis. Obtaining a history of a rash or skin lesion may also provide an important clue to the proper diagnosis.

Stiffness is usually an indication of synovitis, which is inflammation of the synovial membrane. An important aspect to ascertain is whether the stiffness is exacerbated or alleviated after prolonged rest or exercise. The stiffness associated with rheumatoid arthritis is worse after sleep and improves with movement.[7] Conversely, stiffness and pain that is worse with continued movement is more consistent with osteoarthritis (OA).

When approaching a patient with joint pain, the emergency physician should also ensure that the joint is the etiology of the pain. There are several disease entities that can mimic articular pain where the pathology is not related to the joint (i.e., bursitis, tendonitis, cellulitis, myositis). This can best be determined on physical exam. Some distinguishing features are listed in Table 3–1. Patients with bursitis have pain to palpation over the bursa itself and do not have pain with range of motion. Tendonitis pain typically occurs along the length of the tendon, not related to the joint itself, and is exacerbated by exercise or repetitive movements. In patients with cellulitis, the involvement is usually not isolated to the joint alone. When this occurs, it can be difficult to differentiate between septic arthritis and overlying cellulitis. Septic arthritis will have decreased range of motion secondary to pain, which may help narrow the differential.

Another key component of the physical exam is to ascertain whether the joint pain is inflammatory (i.e., arthritis)

▶ **TABLE 3–1. CHARACTERISTIC FEATURES OF INJURY TO INTRA-ARTICULAR VERSUS PERIARTICULAR STRUCTURES**

Intra-articular	Periarticular
ROM restricted in all directions	ROM restricted in some directions
Pain with active and passive ROM	Pain with active ROM
Joint effusion	No joint effusion
Pain most severe at limits of motion	Pain most severe with movement against resistance
Pain with distraction of the joint	No pain when the joint is distracted

ROM, range of motion.

▶ TABLE 3–2. DIFFERENTIAL DIAGNOSIS OF ACUTE MONOARTHRITIS

Classification	Differential Diagnosis
Infections	Bacteria
	Virus
	Lyme disease
	Mycobacteria, fungi
Crystal-induced	Gout
	Pseudogout
Trauma	Intra-articular fracture
	Meniscus tear
	Hemarthrosis
	Avascular necrosis
Osteoarthritis	
Tumor	Metastasis
	Osteoid osteoma
	Villonodular synovitis

or noninflammatory (i.e., arthralgia). Inflammatory conditions, such as septic arthritis and gout, will cause swelling, erythema, effusions, and warmth. Although there is some overlap in presentations, a noninflammatory condition will typically not have those features. Compare the affected joints to the unaffected side to get a better sense for the acute abnormalities.

Acute Monoarthritis

The three most common causes of acute monoarthritis in adults are infections, crystals, and acute trauma.[8] Table 3–2 lists the differential diagnosis.

Approximately 80% to 90% of nongonococcal bacterial infections are monoarticular, often affecting the large joints such as the knees and hips.[9] Other pathogens also infect the joints in a monoarticular pattern. Fungal arthritis is usually insidious in onset and may be seen in an immunocompromised host. Viral arthritis can occur although this diagnosis is one of exclusion. Human immunodeficiency virus (HIV) may be seen in patients presenting with monoarticular (or oligoarticular) arthritis. These patients may have a nonreactive synovial fluid. Infection with HIV increases one's risk for septic arthritis.[10]

Acute monoarticular arthritis in patients with prosthetic joints is a specific concern as it may indicate infection. Having a prosthetic joint (especially a knee or hip) puts patients at a higher risk for having an infectious etiology. A prosthetic joint becomes infected from the surgery itself or from hematogenous spread (which is the most common).[11] One physical exam finding that will increase the risk of infection is an overlying skin infection. Although the likelihood ratio of septic arthritis in a patient with a prosthetic joint is 3.5, if there is an overlying skin infection the likelihood ratio jumps to 15.[12]

Many systemic diseases can initially present with a monoarthritis. This is an uncommon presentation of systemic diseases; however, it should be considered when the other conditions have been ruled out. Systemic diseases that can present with a monoarthritis include systemic lupus erythematosus (SLE), rheumatoid arthritis (RA), arthritis of inflammatory bowel, Behcet's disease, and Reiter syndrome.

Polyarthritis

In polyarthritis, four or more joints are involved. Three patterns of polyarthritis exist:

* *Additive.* Examples include RA, SLE, and psoriatic arthritis, all of which have joint involvement that progresses to include additional joints over time.
* *Migratory.* With gonococcal arthritis or acute rheumatic fever, symptomatic joints subside and then different joints become involved. A migratory pattern may also be seen in viral arthritis, Lyme arthritis, and SLE.
* *Intermittent.* In gout and pseudogout, one sees a picture of arthritis with signs and symptoms that come, last a few days, and then remit.

A differential diagnosis and diagnostic features of some of the more common causes of polyarthritis are listed in Table 3–3.[13] Other less common causes of polyarthritis include endocarditis, vasculitis, and occult malignancy. In one large series, 44% of patients with bacterial endocarditis had a polyarthritis. Some of the joints have an asymptomatic effusion, whereas others are warm, erythematous, and painful.[14] Systemic vasculitis can present with polyarthritis and fever. These patients will also have concurrent skin lesions (purpura and/or petechiae), neuropathy, or microscopic hematuria.

Polyarthritis associated with fever must trigger the clinician to think of infection first and foremost. In patients with polyarthritis, synovial fluid examination can be useful. Unfortunately, overlap exists between inflammatory fluid and infectious synovial fluid. Elevated synovial fluid leukocyte counts increase the likelihood that the etiology is infectious. A white blood cell (WBC) count of ≥25,000 has a likelihood ratio (LR) of 2.9 that the etiology is infectious, as it climbs to >50,000 the LR rises to 7.7, and at WBC counts >100,000 the LR is 28.0.[15] A variety of inflammatory etiologies can cause similar leukocytosis, including RA and crystal-induced arthritis. An elevated erythrocyte sedimentation rate (ESR) and/or C-reactive protein (CRP) is of some diagnostic value. Studies looking at ESR and CRP showed that they had a sensitivity and a specificity of 95% and 29% for ESR and 77% and 53% for CRP, respectively, when evaluating for infection.[16,17]

Arthrocentesis

The clinician ought to have a low threshold to perform an arthrocentesis on joints where the diagnosis of septic arthritis is a possibility because of the morbidity and mortality risk associated. Sterile technique and local anesthetic

▶ TABLE 3–3. **DIFFERENTIAL DIAGNOSIS OF POLYARTHRITIS**

Disease	Characteristic Features
Rheumatoid arthritis	Symmetric, small joints initially, morning stiffness
Systemic lupus erythematosus	Symmetric (hands, wrists, knees), relapsing/remitting, systemic involvement
Gonococcal arthritis	May be mono-, oligo-, or migratory. Wrist is common site. Rash and tenosynovitis
Osteoarthritis	Most common in hand, knee, and hip. Worse with activity. Gradual onset
Viral arthritis	Migratory or symmetric (fingers, wrists, knees); Hepatitis, parvovirus B19, rubella, HIV
Acute rheumatic fever	Migratory polyarthritis. Fevers. Children. Associated carditis, skin nodules, erythema marginatum, and chorea
Lyme arthritis	Migratory arthralgias; Recurrent, knees (common), characteristic rash, cardiac and neurologic involvement
Seronegative spondyloarthropathies	Asymmetric, additive type of polyarthritis predominantly in the large joints of the lower extremities
Gout	10% of cases are polyarticular; may present with fever

HIV, human immunodeficiency virus.

should be used in all cases. The patient should be consented for the procedure. Contraindications include an overlying cellulitis or lack of an effusion seen on ultrasound. When prosthetic material is in the joint due to prior surgery, consultation with an orthopedist prior to aspiration is recommended. The general principles of arthrocentesis include using the extensor surface, distraction, and approximately 20 to 30 degrees of flexion (Video 3–1). Because the synovial fluid is frequently thick and, in the case of inflammatory arthritis, full of cellular debris, a large needle should be used. In larger joints such as the shoulder and knee, an

18-gauge needle is appropriate (Table 3–4). Poor technique or a large amount of movement of the needle during the procedure can damage the articular cartilage. The infection rate secondary to arthrocentesis is 1:10,000 aspirations. Videos 3–2 to 3–10 illustrate the recommended technique for performing arthrocentesis on the joints most commonly requiring the procedure.

Ultrasound-Guided Arthrocentesis

Ultrasonography serves as a valuable tool for guidance in assessing a swollen, painful joint. Confirmation of effusion

▶ TABLE 3–4. **RECOMMENDED NEEDLE SIZE AND TECHNIQUE FOR JOINT ARTHROCENTESIS**

Joint	Needle Size (Gauge)	Important Anatomy for Needle Insertion
IP and MCP of digit	22	On the dorsal surface of the joint, needle directed under the extensor tendon and into the joint space
Intercarpal joint	20	Palpate the lunate fossa and direct needle perpendicular to the skin between the lunate and the capitate
Radiocarpal joint	20	Palpate the lunate fossa and distal radius and direct needle perpendicular to the skin between these structures
Elbow joint	20	On lateral surface of the elbow, in the center of the triangle made by the olecranon, lateral epicondyle, and radial head
Shoulder joint	18	*Anterior approach:* Between the coracoid process and the lesser tuberosity of the proximal humerus (rare complication of neurovascular injury)
		Posterior approach: Insert needle 1–2 cm below the posterolateral portion of the scapular spine aiming toward the coracoid process anteriorly and to a depth of 2–3 cm
MTP joint	22	Lateral aspect of the joint under the extensor tendon
Ankle joint	20	On either side of the extensor hallucis longus tendon between the tibia and talus. Needle directed perpendicular to the tibia
Knee joint	18	Infrapatellar approach on either side of the patellar tendon aiming tip of needle between the femoral condyles
		Suprapatellar approach 1 cm from patella at the superior/medial portion aiming below the posterior surface of the patella

IP, interphalangeal; MCP, metacarpophalangeal; MTP, metatarsophalangeal.

prior to aspiration can avoid an unnecessary invasive procedure for patients without an effusion. When performing arthrocentesis, ultrasound allows for improved delineation of anatomic boundaries, along with accounting for structural variations in patients. Dynamic guidance allows the clinician to visualize the needle tip in the effusion, thus ensuring procedural success. Procedural complication rate is also reduced by visually avoiding important structures within the vicinity of the joint (e.g., vessels and tendons/ligaments), resulting in improved outcomes.[18]

The procedure is best performed under dynamic ultrasound guidance, ensuring precision in joint access and aspiration. Knowledge of the relevant anatomy for the blind technique is important in guiding probe position. Sterile technique should be used with an ultrasound probe sheath, chlorhexidine prep, sterile drape, and gloves. In general, a high-frequency linear transducer provides optimal results in image acquisition. The exceptions to this are deeper joints such as shoulder and hip joints, that are more easily visualized with a curvilinear probe. Positioning the joint of interest between the provider and the ultrasound machine allows for improved maneuverability and ease of execution. Sterile gel should be used for image acquisition, and the site of needle insertion marked and locally anesthetized with a small-bore needle.

Solid structures such as bone appear as a hyperechoic stripe with shadowing posteriorly. Joint fluid will appear anechoic, with all other forms of soft tissue appearing with varying echogenicity. Needle guidance can take place in both an in-plane or an out-of-plane approach. Constant visualization of the entire length of the needle is an advantage of the in-plane approach, but consequently, none of the neighboring structures of the catheter can be identified on either side of the catheter. Alternatively, the out-of-plane approach allows for better understanding of vital structures in the vicinity of the needle, but identifying the location of the needle tip may be challenging. Choice between either approach varies depending on depth of joint and provider preference.

Wrist (Radiocarpal) Arthrocentesis

Position the patient's arm in abduction with the wrist pronated and slightly flexed. While standing on the ulnar side of the forearm, place the ultrasound machine on the opposite (radial) side so the needle, probe, and joint can be within the same field of view as the machine. Always scan prior to the procedure to affirm the optimal site of penetration.

A high-frequency linear transducer provides the optimal imaging characteristics. Place the probe in the sagittal plane over the distal radius. The bony cortex appears as a hyperechoic line with shadowing posteriorly. Slide the probe distally until you arrive at the radiocarpal joint (Fig. 3–1A). A joint effusion will appear as a hypoechoic space between both bones. On identification of the injection site, anesthetize with a local subcutaneous wheal. Given the relative lack of subcutaneous tissue, this procedure is best performed in

an out-of-plane approach. However, make sure the tip of the needle is identified as the short-axis appearance of any point along the shaft of the needle will appear very similar.

Elbow Arthrocentesis

Elbow effusions can be aspirated from both the posterior and lateral approaches. While the lateral approach has traditionally been used in the landmark technique, the posterior approach to the radiocapitellar joint is our preference for the ultrasound-guided technique. Position the patient so he/she is sitting comfortably with the forearm resting on a table, with the elbow flexed 90 degrees and the wrist supinated. Place a linear probe with the probe marker pointing cephalad on the distal posterior humerus off the midline so as to not be directly over the tricep tendon. Slide the probe distally until the posterior olecranon fossa is visualized. In patients with no elbow effusion, the bright soft-tissue structure is the posterior fat pad (Fig. 3–1B). In cases where an elbow effusion exists, the fat pad is displaced superficially and the anechoic effusion is seen (Fig. 3–1C).

Ankle Arthrocentesis

Ankle effusions can be assessed using an anterior approach. The patient should be reclined on stretcher with the knee flexed and foot plantar flexed and resting. The key landmarks are the medial malleolus, the tibialis anterior tendon, and extensor hallicus longus (EHL) tendon.

Place a linear probe on the ankle medial to the tibialis anterior tendon with the probe marker pointing toward the patient's head. Identify the tibia and slide the probe distally until the joint space between the tibia and talus is visualized (Fig. 3–1D). In the presence of an effusion, the joint space will have anechoic fluid (Fig. 3–1E). Due to the superficial nature of the joint space, an out-of-plane needle technique is easiest. After local anesthetic infiltration of the overlying skin, insert the needle medial to the probe at a steep angle of entry (60–90 degrees). Aspirate as the needle approaches and enters the joint space, avoiding puncture of tendons (tibialis anterior and extensor hallicus longus) and the dorsalis pedis artery, which is laterally located to extensor hallicus longus tendon.[21]

Finger Arthrocentesis

Due to the small surface area of finger joints, it will be easier to perform the arthrocentesis without ultrasound guidance; however, ultrasound guidance can be invaluable in confirming joint effusion. Evaluation of the distal interphalangeal (DIP), proximal interphalangeal (PIP), and metacarpophalangeal (MCP) joints is best facilitated by placing the patient's hand in a water bath. By holding the waterproof ultrasound probe approximately 1 to 2 cm above the submerged digit, the water allows the user to ultrasound the finger without putting pressure on the skin, which can obscure the diagnosis of joint effusion[22] (Fig. 3–1F). Effusions will appear as anechoic in those joint spaces.

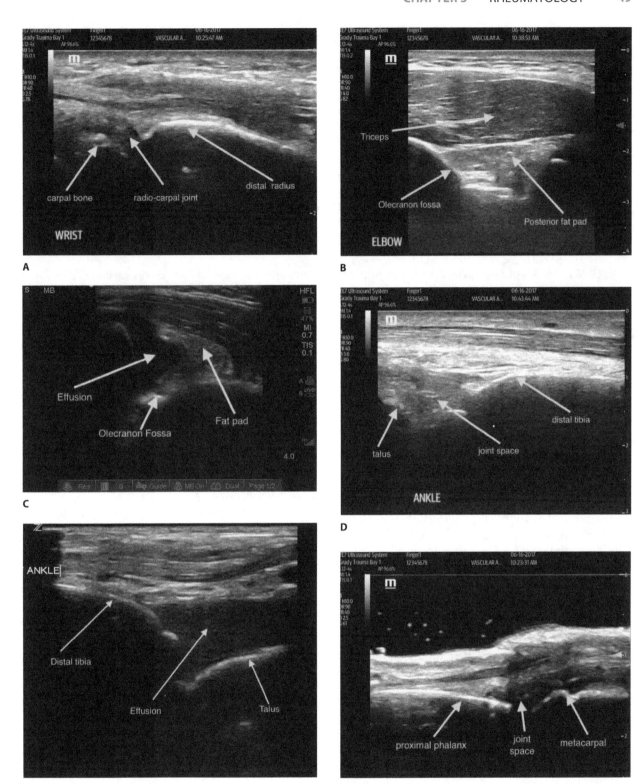

Figure 3–1. Ultrasound guided arthrocentesis. **A.** Ultrasound image of radiocarpal joint using linear probe with marker pointing toward the fingers. **B.** Ultrasound image of posterior olecranon fossa using linear probe with marker pointing toward shoulder showing olecranon fossa and posterior fat pad. **C.** Ultrasound image showing elbow effusion and displaced posterior fat pad. **D.** Ultrasound image of ankle joint showing distal tibia and talus, with linear probe marker pointing to toes. **E.** Ultrasound image of ankle effusion using linear probe with marker pointing to the patient's head. **F.** Ultrasound image of metacarpophalangeal (MCP) joint using linear probe and water-bath technique, with the probe marker pointing to fingertips. (**B** and **C:** Used with permission from Dr. A Nagdev, Highland General Hospital, Department of Emergency Medicine. **D** and **E:** Used with permission from Dr. Srikar Adhikari, University of Arizona, Department of Emergency Medicine.)

▶ TABLE 3–5. **SYNOVIAL FLUID CHARACTERISTICS**

	Noninflammatory	Inflammatory	Septic	Hemorrhagic
Joint Fluid Characteristics				
Viscosity	High	Low	Low	Variable
Appearance	Yellow, transparent	Yellow, transparent	Opaque	Bloody
WBC/mm³	200–2000, mostly lymphocytes	2000–100,000	>50,000[a], mostly PMNs	Variable
Differential Diagnosis	Traumatic arthritis	Crystal-induced (e.g., gout)	Bacterial infection	Trauma
	Osteoarthritis	Immunologic (e.g., rheumatoid arthritis)		Bleeding disorder (e.g., hemophilia, warfarin)
	Osteochondritis dissecans			
	Early or resolving inflammatory arthritis	Infectious (e.g., tuberculosis)		Joint neoplasm

WBC, white blood cell count; PMNs, polymorphonuclear neutrophils.
[a]>50,000 WBC/mm³ is septic arthritis until proven otherwise. Septic arthritis may also occur with WBC counts less than this number.

Synovial Fluid Analysis

Table 3–5 presents some of the common findings of synovial fluid analysis in patients with arthritis. Fluid is sent for differential leukocyte count, culture, Gram stain, and crystals. Other studies to consider are ESR, CRP, and lactic acid. If only a few drops of synovial fluid are obtained, the order of importance for testing is as follows: culture, Gram stain, crystal determination, and cell count. Because the most important diagnosis to rule out is septic joint, the culture is vital and the Gram stain can help with initial antibiotic selection. Getting a leukocyte differential can assist in making a diagnosis of infection. When the polymorphonuclear neutrophils >90%, the odds that the patient has septic arthritis are increased (LR 3.4). Although helpful, a definitive diagnosis from analysis of the joint aspirate is obtained in only 44% of the cases.

The presence of crystals does not exclude infection. In a retrospective study of 1612 joint aspirates, the frequency of septic arthritis with the presence of crystals was 5%. Chronic joint injury in patients with crystal-induced arthropathy makes these patients more susceptible to septic arthritis. Although there is a low likelihood of these conditions occurring concomitantly, when doubt exists, antibiotics should be administered until culture results have returned.

SEPTIC ARTHRITIS

Inflammation of a joint caused by the presence of a microorganism is an uncommon but, perhaps, the most serious arthritic condition presenting to the ED. If it is not recognized, septic arthritis will lead to rapid joint destruction and irreversible loss of function. More than 30% of patients with septic arthritis develop residual joint damage, and mortality rates are approximately 10%. In monoarticular arthritis, the knee is the most frequently affected joint accounting for 50% of cases. The most common agents are gram-positive aerobes,

usually *Staphylococcus aureus (S aureus)*, which accounts for approximately 50% of these infections. In patients with RA, diabetes, or polyarticular septic arthritis, the percentage of cases due to *S aureus* increases to 80%. Note that patients with HIV also have an increased risk for fungal etiologies. In the United States, the most common cause in young sexually active patients is disseminated gonococcal infection.

A prerequisite for the development of septic arthritis is that bacteria must reach the synovial membrane. This may occur in the following ways:

1. *Hematogenous spread*
   * As a result of implantation of the organism within the perivascular synovium or rich vascular beds at the articular surfaces. This typically occurs during a period of bacteremia.
2. *Contiguous spread*
   * A route particularly common in small children is dissemination of bacteria from acute osteomyelitis in the metaphysis or epiphysis.
   * An infection near the joint can progress to the joint or spread through the lymphogenic route. This is most often seen in nonpenetrating traumatic and postoperative wound infections and skin and soft-tissue infections around the joint, particularly the knee.
3. *Direct joint penetration*
   * Iatrogenic infections caused by joint puncture for a diagnostic or therapeutic purpose (rare, incidence of 1:10,000).
   * Penetrating trauma caused by dirty objects or by animal or human bites gives rise to an infection because of the high inoculate of bacteria.

Risk Factors

Although it is true that septic arthritis may occur in any joint and in any individual, there are some clinical situations in which it is more likely. Identified risk factors include age older than 80, diabetes mellitus, RA, joint prosthesis, repeated intra-articular steroid injections, joint surgery, HIV, and a skin infection.[3,10,11,13,17,24,25] Fifty-nine percent of all cases of septic arthritis occur in patients with a previous joint disorder.[26,27] This is significant because of the potential misdiagnoses that can occur if the clinician falsely attributes new joint pain to a "rheumatoid flare" when it is secondary to bacterial infection. In one study, synthetic joint material existed in 29% of infected joints.[27] Systemic conditions associated with bacterial arthritis include liver disease, alcoholism, renal failure, malignancies, acquired immunodeficiency syndrome (AIDS), and immunosuppression. Intravenous drug use predisposes to septic arthritis.

Clinical Presentation

Although septic arthritis usually presents as a monoarthritis, 10% to 20% of patients have polyarthritis at the onset, involving several large joints. When the condition occurs in multiple joints, it presents as an additive type of arthritis. The lower extremities are most often affected, particularly the hip and knee joints.[28] The knee is involved in 50% of cases. The hip is more commonly infected in children. The sacroiliac (SI) joint can be affected in approximately 1% of cases.[29] This is a particularly difficult diagnosis to make. These patients present with gluteal pain and fevers.

A septic joint is, by definition, inflammatory in nature, and therefore is erythematous, warm, and tender. Distention of the joint capsule and increased intra-articular pressure contribute to pain. Patients are reluctant to move or put weight on the joint. Range of motion is severely limited due to pain and joint effusion. Joint effusion is present in 90% of these patients, but is less apparent in joints like the shoulder. Rarely, these findings are less evident if the patient presents early in the clinical course. Multiple studies have looked at the sensitivity of the physical exam findings, with pain (sensitivity 85%) and swelling (sensitivity 78%) being the most common. Fever is less helpful than one would think (sensitivity 57%).[12] There are little to no studies on specificity of physical examination findings in the diagnosis of septic arthritis.[12]

In infants, the symptoms are usually systemic rather than local. Small children develop high fevers and are usually ill-appearing. The clinical features are more often characteristic of sepsis rather than local arthritis. Older children are also febrile and unwell, but the local signs of joint infection are more prominent. Children typically refuse to bear weight and hold the joint in a position that provides for maximum intracapsular volume. The typical workup for children should include fever >38.5°C, ESR >40 mm/h, and peripheral WBC count >12.0 × 10^9.[30] Kocher devised a clinical prediction model with the previous criteria. Patients that didn't have any of the preceding criteria had a probability of septic arthritis of 0.2%.[31] A study done by Caird looked at CRP and showed that a level of >2.0 mg/dL was an independent risk factor.[32] If any of the preceding (and especially if more than one) are positive, then the diagnosis of septic arthritis should be considered.

Gonococcal arthritis is part of a clinical triad of disseminated gonococcal infection (DGI), including dermatitis and tenosynovitis. DGI occurs in 0.5% to 3% of cases of mucosal infection.[33] The arthritis of DGI is polyarticular in 40% to 70% of cases and is usually migratory.[15] It is most common in young, sexually active adults, with a female-to-male ratio of 3:1.[34] A possible explanation for this is that women who have a gonococcal infection tend to be less symptomatic and therefore might not get treatment immediately, thereby allowing the infection to spread.[33] The most common joints involved are the knees and wrists. Characteristic skin lesions are present in two-thirds of cases and include multiple, painless macules, papules, and pustules on an erythematous base.[15] Typically, the rash occurs on the arms, palms, soles, legs, or trunk. Tenosynovitis of the tendons of the wrist and ankle may be associated, and is also present in two-thirds of patients. If the diagnosis is in question, Gram stain from urethral smear or cervical swab should also be obtained in addition to synovial fluid. Synovial fluid alone is not sensitive enough to rule out the disease. In one study, only 44% of patients with gonococcal arthritis had positive synovial fluid cultures.[35]

Diagnosis

A clinical suspicion of infectious arthritis should be followed up by an arthrocentesis of the joint. Arthrocentesis is performed by the emergency physician unless prosthetic material is present within the joint (see Videos 3–1 to 3–10). Hip arthrocentesis is difficult and is best performed with either ultrasound or fluoroscopy by an orthopedic surgeon.

Synovial fluid should be sent for Gram stain, CRP, ESR, culture, lactate, leukocyte and differential counts, and crystal examination. Blood cultures should be obtained as they are positive in 50% of cases of nongonococcal septic arthritis.[36] The peripheral WBC count is elevated in only half of the patients and therefore cannot be relied on to exclude the diagnosis.[37] As noted in Table 3–5, the synovial fluid leukocyte count is usually >50,000 cells/mm^3 with a predominance of polymorphonuclear cells. However, this cutoff is not sensitive enough to exclude the diagnosis.[32] In patients with culture-proven septic arthritis, more than one-third had synovial leukocyte counts <50,000 cells/mm^3 and 10% had counts <10,000 cells/mm^3. Synovial lactic acid can also be drawn. A value of >10 mmol/L has a high likelihood ratio with specificities greater than 95%.[38-41]

As stated previously, the finding of crystals does not exclude the diagnosis of septic arthritis as these two entities can coexist.[42] Diagnosis is further confounded by the fact that both conditions may present with fever, inflammatory arthritis, and high synovial leukocyte counts. In many cases, the Gram stain and good clinical judgment must guide the emergency physician until the culture result is available

2 days later. It is our recommendation that a patient with a history of gout and similar attacks in the past, low CRP (<100 mg/L), low synovial WBC counts (<10,000 μ/L), crystals in the synovial fluid, low clinical suspicion, and a negative Gram stain can be treated for gout alone with close follow-up of the culture results. However, when doubt about the diagnosis exists, the patient should be treated for septic arthritis with antibiotics and an orthopedic consultation.

Bacteria are identified by a Gram stain of the synovial fluid in 50% of cases and on culture in more than 90% of cases. Previous administration of antibiotics can create an increase in false-negative Gram stains and cultures. Conversely, the use of blood culture bottles and a higher volume of synovial fluid may increase the chance of a true-positive culture. Diluting the synovial fluid in a blood culture bottle inhibits the bactericidal components of the synovial fluid and increases the yield.

Laboratory results unique to gonococcal arthritis include a lower yield from synovial fluid cultures (50%). A much higher yield is obtained from mucosal culture (80%). Blood cultures are positive in only 20% to 30% of cases.

Although radiographs are frequently not helpful in making the diagnosis of septic arthritis, they typically show symmetric soft-tissue swelling around the involved joint; marginal erosion or erosions of the bone occur later. The hallmark of septic arthritis is the loss of the white cortical line over a long contiguous segment. Unfortunately, radiographs have limited diagnostic value in the early stages of this disease. Radionuclide scanning and magnetic resonance imaging (MRI) may identify juxta-articular osteomyelitis and effusions in deep locations such as the hip and SI joint.

The difficulty in making this diagnosis is that the peripheral WBC count, synovial WBC count, ESR, CRP, and Gram stain are not sensitive enough to rule out septic arthritis in patients with a high clinical suspicion. If the synovial WBC count, polymorphonuclear cell count, lactic acid, CRP, ESR, and Gram stain are equivocal, and the patient's clinical picture is worrisome for septic arthritis, antibiotics should be started along with an orthopedic consult. The emergency physician should have a low threshold to perform arthrocentesis, initiate antibiotics, and admit these patients as the morbidity and mortality is correlated with the delay in treatment.

Treatment

Therapy consists of systemic antibiotics and closed or open drainage of the septic joint. Initiate antibiotic treatment as soon as possible after arthrocentesis and a set of blood cultures are obtained. Ideally, antibiotic selection is tailored to the Gram stain. Empiric antibiotic treatment for non-gonococcal septic arthritis in the era of methicillin-resistant S aureus (MRSA) consists of vancomycin plus either a third-generation cephalosporin (ceftriaxone) or, for the immuno-compromised patient, a fourth-generation cephalosporin

(cefepime). For prosthetic joints, if possible, antibiotics should be started after synovial fluid has been obtained. A reasonable empiric regimen would include vancomycin and a fourth-generation cephalosporin. Gonococcal arthritis is treated with a third-generation cephalosporin (ceftriaxone).

Orthopedic consultation and admission is warranted for all patients. Currently, the mainstay of treatment is open or closed drainage. If fluid cannot be obtained from the joint or there is a poor response to antibiotic therapy, then open drainage or arthroscopy is required. Open drainage is usually necessary when the hip is affected. Arthroscopy is preferred in the knee and shoulder because of easier irrigation.

Infections that occur with prosthetic material are more difficult to treat, and there is no widely accepted strategy. The options are as follows: debridement with retention of the hardware, removal and replacement of hardware in one operation, removal of hardware with replacement later (with or without use of antimicrobial impregnated spacer), and permanent removal of hardware. These choices are specialist specific and will depend on your consultant's practice pattern.

CRYSTAL-INDUCED ARTHROPATHY

Gout and pseudogout are inflammatory syndromes caused by crystal deposition in the joints and soft tissues. Features of these two syndromes are compared in Table 3-6.

Gout

Gout is caused by the precipitation of uric acid crystals in the joints and soft tissues. Uric acid precipitates from solution at approximately 7 mg/dL, so a slight rise in the serum concentration of urate from the normal range of 4 to 5 mg/dL may lead to gouty arthritis. The long-term goal of treatment of gout is reduction of serum urate to a target of <6 mg/dL. Levels of uric acid are normally higher in men than in premenopausal women and rise with age in both sexes. Hence, the typical patient afflicted with gout is a middle-aged man. In the United States, in patients older than 65, 73.5% of patients with gout are males. Gout is unusual in men younger than 30 years and in premenopausal women. Patients with obesity, diets high in meats, and excessive alcohol intake tend to have higher levels of uric acid. Patients with diets rich in dairy tend to have lower uric acid levels.

Although up to 5% of adults have some degree of hyperuricemia, only one-fifth (1% overall) will develop gout. Among patients with serum uric acid levels of 9 mg/dL, 5% will develop an acute gout attack per year. Hyperuricemia may be caused by either overproduction of uric acid or decreased uric acid excretion. A few of the more common causes of decreased urate excretion that may precipitate an attack of gouty arthritis are loop diuretics (furosemide, thiazides), salicylates, and ethanol.

▶ TABLE 3–6. **CLINICAL FEATURES OF GOUT AND PSEUDOGOUT**

	Gout	Pseudogout
Joints affected	First MTP, foot, ankle, knee	Knee
Initial attack	90% monoarticular	90% Monoarticular
Distribution	Asymmetric, additional joints added with subsequent attacks	Usually monoarticular, more than three joints unusual
Onset	Hyperacute, within a few hours	Acute, within 6–24 h
Tophi	Present in chronic gout	May develop tophi-like deposits
Provocants	Disorders of urate metabolism	Joint trauma
	Diuretics	Systemic illness
	Ethanol	Endocrine disorders
	Cold	
Crystals	Monosodium urate	Calcium pyrophosphate dehydrogenate
	Needle-shaped	Rod-shaped, or rhomboidal
	Negatively birefringent	Positively birefringent
Cell count	Inflammatory, usually >50,000, mostly PMNs	Usually inflammatory, may be <50,000, mostly PMNs
Viscosity	Markedly decreased	Decreased, but variably
Treatment	NSAIDs	Joint aspiration and injection
	Analgesics	NSAIDs
	Colchicine	Early mobilization

MTP, metatarsophalangeal; PMNs, polymorphonuclear neutrophils; NSAIDs, nonsteroidal anti-inflammatory drugs.

Clinical Presentation

The presentation of gout is divided into four stages:

* *Stage 1 (asymptomatic hyperuricemia).* Symptoms are usually not present, although a small percentage of patients develop urinary calculi.
* *Stage 2 (acute gouty arthritis).* This stage is heralded by the rapid onset of severe pain and swelling of the affected joints. The first metatarsophalangeal (MTP) joints are affected in more than half of initial attacks and eventually in up to 90% of patients with gout. Other sites commonly affected are other joints in the foot, ankle, and knee. When the hand is affected, the swelling may be quite significant (Fig. 3–2). Almost 90% of initial attacks are monoarticular. The affected joints are markedly erythematous, more

so than in other types of noninfectious arthritis. Tendons and bursae may be affected. Although mild attacks resolve within a few days, more severe attacks require several weeks to resolve completely. Patients are occasionally systemically ill, and may even appear septic.[53]

* *Stage 3 (intercritical gout).* Between attacks the patient is asymptomatic but may still have urate crystals present in both previously affected and unaffected joints.
* *Stage 4 (chronic gout).* Approximately half of patients who have had attacks of gout for a period of 10 years or more develop tophi, nodules in the skin and soft tissues containing precipitated uric acid crystals (Fig. 3–3). Tophi and the associated inflammatory reaction to urate crystals can damage to cartilage, subchondral bone, tendons, and skin, leading to cosmetic and functional deformities.

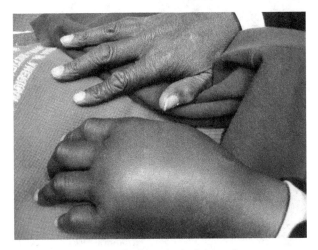

Figure 3–2. Acute attack of gout in the left hand.

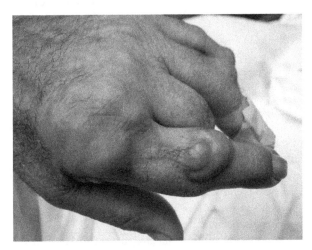

Figure 3–3. Gouty tophi of the hand.

Diagnosis

Serum uric acid levels are usually elevated between attacks in patients with gout. However, during an acute attack, uric acid precipitates into the affected tissues and the serum uric acid level may normalize. Thus, serum uric acid levels are of little utility during an acute attack of gout.

There have been proposals for using clinical criteria only as the diagnostic modality of making the diagnosis. This is an attractive method because it would obviate the need for arthrocentesis. One review article looked at three of these methods and illustrated that none had a sensitivity or a specificity of greater than 70% and 88%, respectively. It remains critical that the emergency physician differentiate crystal-induced arthropathy from septic arthritis, and therefore, arthrocentesis remains the cornerstone of the diagnosis.

Aspiration of the inflamed joint is the key to the diagnosis of gout. Synovial fluid from a gouty joint reveals:

- *Needle-shaped urate crystals.* If polarized light microscopy is available, they will appear yellow when oriented parallel to the axis of slow vibration marked on the microscope's compensator (i.e., negatively birefringent). The crystals are found intracellularly (within neutrophils) during an acute attack of gout.
- *Low viscosity.*
- *High leukocyte count, occasionally >50,000/mm³.* Seventy percent or more will be neutrophils.
- *Absence of bacteria on Gram stain and culture.*

Because little fluid is usually obtained from aspiration, especially from the small joints of the foot, a few guidelines for the use of synovial fluid are in order:

- Often, only two drops of fluid, one for microscopy and one for culture, are necessary.
- Do not discard the small amount of fluid remaining in the needle or its hub. This may be enough to make the diagnosis.
- If only a small amount of fluid is available, the preferred order of analysis is culture, and then Gram stain, crystal examination, and cell count. Additional studies can be performed if sufficient fluid has been obtained.

Radiographic changes, such as joint erosion, occur long after the diagnosis of gout is made and therefore may not help in diagnosis of the acute gout attack (Figs. 3–4 to 3–7).

Treatment

Strategies for managing gout vary, depending on the acuity of the disease. For the patient who has had three or fewer attacks, with recovery between attacks, treatment is aimed at decreasing the pain and inflammation during the acute attacks. Plasma urate concentrations are not treated at this point in the disease as most patients do not go on to develop chronic gout.

Nonsteroidal anti-inflammatory drugs (NSAIDs) are the mainstay of treatment. Guidelines recommend naproxen,

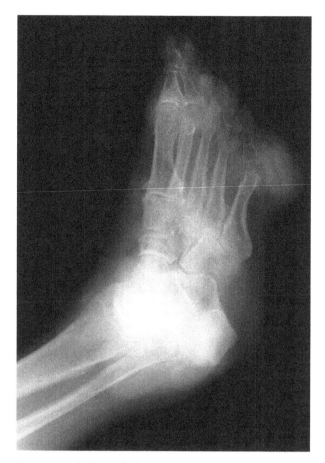

Figure 3–4. Radiograph demonstrating gouty tophi of the foot. *(Used with permission from J. Fitzpatrick, MD, Cook County Hospital.)*

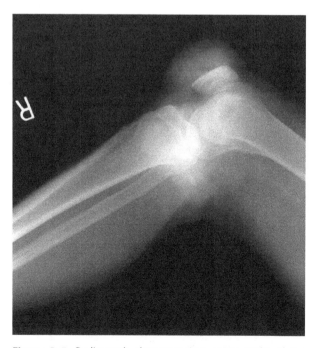

Figure 3–5. Radiograph demonstrating gouty tophi of the knee. *(Used with permission from J. Fitzpatrick, MD, Cook County Hospital.)*

indomethacin, or sulindac as appropriate treatment options. Whichever NSAID is chosen, it should be continued until complete resolution of the gout attack. The provider should be cautious of NSAID use in patients with renal impairment, gastrointestinal (GI) side effects, or other contraindications.

Colchicine is effective treatment for the acute attack, but the side effects of vomiting and diarrhea limit its utility. Colchicine is administered orally, 1.2 mg dose initially, with 0.6 mg given 1 hour later. Subsequent dosing of 0.6 mg daily or two times a day can be prescribed until the attack resolves. Decrease the dose in patients with renal insufficiency. Intravenous colchicine should be given only in conjunction with a consultant.

Intra-articular steroid injection may be performed, but the clinician should avoid its use if there is any doubt about the diagnosis, especially if septic arthritis is a consideration. Oral prednisone at 0.5 mg/kg/d for a duration of 5 to 10 days may be useful, especially if other treatments are ineffective or contraindicated.

Other analgesics, such as acetaminophen and opiates, may further alleviate pain and should not be forgotten. Finally, eliminate any medications such as diuretics that

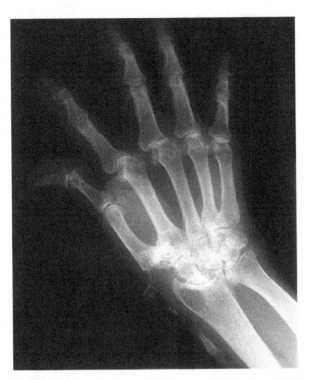

Figure 3–6. Gouty degenerative changes of the hand and wrist.

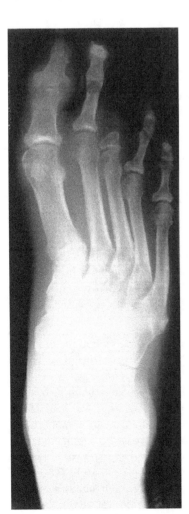
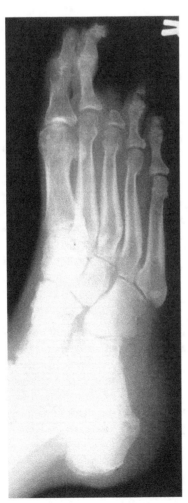

Figure 3–7. Gouty destruction of the foot. *(Used with permission from J. Fitzpatrick, MD, Cook County Hospital.)*

precipitated the attack. The sooner treatment is initiated after an attack begins, the better the response.

Complications

Patients with long-standing gout have a higher incidence of nephrolithiasis, proteinuria, and hypertension.

Septic arthritis may occur in the same joint as crystal-induced arthritis. In these cases, the inflammatory response caused by the joint infection leads to precipitation of urate or calcium pyrophosphate crystals and thus an attack of gout or pseudogout. Because the synovial fluid cell counts of patients with crystal-induced arthritis and infectious arthritis are similar, synovial fluid obtained from patients with acute arthritis should always be sent for Gram stain and culture, even if crystals are seen. Any patient with gout who is systemically ill in the setting of an acute attack of arthritis, or whose arthritis seems worse or different than usual, should have his/her joint fluid cultured and the emergency physician should have a low threshold to start empiric antibiotic treatment.

Finally, RA and gout rarely occur together, so if a patient with RA presents with what appears clinically to be an acute case of gout, an infected joint should be strongly suspected and arthrocentesis performed.

Pseudogout

Calcium pyrophosphate dihydrate (CPPD) crystal deposition in joints occurs primarily in elderly patients. Although historically this has been called pseudogout, many rheumatologists now refer to this entity as acute calcium pyrophosphate crystal arthritis (alternatively, acute CPP crystal arthritis). It may present as acute monoarticular arthritis or as chronic arthritis (usually complicating underlying OA). CPPD crystals are found incidentally at arthrocentesis in more than 40% of patients with OA.

For simplicity, one may want to think of this as gout, with only the real difference being in the synovial fluid results. The clinical presentation, diagnostic approach, and treatment modalities are the same as gout. The difference is that the synovial fluid will have positive birefringent rhomboid or rod-shaped crystals as opposed to the negative birefringent rod-shaped crystals of gout.

Radiographic studies may be normal; may show changes of OA; or may reveal calcification of cartilage, synovial tissues, and tendons. Calcification of joint cartilage, chondrocalcinosis, occurs most commonly in the hand and knee (Fig. 3–8).

Although any joint may be involved, the knee is most commonly affected, followed by the wrist, shoulder, ankle, and elbow. Pain and inflammation are severe and develop rapidly over 6 to 24 hours. As with gout, overlying erythema is common, and the patient may be febrile.

More than 90% of cases affect a single joint; involvement of more than a few joints is rare and should prompt a search for another etiology. Joint trauma; concurrent

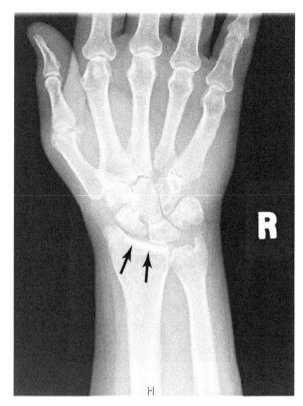

Figure 3–8. Chondrocalcinosis of the wrist (*arrows*).

severe illness; surgery; initiation of thyroid replacement therapy; or other systemic diseases such as Wilson disease, hemochromatosis, and hyperparathyroidism may precipitate attacks. Most attacks, however, are idiopathic.

Diagnosis is made by joint aspiration, which reveals:

- Rhomboidal or rod-shaped CPPD crystals that are weakly positively birefringent and appear blue when oriented parallel to the axis of slow vibration marked on a polarizing microscope's compensator.
- Bloodstained or cloudy synovial fluid.
- Decreased viscosity.
- Elevated leukocyte count, occasionally WBC counts >50,000/mm^3, primarily neutrophils. However, cell counts vary more than in gout and may be much lower.

Treatment

Treatment of acute pseudogout is identical to the treatment of acute gout. NSAIDs are effective, but may have gastric and renal toxicities. Colchicine is appropriate as well as a short course of steroids. Complete joint drainage by aspiration is both therapeutic and diagnostic, and may resolve the attack of pseudogout. The affected joint is mobilized as soon as the patient can tolerate. Ice has been found to relieve the symptoms significantly better than warm packs used for other forms of arthritis. Because patients are usually elderly and have preexisting OA, prolonged immobility should be avoided as it can lead to permanent functional disability.

Hydroxyapatite Crystal Arthropathy

In addition to urate and calcium pyrophosphate crystals, hydroxyapatite crystals can also provoke an acute arthritis. Apatite crystals are found in nearly half of osteoarthritic joints, usually in combination with CPPD crystals.

Although hydroxyapatite crystals are often incidental findings at arthrocentesis, they can occasionally provoke an acute inflammatory reaction resembling gout or pseudogout. The apatite crystals may also lead to rapid erosion of joint cartilage in the setting of OA, with pain and loss of joint function. Apatite crystals are often found with CPPD and urate crystals in the setting of gout or pseudogout. In these cases, the role of the apatite crystals is unclear.

NSAIDs, analgesics, and referral to an orthopedic or rheumatologic specialist are indicated if apatite arthropathy is suspected. Joint aspiration may be therapeutic as well as diagnostic.

OSTEOARTHRITIS

OA is the most common form of arthritis in older patients, causing pain that can significantly reduce function and the quality of life. It is more commonly found in women than men. OA is such a common condition at midlife and in elderly patients that it is safe to say that it is ubiquitous.

Pathologic Features

The pathologic features of OA include the sum of a dysregulation of tissue turnover in weight-bearing joints. The cartilage is broken down over time due to mechanical forces, and because of its avascular nature, is difficult to repair. Focal areas of damage to articular cartilage occur, and there is an increased activity of subchondral bone. Although historically it has been thought of solely as a cartilage repair problem, recent research suggests that there are a host of factors involved, including biomechanical, genetic, and immunologic components that contribute to the formation of OA.

Risk Factors

Risk factors for OA include age, family history, obesity, joint trauma, abnormal joint shape, occupational activity, and the female gender. Obesity is a major risk factor, particularly for OA of the knee in women. Weight loss can prevent the onset of symptomatic OA, delay radiographic progression, and lessen symptoms.

Reproductive and hormonal variables also predispose to generalized OA in women. Genetic factors contribute, as there is a strong familial link, particularly in women. Trauma and overuse are other major causes of joint involvement, particularly in the knee and in the hand. Repeated minor trauma may cause increased OA with occupational overuse. Recreational overuse or habitual physical activity is not associated with symptomatic knee OA; however, there is an increased risk of this disorder in elite athletes.

Clinical Presentation

Pain is undoubtedly the most prominent and important symptom of OA. This pain typically gets worse with the duration and intensity of activity. The most commonly affected joints include the thumb base, DIP, knee, hip, first metatarsal phalangeal, and spinal apophyseal. Symptoms of OA include use-related exacerbations of pain, stiffness with inactivity (gelling) that improves in minutes, loss of movement, feelings of instability, and functional handicaps. The difference between the stiffness in OA and RA is that the stiffness in OA gets better in a few minutes, whereas the stiffness in RA can sometimes take up to an hour to show any improvement.

On examination, the patient has tender spots around the joint margin, and there is firm swelling of the joint margin. The patient has coarse crepitus most easily identified during passive movements. Movements are painful and restricted, and there is tightness in the joint.

Hand Osteoarthritis

The first carpometacarpal joint and the DIP and PIP joints are the most commonly affected joints. Patients have pain and bony swelling at the base of the thumb with Heberden's nodes (small bony growths found at the DIP joints). Loss of function in the hands may be quite marked in the beginning, as the joints go through phases of inflammation, perhaps lasting for months. The long-term outlook for function, however, is generally good despite residual bony deformities.

Knee Osteoarthritis

Symptoms tend to have a gradual onset and deteriorate with time. Mechanical abnormalities, obesity, and poor quadriceps muscle strength contribute to progression and associated disability. The knee may be affected in any or all of its three compartments (medial and lateral tibiofemoral and patellofemoral). Joint-line pain, tenderness, and loss of articular cartilage lead to joint-space narrowing and gradual varus deformity. In approximately 15% to 20% of patients with knee OA, there are effusions that may be long-standing and result in synovial cyst development, particularly in the popliteal fossa (Baker cyst). The Baker cyst may occasionally rupture and mimic deep vein thrombosis with pain, swelling, and inflammation in the calf and lower leg.

Hip Osteoarthritis

Hip OA often occurs in the elderly population and tends to be more common in men. Pain is characteristically present in the groin. Involvement may be unilateral or bilateral. Symptoms of pain or tenderness around the pelvic girdle region (e.g., in the buttocks or lateral aspect of the thigh) may indicate OA of the hip, but other possibly coexisting conditions should be considered, such as referred pain from the spine or trochanteric bursitis. In the early stages, patients may experience pain with extremes of motion, with internal rotation usually being the earliest movement affected. Patients with advanced disease may experience referred pain in the knee.

Diagnosis

The diagnosis is largely clinical, but is supported by the findings on radiographs (Figs. 3–9 and 3–10). Radiographs are normal early in the disease, but narrowing of the joint space develops as the disease progresses. Ninety percent of

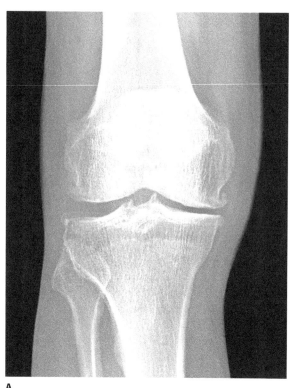

A

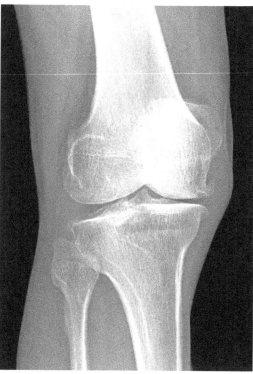

B

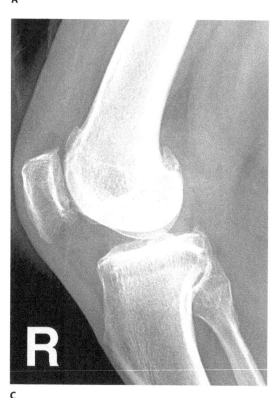

C

Figure 3–9. Osteoarthritis of the knee with osteophyte formation and a decreased joint space of the medial compartment. *A.* Anteroposterior (AP); *B.* Oblique; *C.* Lateral.

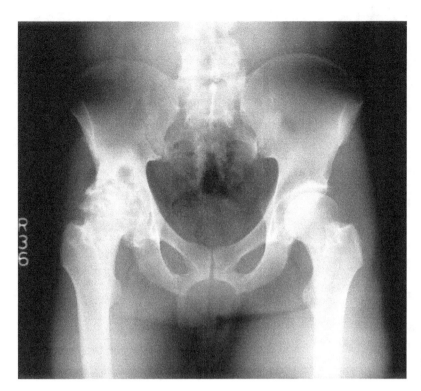

Figure 3–10. Osteoarthritis of the hip. *(Used with permission from J. Fitzpatrick, MD, Cook County Hospital.)*

individuals older than 40 years have radiographic changes characteristic of OA; however, only 30% have symptoms. Other x-ray features include subchondral sclerosis, marginal osteophytes, and joint narrowing. Laboratory features in arthritis are not helpful in making the diagnosis. If arthrocentesis is performed, the fluid results should be noninflammatory in nature with a low WBC count (<2000), no crystals, and appear as a transparent (not cloudy) yellow color.

Treatment

The aim of treatment in OA is to relieve pain and allow the patient to be as active and independent as possible. The drugs used in the management of OA are simple analgesics to relieve pain and NSAIDs to reduce symptoms. In hand OA, thermal modalities, topical and oral NSAIDs, and tramadol are used. For knee and hip OA, the recommendations are the same but also include aerobic exercise, and for patients who are obese, weight loss.[62] Intra-articular corticosteroids provide local relief of symptoms and can be added to the regimen of patients with knee and hip OA. Exercise therapy, hydrotherapy, and walking aids and appliances are all adjuncts that can be used.[63] A Cochrane Review of glucosamine treatment for OA showed that patients may get a small reduction in pain and improvement in function, but that the results were marginal. The American College of Rheumatology (ACR) conditionally recommends the use of either glucosamine or chondroitin for knee OA.[62] Ultimately, many patients need joint replacement surgery, particularly in cases of advanced hip and knee OA. Indications for surgery include substantial disability, the presence of significant night pain or rest pain, and inadequate control of symptoms with nonoperative interventions.[64]

RHEUMATOID ARTHRITIS

RA is an autoimmune disease that affects approximately 1% of the world's population. It is characterized by a symmetric, progressive polyarthritis. Unlike OA, RA often has systemic manifestations. Although the cause of RA is unclear and its course in each patient can be unpredictable, the symptoms can range from mild to tremendous pain, suffering, and disability.[65,66]

RA has varying onset, severity, and progression. It is twice as common in women as in men, and its usual onset in the fourth and fifth decades of life. It is believed that there is a genetic predisposition to RA and prevalence of RA increases with age. (Note: Juvenile rheumatoid arthritis [JRA] is a distinct syndrome and discussed separately.) RA is characterized by an autoimmune attack on synovial tissue, leading to marked (up to 100-fold) proliferation of synovium. Adjoining tissues are affected by this synovial neoplasia, including cartilage, bone, ligaments, tendons, and bursae. This inflammation, combined with physical stress, destroys joint structure and function. In addition, extra synovial manifestations may affect almost any organ.

The emergency physician will encounter two main groups of patients with RA: (1) those who have not yet been diagnosed as having RA and present with polyarticular arthritis; and (2) those who have been previously diagnosed and present with an acute flare, systemic manifestations of the disease, or an unrelated medical problem.

New-Onset Rheumatoid Arthritis

Although etiology of RA is unclear, the current thinking is that it is a combination of environmental and genetic factors. Onset is usually but not always symmetric and gradual. The variability of symptoms and progression in RA often makes initial diagnosis difficult: onset may be over weeks to months, duration of illness may last weeks or decades, and severity may vary from mild arthritis to crippling deformity. It should be noted that the initiation of RA probably begins years before any clinical symptoms are apparent.   This is important to realize because early referral to a rheumatologist and initiation of therapy can greatly improve long-term outcomes.

RA is an autoimmune disease, and 70% to 80% of patients have rheumatoid factor (RF), an immune complex, circulating in their serum. RF is not specific for RA and may be found in other diseases. Anti-citrullinated protein antibodies (ACPA) are also found in patients with RA.

The diagnosis of RA is still based primarily on clinical criteria. The ACR has a scoring system that includes number of joints involved; presence of RF and/or ACPA, CRP, and/or ESR; and duration of symptoms. The higher the score, the more likely the patient has RA. The classification system requires observation of the patient over time (at least 6 weeks), so the initial diagnosis of RA is unlikely to be made in the acute care setting. The goal in the acute care setting is, therefore, to suspect rheumatologic disease, alleviate any acute symptoms, rule out other urgent/emergent conditions (septic arthritis), and then refer the patient to the appropriate provider for definitive diagnosis and long-term management.

Treatment

A variety of agents with varying therapeutic and side effects are used, and must often be combined for optimal results. A treatment regimen should be tailored for each individual patient. Therapy with agents other than NSAIDs, and perhaps a brief course of steroids, should only be undertaken after consultation with the physician who will be following the patient.

NSAIDs are used to treat symptomatic pain and inflammation of RA. Numerous agents are available, with variable dosage and cost. Unfortunately, a given patient's therapeutic response to each drug is not predictable, and neither are the exact side effects the patient will experience.

Disease-modifying antirheumatic drugs (DMARDs) are the mainstay of treatment in RA. DMARDs may alter the destructive course of RA. For this reason, and despite the potential for toxicity, these agents are recommended early in the course of RA. The most commonly used DMARD in the initial phase of treatment is methotrexate. DMARDs are expensive and require several weeks of use for maximal benefit. They are usually combined with NSAID therapy, and rarely corticosteroids. One-third of patients take more than one DMARD.

DMARDs have the potential for severe side effects, and their use requires close follow-up and careful dose titration. Initiation of DMARD treatment without consultation is beyond the acute care scope of practice. Because patients may present with iatrogenic complications, the emergency physician should have some familiarity with the major agents used and their side effects.

Systemic corticosteroids can improve the symptoms of an acute RA flare. The most recent ACR guidelines recommend that they should be started at the lowest dose for the shortest duration.   Systemic corticosteroids do not prevent joint destruction and thus have no sustained benefit for patients with RA. Chronic use of systemic corticosteroids (e.g., prednisone 5–7.5 mg/d) should be limited to severe, unremitting disease and should be initiated by a consultant.

Other therapeutic modalities for the treatment of RA include:

- Joint immobilization or bed rest, or both; these may be useful for patients with an acute flare, but joint rest must be weighed against the effects of deconditioning.
- Physical therapy
- Reconstructive surgery; this is sometimes necessary to correct deformities, particularly in the hand.

Preexisting Rheumatoid Arthritis

The goals in the acute care setting are to treat the patient's pain and inflammation, limit tissue destruction, and improve daily functioning. These patients are often on immunosuppressive drugs (Table 3–7), which predispose them to infections and may obscure signs of serious infection. Both RA and the medications used to treat it may cause systemic complications.

Articular Disease

Usually, symmetric and progressive joint deterioration are seen, with exacerbations and remissions over the course of the disease (Figs. 3–11 and 3–12). Function is worse after immobility or sleep and improves with activity during the day. Patients report morning stiffness, usually lasting more than 30 minutes.

Clinical findings include pain in the affected joints, both at rest and with motion, along with joint swelling, warmth, and tenderness (Table 3–8). Erythema may be present with acute onset or flare; if present, the physician should consider infection. Pain, inflammation, and disuse atrophy of muscles lead to progressive functional impairment and loss of range of motion. Radiologic signs of soft-tissue swelling, symmetric joint-space narrowing, and osteopenia of adjoining bones are present.

▶ **TABLE 3–7. DRUGS USED IN THE TREATMENT OF RHEUMATOID ARTHRITIS**

Agent	Major Side Effects
Hydroxychloroquine (Plaquenil)	Retinal lesions
Sulfasalazine	Gastrointestinal (GI) upset, rash
Methotrexate (MTX)	Rash, GI upset, pulmonary toxicity, hepatitis, immunosuppression, teratogenesis
Azathioprine (Imuran)	GI upset, abdominal pain, leukopenia, immunosuppression, hepatitis
Leflunomide (Arava)	Myelosuppression, hepatic fibrosis, teratogenesis
Cyclosporine	Renal insufficiency, anemia, hypertension
Tumor necrosis factor (TNF) inhibitors	
Infliximab (Remicade)	Infections
Etanercept (Enbrel)	Infections
Adalimumab (Humira)	Infections
Interleukin-1 inhibitor	
Anakinra	Pneumonia, neutropenia

The "rheumatic hand" is characteristic: the PIP, MCP, and wrist joints are inflamed, whereas the DIP joints are spared. Initial treatment is with NSAIDs and modification of activity. Rest, splinting, and preferential use of large rather than small joints (e.g., carrying a bag on the shoulder rather than in the hand) can delay joint destruction.

DMARDs are added, with consultation, for progressive disease.

Acute Rheumatoid Arthritis Flare

In this presentation, the patient has acutely increased synovial inflammation with variable systemic and constitutional symptoms. Joint involvement is symmetric, usually with six or more painful, tender, swollen joints. Morning stiffness worsens, typically lasting longer than 1 hour. ESR >30 mm/h and elevated CRP levels are often present.[69]

The immediate goal of treatment is alleviation of the acute pain and inflammation, followed by prompt referral to the patient's primary care provider or rheumatologist. Joint infection must always be considered, particularly with mono- or pauciarticular flares (see later discussion).

Bed rest may be sufficient in some patients. NSAIDs are prescribed unless contraindicated. The patient should be referred promptly to a specialist for DMARD treatment.

A systemic steroid bolus given after consultation can help control a severe, generalized flare. Some patients may require up to 1 month of daily, low-dose systemic steroid therapy. Local steroid injection into the most acute joints, after infection is ruled out, can decrease local inflammation. The patient's rheumatologist or primary care provider generally performs injection.

Finally, the emergency physician should be alert for signs of new systemic disease, either rheumatic or iatrogenic.

Septic Rheumatic Joint

Patients with RA are at increased risk of joint infection as a result of inflammation and immunosuppression. Furthermore, anti-inflammatory and immunosuppressive medications may suppress clinical signs of infection and delay the diagnosis.

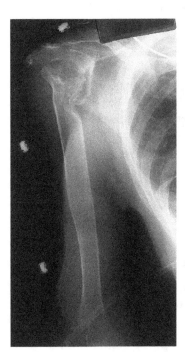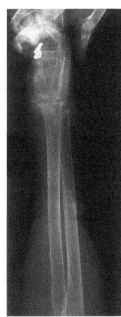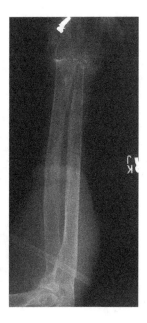

Figure 3–11. Rheumatoid arthritis of the wrist, elbow, and shoulder.

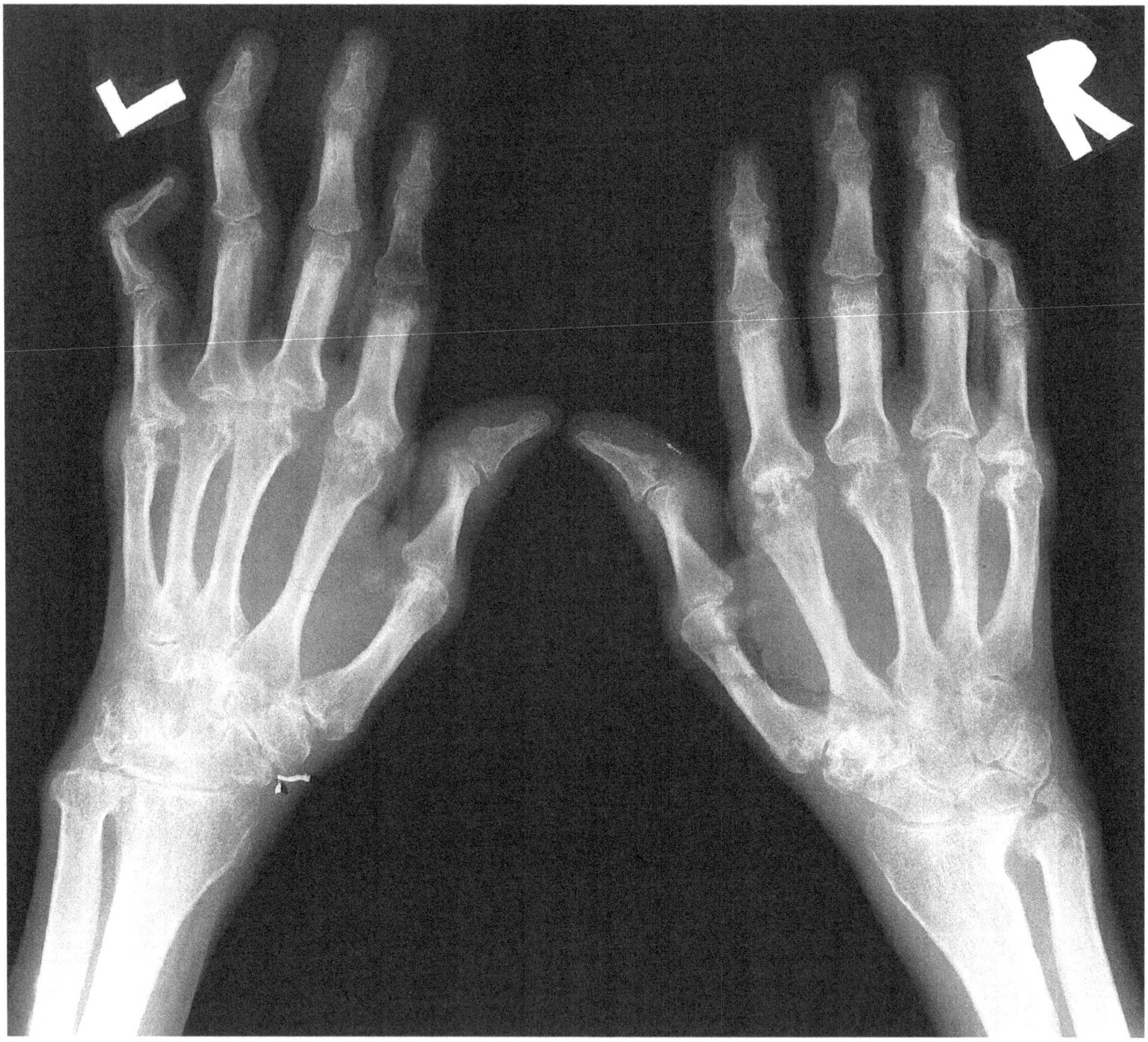

Figure 3–12. Rheumatoid arthritis of the hand. *(Used with permission from J. Fitzpatrick, MD, Cook County Hospital.)*

Unfortunately, these two entities can present in very similar ways, and given the high morbidity of septic arthritis, the clinician should have a low threshold for performing arthrocentesis when septic arthritis is a possibility. A number of findings can guide the clinician's diagnosis and treatment decisions.

Joint infection is usually monoarticular. Diagnosis is much more difficult if the infection is polyarticular. Infection may be indicated by pain greater than the patient's usual flare, fever, and systemic toxicity. Polyarticular infection is usually asymmetric because of hematogenous spread.

Diagnosis necessitates joint aspiration for culture, Gram stain, and cell count. The physician should attempt to obtain synovial fluid for culture before starting antibiotic therapy.

Empiric antibiotic treatment should be started if clinical suspicion is high or if the aspirate demonstrates positive Gram stain, leukocyte count >50,000 mm³ (unusual in RA, but possible), or PMNs >90%. Blood and other specimens, such as urine, should be cultured to increase the yield of any infecting organism and to search for a site of initial infection. Empiric treatment without the proper diagnostic workup may commit the patient to an unnecessary course of antibiotics and may delay initiation of appropriate anti-inflammatory therapy.

Popliteal (Baker) Cyst
Popliteal cysts are common because of the synovial proliferation that characterizes RA. A cyst may rupture spontaneously or as a result of physical activity, leading to acute calf pain and swelling. The most important task is in this clinical scenario is ruling out an acute deep venous thrombosis (DVT). Heparinization following a misdiagnosis of DVT can lead to continuing hemorrhage into the calf, with

▶ TABLE 3–8. **SPECIFIC SYNDROMES IN RHEUMATOID ARTHRITIS**

Region	Diagnostic Findings (Synovial Inflammation)	Frequency	Treatment Considerations
Upper Extremities			
Hand tendons	*Flexors:* Decreased ROM, tendon rupture, trigger effect, CTS	Common	Immobilization for 2–3 wk
	Extensors: Dorsal hand mass, tendon rupture		Medications, splint, physical therapy, reconstructive surgery
PIP	Fusiform swelling, boutonniere deformity, swan-neck deformity, flail joint	Usual, early	Reconstructive surgery sometimes needed
DIP	Swelling	Rare, never initial or isolated finding	
MCP	Swelling, ulnar drift, volar subluxation (fixed)	Usual, early	
Thumb	Boutonniere deformity, CMC dislocation ("duckbill thumb"), flail IP joint	Common, except duckbill thumb	
Wrist	Carpal subluxation, radiocarpal dislocation, synovial cysts, CTS, fracture due to osteoporosis	Almost universal, early CTS may be initial complaint	
Elbow	Subcutaneous nodules, synovial cysts, CTS, fracture due to osteoporosis	Common, late	Same as above; nerve compression at elbow may require decompression
Shoulder	Synovitis, bursitis, rotator cuff inflammation, AC joint pain, biceps rupture	Variable, late	Joint injection
Lower Extremities			
Foot	Synovitis, bone erosion, valgus deformity, "claw foot," ulcers or MTP–cutaneous fistulae	Common (90%), especially first and fifth MTPs	Immobilize for 6–8 wks Local wound care
Ankle	Tendonitis, may lead to Achilles tendon rupture, may compress posterior tibial nerve	Common, but not as sole joint involved	Medications, rest
Knee	Effusion; ligament destruction, which may cause instability; valgus deformity; popliteal (Baker) cyst formation and rupture (crescent-shaped hemorrhage below malleolus with cyst rupture)	Most common single joint early in disease	Medications, bed rest, injection Be alert for ligamentous instability Ruptured cyst: rule out DVT, occasionally requires decompression
Hip	Synovitis, bursitis	Less common	Medications, bed rest, injection
Spine			
Cervical	C1-C2 subluxation: odontoid–C1 arch space over 3 mm (can cause cord compression and vertebrobasilar insufficiency); discitis; nerve root compression	Spine involvement common in patients with severe disease, although actual subluxation is approximately 5% overall, and cord or vessel compression is rare	Use caution during airway maneuvers Immobilization and spinal fusion, if needed
Thoracic	Synovitis, spinal stenosis, osteoporotic disease	Rare—consider other diagnoses	
TMJ	Pain with chewing, limited opening, posterior subluxation	Common	

ROM, range of motion; PIP, proximal interphalangeal; DIP, distal interphalangeal; MCP, metacarpophalangeal; CMC, carpometacarpal; IP, interphalangeal; CTS, carpal tunnel syndrome; AC, acromioclavicular; MTP, metatarsophalangeal; DVT, deep venous thrombosis; TMJ, temporomandibular joint.

subsequent compartment syndrome. Ultrasound is the least invasive test and is widely available. Note that often patients with ruptured cysts will have a crescent-shaped hemorrhage in the lower calf.

Rest, elevation, and analgesia are usually all that is required. Actual compartment syndrome is rare, and residual calf swelling usually lasts several weeks, but may persist as long as 3 years.

Atlanto-Axial Subluxation

Although spinal arthritis is common in RA, actual C1-C2 subluxation is uncommon. The incidence increases with increasing severity of the patient's overall disease. Actual cord or vascular compromise is rare, but it does occur and can be iatrogenic, resulting from manipulation, such as intubation.

Symptoms and signs of cord compression include severe neck pain, usually radiating to the occiput; extremity weakness, which may be upper or lower, or both (often difficult to assess because of the patient's severe and long-standing arthritis); numbness or tingling in the fingers or feet; loss of vibration sense, with preservation of proprioception; "jumping legs," caused by spinal reflex disinhibition; and bladder dysfunction. Patients may also have vertebral artery insufficiency, which can result in syncope or vertigo.

An atlanto-dens interval >2.5 mm in adults and >5 mm in children is diagnostic. Although an emergent computed tomography (CT) can help if cord compression is suspected, MRI will give much more information and is the test of choice.

Treatment is generally medical until there are signs of cord compression, at which point surgical options become the mainstay of therapy. For the emergency physician, emergent airway management is of particular importance. The clinician should avoid any aggressive airway maneuvers in patients with signs of RA, or a history of RA, if at all possible.

Systemic Disease

RA may affect nearly any organ. Systemic disease is common and may be life threatening. Systemic complications may be caused by the primary rheumatic disease process, a medication, or a combination of both. The organs that are most often affected include the lungs, heart, liver, and spleen. Blood vessel involvement is also common.

Pulmonary Disease. Mild and asymptomatic pulmonary disease is common in RA. Patients may have pulmonary nodules, pleural effusion, or fibrosis. They occasionally present with restrictive, chronic obstructive pulmonary disease-like symptoms. Acute obliterative bronchiolitis is uncommon, but may be fatal; it is unclear if it is caused by the RA itself or by the medications (DMARDs) used to treat RA.

Cardiac Disease. Pericarditis is the most common cardiac disorder. Usually, asymptomatic chronic inflammation is

detected only at autopsy, but inflammation may be acute and constrictive. Rheumatic myocarditis and endocarditis occasionally occur. With endocarditis, the physician must rule out bacterial endocarditis as these patients are predisposed to bacteremia due to open wounds and immunosuppression.

Hepatic Disease. Hepatitis is often subclinical but may be overt. Liver abnormalities typically occur as a result of drug side effects.

Spleen. Felty syndrome is RA that occurs in association with an enlarged spleen and leukopenia. Patients are subject to neutropenia and severe bacterial infections, as well as thrombocytopenia. Any patient suspected of having Felty syndrome requires emergent consultation, admission, and aggressive treatment of any suspected bacterial infections. Treatment of RA may improve the manifestations of Felty syndrome, but plasmapheresis or splenectomy may be required.

Blood Vessel Disease. Small vessel inflammation is integral to the pathophysiology of RA. Clinically diagnosable vasculitis may be chronic or acute. With chronic vasculitis, leg ulcers and nail fold infarcts are common. Distal sensory neuropathy may also be seen. Acute systemic vasculitis is rare and usually occurs in patients with long-standing disease.

JUVENILE IDIOPATHIC ARTHRITIS

Juvenile idiopathic arthritis (JIA) is the current terminology for JRA (or Still disease). It may develop at any age and is characterized as a chronic synovial inflammation without a known cause. No laboratory tests are diagnostic of this condition. The clinical manifestations include spiking fever for 3 days or greater, a salmon-pink rash, generalized lymphadenopathy, and hepatomegaly and/or splenomegaly. In 50% of patients, the temperature is higher than 40°C, and there is polyarticular involvement. The evanescent pink rash blanches and may be pruritic, and thus can be confused with a drug-sensitivity reaction. The polyarthritis is initially a migratory arthritis that eventually becomes a persistent arthritis (Fig. 3–13). This is a very difficult diagnosis to make, and the emergency clinician—rather than trying to make the diagnosis—should focus on excluding more emergent causes of arthritis (i.e., Lyme disease, infection, avascular necrosis, osteomyelitis, tumors, Kawasaki disease), and then refer the patient to a rheumatologist.

In a similar fashion to adult RA, the treatment of JIA has made many advances. Methotrexate, intra-articular corticosteroid injections, and the biologic modifier etanercept (Enbrel) are all being used to treat JIA. In the acute setting, NSAIDs may be used while awaiting rheumatology follow-up.

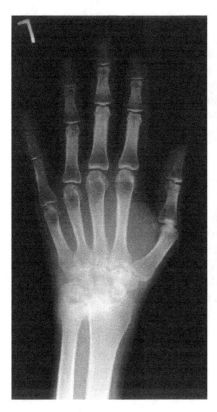
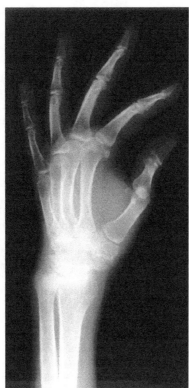

Figure 3–13. Juvenile rheumatoid arthritis of the wrist. *(Used with permission from J. Fitzpatrick, MD, Cook County Hospital.)*

SYSTEMIC LUPUS ERYTHEMATOSUS

Although SLE is not usually thought of as a joint disorder, inflammatory arthritis occurs in most patients. SLE is, similar to RA, an autoimmune disorder whereby there is a production of pathogenic autoantibodies with subsequent tissue destruction.[75] Lupus has a wide variety of presentations due to the fact that it can affect almost any organ system.

Clinical Presentation

SLE follows a relapsing and remitting course. It typically affects multiple organ systems, with different systems affected at different times over the course of the disease. Onset early in life is associated with more severe disease than is late onset.

Arthritis and arthralgias are commonly present at the onset of SLE in 50% and 75% of patients, respectively. Throughout the course of their disease, more than 90% of patients suffer musculoskeletal involvement. Symmetric synovitis affecting the hands, wrists, and knees is typical, and is clinically indistinguishable from RA. The arthritis can vary greatly in duration from days to months.[76] Bone destruction is not usually present in SLE, unlike RA. The combination of synovial inflammation and tendonitis along with chronic corticosteroid usage can result in tendon and ligament damage. Typical musculoskeletal deformities are summarized in Tables 3–9 and 3–10.

Although musculoskeletal involvement in SLE is generally symmetric, it is not always the case. However, if only a single joint is involved, or if one joint is much more acutely inflamed

▶ TABLE 3–9. **JOINT DEFORMITIES ASSOCIATED WITH SLE**

Joints Affected[a]	Deformities	Comments
Fingers	Subluxations, swan-neck deformity, contractures	Subluxation initially reducible, later fixed; usually ulnar deviation
Thumb	Hyperextension of interphalangeal joint (hitchhiker's thumb)	Seen in 30% of patients
Elbow	Flexion contractures	
Hips	Avascular necrosis (osteonecrosis)	May be due to long-term steroid usage; in approximately 10% of patients
Knees	Patellar tendon laxity	
Feet	Gangrene of toes (vasculitis), arthritic deformities	

SLC, systemic lupus erythematosus.
[a]Nonerosive arthritis and synovitis.

▶ TABLE 3–10. **OTHER MUSCULOSKELETAL FINDINGS ASSOCIATED WITH SLE**

Associated Tissues	Deformities	Comments
Muscles	Myositis, myalgias, atrophy (may include diaphragm)	Myositis occurs in approximately 5%–10% of patients with SLE
Tendons	Tenosynovitis, rupture	Often seen early in disease; rupture may be due to SLE or steroid use
Skin	Rheumatoid nodules, other manifestations (see text discussion)	Occurs in approximately 10% of patients with SLE

SLC, systemic lupus erythematosus.

than others, intra-articular infection should be ruled out. The clinician should also be on the lookout for avascular necrosis as it can occur in approximately 5% of patients with SLE.

SLE can affect any organ in the body. Although a complete discussion is beyond the scope of this chapter, the provider should be alert for signs of systemic illness in any patient presenting with inflammatory arthritis.

A number of laboratory abnormalities can occur in patients with SLE, including autoantibodies, but most tests are not available emergently, and no single antibody is completely sensitive or specific for SLE. If an arthrocentesis is performed, the fluid should be consistent with inflammatory results. The ESR is usually elevated, but does not correlate with clinical disease activity.

Treatment

Most patients will be on hydroxychloroquine as this is the drug of choice in the treatment of lupus. Patients maybe on low dose steroids (5–7.5 mg of prednisone daily), but recent recommendations are to use the lowest dose of steroids possible or to stop steroids completely if possible. Systemic corticosteroids are the mainstay of treatment for SLE flares. Both low-dose (<0.5 mg/kg/d) and high-dose (1.0 mg/kg/d) short-course regimens (3–4 days) of prednisone are used. In the acute care setting, NSAIDs are also appropriate for pain control. As with RA, antimalarials and immunosuppressive drugs are commonly prescribed, but this should be done by a specialist.

VIRAL ARTHRITIS

Arthritis is a sequela to several common viral infections. The following is a discussion of arthritis secondary to viral hepatitis, HIV, rubella, and parvovirus.

Hepatitis

In hepatitis B virus infection, during the 1- to 3-week prodromal phase, polyarthritis may be accompanied by moderate fever and, sometimes, by an urticarial or a maculopapular rash. Usually, the small joints are affected symmetrically with arthralgias or arthritis. Aminotransferase levels are usually elevated at this stage, and hepatitis B surface antigen is detectable.

Hepatitis C virus may also induce rheumatologic symptoms. In one study, arthralgias and arthritis were found in 4% to 9% of patients. The arthritis presents as either a symmetric polyarthritis (very similar to RA) or a mono-oligoarthritis. Corticosteroids and NSAIDs are usually avoided due to their potential to worsen the infection or cause hepatotoxicity.

Human Immunodeficiency Virus

Several patterns of arthropathy have been described in patients infected with HIV, including brief episodes of severe arthralgia, acute episodic oligoarthritis, and persistent symmetric polyarthritis. Arthritis may be an early feature of AIDS. Arthritis associated with AIDS infrequently presents with a fever, but the picture may be confounded by coincidental infection, and the clinician should have a low threshold for arthrocentesis. Both a Reiter-like syndrome and a Sjögren-like syndrome occur with increased frequency in this disease.

Most patients with HIV who exhibit rheumatic complaints are ill as a consequence of other clinical features of HIV. In general, most patients exhibit a mild-to-severe rheumatic disorder that is self-limiting and experience a good response to a combination of analgesics and NSAIDs.

Rubella

Arthralgias and arthritis are reported to occur in up to 70% of infected women. Joint symptoms usually start within 1 week of the skin rash in natural infection or within 10 to 28 days of immunization. Finger, wrist, elbow, hip, knee, and toe joints are most frequently affected, usually asymmetrically. Arthralgia and joint stiffness, as well as arthritis, may be accompanied by tenosynovitis and even carpal tunnel syndrome. Usually, both the natural and the vaccine-induced arthritis resolve within 30 days; however, some patients experience recurrent arthralgias and episodes of arthritis for up to 2 years or longer. There are no abnormal laboratory findings in analysis of synovial fluid.

Parvovirus

Parvovirus B19 is most commonly associated with erythema infectiosum (fifth disease) in children or aplastic anemia. Arthritis occurs in up to 8% of children and up to 50% of adults infected with parvovirus B19.

In adults, a rheumatoid-like polyarthritis may occur. It is characterized by a symmetric polyarthropathy with pain, swelling, and morning stiffness in the affected joints. The finger joints, wrists, and knees are most often affected. Although the median duration of joint symptoms is approximately 10 days and most resolve by this time; rarely, the pain and stiffness may persist longer.

Treatments with immunoglobulin preparations have been reported to be successful in patients with parvovirus B19-induced red cell aplasia. NSAIDs have been used to treat myalgias and arthralgias.

LYME DISEASE

Lyme disease is caused by the spirochete *Borrelia burgdorferi* (*B burgdorferi*) and is transmitted by the *Ixodes* tick. Lyme disease is endemic in the northern Atlantic states, upper Midwest, and Pacific Northwest. Lyme arthritis is differentiated from other forms of arthritis due to the characteristic joint involvement and nearly universal correlation with an immune response.[82]

Clinical Presentation
The clinical progression of Lyme disease is generally described in three stages. Dissemination of *B burgdorferi*, the causative agent, is accompanied by fever and migratory arthralgia, with little or no joint swelling, but frank arthritis appears weeks or months later. Arthritis is usually episodic, affecting primarily large, but also some small joints.

Stage 1 (Early Infection)
The first sign of infection occurs within 3 to 30 days of the tick bite. It is characterized by erythema chronicum migrans. This rash occurs in 60% to 80% of patients and usually fades within 3 to 4 weeks regardless of the treatment, although the lesions may recur.[83] Other signs and symptoms include fatigue, malaise, fever, arthralgia, headache, sore throat, and lymphadenopathy.

Stage 2 (Disseminated Infection)
This stage of infection begins weeks to months later and is associated with cardiac, neurologic, skin, and musculoskeletal abnormalities. Predominant symptoms in stage 2 are debilitating fatigue and malaise. Fluctuating symptoms of meningitis accompanied by facial palsy and peripheral radiculopathy are the usual pattern. At this stage, musculoskeletal pain is common and migratory. The pain can be located in joints, bursae, tendons, muscles, and bones. If the pain occurs in the joints, it is without swelling and lasts hours or days.

During stage 2, approximately 70% of patients develop brief attacks of asymmetric monoarticular or oligoarticular arthritis, primarily in large joints.[84] The knee joint is affected in approximately 80% of these patients. These attacks occur within 2 weeks to 2 years (average 6 months) after the onset of the disease and usually follow intermittent episodes of arthralgia or migratory musculoskeletal pain.

Stage 3 (Late Infection)
This stage occurs in approximately 60% of untreated patients. Of the patients that reach this stage, only 10% will suffer with arthritis.[84] In patients who do have arthritis, the duration of attacks increases to months, but individual attacks may be separated by remission of months or even years. Chronic arthritis leads to loss of cartilage, subchondral sclerosis, periarticular soft-tissue ossification, bony erosion, osteopenia, osteophyte formation, and even permanent joint disability. In this stage, spirochetes have been found in joint fluid, synovial tissue, and blood vessels.

Diagnosis
The diagnosis may be difficult in early or disseminated stages before seroconversion, unless one identifies the characteristic erythema migrans lesion. Patients with an erythema migrans lesion can be seronegative as the patient has not yet had time to mount an immune response. Therefore, a patient with a history of travel to a Lyme endemic area and an erythema migrans rash is sufficient to make the diagnosis of Lyme disease. For these patients, treatment is initiated with repeat serological testing in 2 to 4 weeks.[85] The initial test of choice is the enzyme-linked immunosorbent assay test, and if negative, then no further testing is needed. If positive, then a Western blot test is sent for confirmation. IgG antibodies often persist in cases of successfully treated inactive disease.

Treatment
Patients may present requesting Lyme prophylaxis. This is appropriate if they live in an endemic area, the tick was attached for ≥36 hours, and treatment is started within 72 hours of tick removal.[86] Prophylaxis for Lyme disease is a single dose of doxycycline 200 mg. In early Lyme disease, the treatment is docycline 100 mg BID × 14 days. Other than uncomplicated early Lyme disease, the antibiotic choice and duration of treatment varies widely. They depend on appropriate disease staging and organs affected; therefore, consultation with an infectious disease specialist is highly recommended to ensure appropriate workup and treatment.

SERONEGATIVE SPONDYLOARTHROPATHY

The seronegative spondyloarthropathies (SNS) are a group of related disorders that lead to inflammation and fusion of the SI joint and, in some cases, of peripheral joints.[44,87,88] The term "seronegative" refers to the lack of IgM-RF in the patient's serum. This group of disorders is, similar to RA, characterized by morning stiffness. Unlike RA, these disorders lack serum RF and rheumatoid nodules, and tend

▶ TABLE 3–11. **COMPARISON OF SERONEGATIVE SPONDYLOARTHROPATHIES**

	Ankylosing Spondylitis	Reactive Arthritis (Reiter Syndrome)	Enterohepatic Spondyloarthropathy (IBD)	Psoriatic Arthropathy
Age at onset (y)	20–40 (average: 25)	20s and older	Adult	Any age
Onset	Gradual	Acute	Usually gradual	Variable
Sacroiliitis/Spondylitis	Symmetric (nearly all)	Asymmetric (common)	Symmetric (<20%)	Asymmetric (20%)
Peripheral joints	Lower limb, hip (~25%)	Lower limb (90%)	Lower > upper extremity (<20%)	Upper > lower extremity (>90%)
Cardiac aortic insufficiency	<5%	5–10%	Rare	Rare
Eye (conjunctivitis uveitis)	Primary uveitis (25%)	Conjunctivitis > uveitis (50%)	Uveitis (<20%)	Conjunctivitis
Skin or nail involvement	None	Common (<40%)	Uncommon	Nearly all (~100%)
HLA-B27	90%	75–90%	50% with SI/spine (5% without)	50% with SI/spine (20% without)

IBD, irritable bowel syndrome; HLA, human leukocyte antigen; SI, sacroiliac.

to affect predominantly the axial skeleton rather than the small joints of the distal extremities. These diseases are compared in Table 3–11.

Although each disease has its own characteristics, there is significant overlap between them. With the exception of Reiter syndrome, patients with SNS usually have a subacute presentation. As long as the emergency physician refers the patient for timely follow-up, a definite diagnosis of a specific SNS need not be made in the ED.

Ankylosing Spondylitis

Ankylosing spondylitis is characterized by inflammation of the SI and intervertebral joints. Inflammation at the sites of ligamentous insertion (enthesopathy) leads to calcification and loss of motion of the joints. It is helpful to differentiate between an inflammatory back pain presentation and a mechanical back pain presentation. Inflammatory back pain has no improvement with rest and pain is better with exercise, whereas mechanical back pain is improved with rest and worse with exercise.

Clinical Presentation

The presence of ankylosing spondylitis is suggested by gradual onset of back discomfort (often dull and difficult to localize) onset before 40 years of age, persistence of discomfort for 3 months or longer, and morning stiffness that improves with exercise. If there is no evidence of Reiter syndrome, psoriasis, or inflammatory bowel disease (IBD, see later discussion), ankylosing spondylitis is the likely diagnosis. Radiographs of the SI joints should show at least some evidence of sacroiliitis. Spinal films show progressive syndesmophytes and kyphosis.

The symptoms of inflammatory back disease are particularly characteristic of ankylosing spondylitis. Some patients continue to have only low back pain related to sacroiliitis, whereas others show progressively more widespread back pain and limitation of motion as a result of involvement of the lumbar, dorsal, and cervical spine. Few patients progress to develop the classic rigid "bamboo" spine. Peripheral joint involvement frequently accompanies the back disease, with hips and shoulders being affected. Other joints affected are the wrist, MCP, and MTP joints. Most typically, involvement is in an asymmetric pattern, but in some patients, the polyarthritis is symmetric, making it clinically indistinguishable from RA.

Other manifestations of ankylosing spondylitis include fatigue, weight loss, and iritis in up to 25% of patients. Acute iritis requires ophthalmologic referral for possible corticosteroid treatment. Pulmonary fibrosis, particularly of the upper lobe, is associated with cough, dyspnea, and sputum production. Patients with severe disease may develop restrictive pulmonary disease because of their stooped posture. Aortic insufficiency caused by fibrosis involving the aortic ring and valve has been recognized for many years. HLA-B27–positive spondyloarthropathies are associated with severe bradyarrhythmias, and these patients may present with symptomatic complete heart block. Less than 10% of patients with severe ankylosing spondylitis will develop cardiac disease (i.e., aortic incompetence and conduction defects).

Physical examination may initially be unremarkable. With progressive disease, the normal lumbar lordosis is lost, and marked kyphosis of the spine may develop. In advanced disease, the patient develops severe flexion deformities of the lumbar spine, with compensatory (and occasionally primary) flexion of the hips and knees.

The diagnosis of ankylosing spondylitis is based primarily on the history, with typical features of inflammatory back disease and other manifestations, as previously described. Standard criteria for the diagnosis of ankylosing spondylitis include the presence of sacroiliitis. Laboratory studies are nonspecific in ankylosing spondylitis. The HLA-B27 marker is usually present, but it is not readily tested in acute care settings. Radiographic changes range from vague loss of definition of the edge of the SI joint with some sclerosis to more definite sclerosis, indistinct margins, erosions, and subsequent fusion. Additional techniques such as radionuclide bone scan, CT scan, and MRI are occasionally helpful in clarifying an uncertain picture. This is not a diagnosis that needs to be made in the ED.

Treatment

The most effective treatment for ankylosing spondylitis is physical therapy, which attempts to reduce pain, improve function, and prevent the progressive spinal kyphosis that characterizes the disease. Analgesic and anti-inflammatory medications are used to allow the patient to participate actively in physical therapy. NSAIDs, including indomethacin and naproxen, can be effective in decreasing morning stiffness and increasing physical activity. NSAIDs without physical therapy are of little benefit. Some of these patients will be placed on steroids, but these should not be started without guidance by a rheumatologist. Since the advent of antitumor necrosis factor therapy, the treatment has improved substantially in this condition.[89] Some patients may go on to require surgical options such as joint replacement or fusion.

Reactive Arthritis

Reactive arthritis is triggered by an infection at a distant site.[90,91] The arthritis occurs several weeks after the initial infection, and the infecting organism is not present in the joints at the time arthritis develops. Hence, the arthritis is reactive rather than infectious (e.g., disseminated gonorrhea). It may occur in a previously healthy patient following an episode of infectious enteritis, cervicitis, urethritis, or less commonly, pneumonia or bronchitis.

The original description of reactive arthritis linked this condition entirely to Reiter syndrome, with the presence of arthritis, urethritis, and conjunctivitis. We now realize that Reiter syndrome is only one example of reactive arthritis.[92]

The mechanism of reactive arthritis remains unclear. Organisms that may cause reactive arthritis include *Chlamydia trachomatis, Streptococcus pneumoniae, Salmonella, Shigella, Campylobacter,* and *Yersinia enterocolitica.* HIV has also been implicated. The incidence of reactive arthritis following infection with a responsible organism varies but is on the order of 1% to 2% or less.

Clinical Presentation

Reactive arthritis should be high on the list of differential diagnoses whenever a young adult presents with acute arthritis affecting the knees and ankles (it is unusual for the upper extremity to be involved). Reactive arthritis is typically accompanied by malaise, fever, and weight loss.

Acute onset of arthritis occurs 2 to 6 weeks after the inciting infection. Distribution of arthritis is asymmetric, primarily affecting the knees and ankles. Inflammation is centered about the sites of ligament and tendon insertion (enthesopathy), including the Achilles tendon and plantar fascia insertions.

Entire fingers or toes are often swollen, leading to dactylitis, or "sausage digits." As with the other SNS disorders, low back pain associated with sacroiliitis may occur.

Nonmusculoskeletal manifestations include sterile conjunctivitis, which occurs in approximately 40% of patients. Iritis occurs in up to 5% of patients and may lead to permanent visual impairment and mucous membrane involvement with oral and genital ulcers. These ulcers occur early in the course of the disease and are usually painless; painful ulcers are most often the result of other disorders or superinfection. Cardiac (conduction system and aortic valve) and neurologic (central or peripheral) involvement occurs, but is uncommon.

Diagnosis

The diagnosis of reactive arthritis is mostly clinical. Synovial fluid analysis shows inflammatory cell counts, with leukocyte counts of 500 to 75,000/mm^3, mostly neutrophils. Human leukocyte antigen testing is useful in making a definitive diagnosis, but is not available on an emergent basis. Radiographs show bony erosion at sites of tendon and fascia insertion. Radiologic sacroiliitis tends to be asymmetric, but may be indistinguishable from the lesions of ankylosing spondylitis.

Treatment

Antibiotics have little effect on established disease process, and this in itself is suggestive that it is triggered by a self-perpetuating inflammatory response.[79,90,91] The arthritis is treated with NSAIDs. Steroids are used in this condition when there is a poor response to NSAIDs. Disease-modifying antirheumatic drugs such as azathioprine and methotrexate have been used in some patients with good results.[92] Corticosteroid injection of a particularly symptomatic joint may also be performed by a specialist after infection is ruled out.

Enteropathic Spondyloarthropathy

Up to 20% of patients with IBD (which includes Crohn's disease and ulcerative colitis) will develop arthritis.[91] This arthritis may be peripheral, affecting primarily the ankles and knees, or central, affecting the SI joints.

IBD-associated spondylitis is unrelated to the stage or course of the patient's IBD and may occur before the onset of IBD symptoms. The joints involved are large and small joints, predominantly in the lower limbs. Frequently, there is a tendonitis with inflammation at the insertion of the tendon, which is the hallmark of this disorder. A peripheral arthritis, mainly asymmetric, appears in 17% to 20% of cases of IBD.[93]

The prevalence of Crohn's disease has increased during the past three decades to approximately 75 per 100,000 population. Peripheral arthritis, mainly articular and asymmetric, appears with an equal gender ratio, as previously indicated. Large and small joints are involved, predominantly those of the lower limb (most commonly, the knees and the ankles but also the MCP and MTP joints). The arthritis is mainly migratory and transient and usually subsides within 6 weeks, but it may become chronic and destructive.

In ulcerative colitis, the pattern of peripheral arthritis is identical to those seen in Crohn's disease, but its prevalence is lower (5%–10%). The disease onset usually precedes the joint symptoms, but a coincidental onset of joint and abdominal symptoms is not uncommon. In the course of the disease, the temporal relationship between attacks of arthritis and the flares of bowel disease is more marked than in Crohn's disease. Surgical removal of the inflamed colon has a therapeutic effect on joint symptoms.

Treatment of enteropathic spondyloarthropathy consists of systemic glucocorticoids and/or DMARDs. These drugs improve symptoms but do not halt joint damage. Patients do best under the care of both a rheumatologist and gastroenterologist, and therefore should be referred to both.

Psoriatic Arthropathy

Psoriasis occurs in approximately 3% of the US population. In patients with psoriasis, anywhere from 1% to 39% will have psoriatic arthritis (the wide variance is probably due to lack of clear diagnostic criteria). The clinical presentation is also difficult to quantify as these patients can have an oligoarticular or polyarticular presentation with peripheral or axial predominance.

Initial treatment of psoriatic arthritis uses NSAIDs. DMARDs and anti-tumor necrosis factor agents are also used but should be initiated by a rheumatologist.

SARCOID ARTHRITIS

Sarcoidosis is a chronic systemic inflammatory condition that is characterized by the presence of noncaseating granulomas. Although pulmonary manifestations are most common, acute arthritis may be the initial presentation and can mimic other forms of arthritis.

Arthritis secondary to sarcoidosis is usually an oligoarthritis, but may be polyarticular or, rarely, monoarticular. The ankle and knee joints are most frequently involved in acute sarcoidosis. Symmetric ankle arthritis at onset is very sensitive and specific for the diagnosis of acute sarcoid arthritis. Most commonly, sarcoid arthritis occurs in conjunction with bilateral hilar lymphadenopathy and erythema nodocusm (Fig. 3–14). This triad is called Löfgren syndrome. The patient generally has an atraumatic, tender, warm, erythematous swelling that is often clearly

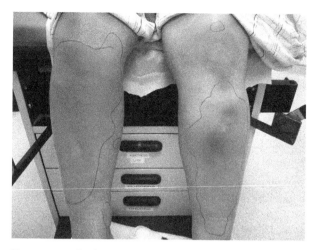
Figure 3–14. Erythema nodosum.

periarticular rather than synovial. Chronic arthritis is uncommon as this condition usually remits after a few weeks to months.

Diagnosis

Patients will have three of the four following clinical features: symmetric ankle arthritis, symptom duration of less than 2 months, erythema nodosum, and age younger than 40. Radiographs show only soft-tissue swelling. If an arthrocentesis is performed the leukocyte counts are <1000/mm^3. Cultures are negative, and crystals are not identified by microscopy.

Treatment

Acute sarcoid arthritis may respond to NSAIDs, and these are used as the initial treatment of choice. Refractory disease is treated with steroids. Other options include antimalarials, methotrexate, azathioprine, cyclosporine, cyclophosphamide, and a tumor necrosis factor inhibitor. This is typically a self-limited disease.

POLYMYALGIA RHEUMATICA

Polymyalgia rheumatica and temporal arteritis represent different manifestations of the same disease process. To this end, many of the symptoms of these conditions overlap. More than half of patients with temporal arteritis have signs of polymyalgia rheumatic, and, conversely, one-third of patients with polymyalgia rheumatica have evidence of temporal arteritis on biopsy. Both conditions occur in women twice as frequently as men. Age at onset is older than 50 years (for both conditions), and the conditions are more common in Caucasian people of northern European ancestry. The most common systemic symptom is fever. Other nonspecific complaints include fatigue, anorexia, and weight loss. ESRs are typically >50 mm/h with normal values being present in only 4% to 13% of patients.[98]

Diagnosis

Polymyalgia rheumatic presents in patients older than 50 years with pain and stiffness in the shoulder, neck, and pelvic girdle. Patients may report difficulty getting out of bed, getting dressed, or combing their hair. Affected muscles are tender to palpation. The diagnosis is largely clinical.

Treatment

Prednisone in an oral dose of 20 to 40 mg is given initially. Steroids are tapered gradually. Polymyalgia rheumatic tends to have a self-limited course, but relapse may occur in up to 25%.[99]

NEUROPATHIC ARTHROPATHY

Neuropathic (Charcot) arthropathy is a progressive deterioration of joints in patients with a neuropathy.[100–102] Charcot described the condition in 1868 in patients with tabes dorsalis. Other associated neurologic conditions include cerebral palsy, leprosy, syringomyelia, meningomyelocele, and alcoholic neuropathy. Today, diabetic neuropathy is by far the leading cause.[103] The reported prevalence of the condition in diabetic populations ranges from 0.1% to 0.4%.[100] The foot and ankle are the most common location for the development of neuropathic arthropathy, with the tarsometatarsal joint being the most common joint affected.

Controversy exists as to the true mechanism. The condition seems to be brought on by trauma, which triggers autonomic dysfunction with an increase in bone blood flow as well as inappropriate inflammation that leads to osteoclastic bone destruction. Injury to bone progresses due to abnormal weight bearing.[100]

Early in the course of this condition, the joint is usually warm and erythematous with hyperemia. With time, the foot becomes swollen, deformed, and unstable. Sensory loss and the absence of deep tendon reflexes are common in this condition.

Two types of neuropathic joints are noted on radiographs—atrophic and hypertrophic.[102] In the atrophic variety, there is rapid destruction and resorption of the joint. It is generally localized to the forefoot and causes osteolysis of the distal metatarsals. A hypertrophic joint develops over time and appears in the midfoot, hindfoot, or ankle. In the hypertrophic variety, there is massive juxta-articular joint inflammation with very large osseous debris accompanied by deformity and subluxation of the joint.

Treatment of this condition involves immobilization of the affected joint and restriction of weight bearing to avoid further injury. Mechanical devices fitted to prevent accelerated bone destruction have been used. When possible, surgical arthroplasty can be tried, but it often fails. In the ED, focus should be made to protect the joint from further injury and refer to a specialist.

REFERENCES

1. Coakley G, Mathews C, Field M, et al. BSR & BHPR, BOA, RCGP and BSAC guidelines for management of the hot swollen joint in adults. *Rheumatology (Oxford)*. 2006;45(8):1039–1041.
2. Towheed TE, Hochberg MC. Acute monoarthritis: a practical approach to assessment and treatment. *Am Fam Physician*. 1996;54(7):2239–2243.
3. Litman K. A rational approach to the diagnosis of arthritis. *Am Fam Physician*. 1996;53(4):1295–1300, 1305–1296, 1309–1210.
4. Baer PA, Tenenbaum J, Fam AG, Little H. Coexistent septic and crystal arthritis. Report of four cases and literature review. *J Rheumatol*. 1986;13(3):604–607.
5. Garcia-De La Torre I. Advances in the management of septic arthritis. *Rheum Dis Clin North Am*. 2003;29(1):61–75.
6. Goldenberg DL. Septic arthritis. *Lancet*. 1998;351(9097):197–202.
7. Pioro MH, Mandell BF. Septic arthritis. *Rheum Dis Clin North Am*. 1997;23(2):239–258.
8. Siva C, Velazquez C, Mody A, Brasington R. Diagnosing acute monoarthritis in adults: a practical approach for the family physician. *Am Fam Physician*. 2003;68(1):83–90.
9. Baker DG, Schumacher HR Jr. Acute monoarthritis. *N Engl J Med*. 1993;329(14):1013–1020.
10. Saraux A, Taelman H, Blanche P, et al. HIV infection as a risk factor for septic arthritis. *Br J Rheumatol*. 1997;36(3):333–337.
11. Kaandorp CJ, Van Schaardenburg D, Krijnen P, Habbema JD, van de Laar MA. Risk factors for septic arthritis in patients with joint disease. A prospective study. *Arthritis Rheum*. 1995;38(12):1819–1825.
12. Margaretten ME, Kohlwes J, Moore D, Bent S. Does this adult patient have septic arthritis? *JAMA*. 2007;297(13):1478–1488.
13. Pinals RS. Polyarthritis and fever. *N Engl J Med*. 1994;330(11):769–774.
14. Jeng GW, Wang CR, Liu ST, et al. Measurement of synovial tumor necrosis factor-alpha in diagnosing emergency patients with bacterial arthritis. *Am J Emerg Med*. 1997;15(7):626–629.
15. O'Brien JP, Goldenberg DL, Rice PA. Disseminated gonococcal infection: a prospective analysis of 49 patients and a review of pathophysiology and immune mechanisms. *Medicine (Baltimore)*. 1983;62(6):395–406.
16. Soderquist B, Jones I, Fredlund H, Vikerfors T. Bacterial or crystal-associated arthritis? Discriminating ability of serum inflammatory markers. *Scand J Infect Dis*. 1998;30(6):591–596.
17. Chong YY, Fong KY, Thumboo J. The value of joint aspirations in the diagnosis and management of arthritis in a hospital-based rheumatology service. *Ann Acad Med Singapore*. 2007;36(2):106–109.

18. Krishnamurthy R, Yoo JH, Thapa M, Callahan MJ. Water-bath method for sonographic evaluation of superficial structures of the extremities in children. *Pediatr Radiol.* 2013;43(1):41–47. doi:10.1007/s00247-012-2592-y.

19. Mantuani D, Nagdev A. Ultrasound-guided elbow arthrocentesis. ACEP Now. September 1, 2013. http://www.acepnow.com/article/ultrasound-guided-elbow-arthrocentesis/. Accessed December 5, 2017.

20. Boniface KS, Ajmera K, Cohen JS, Liu YT, Shokoohi H. Ultrasound-guided arthrocentesis of the elbow: a posterior approach. *J Emerg Med.* 2013;45(5):698–701. doi:10.1016/j.jemermed.2013.04.053.

21. Cunningham A, Eston V. Owning the Ankle Arthrocentesis (NUEM Blog). June 14, 2016. http://www.nuemblog.com/blog/ankle-arthrocentesis. Accessed December 5, 2017.

22. Jeong HY, Krishnamurthy R. 1012: Water-bath method for sonographic evaluation of superficial structures of the extremities. *Ultrasound Med Biol.* 2009;35(8 suppl):S101-S102. doi:10.1016/j.ultrasmedbio.2009.06.394.

23. Papanicolas LE, Hakendorf P, Gordon DL. Concomitant septic arthritis in crystal monoarthritis. *J Rheumatol.* 2012; 39(1):157–160.

24. Brower AC. Septic arthritis. *Radiol Clin North Am.* 1996; 34(2):293–309, x.

25. Ho G, Jr. Bacterial arthritis. *Curr Opin Rheumatol.* 1993;5(4): 449–453.

26. Kaandorp CJ, Dinant HJ, van de Laar MA, Moens HJ, Prins AP, Dijkmans BA. Incidence and sources of native and prosthetic joint infection: a community based prospective survey. *Ann Rheum Dis.* 1997;56(8):470–475.

27. Kaandorp CJ, Krijnen P, Moens HJ, Habbema JD, van Schaardenburg D. The outcome of bacterial arthritis: a prospective community-based study. *Arthritis Rheum.* 1997; 40(5):884–892.

28. Kumar A, Marwaha V, Grover R. Emergencies in rheumatology. *J Indian Med Assoc.* 2003;101(9):520, 522, 524 passim.

29. Hermet M, Minichiello E, Flipo RM, et al. Infectious sacroiliitis: a retrospective, multicentre study of 39 adults. *BMC Infect Dis.* 2012;12:305.

30. Howard A, Wilson M. Septic arthritis in children. *BMJ.* 2010;341:c4407.

31. Kocher MS, Zurakowski D, Kasser JR. Differentiating between septic arthritis and transient synovitis of the hip in children: an evidence-based clinical prediction algorithm. *J Bone Joint Surg Am.* 1999;81(12):1662–1670.

32. Caird MS, Flynn JM, Leung YL, Millman JE, D'Italia JG, Dormans JP. Factors distinguishing septic arthritis from transient synovitis of the hip in children. A prospective study. *J Bone Joint Surg Am.* 2006;88(6):1251–1257.

33. Cucurull E, Espinoza LR. Gonococcal arthritis. *Rheum Dis Clin North Am.* 1998;24(2):305–322.

34. Garcia-De La Torre I, Nava-Zavala A. Gonococcal and nongonococcal arthritis. *Rheum Dis Clin North Am.* 2009;35(1): 63–73.

35. Wise CM, Morris CR, Wasilauskas BL, Salzer WL. Gonococcal arthritis in an era of increasing penicillin resistance. Presentations and outcomes in 41 recent cases (1985–1991). *Arch Intern Med.* 1994;154(23):2690–2695.

36. Esterhai JL Jr, Gelb I. Adult septic arthritis. *Orthop Clin North Am.* 1991;22(3):503–514.

37. Li SF, Henderson J, Dickman E, Darzynkiewicz R. Laboratory tests in adults with monoarticular arthritis: can they rule out a septic joint? *Acad Emerg Med.* 2004;11(3): 276–280.

38. Carpenter CR, Schuur JD, Everett WW, Pines JM. Evidence-based diagnostics: adult septic arthritis. *Acad Emerg Med.* 2011;18(8):781–796.

39. Gratacos J, Vila J, Moya F, et al. D-lactic acid in synovial fluid. A rapid diagnostic test for bacterial synovitis. *J Rheumatol.* 1995;22(8):1504–1508.

40. Mossman SS, Coleman JM, Gow PJ. Synovial fluid lactic acid in septic arthritis. *N Z Med J.* 1981;93(678): 115–117.

41. Riordan T, Doyle D, Tabaqchali S. Synovial fluid lactic acid measurement in the diagnosis and management of septic arthritis. *J Clin Pathol.* 1982;35(4):390–394.

42. Ilahi OA, Swarna U, Hamill RJ, Young EJ, Tullos HS. Concomitant crystal and septic arthritis. *Orthopedics.* 1996;19(7): 613–617.

43. Swan A, Amer H, Dieppe P. The value of synovial fluid assays in the diagnosis of joint disease: a literature survey. *Ann Rheum Dis.* 2002;61(6):493–498.

44. Kortekangas P, Aro HT, Lehtonen OP. Synovial fluid culture and blood culture in acute arthritis. A multi-case report of 90 patients. *Scand J Rheumatol.* 1995;24(1): 44–47.

45. von Essen R. Culture of joint specimens in bacterial arthritis. Impact of blood culture bottle utilization. *Scand J Rheumatol.* 1997;26(4):293–300.

46. Goldenberg DL, Sexton DJ. Septic arthritis in adults. UpToDate. 2016. https://www.uptodate.com/contents/septic-arthritis-in-adults?source=search_result&search=Septic+arthritis+in+adults&selectedTitle=1-150. Accessed December 5, 2017.

47. Sharff KA, Richards EP, Townes JM. Clinical management of septic arthritis. *Curr Rheumatol Rep.* 2013;15(6):332.

48. Trampuz A, Zimmerli W. Diagnosis and treatment of implant-associated septic arthritis and osteomyelitis. *Curr Infect Dis Rep.* 2008;10(5):394–403.

49. Khanna D, Fitzgerald JD, Khanna PP, et al. 2012 American College of Rheumatology guidelines for management of gout. Part 1: systematic nonpharmacologic and pharmacologic therapeutic approaches to hyperuricemia. *Arthritis Care Res (Hoboken).* 2012;64(10):1431–1446.

50. Smith EU, Diaz-Torne C, Perez-Ruiz F, March LM. Epidemiology of gout: an update. *Best Pract Res Clin Rheumatol.* 2010;24(6):811–827.

51. Choi HK, Liu S, Curhan G. Intake of purine-rich foods, protein, and dairy products and relationship to serum levels of uric acid: the Third National Health and Nutrition Examination Survey. *Arthritis Rheum.* 2005;52(1): 283–289.

52. Emmerson BT. The management of gout. *N Engl J Med.* 1996;334(7):445–451.

53. Lawry GV II, Fan PT, Bluestone R. Polyarticular versus monoarticular gout: a prospective, comparative analysis of clinical features. *Medicine (Baltimore).* 1988;67(5): 335–343.

54. Malik A, Schumacher HR, Dinnella JE, Clayburne GM. Clinical diagnostic criteria for gout: comparison with the gold standard of synovial fluid crystal analysis. *J Clin Rheumatol.* 2009;15(1):22–24.

55. Schlesinger N. Response to application of ice may help differentiate between gouty arthritis and other inflammatory arthritides. *J Clin Rheumatol.* 2006;12(6):275–276.

56. Klippel JH DP, Arnett FC. Rheumatology. In: Klippel JH, Dieppe PA, eds. *Rheumatology.* Vol 1. London: Mosby; 1998.

57. Chui CH, Lee JY. Diagnostic dilemmas in unusual presentations of gout. *Aust Fam Physician.* 2007;36(11):931–934.

58. Doherty M, Chuck A, Hosking D, Hamilton E. Inorganic pyrophosphate in metabolic diseases predisposing to calcium pyrophosphate dihydrate crystal deposition. *Arthritis Rheum.* 1991;34(10):1297–1303.

59. Gibilisco PA, Schumacher HR, Jr., Hollander JL, Soper KA. Synovial fluid crystals in osteoarthritis. *Arthritis Rheum.* 1985;28(5):511–515.

60. Zhang W, Doherty M, Pascual E, et al. EULAR recommendations for calcium pyrophosphate deposition. Part II: management. *Ann Rheum Dis.* 2011;70(4):571–575.

61. Buskila D. Hepatitis C-associated arthritis. *Curr Opin Rheumatol.* 2000;12(4):295–299.

62. Hochberg MC, Altman RD, April KT, et al. American College of Rheumatology 2012 recommendations for the use of nonpharmacologic and pharmacologic therapies in osteoarthritis of the hand, hip, and knee. *Arthritis Care Res (Hoboken).* 2012;64(4):465–474.

63. Hunter DJ, Lo GH. The management of osteoarthritis: an overview and call to appropriate conservative treatment. *Rheum Dis Clin North Am.* 2008;34(3):689–712.

64. Carr AJ, Robertsson O, Graves S, et al. Knee replacement. *Lancet.* 2012;379(9823):1331–1340.

65. O'Dell JR. Therapeutic strategies for rheumatoid arthritis. *N Engl J Med.* 2004;350(25):2591–2602.

66. Olsen NJ, Stein CM. New drugs for rheumatoid arthritis. *N Engl J Med.* 2004;350(21):2167–2179.

67. Wollheim F, Firestein, GS, Panayi, GS. *Rheumatoid Arthritis.* Oxford University Press; 2006.

68. Singh JA, Saag KG, Bridges SL Jr, et al. 2015 American College of Rheumatology Guideline for the Treatment of Rheumatoid Arthritis. *Arthritis Rheumatol.* 2016;68(1):1–26.

69. Raza K, Falciani F, Curnow SJ, et al. Early rheumatoid arthritis is characterized by a distinct and transient synovial fluid cytokine profile of T cell and stromal cell origin. *Arthritis Res Ther.* 2005;7(4):R784–R795.

70. Prince FH, Otten MH, van Suijlekom-Smit LW. Diagnosis and management of juvenile idiopathic arthritis. *BMJ.* 2010;341:c6434. doi:10.1136/bmj.c6434.

71. Cleary AG, Murphy HD, Davidson JE. Intra-articular corticosteroid injections in juvenile idiopathic arthritis. *Arch Dis Child.* 2003;88(3):192–196.

72. Culy CR, Keating GM. Spotlight on etanercept in rheumatoid arthritis, psoriatic arthritis and juvenile rheumatoid arthritis. *BioDrugs.* 2003;17(2):139–145.

73. Ramanan AV, Whitworth P, Baildam EM. Use of methotrexate in juvenile idiopathic arthritis. *Arch Dis Child.* 2003;88(3):197–200.

74. Wilkinson N, Jackson G, Gardner-Medwin J. Biologic therapies for juvenile arthritis. *Arch Dis Child.* 2003;88(3):186–191.

75. Choi J, Kim ST, Craft J. The pathogenesis of systemic lupus erythematosus—an update. *Curr Opin Immunol.* 2012;24(6):651–657.

76. Ruiz-Irastorza G, Khamashta MA, Castellino G, Hughes GR. Systemic lupus erythematosus. *Lancet.* 2001;357(9261):1027–1032.

77. Asherson RA, Liote F, Page B, et al. Avascular necrosis of bone and antiphospholipid antibodies in systemic lupus erythematosus. *J Rheumatol.* 1993;20(2):284–288.

78. van Vollenhoven RF, Mosca M, Bertsias G, et al. Treat-to-target in systemic lupus erythematosus: recommendations from an international task force. *Ann Rheum Dis.* 2014;73(6):958–967.

79. Palazzi C, D'Angelo S, Olivieri I. Hepatitis C virus-related arthritis. *Autoimmun Rev.* 2008;8(1):48–51.

80. White SJ, Boldt KL, Holditch SJ, Poland GA, Jacobson RM. Measles, mumps, and rubella. *Clin Obstet Gynecol.* 2012;55(2):550–559.

81. Moore TL. Parvovirus-associated arthritis. *Curr Opin Rheumatol.* 2000;12(4):289–294.

82. Puius YA, Kalish RA. Lyme arthritis: pathogenesis, clinical presentation, and management. *Infect Dis Clin North Am.* 2008;22(2):289–300, vi–vii.

83. Jouben LM, Steele RJ, Bono JV. Orthopaedic manifestations of Lyme disease. *Orthop Rev.* 1994;23(5):395–400.

84. Stanek G, Strle F. Lyme borreliosis. *Lancet.* 2003;362(9396):1639–1647.

85. Hu L. Diagnosis of Lyme disease. UpToDate. http://www.uptodate.com/contents/diagnosis-of-lyme-disease. Accessed May 21, 2017.

86. Wormser GP, Dattwyler RJ, Shapiro ED, et al. The clinical assessment, treatment, and prevention of Lyme disease, human granulocytic anaplasmosis, and babesiosis: clinical practice guidelines by the Infectious Diseases Society of America. *Clin Infect Dis.* 2006;43(9):1089–1134.

87. Khan MA. Spondyloarthropathies. *Curr Opin Rheumatol.* 1994;6(4):351–353.

88. Romano TJ. The fibromyalgia syndrome. It's the real thing. *Postgrad Med.* 1988;83(5):231–232, 237–243.

89. Nghiem FT, Donohue JP. Rehabilitation in ankylosing spondylitis. *Curr Opin Rheumatol.* 2008;20(2):203–207.

90. Carter JD. Reactive arthritis: defined etiologies, emerging pathophysiology, and unresolved treatment. *Infect Dis Clin North Am.* 2006;20(4):827–847.

91. Hamdulay SS, Glynne SJ, Keat A. When is arthritis reactive? *Postgrad Med J.* 2006;82(969):446–453.

92. Palazzi C, Olivieri I, D'Amico E, Pennese E, Petricca A. Management of reactive arthritis. *Expert Opin Pharmacother.* 2004;5(1):61–70.

93. Rodriguez-Reyna TS, Martinez-Reyes C, Yamamoto-Furusho JK. Rheumatic manifestations of inflammatory bowel disease. *World J Gastroenterol.* 2009;15(44):5517–5524.

94. Peluso R, Di Minno MN, Iervolino S, et al. Enteropathic spondyloarthritis: from diagnosis to treatment. *Clin Dev Immunol.* 2013, Article ID 631408. doi:10.1155/2013/631408.

95. Chandran V, Raychaudhuri SP. Geoepidemiology and environmental factors of psoriasis and psoriatic arthritis. *J Autoimmun.* 2010;34(3):J314–J321.

96. Cantini F, Niccoli L, Nannini C, Kaloudi O, Bertoni M, Cassara E. Psoriatic arthritis: a systematic review. *Int J Rheum Dis.* 2010;13(4):300–317.

97. Visser H, Vos K, Zanelli E, et al. Sarcoid arthritis: clinical characteristics, diagnostic aspects, and risk factors. *Ann Rheum Dis.* 2002;61(6):499–504.

98. Brooks RC, McGee SR. Diagnostic dilemmas in polymyalgia rheumatica. *Arch Intern Med.* 1997;157(2):162–168.

99. Epperly TD, Moore KE, Harrover JD. Polymyalgia rheumatica and temporal arthritis. *Am Fam Physician.* 2000;62(4):789–796, 801.

100. Rajbhandari SM, Jenkins RC, Davies C, Tesfaye S. Charcot neuroarthropathy in diabetes mellitus. *Diabetologia.* 2002;45(8):1085–1096.

101. Sinacore DR, Withrington NC. Recognition and management of acute neuropathic (Charcot) arthropathies of the foot and ankle. *J Orthop Sports Phys Ther.* 1999;29(12):736–746.

102. Sommer TC, Lee TH. Charcot foot: the diagnostic dilemma. *Am Fam Physician.* 2001;64(9):1591–1598.

103. Klenerman L. The Charcot joint in diabetes. *Diabet Med.* 1996;13(suppl 1):S52–S54.

CHAPTER 4

Complications

Erik K. Nordquist, MD

COMPARTMENT SYNDROME

Nearly 200,000 people are affected with compartment syndrome each year in the United States.¹ Although there are many causes, the clinical pathway in the development of this syndrome is the same.

Muscle groups in the body are surrounded by fascial sheaths that enclose the muscles within a defined space or compartment. When an injury occurs to the muscles within a compartment, swelling ensues. Because the tight fascial sheaths allow little room for expansion, the pressure within the compartment begins to increase. Eventually, blood flow is compromised, and irreversible muscle injury follows. One must suspect a compartment syndrome early to prevent contracture deformities (e.g., Volkmann ischemic contractures) that result from ensuing muscle and nerve necrosis.

The most common locations for compartment syndrome are the forearm and leg.¹ Other sites that have been implicated include the hand, shoulder, back, buttocks, thigh, abdomen, and foot. A discussion specific to these muscle compartments is included elsewhere in the text.

In approximately 70% of cases, compartment syndrome develops after a fracture and half of those are caused by tibia fractures.² Other commonly associated fractures include the humeral shaft, the bones of the forearm, and supracondylar fractures in children.³⁴ Other causes of acute compartment syndrome include crush injury, constrictive dressings/casts, seizures, intravenous infiltration, snakebites, infection, prolonged immobilization, burns, acute arterial occlusion or injury, and exertion.²⁵ A venous tourniquet can produce compartment syndrome in as little as 90 minutes if it is accidentally left in place.⁶ Patients with a coagulopathy (e.g., oral anticoagulant use, hemophilia) are at increased risk and may develop compartment syndrome after minimal trauma.

Clinical Features

The diagnosis of compartment syndrome is primarily a clinical one. Patients will exhibit pain out of proportion to the underlying injury, sensory symptoms, and muscle weakness. Pain is the earliest and most consistent sign. It is usually persistent and not relieved by immobilization. It is critical that the emergency physician recognizes this condition by its early features, before other signs and symptoms develop, to prevent permanent injury.

Pain that is aggravated by passive stretching is the most reliable sign of compartment syndrome.⁷ Diminished sensation is the second most sensitive examination finding for compartment syndrome. Sensory examination of the nerves coursing through the affected compartments will reveal diminished two-point discrimination or light touch. Both of these tests are more sensitive than pinprick. Palpation of the compartment will disclose tenderness and "tenseness" over the ischemic segments. The distal pulses and capillary filling may be entirely normal in a patient with significant muscle ischemia; therefore, these findings should not be used to rule out the existence of compartment syndrome.

To summarize, disproportionate pain is the earliest symptom, whereas pain with passive stretching of the involved muscles is the most sensitive sign of compartment syndrome. Paresthesias or hypesthesias in nerves traversing the compartment are also important signs of a developing compartment syndrome. A complete neurologic examination of any injured extremity should be performed. Orthopedic consultation should be obtained as soon as compartment syndrome is a consideration.

Compartment Pressure Measurement

The decision to perform a fasciotomy is often based on a combination of concerning clinical findings and possibly the measurement of compartment pressures. If one suspects a compartment syndrome, surgical consultation must be carried out and measurement of compartment pressures can be considered. Compartment pressures are most commonly performed using the commercially developed Stryker STIC device (Fig. 4–1 and Videos 4–1 and 4–2).²⁷⁻⁹

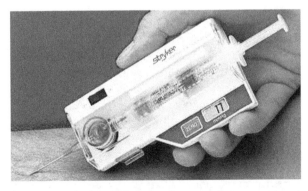

Figure 4–1. Stryker STIC device for measuring compartment pressure. (Reproduced with permission from Reichman EF, Simon RR: *Emergency Medicine Procedures.* New York: McGraw-Hill; 2004.)

Normal compartment pressures are below 10 mm Hg. At pressures >20 mm Hg, capillary blood flow within the compartment may be compromised. Traditional teaching had been to perform fasciotomy at pressures >30 mm Hg. However, in experimental studies, patients with higher diastolic blood pressures have shown a reduced likelihood of ischemic necrosis because of higher perfusion pressures. For this reason, many experts recommended fasciotomy when the compartment pressure reaches a point that is 20 to 30 mm Hg below the diastolic pressure (i.e., perfusion pressure = diastolic pressure − compartment pressure). More recently, a perfusion pressure <30 mm Hg has also been challenged for a lack of specificity with false positive rates ranging from 18% to 84%.

If the decision to perform compartment pressures is made with the input of the consulting orthopedic surgeon, measurements are made in all compartments of the extremity in question. Multiple measurements within a single compartment may be necessary as evidence suggests that pressures at different locations within the same compartment are not uniform. Distances as short as 5 cm result in significantly different pressure readings that will alter clinical decision making. The highest pressure recorded should be used. Also given that the highest compartment pressures are often found after 12 to 36 hours, multiple measurements over time may be necessary.

Several noninvasive methods of measuring compartment pressures are under investigation. Promising technology includes ultrasound with a pulsed phase-locked loop, laser Doppler flowmetry, and near-infrared spectroscopy.

To summarize, diagnosing compartment syndrome is challenging. Compartment pressure measurement may be used as an adjunct to clinical examination, but generally in consultation with an orthopedic surgeon. Controversy exists over cutoffs of compartment pressure that require immediate fasciotomy, and there is concern that traditional cutoff pressures are increasing the fasciotomy rate unnecessarily. For this reason, the patient with a concerning presentation requires at a minimum prompt orthopedic consultation and possibly clinical observation with serial examinations.

Treatment

The treatment of compartment syndrome requires immediate fasciotomy. Delays may result in irreversible damage to muscles and nerves. In general, nerves and muscles can tolerate up to 4 hours of total ischemia. After 8 hours, damage is irreversible. However, there is evidence that pediatric patients may still have reasonably good outcomes despite delayed presentations.

In addition to arranging for fasciotomy, the emergency physician must remove all circular constrictive dressings and splints and relieve flexion if the elbow and forearm are involved. The affected limb should be placed at the level of the heart to avoid reduction in arterial flow and increase in compartment pressure due to dependent edema. Hypotension must be avoided and treated aggressively. In partially reduced supracondylar fractures, skeletal traction is recommended. If relief is not obtained within 30 minutes, then surgery is indicated. One must not "watch and wait" as the goal is to restore circulation before irreparable damage ensues. Rhabdomyolysis may complicate compartment syndrome, thus adequate hydration to maintain urinary output is essential.

OSTEOMYELITIS

Osteomyelitis is a suppurative process in bone caused by pyogenic organisms. It is most common in patients younger than 20 years or older than 50 years. Bone infection occurs secondary to bacteria that are spread (1) hematogenously, (2) from a contiguous focus, or (3) secondary to vascular insufficiency. Osteomyelitis is accompanied by bone destruction that may be limited to a single portion of bone or may involve several regions, including the marrow, cortex, periosteum, and surrounding soft tissues.

Hematogenous osteomyelitis occurs most commonly in children. The infection is acute in nature and is localized to the bony metaphysis, and then spreads into the subperiosteal space. The most frequently affected bones are the proximal tibia and distal femur. In adult patients, the vertebrae are the most common sites infected due to hematogenous spread of bacteria.

Osteomyelitis that develops from a contiguous source of infection most commonly follows trauma (e.g., open fracture or puncture wound) or surgery (e.g., joint replacement or fracture fixation). The hand and the foot are the most common sites for this type of osteomyelitis. Vascular insufficiency, as a cause of osteomyelitis, is most often due to diabetes. In this scenario, a soft-tissue infection of the foot is the nidus for the spread of infection to the bone. In adults with contiguous osteomyelitis or osteomyelitis in the presence of vascular insufficiency, the process is usually subacute or chronic in nature.

Bacteriology

The bacterium most often isolated in cases of osteomyelitis is *Staphylococcus aureus* (*S aureus*). Infecting organisms differ according to the age of the patient. *S aureus* and streptococci are common causes in neonates. *Haemophilus influenzae* and *Escherichia coli* also occur in neonatal osteomyelitis. Gram-negative rods are seen in elderly patients, whereas fungal osteomyelitis is a complication of immunocompromised patients. Patients with sickle cell disease frequently have infection due to *S aureus* or *Salmonella* species. A mixed flora (*S aureus*, streptococci, and anaerobic bacteria) may be noted when osteomyelitis is secondary to spread directly from an adjacent wound, as in the diabetic patient with a foot ulcer.

Clinical Presentation

The typical clinical features in all forms of osteomyelitis are chills, fever, malaise, local pain, and swelling. Constitutional symptoms are more common in children than in adults and generally absent in patients with chronic osteomyelitis. In the contiguous form, pain and edema as well as erythema are noted around the wound and drainage occurs in most cases. As the process progresses, the involved extremity is held in slight flexion and passive movement is resisted secondary to pain. Initially, there is no swelling; however, the soft tissues later become edematous as a subperiosteal abscess develops. Eventually, as chronic osteomyelitis develops, a sinus tract breaks through the skin and drains infectious material.

In diabetic patients with an infected foot ulcer, osteomyelitis can be assumed to be present whenever bone is exposed in the ulcer bed or gentle advancement of a sterile probe contacts bone.[20,21] Probe-to-bone has a sensitivity of 87% and a specificity of 83% in diabetic patients with foot ulcers.[22]

Diagnosis

Isolating causative organisms is the most important step in diagnosis and treatment; however, this information is rarely available to the emergency physician. Blood cultures should be obtained and are positive in 50% of cases of hematogenous osteomyelitis.[18] Cultures of material from the wound or sinus tract can be performed, but may be misleading as many of the cultured microorganisms will represent colonizing bacteria.[20] Surface swab cultures of infected diabetic feet have no diagnostic utility.[21]

Laboratory tests are usually not helpful. The leukocyte count is not a sensitive marker for osteomyelitis. The erythrocyte sedimentation rate (ESR) is elevated in 90% of patients with osteomyelitis, but this test lacks specificity.[18] A normal ESR in a patient with a low clinical suspicion may help the clinician rule out the diagnosis. The C-reactive protein (CRP) is another nonspecific inflammatory marker that has the advantage of increasing within the first 24 hours of the disease course and returning to normal levels within 1 week of effective treatment. Ultimately, a needle aspiration of the bone is required to reveal the infecting organism in almost 90% of cases.[21] An open biopsy may be required to obtain sufficient material.

Plain radiographs are the initial study of choice in patients with osteomyelitis, although they are of little value early in the disease process. A negative radiograph, therefore, does not rule out osteomyelitis. Less than one-third of patients with symptomatic osteomyelitis for 7 to 10 days will have radiographic findings. Rarefaction, indicating diffuse demineralization, requires 30% to 50% of the bone mineral to be lost before it is seen on a radiograph. Demineralization and periosteal elevation followed by sclerosis is rare until after 10 to 21 days of infection, but by 28 days, 90% of patients will demonstrate plain-film abnormalities (Fig. 4–2). The most common finding in early infection is

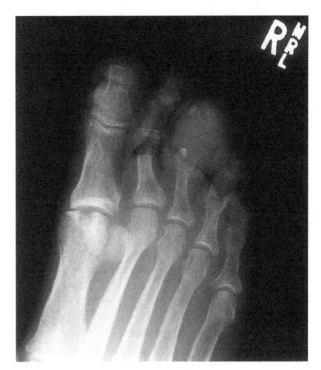

Figure 4–2. Osteomyelitis in the foot.

soft-tissue swelling, followed by periosteal elevation. Periosteal elevation is less commonly seen in adults due to a more fibrous and adherent periosteum. Late findings of osteomyelitis on plain films are lytic areas surrounded by sclerotic bone.[19,21]

Alternate methods for diagnosing osteomyelitis include radionuclide bone scanning, computed tomography (CT), and magnetic resonance imaging (MRI). A bone scan typically turns positive within 24 to 48 hours after onset of symptoms.[19,20] A normal bone scan makes the diagnosis very unlikely. CT is more sensitive than plain radiography. It is helpful in detecting necrotic bone (i.e., sequestra) in patients with chronic osteomyelitis and this may help the orthopedic surgeon plan treatment. Of all imaging studies, MRI has the highest sensitivity for diagnosing osteomyelitis.[23] MRI is also favored for any patient suspected of having vertebral involvement.[19-25]

Treatment

Antibiotics, used alone, have the potential to be curative only in patients with hematogenous osteomyelitis. Empiric intravenous antibiotics should be administered by the emergency physician in patients with (1) hematogenous osteomyelitis, (2) a toxic appearance, (3) suspicion of vertebral osteomyelitis, or (4) partially treated or recurrent disease at the request of a consulting orthopedist. Antibiotic regimens should be tailored to culture sensitivities. Methicillin-susceptible *S aureus* may be treated with penicillinase-resistant penicillin, such as nafcillin. Methicillin-resistant *S aureus* and coagulase-negative staphylococcus are treated with vancomycin. Gram-negative organisms, including *Pseudomonas*, may be treated with a fluoroquinolone or a third-generation cephalosporin. Patients with sickle cell disease and osteomyelitis should receive a fluoroquinolone or a third-generation cephalosporin to cover *Salmonella*. Typical empiric coverage includes vancomycin plus coverage for gram-negative organisms.

In adults with contiguous spread or vascular insufficiency (e.g., diabetic foot), cure cannot be achieved without debridement of infected bone. In the case of a patient with prosthesis or other foreign material, removal is generally required. Patients are treated with antibiotic therapy for a total of 4 to 6 weeks following the final debridement surgery.

Prevention

The prevention of possible future complications, such as osteomyelitis, in patients presenting with trauma is a vital task of the emergency physician. Open fractures require thorough irrigation and debridement, commonly in the operating room. Prophylactic antibiotics and tetanus immunization should be administered promptly. Antibiotic therapy directed against gram-positive and gram-negative organisms should be administered within 6 hours after open trauma to reduce the risk of osteomyelitis.

SOFT-TISSUE INFECTIONS

Cellulitis

This infection affects the skin and subcutaneous tissues and is most often caused by *S aureus* and beta-hemolytic streptococci. Other organisms may be present and polymicrobial infection is especially common in diabetic patients. *Pseudomonas* should be suspected after puncture wounds to the foot.

Clinical features are consistent and include pain, tenderness, warmth, induration, and erythema (Fig. 4–3). Lymphangitis and lymphadenopathy are often associated with

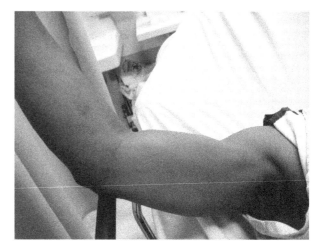

Figure 4–4. Lymphangitis.

infection (Fig. 4–4). The clinician should consider the possibility of an abscess cavity and palpate for the presence of a fluctuant area. Ultrasound or needle aspiration may be necessary if an abscess is suspected (Fig. 4–5).

Treatment with an oral antibiotic to cover methicillin-resistant *S aureus* and beta-hemolytic streptococci for 7 to 10 days is appropriate in nonimmunocompromised, nontoxic patients with mild infection. For animal or human bites, amoxicillin clavulanate (Augmentin) is the agent of choice for outpatient treatment. Cellulitis originating from a puncture wound to the foot is treated with ciprofloxacin or ceftazidime to cover *Pseudomonas*.

Necrotizing Infections

Patients with necrotizing soft-tissue infections typically present with a short clinical course that rapidly deteriorates to septic shock and death if not treated promptly. The initial management of all necrotizing soft-tissue infections is the same. Important treatment principles include high clinical

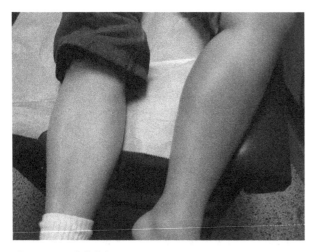

Figure 4–3. Cellulitis.

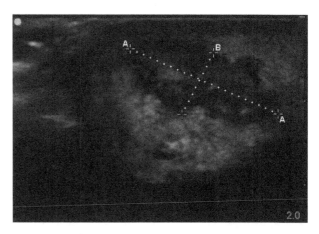

Figure 4–5. Ultrasound demonstrating an abscess cavity.

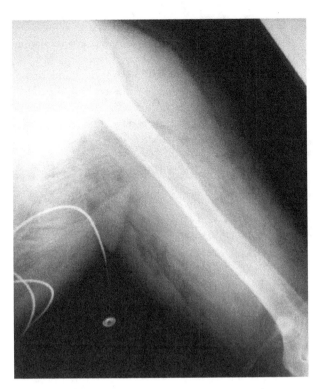

Figure 4–6. Plain film of left shoulder in a patient with a necrotizing soft-tissue infection.

suspicion, early surgical debridement, and broad-spectrum antibiotics.[30] Plain radiography may reveal the presence of gas (Fig. 4–6). CT will better delineate the extent of the infection, but should not delay treatment (Fig. 4–7).

Two examples of necrotizing soft-tissue infections—necrotizing fasciitis and clostridial myonecrosis—are considered subsequently. These entities differ in the depth of the infectious process and the pathogens that cause disease.

Necrotizing Fasciitis

This condition is a rare, but often fatal, soft-tissue infection that involves the superficial fascial layers of the extremities, abdomen, or perineum.[31,32] Risk factors include the immunocompromised host (e.g., diabetes), peripheral vascular disease, intravenous drug use, older age, and recent trauma or surgery. Two types are considered, depending on the infectious agents involved.

Type I necrotizing fasciitis accounts for the majority of cases of necrotizing fasciitis. The causative agents are polymicrobial. Gram-positive, gram-negative, and anaerobic bacteria act synergistically to produce extensive tissue destruction. In the early stages, it may be mistaken for a simple cellulitis or abscess. The appearance of the skin may range from mild erythema early on to red-purple blebs with foul-smelling, watery drainage. Pain is almost universally present and is often out of proportion and beyond the visible signs of skin infection.[31,32] Gas may or may not be present in the subcutaneous tissues. One commonly recognized form of this entity occurs in the perineum and is termed "Fournier gangrene" (Fig. 4–8).

Type II necrotizing fasciitis is mono-microbial, most often caused by group A *Streptococcus*. This infection represents 25% to 45% of cases of necrotizing fasciitis. Particularly virulent subtypes have given this pathogen the distinction of the title "flesh-eating bacteria" by the lay press. Type II necrotizing fasciitis is more likely to occur in younger, healthier patients without predisposing illnesses. In more than a third of patients, no portal of entry is identified.[31,32] Characteristic findings of this infection include a rapidly progressive necrosis, the rare presence of gas, and a high incidence of streptococcal toxic shock syndrome.

Necrotizing fasciitis is a clinical diagnosis. A high index of suspicion must be maintained to avoid a delay due to nonspecific findings. Adjunctive tests are available to support clinical suspicion; however, currently, the only way to completely confirm or rule out the diagnosis is surgical

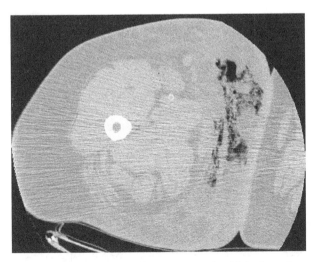

Figure 4–7. CT scan with soft-tissue gas in the thigh of a patient with a necrotizing soft-tissue infection.

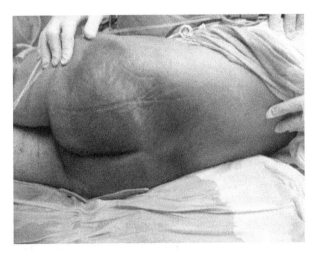

Figure 4–8. Fournier gangrene.

exploration. CT may identify signs of necrotizing fasciitis, such as deep fascial thickening, enhancement, and fluid and gas in the soft-tissue planes in and around the superficial fascia. Although much better than plain radiography, the sensitivity may be as low at 80%, whereas more recent data suggests the sensitivity of the newer generation CT scanners is much better. MRI sensitivity is believed to be quite high, but its usefulness is limited due to test availability, time required to obtain the study, and controversy regarding its low specificity. Ultrasound has not been well studied in necrotizing fasciitis. A scoring system (laboratory risk indicator for necrotizing fasciitis [LRINEC]) was developed to place patients in low-, intermediate-, and high-risk categories for necrotizing fasciitis. The calculation is based on CRP, white blood cell count, hemoglobin, Na$^+$, serum creatinine, and serum glucose levels. Initial findings appeared promising. However, subsequent data demonstrated inadequate sensitivity, thereby limiting the clinical utility of the LRINEC score.

Treatment of necrotizing fasciitis consists of early debridement of necrotic tissue and antibiotic therapy. Antibiotic agents of choice include carbapenem or beta-lactam/beta-lactamase inhibitor and clindamycin in combination with coverage against methicillin-resistant *S aureus* until culture results are available.

Clostridial Myonecrosis (Gas Gangrene)

This is a distinct necrotizing infection of muscle caused by *Clostridium perfringens* or *septicum*. The most common predisposing factors include trauma and surgery. As the name implies, gas formation and crepitus are prominent features. This condition can present in a similar manner to other forms of necrotizing soft-tissue infections, but distinctive features include a bronze-brown skin discoloration, bullae formation, and copious foul-smelling drainage. The course of clostridial myonecrosis is rapid, with an incubation period of less than 24 hours.

Initial treatment is prompt surgical decompression and debridement and broad-spectrum antibiotics. After definitive bacterial diagnosis, antibiotic agents of choice are penicillin and clindamycin. Hyperbaric oxygen is believed to be of greater benefit in clostridial infections than other forms of necrotizing soft-tissue infections, although randomized controlled trials are lacking.

COMPLEX REGIONAL PAIN SYNDROME

Complex regional pain syndrome (CRPS), formerly known as reflex sympathetic dystrophy, is a painful condition of an extremity that follows trauma, infection, or surgery. The peak incidence is in people 55 to 75 years of age and occurs in women more frequently than in men by a ratio of 3.5:1. The syndrome is more common in the upper extremity, but the lower extremity also may be affected. In some cases, the traumatic event is minimal in severity, such as following venipuncture or an intramuscular injection. A precipitating event is not identified in 10% of cases.

The pathophysiology of CRPS is not fully understood. Three major pathophysiological pathways have been identified: aberrant inflammatory mechanisms, neurogenic inflammation, and maladaptive changes in pain perception in the central nervous system. A detailed description of these pathways is outside the scope of this text.

The diagnosis of CRPS is based primarily on history and physical examination. A history of recent or remote trauma followed by the characteristic triad of symptoms is suggestive of CRPS. The triad includes autonomic, sensory, and motor disturbances. In the acute phase, the injured limb is usually painful, commonly described as "burning" or "tearing." The limb is also red, warm (although occasionally it may be cool), and swollen. Allodynia and hyperalgesia; changes in sweating; changes in skin, hair, and nail growth; and muscle weakness may also be present. Over time, if the disorder persists, symptoms change. Pain continues and may spread. However, patients may also experience numbness. Voluntary motor control may be reduced. The warm limb often becomes cold. Dystonia, tremor, and myoclonus may develop. The Budapest criteria are used to score the signs and symptoms to determine a diagnosis of CRPS. Radiographs commonly show demineralization of the bone.

Approximately 80% of those with CRPS who begin treatment within 1 year of injury have considerable improvement in their symptoms, but only approximately 50% of those treated after 1 year improve substantially. Early treatment is paramount to allow for improved prognosis.

Multiple modalities are used in the treatment of CRPS. Physical therapy is considered a first-line treatment and may be more important than drug therapy. Medications that are commonly used to treat CRPS include nonsteroidal anti-inflammatory drugs, anticonvulsants (gabapentin, pregabalin), bisphosphonates/calcitonin, oral glucocorticoids, tricyclic antidepressants (amitriptyline, nortriptyline), alpha-adrenergic blocking agents, and calcium channel blockers. Of note, opioids have minimal effect on pain. Patients who do not respond to initial therapy may require more invasive treatment, such as intrathecal injections, sympathectomy, and spinal cord stimulation. Cognitive behavior techniques are also employed. No emergency treatment is required. However, it is incumbent on the emergency physician to recognize this condition and refer the patient appropriately so the patient receives early treatment.

Emergency physicians are in a unique position to aid in the prevention of CRPS. Studies suggest that, when appropriate, early immobilization reduces the risk of CRPS. Also, vitamin C in higher doses (500 mg/day for 50 days) has been shown to decrease the risk of CRPS in patients after a distal radius fracture.

FAT EMBOLISM SYNDROME

Fat embolism occurs in almost all patients who sustain a pelvic or long bone fracture. However, clinical signs and symptoms of fat embolism syndrome (FES) occur in only 0.5% to 10% of patients.[45] Mortality rates of FES are currently believed to be about 10%.[46] FES is characterized by a classic triad of respiratory insufficiency, cerebral involvement, and a petechial rash that typically develops within 72 hours of injury. The incidence increases in young adults with multiple injuries and rarely occurs in children or patients with upper-extremity fractures.[47] Open fractures are less likely to develop FES compared with closed fractures, as higher pressures are more likely to develop in the latter.[46]

There are two main theories concerning the etiology of FES.[48] Following a fracture, intramedullary fat is released into the venous circulation. These fat globules subsequently embolize to end organs such as the lungs, brain, and skin. Mechanical obstruction of the end-organ capillary beds has been proposed as a potential source of injury in FES. However, the 24- to 72-hour delay between injury and the emergence of symptoms cannot be explained by mechanical obstruction alone. This fact has given rise to a second theory that fat emboli cause an inflammatory cascade that damages end-organ tissues. In this theory, fat emboli are metabolized to free fatty acids that, when present in high concentrations, induce an inflammatory reaction that damages end organs. It is still unclear why this syndrome develops in some patients and not in others, although the likelihood does seem to increase in patients with more significant fractures.

Clinical Manifestations

All cases have a latent period that ranges from 12 to 48 hours after the injury.[48] Pulmonary involvement is the earliest feature and is present in 75% of patients.[49] It manifests as tachypnea and dyspnea that may be confused with pulmonary embolism. Hypoxia is present and the PaO$_2$ is often <60 mm Hg.[46] Moist rales may be noted over the lung fields on examination. The chest radiograph is normal in mild-to-moderate cases, but after an initial delay, bilateral diffuse pulmonary edema develops in severe cases.[49] The findings of high-resolution CT in mild cases of FES demonstrate ground-glass opacities.[50] Mechanical ventilation will be necessary in 10% of patients.[49] Pulmonary function recovers completely within 1 week.

Neurologic symptoms range from restlessness to confusion to convulsions. Prolonged coma due to cerebral fat embolism has been reported, but in the majority of cases, symptoms resolve spontaneously.[46] Recovery of higher cortical function may be delayed. A CT scan of the brain may reveal cerebral edema or be entirely normal, but MRI may help in diagnosing cerebral fat embolism by revealing high-intensity signal abnormalities in watershed areas.

Petechiae are observed in 20% to 50% of patients with FES.[49] The low specific gravity of fat globules is believed to predispose to embolization in nondependent areas of the skin. Therefore, petechiae are initially observed over the anterior axillary folds and the anterior surface of the neck and chest. They are also found in the buccal mucosa and conjunctiva. The distribution and intensity of the rash varies, and resolution is usually noted within 1 week.

FES is a clinical diagnosis. The diagnosis should be suspected when hypoxia and neurologic findings appear together in the proper clinical context with or without the less prevalent petechial rash. Given that the signs and symptoms of FES are nonspecific, alternative diagnoses should be considered and excluded while providing care for suspected FES.[43,51] Several diagnostic criteria, such as those from Gurd and Wilson,[52] have been developed, but none are widely used due to a lack of validated studies. Laboratory findings such as anemia, thrombocytopenia, or an elevated ESR are nonspecific.

Treatment

The cornerstone of treatment is prevention and early detection. Early resuscitation, stabilization, and operative treatment are believed to have decreased the incidence of FES in recent years. Immobilization with no excessive motion permitted has been shown to decrease the incidence of FES. In addition, open reduction with internal fixation within 24 to 48 hours of injury will decrease fat embolism.[46] Of patients who develop FES, one-third of cases are mild and require only supportive treatment. The management of respiratory failure secondary to fat embolism is similar to the management of the adult respiratory distress syndrome. Respiratory support with oxygen is employed to keep the PaO$_2$ above 70 mm Hg. There is insufficient controlled data to confirm the benefit of steroids in the treatment of this inflammatory condition; nonetheless, some experts recommend systemic corticosteroids in cases of life-threatening FES.[51] The mainstay of treatment, however, is respiratory support and fluid resuscitation, which must be started early.

REFERENCES

1. Konstantakos EK, Dalstrom DJ, Nelles ME, Laughlin RT, Prayson MJ. Diagnosis and management of extremity compartment syndromes: an orthopaedic perspective. *Am Surg*. 2007;73(12):1199–1209.
2. Newton EJ, Love J. Acute complications of extremity trauma. *Emerg Med Clin N Am*. 2007;25(4):751–761.
3. Kalyani BS, Fisher BE, Roberts CS, Giannoudis PV. Compartment syndrome of the forearm: a systematic review. *J Hand Surg Am*. 2011;36(3):535–543.
4. Hosseinzadeh P, Hayes CB. Compartment syndrome in children. *Orthop Clin N Am*. 2016;47(3):579–587.
5. Frink M, Hildebrand F, Krettek C, Brand J, Hankemeier S. Compartment syndrome of the lower leg and foot. *Clin Orthop Relat Res*. 2010;468(4):940–950.

6. O'Neil D, Sheppard JE. Transient compartment syndrome of the forearm resulting from venous congestion from a tourniquet. *J Hand Surg Am.* 1989;14(5):894–896.

7. Von Keudell AG, Weaver MJ, Appleton PT, et al. Diagnosis and treatment of acute extremity compartment syndrome. *Lancet.* 2015;386(10000):1299–1310.

8. Simon RR, Ross C, Bowman SH, Wakim PE. *Cook County Manual of Emergency Procedures.* Philadelphia, PA: Lippincott Williams & Wilkins; 2012.

9. Whitesides TE, Heckman MM. Acute compartment syndrome: update on diagnosis and treatment. *J Am Acad Orthop Surg.* 1996;4(4):209–218.

10. Nelson JA. Compartment pressure measurements have poor specificity for compartment syndrome in the traumatized limb. *J Emerg Med.* 2013;44(5):1039–1044.

11. Heckman MM, Whitesides TE Jr, Grewe SR, Rooks MD. Compartment pressure in association with closed tibial fractures. The relationship between tissue pressure, compartment, and the distance from the site of the fracture. *J Bone Joint Surg Am.* 1994;76(9):1285–1292.

12. Shuler MS, Reisman WM, Whitesides TE Jr, et al. Near-infrared spectroscopy in lower extremity trauma. *J Bone Joint Surg Am.* 2009;91(6):1360–1368.

13. Shadgan B, Menon M, O'Brien, PJ, Reid WD. Diagnostic techniques in acute compartment syndrome of the leg. *J Orthop Trauma.* 2008;22(8):581–587.

14. Flynn JM, Bashyal RK, Yeger-McKeever M, Garner MR, Launay F, Sponseller PD. Acute traumatic compartment syndrome of the leg in children: diagnosis and outcome. *J Bone Joint Surg Am.* 2011;93(10):937–941.

15. Schmitt SK. Osteomyelitis. *Infect Dis Clin North Am.* 2017; 31(2):325–338.

16. Lipsky BA, Berendt AR, Cornia PB, et al. 2012 Infectious Diseases Society of America clinical practice guideline for the diagnosis and treatment of diabetic foot infections. *Clin Infect Dis.* 2012;54(12):e132–e173.

17. Lazzarini L, Mader JT, Calhoun JH. Osteomyelitis in long bones. *J Bone Joint Surg Am.* 2004;86-A(10):2305–2318.

18. Lew DP, Waldvogel FA. Osteomyelitis. *Lancet.* 2004;364 (9431):369–379.

19. Pineda C, Vargas A, Vargas Rodriguez A. Imaging of osteomyelitis: current concepts. *Infect Dis Clin North Am.* 2006;20(4): 789–825.

20. Calhoun JH, Manring MM, Shirtliff M. Osteomyelitis of the long bones. *Infect Dis Clin North Am.* 2006;20(4):789–825.

21. Butalia S, Palda VA, Sargeant RJ, Detsky AS, Mourad O. Does this patient with diabetes have osteomyelitis of the lower extremity? *JAMA.* 2008;299(7):806–813.

22. Lam K, van Asten SA, Nguyen T, et al. Diagnostic accuracy of probe to bone to detect osteomyelitis in the diabetic foot: a systematic review. *Cain Infect Dis.* 2016;63(7):944–948.

23. Kapoor A, Page S, Lavalley M, Gale DR, Felson DT. Magnetic resonance imaging for diagnosing foot osteomyelitis: a meta-analysis. *Arch Intern Med.* 2007;167(2):125–132.

24. Zimmerli W. Clinical practice. Vertebral osteomyelitis. *N Engl J Med.* 2010;362(11):1022–1029.

25. Liu C, Bayer A, Cosgrove SE. Clinical practice guidelines by the infectious diseases society of America for the treatment of methicillin-resistant *Staphylococcus aureus* infections in adults and children: executive summary. *Clin Infect Dis.* 2011;52(3):285–292.

26. Hoff WS, Bonadies JA, Cachecho R, Dorlac WC. EAST practice management guidelines work group: update to practice management guidelines for prophylactic antibiotic use in open fractures. *J Trauma.* 2011;70(3):751–754.

27. Raff AB, Kroshinsky D. Cellulitis: a review. *JAMA.* 2016;316(3): 325–337.

28. Stevens DL, Bisno AL, Chambers HF, et al. Practice guidelines for the diagnosis and management of skin and soft tissue infections: 2014 update by the Infectious Diseases Society of America. *Clin Infect Dis.* 2014;59(2):147–159.

29. Adhikari S, Blaivas M. Sonography first for subcutaneous abscess and cellulitis evaluation. *J Ultrasound Med.* 2012; 31(10):1509–1512.

30. Ustin JS, Malangoni MA. Necrotizing soft-tissue infections. *Crit Care Med.* 2011;39(9):2156–2162.

31. Lancerotto L, Tocco I, Salmaso R, Vindigni V, Bassetto F. Necrotizing fasciitis: classification, diagnosis, and management. *J Trauma Acute Care Surg.* 2012;72(3):560–566.

32. Sultan HY, Boyle AA, Sheppard N. Necrotising fasciitis. *BMJ.* 2012;345:e4274.

33. Wong CH, Wang YS. The diagnosis of necrotizing fasciitis. *Curr Opin Infect Dis.* 2005;18(2):101–106.

34. Zacharias N, Velmahos GC, Salama A, et al. Diagnosis of necrotizing soft tissue infections by computed tomography. *Arch Surg.* 2010;145(5):452–455.

35. Wong CH, Khin LW, Heng KS, Tan KC, Low CO. The LRINEC (Laboratory Risk Indicator for Necrotizing Fasciitis) score: a tool for distinguishing necrotizing fasciitis from other soft tissue infections. *Crit Care Med.* 2004;32(7): 1535–1541.

36. Wilson MP, Schneir AB. A case of necrotizing fasciitis with a LRINEC score of zero: clinical suspicion should trump scoring systems. *J Emerg Med.* 2013;44(5):928–931.

37. Holland MJ. Application of the Laboratory Risk Indicator in Necrotizing Fasciitis (LRINEC) score in patients in a tropical tertiary referral centre. *Anaesth Intensive Care.* 2009: 37(4):588–592.

38. Marinus J, Moseley GL, Birklein F, et al. Clinical features and pathophysiology of complex regional pain syndrome. *Lancet Neurol.* 2011;10(7):637–648.

39. Bussa M, Guttilla D, Lucia M, et al. Complex regional pain syndrome type I: a comprehensive review. *Acta Anaesthesiol Scand.* 2015;59(6):685–697.

40. Maihofner, C, Seifert F, Markovic K. Complex regional pain syndromes: new pathophysiological concepts and therapies. *Eur J Neurol.* 2010;17(5):649–660.

41. Harden RN, Oakland AL, Burton AW, et al. Complex regional pain syndrome: practical diagnostic and treatment guidelines, 4th edition. *Pain Med.* 2013;14(2):180–229.

42. Patterson RW, Li Z, Smith BP, Smith TL, Koman LA. Complex regional pain syndrome of the upper extremity. *J Hand Surg Am.* 2011;36(9):1553–1562.

43. Zollinger PE, Tuinebreijer WE, Breederveld RS, Kreis RW. Can vitamin C prevent complex regional pain syndrome in patients with wrist fractures? A randomized, controlled, multicenter dose-response study. *J Bone Joint Surg.* 2007;89(7): 1424–1431.

44. Shibuya N, Humphers JM, Agarwal MR, Jupiter DC. Efficacy and safety of high-dose vitamin C on complex regional pain syndrome in extremity trauma and surgery-systematic review and meta-analysis. *J Foot Ankle Surg.* 2013;52(1):62–66.

45. Repesse X, Bodson L, Au SM, et al. An unusual cause of fat embolism syndrome. *Anesthesiology*. 2012;117(1):216–218.

46. Akhtar S. Fat embolism. *Anesthesiol Clin*. 2009;27(3): 533–550.

47. Stein PD, Yaekoub AY, Matta F, Kleerekoper M. Fat embolism syndrome. *Am J Med Sci*. 2008;336(6):472–477.

48. Taviloglu K, Yanar H. Fat embolism syndrome. *Surg Today*. 2007;37(1):5–8.

49. Shaikh N. Emergency management of fat embolism syndrome. *J Emerg Trauma Shock*. 2009;2(1):29–33.

50. Erba P, Farhadi J, Johannes D, Pierer G. Fat embolism syndrome after combined aesthetic surgery. *J Plast Surg Hand Surg*. 2011;45(1):51–53.

51. Fat embolism syndrome: state of-the-art review focused on pulmonary imaging findings. *Respir Med*. 2016;113: 93–100.

52. Gurd AR, Wilson RI. The fat embolism syndrome. *J Bone Joint Surg Br*. 1974;56(3):408–416.

CHAPTER 5

Special Imaging Techniques

Joy L. English, MD

Plain radiographs are a sufficient adjunct to the history and physical examination for the evaluation of most acute extremity complaints. It must be stressed that this statement is true assuming that the quality of views is adequate. A minimum of two perpendicular views are required to adequately visualize and describe fractures. Oblique views are commonly included when imaging the small joint of the wrist, hand, ankle, and foot. In addition, radiographs of the joints above and below a fracture should be considered to exclude the presence of a subluxation, dislocation, or second fracture.

Several other imaging techniques exist that offer additional information not readily available when imaging with plain radiography. These techniques, which include ultrasound, computed tomography (CT), magnetic resonance imaging (MRI), and fluoroscopy, may be used in conjunction with plain radiographs and may be superior to plain radiographs for certain musculoskeletal disorders. These studies and the clinical situations in which they are useful are discussed in this chapter.

ULTRASOUND

Ultrasonography is gaining an increasing role within the specialty of emergency medicine, and this role continues to grow for orthopedic conditions. Soft-tissue and musculoskeletal ultrasound is now recognized as one of the 11 core emergency ultrasound applications. This modality offers several advantages over traditional imaging methods, including portability, the ability to perform dynamic imaging of the affected body part, the ability to easily compare findings on the affected side with those on the unaffected side, and lack of exposure to the harmful effects of radiation. The last advantage mentioned is particularly important when evaluating the pediatric population who are more susceptible to ionizing radiation, which is delivered in large doses with imaging techniques such as CT.

Common musculoskeletal ultrasound applications in the emergency department (ED) include tendon evaluation, muscle evaluation, joint evaluation for effusion, foreign body identification, and procedural guidance. There are several studies documenting the usefulness of ultrasound in trauma, especially with regard to the evaluation of bony trauma. It may be used in conjunction with plain radiographs to evaluate for fractures and may even be superior to plain radiographs in certain types of fractures, including rib and scaphoid fractures (Fig. 5-1). In addition, recent research has also suggested that this modality is useful in diagnosing extremity fractures in military or

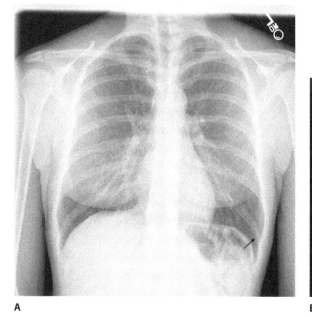
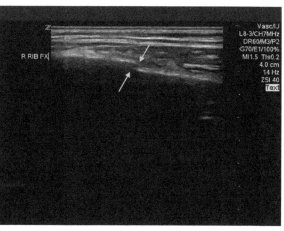

Figure 5-1. Comparison of plain radiography and ultrasound in rib fractures. **A.** Normal chest radiograph in a patient with left-sided pleuritic chest pain after trauma (*arrow* notes the location of an occult rib fracture). **B.** Ultrasound showing cortical disruption of the rib (*arrows*).

sideline settings where other imaging capabilities are not readily available.[10,11] This role of ultrasound in the acute setting is also expanding to include evaluation of musculoskeletal infections. The localization of soft-tissue collections by ultrasound helps narrow the differential diagnosis based on the finding of fluid in the dermis, joint, bursa, or muscle. For this reason, ultrasound can be used to detect simple abscesses, pyomyositis, septic bursitis, tenosynovitis, joint effusions, and subperiosteal fluid associated with osteomyelitis.[12]

Musculoskeletal Ultrasound Techniques

The following is an overview of the basic musculoskeletal imaging that may be useful and can be easily performed in the ED. There is a focus on normal imaging findings, as well as how to obtain the images for evaluation and how to identify deviations from the normal patterns. If your findings deviate from the normal appearance of the structure,

pathology should be expected, and further investigation should be pursued with appropriate imaging techniques, lab studies, or expert consultation.

Most EDs use ultrasound imaging systems with a high-frequency 7- to 12-MHz linear transducer. This transducer is ideal for superficial (<3–4 cm deep) musculoskeletal imaging. It provides good resolution in the near field with less penetration into deeper structures (Fig. 5–2A and B). For imaging that requires deeper penetration (>3–4 cm deep), such as hip ultrasound, a lower-frequency 2- to 5-MHz curvilinear transducer should be used (Fig. 5–2C and D). The typical width of an ultrasound beam is 0.2 to 1 mm thick; therefore, careful interrogation of musculoskeletal structures is imperative so as not to overlook a small abnormality. Ultrasound imaging, regardless of the structure being evaluated, should be performed in both the longitudinal and short axes of the structure. When evaluating small parts or parts with abnormal contours, a water bath or

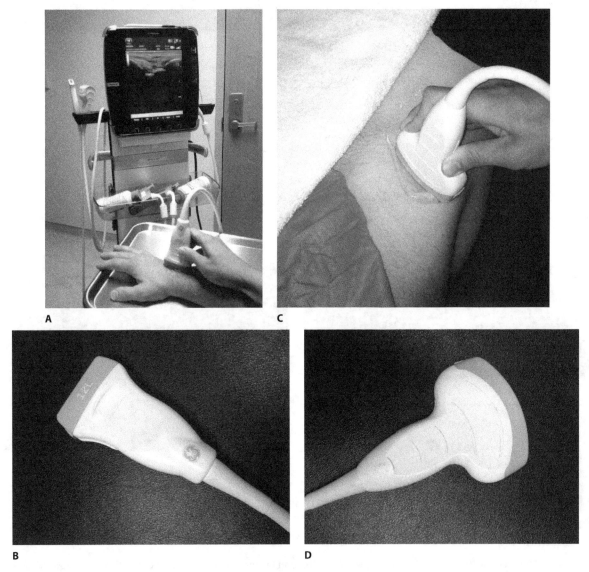

A   **C**   **B**   **D**

Figure 5–2. Transducer selection. ***A, B.*** Linear transducer for superficial imaging. ***C, D.*** Curvilinear transducer for deeper imaging.

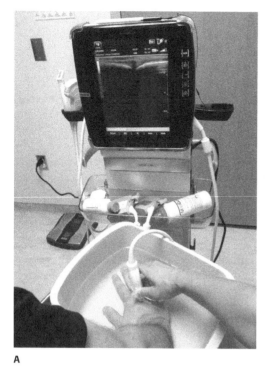
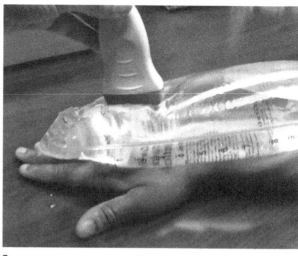

A **B**

Figure 5–3. Adjuncts for musculoskeletal imaging. **A.** Water bath and associated ultrasound image showing the metacarpal phalangeal joint. **B.** Stand-off pad using a liter of normal saline.

a stand-off pad may help increase through transmission of the ultrasound waves being transmitted and improve image quality (Fig. 5–3).[13]

Tendon Evaluation

Ultrasonographic evaluation of tendons is used to identify traumatic tendon rupture and infections of the tendon and

tendon sheath. Tendons are best evaluated with the linear transducer in both the long and short axes. In long axis, tendons exhibit an echogenic fibrillar pattern that is linear in nature without disruption (Fig. 5–4A).[13] Disruption of the normal linear pattern, often evidenced by a hypoechoic region, should prompt further evaluation for an acute tear (Fig. 5–4B). Dynamic evaluation is helpful when imaging

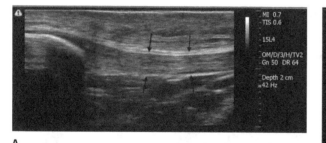

A

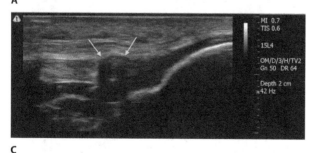

C

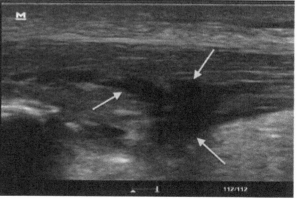

B

Figure 5–4. Tendon evaluation for trauma. **A.** Normal patellar tendon in long axis. **B.** Patellar tendon with a large (50%–60%) tear in long axis. **C.** Patellar tendon exhibiting anisotropy when imaged in full extension.

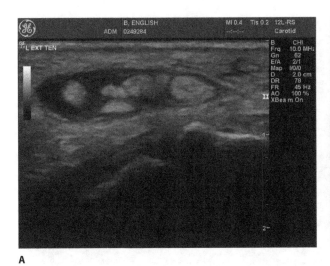
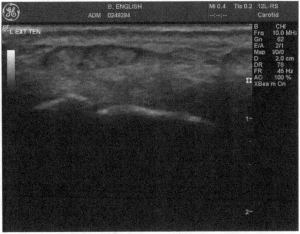

A   B

Figure 5-5. Tendon evaluation for infection. **A.** Wrist extensor tenosynovitis with anechoic areas of fluid surrounding the individual extensor tendons. **B.** Normal contralateral tendon for comparison.

tendons as this may enlarge an area of hematoma or rupture not previously visualized on static imaging.

Of note, it is important to maintain a perpendicular angle between the ultrasound beam and the tendon being imaged because tendons demonstrate anisotropy. In other words, the footprint of the ultrasound probe should remain parallel to the structure of interest. Anisotropy is an artifact that occurs when the ultrasound beam and the tendon are not perpendicular to each other. It may create a dark area within the tendon that can be easily be mistaken for pathology (Fig. 5–4C).[15]

When there is concern for an infectious process involving the tendon, any amount of fluid within a tendon sheath (>2 mm) should be considered abnormal and may suggest a tenosynovitis (Fig. 5–5).

Muscle Evaluation

Ultrasound is used to detect muscle tears and infections such as myositis or abscess. Muscles may be evaluated with either the linear or the curvilinear transducer, depending on how deeply situated the muscle in question lies within the body. Again, the muscular tissue should be evaluated in the long and short axes. On ultrasound, muscle appearance ranges from hypoechoic to echoic in nature and is encased in a hyperechoic fascial sheath (Fig. 5–6).[16] Dynamic imaging will provide important information regarding muscle structure and function. Disruption of the normal fiber organization or the inability to contract the muscle under ultrasound is suggestive of a tear (Fig. 5–7).[5] Enlargement of the muscle belly as a whole, loss of the normal architecture, and diffuse hypoechogenicity when compared to the contralateral muscle is suggestive of myositis (Fig. 5–8A).[12] A well-circumscribed anechoic area or an area of hypoechogenicity within the muscle belly should be concerning for an abscess or hematoma depending on patient history (Fig. 5–8B).[17]

Joint Evaluation

Ultrasonic evaluation of the joint is useful to identify joint effusions. For most joints, the linear transducer can be used, but evaluation of the hip joint will likely require the curvilinear transducer. Every joint contains a small, physiologic amount of joint fluid. Any joint fluid in excess of normal should prompt further evaluation with joint aspiration and

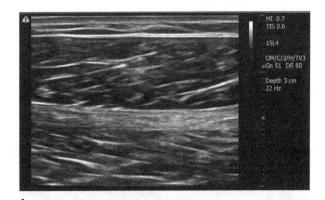

A

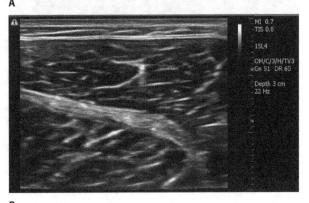

B

Figure 5-6. Muscle. **A.** Normal muscle tissue in long axis. **B.** Normal muscle tissue in short axis.

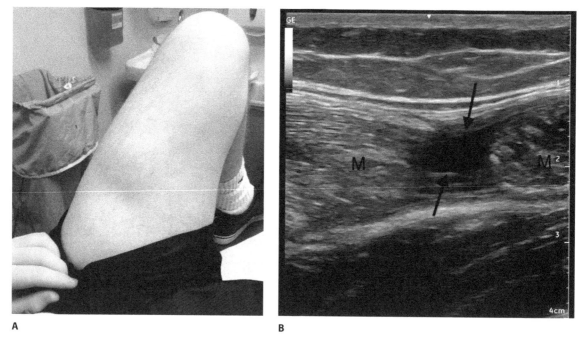

Figure 5–7. Muscle evaluation in trauma. **A.** Physical examination findings suggestive of muscular tear. **B.** Chronic muscle tear with muscle bellies (M) located laterally and hematoma (*arrows*) located medially.

fluid analysis if there is any concern for infection or other inflammatory processes (Fig. 5–9). The suggested norms for joint fluid, measured in millimeters, are provided in Table 5–1. Ultrasound is not only useful for identifying joint effusions, but it is also useful for distinguishing their presence from other soft-tissue abnormalities.

Bone Evaluation

Ultrasound is used to detect fractures or the secondary signs of fractures. The high-frequency linear transducer should be used for bony evaluation, and the bone should be evaluated in both the long and short axes. In both the long and short axes, the cortex of the bone should appear as a continuous hyperechoic linear structure with posterior acoustic shadowing (Fig. 5–10). When there is any disruption or buckling of the cortex, a fracture should be suspected. Ultrasound is also useful for identifying secondary signs of fracture that are not readily visualized with plain radiography. These include soft-tissue edema overlying the bone and hematoma formation adjacent to the fracture site (Fig. 5–11).

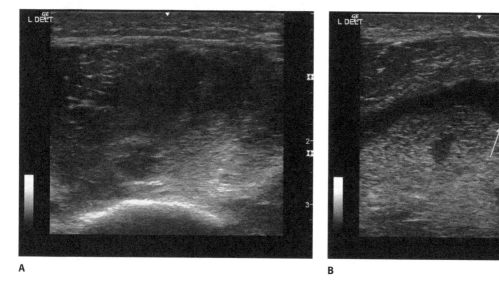

Figure 5–8. Muscle evaluation for infection. **A.** Biceps muscle in short axis showing blurring of the margins and generalized hypoechogenicity, suggestive of myositis. **B.** Biceps myositis with a focal area of abscess (*arrows*).

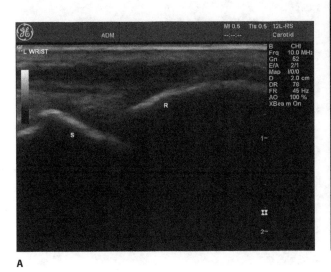

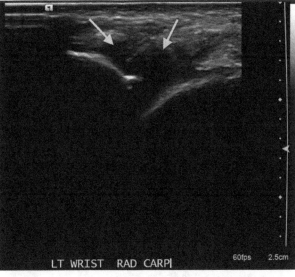

Figure 5–9. Joint. **A.** Normal wrist ultrasound (S, scaphoid; R, radius). **B.** Wrist effusion with anechoic distention of the joint space (*arrows*).

Foreign Body Identification

Ultrasound may be employed to identify foreign bodies within soft tissues. Using a high-frequency probe, ultrasound is better equipped to detect radiolucent foreign bodies (plastic and wood) than conventional radiography and fluoroscopy.[19] In one experimental model, ultrasound identified wood and plastic foreign bodies with a sensitivity of 83% and a specificity of 59%.[20] Emergency physicians trained in this technique exhibit a similar rate of detection as ultrasound technologists and radiologists.[21]

Procedural Guidance

There is an increasingly large role for ultrasound when performing procedures of the musculoskeletal system. The procedures in which ultrasound may be useful include fracture reduction, joint aspiration, joint injection, hematoma blocks, and peripheral nerve blocks. A few recent studies have shown ultrasound to be useful in forearm fracture reduction in the pediatric population.[22–24] Ultrasound guidance of hematoma blocks has also been shown to be superior to a landmark-based approach, which should help

▶ TABLE 5–1. **NORMAL JOINT SPACE ON ULTRASOUND**

Joint	Normal Joint Space (mm)[a]
Upper extremity	
Shoulder	
Posterior joint recess	2–5
Elbow	
Anterior or posterior joint recess	1–2
Wrist	
Volar or dorsal joint recess	<1
Lower extremity	
Hip	
Anterior joint recess	5 (or <2 mm difference than the contralateral side)
Knee	
Suprapatellar joint recess	1–2
Ankle	
Anterior joint recess	1.8–3.5

[a]Higher measurements suggest an effusion.

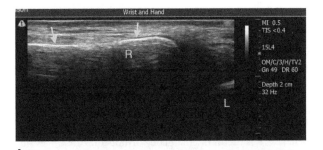

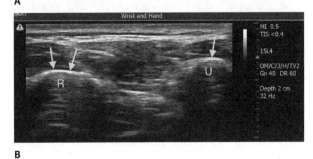

Figure 5–10. Bone. **A.** Normal cortical bone in long axis (R, radius). **B.** Normal cortical bone in short axis (R, radius; U, ulna).

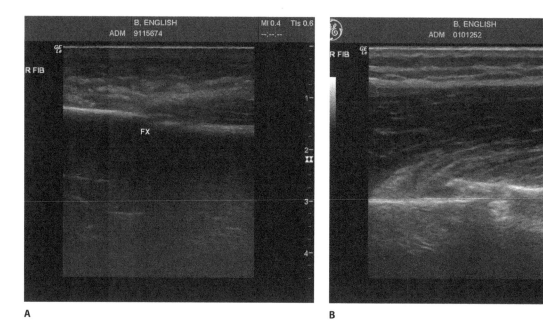

Figure 5–11. Bone evaluation in trauma. **A.** Fibula fracture with cortical disruption and soft-tissue edema (FX, fracture). **B.** Fibular fracture with cortical disruption and soft-tissue edema.

facilitate adequate fracture reduction. When ultrasound guidance has been studied for joint aspiration at the level of the knee, it was shown to cause less procedural pain, improve physician's confidence with the procedure, and provide greater synovial fluid for analysis. Peripheral nerve blocks under ultrasound guidance for acute bony trauma and joint dislocation are also becoming more widely used as they have been shown to decrease ED length of stay when compared with procedural sedation for upper-extremity injuries.

COMPUTED TOMOGRAPHY

Numerous advances in CT have expanded its uses for bone and soft-tissue injuries. With the advent of spiral CT scanning with multiple detectors, both speed and resolution have improved, and three-dimensional computer reconstructions make diagnosis easier. The two major areas where CT is useful in emergency orthopedics are the evaluation of trauma and the evaluation of soft-tissue infections and tumors.

Trauma

CT has two major applications for the evaluation of a traumatized extremity: to detect a fracture that is suspected clinically but not visualized on plain radiographs and to determine the extent of a previously identified fracture. Table 5–2 outlines specific areas where spiral CT is useful in the setting of trauma. In addition, CT is useful for the detection of radiolucent bodies within the soft tissues of the extremities (Fig. 5–12).

CT has proved to be useful in the evaluation of pelvic fractures. The axial format allows better visualization of anterior and posterior displacement than do plain radiographs. The acetabulum is well visualized by this technique, and the data provided by the CT scan may influence the decision to proceed with open reduction and the type of procedure needed. The cost and radiation exposure of this technique, however, should be borne in mind, and it should not be used routinely on all pelvic fractures. Simple fractures not involving the acetabulum, which are stable on clinical examination, are usually adequately evaluated on plain films.

CT can evaluate nondisplaced fractures of the femoral head and neck. The axial projection allows good visualization of the head of the femur and its relationship to the acetabulum. Bone fragments or distortions of the joint surface, which are not appreciated on plain films, are seen routinely on high-resolution CT.

The introduction of CT and MRI has led to improved assessment of the Salter injuries to the physis, epiphysis, and metaphysis. In addition, the analysis of growth disturbances and injuries to these structures has clearly become much easier using these two imaging techniques.

Soft-Tissue Infections and Tumors

The advent of spiral CT has increased the sensitivity for detecting inflammatory and infectious processes in the soft tissues because the entire examination can be obtained at the peak of the intravenous contrast bolus. CT will aid the clinician by demonstrating the extent of the process, including the compartments involved. This information will impact the need for surgical versus medical management. CT will

▶ TABLE 5–2. **SPECIFIC AREAS WHERE CT IS USEFUL IN SETTING OF ORTHOPEDIC TRAUMA**

Area of Interest	Advantages of CT
Shoulder	Improved diagnosis of fractures associated with shoulder dislocations
	Detection of subtle scapular fractures
	Determine fragment rotation and displacement of proximal humerus fractures that impact decision to operate
Sternoclavicular joint	Detection of great vessel injuries after posterior dislocation[a]
	Diagnosing common associated injuries such as rib and shoulder fractures
Elbow	Detecting occult fractures
Wrist	Detection of occult fractures superior to plain films for diagnosing scaphoid and lunate fractures
Pelvis	Detecting subtle acetabular fractures
	Detecting associated vascular injury (84% sensitive and 85% specific for diagnosing active bleeding)[a]
	Better delineation of posterior injuries
Hip	Diagnosing intra-articular fragments and lesions of articular surface of femoral head
	Diagnosing occult nondisplaced fractures
Knee	Better able to determine fracture fragment depression (e.g., tibial plateau, femoral condyle)
	Changes treatment plan in up to one-half of patients
Ankle and calcaneus	Improved sensitivity over plain films when suspicion of joint space extension
	Useful for operative indications and planning in select cases[a]
Cervical spine	Greatly improved sensitivity over plain radiography for clinically significant fractures

CT, computed tomography.
[a]Consider using an IV contrast agent for these studies.

assist in the diagnosis of necrotizing fasciitis, intramuscular abscess, myositis, pyomyositis, and osteomyelitis.[36]

CT has been demonstrated to be an extremely valuable tool in the evaluation of bone and soft-tissue neoplasms in the extremities.[37,46,47] Ordinarily, the emergency physician will refer patients with suspected bone tumors, but the increasing availability of CT may make this a routine part of the initial evaluation. Although the CT scan may not be diagnostic, it often provides important information about the density of the mass, its relation to normal bone, nerves, and vessels, and the presence or absence of recurrence in patients who have been treated surgically.[48,49] The radionuclide scan and MRI are more sensitive tools for the detection of neoplasms of the extremities, whereas CT scan is superior in the detection of cortical destruction and lesion calcification.

MAGNETIC RESONANCE IMAGING

In patients with extremity injuries, MRI remains a rarely ordered study from the ED. However, MRI in patients with acute musculoskeletal trauma has an increasing application that should be understood by the emergency physician.

MRI of bone identifies occult traumatic lesions, such as fractures of the scaphoid and femoral neck, not always seen with other imaging techniques.[50–52] The types of injury detected by MRI include bone bruises, stress or insufficiency fractures, and osteochondral fractures.[53] Increasing evidence suggests that occult fractures are detected by MRI sooner and with greater specificity than with bone scan.[51]

In addition, MRI is indispensable in the diagnosis of a number of soft-tissue diagnoses. MRI is sensitive and therefore routinely used following knee trauma to detect ligamentous and meniscal injuries. At the shoulder, MRI is used to evaluate the integrity of the rotator cuff, glenoid

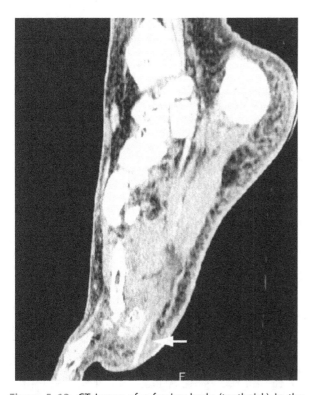

Figure 5–12. CT image of a foreign body (toothpick) in the forefoot (*arrow*).

labrum, and biceps tendon. And, at the ankle, it is used to detect ligamentous and syndesmotic injuries that are not as readily visualized with x-ray or ultrasound imaging.

Of note, it is not commonplace to obtain an MRI in the ED setting for the diagnoses listed above unless there is a fair amount of diagnostic uncertainty and concern exists for other pathology such as vascular or nerve injury.

FLUOROSCOPY

Fluoroscopy uses x-ray beams that strike a fluorescent plate that is coupled to an image intensifier and monitor. For ED use, a fluoroscope, or "C-arm," can be purchased for $30,000 to $60,000 (Fig. 5–13). The primary advantage of fluoroscopy is the ability to view anatomic structures in real time. Fluoroscopic films have been shown to be equal to plain radiographs in evaluating skeletal injuries. They may offer an advantage because they demonstrate motion of fracture fragments and because the examiner can obtain multiple views. In addition, fluoroscopy decreases the length of patient stay within the ED by eliminating the need to have a radiograph performed outside the department.

The advantage of real-time viewing using fluoroscopy is for foreign body removal, fracture reduction, and difficult arthrocentesis. In a similar manner to conventional radiography, fluoroscopy will reliably detect gravel, metal, and glass, but it cannot be used to identify plastic or wood. The technique is easily learned by clinicians, and retention rates are high. For radiopaque foreign materials, removal is aided because the clinician can visualize both the instrument and the foreign body. Although the fluoroscope is turned on, the extremity can easily be manipulated to give a three-dimensional picture that allows the object to be located and removed.

The use of fluoroscopy is also advantageous for fracture reduction. Rather than sending the patient back to the radiology suite, confirmation of adequate reduction can be obtained immediately with a portable fluoroscope. Fracture reduction using a portable ED fluoroscope is more successful, thereby decreasing extra trips to radiology for postreduction films by 30%. This technique will also reduce procedural sedation requirements by ensuring the reduction is done correctly the first time.

The dose of radiation received from fluoroscopy is not negligible, but the patient receives a greater dose from a conventional radiograph than from a "spot film" taken by a fluoroscope by a ratio of 2:1. Estimates of whole-body radiation suggest that the clinician using a portable ED fluoroscope could work with the instrument at 1-m distance continuously for 2 hours every day and still be under the maximum permissible dose equivalent for radiation workers. Although this statistic is encouraging, most work is performed at a distance closer than 1 m; therefore, lead aprons are recommended as they reduce the radiation exposure by 85%.

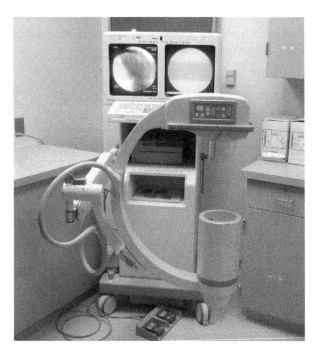

Figure 5–13. Portable fluoroscope ("C-arm") used in the emergency department.

REFERENCES

1. American College of Emergency Physicians (ACEP). Emergency Ultrasound Guidelines, ACEP Policy Statement, October 2008. https://www.emra.org/uploadedFiles/EMRA/committees-divisions/ultrasound/ACEP-2008-EUS-Guidelines.pdf. Accessed December 9, 2017.
2. Fornage BD, Touche DH, Edeiken-Monroe BS. The tendons. In: Rumack CM, Wilson SR, Charboneau JW, eds. *Diagnostic Ultrasound.* 4th ed. Philadelphia, PA: Elsevier; 2011:902–934.
3. Pasta G, Nanni B, Molini L, Bianchi S. Sonography of the quadriceps muscle: examination technique, normal anatomy, and traumatic lesions. *J Ultrasound.* 2010;13(2):76–84.
4. Fessell DP, Jacobson JA, Craig J, et al. Using sonography to reveal and aspirate joint effusions. *Am J Roentgenol.* 2000; 174(5):1353–1362.
5. Brenner D, Elliston C, Hall E, Berdon W. Estimated risks of radiation-induced fatal cancer from pediatric CT. *Am J Roentgenol.* 2001;176(2):289–296.
6. Cross KP, Warkentine FH, Kim IL, Gracely E, Paul RI. Bedside ultrasound diagnosis of clavicle fractures in the pediatric emergency department. *Acad Emerg Med.* 2010;17(7):687–693.
7. Griffith JF, Rainer TH, Ching AS, Law KL, Cocks RA, Metreweli C. Sonography compared with radiography in revealing acute rib fracture. *Am J Roentgenol.* 1999;173(6):1603–1609.
8. Turk F, Kurt AB, Saglam S. Evaluation by ultrasound of traumatic rib fractures missed by radiography. *Emerg Radiol.* 2010;17(6):473–477.
9. Herneth AM, Siegmeth A, Bader TR, et al. Scaphoid fracture: evaluation with high-spatial-resolution US—initial results. *Radiology.* 2001;220(1):231–235.

10. Dulchavsky SA, Henry SE, Moed BR, et al. Advanced ultrasonic diagnosis of extremity trauma: the FASTER examination. *J Trauma*. 2002;53(1):28–32.

11. Marshburn TH, Legome E, Sargsyan A, et al. Goal-directed ultrasound in the detection of long-bone fractures. *J Trauma*. 2004;57(2):329–332.

12. Cardinal E, Bureau NJ, Aubin B, Chhem RK. Role of ultrasound in musculoskeletal infections. *Radiol Clin North Am*. 2001;39(2):191–201.

13. Blaivas M, Lyon M, Brannam L, Duggal S, Szierznski P. Water bath evaluation technique for emergency ultrasound of painful small parts. *Am J Emerg Med*. 2004;22(7):589–593.

14. Robinson P. Sonography of common tendon injuries. *Am J Roentgenol*. 2009;193(3):607–618.

15. Crass JR, van de Vegte GL, Harkavy LA. Tendon echogenicity: ex vivo study. *Radiology*. 1998;167(2):499–501.

16. Jacobsen JA, van Holsbeeck MT. Musculoskeletal ultrasonography. *Orthop Clin North Am*. 1998;29(1):135–167.

17. Bureau NJ, Chhem RK, Cardinal E. Musculoskeletal infections: US manifestations. *Radiographics*. 1999;19(6):1585–1592.

18. Adhikari S, Blaivas M. Utility of bedside sonography to distinguish soft tissue abnormalities from joint effusions in the emergency department. *J Ultrasound Med*. 2010;29(4):519–526.

19. Dean AJ, Gronczewski CA, Costantino TG. Technique for emergency medicine bedside ultrasound identification of a radiolucent foreign body. *J Emerg Med*. 2003;24(3):303–308.

20. Hill R, Conron R, Greissinger P, Greissinger P, Heller M. Ultrasound for the detection of foreign bodies in human tissue. *Ann Emerg Med*. 1997;29(3):353–356.

21. Orlinsky M, Knittel P, Feit T, Chan L, Mandavia D. The comparative accuracy of radiolucent foreign body detection using ultrasonography. *Am J Emerg Med*. 2000;18(4):401–403.

22. Chen L, Kim Y, Moore CL. Diagnosis and guided reduction of forearm fractures in children using bedside ultrasound. *Pediatr Emerg Care*. 2007;23(8):528–531.

23. Ang SH, Lee DW, Lam KY. Ultrasound-guided reduction of distal radius fractures. *Am J Emerg Med*. 2010;28(9):1002–1008.

24. Chinnock B, Khaletskiy A, Kuo K, Hendey GW. Ultrasound-guided reduction of distal radius fractures. *J Emerg Med*. 2011;4(3):308–312.

25. Kiley PD, O'Farrell D, Riordan J, Harmon D. The use of ultrasound-guided hematoma block for wrist fractures. *J Clin Anesth*. 2009;21(7):540–542.

26. Wiler JL, Constantino TG, Filippone L. Comparison of ultrasound guided and standard landmark techniques for knee arthrocentesis. *J Emerg Med*. 2010;39(1):76–82.

27. Sibbitt WL, Kettwich LG, Band PA, et al. Does ultrasound guidance improve outcomes of arthrocentesis and corticosteroid infection of the knee? *Scand J Rheumatol*. 2012;41(1):66–72.

28. De Buck F, Devroe S, Missant C, Missant C, Van de Velde M. Regional anesthesia outside the operating room: indications and techniques. *Curr Opin Anaesthesiol*. 2012;25(4):501–507.

29. Bhoi S, Chandra A, Galwankar S. Ultrasound-guided nerve blocks in the emergency department. *J Emerg Trauma Shock*. 2010;3(1):82–88.

30. Stone MD, Price DD, Wang R. Ultrasound-guided supraclavicular block for the treatment of upper extremity fractures, dislocations, and abscesses in the ED. *Am J Emerg Med*. 2007;25(4):472–475.

31. Liebmann O, Price D, Mills C, et al. Feasibility of forearm ultrasonography-guided nerve blocks for the radial, ulnar, and median nerves for hand procedures in the emergency department. *Ann Emerg Med*. 2006;48(5):558–562.

32. Stone MB, Wang R, Price DD. Ultrasound-guided supraclavicular brachial plexus nerve block vs procedural sedation for the treatment of upper extremity emergencies. *Am J Emerg Med*. 2008;26(6):706–710.

33. Albrechtsen J, Hede J, Jurik AG. Pelvic fractures. Assessment by conventional radiography and CT. *Acta Radiol*. 1994;35(5):420–425.

34. Wechsler RJ, Schweitzer ME, Karasick D, Deely DM, Morrison W. Helical CT of calcaneal fractures: technique and imaging features. *Skeletal Radiol*. 1998;27(1):1–6.

35. Chan PS, Klimkiewicz JJ, Luchetti WT, et al. Impact of CT scan on treatment plan and fracture classification of tibial plateau fractures. *J Orthop Trauma*. 1997;11(7):484–489.

36. Pretorius ES, Fishman EK. Spiral CT and three-dimensional CT of musculoskeletal pathology. Emergency room applications. *Radiol Clin North Am*. 1999;37(5):953–974, vi.

37. Pretorius ES, Fishman EK. Volume-rendered three-dimensional spiral CT: musculoskeletal applications. *Radiographics*. 1999;19(5):1143–1160.

38. Liow RY, Birdsall PD, Mucci B, Greiss ME. Spiral computed tomography with two- and three-dimensional reconstruction in the management of tibial plateau fractures. *Orthopedics*. 1999;22(10):929–932.

39. Wicky S, Blaser PF, Blanc CH, Leyvraz PF, Schnyder P, Meuli RA. Comparison between standard radiography and spiral CT with 3D reconstruction in the evaluation, classification and management of tibial plateau fractures. *Eur Radiol*. 2000;10(8):1227–1232.

40. Linsenmaier U, Brunner U, Schoning A, et al. Classification of calcaneal fractures by spiral computed tomography: implications for surgical treatment. *Eur Radiol*. 2003;13(10):2315–2322.

41. Chapman CB, Herrera MF, Binenbaum G, et al. Classification of intertrochanteric fractures with computed tomography: a study of intraobserver and interobserver variability and prognostic value. *Am J Orthop*. 2003;32(9):443–449.

42. Erb RE. Current concepts in imaging the adult hip. *Clin Sports Med*. 2001;20(4):661–696.

43. Bauer AR Jr, Yutani D. Computed tomographic localization of wooden foreign bodies in children's extremities. *Arch Surg*. 1983;118(9):1084–1086.

44. Manco LG, Berlow ME. Meniscal tears—comparison of arthrography, CT, and MRI. *Crit Rev Diagn Imaging*. 1989;29(2):151–179.

45. Rogers LF, Poznanski AK. Imaging of epiphyseal injuries. *Radiology*. 1994;191(2):297–308.

46. Struk DW, Munk PL, Lee MJ, Ho SG, Worsley DF. Imaging of soft tissue infections. *Radiol Clin North Am*. 2001;39(2):277–303.

47. Woertler K. Benign bone tumors and tumor-like lesions: value of cross-sectional imaging. *Eur Radiol*. 2003;13(8):1820–1835.

48. Magid D. Computed tomographic imaging of the musculoskeletal system. Current status. *Radiol Clin North Am*. 1994;32(2):255–274.

49. Watt I. Radiology in the diagnosis and management of bone tumours. *J Bone Joint Surg Br*. 1985;67(4):520–529.

50. Yin ZG, Zhang JB, Kan SL, Wang XG. Diagnosing suspected scaphoid fractures: a systematic review and meta-analysis. *Clin Orthop Relat Res.* 2010;468(3):723–734.

51. Eustace S, Adams J, Assaf A. Emergency MR imaging of orthopedic trauma. Current and future directions. *Radiol Clin North Am.* 1999;37(5):975–994, vi.

52. Newberg AH, Wetzner SM. Bone bruises: their patterns and significance. *Semin Ultrasound CT MR.* 1994;15(5):396–409.

53. Dalinka MK, Meyer S, Kricun ME, Vanel D. Magnetic resonance imaging of the wrist. *Hand Clin.* 1991;7(1):87–98.

54. Horton MG, Timins ME. MR imaging of injuries to the small joints. *Radiol Clin North Am.* 1997;35(3):671–700.

55. Lee SM, Orlinsky M, Chan LS. Safety and effectiveness of portable fluoroscopy in the emergency department for the management of distal extremity fractures. *Ann Emerg Med.* 1994; 24(4):725–730.

56. Choplin RH, Gilula LA, Murphy WA. Fluoroscopic evaluation of skeletal problems. *Skeletal Radiol.* 1981;7(3):191–196.

57. Cohen DM, Garcia CT, Dietrich AM, Hickey RW Jr. Miniature C-arm imaging: an in vitro study of detecting foreign bodies in the emergency department. *Pediatr Emerg Care.* 1997; 13(4):247–249.

58. Wyn T, Jones J, McNinch D, Heacox R. Bedside fluoroscopy for the detection of foreign bodies. *Acad Emerg Med.* 1995;2(11):979–982.

59. Levine MR, Yarnold PR, Michelson EA. A training program in portable fluoroscopy for the detection of glass in soft tissues. *Acad Emerg Med.* 2002;9(8):858–862.

CHAPTER 6

Pediatrics

Ghazala Q. Sharieff, MD

GENERAL PRINCIPLES

Children present with different musculoskeletal injuries than are commonly seen in adults. Because ligamentous attachments are stronger than bony attachments in children, fractures are more prevalent than sprains, dislocations, and strains. This chapter discusses orthopedic injuries that are unique to the pediatric population.

The following terms are typically used in pediatric orthopedics:

- *Physis:* The cartilaginous growth plate that appears lucent on radiographs.
- *Epiphysis:* A secondary ossification center at the ends of long bones that is separated by the physis from the remainder of the bone.
- *Apophysis:* A secondary ossification center at the insertion of tendons onto bones.
- *Diaphysis:* The shaft of a long cortical bone.
- *Metaphysis:* The widened portion at the ends of a bone adjacent to the physis.

Evaluation of the Child

It is important to carefully palpate the uninjured extremity first to obtain the child's confidence. It is also important to determine whether the history that is given by the parents or guardians is consistent with the observed injuries or whether there is a suggestion of child abuse.

A subtle fracture may be difficult to find in an injured child who is crying. On physical examination, palpation of areas that are not fractured will generally hurt less than areas that are injured. Palpation should be gentle, but with enough pressure so as to make a comparison between the normal and abnormal.

Neurologic evaluation of the extremity is often difficult. A generalized withdrawal response can be evaluated by using pinprick. Two-point discrimination testing is also useful in determining distal neurologic function in hand and finger injuries. In addition, wrinkling of the skin when the digit is submerged in warm water for approximately 10 minutes suggests that the nerve is intact. In assessing the vascular status of the extremity, palpation of pulses may be difficult because of the subcutaneous fat, and therefore, it is important to assess and document capillary refill time.

Radiologic Examination

When performing plain radiographs of children, at least two views that are perpendicular to one another must be obtained. In addition, views of the entire extremity, including both joints at the end of the long bones, are integral to the patient's evaluation. Comparison views are invaluable, particularly when looking for a subtle fracture. The growth plates in comparison views taken in exactly the same position should be closely evaluated. Anterior and posterior fat pad signs will help identify subtle fractures (Fig. 6–1). The epiphyseal centers can often be a challenge when reading plain films and therefore it is

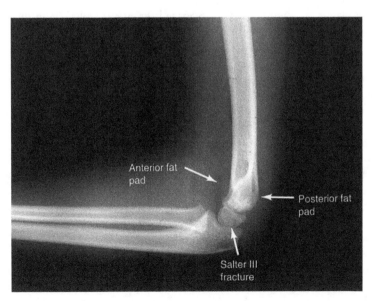

Figure 6–1. A subtle Salter III fracture of the elbow is shown on the lateral view. Notice the anterior fat pad and posterior fat pad.

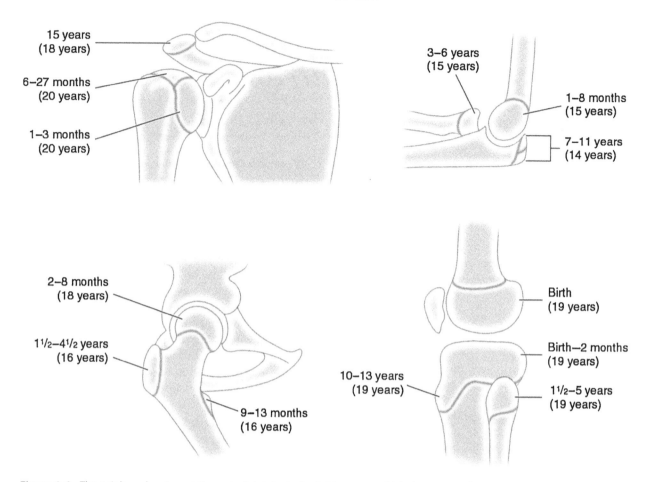

Figure 6–2. The epiphyseal regions at the major joints in the body. The age at which the centers of ossification appear on roentgenograms is shown in months or years. The age at which union occurs is shown in parentheses.

imperative that the practitioner knows when these centers begin to appear (Fig. 6–2).

Salter–Harris Classification

The Salter–Harris classification refers to physeal fractures (Figs. 6–3 and 6–4). This classification is a radiologic classification and is not anatomic, or related to the mechanism or severity of injury.

A *Salter I* fracture is a fracture through the physis. These fractures may be displaced or nondisplaced; however, there is no extension proximally or distally. A nondisplaced Salter I fracture may not be obvious on x-ray acutely; therefore, clinical suspicion is the key to making the diagnosis. Patients will typically present with circumferential tenderness along the physeal area. These fractures commonly occur in the distal tibia and fibula, and may present with the same mechanism as a sprained ankle without any ligamentous tenderness. In addition, these fractures occur in the hands and fingers of children.

A *Salter II* fracture is a fracture through the physis that continues on into the metaphysis. These fractures account for the majority of all physeal fractures. Undisplaced fractures generally do not cause growth disturbances.

In a *Salter III* fracture, the fracture extends through the physis and continues into the epiphysis. These fractures typically occur in children who are older with a partially closed physis. These fractures should be referred early to have careful and accurate reduction.

Salter IV fractures extend through the physis and into both the epiphysis and the metaphysis. Salter IV fractures need accurate reduction to prevent bone bridging between the epiphysis and the metaphysis because these fractures involve fracture through the physis and extend both proximally and distally. This fracture and the subsequent bridging can lead to partial or complete growth arrest.

Salter V fractures are crush injuries of the physis and are the most serious type of fracture. Fortunately, Salter V fractures only account for 1% of physeal fractures. Salter V fractures may not be clearly visible at the time of injury and are often diagnosed in retrospect when growth arrest is noted. Comparison views of the contralateral limb may be helpful in making the diagnosis acutely.

A major concern with fractures involving the physis is the potential for growth arrest or growth retardation. Salter I and II fractures have the lowest risk of growth disturbance, whereas Salter IV and V fractures have the most

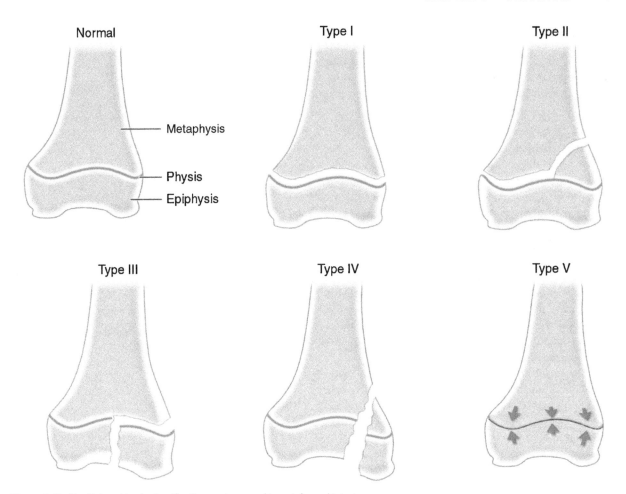

Figure 6–3. The Salter–Harris classification system used in epiphyseal injuries.

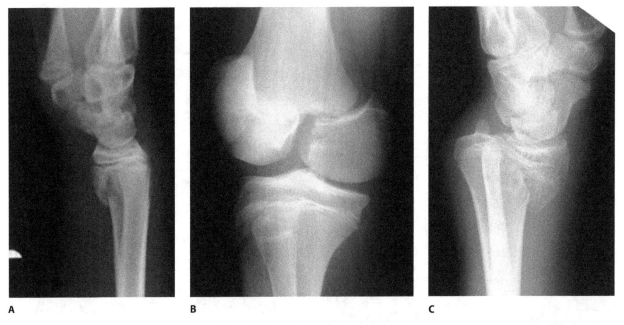

Figure 6–4. **A.** Salter II fracture of the distal radius. **B.** Salter III medial femoral condyle fracture. **C.** Salter IV distal radius fracture.

significant likelihood of growth disturbance. Fractures in children can result in subsequent disturbance of growth, and this is not confined to only those fractures involving the growth plates. In general, the greater the mechanism and force generated, the greater the likelihood of growth disturbance, regardless of the fracture type.

Fractures Unique to Children

The bone in children is more porous than that of adults, and thus fractures may not appear as readily. The bones of children undergo greater plastic deformation, and micro-fractures may occur that are not seen in adults. These microfractures may not be visualized on routine x-rays, the patient may present with tenderness, and the mechanism may suggest significant trauma to the bone or joint, but the radiograph will appear normal.

Torus fractures (buckle) involve a failure of bone with a compressive mechanism. These fractures occur over the metaphyseal region (Fig. 6–5). Torus or buckle fractures are very common, stable, and heal readily when immobilized. Complications are quite rare.

Greenstick fractures are incomplete fractures that result in a fracture through the tension side of a bone undergoing a deforming stress (Figs. 6–6 and 6–7). These fractures are typically angulated and may require conversion to a complete fracture to correct the deformity.

Bowing occurs when the bone undergoes plastic deformation after an injury and does not recoil back to its original position. The fibula and ulna are most commonly involved. If there is a fracture of the adjacent bone, bowing can inhibit reduction of the fractured bone.

A minimally displaced fracture may result in serious associated soft-tissue injury and visceral injuries caused by displacement of the bone during the fracture mechanism. Thus, a minimally displaced pelvic fracture may be

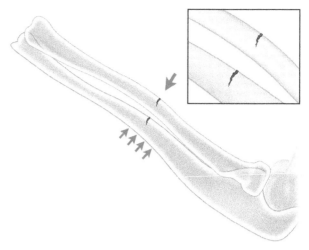

Figure 6–6. Schematic of the mechanism that causes a green-stick fracture.

associated with a more significant bladder, sacral plexus, or urethral injury than is seen with a similarly displaced fracture in an adult.

Joint Injuries in Children

Traumatic joint dislocations are quite unusual in children with the exception of the patellofemoral joint. The ligaments are attached to the epiphysis and are stronger than the bone. Excessive force on a child's joint usually results in epiphyseal injury, rather than ligamentous injury or dislocation.

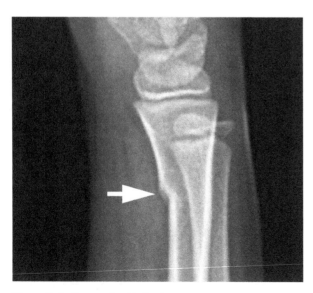

Figure 6–5. Torus or buckle fracture.

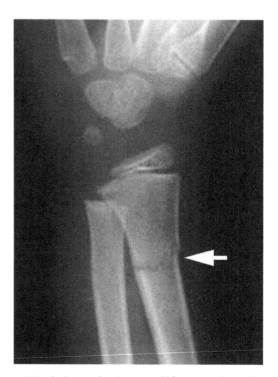

Figure 6–7. An incomplete (greenstick) fracture is shown through the distal radius. Notice the bowing of the ulna.

THE SPINE

Neck Injuries

The level of cervical spine injury varies with age because of the effect of the relatively large head of the child and ligamentous laxity. Therefore, when injury occurs in young children, high torques and shear forces are typically applied to the C1 to C3 region.[2] In children, the most common cause of injury is falls, whereas in adolescents, sports injuries and motor vehicle accidents become more common. Leonard et al. identified eight factors associated with cervical spine injury: altered mental status, focal neurologic findings, neck pain, torticollis, substantial torso injury, conditions predisposing to cervical spine injury, diving, and high-risk motor vehicle crash. Furthermore, the presence of one or more factors was 98% (95% confidence interval, 96%–99%) sensitive and 26% (95% confidence interval, 23%–29%) specific for cervical spine injury.[3] Although C-spine injuries account for less than 1% of children seen in emergency department (ED) trauma cases, the mortality rate in children younger than 8 years may be as high as 60%.[3]

Pseudosubluxation

The extreme laxity of the cervical ligaments can increase the vertebral override of adjacent vertebrae of children younger than 8 years. This finding, known as pseudosubluxation, is most commonly found at the C2 to C3 level (Fig. 6–8). To distinguish pseudosubluxation from true subluxation,

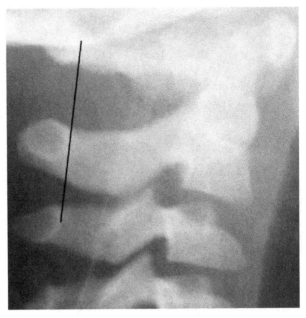

Figure 6–9. Posterior cervical line of Swischuk. (Reproduced with permission from Yamamoto LG. Cervical spine malalignment—true or pseudosubluxation? In: Yamamoto LG, Inaba AS, DiMauro R, eds. *Radiology Cases in Pediatric Emergency Medicine*. Vol. 1, Case 5. Honolulu: University of Hawaii John A. Burns School of Medicine, Department of Pediatrics, 1994. http://www.hawaii.edu/medicine/pediatrics/pemxray/v1c05.html. Accessed March 28, 2018)

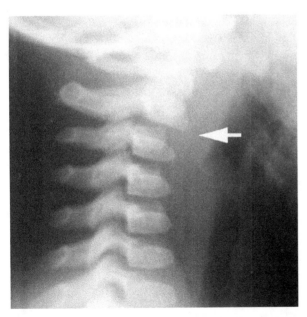

Figure 6–8. Pseudosubluxation. (Reproduced with permission from Yamamoto LG. Cervical spine malalignment—true or pseudosubluxation? In: Yamamoto LG, Inaba AS, DiMauro R, eds. *Radiology Cases in Pediatric Emergency Medicine*. Vol. 1, Case 5. Honolulu: University of Hawaii John A. Burns School of Medicine, Department of Pediatrics, 1994. http://www.hawaii.edu/medicine/pediatrics/pemxray/v1c05.html. Accessed March 28, 2018)

Swischuk defined the posterior cervical line (Fig. 6–9).[4] This line is drawn by connecting the anterior aspects of the spinous processes of C1 and C3. If the anterior aspect of the spinous process of C2 misses this line by 2 mm or more, a true subluxation or hangman's fracture of the neural arches of C2 should be suspected.

Spinal Cord Injury without Radiographic Abnormality

In addition to vertebral injuries seen on plain x-rays, children may also suffer spinal cord injury without radiographic abnormality (SCIWORA). These injuries cause cord traction or ischemia without anatomic defects. Mechanisms that result in SCIWORA include spinal cord traction, spinal cord concussion, vertebral artery spasm, hyperextension with inward bulging of the interlaminar ligaments, and flexion compression of the cord.

In a study by Cirek et al.,[5] the incidence of SCIWORA was 6%. However, other studies show ranges between 18% and 38%, with most cases occurring in children younger than 8 years.[6] The upper cervical spine is involved in up to 80% of cases.[7] Most cases of SCIWORA present with some type of neurologic symptom, most commonly, paresthesias and partial cord syndromes. However, delayed onset of neurologic deficit and complete cord transection can occur.

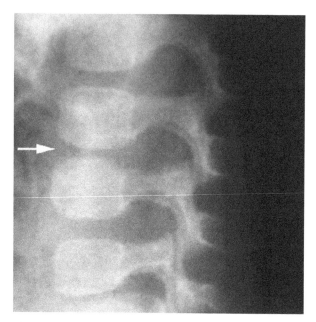

Figure 6–10. Diskitis. Note the narrowed disk spaces between L3 and L4 (*arrow*). (Used with permission from Michael P. D'Alessandro, MD. www.pediatricimaging.org.)

Treatment of suspected spinal cord injuries with methylprednisolone is no longer recommended.

Diskitis

Diskitis is inflammation or infection of an intervertebral disk space or a vertebral end plate. The lumbar spine is typically involved and the most common age of presentation is between 4 and 10 years. Patients present with nonspecific complaints such as refusal to walk or back pain with inability to flex the lower back. Fever is present in less than 50% of cases. On examination, percussion pain over the affected area helps localize the site of involvement. Laboratory data are not always helpful as the white blood cell (WBC) count and blood cultures may be normal; however, the C-reactive protein (CRP) and sedimentation rate are typically elevated. *Staphylococcus aureus* is the organism that is most commonly involved. Although, initial x-rays of the spine may be negative, the characteristic finding is of a narrowed disk space in the involved area (Fig. 6–10). However, if plain films are nondiagnostic, an MRI can help localize the lesion. Treatment involves IV antibiotics and bed rest. Some experts also recommend immobilization of the spine.

UPPER EXTREMITY

Clavicle Fractures

The clavicle is the most commonly injured bone during delivery (Fig. 6–11). Although there is a higher incidence following deliveries that require oxytocin, instrumental extraction, maneuvers for dystocia, or prolonged

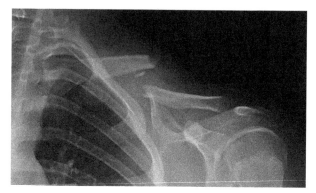

Figure 6–11. Clavicle fracture.

second-stage labor, clavicle fractures can occur during normal deliveries and Cesarean sections. In older children, fractures usually result from falls or direct blows, and most commonly involve the middle third of the bone. The majority of these fractures can be managed without orthopedic referral. Fractures of the clavicle are treated with an arm sling, which is more comfortable than a figure-of-eight splint.

Elbow

The elbow is a common site for fractures in children. The typical history is a fall on the outstretched arm with hyperextension at the elbow and resultant injury to the distal humerus.

Radiologic evaluation of a child's elbow is made more complicated due to the six ossification centers around the elbow, which appear at different ages. Comparison views of the opposite elbow should be obtained if there is any question about a possible fracture. Knowledge of the timing of the ossification centers about the elbow aids in determining whether a small piece of bone represents an avulsion fracture or an ossification center (Figs. 6–12 and 6–13).

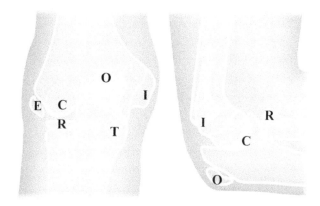

Figure 6–12. Ossification centers of the elbow. C, capitellum (1–8 mo); R, radial head (3–5 yr); I, internal epicondyle (5–7 yr); T, trochlea (7–9 yr); O, olecranon (8–11 yr); E, external epicondyle (11–14 yr).

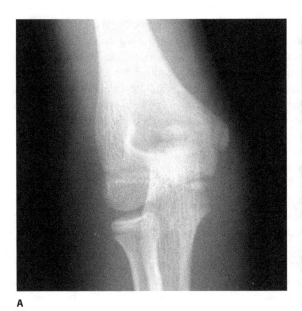
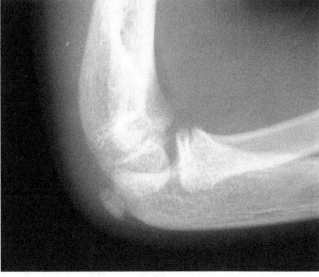

A

B

Figure 6–13. Normal (**A**) anteroposterior (AP) and (**B**) lateral radiographs of the elbow of a 10-year-old. As would be expected, all ossification centers are visible except the external (lateral) epicondyle.

"CRITOE"	
Capitellum	1–8 mo
Radial head	3–5 yr
Internal (medial) epicondyle	5–7 yr
Trochlea	7–9 yr
Olecranon	8–11 yr
External (lateral) epicondyle	11–14 yr

In general, four radiographic views should be obtained to accurately assess the elbow in children. These four views obtained in the flexed elbow include the anteroposterior (AP) view of the forearm, AP view of the humerus, lateral view of the forearm, and lateral view of the humerus.

Supracondylar Fractures

Horizontal fractures of the distal humerus are divided into two broad categories: supracondylar and transcondylar. Supracondylar fractures are further subdivided, based on the position of the distal humeral segment, and also on the type of injury—extension type (posterior displacement) or flexion type (anterior displacement) (Fig. 6–14). Transcondylar fractures involve the joint capsule and are also of the extension or flexion type.

Supracondylar fractures are generally extra-articular, account for 50% to 70% of all elbow fractures, and are most commonly seen in children between the ages of 3 and 11 years. The most common mechanism encountered is a fall on the outstretched arm with the elbow in extension

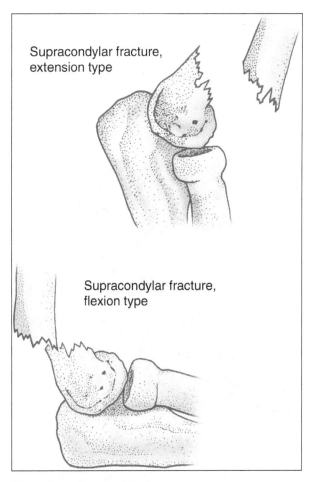

Supracondylar fracture, extension type

Supracondylar fracture, flexion type

Figure 6–14. Supracondylar fractures.

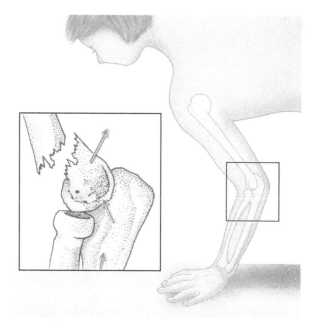

Figure 6–15. Mechanism of injury for supracondylar fractures in children.

(Fig. 6–15). In children, the surrounding anterior capsule and collateral ligaments are stronger than the bone, and fractures rather than ligamentous tears usually result. Extension-type supracondylar fractures account for 95% to 98% of all supracondylar fractures, and 20% to 30% of supracondylar fractures will have little or no displacement. In children, 25% of supracondylar fractures are of the greenstick type. Radiographic diagnosis in these cases may be exceedingly difficult.

There are three types of supracondylar extension fractures. Type I supracondylar fractures are nondisplaced or minimally displaced. Type II supracondylar fractures have angulation of the distal fragment–posterior displacement with extension-type injuries and anterior displacement with flexion-type injuries. Type III supracondylar fractures involve fractures of both cortices and are completely displaced.

Examination. With nondisplaced fractures, there may be little swelling (Fig. 6–16A). When displaced, the deformity is usually more obvious, and the distal humeral fragment can often be palpated posteriorly and superiorly due to the pull of the triceps muscle (Fig. 6–17A). As swelling increases, this injury can be confused with a posterior dislocation of the elbow resulting from the prominence of the olecranon and the presence of a posterior concavity. In addition, the involved forearm may appear shorter when compared with the uninvolved side.

Imaging. Routine views must include AP and lateral projections in comparison with the uninvolved extremity in children. Oblique views may also be helpful (Fig. 6–17B).

Subtle changes, such as the presence of a posterior fat pad or an abnormal *anterior humeral line*, may be the only radiographic clues to the presence of a fracture (Figs. 6–16B and 6–18). The anterior humeral line (Fig. 6–18) is a line drawn on a lateral radiograph along the anterior surface of the humerus through the elbow. Normally, this line transects the middle third of the capitellum. With a supracondylar extension fracture, this line will either transect the anterior third of the capitellum or pass entirely anterior to it

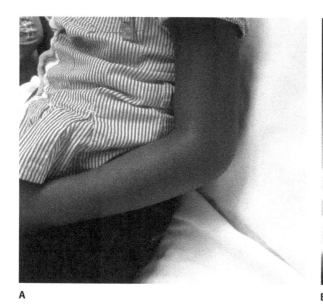

A

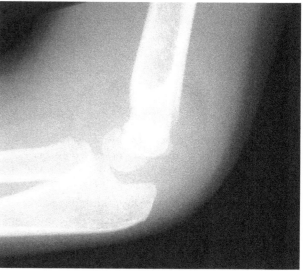

B

Figure 6–16. Nondisplaced occult supracondylar fracture. **A.** Appearance of the elbow reveals edema without deformity. **B.** Lateral radiograph with fat pads and a normal anterior humeral line.

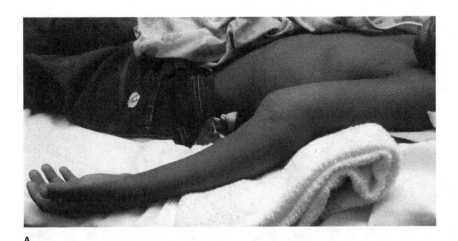

A

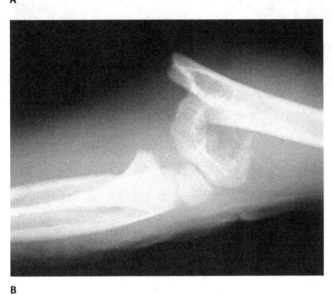

B

Figure 6-17. Displaced supracondylar fracture. **A.** Gross deformity of the elbow. **B.** Displaced fracture is evident on the lateral radiograph.

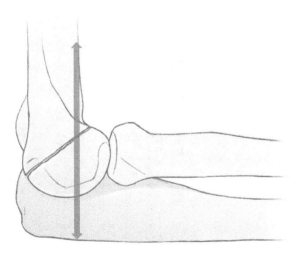 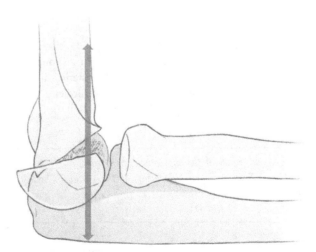

Figure 6-18. The anterior humeral line is a line drawn on the lateral radiograph along the anterior surface of the humerus through the elbow. Normally this line transects through the middle of the capitellum. With an extension fracture of the supracondylar region, this line will either transect the anterior third of the capitellum or pass entirely anterior to it.

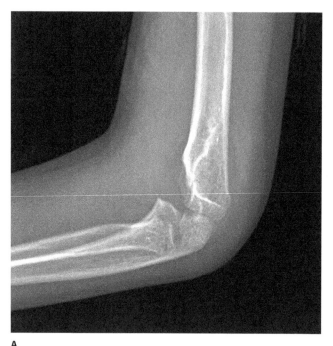
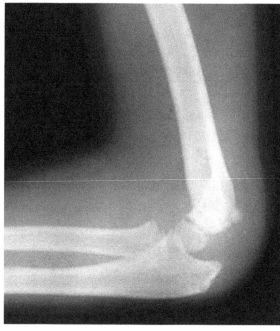

A   **B**

Figure 6–19. Supracondylar epiphyseal fractures detected by noting an abnormal anterior humeral line. **A.** Extension type. **B.** Flexion type.

(Fig. 6–19A). The anterior humeral line of a flexion injury passes posterior to the capitellum (Fig. 6–19B).

Another diagnostic aid in evaluating radiographs of suspected supracondylar fractures in children is to determine the carrying angle. The intersection of a line drawn through the midshaft of the humerus and a line through the midshaft of the ulna on an AP extension view determines the carrying angle (Fig. 6–20). Normally, the carrying angle is between 0 and 12 degrees. Traumatic or asymmetric carrying angles of greater than 12 degrees are often associated with fractures.

Elevation of the fat pad in the coronoid fossa (anterior fat pad sign) and olecranon fossa (posterior fat pad sign) occurring due to an effusion from trauma or an infection is an important feature to investigate. A posterior fat pad is always pathologic and raises the index of suspicion for a fracture. An anteriorly displaced fat pad, the "sail sign" may also be an indication of an occult fracture.

Axiom: *A posterior fat pad sign in the child or adolescent indicates a fracture or dislocation of the elbow. Therapy must be initiated until fracture or dislocation is absolutely ruled out.*

Associated Injuries. Distal humeral fractures are frequently associated with neurovascular complications, even in the absence of displacement. The most commonly injured structures are the median nerve and the brachial artery. Initially, document the presence and strength of the

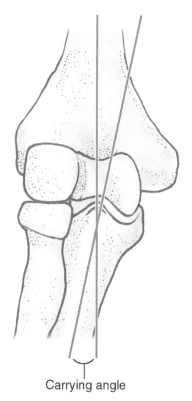

Carrying angle

Figure 6–20. The carrying angle demonstrated by a line drawn through the midshaft of the ulna and another line through the midshaft of the humerus. The normal carrying angle is between 0 and 12 degrees. A carrying angle of greater than 12 degrees is often associated with fractures of the distal humerus.

radial, ulnar, and brachial pulses. The presence of a pulse, however, does not exclude a significant arterial injury. Also examine and document the motor and sensory components of the radial, ulnar, and median nerves. The three types of nerve injuries are contusion, partial severance, and complete severance.

Caution: Subsequent manipulation may result in serious neurovascular compromise.

Brachial artery compromise is not an uncommon complication and can lead to compartment syndrome, which in turn leads to diminished perfusion and loss of function of the muscles within the forearm. An intact radial pulse at the wrist has no merit in ruling out the evolution of a compartment syndrome or in evaluating the perfusion to the forearm.

Treatment. Nondisplaced (type I) fractures are treated with cast immobilization. The extremity is placed in a posterior long-arm splint extending from the axilla to a point just proximal to the metacarpal heads. The splint should encircle three-fourths of the circumference of the extremity (Appendix A–9). The elbow should be between 90 and 100 degrees of flexion. The distal pulses should be checked and, if absent, the elbow is to be extended 5 to 15 degrees or until the pulses return. A sling for support and ice to reduce swelling are applied.

Although nondisplaced fractures are rarely associated with complications, even a radiographically occult fracture can result in compartment syndrome, a pulse deficit, or neuropathy. Only the most stable fractures with minimal swelling after a period of 6 to 12 hours of observation can be safely discharged. Consultation with an orthopedic surgeon who will take responsibility for the care of the patient should be obtained before the patient leaves the ED.

All displaced fractures require emergent consultation with an experienced orthopedic surgeon and admission for neurovascular monitoring. Manipulative reductions are at times difficult to perform and fraught with complications. Emergent reduction by the emergency specialist is indicated only when the displaced fracture is associated with vascular compromise, which immediately threatens the viability of the extremity.

Definitive management of flexion type II fractures includes reduction and casting in extension. Percutaneous pinning may be necessary. Closed reduction and pinning has been found to be effective for the treatment of pediatric supracondylar humerus fractures.[13,14] Extension type II fractures are also treated with reduction and percutaneous pinning.

Extension type III fractures often require open reduction and pinning because of difficulty with closed reduction attempts. Flexion type III supracondylar fractures may also require open reduction and percutaneous pinning.

Open reduction with internal fixation is indicated under the following circumstances:

- Inability to achieve a satisfactory closed reduction
- Complicating fractures of the forearm
- Inability to maintain a closed reduction
- Vascular compromise

Axiom: *A cylinder cast should never be applied initially on any supracondylar fracture.*

Delayed swelling with subsequent neurovascular compromise is frequently noted following displaced supracondylar fractures, and therefore, admission for close monitoring is recommended.

Complications. Complications of supracondylar fractures include neurovascular injuries, compartment syndrome, ulnar nerve palsy, joint stiffness, and cubitus varus and valgus deformities (because of malposition of the distal humeral fragment after reduction). Diminished range of motion may be secondary to inadequate reduction or callus formation within the joint. The median nerve and radial nerve are injured commonly. When the anterior interosseous nerve is injured, there is loss of thumb interphalangeal joint flexion and the index distal interphalangeal joint flexion.

Medial Epicondylar Fractures

Epicondylar fractures are most commonly seen in children (Fig. 6–21). Medial epicondylar fractures are seen more often than lateral epicondyle fractures.

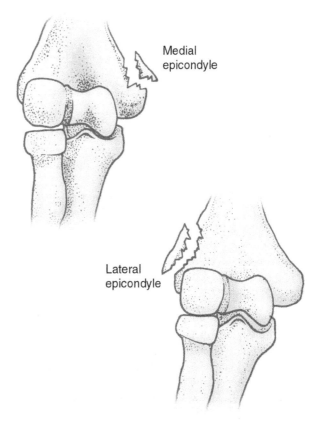

Figure 6–21. Epicondylar fractures.

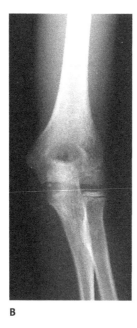

A   **B**

Figure 6–22. A medial epicondylar fracture in a child. Notice the displacement in (**A**) that may be difficult to recognize without the comparison view of the uninjured elbow (**B**).

The ossification center for the medial epicondyle appears by age 5 to 7 years and fuses to the distal humerus by age 20 years. Medial epicondylar displacement as an isolated injury is uncommon. More often seen is the palpable avulsion fracture associated with a posterolateral dislocation of the elbow (Fig. 6–22). The typical age of presentation is 7 to 15 years, with medial epicondyle fractures accounting for 10% of elbow fractures in children.

There are three mechanisms commonly associated with fractures of the medial epicondyle:

- The more common avulsion fracture is associated with childhood or adolescent posterior dislocations. This fracture is rarely associated with posterior dislocations in those older than 20 years.
- The flexor pronator tendon is attached to the medial epicondylar ossification center. Repeated valgus stress on the elbow may result in a fracture with fragment displacement distally. This is commonly seen in adolescent baseball players and is called "Little League elbow."
- Isolated medial epicondylar fractures in adults are usually due to a direct blow.

If this fracture is associated with a posterior dislocation, the elbow will be in flexion, and there will be a prominence of the olecranon. The elbow dislocation is reduced (see Chapter 14) and fracture fragments assessed. If the epicondyle is within the joint, open reduction is indicated. Isolated fractures produce localized pain over the medial epicondyle. Pain is increased with flexion of the elbow and the wrist, or with pronation of the forearm.

When assessing this fracture, the physician must examine and document ulnar nerve function before initiating therapy. Displaced fragments may migrate and become intra-articular.

Caution: Radiographically, if the fragment has migrated to the joint line, it should be considered intra-articular.

Fragments that are displaced less than 5 mm, as determined by measuring the clear space between the fracture fragment and the humerus, can be immobilized in a long-arm posterior splint (Appendix A–9). The elbow should be flexed with the forearm pronated and the wrist held in a flexed position. The splint should remain in place, and the patient is referred. Fragments of 5 mm or more are often controversial, with some experts advocating for open reduction and internal fixation and others supporting an initial trial of closed management. The individual case should therefore be discussed with the consulting orthopedist.

Medial Condyle Fractures

In young children, medial condylar fractures are often difficult to diagnose radiographically, especially if the injury occurs before the trochlea ossifies. For this reason, it is easy to assume that the fracture is of the medical epicondyle. In older children, a metaphyseal fragment may be visualized, and this helps identify condylar involvement. Comparison views of the uninjured elbow may be helpful in differentiating a fracture from a secondary ossification center.

One of the most serious complications of a medial condyle fracture is bleeding and swelling of the closed fascial space leading to the development of compartment syndrome. Fractures with more than 2 mm of displacement generally require surgical fixation.

Lateral Condyle Fractures

Lateral condyle fractures frequently require open reduction and fixation as they are transphyseal and intra-articular. These fractures typically occur from a fall onto an outstretched arm. Oblique views of the elbow may help determine whether the fracture is displaced. The lateral epicondyle is the last ossification center to appear. One classification of lateral condyle fractures describes the fractures as nondisplaced (<2 mm), minimally displaced (2–4 mm), or displaced (>4 mm).

The management of minimally displaced lateral condyle fractures is controversial—casting, percutaneous fixation, and open reduction have all been used with success. However, displaced lateral epicondyle fractures should undergo open reduction and pinning. Complications of lateral epicondyle fractures include cubitus valgus deformity, lateral transposition of the forearm, arthritis because of joint capsule and articular disruption, ulnar nerve palsy, and overgrowth with subsequent cubitus varus deformity.

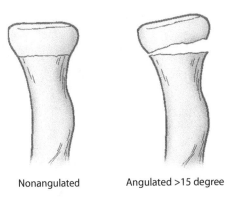

Nonangulated   Angulated >15 degree

Figure 6–23. Epiphyseal radial head fractures.

Radial Head and Neck Fractures

Epiphyseal fractures of the radial neck are classified on the basis of the degree of angulation (Fig. 6–23). When the epiphysis is not yet ossified and one suspects a nondisplaced radial head fracture, look at the *radiocapitellar line* (Fig. 6–24). A line drawn through the midportion of the radius normally passes through the center of the capitellum on the lateral view of the elbow. In a subtle fracture at the epiphysis of the radial head, this line will be displaced away from the center of the capitellum. This may be the only finding suggesting a fracture in a child.

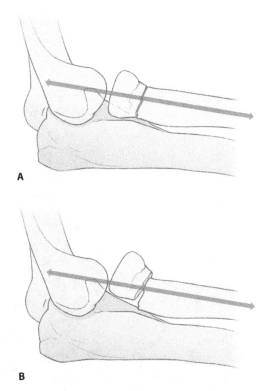

A

B

Figure 6–24. A. The radiocapitellar line drawn through the center of the radius should pass through the center of the capitellum of the humerus on the lateral view. **B.** It is useful in making the diagnosis in patients with a fracture of the radial neck in whom the epiphysis has not closed.

Radial head and neck fractures often require oblique views for radiographic visualization. Impact fractures of the neck are best seen on the lateral projection. The presence of a bulging anterior fat pad or a posterior fat pad sign is indicative of significant joint capsule distension.

Fractures with angulation of less than 15 degrees are best treated with immobilization for 2 weeks in a long-arm posterior splint (Appendix A–9). This should be followed by active exercises with a sling for support. Remodeling will generally correct this degree of angulation. With angulation of greater than 15 degrees, the arm should be immobilized in a posterior splint and the patient admitted for reduction under general anesthesia. Reduction attempts in children without good anesthesia are difficult to perform and fraught with complications.

Angulation of greater than 60 degrees is regarded as complete displacement and usually requires open reduction. Limited success has been achieved with manipulative reductions.

Osteochondritis Dissecans

Osteochondritis dissecans occurs in young athletes who overload and hyperextend the elbow. Gymnasts, who are constantly loading their elbows as they balance on beams and high bars, are particularly susceptible to this condition. The symptoms that occur are locking, giving way, and crepitus on range of motion. Radiographs may reveal a loose body within the joint or demonstrable osteochondritis dissecans. MRI is often helpful in suspicious cases when the x-ray is negative.

Treatment is conservative unless there are loose bodies within the joint that require mechanical removal. Conservative treatment for acute exacerbations consists of splinting the elbow for 3 to 4 days, anti-inflammatory medications, and the application of heat. If mechanical symptoms occur and persist, arthroscopic intervention to remove and debride loose bodies is necessary.

Little League Elbow

Little League elbow occurs when young throwers, typically between the ages of 9 and 11 years, have repetitive microtrauma at the ossification center along the radial head. Osteochondral changes in the capitellum, premature proximal radial epiphyseal closure, and fragmentation of the medial epicondyle are collectively known as Little League elbow. The condition is predominantly a result of forces applied during a late phase of throwing causing a valgus strain of the elbow. Comparison views on x-rays show that the apophysis has become separated. Bony fragments can ultimately lodge in the joint and require open reduction and removal. Loss of extension occurs as a result of tightening of the ulnar collateral ligament, producing pain and varus stress. Ulnar neuritis may present because of subluxation or compression of the fascial planes. Arthroscopy may be required, particularly if a bone fragment is noted. Treatment includes rest, ice, and the institution of routine stretching and range-of-motion exercises prior to overhand pitching.

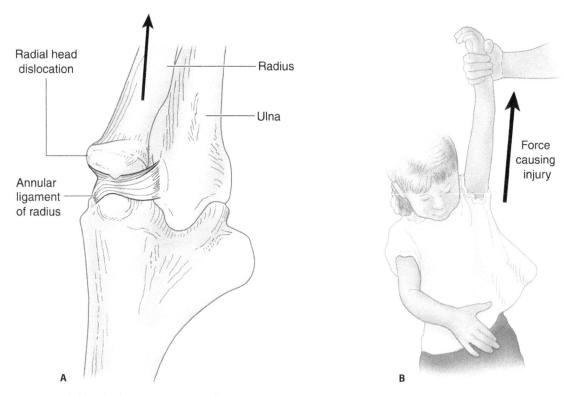

Figure 6-25. Radial head subluxation (nursemaid's elbow). **A.** Anatomy. **B.** Mechanism.

Radial Head Subluxation (Nursemaid's Elbow)

Nursemaid's elbow (radial head subluxation) is a common orthopedic injury occurring in early childhood. The peak incidence is in the toddler years; however, the condition does occur in the first year of life and has been described to occur as late as 31 years of age.   The annular ligament provides support for the radial head, maintaining the head in its normal relationship with the humerus and the ulna. In children, there is little structural support between the radius and the humerus. With sudden traction of the hand or the forearm, nursemaid's elbow occurs when a parent pulls a child up by the arm to prevent a fall; the annular ligament is pulled over the radial head and is interposed between the radius and the capitellum (Fig. 6-25).

Children with nursemaid's elbow present because of disuse of the affected arm and will be noted to hold the arm at their side with the forearm in a pronated position (Fig. 6-26). It is important to note that patients with nursemaid's elbow do not have swelling, warmth, or ecchymosis about the elbow. Radiographs should be performed prior to reduction attempts in cases in which aspects of the history (e.g., witnessed direct trauma to the upper extremity) and examination findings (e.g., swelling, bruising, warmth over the joint) suggest that infection or fracture is more likely than radial head subluxation. Patients who present with a history and examination findings consistent with nursemaid's elbow need not undergo radiography prior to reduction attempts.

Treatment. Two different methods are commonly used for reducing a nursemaid's elbow. Prospective studies comparing the two methods reveal that the hyperpronation technique has a higher initial success rate (95%) than the supination/flexion technique (77%).[16-18]

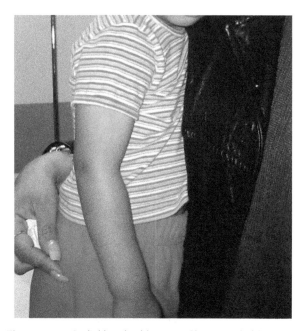

Figure 6-26. Radial head subluxation. The arm is held in slight flexion and pronation. Any movement from this position is resisted by the patient.

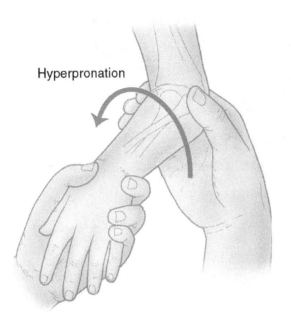

Figure 6–27. Hyperpronation technique for radial head subluxation reduction.

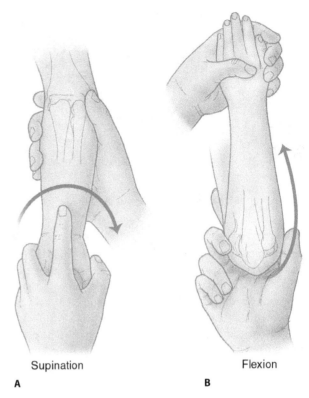

Supination   Flexion

A   B

Figure 6–28. Supination/flexion technique for radial head subluxation reduction.

Hyperpronation Technique. The hyperpronation method involves the examiner cradling the child's elbow with one hand (with thumb or forefingers overlying the radial head) while the other hand is used to hyperpronate the child's forearm by holding and turning the child's hand into a hyperpronated position. With successful reduction, a "click" will be felt about the child's elbow by the examiner (Fig. 6–27 and Video 6–1).

Supination/Flexion Technique. The supination/flexion technique involves the examiner cradling the child's elbow with one hand (again, with thumb or forefingers over the radial head) and supinating the patient's hand completely. The examiner then fully flexes the child's elbow by bringing the supinated hand up toward the shoulder. With successful reduction, a "click" will be felt near the elbow (Fig. 6–28 and Video 6–2).

Regardless of which reduction technique is used, the child will typically begin to use the arm normally within 10 to 15 minutes. A failed reduction attempt should be followed by a second attempt using either the same or an alternate technique. The second attempt often meets with success. If the reduction is unsuccessful after two or three attempts, radiographs of the upper extremity should be obtained to help exclude fracture or other pathology as the cause of the child's symptoms.

The child with a successfully reduced nursemaid's elbow does not need specific follow-up with the primary caregiver unless symptoms (pain or disuse of the arm) return. Parents and caregivers should be cautioned about refraining from any activity that involves pulling on the child's arm, as the condition recurs in approximately 25% of children who have experienced at least one episode.[19]

A patient who does not respond to nursemaid's elbow reduction attempts will require close primary care follow-up and possibly orthopedic consultation.

Forearm
Radius and Ulna Shaft Fractures
The most common childhood fractures are those involving the radius and ulna (Fig. 6–29 and Video 6-3). In most children with forearm fractures, both bones are usually fractured. When only one forearm bone is fractured, the emergency physician should look for evidence of dislocation of the proximal or distal radioulnar joints. Monteggia fractures involving the proximal ulna associated with a radial head dislocation are sometimes missed. The radial head should always be in good alignment with the capitellum. Galeazzi fractures involve a distal radius fracture associated with a distal radioulnar dislocation. For more information on these fractures, the reader is referred to Chapter 13.

Wrist
Distal Radius and Ulna Fractures
The distal radial physis is the most commonly fractured growth plate. Salter II injuries are the most common, accounting for 58% of these fractures.[20]

Ulnar physeal injuries are less common and occur in only 5% of distal forearm fractures. The thick, triangular fibrocartilage complex protects the distal ulnar physis, but

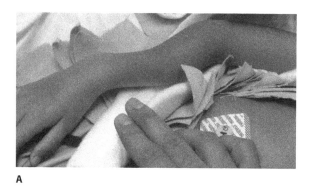
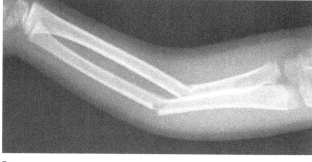

A   **B**

Figure 6–29. Both bone forearm fracture. **A.** Clinical photo. **B.** Radiograph.

concentrates force on the attachment to the styloid. Unfortunately, distal ulnar growth arrest occurs in approximately 55% of these fractures when they are associated with distal radius fractures. Salter I injuries are the most common pattern occurring in half of patients. Approximately 70% to 80% of the longitudinal growth of the ulna comes from the distal physis. Thus, growth arrest can cause significant shortening as well as a milder radial shortening because of a tethering effect.

Displaced or angulated distal forearm fractures in children, unlike adults, have a great ability to remodel. They rarely lead to dysfunction. Thus, angulation of a distal forearm fracture of at least 20 degrees can be accepted in the younger child, especially those younger than 10 years. In children with minimally angulated fractures of the distal radius, Boutis et al. found that the use of a removable splint was as effective as a cast with respect to the recovery of physical function. In addition, the devices were comparable in terms of the maintenance of fracture stability and the occurrence of complications.

Distal Radius Epiphyseal Separation—Extension Type. This injury usually results from a fall on an outstretched hand with forced dorsiflexion of the hand and epiphyseal plate. The typical result is a Salter I or II fracture of the epiphysis (Fig. 6–30). Growth arrests are uncommon but may occur, and therefore, these fractures require orthopedic referral. It is important to exclude the diagnosis of epiphyseal slip as these fractures require emergent reduction (Fig. 6–31).

In treating these injuries, more angulation and displacement can be accepted. Reduction is recommended for angulation of greater than 25 degrees or displacement of greater than 25% of the radial diameter. Immobilization is accomplished by one of two means. For stable fractures, a short-arm AP splint should be applied with the forearm in supination and the wrist in slight extension. For unstable fractures, immobilization in a long-arm AP splint (Appendix A–10) is recommended with the forearm in supination and the wrist in flexion. Some authors advocate placing the wrist in extension. Others believe that extension of the wrist should be avoided as it places a volar distracting force against the fracture. Therefore, an orthopedic

consultation by the treating clinician is recommended. If the fracture is unstable after a closed reduction, pin fixation or open reduction with internal fixation is advocated.

LOWER EXTREMITY

Pelvis
Iliac Crest Apophysitis
Iliac crest apophysitis is an overuse injury commonly seen in runners and hockey, soccer, and football players. The main symptom is pain over the affected iliac crest that is worsened with running. Plain radiographs are normal. Treatment is conservative and includes anti-inflammatory medication.

Hip
Developmental (Congenital) Hip Dislocation
Developmental hip dislocation, previously known as congenital hip dislocation, is an intra-articular displacement

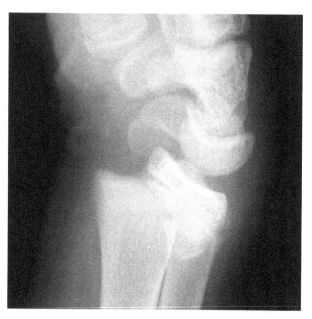

Figure 6–30. Salter II fracture of the distal radius in a child. This fracture requires reduction in the emergency department (ED).

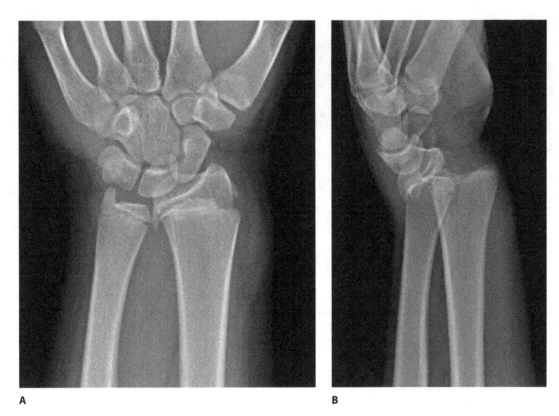

A   **B**

Figure 6–31. Fracture of the radial epiphysis with displacement. ***A.*** AP. ***B.*** Lateral.

of the femoral head from its normal position within the acetabulum. This leads to an interruption in the normal development of the joint occurring before or shortly after birth. At birth, the acetabular fossa is shallow with the superior portion of the acetabulum poorly developed, offering little resistance to the upward movement of the head by muscle pull or weight bearing. This leads to a condition called *congenital subluxation of the femoral head*, in which the femoral head is displaced laterally and proximally and articulates with the outer portion of the acetabulum. In *complete dislocation* of the hip, the femoral head is located completely outside the acetabulum and rests against the lateral wall of the ilium. Later, a false acetabulum forms with a capsule interposed between the femoral head and the ilium.

In the normal infant, one sees folds in the groin, below the buttocks, and several along the thigh, which are symmetrical. In subluxation or dislocation, these folds will be asymmetrical. When the examiner places the infant on the table, the pelvis and the limb on the affected side will be pulled proximally by muscle action. This proximal displacement causes apparent shortening of the limb.

The *Ortolani click test* is performed as a routine part of the examination on infants before 1 year of age. In the normal infant, when the hip is flexed 90 degrees and the thigh is abducted, the lateral aspect of both thighs will nearly touch the table. In subluxation or dislocation, abduction is restricted and the involved hip is unable to be abducted as far as the opposite one, producing an audible or palpable click as the femoral head slips over the acetabular rim (Fig. 6–32).

The *Barlow provocative test* is performed with the newborn positioned supine and the hips flexed to 90 degrees. The leg is then gently adducted while posteriorly directed pressure is placed on the knee. A palpable clunk or sensation of movement is felt as the femoral head exits the acetabulum posteriorly. The Ortolani and Barlow maneuvers are performed one hip at a time.

Repeat examination of the infant is mandatory until the child starts walking because the lack of symptoms and subtle physical findings make early diagnosis difficult. Patients with late-presenting developmental dysplasia of the hip (DDH) will typically present with a painless limp. There is

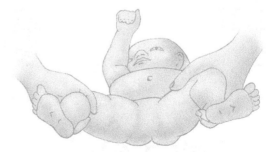

Figure 6–32. The Ortolani click test. In subluxation or dislocation, abduction is restricted, and the involved hip is unable to be abducted as far as the opposite one, producing an audible or palpable click as the femoral head slips over the acetabular rim.

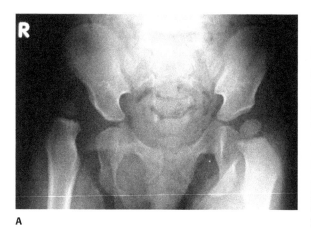
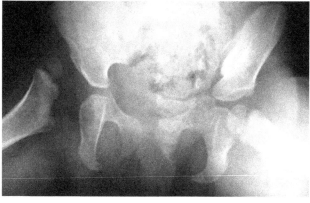

A   **B**

Figure 6–33. Developmental hip dislocation of the right hip. **A.** AP. **B.** Frog leg lateral.

usually a history of a delay in walking, with the age of onset being between 14 and 15 months instead of 12 months. The affected lower leg may be shortened. If the DDH is bilateral, the toddler may walk with a waddle. A radiograph of the pelvis after 4 months of age will help confirm the diagnosis (Fig. 6–33). Ultrasound may be effective for early diagnosis of this disorder in infants younger than 4 to 6 months. However, the use of screening ultrasounds is not recommended. Close physical examination and referral to orthopedics for suspected cases is appropriate.

Legg–Calvé–Perthes Disease (Coxa Plana)

Legg–Calvé–Perthes disease (LCPD) is an idiopathic form of avascular necrosis of the femoral head occurring in children (Fig. 6–34). This condition, which affects boys three to five times more often than girls, occurs most often in children between 4 and 9 years.

The definitive cause of the vascular disturbance resulting in LCPD is unknown. The condition results in necrosis of the head and all or part of the epiphysis. An almost constant early sign is a limp, which is caused by limited abduction

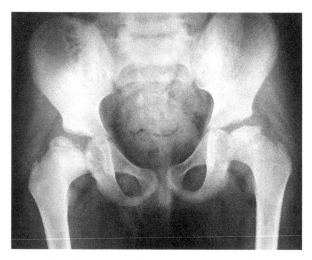

Figure 6–34. Legg–Calvé–Perthes disease is present bilaterally.

of the hip and limited internal rotation in both flexion and extension. The patient complains of a vague ache in the groin that radiates to the medial thigh and inner aspect of the knee. This is aggravated by activity and relieved by rest. The patient may also complain of stiffness in a joint, and tenderness is noted over the anterior aspect of the joint. Muscle spasm is another common complaint in the early stages of the disease.

The early signs on x-ray are of joint space widening and prominence of the soft tissues over the capsule with a minimal joint effusion. The femoral head may be slightly shifted laterally in the acetabulum. A few weeks later, the femoral head will appear denser than the rest of the bone. Later, a fragmented appearance on the radiograph is evidence of necrosis; ingrowth of new vessels initiates the process of reabsorption. This results in a decreased density of the proximal end of the metaphysis because of increased vascularity. Osteosclerosis with broadening and shortening of the femoral neck and an increased density of the head is also seen. Eventually, osteoarthritis develops.

Initial therapy includes minimal weight bearing and protection of the joint, which is accomplished by maintaining the femur abducted and internally rotated. This will keep the femoral head well inside the rounded portion of the acetabulum. Abduction and rotation of the femur is accomplished either by the use of orthotic devices (bracing) or surgery (osteotomy).

The Scottish Rite brace achieves containment by abduction, while allowing free knee motion. This brace allows the hip to flex to 90 degrees, but it cannot control the rotation of the hip. In older patients with more extensive femoral head involvement, surgical repair results in improved outcome when compared with nonsurgical management.

Slipped Capital Femoral Epiphysis

Slipped capital femoral epiphysis (SCFE) is a physeal injury where the proximal femoral epiphysis slips posterior and medial in relation to the femoral neck metaphysis. It occurs in children typically between the ages of 10 and 16 years, with a male predominance. Patients are often overweight with more than 80% of patients having a body mass index above the 95th percentile.[26] In approximately one-fourth of the cases, both hips are affected. There is an increased frequency of this disorder in patients with endocrine disorders, including hypothyroidism, growth hormone deficiency, and hypogonadism. The end result if left untreated is a very disabling external rotation deformity of the lower extremity that later goes on to develop into degenerative arthritis and avascular necrosis of the hip.

SCFE is classified based on the ability to bear weight, temporally or radiographically, by the percentage of slippage. Patients with a stable SCFE are able to bear weight while unstable patients are not even able to ambulate with crutches. This classification has prognostic significance as patients with unstable SCFE have a much higher incidence of developing osteonecrosis of the femoral head. In the temporal classification, patients with acute SCFE present within 3 weeks of the onset of symptoms, chronic SCFE greater than 3 weeks, and acute on chronic SCFE when more than 3 weeks of symptoms are present with an acute exacerbation. The temporal classification does not have prognostic significance and is rarely used. Radiographically, SCFE of 0% to 33% slippage is considered grade I; 33% to 50%, grade 2; and >50%, grade 3.

The patient will present to the ED with pain and altered gait. There may be a history of minor trauma or strain, but persistent symptoms. Pain is typically present in the groin, but some children present with thigh or knee pain. This is particularly true in young athletes between the ages of 8 and 12 years, where knee discomfort and no effusion should be investigated for SCFE.

On examination, the hip is externally rotated, and there is pain and diminished range of motion to internal rotation, abduction, and flexion. When this occurs, the patient's diagnosis is clear, and the approach is fairly straightforward. Often, clinical findings are subtle and may be missed.[27]

Three clinical stages exist. In the *preslipping stage*, there is slight discomfort about the groin, which usually occurs after activity and subsides with rest. The patient may complain of stiffness and an occasional limp. Discomfort may radiate along the anterior and medial aspect of the thigh to the inner aspect of the knee. The symptoms are usually vague, and no objective findings are noted on physical examination. The second stage is the *chronic slipping stage*, where the epiphysis is separated and gradually shifts backward, as is usually noted on x-rays taken during that time. In this stage, a patient has tenderness around the hip joint and limitation of motion (particularly abduction and internal rotation). The limb develops an adduction and external rotation deformity. As the hip is flexed and externally rotated, the slipping is accentuated, and the gluteus medius becomes inadequate. The patient develops a positive Trendelenburg test. When the condition is bilateral, the patient has a waddling gait. This is followed by a stage of *fixed deformity* in which pain and muscle spasm disappear. The limp and external rotation and adduction deformity persist, as does the limitation of internal rotation and abduction.

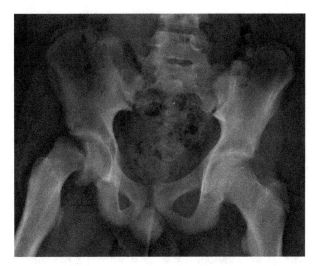

Figure 6–35. Slipped capital femoral epiphysis. AP view demonstrates obvious slip of the right hip.

AP and lateral views of both hips should be taken (Fig. 6–35). The lateral view with the hip flexed 90 degrees and abducted 45 degrees (frog-leg lateral) is best for demonstrating the displaced capital femoral epiphysis (Fig. 6–36). There is some controversy over whether the frog-leg lateral view should be obtained in patients with an acute unstable slip as the positioning may increase the slip. In these patients, a cross-table (true) lateral can be obtained.

In the preslipping stage, widening of the epiphysis and decalcification of the metaphysis at the epiphyseal border are the prominent radiographic features. At this stage, MRI may aid in the diagnosis. When the epiphysis begins to slip, the initial direction is usually posterior, making the lateral view the more likely view to demonstrate SCFE early on. A line drawn through the center of the femoral neck on the lateral view should bisect the femoral head in a patient

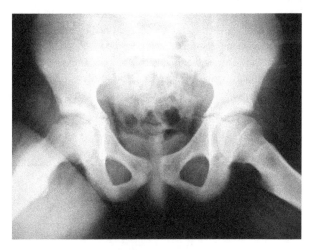

Figure 6-36. A frog leg lateral view in a different patient demonstrating a more subtle slip of the right hip. On this view, a line drawn through the femoral neck should bisect the head on a normal radiograph.

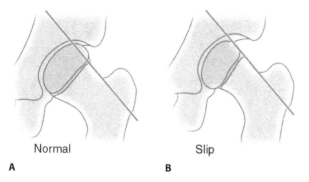

Figure 6-37. Klein's line. A normal Klein's line should intersect the epiphysis of the femoral head. **A.** Normal hip. **B.** SCFE.

without slip. Additionally, a line drawn along the inferior border of the femoral neck should smoothly lead to the femoral head, without disruption.

As the slip progresses, medial displacement occurs, which is picked up on the AP view. On the AP projection, Klein's line, a line drawn through the superior border of the proximal femoral metaphysis should intersect part of the proximal femoral epiphysis. If this does not occur, SCFE should be suspected (Fig. 6-37). Unfortunately, Klein's line has a sensitivity of only 40%. A modification of Klein's line proposed a comparison of the width of the epiphysis lateral to Klein's line to the opposite hip. A difference of 2 mm between hips indicated a slip with increased sensitivity (79%).

Patients with SCFE should be kept from weight bearing, and an orthopedic surgeon should be consulted. Patients with acute or unstable SCFE are usually admitted to the hospital, although this decision should be made in conjunction with the consulting orthopedist. Definitive treatment of a SCFE is often best performed within a few days (or as soon as possible) to prevent further slipping, which can occur even in the non–weight-bearing patient. Patients will most frequently be treated with in situ percutaneous fixation with a single central screw. Occasionally, two screws are used. Open reduction of the severe and unstable slipped epiphysis before screw placement is sometimes performed but remains controversial. The priorities in treating an unstable (acute) slip are to avoid avascular necrosis and chondrolysis (joint space narrowing and loss of articular cartilage), prevent further slip, and correct the deformity. Because of the frequency of this condition being bilateral, screw fixation of the contralateral hip may be performed, but this is also controversial.

Axiom: *A child who presents with knee pain who has a normal knee examination must have the hip examined for possible etiology.*

Transient Synovitis

Transient synovitis is the most common cause of acute hip pain in children between 3 and 10 years of age. Typically,

these children present with hip pain of 1 to 3 days' duration, accompanied by a limp or a refusal to bear weight. The extremity is held in *flexion, adduction,* and *internal rotation,* while the child resists all attempts at passive motion resulting from muscle spasm. The temperature is usually normal to slightly elevated and is rarely high. This condition has an uncertain etiology and is diagnosed through a process of exclusion. Patients often report a preceding viral or bacterial infection. The disorder is usually unilateral, although it can be bilateral. The treatment for transient synovitis is rest and anti-inflammatory medication with close follow-up.

Septic arthritis must first be ruled out because femoral head destruction and degenerative arthritis will result if septic arthritis is not treated promptly. These patients, unlike patients with transient synovitis, are toxic in appearance and generally have high fevers. The patient resists any attempts at range of motion. When the diagnosis is unclear (temperature <102°F, limited range of motion, and negative ultrasound), a brief period of observation after a dose of ibuprofen may help differentiate the two entities, as the child with transient synovitis will improve.

However, if any doubt exists as to the etiology of the pain, blood cultures, antibiotics, aspiration of the hip joint, and culture of the synovial fluid are mandatory.

Septic Arthritis and Osteomyelitis

Septic arthritis and osteomyelitis are not uncommon in children. The pathologic origin is hematogenous seeding, local invasion from contiguous infection, or direct inoculation of the bone, either surgically or after trauma.

The presentation of septic arthritis is usually that of a fever, which may be low grade, and what is called *pseudoparalysis,* which is essentially a refusal of the child to use that limb. Gentle passive motion, however, is usually allowed. Presenting symptoms in neonates may be as vague as increased irritability, fever, or poor feeding. Children with osteomyelitis have tenderness to palpation particularly over the metaphysis, which is commonly affected. When the hip and shoulder are involved in osteomyelitis, the pus can track under the periosteum of the metaphysis into the adjacent joint, and thus the patient may have findings of both osteomyelitis and septic arthritis. The diagnosis of osteomyelitis can be made by the presence of any two of the following diagnostic criteria:

- Purulence of the bone
- A positive bone or blood culture
- Localized erythema, edema, or both
- A positive imaging study on radiography, scintigraphy, or MRI

Cultures taken from bone result in a culture yield of 80%. Blood cultures should be drawn on all patients suspected of having osteomyelitis as they are positive in up to 50% of patients. The most common organisms involved in newborns include staphylococci, *Haemophilus influenzae*, and gram-negative bacilli. In infants and children, *S aureus* is the most common major organism. However, Goergens et al.[30] found methicillin-resistant *S aureus* (MRSA) to be an emerging organism contributing to 6% of septic arthritis cases. *H influenza* disease is no longer a threat due to universal vaccination, except in neonates and unimmunized children. *Neisseria gonorrhoeae* should be suspected in sexually active teenagers. Patients with sickle cell disease are also at risk for *Salmonella*-related osteomyelitis.

In a univariate analysis, Jung et al. showed significant differences in body temperature, serum WBC count, erythrocyte sedimentation rate (ESR), and CRP levels between patients with septic arthritis versus transient synovitis. Plain radiographs showed a displacement or blurring of periarticular fat pads in patients with acute septic arthritis, and multivariate regression analysis revealed that a fever, ESR greater than 20 mm/h, CRP greater than 1 mg/dL, WBC greater than 11,000/mL, and an increased hip joint space of greater than 2 mm were independent predictors of acute septic arthritis.[31] In a prospective study of patients with suspicious physical examination findings, Caird et al.[32] found that fever (an oral temperature >38.5°C) was the best predictor of septic arthritis followed by an elevated CRP level, an elevated ESR, refusal to bear weight, and an elevated serum WBC count. In their study group, a CRP level greater than 2 mg/dL (>20 mg/L) was a strong independent risk factor for having septic arthritis of the hip.

The femur and tibia are by far the most common bones affected. Plain films are generally normal, and it takes 7 to 10 days for radiographic changes to appear in either osteomyelitis or septic arthritis.[33] Soft tissue, however, may show changes earlier. The younger the child, the more likely one is to see widening of the joint space. Abnormal subluxation of the hip with widening of the joint space is the most common x-ray finding. Because plain x-rays are usually not helpful early in the course of this disease, a low threshold should be used for skeletal scintigraphy. Guided aspiration of the hip evacuates pus, decreases damage to periarticular surfaces, differentiates joint sepsis from other effusions, and helps direct antibiotic therapy. CT scans are not useful in establishing a diagnosis of acute musculoskeletal sepsis.[34]

In treating children with osteomyelitis and septic arthritis, β-lactamase–resistant antibiotics should be included, particularly due to the prevalence of MRSA. In patients who are allergic to penicillin, clindamycin 24 mg/kg in divided doses over 24 hours, or vancomycin, is indicated.[35]

Knee and Leg

Osgood–Schlatter Disease

Osgood–Schlatter disease represents a disturbance in the development of the tibial tuberosity caused by repeated and rapid application of tensile forces by the quadriceps muscles at its tendinous insertion on the tuberosity.[36,37] The most widely accepted cause of Osgood–Schlatter disease is chronic repetitive trauma to the anterior portion of the maturing proximal tibial growth plate.

This disease is typically seen in girls between 8 and 13 years of age and in boys between 10 and 15 years. The disorder has been associated with inflexibility of the quadriceps muscle. The condition is usually unilateral, but it may be bilateral in 35% to 56% of boys and approximately 18% of girls.[38] In addition, boys are affected more often than girls.

On examination, there is typically pain, swelling, and tenderness localized over the tibial tubercle (Video 6–4). Joint effusion should not be present. Quadriceps used against resistance aggravates the pain, particularly during step climbing, squatting, or kneeling. These symptoms are secondary to incomplete separation of the cartilaginous link between the patellar tendon and the tibia. The separation interrupts the blood supply, resulting in aseptic necrosis, fragmentation, and eventually new bone formation (Fig. 6–38). Fusion of the tubercle to the tibia occurs by 18 years of age, thus eliminating any further symptoms. MRI and ultrasound of the knee have been shown to be superior to plain radiographs in diagnosing Osgood–Schlatter disease.[39] However, neither of these studies is immediately necessary in the ED.

The treatment includes a reduction of activity (i.e., sprinting, jumping, kicking) for 2 to 4 months, ice after exercise, and a short course of nonsteroidal anti-inflammatory medications.[40] Resolution of symptoms may take up to 12 to 18 months.[41] Stretching exercises for the quadriceps and hamstrings are also helpful. Complete restriction of all athletic activities is generally not necessary. Corticosteroid injections are not recommended due to the risk

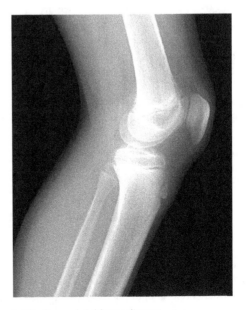

Figure 6–38. Osgood–Schlatter disease.

of subcutaneous atrophy and degenerative changes. Some patients develop chronic pain, which is associated with a discrete ossicle in the patellar tendon. Surgical treatment can provide relief in these patients. Immobilization is not generally recommended except in severe or persistent cases.

Patella Apophysitis

Apophysitis of the inferior pole of the patella is referred to as Sinding–Larsen–Johansson disease. This condition is also called *inferior pole patellar chondropathy* and is nine times more prevalent in boys between the ages 10 and 14 years than it is in girls. Patients present with lower-pole patellar pain exacerbated by running or kneeling. On examination, pain is noted with extension against resistance, along with localized tenderness on the inferior pole of the patella. With protracted symptoms, there is an elongation of the involved pole, which may develop a stress fracture and eventually an avulsion fracture if not diagnosed. Radiographs are usually normal, although blurring of the poles may be seen in chronic cases. The treatment is similar to Osgood–Schlatter disease. Nonsteroidal agents and rest are recommended. This condition is self-limited and usually resolves completely within 12 to 18 months. In rare cases, a 2- to 3-week trial of crutches is necessary.

Patellofemoral Stress Syndrome

Patellofemoral stress syndrome is the most common complaint in young female athletes. The common presentation is of aching knees, with pain increased by jumping or climbing. Physical findings usually include pain on compression of the patellar region; joint effusion and swelling are rare. Plain films are normal. Treatment includes relative rest and physical therapy.

Ligamentous Injuries

Ligamentous injuries involving the knee are uncommon in children because the bone is weaker than the ligaments. In the knee, an adult will experience a talofibular ligament rupture, whereas a child more frequently suffers a Salter I or II fracture of the proximal tibia or distal femur. Following a rotational injury or varus stress to the knee in a child, an avulsion of the tibial spine occurs more frequently than an anterior cruciate ligament rupture. By the same token, it is more common in the adult to have a rupture of the patellar tendon or quadriceps tendon from an extension-block injury to the quadriceps apparatus, whereas a child is more likely to suffer an avulsion of the tibial tubercle. Subtle and occult fractures are common in children. For this reason, a child with an effusion following a knee injury and negative plain radiographs should be immobilized and referred.

In dealing with a patellar injury or dislocation, always remember to examine the undersurface of the patella because osteochondral chip fractures are more common in children than in adults.

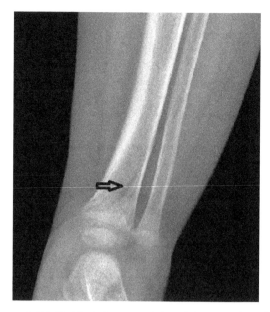

Figure 6–39. Toddler's fracture of the tibia. Note the subtle oblique fracture line (*arrow*).

Toddler's Fracture

A toddler's fracture is a nondisplaced spiral or oblique fracture of the lower third of the tibial shaft. This fracture occurs in patients between the ages of 9 months and 3 years. This injury results from torsion of the lower leg (Fig. 6–39). A fibula fracture is not present. Often, the parents do not recall any trauma, and the only complaint is difficulty walking or resistance to weight bearing. Physical examination often fails to reveal swelling, but may show increased warmth and pain with palpation of the lower third of the tibia.

AP and lateral films may reveal an obvious fracture; however, oblique films may help confirm the fracture. Initial radiographs may appear normal; however, 2 to 3 weeks later, subperiosteal bone formation may be seen.

The treatment of radiographically confirmed toddler's fracture consists of a below-knee walking cast for approximately 3 weeks. The treatment of a presumed toddler's fracture, in which no fracture is visualized on the initial radiograph, is somewhat controversial. Some advocate splinting for comfort and repeat radiographs in 10 days, whereas others recommend casting all children with a history of acute injury, inability to walk or limp, no constitutional signs, and negative radiographs to avoid a delay in treatment.

Ankle and Foot
Ankle Fractures

Children do not sustain "sprains," and therefore this diagnosis should be used with caution, if at all. Salter type I and II fractures can usually be managed conservatively with closed reduction followed by short-leg splint immobilization for 3 to 4 weeks. Nondisplaced distal fibular fractures may also be treated with a removable brace as return

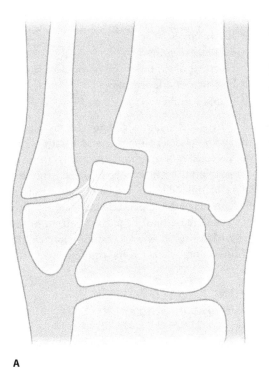
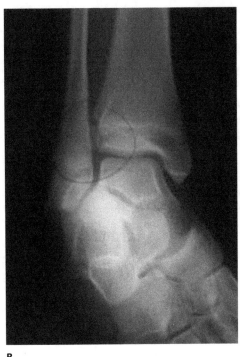

A   **B**

Figure 6–40. Tillaux fracture. The anterior talofibular ligament pulls on the unfused epiphysis of the tibia and results in a Salter III fracture. **A.** Schematic. **B.** Radiograph.

to functionality appears to be faster with this treatment approach. Salter types III, IV, and V will likely require operative intervention some time during their management. Pain over the distal fibula physis with a normal radiograph in a child should be managed as a Salter type I fracture.

The fracture pattern varies with age. An example of this age variation is the distal tibia fracture called a "Tillaux fracture," which is unique to adolescents (Fig. 6–40). As skeletal maturity is achieved and growth plates are beginning to close, the medial distal tibial epiphysis closes prior to the lateral. This creates a fulcrum through which a Salter type III fracture may occur, just lateral to the point of fusion. Because of growth plate involvement and a potential need for open fixation, a prompt orthopedic consultation is indicated. Intra-articular injury is common. CT scans are useful in evaluating complex fracture patterns. Comparison views may help in difficult cases.

Talar dome fractures are far more common in children than in adults. An osteochondral fracture of the talar dome should be highly suspected when evaluating a child who presents with a nonhealing "ankle sprain" or recurrent effusions after an ankle sprain.

Tarsal Coalition

Tarsal coalition should be suspected in any child with a history of multiple ankle sprains who demonstrates subtalar stiffness on a physical examination. Tarsal coalition is the abnormal union of two or more bones in the hindfoot and midfoot. This condition may be congenital or acquired because of infection, trauma, or articular disorders. Patients typically present between 8 and 16 years of age. A family history of tarsal coalition may exist. Of all the coalition syndromes, talocalcaneal and calcaneonavicular are the most frequent type. The initial treatment is conservative, consisting of rest and a short-leg cast for 2 to 4 weeks, or the use of a well-molded orthotic and physical therapy. These patients should be referred for appropriate care and follow-up.

Pes Planus

Pes planus occurs quite commonly, and most patients are asymptomatic. Treatment of symptomatic flat feet with an accessory navicular consists of the use of an orthotic and an exercise program to strengthen the posterior tibial muscles and the peroneal tendons of the foot. Surgery is indicated in some cases.

Freiberg Disease

Freiberg disease involves collapse of the articular surface and subchondral bone of the second metatarsal, presumably from a vascular insult. Although this is most commonly seen in the second metatarsal, it can occur in the third metatarsal. Symptoms are pain and tenderness over the metatarsal head, with swelling in this area on clinical examination. Radiographs confirm the diagnosis and treatment consists of decreased weight bearing to the area and a metatarsal pad or orthotic. Surgical excision of loose bodies because of fragmentation of the head is occasionally required.

Osteochondritis Dissecans of the Talus

Most of these lesions are in the middle third of the lateral border of the talus. Lesions are classified into four different stages.

- *Stage 1*: A small area of compression of subchondral bone
- *Stage 2*: A partially detached osteochondral fragment
- *Stage 3*: A completely detached osteochondral fragment remaining in the crater
- *Stage 4*: A displaced osteochondral fragment

Stage 1 and 2 lesions are treated without surgery using a cast, brace, or strap. Stage 3 medial lesions initially should be treated without surgery, but if symptoms persist, surgical excision and curettage is recommended. Stage 3 lateral lesions and all stage 4 lesions are treated surgically with removal of the lesion.

Sever's Disease

Sever's disease, or calcaneal apophysitis, is a common entity occurring in patients between 9 and 11 years of age. The child presents with heel pain, particularly with running, and may use a tiptoe gait or limp. Radiographs are often not helpful; however, the patient is tender on palpation of the calcaneal apophysis. Treatment depends on the severity of the symptoms, the primary role being to rest the heel. In very symptomatic patients, a short-leg walking cast for 10 to 14 days is the treatment of choice.

CHILD ABUSE

Whenever there is delay in seeking treatment for an orthopedic injury, suspect the possibility of child abuse. If the history is inconsistent with the examination, this should also be a sign that increases the suspicion of abuse.

Radiographic Evidence of Child Abuse

Fractures of the ribs or sternal area suggest child abuse. Any fractures seen in a child younger than 3 years should be suspect, particularly those seen in a child who is handicapped or premature. Metaphyseal corner (bucket handle) fractures are also suspect as these fractures are rarely accidental and are due to traction of the extremity or a shearing force across the end of the bone (Fig. 6–11). Humerus fractures, particularly spiral fractures, in children younger than 3 years are strongly suggestive of abuse because spiral fractures occur in response to a torsional force. Scapular fractures are difficult to obtain and should also be suspected. Fractures of the femur, and particularly fractures of the distal femur, are highly suspicious injuries in the nonambulatory child. However, spiral femur fractures can occur accidentally in nonambulatory patients if the mechanism is appropriate.

The most critical features to look for when examining the radiograph of a potentially abused child are the following:

- Bilateral fractures
- Multiple fractures
- Metaphyseal fractures
- Rib fractures
- Scapular fractures
- Fractures of the outer end of the clavicle
- Fractures of different ages
- Skull fractures

Physicians treating children in the ED must have a basic knowledge of the stages of fracture healing that can be detected radiographically. Table 6–1 provides a general timetable of the various phases of fracture healing. The data in this table are estimates only because very young infants may exhibit an accelerated rate of repair.

Child abuse must be at the forefront of the emergency physician's mind when examining any child, particularly those younger than 3 years with fractures.

BONE AND SOFT-TISSUE TUMORS IN CHILDREN

The most common site for childhood malignant tumors is around the knee. One must be suspicious whenever there is unilateral knee pain without any associated trauma. Pathologic fractures are also suspect, particularly when they occur through weakened bone, which may be a bone cyst. A number of benign tumors occur in children as incidental findings; these include osteochondromas and fibrous cortical defects (FCDs).

Fibroxanthomas

Fibroxanthoma, nonossifying fibroma (NOF); FCD; and, less commonly, benign fibrous histiocytoma have all been used interchangeably in the radiology literature. However, NOF and FCD are considered to be two distinct lesions, with respect to size and natural history. Fibroxanthoma is the preferred term for the NOF lesion. FCDs are asymptomatic, small (<3 cm), eccentrically located, metaphyseal cortical defects. Most FCDs spontaneously disappear. However, some evolve and enlarge into fibroxanthomas.

Conversely, fibroxanthomas (>3 cm) are larger, eccentric, intramedullary lesions. They have a typical superficial scalloping pattern in the adjacent cortex (Fig. 6–12). Both lesions occur in the developing skeleton. Approximately 90% of cases of both lesions involve the tubular long bones, with the most common sites being the femur (particularly, the distal femur), the proximal and distal tibia, and the knee. FCDs occur in younger patients (4–8 years) and are typically incidental findings on radiographs that are obtained for other indications. The peak incidence for fibroxanthomas is 10 to 15 years.

Fibroxanthomas also are characteristically asymptomatic. In larger lesions, however, mild pain may occur secondary to radiographically undetected microfractures that can eventually lead to painful and radiographically evident pathologic fractures. With larger lesions, careful radiographic observation and decreased vigorous activity of the

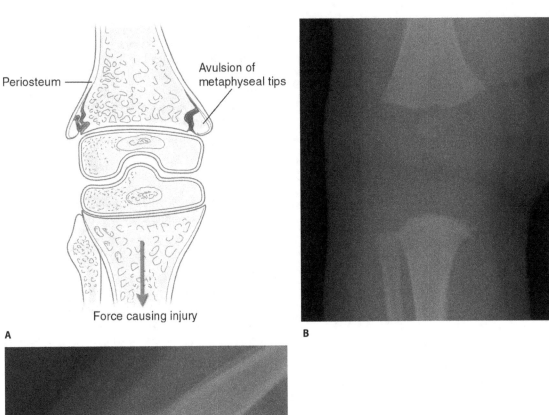

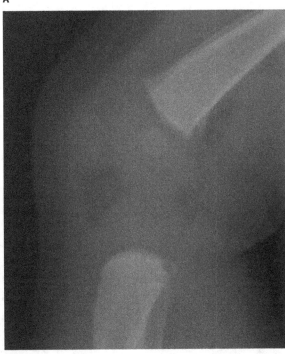

Figure 6–41. Metaphyseal corner fractures are due to traction or shear forces and are highly suspicious of child abuse. *A.* Schematic. *B.* AP. *C.* Lateral radiographs. *(Radiographs used with permission from Robert Tubbs, MD.)*

▶ TABLE 6–1. **TIMETABLE OF RADIOGRAPHIC CHANGES IN PEDIATRIC FRACTURES**

Stage	Radiographic Changes	Time Line
Stage I: Induction	Fracture gap widening	0–3 weeks
Stage II: Inflammation		
Stage III: Soft callus	Periosteal reaction	2–6 weeks
Stage IV: Hard callus	Callus density greater than cortex	2–13 weeks
Stage V: Remodeling	Remodeling occurs	3 months–2 years

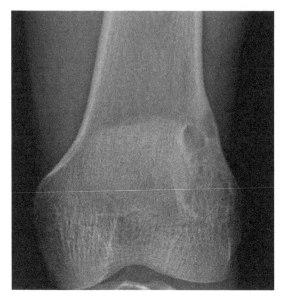

Figure 6–42. Fibroxanthoma (nonossifying fibroma).

patient are recommended. Surgical treatment is generally determined by four criteria, which include the following: the patient's skeletal maturity, where it is localized, initial diagnosis, and amount of bone loss in the femoral neck and lateral proximal femur. Surgical procedures include curettage, bone grafting, and internal fixation when required.

Ewing Sarcoma

Ewing sarcoma, also known as peripheral primitive neuroectodermal tumors of bone, is a type of cancer usually found in children and young adults. The peak incidence is between ages 10 and 20 years. It is less common in children younger than 5 or in adults older than 30 years. Sarcomas can develop in any of the bones of the skeleton, but may also develop in the soft tissue near bones.

The most common symptom is pain in the bone in the area of the tumor. Some swelling may eventually be seen in the area, and it may become tender to touch. Children may also present with a fever.

Ewing sarcomas are graded from 1 to 3. Grade 1 indicates a low-grade cancer, and grades 2 to 3 indicate a high-grade cancer. High-grade tumors grow more quickly and are more likely to spread. Ewing sarcomas tend to be high-grade cancers.

Ewing sarcomas are staged as follows:

- *Stage 1A*: The cancer is a low-grade type found only within the hard coating of the bone.
- *Stage 1B*: A low-grade type of cancer extending outside the bone and into the soft-tissue space.
- *Stage 2A*: The cancer is a high-grade type found only within the hard coating of the bone.
- *Stage 2B*: A high-grade type of cancer extending outside the bone and into the soft-tissue space.
- *Stage 3*: The cancer can be a low-grade or high-grade type, and it is found either within the bone or outside the bone. The cancer has spread to other parts of the body or to other bones not directly connected to the bone where the tumor started.

On plain films, a high-grade Ewing sarcoma is associated with significant periosteal reaction (Fig. 6–43).

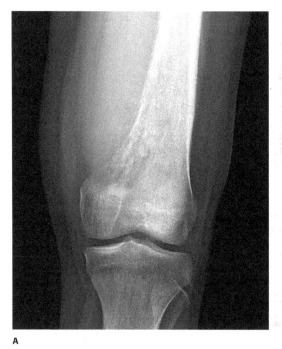

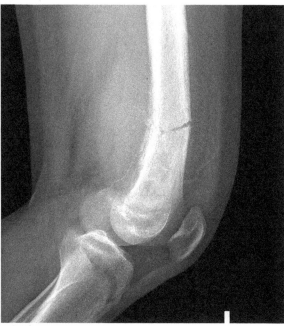

A   B

Figure 6–43. Ewing sarcoma. This 16-year-old boy presented with 2 weeks of knee pain after playing football. **A.** AP. **B.** Lateral radiographs reveal a malignant periosteal reaction with a "sunburst" pattern. A pathologic fracture of the distal femur is also noted.

A sunburst appearance is used to describe the multiple interrupted linear areas of periosteal reaction that run perpendicular to the bone. When the lines of periosteal reaction run parallel to the bone, an "onion skin" appearance is used. Codman triangle refers to a short spicule of bone seen at the edge of the lesion where the periosteum is lifted off the cortex. CT delineates the extent of cortical involvement and provides some information about the amount of soft-tissue component. MRI reveals a large, highly vascular soft-tissue mass with extensive intramedullary spread.

Ewing sarcoma can occur in any bone in the body; however, the most common sites are the pelvis, thigh, lower leg, upper arm, and rib. Treatment consists of chemotherapy, radiotherapy, and possible limb-sparing surgery or amputation.

Osteoid Osteomas

Osteoid osteomas are benign bone-forming lesions typically found in children older than 5 years. The most common complaint is limp and localized pain. Radiographs reveal a small lucent lesion, which is less than 1 cm, surrounded by reactive sclerosis (Fig. 6–44).

Osteoid osteomas account for 12% of benign tumors and 3% of all tumors. The most common skeletal sites are the metaphysis or diaphysis of long bones, which are affected in 73% of patients. The spine is affected in 10% to 14% of patients. The classic presentation includes focal skeletal bone pain, which worsens at night and is frequently relieved with small doses of anti-inflammatory medication. In most patients with spinal tumors, the pain increases with activity and also occurs at night. The site of involvement may be tender to touch or pressure. Constitutional symptoms are usually absent. The tumor can be percutaneously

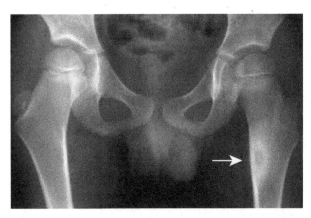

Figure 6–44. Osteoid osteoma. Note the reactive sclerosis (*arrow*). (Reproduced with permission from Yamamoto LG. Osteoid osteoma. In: Yamamoto LG, Inaba AS, DiMauro+H32 R, eds. *Radiology Cases in Pediatric Emergency Medicine.* Vol. 4, Case 15. Honolulu: University of Hawaii John A. Burns School of Medicine, Department of Pediatrics, 1994. http://www.hawaii.edu/medicine/pediatrics/pemxray/v4c15.html. Accessed March 28, 2018.)

ablated by using radiofrequency, ethanol, laser, or thermocoagulation therapy under CT guidance.

ACKNOWLEDGMENT

Special thanks to Mariyah S. Shad for her assistance in the revision of this chapter.

REFERENCES

1. Salter R, Harris W. Injuries involving the epiphyseal plate. *J Bone Joint Surg Am.* 2001;83(11):1753.
2. Leonard JC, Kuppermann N, Olsen C, et al. Pediatric Emergency Care Applied Research Network. Factors associated with cervical spine injury in children after blunt trauma. *Ann Emerg Med.* 2011;58(2):145–155. doi:10.1016/j.annemergmed.2010.08.038.
3. Patel JC, Tepas JJ III, Mollitt DL, Pieper P. Pediatric cervical spine injuries: defining the disease. *J Pediatr Surg.* 2001; 36(2):373–376.
4. Swischuk LE. *Emergency Imaging of the Acutely Ill or Injured Child.* 4th ed. Baltimore, MD: Lippincott Williams & Wilkins; 2000.
5. Cirak B, Ziegfeld S, Knight VM, Chang D, Avellino AM, Paidas CN. Spinal injuries in children. *J Pediatr Surg.* 2004; 39(4):607–612.
6. Proctor MR. Spinal cord injury. *Crit Care Med.* 2002;30(suppl 11):S489–S499.
7. Kokoska ER, Keller MS, Rallo MC, Weber TR. Characteristics of pediatric cervical spine injuries. *J Pediatr Surg.* 2001; 36(1):100–105.
8. Parent S, Mac-Thiong JM, Roy-Beaudry M, Sosa JF, Labelle H. Spinal cord injury in the pediatric population: a systematic review of the literature. *J Neurotrauma.* 2011;28(8):1515–1524.
9. Fucs PM, Meves R, Yamada HH. Spinal infections in children: a review. *Int Orthop.* 2012;36(2):387–395. doi: 10.1007/s00264-011-1388-2.
10. Brown R, Hussain M, McHugh K, Novelli V, Jones D. Discitis in young children. *J Bone Joint Surg Br.* 2001;83(1):106–111.
11. Cekanauskas E, Degliute R, Kalesinskas RJ. Treatment of supracondylar humerus fractures in children, according to Gartland classification. *Medicina (Kaunas).* 2003;39(4):379–383.
12. Perron A. *Harwood-Nuss' Clinical Practice of Emergency Medicine.* 4th ed. Philadelphia, PA: Lippincott Williams & Wilkins; 2005.
13. Ozkoc G, Gonc U, Kayaalp A, Teker K, Peker TT. Displaced supracondylar humeral fractures in children: open reduction vs. closed reduction and pinning. *Arch Orthop Trauma Surg.* 2004;124(8):547–551.
14. Yu SW, Su JY, Kao FC, Ma CH, Yen CY, Tu YK. The use of the 3-mm K-wire to supplement reduction of humeral supracondylar fractures in children. *J Trauma.* 2004;57(5):1038–1042.
15. Pearson BV, Kuhns DW. Nursemaid's elbow in a 31-year-old female. *Am J Emerg Med.* 2007;25(2):222–223.
16. Green DA, Linares MY, Garcia Peña BM, Greenberg B, Baker RL. Randomized comparison of pain perception during radial head subluxation reduction using supination-flexion or forced pronation. *Pediatr Emerg Care.* 2006;22(4):235–238.

17. Macias CG, Bothner J, Wiebe R. A comparison of supination/flexion to hyperpronation in the reduction of radial head subluxations. *Pediatrics.* 1998;102(1):e10.

18. McDonald J, Whitelaw C, Goldsmith LJ. Radial head subluxation: comparing two methods of reduction. *Acad Emerg Med.* 1999;6(7):715–718.

19. Teach SJ, Schutzman SA. Prospective study of recurrent radial head subluxation. *Arch Pediatr Adolesc Med.* 1996;150(2):164–166.

20. Pannu GS, Herman M. Distal Radius-Ulna Fractures in Children. *Orthop Clin North Am.* 2015;46:235–248.

21. Boutis K, Willan A, Babyn P, Goeree R, Howard A. Cast versus splint in children with minimally angulated fractures of the distal radius: a randomized controlled trial. *CMAJ.* 2010;182(14):1507–1512. doi:10.1503/cmaj.100119.

22. Roovers EA, Boere-Boonekamp MM, Castelein RM, Zielhuis GA, Kerkhoff TH. Effectiveness of ultrasound screening for developmental dysplasia of the hip. *Arch Dis Child Fetal Neonatal Ed.* 2005;90(1):F25–F30.

23. Committee on Quality Improvement, Subcommittee on Developmental Dysplasia of the Hip, American Academy of Pediatrics. Clinical practice guideline: early detection of developmental dysplasia of the hip. *Pediatrics.* 2000;105(4 pt 1):896–905.

24. Frick SL. Evaluation of the child who has hip pain. *Orthop Clin North Am.* 2006;37(2):133–140, v.

25. Herring JA, Kim HT, Browne R. Legg-Calvé-Perthes disease. Part II: prospective multicenter study of the effect of treatment on outcome. *J Bone Joint Surg Am.* 2004;86-A(10):2121–2134.

26. Manoof EM, Banffy MB, Winell JJ. Relationship between body mass index and slipped capital femoral epiphysis. *J Pediatr Orthop.* 2005;25:744–746.

27. Kocher MS, Bishop JA, Weed B, et al. Delay in diagnosis of slipped capital femoral epiphysis. *Pediatrics.* 2004;113(4):e322–e325.

28. A. Green DW, Ngozi M, Scher DM, Sheryl H, Peter C, Widmann RF. A modification of Klein's line to improve sensitivity at the anterior-posterior radiograph in slipped capital femoral epiphysis. *J Pediatr Orthop.* 2009;29(5):449–453.

29. Kermond S, Fink M, Graham K, Carlin JB, Barnett P. A randomized clinical trial: should the child with transient synovitis of the hip be treated with nonsteroidal anti-inflammatory drugs? *Ann Emerg Med.* 2002;40(3):294–299.

30. Goergens ED, McEvoy A, Watson M, Barrett IR. Acute osteomyelitis and septic arthritis in children. *J Paediatr Child Health.* 2005;41(1-2):59–62.

31. Jung ST, Rowe SM, Moon ES, Song EK, Yoon TR, Seo HY. Significance of laboratory and radiologic findings for differentiating between septic arthritis and transient synovitis of the hip. *J Pediatr Orthop.* 2003;23(3):368–372.

32. Caird MS, Flynn JM, Leung YL, Millman JE, D'Italia JG, Dormans JP. Factors distinguishing septic arthritis from transient synovitis of the hip in children. A prospective study. *J Bone Joint Surg Am.* 2006;88(6):1251–1257.

33. Barkin RM, Barkin SZ, Barkin AZ. The limping child. *J Emerg Med.* 2000;18(3):331–339.

34. Connolly LP, Connolly SA. Skeletal scintigraphy in the multimodality assessment of young children with acute skeletal symptoms. *Clin Nucl Med.* 2003;28(9):746–754.

35. Kaplan SL, Hulten KG, Gonalez BE, et al. Three-year surveillance of community-acquired *Staphylococcus aureus* infections in children. *Clin Infect Dis.* 2005;40(12):1785–1791.

36. Lau LL, Mahadev A, Hui JH. Common lower limb sport-related overuse injuries in young athletes. *Ann Acad Med Singapore.* 2008;37(4):315–319.

37. DeBerardino TM, Branstetter JG, Owens BD. Arthroscopic treatment of unresolved Osgood–Schlatter lesions. *Arthroscopy.* 2007;23(10):1127–1123.

38. Gholve PA, Scher DM, Khakharia S. Osgood–Schlatter syndrome. *Curr Opin Pediatr.* 2007;19(1):44–50.

39. Hirano A, Fukubayashi T, Ishii T, Widmann RF, Green DW. Magnetic resonance imaging of Osgood–Schlatter disease: the course of the disease. *Skeletal Radiol.* 2002;31(6):334–342.

40. Bloom OJ, Mackler L, Barbee J. Clinical inquiries. What is the best treatment for Osgood–Schlatter disease? *J Fam Pract.* 2004;53(2):153–156.

41. Duri ZA, Patel DV, Aichroth PM. The immature athlete. *Clin Sports Med.* 2002;21(3):461–482, ix.

42. Orava S, Malinen L, Karpakka J, et al. Results of surgical treatment of unresolved Osgood–Schlatter lesion. *Ann Chir Gynaecol.* 2000;89(4):298–302.

43. Halsey MF, Finzel KC, Carrion WV, Haralabatos SS, Gruber MA, Meinhard BP. Toddler's fracture: presumptive diagnosis and treatment. *J Pediatr Orthop.* 2001;21(2):152–156.

44. Perron AD, Miller MD, Brady WJ. Orthopedic pitfalls in the ED: pediatric growth plate injuries. *Am J Emerg Med.* 2002;20(1):50–54.

45. Islam O, Soboleski D, Symons S, et al. Development and duration of radiographic signs of bone healing in children. *AJR Am J Roentgenol.* 2000;175(1):75–78.

46. Erol B, Topkar MO, Aydemir AN, et al. A treatment strategy for proximal femoral benign bone lesions in children and recommended surgical procedures: retrospective analysis of 62 patients. *Arch Orthop Trauma Surg.* 2016;136(8):1051–1061. doi:10.1007/s00402-016-2486-9.

47. Cantwell CP, Obyrne J, Eustace S. Current trends in treatment of osteoid osteoma with an emphasis on radiofrequency ablation. *Eur Radiol.* 2004;14(4):607–617.

PART II

Spine

CHAPTER 7

Approach to Neck and Back Pain

Zheng Ben Ma, MD and Emily Senecal Miller, MD

INTRODUCTION

Neck and back pain are among the most common presenting complaints in emergency department (ED) patients. While the quoted lifetime prevalence of back pain varies within medical literature, approximate figures range up to 84%, suggesting the vast majority of individuals will experience an episode of back pain at some point in their lifetime.[1] On a global scale, neck and lower back pain remained the leading cause of disability in the world from 1990 to 2015.[2] In a US-based survey involving more than 31,000 individuals, low back pain lasting at least a whole day in the past 3 months was reported by 26.4% of respondents, and neck pain was reported by 13.8%.[3]

Back pain is not only common but also costly, with total costs in the United States exceeding $100 billion per year. Two-thirds of these costs are indirect, attributed to lost wages and reduced workplace productivity.[4] Lower back pain accounts for one-third of all occupational musculoskeletal injuries and illnesses resulting in work disability.[5] Although two-thirds of lower back pain cases return to work within 1 month, 17% of patients experience work disability between 1 and 6 months while 7% of cases require more than 6 months to return to work.[6]

Literature reports an estimated 85% of patients have back pain secondary to muscle or ligamentous injury and only a minority of patients have pain originating from nerve roots (e.g., herniated disk), facet joints (e.g., arthritis), or the bone (e.g., osteomyelitis). However, this imbalance is likely exaggerated as the majority of muscle spasm and strain is the result of a different injury or disease process, which is the primary cause of pain. This chapter aims to provide the reader with tools to ascertain the differences between these entities. Chapter 8 delves into further details regarding each disease while Chapters 9 and 10 focus on traumatic injuries of the cervical and thoracolumbar spines, respectively.

Regardless of whether the exact etiology of the patient's pain can be determined, the ability to differentiate life-threatening from benign causes of back pain is of paramount importance to the emergency physician. When evaluating a patient with back pain, two important questions need to be considered:

- Is there a serious underlying systemic disease responsible for the pain?
- Is there evidence of neurologic compromise that indicates spinal cord injury and necessitates emergent imaging and surgical consultation?

ANATOMY

The spinal column consists of 33 vertebrae: 7 cervical, 12 thoracic, and 5 lumbar (Fig. 7–1). The sacrum consists of five fused vertebrae and the coccyx. The first two cervical vertebrae, the atlas (C1) and axis (C2), are unique from the remainder

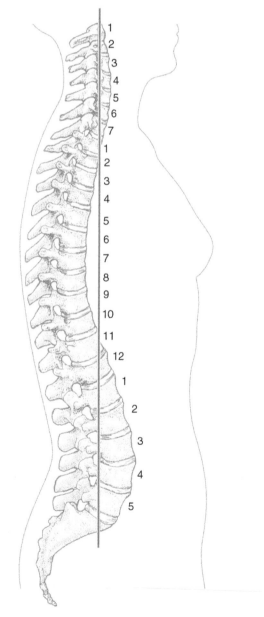

Figure 7–1. The spine consists of 7 cervical, 12 thoracic, and 5 lumbar vertebrae.

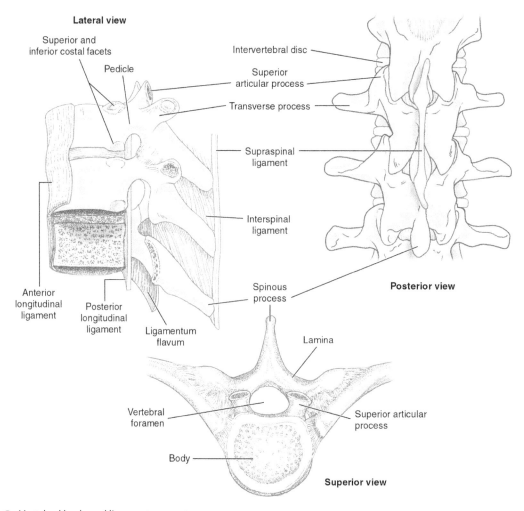

Lateral view

Superior and inferior costal facets

Pedicle

Intervertebral disc

Superior articular process

Transverse process

Supraspinal ligament

Interspinal ligament

Anterior longitudinal ligament

Posterior longitudinal ligament

Ligamentum flavum

Spinous process

Posterior view

Lamina

Vertebral foramen

Superior articular process

Body

Superior view

Figure 7-2. Vertebral body and ligamentous anatomy.

of the cervical spine. The atlas is a ring-shaped structure that articulates with the skull, and is responsible for 50% of the neck's mobility in flexion and extension. The odontoid process of the axis is secured to the anterior portion of the atlas and allows rotational movement of the skull.

The vertebral bodies gradually increase in size as they descend down the spine. The posterior arch encases the spinal cord and consists of the broad pedicles, flat laminae, and pointy spinous processes (Fig. 7–2). The transverse processes extend laterally near the junction of the pedicles and laminae. The posterior arch has four facets that articulate with the superior and inferior vertebrae forming synovial joints. Depending on their location, the transverse processes may also articulate with the ribs.

The spinal column is enmeshed in a network of ligaments. The anterior and posterior longitudinal ligaments interconnect the vertebral bodies and run down the entire length of the spine. Posteriorly, the ligamentum flavum, interspinous ligament, and supraspinous ligament provide further stability.

Although the vertebrae provide support and protection for the spinal cord, ligaments and intervertebral disks account for the spine's flexibility. Flexibility is greatest in the cervical and lumbar spine, whereas the thoracic spine, which articulates with the ribs, is more restricted in motion. The sections of the vertebral column with the greatest mobility are also most susceptible to injury. The most common location for spinal cord injury is in the cervical spine between C5 and C6.

Intervertebral discs are fibrocartilaginous structures situated between adjacent vertebral bodies that are crucial for flexibility and shock absorption for the spine. These discs are composed of the nucleus pulposus at the center surrounded by the annulus fibrosus. Discs located in the cervical and lumbar spine are thicker than those located in the thoracic spine, and they further promote increased flexibility in these regions. With age and repetitive use, small tears occur in the annulus fibrosus that begin centrally and radiate to the periphery. With a sudden increase in pressure, the annulus fibrosus can completely tear and cause the nucleus pulposus to herniate. Herniation is less common in individuals older than 50 years because the nucleus pulposus is desiccated and fibrotic.

The spinal canal and cord are widest in diameter in the cervical region. In the thoracic spine, the spinal canal is very narrow, and therefore, small displacement can lead to significant neurologic injury (i.e., cord transection). Nerve roots extending from the spinal cord exit the spinal foramina laterally. Cervical nerve roots emerge above the corresponding vertebrae, whereas the opposite is true of thoracolumbar nerve roots. This is because there are eight cervical nerve roots and only seven cervical vertebrae (Fig. 7–3). In the adult, the spinal cord ends at the L1-L2 interspace, where the remaining nerve roots form a bundle referred to as the cauda equina, which then loosely fills the remainder of the spinal canal. The cauda equina tolerates compression better than the spinal cord itself.

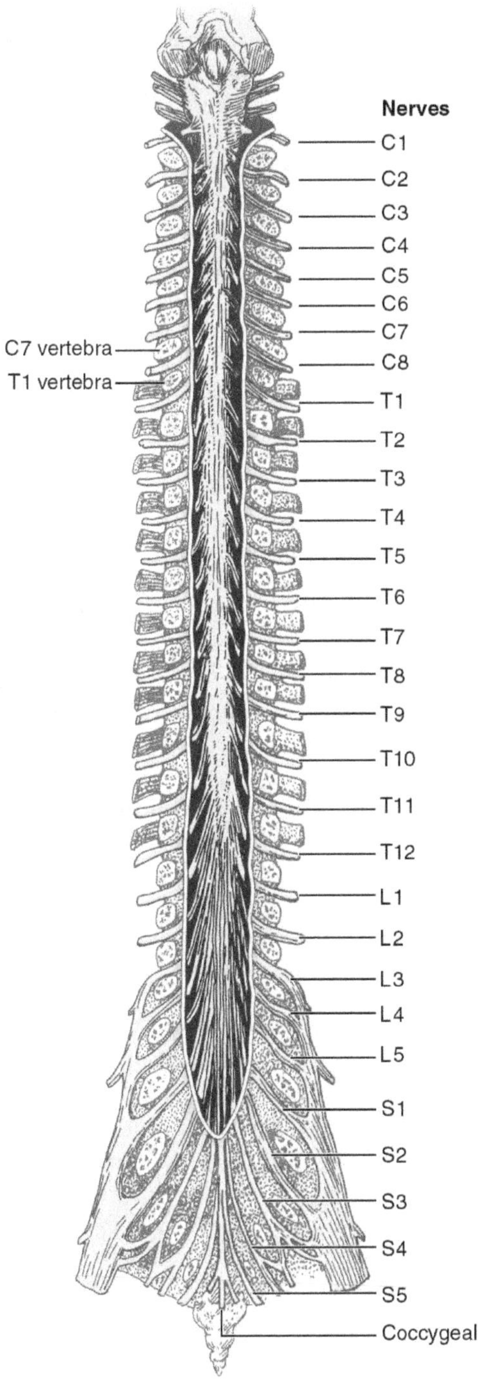

HISTORY

Although the differential diagnosis for back pain is broad, identifying patients who may be suffering from conditions that produce significant morbidity and mortality is of utmost importance. Disorders such as spinal epidural abscess, epidural hematoma, malignancy with spinal metastasis, spinal fracture, aortic dissection, aortic aneurysms, spinal cord compression, and cauda equine syndrome, although less common, frequently require emergent treatment. As such, a delay in diagnosis can be problematic. A systematic approach is therefore useful to avoid missing these and other critical diagnoses. One such approach is to categorize the source of pain as vascular, visceral, infectious, mechanical, or rheumatologic.

Approximately 85% to 90% of patients evaluated for back pain are ultimately diagnosed as having nonspecific low back pain, which is not attributed to a specific disease or spinal abnormality.[8,9] Therefore, there is a high "noise-to-signal ratio" that complicates the clinician's responsibility in differentiating life-threatening from benign causes of back pain. This section discusses a general approach to aid the clinician in diagnosing these potentially life-threatening conditions. It will highlight the importance of recognizing "red flag" symptoms that can hint at the presence of diseases requiring urgent or emergent diagnosis and treatment (Table 7–1).

The patient's age is the first clue in differentiating the etiology of back pain because the natural history of each

Figure 7–3. The spinal canal and cord.

▶ TABLE 7–1. RED FLAG SIGNS AND SYMPTOMS OF SERIOUS UNDERLYING CAUSE OF BACK PAIN

Diagnosis	Red Flag Signs and Symptoms
Infection	Immunocompromised (e.g., DM, HIV, steroids, transplant), fever, neurologic deficit, pain persists at rest and worse at night, history of IV drug use, recent infection
Malignancy	Elderly, history of malignancy, neurologic deficit, weight loss, pain persists at rest and worse at night, pain >6 wk
Fracture	Elderly, trauma, steroids, history of osteoporosis
Cauda equina syndrome	Bowel or bladder problems, bilateral leg symptoms, saddle anesthesia, motor deficits at multiple levels
Abdominal aortic aneurysm	Age >60 y, pulsating abdominal mass, vasculopathic risk factors

disease tends to favor specific age groups. In patients younger than 20 years, back pain in the absence of trauma suggests spondylolisthesis or spondylolysis. Onset of back pain before the age of 40 should also raise concern for inflammatory and rheumatologic etiologies such as spondyloarthritis and ankylosing spondylitis. The prevalence of herniated intervertebral discs increases with age, from 30% of those 20 years of age to 84% of those 80 years of age, although this condition is not always symptomatic. Elderly patients are at increased risk for malignancy, aneurysm, and fracture. Patients older than 50 years account for over three-quarters of malignancy-related causes of back pain. Patients older than 65 are also at increased risk for vertebral compression fractures.

The clinician should ask the patient to describe the onset and duration of the pain, their activity at the time of onset, whether they have had any prior episodes of similar pain and any reproducibility of the pain. Clear inciting events such as heavy lifting, twisting, prolonged sitting, motor vehicle collision, or fall would suggest muscular strain, disc herniation, or vertebral fracture. Pain following a fall, especially in an elderly patient, suggests a possible fracture. In patients who have sustained a traumatic injury, a fracture should be considered until proven otherwise. In certain patient populations such as the elderly, patients with history of osteoporosis, steroid use, known malignancy or multiple comorbidities, or vertebral compression fractures should be considered, even in the absence of trauma.

A slower onset of pain with gradual progression in intensity over longer periods of time should raise concern for infection or malignancy. Because the majority of patients with back pain improve over a 4- to 6-week period, pain persisting longer than 6 weeks should raise concern for malignancy or other systemic illness.

The location of pain is of obvious importance. Pain in the paraspinal area suggests muscular injury, while midline pain is more frequently seen in fracture, malignancy, or infection. Caution is required, however, as serious nonmuscular diseases may also present with paraspinal muscle spasm. Back pain in the lumbar region is most common, but thoracic back pain is potentially more concerning to suggest etiologies such as aortic dissection, expanding aortic aneurysm, retroperitoneal hemorrhage, primary or metastatic malignancy, or spinal infections.

It is particularly important to elicit "red flag" symptoms from the history to risk stratify for etiologies of back pain that are surgical emergencies, specifically spinal cord compression or cauda equina syndrome. It is vitally important to document the presence or absence of bowel or bladder dysfunction, which may be a symptom of severe compression of the spinal cord by a tumor, abscess, hemorrhage, or large midline disk herniation. In this condition, urinary retention with overflow incontinence is typically present (90% sensitivity), and can often be associated with saddle anesthesia, bilateral sciatica, or leg weakness. Studies quote various predictive value for each sign and symptom

of this surgical emergency. However, because of the high-risk nature of this disease, any patient in whom a reasonable suspicion of cauda equine syndrome exists should undergo an urgent magnetic resonance imaging (MRI) to assess for this diagnosis.

Axiom: *Pain at night, at rest, or unrelated to patient position are key "red flags" that suggest tumor, infection, or referred pain from another source.*

Exacerbating and alleviating factors also provide clues to the etiology. Pain that persists despite rest or worsens during the night may herald an underlying malignancy or spinal infection as musculoskeletal pain is expected to improve with rest. Specific positions that trigger the pain may also point toward an etiology. Increased intensity of pain in the prone position or extended position can be seen with facet syndrome, central stenosis, or lateral disc herniation. Pain increased by sitting is usually suggestive of an annular tear in the disk or a paramedian herniation. Standing up from a seated position will often worsen pain in patients with discogenic pain. Ambulation usually exacerbates the pain of spinal stenosis, whereas flexion or bending would improve the pain. If coughing or other Valsalva maneuvers exacerbate the pain, disc herniation should again be considered.

Radiation of pain along an extremity, often with associated numbness or tingling, is suggestive of a radiculopathy, that is, a compression of the nerve or nerve root along the spine. The most common cause is a herniated disc compressing the nerve root, but spinal stenosis, malignancy, and infection can also cause a compressive radiculopathy. Lumbar radiculopathy can often be exacerbated by sitting, coughing, or straining, whereas lying flat improves the pain.

The majority of symptomatic lumbar disc herniations occur at the L4-L5 and L5-S1 levels, resulting in pain that radiates down the leg and past the knee (sciatica). Although radiculopathy is present in only a minority of patients with low back pain, its absence makes a clinically important disc herniation unlikely. A patient with unilateral lower extremity weakness should raise particular concern. Differentiating true loss of muscular strength from the decreased ability to perform muscle function secondary to pain is challenging, but crucial. This distinction starts with the history but also requires observing the patient's movements. Did the patient ambulate into the ED or to the bathroom?

During the review of symptoms and past medical history, the physician should specifically assess for symptoms and predisposing conditions that may raise suspicion for a significant underlying systemic illness. Weight loss, fevers, immunocompromised status (e.g., HIV, chronic steroid use), or a history of intravenous drug use should raise concern for both focal and systemic infectious causes of the pain. Up to 51% of vertebral osteomyelitis have a primary focus of infection elsewhere in the body such as urinary tract, skin, soft tissue, vascular access site, endocarditis, or joint infection.[17] The spine is the most frequent location for skeletal metastases of malignant disease, found in up to 40% of patients with cancer.[18] Metastatic spine disease accounts for 10% to 30% of new cancer diagnoses annually.[19] The most common cancers that metastasize to spine include breast, lung, prostate, kidney, and thyroid carcinomas; therefore, patients with a history of one of these malignancies should elicit heightened alarm for a nonmechanical etiology of back pain.[20]

The clinician should also consider a referred source of back pain from the abdominal cavity and retroperitoneum (Tables 7–2 and 7–3). Identification of these entities by eliciting key clues from the patient's history requires a high index of suspicion by an astute clinician.

▶ **TABLE 7-2. NONMUSCULOSKELETAL CAUSES OF BACK PAIN**

Neoplasm
- Lung cancer
- Liver metastasis
- Pancreatic cancer
- Renal cancer
- Prostate cancer
- Testicular cancer
- Ovarian neoplasm
- Uterine fibroids

Infection
- Pneumonia
- Pleural effusion
- Chronic prostatitis
- Pyelonephritis
- Pelvic inflammatory disease

Vascular Causes
- Thoracic or abdominal aortic aneurysm
- Aortic dissection
- Pericarditis
- Pulmonary embolism
- Renal infarction
- Cardiac ischemia
- Retroperitoneal hemorrhage

Miscellaneous Causes
- Kidney stones
- Diabetic radiculopathy
- Osteoporosis
- Osteomalacia
- Gout and pseudogout
- Prolapsed uterus
- Endometriosis
- Ovarian torsion
- Pancreatitis
- Cholecystitis
- Peptic ulcer disease
- Herpes zoster
- Hip disorders

▶ **TABLE 7-3. NONMUSCULOSKELETAL CAUSES OF NECK PAIN**

Cardiac
- Myocardial infarction
- Angina pectoris

Gastrointestinal
- Hiatal hernia
- Esophageal spasm
- Biliary colic, cholecystitis, and choledocholithiasis
- Pancreatitis

Chest
- Mediastinal lesions
- Apical pulmonary lesions (Pancoast tumor)

Miscellaneous Causes
- Herpes zoster
- Temporomandibular joint syndrome
- Costochondritis

PHYSICAL EXAMINATION

Axiom: *In the setting of trauma or neurologic deficit, any motion in the spine should be avoided until after imaging to evaluate spinal stability.*

As with all patients in the ED, the examination of a patient with back pain begins with an assessment of the vital signs, with particular attention to acute life-threatening etiologies. Hypertension should raise suspicion for aortic dissection, while hypotension in the presence of back pain suggests an abdominal aortic aneurysm until proven otherwise. In the setting of trauma with potential spinal cord injury, consider neurogenic shock as a possible cause of hypotension once hemorrhage has been excluded. A fever is important to note; however, its absence does not exclude a significant infection. Only 35% to 60% of patients with vertebral osteomyelitis are found to have fevers, possibly due to use of analgesic medications that may also have antipyretic effects.[21]

A complete physical examination should be performed with particular attention to the heart, peripheral pulses, lungs, abdomen, and skin, followed by detailed musculoskeletal and neurologic examinations. Decreased breath sounds may suggest a malignancy-related effusion, while rales or rhonchi may suggest pneumonia or other active infection. Cardiovascular examination including peripheral pulse examination should be completed to assess for asymmetry of peripheral pulses or upper-extremity blood pressures, raising concern for aortic dissection. The abdominal examination should assess for the presence of a pulsatile mass, which would suggest an abdominal aortic aneurysm. In patients with concern for cord compression or cauda equine syndrome, it is important to perform a rectal examination to assess for loss of rectal tone or perianal anesthesia. A thorough examination of the skin may reveal evidence of the early lesions of herpes zoster or other potentially painful dermatologic conditions. Neurologic examination should include full assessment of strength, sensation, and reflexes, as well as rectal tone and perianal sensation in appropriate patients. Gait assessment should also be performed.

Cervical Spine Examination

Inspection starts by looking for scars, ecchymoses, or erythema. In the nontraumatic setting, the normal lordosis of the cervical spine is best seen from the side of the patient. If Valsalva or axial loading by applying a compressive force from the top of the head reproduces pain, there is likely a herniated disk or spinal stenosis affecting the diameter of the spinal canal or foramina.

In the cervical spine, the muscles are relaxed in the supine position, making the deeper bony and ligamentous structures more readily palpable in this position. In the patient who has suffered traumatic injuries with cervical immobilizing collar placed in the prehospital setting, careful attention should be paid to applying inline stabilization while the collar is carefully removed to examine for midline cervical spinal step-offs or tenderness. The examiner begins by palpating the occiput and the base of the skull in the midline. The posterior bony structures are best palpated if the examiner stands behind the patient's head and cups the hands under the neck so the fingertips meet at the midline (Fig. 7–4). The first structure noted is the spinous process of the axis (C2). The posterior arch of C2 is not palpable. In the thin patient, the examiner should be able to feel all the spinous processes of the cervical spine. Loss of alignment is seen in unilateral facet joint dislocation or with a fracture.

C7 (and sometimes T1) has the largest spinous process in most individuals and is a helpful landmark. Other landmarks in the cervical spine include the thyroid cartilage, which overlies C4 and C5, and the cricoid cartilage at the level of C6. The facet joints are palpated lateral to and between the spinous processes on each side. In the relaxed neck, they feel like a small dome. Tenderness over the facet joints suggests arthritis, fracture, or ligamentous injury.

The neurologic examination should include an assessment of motor strength, sensation, and reflex testing of the bilateral upper extremities. The location of cord injury can be localized based on the knowledge of specific motor function and sensory levels of each cervical

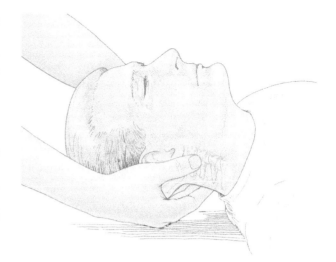

Figure 7–4. Examine the posterior cervical spine from behind the patient's head with the hands cupped so that the fingertips meet at the midline.

nerve root. Up to 20% of spinal injuries affect more than one level, and the cervical spine is more vulnerable to displacement than the thoracolumbar spine as it lacks the support of the rib cage and its relatively smaller size of facet joints. In the cervical spine, C5 to C8 are most commonly affected by traumatic injuries (Table 7–4 and Figs. 7–5 to 7–8).

Thoracolumbar Spine Examination

The thoracolumbar examination should proceed in a systematic manner for both efficiency and completeness. The complete examination of the spine in the nontraumatized patient is reviewed in this section, but different portions of the reviewed maneuvers should be employed based on the clinical scenario.

Standing

If the patient is able to stand, the examination begins in this position with inspection. Note the normal lordosis of the lumbar spine. Difficulty with straightening of the lumbar spine might suggest ankylosing spondylitis or paravertebral muscle spasm. Next, check the alignment of the back from behind the patient. More than half of patients will have abnormalities of alignment that may contribute to back

▶ TABLE 7–4. **PHYSICAL EXAMINATION TO TEST CERVICAL NERVE ROOTS**

	C5	C6	C7	C8
Sensory	Lateral arm	Lateral forearm and thumb	Middle finger	Ulnar forearm or little finger
Motor	Shoulder abduction and elbow flexion	Elbow flexion and wrist extension	Elbow extension and wrist flexion	Finger flexion
Reflex	Biceps	Brachioradialis	Triceps	None

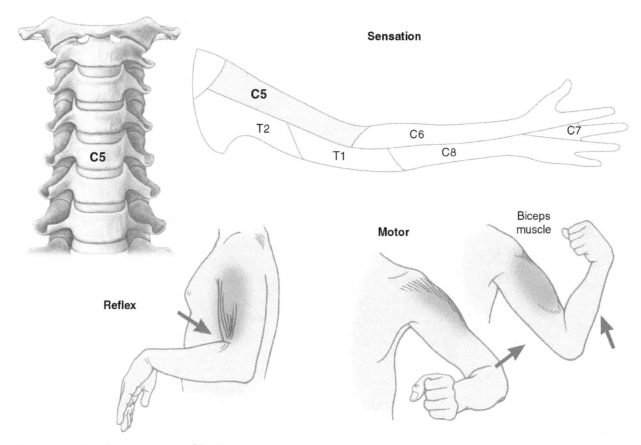

Figure 7–5. Neurologic assessment of the C5 nerve root.

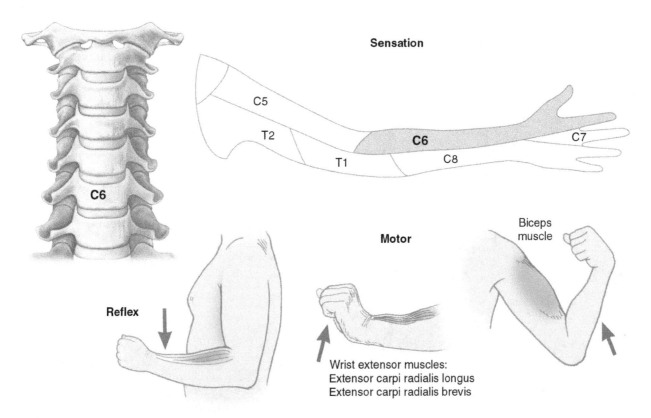

Figure 7–6. Neurologic assessment of the C6 nerve root.

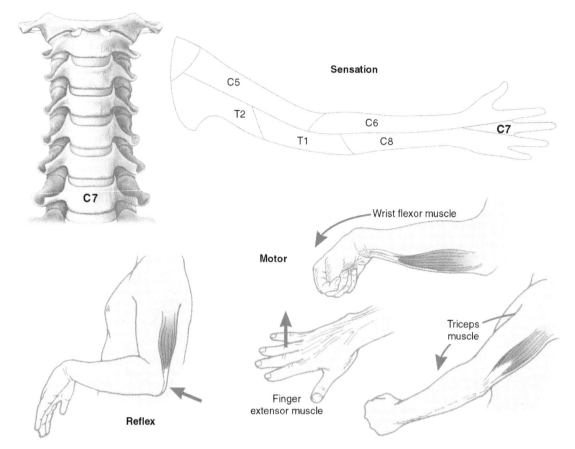

Figure 7–7. Neurologic assessment of the C7 nerve root.

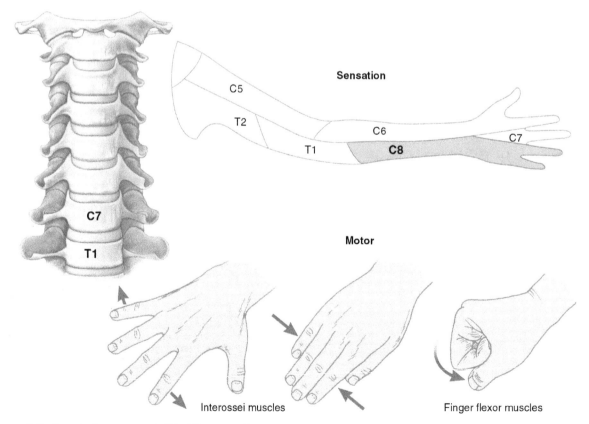

Figure 7–8. Neurologic assessment of the C8 nerve root.

strain. The first thoracic vertebrae should be centered over the sacrum, and the posterior superior iliac spines (PSISs) should be equal in height.

The sacroiliac (SI) joint is assessed by placing one thumb on the PSIS and the other on the spine of the sacrum. After asking the patient to raise the ipsilateral leg off the ground, determine if the PSIS moves downward in a normal fashion or upward to suggest potential SI joint pathology. In addition to assessing the SI joint, raising one leg while extending the back will exacerbate back pain in patients with facet joint disease or spondylolisthesis. If the patient prefers to stand while leaning over slightly to one side with the hip and knee flexed, this suggests sciatic nerve irritation, commonly from a herniated disk.

Range of motion in flexion and extension does not reliably distinguish among pathologic causes but can provide a baseline from which to evaluate for therapeutic response. Normal range of motion of the back involves 40 to 60 degrees of flexion. If the lumbar spine maintains its lordosis and flexion occurs at the hips when the patient bends forward, pathology of the lumbar spine, usually at the L4-L5 or L5-S1 interspaces, should be suspected. Pain with flexion is consistent with sciatica, disk herniation, or lumbar strain. Normal extension of the lumbar spine is 20 to 35 degrees. Extension stresses the facet joints and narrows the foramina through which the nerve roots exit. Painful extension, therefore, is characteristic of facet joint pathology and arthritis.

Palpation of the spine is ideally performed in flexion. The spinous processes of the thoracolumbar spine are easily palpated, except in extremely obese patients. Any lateral deviation of these processes suggests rotational deformity such as scoliosis or fracture. The distance between the spinous processes should be equivalent from one segment to the next. The supraspinous and interspinous ligaments are palpated in the recesses between the spinous processes (Fig. 7–9). Some helpful landmarks to remember include the iliac crests at the level of the L4 and L5 interspace and the S2 spinous process at the level of the PSIS (Fig. 7–10).

Pressure on the spinous processes is transmitted anteriorly to the arches and toward the vertebral bodies. For that reason, percussion of the spinous processes with a reflex hammer may aid in differentiating pain from the vertebral column versus deeper retroperitoneal structures. Percussion along the spinal column is a frequent deficiency in examining the spine but may be helpful in revealing metastatic disease, occult fracture, or infection.

The facet joints are located approximately 3 cm lateral to the spinous processes in the thoracolumbar region. Like the cervical spine, the facet joints are both lateral to and between the spinous processes. Direct palpation of the facet joints is not possible in the thoracolumbar spine because they are deep to the paraspinous muscles.

Lastly, while the patient is still standing, have the patient stand on his/her heels to test the motor function of the L5 root and stand on tiptoes to test the S1 root.

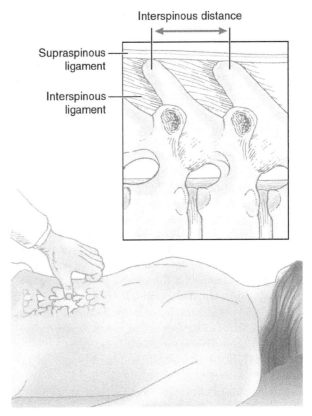

Figure 7–9. The supraspinous and interspinous ligaments are palpated between the spinous processes.

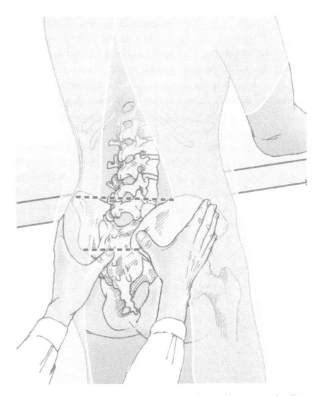

Figure 7–10. The L4-L5 interspace is palpated between the iliac crests, while S2 is palpated at the level of the posterior superior iliac spines.

▶ TABLE 7–5. **PHYSICAL EXAMINATION TO TEST LUMBOSACRAL NERVE ROOTS**

	L3	L4	L5	S1
Sensory	Anterior and medial thigh	Medial foot	Web space of 1st and 2nd digit	Lateral foot
Motor	Hip flexion	Knee extension	Big toe and ankle dorsiflexion	Ankle plantar flexion

Supine

With the patient supine, the straight-leg raise and crossed straight-leg raise tests can be performed. With the knee in extension, the leg is raised gradually. Pain before 30 degrees of elevation is not consistent with nerve root irritation because only the dura is being stretched until this point. Elevation from 30 to 60 degrees stretches the nerve root and reproduces pain in the presence of a herniated disk (Lasègue sign). For either test to be considered positive, the pain must radiate beyond the knee. A positive straight-leg test is sensitive, but not specific, for herniated disc. The crossed straight-leg test is less sensitive for herniated disks, but 90% specific.   An increase of pain with the Valsalva maneuver is also sensitive for sciatic nerve irritation.

The FABER (flexion, abduction, and external rotation of the hip) test for pathology of the hip and SI joints can also be performed while the patient is supine. The foot of the affected side is placed on the opposite knee. Pain in the groin suggests pathology of the hip, not the spine. Gentle, but firm, downward pressure on the flexed knee and opposite anterior superior iliac crest produces SI joint pain in patients with joint pathology.

The majority of the neurologic assessment can be performed while the patient is lying supine. The neurologic examination should include an assessment of motor strength, sensation, and reflex testing. Similar to the neurologic exam of the cervical spine, location of cord injury in the lumbosacral spine can be localized by testing motor and sensory function in specific nerve roots. In the

lumbar spine, the L3, L4, L5, and S1 nerve roots are tested (Table 7–5 and Figs. 7–11 to 7–13). L5 motor nerve root testing evaluates strength of ankle and great toe dorsiflexion. L5 sensory nerve root damage would result in numbness in the medial foot and the web space between the first and second toe. The S1 nerve root is tested by evaluating ankle reflexes and sensation at the posterior calf and lateral foot. S1 radiculopathy may cause weakness of plantar flexion. The ability to squeeze the buttocks together (i.e., gluteus maximus) is an additional reliable motor finding of the S1 nerve root.

One neurologic test that is frequently overlooked, but often diagnostic, is vibratory sensation. This test involves placement of a tuning fork over a bony prominence supplied by the nerve root (e.g., medial malleolus for L4, patella for L3). The vibration will elicit discomfort that radiates upward to the back in the sensory distribution of the irritated nerve root. Vibratory sense is the most superficial layer of the nerve and thus is the most sensitive for early compression.

When attempting to determine the location of neurologic injury, several general principles are useful. Unilateral weakness suggests a radiculopathy, whereas bilateral weakness or spasticity is characteristic of a lesion within the spinal cord (i.e., myelopathy). Cauda equina syndrome should be suspected in patients with lower motor neuron findings, bilateral leg weakness, loss of rectal tone, saddle anesthesia, and urinary retention. Sensory deficits within a single dermatome support a radicular source of pain, whereas

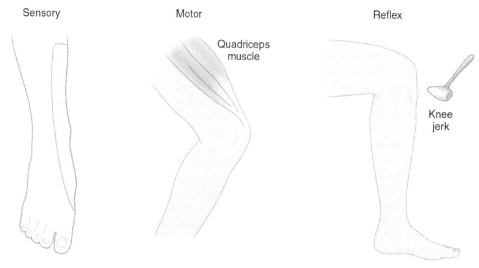

Figure 7–11. Neurologic assessment of the L4 nerve root.

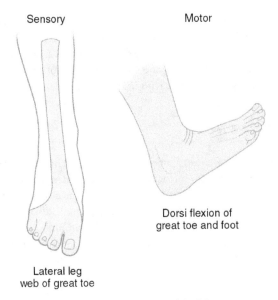

Figure 7–12. Neurologic assessment of the L5 nerve root.

involvement of multiple dermatomes is more likely to be due to pathology within the spinal cord (Fig. 7–14).

Prone

The S1 nerve root can be tested by assessing the function of the gluteus maximus muscle. Ask the patient to clench the buttocks together. If one side is weaker, there is likely a deficit of the S1 nerve root. The *femoral stretch test* is performed by extending the hip in the prone position. This maneuver produces pain lateral to the midline in patients with facet joint pathology. Pain produced in the anterior thigh, however, suggests irritation of the L2-L3 nerve roots.

The sciatic nerve may be palpated as it courses between the ischial tuberosity and the greater trochanter. If this produces tenderness, irritation of the nerve in this location should be suspected as opposed to irritation in the back. Piriformis syndrome is a cause of sciatic nerve irritation in this position and is covered in further detail in Chapter 17.

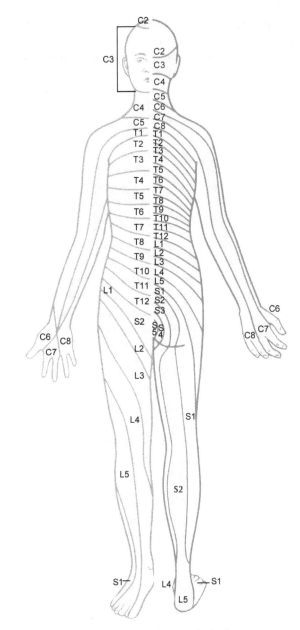

Figure 7–14. Dermatome distribution of spinal nerves.

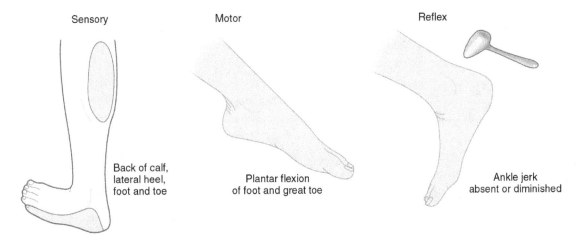

Figure 7–13. Neurologic assessment of the S1 nerve root.

A sheet placed under the umbilicus in the prone patient will flex the lumbar spine and make the facet joints more apparent. The spinous processes should be equidistant. A step-off between L5-S1 and L4-L5 suggests spondylolisthesis. As in the standing patient, tenderness 3 cm lateral to the spinous process suggests facet joint pathology.

IMAGING

Because the majority of patients with back pain recover uneventfully, advanced imaging studies are not routinely recommended. The American College of Physicians (ACP) provided guidelines in 2011 that recommended that diagnostic imaging is only indicated for patients with low back pain if they have "severe progressive neurologic deficits or signs or symptoms that suggests a serious or specific underlying condition." Furthermore, the same ACP guidelines suggest that routine imaging of uncomplicated back pain is not clinically beneficial and may also lead to harm. Table 7-6 identifies eight "red flags" that may be helpful in identifying patients in whom imaging should be considered.

Plain films radiographs may be used to assess lower back pain in patients with a history of osteoporosis or steroid use in whom pathologic or vertebral compression fractures are suspected.

In the spine, the anteroposterior, lateral, and oblique views are routine. The odontoid (open-mouth) view is unique to the cervical spine and allows for better visualization of C1 and C2, although it is not commonly used. Any patient with high risk for a traumatic vertebral injury should undergo computed tomography (CT) as it provides a detailed analysis of fractures extending to the posterior column, detects subtle fractures, and evaluates the integrity of pedicles and the posterior cortex.

MRI or CT imaging is recommended in patients who have severe or progressive neurologic deficits or who are suspected of having a serious underlying condition such as vertebral infection, cauda equina syndrome, or malignancy with impending cord compression. CT scan may demonstrate intervertebral disk disease or sizeable tumors, although it is not sensitive enough to diagnose spinal cord malignancy. MRI, which is the diagnostic test of choice for visualizing the spinal cord, vertebral marrow, and soft tissue, is emergently indicated when cord compression is suspected. MRI provides good definition of the disks, spinal cord, and nerve roots. It has a sensitivity of 97%, a specificity of 93%, and an accuracy of 94% in diagnosing vertebral osteomyelitis.

TREATMENT

The 2017 American College of Physicians clinical guidelines for treatment of acute, subacute, and chronic low back pain emphasizes the use of nonpharmacologic therapies, including superficial heat, massage, multidisciplinary rehabilitation, acupuncture, and exercise, among others. In those who have failed nonpharmacologic therapy, clinicians are encouraged to consider nonsteroid anti-inflammatory drugs as first-line therapy.

Any patient with significant trauma, impaired consciousness, or neurologic deficits should have spinal protection instituted with a cervical collar and logroll precautions in the ED, if not already performed in the prehospital setting. These precautions should be maintained until definitive imaging and repeat assessments are performed to rule out significant fractures or structural instability.

For information regarding the specific treatments of emergent conditions that cause back pain in the absence of trauma, refer to Chapter 8. Further treatment guidelines for patients with cervical and thoracolumbar trauma are presented in Chapters 9 and 10.

REFERENCES

1. Balagué F, Mannion AF, Pellisé F, Cedraschi C. Non-specific low back pain. *Lancet.* 2012;379(9814):482–491. doi:10.1016/S0140-6736(11)60610-7.
2. GBD 2015 Disease and Injury Incidence and Prevalence Collaborators. Global, regional, and national incidence, prevalence, and years lived with disability for 310 diseases and injuries, 1990–2015: a systematic analysis for the Global Burden of Disease Study 2015. *Lancet.* 2016;388(10053):1545–1602. doi:10.1016/S0140-6736(16)31678-6.
3. Deyo RA, Mirza SK, Martin BI. Back pain prevalence and visit rates: estimates from U.S. national surveys, 2002. *Spine.* 2006;31:2724–2727
4. Katz JN. Lumbar disc disorders and low-back pain: socioeconomic factors and consequences. *J Bone Joint Surg Am.* 2006; 88(suppl 2):21–24.
5. Bureau of Labor Statistics. Nonfatal occupational injuries and illnesses requiring days away from work 2013. http://www.bls.gov/news.release/pdf/osh2.pdf. Accessed December 11, 2017.
6. Wynne-Jones G, Cowen J, Jordan JL, et al. Absence from work and return to work in people with back pain: a systematic review and meta-analysis. *Occup Environ Med.* 2014;71:448–456
7. Deyo RA, Rainville J, Kent DL. What can the history and physical examination tell us about low back pain? *JAMA.* 1992; 268(6):760–765.

▶ **TABLE 7-6. RED FLAGS TO CONSIDER IMAGING STUDIES**

History of recent trauma
Age <18 or >50 yr
History of cancer
Pain at night
Fever, immunocompromised, IV drug abuse
Symptoms longer than 4–6 wk
Neurologic complaints or incontinence
Neurologic deficits on examination

8. van Tulder MW, Assendelft WJ, Koes BW, Bouter LM. Spinal radiographic findings and nonspecific low back pain. A systematic review of observational studies. *Spine*. 1997;22:427–434.

9. Koes BW, van Tulder MW, Thomas S. Diagnosis and treatment of low back pain. *BMJ*. 2006;332(7555):1430–1434. doi: 10.1136/bmj.332.7555.1430.

10. Winters ME, Kluetz P, Zilberstein J. Back pain emergencies. *Med Clin North Am*. 2006;90(3):505–523.

11. Sieper J, van der Heijde D, Landewé R, et al. New criteria for inflammatory back pain in patients with chronic back pain: a real patient exercise by experts from the Assessment of Spondylo-Arthritis International Society (ASAS). *Ann Rheum Dis*. 2009;68(6):784–788. doi:10.1136/ard.2008.101501. Epub 2009 Jan 15.

12. Brinjikji W, Luetmer PH, Comstock B, et al. Systematic literature review of imaging features of spinal degeneration in asymptomatic populations. *AJNR Am J Neuroradiol*. 2015;36(4):811–816. doi:10.3174/ajnr.A4173. Epub 2014 Nov 27.

13. Deyo RA, Diehl AK. Cancer as a cause of back pain: frequency, clinical presentation, and diagnostic strategies. *J Gen Intern Med*. 1988;3(3):230–238.

14. Alexandru D, So W. Evaluation and management of vertebral compression fractures. *Permanente J*. 2012;16(4):46–51.

15. Rudwaleit M, Metter A, Listing J, Sieper J, Braun J. Inflammatory back pain in ankylosing spondylitis: a reassessment of the clinical history for application as classification and diagnostic criteria. *Arthritis Rheum*. 2006;54:569–578.

16. Balasubramanian K, Kalsi P, Greenough CG, Kuskoor Seetharam MP. Reliability of clinical assessment in diagnosing cauda equina syndrome. *Br J Neurosurg*. 2010;24(4):383–386. doi:10.3109/02688697.2010.505987.

17. McHenry MC, Easley KA, Locker GA. Vertebral osteomyelitis: long-term outcome for 253 patients from 7 Cleveland-area hospitals. *Clin Infect Dis*. 2002;34:1342–1350.

18. Singh K, Samartzis D, Vaccaro AR, Andersson GB, An HS, Heller JG. Current concepts in the management of metastatic spinal disease. The role of minimally-invasive approaches. *J Bone Joint Surg Br*. 2006;88:434–442.

19. White AP, Kwon BK, Lindskog DM, Friedlaender GE, Grauer JN. Metastatic disease of the spine. *J Am Acad Orthop Surg*. 2006;14:587–598.

20. Deyo RA, Weinstein JN. Primary care: low back pain. *N Engl J Med*. 2001;344:363–370.

21. Zimmerli W. Vertebral osteomyelitis. *N Engl J Med*. 2010;362(11):1022–1029. doi:10.1056/NEJMcp0910753.

22. Theodore N, Hadley MN, Aarabi B, et al. Prehospital cervical spinal immobilization after trauma. *Neurosurgery*. 2013;72(suppl 2):22–34. doi:10.1227/NEU.0b013e318276edb1.

23. Holdsworth F. Review article fractures, dislocations, and fracture-dislocations of the spine. *J Bone Joint Surg Am*. 1970;52(8):1534–1551.

24. van der Windt DA, Simons E, Riphagen II, et al. Physical examination for lumbar radiculopathy due to disc herniation in patients with low-back pain. *Cochrane Database Syst Rev*. 2010;17(2):CD007431.

25. Chou R, Qaseem A, Owens DK, Shekelle P; Clinical Guidelines Committee of the American College of Physicians. Diagnostic imaging for low back pain: advice for high-value health care from the American College of Physicians. *Ann Intern Med*. 2011;154(3):181–189. doi:10.7326/0003-4819-154-3-201102010-00008.

26. Patel ND, Broderick DF, Burns J, et al. *American College of Radiology ACR Appropriateness Criteria®: low back pain*. Date of origin: 1996; Last review date: 2015. https://acsearch.acr.org/docs/69483/Narrative/. Accessed December 19, 2017.

27. Daffner RH, Weissman BN, Wippold FJ II, et al. *American College of Radiology ACR Appropriateness Criteria®: suspected spine trauma*. Date of origin: 1999; Last review date: 2012. https://acsearch.acr.org/docs/69359/Narrative/. Accessed December 19, 2017.

28. Jarvik JG, Deyo RA. Diagnostic evaluation of low back pain with emphasis on imaging. *Ann Intern Med*. 2002;137:586–597.

29. Berbari EF, Kanj SS, Kowalski TJ, et al. 2015 Infectious Diseases Society of America (IDSA) clinical practice guidelines for the diagnosis and treatment of native vertebral osteomyelitis in adults. *Clin Infect Dis*. 2015;61(6):e26–46. doi:10.1093/cid/civ482. Epub 2015 Jul 29.

30. Qaseem A, Wilt TJ, McLean RM, Forciea MA; Clinical Guidelines Committee of the American College of Physicians. Noninvasive treatments for acute, subacute, and chronic low back pain: a clinical practice guideline from the American College of Physicians. *Ann Intern Med*. 2017;166(7):514–530. doi:10.7326/M16-2367. Epub 2017 Feb 14.

CHAPTER 8

Specific Disorders of the Spine

Andrew D. Perron, MD and Carl A. Germann, MD

INTRODUCTION

Chapter 7 covered a general approach to and a detailed examination of the patient with back or neck pain. In this chapter, a more extensive discussion of specific conditions of the spine is presented. For a review of seronegative spondyloarthropathy (e.g., ankylosing spondylitis), the reader is referred to Chapter 3. Fractures of the spine are addressed in Chapters 9 and 10.

It should be noted that in an unselected emergency department (ED) population presenting with back pain, between 1 and 5 patients will have a specific diagnosis and approximately 1 in 200 patients will need surgery. The challenge for the clinician is to identify these small patient populations from among the larger group with a complaint of "back pain." The clinician, armed with a history and physical examination, must frequently decide who needs further emergent workup and who can be safely observed. Further challenges the clinician faces are that spinal syndromes can present in a subtle fashion and that a great deal of clinical overlap occurs between many of the pathophysiologic processes.

The imaging of most patients presenting with spinal disorders is driven by the search for "red flags" in the history or physical examination. Generally, there is higher concern and hence a lower threshold to image those younger than 18 and those older than 50. Also included in this group are those with immunocompromise, those who use IV drugs, those with histories of primary cancers known to metastasize to the spine, those with recurrent infections (e.g., GU infections), those with significant trauma, and those exhibiting neurologic dysfunction. Regarding the search for red flags, a recent systematic review of the literature found that there were currently 26 different "red flags" identified in the literature, and there was very little evidence for any of them beyond common sense and anecdote. The review noted that of the 26 possible red flags, the 3 that were the most likely to predict pathology were older age, prolonged steroid use, and a history of malignancy. In the absence of red flags, it is generally recommended that imaging be avoided in the first 4 to 6 weeks of the back pain syndrome, as the vast majority of patients will resolve within this time frame.

CAUDA EQUINA SYNDROME

Cauda equina syndrome refers to nerve compression within the spinal canal that occurs below the L1-L2 interspace after the termination of the spinal cord. The clinical picture is that of a lower motor neuron lesion with weakness or paralysis, loss of rectal tone, sensory loss in a dermatomal pattern, decreased deep tendon reflexes, and bladder dysfunction. The classic sensory description is "saddle" anesthesia, with loss of sensation in the buttocks and perineal areas. It should be noted that within the first few days, a complete cord syndrome may present similarly until upper motor neuron symptoms develop.

The most common cause of cauda equina syndrome is a large midline disc herniation, usually at the L4-L5 or L5-S1 interspaces. Other causes include spinal metastases, spinal hematoma, epidural abscess, vertebral fracture, or transverse myelitis. Although anal sphincter tone is decreased in up to 80% of patients, an elevated urinary postvoid residual is the most consistent finding to make the diagnosis. A postvoid residual of more than 100 to 200 mL of urine is 90% sensitive and 95% specific for the diagnosis in patients suspected of cauda equina syndrome. The diagnosis is confirmed by an emergent magnetic resonance imaging (MRI) or computed tomography (CT)-myelography in those who cannot have an MRI. Treatment consists of high-dose IV steroids (recommended range, 4–100 mg of dexamethasone) and surgical consultation. Surgical intervention is recommended on an urgent basis to increase the likelihood of neurologic recovery.

DISC HERNIATION

With aging, degeneration develops in the annulus fibrosis that can lead to herniation of the nucleus pulposus following an acute increase in pressure within the disc. Herniation usually progresses gradually as the posterior longitudinal ligament acts to restrain the nucleus. Eventually, as the ligament weakens, the nucleus migrates into the intravertebral foramen, most commonly in a posterolateral direction (i.e., paramedian herniation). In this location, the disc comes into contact with the nerve root, causing pain and potentially a radiculopathy. A large central herniation can compress the spinal cord or cauda equina.

Approximately 4% to 6% of the population will suffer from a clinically significant disc herniation. The vast majority occurs in the lumbar spine and causes low back and leg pain. In patients with sciatica, 90% of cases are due to a herniated disc, whereas lumbar stenosis and less often a tumor are other possible causes. Approximately 98% of clinically important lumbar disc herniations occur at the L4-L5 or L5-S1 intervertebral level. In the cervical spine, the C6-C7 and C5-C6 discs account for 70% and 20% of cases, respectively. Cervical radiculopathy is more likely to be due to degenerative changes than disc herniation by a factor of 3:1.

Clinical Features

Most commonly, the patient is between the ages of 30 and 50 because in older individuals the nucleus is desiccated and fibrotic and less likely to herniate. Men are affected three times more frequently than women.

The pain usually originates in the general location of the herniation (i.e., low back), but frequently the pain from radiculopathy (i.e., sciatica) predominates. Sciatica is 95% sensitive for lumbar disc herniation. The absence of sciatica makes a clinically important disc herniation unlikely, estimated to be present in 1 of 1000 patients.

The patient might report a history of recurrent episodes of back pain that have resolved spontaneously. With an acute rupture, severe low back pain occurs either instantaneously or several hours after an injury (e.g., lifting). Any movement exacerbates the pain, and it is worse on sitting than on standing. Arising from a seated position markedly exaggerates the pain. The first 30 minutes after awakening are characterized by the worst pain, which later improves. Prolonged driving will exacerbate the pain, and it can be greatly increased after coughing or sneezing (i.e., Valsalva).

The back examination may reveal significant muscle spasm and flattening of the lumbar lordosis. The patient with a paramedian herniation (most common) will frequently be in the lateral decubitus position with flexion of the lumbar spine, hips, and knees. This position, which is more comfortable for such patients, is virtually pathognomonic of disc disease. The physical examination should include an examination of the neurologic function in the legs. Each nerve root should be tested as described in Chapter 7. Depending on the nerve root involved, weakness and sensory loss can occur. Sensory loss in a dermatomal distribution is the most reliable predictor of the location of the affected nerve root.

The straight-leg raise test (Lasègue sign) exacerbates pain in a patient with a herniation at the L5 or S1 nerve root by stretching the compressed nerve. This test is performed in the supine patient by cupping the heel in one hand and slowly raising the affected leg while the knee remains extended (Fig. 8–1). A positive test is present if sciatica is reproduced between 30 and 60 degrees of leg elevation. The lower the angle that produces a positive test, the more specific the test and the more likely that a significant herniation will be found at surgery. Dorsiflexion of the foot may further exacerbate the pain. It should be emphasized that pain reproduced in the back does not constitute a positive test. When positive, this test is 80% sensitive and 40% specific for lumbar disc herniation. The crossed straight-leg raise test involves the same maneuver on the unaffected side. It is 25% sensitive, but the specificity is higher at 90%.

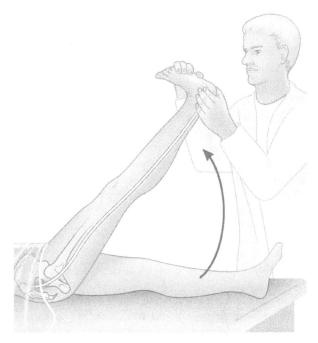

Figure 8–1. The supine straight-leg raise test.

The straight-leg raise test can also be performed in a seated position (Fig. 8–2). This test has been used as a way of differentiating patients with nonorganic causes of pain because it should theoretically produce the same results. However, when compared with the supine version using MRI as the gold standard, the seated straight-leg raise test was found to be less sensitive.

In the case of a cervical disc herniation, pain is felt in the neck and may radiate to the shoulder and into the arm in the spinal root distribution. Headache may be associated with herniations of C3-C4 and C4-C5. There is usually a noted decreased range of motion in the neck and point tenderness over the spinal level of the involved disc.

The location of radiated pain depends on the nerve root affected. The C4 nerve root causes radiation of pain to the

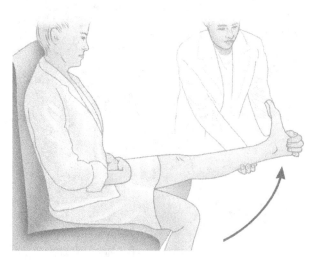

Figure 8–2. The sitting straight-leg raise test.

scapula, whereas the C5 nerve root refers pain to the shoulder. Both the C4 and C5 nerve roots may radiate pain to the anterior chest and be confused with cardiac ischemia. When the C6 or C7 nerve root is affected, pain is radiated to the lateral arm and dorsal forearm. The C8 nerve root radiates pain to the medial forearm. When pain radiates to both arms (± legs), consider a cervical myelopathy from a centrally protruding disc.

Spurling sign is positive in the presence of a cervical disc herniation when hyperextension and lateral flexion of the neck to the symptomatic side reproduce the pain. The shoulder abduction test is performed by placing the symptomatic hand on top of the head. A positive test is present when this action results in the relief of pain.

Imaging

In the setting of back pain with radiculopathy likely due to a herniated disc, diagnostic imaging is only useful if the results will alter the management. Therefore, in the ED, imaging is indicated if an alternate diagnosis such as infection or malignancy is suggested on the basis of the history and physical examination. Imaging may also be appropriate in patients with severe symptoms who fail conservative treatment for a period of 6 to 8 weeks. In these patients where surgery might be considered, confirmation of the location of a herniated disc will be necessary, but it does not need to occur emergently. Emergent imaging should be performed in patients with cauda equina syndrome or acute severe/progressive weakness.

Plain films are not recommended because identification of a herniated disc is not possible. Both CT and MRI are equally accurate at diagnosing disc herniation. MRI is usually favored because it lacks ionizing radiation and has better soft-tissue visualization (Fig. 8–3). The major disadvantage

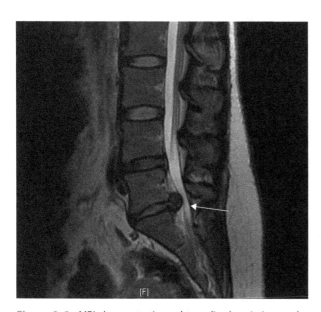

Figure 8–3. MRI demonstrating a large disc herniation at the L5-S1 interspace.

of MRI is availability, especially for the ED. Of note, approximately 20% to 36% of asymptomatic individuals will have evidence of a lumbar disc herniation on CT or MRI.

Treatment

Treatment of both cervical and lumbar radiculopathy is usually conservative with nonsteroidal anti-inflammatories and acetaminophen. Muscle relaxants are frequently prescribed but are no better than nonsteroidal anti-inflammatories. Narcotics provide no quicker return to normal activity, but may be prescribed in the setting of severe pain for a short time. Bed rest is no longer recommended. Physical therapy, acupuncture, and spinal manipulation have an unknown effectiveness.

The literature is conflicting on the use of systemic corticosteroids. Recent randomized-controlled trials have demonstrated transient pain reduction with IV glucocorticoids for radicular pain, whereas no measurable benefit is found from the use of oral steroids. In practice, many physicians still favor a short course of tapered steroids for radicular symptoms. Multiple studies have shown no specific benefit for this regimen in back pain patients without radiculopathy.

Epidural steroid injection is sometimes effective in the treatment of early symptoms (within 3 months), but there is no difference at 1 year. Repeated injections, a common practice, are not supported by the current literature. Although epidural injection can offer some short-term relief for some patients with sciatica, it does not provide functional improvement, nor does it alter the need for surgery. The procedure does not confer benefit on patients without radicular symptoms.

Lumbar discectomies are among the most common elective procedures performed; however, there is significant controversy regarding both the need for surgery and the optimal timing of the procedure. Most acute attacks of sciatica resolve on their own with nonsurgical management. Approximately half of patients start to improve within 10 days, 60% recover within 3 months, and 70% recover within 12 months. Among patients seeking specialty care, approximately 15% undergo surgery within 6 months.

Surgery is an option for more rapid relief in patients whose recovery is slow or too debilitating. These patients are usually able to get back to work faster, making the cost of the surgery equal to the societal costs of the conservative approach. In general, surgery is not considered unless symptoms do not improve over 6 to 8 weeks, or there is rapid progression with motor dysfunction. Immediate surgery is indicated when cauda equina syndrome is present.

Open microdiscectomy is the most common technique. Minimally invasive endoscopic discectomies are becoming more common and are theoretically desirable because they reduce tissue damage. Evidence for their superiority is still lacking. Although patients undergoing surgery tend to have improved function and fewer symptoms at 1 and 2 years postoperation, results are comparable beyond 4 years.

SCIATIC NEUROPATHY

In patients with sciatica (neuropathic pain in the L5-S1 distribution), a herniated disc or spinal stenosis is often assumed to be the cause and other diagnoses are not considered. However, direct compression of the sciatic nerve can occur from blunt trauma or a tumor that can produce a neuropathy of the sciatic nerve.

Another form of sciatic neuropathy occurs following injury to the piriformis muscle, where hematoma formation and subsequent scarring causes mechanical irritation of the anatomically adjacent sciatic nerve. Patients may present with low back, buttocks, or posterior thigh pain. Prolonged hip flexion, adduction, and internal rotation aggravate the pain. The patient will hold the leg in external rotation when supine. Forceful internal rotation of the flexed thigh will reproduce symptoms (Freiberg sign). There is weakness and pain on resisted abduction and external rotation. For more information on piriformis syndrome, the reader is referred to Chapter 17.

In this setting, neurologic complaints are more common than pain. The peroneal division of the sciatic nerve is most susceptible to trauma because of its peripheral location. Sciatic neuropathy is more likely when changes in position or Valsalva do not cause an exacerbation of symptoms.

SPINAL STENOSIS

Spinal stenosis refers to a narrowing of the spinal canal. It occurs in the area of the central canal or neural foramina, which puts pressure on the nerve roots causing pain and radiculopathy. Age-associated degeneration of the lumbar discs and facet joints is the most common etiology. Pathologic features include loss of disc height, disc bulging, ligamentum flavum hypertrophy, facet osteophyte formation, and joint capsule thickening (Fig. 8–4). Narrowing from a prior surgical procedure (e.g., spinal fusion or laminectomy) can also be causative. Stenosis may also arise from spondylolisthesis, Paget disease, acromegaly, and excess corticosteroids. Congenital spinal stenosis affects individuals in their 20s to 40s and is due to developmentally shortened pedicles.[28]

Clinical Features

Because degenerative changes are the primary cause, spinal stenosis occurs in older individuals and is the most frequent indication for spinal surgery in patients older than 65 years.[29] Approximately 85% of patients experience radiation of pain in the buttocks, thighs, and legs. Numbness, tingling, or cramping of the legs may occur. Bowel or bladder dysfunction is rare. Symptoms may be unilateral or bilateral.

The symptoms of spinal stenosis bear similarity with vascular claudication, thus earning the name neurogenic claudication or pseudoclaudication. In both conditions, pain is exacerbated by ambulation, yet the pain from spinal stenosis persists while a patient remains standing in an upright position. Symptoms are relieved with sitting and other positions of increased lumbar flexion. In one systematic review, neurogenic claudication was present in 82% of patients with lumbar spinal stenosis.[30] The most specific findings were absence of pain with sitting, leaning forward,

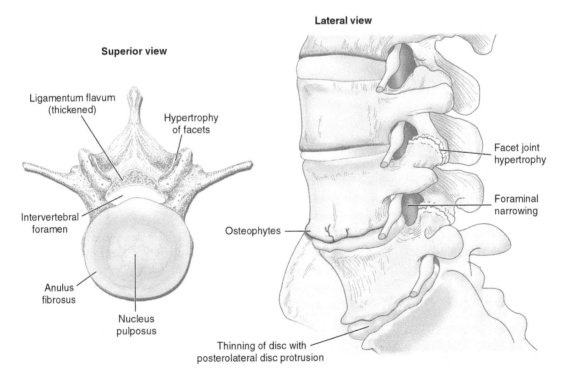

Figure 8–4. Pathologic features of spinal stenosis.

or squatting. Many patients can tolerate vigorous activity such as bike riding or walking uphill, yet simply standing upright proves to be unbearable. Similar to disc herniation, pain may also increase with coughing, sneezing, or other forms of Valsalva maneuvers.

On physical examination, there is increased pain with spine extension, as this position further reduces the cross-sectional area of the spinal canal. As a result, the patient with spinal stenosis will ambulate with a slightly stooped posture. This is in contrast to disc herniation, where flexion is usually most painful. Closing the eyes may produce unsteadiness (Romberg maneuver) if the proprioceptive fibers in the posterior column are involved. For this reason, patients with spinal stenosis frequently walk with a wide-based gait. A wide-based gait or positive Romberg in the setting of low back pain has a specificity of greater than 90% for lumbar spinal stenosis. Thigh pain following brief periods of lumbar extension may also occur. Approximately 60% of patients will develop neurologic deficits, which may be bilateral or polyradicular. The most commonly involved nerve root is L5 (75%) followed by L4 (15%). Motor findings are mild in most cases, and weakness that inhibits activity is unusual.

Imaging

Plain films can be useful if they show evidence of degenerative disease of the spine or spondylolisthesis, but they are not routinely indicated. CT or MRI will reveal the pathologic features of spinal stenosis in more than 70% of affected patients. Advanced imaging is usually only obtained when surgery is being considered. Interestingly, CT and MRI findings consistent with spinal stenosis are present in 20% of patients older than 60 years who have no symptoms. In addition, actual measurements of the degree of spinal stenosis on MRI are only loosely correlated with the clinical syndrome of spinal stenosis. In other words, patients may be symptomatic despite minimal compression, and conversely, others with a high degree of compression may be asymptomatic.

Other diagnostic tests not routinely obtained include CT-myelography, electromyography (EMG), and nerve conduction studies (NCS). CT-myelography improves visualization of nerve root compression over CT alone, but is invasive and is performed only when MRI is contraindicated. EMG and NCS aid the clinician in distinguishing other forms of peripheral neuropathy and increase the overall specificity for lumbar spinal stenosis. The most common finding is bilateral multilevel radiculopathies.

Treatment

Nonoperative treatment can provide long-lasting relief from pain and improved quality of life. The pain of spinal stenosis is managed with acetaminophen initially, and then nonsteroidal anti-inflammatory drugs. Mild narcotic analgesics are not routine, but can be used. Calcitonin has been useful in many patients with neurogenic claudication and pain. The North American Spine Society's most recent guidelines indicated little evidence to support any long-term benefits from pharmacotherapy.

Physical therapy is the mainstay of conservative treatment, with the aim of strengthening core musculature and correcting posture. Aerobic activities such as bicycling are typically well tolerated, with the added benefit of weight loss to decrease lumbar lordosis. Lumbar supports (i.e., corsets) can help patients maintain a flexed posture. Traction provides segmental unloading and relief when there is foraminal compression. The use of epidural corticosteroid injections is becoming increasingly common, but data on their effectiveness are limited.

Operative management should be considered when conservative measures have failed. Laminectomy or partial facetectomy are used to decompress the central spinal canal and neural foramina. Minimally invasive operative techniques have been developed and are proving useful.

Studies comparing operative to conservative management suggest an improvement in symptoms for the operative group that lasts several years. Surgery is currently recommended for patients with severe or rapidly progressive symptoms. Patients with moderate symptoms also tend to have less pain and functional improvement compared to nonoperative management. Reoperation is necessary in less than a quarter of patients over the course of 10 years.

SPONDYLOLISTHESIS

The pars interarticularis is the portion of the posterior vertebral arch between the inferior and superior articular processes. Disruption of the pars interarticularis is termed *spondylolysis*. It is usually bilateral, and 90% of cases affect the L5 vertebra.

When spondylolysis is present, the vertebra can move, most commonly with the superior vertebra shifting forward relative to the inferior vertebra. Forward translation of the vertebra is termed *spondylolisthesis*, Greek for "vertebral slippage down a slope" (Fig. 8–1). Spondylolysis is the most common precipitant of spondylolisthesis, accounting for 80% of cases. Other causes of spondylolisthesis are listed in Table 8–1.

A stress fracture is the most common cause of spondylolysis, usually occurring in young patients with sports that require extension (e.g., gymnastics) or rotation (e.g., tennis). Lumbar extension results in the inferior articular process of the superior vertebra coming into contact with the pars interarticularis of the inferior vertebra. Repetitive impact is believed to lead to the fracture.

There is a genetic predisposition to spondylolysis. It occurs in 15% to 70% of first-degree relatives of patient with spondylolysis. Approximately 3% to 6% of Caucasians have spondylolysis, a rate that is two to three times higher than African Americans. There is a higher rate of spondylolysis in males, but slippage is more common in females. Progression to spondylolisthesis occurs in 15%

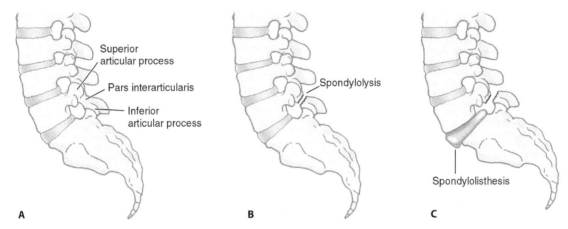

Figure 8–5. **A.** The pars interarticularis. **B.** Spondylolysis. **C.** Spondylolisthesis.

of individuals and is usually seen by age 16. Up to 6% of 14-year-olds in the United States have spondylolisthesis.[53]

The severity of spondylolisthesis is graded on the basis of the percentage of translation of the superior vertebra in relation to the caudal one (Fig. 8–6). Grade I is present if <25% translation is present, grade II if 26% to 50%, grade III if 51% to 75%, and grade IV if 76% to 100%. Grade V spondylolisthesis, also termed *spondyloptosis*, is present when there is greater than a 100% slip. When less than 50% translation has occurred, the spondylolisthesis is considered low-grade and is stable. Slips greater than 50% are considered unstable.

Clinical Features

Although many patients with spondylolisthesis remain asymptomatic, the most common complaint is low back pain that may radiate to the buttock or posterior thigh. The onset may be acute, but a gradual onset is more common. Pain is worse with hyperextension and rotation and is improved with rest. On examination, tenderness in the lumbar region is typical, and an associated step-off may be palpable if spondylolisthesis is significant (Fig. 8–7). Ambulation is characterized by a short stride length and crouching in severe cases. When high-grade spondylolisthesis has occurred, neurologic deficits from pressure on a nerve root or the cauda equina may occur.

Imaging

Plain films are a good screening test. Oblique lumbar radiographs demonstrate the "Scotty dog" appearance (Fig. 8–8). The neck of the dog corresponds to the pars interarticularis and a broken neck or a collar represents spondylolysis.[54,55] Plain films are 84% sensitive.[49] A stress fracture may not be visible on oblique radiographs, and further imaging may be necessary on an outpatient basis. The lateral radiograph is best to diagnose spondylolisthesis (Fig. 8–9).

CT scans may also miss a stress fracture of the pars, but the sensitivity is higher than plain radiographs, particularly when SPECT imaging is used.[49] MRI has the highest sensitivity. MRI is indicated for patients with high-grade spondylolisthesis and patients with neurologic symptoms (e.g., radiculopathy).[56–58]

Treatment

Spondylolysis and low-grade spondylolisthesis are treated conservatively with physical therapy and pain medications. Back exercises increase spinal stability and reduce pain and disability.[59,60] Steroid injections at the nerve root or pars interarticularis can be both diagnostic and therapeutic.[52] A rigid or elastic orthotic brace to reduce lumbar lordosis may be indicated for children, along with the recommendation not to participate in sports. More than 90% of children with spondylolysis treated nonoperatively have resolution of their

▶ TABLE 8-1   **FIVE TYPES OF SPONDYLOLISTHESIS**

Type	Name	Criteria
I	Dysplastic	Congenital malformed facet joints allow translation
II	Isthmic	Three causes of spondylolysis: stress fracture (lytic), elongation of the pars due to a healing stress fracture, acute traumatic fracture
III	Degenerative	Osteoarthritis and disc degeneration lead to facet incompetence
IV	Traumatic	Fracture of posterior elements other than the pars interarticularis
V	Pathologic	Changes in the posterior elements secondary to malignancy or primary bone diseases

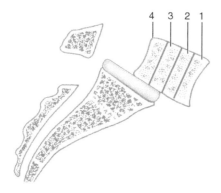

Figure 8–6. The grade of spondylolisthesis is calculated by the percentage shift of the superior vertebra on the inferior one.

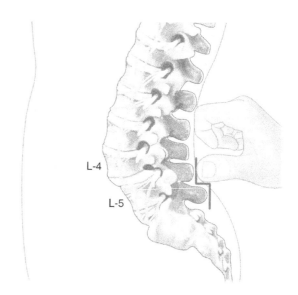

Figure 8–7. A step-off may be appreciated in a patient with spondylolisthesis.

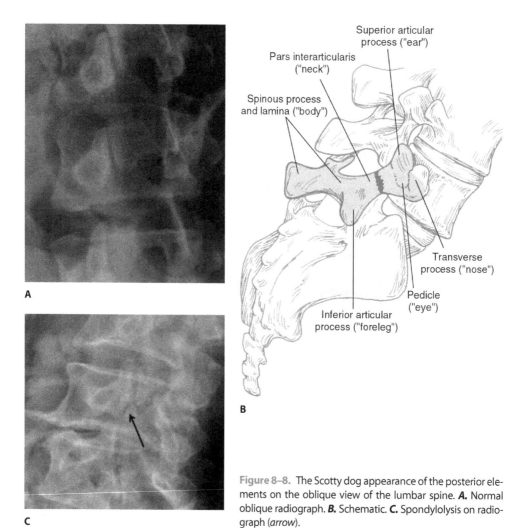

Figure 8–8. The Scotty dog appearance of the posterior elements on the oblique view of the lumbar spine. **A.** Normal oblique radiograph. **B.** Schematic. **C.** Spondylolysis on radiograph (*arrow*).

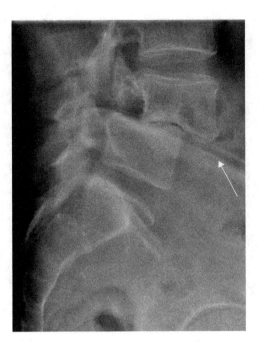

Figure 8–9. A 50% spondylolisthesis of L4 on L5.

symptoms.[61] Adults with degenerative spondylolisthesis also fair well with conservative treatment unless they present with neurologic deficits.[62,63] Indications for surgery in patients with low-grade spondylolisthesis include significant low back pain or radicular pain refractory to nonoperative treatment. Decompression (in patients with neural compression) and spinal fusion are the operative treatments of choice.[50,64]

The definitive treatment of high-grade spondylolisthesis depends on the age of the patient. Children should be considered for surgical stabilization because they are at a high risk of further slippage, whereas adults should undergo operative treatment only after conservative measures have proven unsuccessful.[52]

SACROILIAC JOINT DISEASE

In patients with low back pain below the belt line, 40% will have a diagnosis of sacroiliac joint disease. Pain is localized to the joint and buttocks area and does not radiate like that of a herniated disc. The onset of pain is gradual and pain is usually unilateral and may radiate to the groin. Most patients feel relief when lying down. This condition is especially common in patients with rheumatoid arthritis, pregnancy, inflammatory bowel disease, or following pelvic trauma. A test for sacroiliac joint disease is the "standing forward flexion test." The examiner places his/her thumbs just under the PSIS with the thumbs facing each other. The patient flexes his/her lumbar spine maximally. The side with SI joint disease moves less and appears to move cephalad. In "Gillet test," the thumb is moved to the sacrum while the other thumb is kept under the PSIS. Now ask the patient to flex the ipsilateral hip.

A positive test is seen when the thumb under the PSIS does not move cephalad.

Treatment of SI joint disease may consist of a combination of bracing, anti-inflammatory medications, and physical therapy. The patient should generally refrain from athletics. Steroid injection may also be of benefit.

SPINAL INFECTIONS

Spinal Epidural Abscess

Spinal epidural abscess (SEA) is a rare infection that may first present with nonspecific findings. These features contribute to SEA being initially misdiagnosed in approximately half of cases (range, 11%–75%).[65] Because the outcome may depend on early treatment, a rapid diagnosis is the goal. Left untreated, irreversible paralysis occurs in 4% to 22% of patients.

Although SEA remains a rare entity (1 in 10,000 hospital admissions), the incidence has increased in the past two decades due to an increase in the number of patients at risk (e.g., increased rate of spinal surgery).[65] Predisposing conditions include immunocompromise (e.g., diabetes, HIV, elderly), spinal abnormality (e.g., arthritis, trauma, surgery), and an outside source of infection (e.g., injection drug use, indwelling catheter).[66-68]

The majority of cases are due to hematogenous spread of infection, whereas contiguous spread is less common. *Staphylococcus aureus* (*S aureus*) is responsible for two-thirds of cases.[68] Less common pathogens include coagulase-negative staphylococcus and gram-negative bacteria. The presence of the abscess in the epidural space is potentially deleterious to the spinal cord due to both physical compression and a localized ischemic mechanism.

Abscesses are more common in the posterior epidural space and within the thoracolumbar spine because there is more adipose tissue in these locations that is prone to infection (Fig. 8–10).

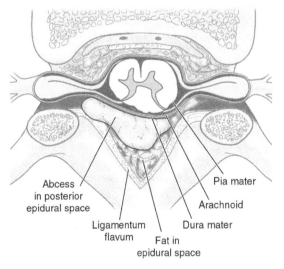

Figure 8–10. Spinal epidural abscess.

Clinical Features

The symptoms of SEA progress in four classical stages. Initially, back pain at the level of the affected portion of the cord is present followed by nerve root pain. Cord dysfunction in the form of motor weakness, sensory loss, and bowel/bladder dysfunction follows. The final stage of untreated disease is paralysis. The rate of progression from one stage to the next varies from as short as hours to as long as days, weeks, and even months.

The most common symptoms at the time of diagnosis are back pain (75%), fever (50%), and neurologic dysfunction (33%). The triad of all three symptoms is seen in only 13% of patients at the time of diagnosis. Nighttime pain is an early indication of infection. The duration of symptoms before presentation ranges from 1 day to several months.

On physical examination, tenderness is common, especially over the spinous processes, but paraspinous muscle spasm and tenderness may also be present. The clinician should be careful not to diagnose a simple muscle strain due to the reproducible muscle tenderness and spasm.

Laboratory and Imaging

An elevated leukocyte count is present in two-thirds of cases. C-reactive protein (CRP) and erythrocyte sedimentation rate (ESR) are elevated in many cases, but these abnormalities are nonspecific and generally cannot be used to rule in or rule out the disease because so many other diseases may elevate these markers. A 2011 study did examine the combined sensitivity and specificity of CRP and ESR is ruling in or out SEA in an ED population. In a group of 86 patients with back pain and a combination of fever, risk factors, neurologic deficit, or radicular pain, the two tests combined had a 100% sensitivity and a 67% specificity in that population. The study has not been replicated on a larger scale, however. Blood cultures should be obtained and will be positive in 60% of cases.

Importantly, a lumbar puncture is relatively contraindicated when SEA is being considered in the differential diagnosis. MRI with intravenous gadolinium is >90% sensitive and is the diagnostic test of choice (Fig. 8–11). CT may reveal narrowing of a disc (i.e., diskitis) and bone lysis (i.e., osteomyelitis), but does not take the place of MRI. The usual extent of a SEA is three to five vertebrae, but some cases involve the entire spine.

Treatment

The treatment of SEA includes surgical drainage and systemic antibiotics. Decompressive laminectomy and debridement are ideally performed within 24 hours of presentation. Empiric antibiotics against *S aureus* (vancomycin) and gram-negative bacilli (third-generation cephalosporin) should be initiated. Surgery is not indicated in several situations: when the patient refuses or is at high operative risk, when paralysis has been present for 24 to 36 hours, or if there is panspinal infection. A nonsurgical route may also be chosen if the patient is neurologically

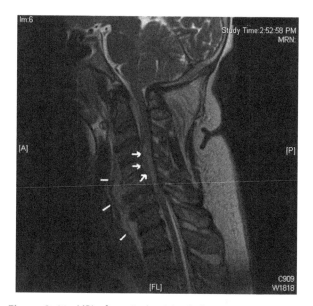

Figure 8–11. MRI of a spinal epidural abscess in the cervical region (*arrows*). *Lines* demonstrate a large prevertebral abscess that is also present.

intact, the microbial etiology is identified, and the patient is monitored closely. If the abscess is small, sometimes CT-guided aspiration alone is all that is needed.

Vertebral Osteomyelitis

Like SEA, the diagnosis of vertebral osteomyelitis is difficult and frequently delayed due to its subacute presentation and the nonspecific laboratory and radiographic findings. Eliciting risk factors for the development of spinal infection (e.g., elderly, immunocompromise) may be the most important clue to lead the astute clinician to the proper diagnosis.

The vertebrae are susceptible to infection because the venous system surrounding the bodies has an extensive venous plexus and lacks valves. Both features contribute to the pooling of blood, increasing the chances for bacteremia to seed the bone. The areas most commonly involved are the lumbar, thoracic, and cervical spine, in that order. Two adjacent vertebrae and the disc (i.e., diskitis) are usually affected, but more extensive spinal involvement is also possible.

Vertebral osteomyelitis can progress to an epidural abscess, psoas muscle abscess, empyema, paraspinal abscess, or retropharyngeal abscess. Spread to the epidural space is uncommon, however, occurring in 15% of cases.

Clinical Features

Typically, patients present with an insidious onset of back pain that is exacerbated by movement. The pain may be described as dull or aching. Malaise, weight loss, and low-grade fevers are all possible associated symptoms. Pain at night and pain unrelated to position may also be signs of infection. A recent infection elsewhere (e.g., urinary tract, lung, or skin) may be elicited during the history. Risk factors are similar to SEA and include immunocompromise, elderly age, and injection drug use.

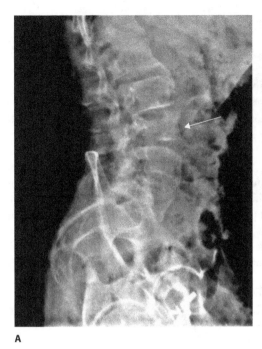
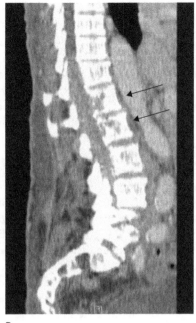

A   **B**

Figure 8–12. Vertebral osteomyelitis. **A.** Initial plain radiograph was misdiagnosed as a compression fracture of L3. **B.** CT scan 2 months later revealed bony destruction of L3 and L4 consistent with infection.

Only a minority of patients with vertebral osteomyelitis appear ill, whereas the majority present in a subacute manner with absent or minimal systemic symptoms. In fact, patients with vertebral osteomyelitis may have symptoms for several months before presentation.[77]

On examination, there is usually tenderness over the involved vertebral segments. Paraspinal muscle spasm and decreased mobility are also common. Neurologic deficits are reported much less frequently than with SEA and, if present, should raise the suspicion for an epidural abscess.

Laboratory and Imaging

Laboratory findings are usually not impressive. The white blood cell count may be mildly elevated or normal. C-reactive protein and sedimentation rate are frequently elevated, but these abnormalities are nonspecific. Blood cultures are positive in 40% of patients. *S aureus* is the most common organism identified, followed by gram-negative rods from gastrointestinal (GI) and urinary sources.

Plain radiographs are normal until bone becomes demineralized over the course of 2 weeks to 2 months. If radiographic abnormalities are present on plain films, bony destruction, vertebral end plate irregularity, and disc space narrowing are most common.[10] One study demonstrated an 82% sensitivity and a 57% specificity for plain radiographs.[78] Occasionally, vertebral osteomyelitis may appear as a spinal compression fracture on the plain radiographs and the diagnosis is missed (Fig. 8–12).[79] CT scan is good for defining bony destruction and may also be used to guide needle aspiration for the causative bacteria (Fig. 8–13). Like SEA, MRI is the gold standard imaging study for diagnosing vertebral

osteomyelitis. It is more sensitive than CT, picks up disease earlier, and better assesses the spinal cord.

Treatment

Treatment of vertebral osteomyelitis usually consists of intravenous antibiotics for 6 weeks followed by an oral course of antibiotics for another 1 to 2 months. Empiric antibiotic choices are similar to SEA. Surgical consultation should be obtained as a core bone biopsy may be desired to identify the causative pathogen.

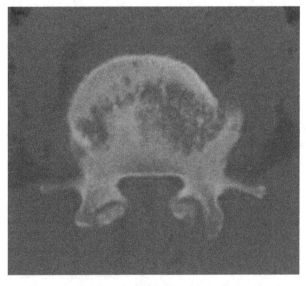

Figure 8–13. CT scan demonstrating bony destruction from osteomyelitis of a lumbar vertebra.

METASTATIC EPIDURAL SPINAL CORD COMPRESSION

Approximately 10% of cancer patients will have epidural spinal cord compression during the course of their disease. Left untreated, the patient will become paralyzed. For the emergency physician, diagnosing this condition early may stop the progression and improve outcomes. Unfortunately, a delay in diagnosis of up to several months is not uncommon and portends a worse prognosis.

Metastatic disease to the spinal column is 25 times more common than primary bone tumors. The most common metastatic tumors to the spine are breast (15%), lung (15%), prostate (10%), lymphoma (10%), kidney (5%), multiple myeloma (5%), and GI (5%). In autopsy studies, the rate of spinal metastases is more than 75% in patients with prostate and breast cancer.

The distribution of metastases within the spinal column depends on the amount of bone in that region of the spine. The 12 vertebrae of the thoracic spine account for 70% of metastatic lesions. The lumbosacral vertebrae, with their larger volume, contribute 20% of metastatic lesions, followed lastly by the cervical vertebrae at 10%.

Clinical Features

Severe, localized back pain of gradually increasing intensity is the earliest and most common symptom of spinal metastases. Pain is often more severe when lying down and with any increase in intra-abdominal pressure. Referred or radicular pain may also occur and depend on the primary location of the spinal metastasis (e.g., cervical compression commonly refers pain to the midscapular region). Pain that occurs at night, awakening the patient from sleep, is common, and pain that is not improved with any position is indicative of tumor. On average, pain occurs 4 to 8 weeks before the onset of neurologic deficits. Asymptomatic lesions occur if they are confined to the insensate bone marrow.

Physical examination should consist of a thorough back and neurologic examination. Patients without the diagnosis of malignancy who have symptoms suspicious for spinal metastasis should also have an examination searching for a primary tumor (e.g., breast, lung, prostate). In examining the back, percussion of the spinous processes will increase the pain associated with a metastatic tumor. Neurologic status at the time of presentation is the most important prognostic factor. Patients who are ambulatory at the time of diagnosis will remain so, at least in the short term, in most cases. However, if paraparesis is present, only 30% to 40% of the patients will regain the ability to walk after treatment. When paraplegia is present on initial evaluation, this number drops to 10%. However, due to frequent delays in diagnosis, two-thirds of patients who have cord compression are nonambulatory due to weakness.

Imaging

Plain radiographs are not sensitive for detecting spinal metastases because approximately 50% of the trabecular bone must be destroyed before a lytic lesion is visible. Plain radiographs are 60% sensitive and 99.5% specific for detecting spinal metastases. There is no good data for the utility of CT (Fig. 8–14). It is likely better than plain radiographs, but in almost all cases should be deferred in favor of an MRI.

MRI is the imaging test of choice and should be done emergently in the setting of suspected spinal malignancy and neurologic deficits (Fig. 8–15). Patients with a known malignancy and a new onset of back pain should also receive an MRI on an urgent basis. In this scenario, more than 50% of patients will have spinal metastases identified. The entire spine should be imaged because half of patients will have multilevel disease. In 45% of cases, this resulted in an alteration in the planned field of radiation. Sensitivity and specificity of MRI are 83% and 92%, respectively.

Treatment

When metastatic epidural compression is suspected, treatment should begin in the ED with steroids. Waiting for the results of an MRI will unnecessarily delay treatment that will decrease vasogenic edema and reduce cord compression. The most commonly recommended initial dose is dexamethasone 10 mg intravenously, although dosing regimens vary widely. A high-dose regimen of dexamethasone 100 mg intravenously initially, followed by 24 mg orally four times daily for 3 days, has also been studied. Not all

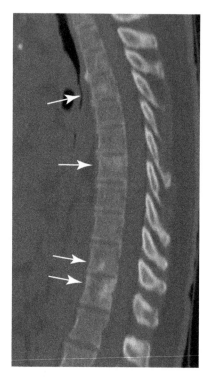

Figure 8–14. CT scan in a patient with lung cancer with vertebral body metastases of T5, T8, T11, and T12 (*arrows*).

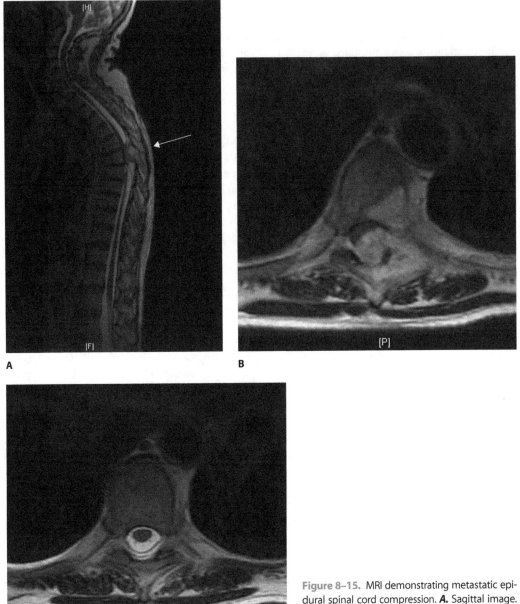

Figure 8–15. MRI demonstrating metastatic epidural spinal cord compression. **_A._** Sagittal image. **_B._** Axial images reveal a lesion at T6. **_C._** The normal appearance of the noncompressed spinal cord in the same patient at T8.

specialists favor the high-dose regimen due to side effects from the steroids, and unfortunately, the available literature does not make clear the optimal dose.[81,92–94]

Radiation therapy is indicated in almost all cases to reduce tumor size and decrease cord compression.[80] When cord compression is present, radiation therapy should be initiated as soon as possible and consultation with a radiation therapist from the ED is ideal.

Surgery is used in some cases to circumferentially remove tumor, decompress the spinal cord, and stabilize the spine. The most common indications include patients with expected survival beyond 3 months with intractable pain, spinal instability, or poorly radiosensitive tumors (e.g., renal cell carcinoma).[81,88,95,96] Patients with progression of neurologic symptoms despite steroids and radiation should also be considered for surgical intervention.[97]

PRIMARY BONE TUMORS

Although metastatic bone tumor is much more common than primary tumors, several primary bone tumors can occur in the spine. The most common benign tumors are osteoid osteoma and osteoblastoma. These tumors affect young men most commonly. Osteoid osteomas present with nighttime pain that is deep and without radiation.

Osteoblastomas present with a dull ache that may radiate to the posterior thigh. In both tumors, there may be localized tenderness over the involved bone. On radiographs, osteoid osteomas appear as a lytic area surrounded by sclerotic bone. Osteoblastomas commonly appear in the posterior vertebral body as an expansile, well-delineated lesion with periosteal new bone formation. Treatment of both tumors is often with excision. Other benign tumors of the spine are osteochondromas, giant cell tumors, aneurysmal bone cysts, hemangiomas, and eosinophilic granulomas.

Malignant primary tumors include multiple myeloma, chondrosarcoma, and chordoma. Multiple myeloma should be considered in patients with back pain older than 40 years. Symptoms are usually mild, but the patient may be prone to fracture. In addition to bone pain, there is usually generalized fatigue, nausea, and vomiting. Radiographs demonstrate diffuse vertebral body osteolysis without reactive sclerosis that spares the posterior elements. CT is more sensitive than plain films. Any patient suspected of multiple myeloma needs timely referral.

Chondrosarcoma is the second most common primary malignant tumor of the bone, representing 25% of cases. A patient with a chondrosarcoma or a chordoma is also usually between 40 and 60 years of age and will present with mild discomfort in the affected bone. On examination, a patient with a chondrosarcoma may have painless swelling. Radiographs of a chondrosarcoma reveal an expansile fluffy or lobular calcification in the medullary bone with a thickened cortex. CT scan is more sensitive and will also show soft-tissue extension. Plain films of a chordoma demonstrate osteolysis with a calcific soft-tissue mass that involves the vertebral body, but not the disc.

SPINAL EPIDURAL HEMATOMA

A spinal epidural hematoma (SEH) is a rare condition that occurs due to rupture of the posterior epidural venous plexus. As blood accumulates, compression on the spinal cord occurs in a similar manner to tumor, abscess, or central disc herniation. Of all spinal space-occupying lesions, epidural hematoma accounts for less than 1%. SEH is spontaneous in 50% of cases. These patients have risk factors for hemorrhage such as anticoagulants and coagulopathies (e.g., hemophilia). Minor trauma, such as sneezing or spinal manipulation, can also precipitate SEH in at-risk individuals. Other causes of spontaneous SEH include vascular malformation and pregnancy. The remaining cases occur after instrumentation or surgery. Spinal surgery is most commonly associated, but SEH has also been reported after spinal anesthesia and even acupuncture.

Clinical Features
Patients with SEH are usually older than 50 years, but the condition can occur at any age. The classic clinical picture is that of sudden onset of severe back or neck pain, frequently with radicular symptoms. Within minutes to hours (rarely days), neurologic symptoms develop that herald compression of the spinal cord. A short course between the onset of pain and neurologic symptoms is more common when the hematoma is in the cervical or thoracic regions because the epidural space is narrowest.

Imaging
MRI is the diagnostic imaging study of choice. The hematoma appears as a hyperintense signal on T2-weighted imaging if done within the first 24 hours after onset of symptoms. Peripheral enhancement is seen with gadolinium contrast and helps differentiate hematoma from other mass lesions within the epidural space.

CT may demonstrate the hematoma, but it is not as sensitive as MRI and will not reveal the extent of the lesion. However, CT can be used if there is delay in obtaining the MRI for whatever reason.

Treatment
Early surgical intervention with decompressive laminectomy is the treatment of choice. A better neurologic recovery is seen when the time from symptom onset to surgery is shorter. A complete recovery is likely if the time to surgery is less than 6 to 8 hours. Patients with coagulopathy should be treated with blood products as needed (e.g., fresh frozen plasma, vitamin K factor). Conservative management is sometimes employed in patients with minimal to no neurologic symptoms.

TRANSVERSE MYELITIS

Transverse myelitis is an acute inflammatory disorder of the spinal cord. The cause is frequently difficult to determine, but a recent infection (e.g., viruses or mycoplasma) or vaccination have all been implicated as possible etiologies. Most patients present with focal neck or back pain followed by neurologic deficits. Motor, sensory, and autonomic dysfunctions occur in different patterns, depending on the portion of the cord affected. For this reason, transverse myelitis can mimic cord compression (e.g., hematoma, metastasis, herniation), cord ischemia from aortic dissection, Guillain–Barré syndrome, and neuromuscular disorders. MRI is the diagnostic tool of choice, and the typical pattern of transverse myelitis is high-intensity signals on T2-weighted images that run longitudinally along the affected portion of the spinal cord. Lumbar puncture will usually demonstrate a lymphocytosis and an elevated protein. Treatment is mostly supportive. Steroids and plasma exchange therapy can be considered, although their utility is unclear. The emergency physician should consider transverse myelitis a diagnosis of exclusion, as other more treatable causes of back pain and neurologic deficits should be considered first.

MUSCLE STRAIN

Muscle strain of the back, usually the lumbosacral portion, is less common than is diagnosed. Even muscle spasms palpated on examination are frequently secondary to posterior facet syndrome or an annular tear of a disc. However, the diagnosis of a muscle or ligament injury is supported in patients after a sudden stress or stretching in the back. The pain is frequently intense. The pain may continue to be severe for the first few days and a dull ache may remain for several weeks. On examination, pain is reproduced by palpation along the paraspinal muscles. There is usually spasm. Radiographs are not indicated. Treatment consists of the avoidance of heavy lifting and nonsteroidal anti-inflammatory agents with muscle relaxants.

Muscle strain of the neck is not uncommon after what may seem like a trivial injury. Exclude fracture or an unstable ligamentous injury first, as discussed in Chapter 9. The mainstays of treatment of a cervical muscle strain are nonsteroidal anti-inflammatory medications and analgesics/muscle relaxants. Sleeping with a roll under the neck may relieve tension and be more comfortable for the patient. Resistance exercises may also aid in muscle relaxation. To perform these exercises, the patient is instructed to gently turn the head to the unaffected (painless) side while providing some resistance with the hand over the face. This causes contraction of the unaffected muscles and a reflexive relaxation of the strained muscles, thus decreasing pain. Performance of these exercises in repetitions of 20, two to three times a day is recommended.

POSTERIOR FACET SYNDROME

Posterior facet syndrome is the term used to describe injury to the capsule or arthritic degeneration of the facet joint. The facet joint is a true synovial joint between the superior and inferior articular processes of adjacent vertebrae. The joint is surrounded by a ligamentous capsule. With sudden movements, particularly hyperextension, or with carrying heavy objects, the capsule may be injured and the joint can become subluxated. In the absence of trauma, arthritic degeneration can also lead to similar symptoms.

The patient will complain of pain that is worse with extension and ipsilateral side bending. Standing is worse than sitting. The pain is confined to the back, however, and does not radiate to the buttocks or legs like a herniated disc.

The neurologic examination is normal. There is frequently severe muscle spasm, but if the facet joint can be palpated (two finger breadths lateral to and between the spinous processes), there will be local tenderness. As pointed out in Chapter 7, the joints are more easily palpated when the patient is in the prone position with a towel or small pillow under the umbilicus. Hyperextension will increase the pain. Imaging is generally not necessary. Treatment consists of the avoidance of heavy lifting and nonsteroidal anti-inflammatory agents with muscle relaxants. Injection of the joint with a local anesthetic can be both diagnostic and therapeutic, usually associated with a rapid relief of symptoms (Fig. 8–16). The patient should avoid hyperextension

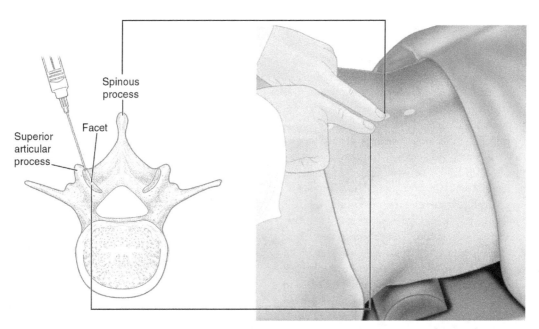

Figure 8–16. Injection of a patient with posterior facet syndrome. Once the facet joint is located (two finger breadths lateral to and between the spinous processes), put an X at this landmark. In the thin patient, you can palpate the bony protuberance of the facet joints, but this is not usually the case due to the erector spinae muscles. Next take a 22-gauge spinal needle without an attached syringe and insert at the X, aiming 20-degree cephalad and slightly medial as shown in the diagram. In the average patient, you will need to insert the needle several centimeters (just as you would if doing a spinal tap) until your needle touches bone. You will be in the joint or the vicinity of the joint. Inject 2 to 3 mL of bupivacaine mixed with triamcinolone 80 mg. This procedure is often done under fluoroscopy, but this is not necessary except in the very obese patient.

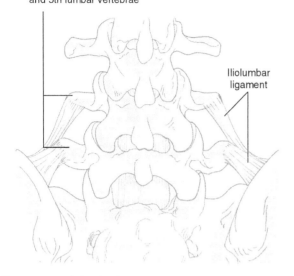

Transverse processes 4th
and 5th lumbar vertebrae

Iliolumbar
ligament

Figure 8–17. Iliolumbar ligament.

(i.e., prone position). Bed rest is not recommended, and the patient should let pain guide their mobility. Spinal manipulation may be helpful in the acute setting if the joint is subluxated. Later, an exercise program to strengthen the abdominal and gluteal muscles will reduce recurrence.

ILIOLUMBAR LIGAMENT SPRAIN

The iliolumbar ligament extends between the transverse process of L5 and the posterior aspect of the iliac crest (Fig. 8–17). Sprain of this ligament is a common source of musculoskeletal back pain presenting to the ED. In fact, when a patient presents with a history of "back strain" and he/she is in extreme pain, it is frequently due to this injury. Fortunately, it is easily diagnosed and treated. On examination, start by palpating the spinous processes, gradually moving down to L5. Next, move laterally to the iliac crest on the side of the pain. Immediately between these two structures is where the iliolumbar ligament is located and where profound tenderness will be present. Treatment of this injury is amendable to injection of triamcinolone 80 mg and approximately 3 mL of 1% bupivacaine. Using a spinal needle, aim 20 degrees inferiorly and insert the needle to a depth of approximately 3 cm before injecting. Move the needle back and forth while injecting to ensure medication is delivered to the entire iliolumbar ligament. Injection frequently results in complete relief of the pain that is sustained for at least a week, during which time the strained ligament usually heals.

REFERENCES

1. Downie A, Williams M, Henschke N, et al. Red flags to screen for malignancy and fracture in patients with low back pain: systematic review. *BMJ*. 2013;347:f7095. doi:10.1136/bmj.f7095.

2. Roohi F, Fox A. Burst fracture of the first lumbar vertebra and conus-cauda syndrome complicating a single convulsive seizure: a challenge of diagnosis in the emergency department. *J Emerg Med*. 2006;31(4):381–385.

3. Small SA, Perron AD, Brady WJ. Orthopedic pitfalls: cauda equina syndrome. *Am J Emerg Med*. 2005;23(2):159–163.

4. Domen PM, Hofman PA, van Santbrink H, Weber WE. Predictive value of clinical characteristics in patients with suspected cauda equina syndrome. *Eur J Neurol*. 2009;16(3):416–419.

5. Deyo RA, Rainville J, Kent DL. What can the history and physical examination tell us about low back pain. *JAMA*. 1992;268(6):760–765.

6. Hussain SA, Gullan RW, Chitnavis BP. Cauda equina syndrome: outcome and implications for management. *Br J Neurosurg*. 2003;17(2):164–167.

7. Koes BW, van Tulder MW, Peul WC. Diagnosis and treatment of sciatica. *BMJ*. 2007;334(7607):1313–1317.

8. Rabin A, Gerszten PC, Karausky P, Bunker CH, Potter DM, Welch WC. The sensitivity of the seated straight-leg raise test compared with the supine straight-leg raise test in patients presenting with magnetic resonance imaging evidence of lumbar nerve root compression. *Arch Phys Med Rehabil*. 2007;88(7):840–843.

9. Lateef H, Patel D. What is the role of imaging in acute low back pain? *Curr Rev Musculoskelet Med*. 2009;2(2):69–73.

10. Jarvik JG, Deyo RA. Diagnostic evaluation of low back pain with emphasis on imaging. *Ann Intern Med*. 2002;137(7):586–597.

11. Roelofs PD, Deyo RA, Koes BW, Scholten RJ, van Tulder MW. Nonsteroidal anti-inflammatory drugs for low back pain: an updated Cochrane Review. *Spine*. 2008;33(16):1766–1774.

12. Hagen KB, Jamtvedt G, Hilde G, Winnem MF. The updated Cochrane Review of bed rest for low back pain and sciatica. *Spine*. 2005;30(5):542–546.

13. Finckh A, Zufferey P, Schurch MA, Balagué F, Waldburger M, So AK. Short-term efficacy of IV pulse glucocorticoids in acute discogenic sciatica. A randomized controlled trial. *Spine*. 2006;31(4):377–381.

14. Holve RL, Barkan H. Oral steroids in initial treatment of acute sciatica. *J Am Board Fam Med*. 2008;21(5):469–474.

15. Friedman BW, Holden L, Esses D, et al. Parenteral corticosteroids for emergency department patients with non-radicular low back pain. *J Emerg Med*. 2006;31(4):365–370.

16. Wilson-MacDonald J, Burt G, Griffin D, Glynn C. Epidural steroid injection for nerve root compression. A randomised, controlled trial. *J Bone Joint Surg Br*. 2005;87(3):352–355.

17. Novak S, Nemeth WC. The basis for recommending repeating epidural steroid injections for radicular low back pain: a literature review. *Arch Phys Med Rehabil*. 2008;89(3):543–552.

18. Pinto RZ, Maher CG, Ferreira ML, et al. Epidural corticosteroid injections in the management of sciatica: a systematic review and meta-analysis. *Ann Int Med*. 2012;157(12):865–877.

19. Staal JB, de Bie R, de Vet HCW, Hildebrandt J, Nelemans P. Injection therapy for subacute and chronic low-back pain: an updated Cochrane Review. *Spine*. 2009;34(1):49–59.

20. Ng LC, Sell P. Predictive value of the duration of sciatica for lumbar discectomy. A prospective cohort study. *J Bone Joint Surg Br.* 2004;86(4):546–549.

21. Fisher C, Noonan V, Bishop P, et al. Outcome evaluation of the operative management of lumbar disc herniation causing sciatica. *J Neurosurg.* 2004;100(suppl 4):317–324.

22. Vroomen PC, de Krom MC, Slofstra PD, Knottnerus JA. Conservative treatment of sciatica: a systematic review. *J Spinal Disord.* 2000;13(6):463–469.

23. Vroomen PC, de Krom MC, Knottnerus JA. When does the patient with a disc herniation undergo lumbosacral discectomy? *J Neurol Neurosurg Psychiatry.* 2000;68(1):75–79.

24. Van Den Hout WB, Peul WC, Koes BW, et al. Prolonged conservative care versus early surgery in patients with sciatica from lumbar disc herniation: cost utility analysis alongside a randomised controlled trial. *BMJ.* 2008;336(7657): 1351–1354.

25. Arts MP, Brand R, van den Akker ME, et al. Tubular diskectomy vs conventional microdiskectomy for sciatica: a randomized controlled trial. *JAMA.* 2009;302(2):149–158.

26. Yeung AT, Yeung CA. Minimally invasive techniques for the management of lumbar disc herniation. *Orthop Clin North Am.* 2007;38(3):363–372.

27. Deyo RA, Weinstein JN. Low back pain. *N Eng J Med.* 2001; 344(5):363–370.

28. Katz JN, Harris MB. Clinical practice. Lumbar spinal stenosis. *N Engl J Med.* 2008;358(8):818–825.

29. Ciol MA, Deyo RA, Howell E, Kreif S. An assessment of surgery for spinal stenosis: time trends, geographic variations, complications, and reoperations. *J Am Geriatr Soc.* 1996; 44(3):285–290.

30. Suri P, Rainville J, Kalichman L, Katz JN. Does this older adult with lower extremity pain have the clinical syndrome of lumbar spinal stenosis? *JAMA.* 2010;304(23):2628–2636.

31. Kim SL, Lim RD. Spinal stenosis. *Dis Mon.* 2005;51(1):6–17.

32. de Graaf I, Prak A, Bierma-Zeinstra S, Thomas S, Peul W, Koes B. Diagnosis of lumbar spinal stenosis: a systematic review of the accuracy of diagnostic tests. *Spine.* 2006;31(10): 1168–1176.

33. Haig AJ, Geisser ME, Tong HC, et al. Electromyographic and magnetic resonance imaging to predict lumbar stenosis, low-back pain, and no back symptoms. *J Bone Joint Surg Am.* 2007; 89(2):358–366.

34. Modic MT, Ross JS. Lumbar degenerative disk disease. *Radiology.* 2007;245(1):43–61.

35. Nardin RA, Patel MR, Gudas TF, Rutkove SB, Raynor EM. Electromyography and magnetic resonance imaging in the evaluation of radiculopathy. *Muscle Nerve.* 1999;22(2): 151–155.

36. Robinson LR. Electromyography, magnetic resonance imaging, and radiculopathy: it's time to focus on specificity. *Muscle Nerve.* 1999;22(2):149–150.

37. Watters WC III, Baisden J, Gilbert TJ, et al. Degenerative lumbar spinal stenosis: an evidence-based guideline for the diagnosis and treatment of degenerative lumbar spinal stenosis. *Spine J.* 2008;8(2):305–310.

38. Atlas SJ, Delitto A. Spinal stenosis: surgical versus nonsurgical treatment. *Clin Orthop Relat Res.* 2006;443:198–207.

39. Rittenberg JD, Ross AE. Functional rehabilitation for degenerative lumbar spinal stenosis. *Phys Med Rehabil Clin N Am.* 2003; 14(1):111–120.

40. Friedly J, Chan L, Deyo R. Increases in lumbosacral injections in the Medicare population: 1994 to 2001. *Spine.* 2007; 32(16):1754–1760.

41. Radcliff K, Kepler C, Hilibrand A, et al. Epidural steroid injections are associated with less improvement in patients with lumbar spinal stenosis: a subgroup analysis of the Spine Patient Outcomes Research Trial. *Spine.* 2013;38(4): 279–291.

42. Cooper G, Lutz GE, Boachie-Adjei O, Lin J. Effectiveness of transforaminal epidural steroid injections in patients with degenerative lumbar scoliotic stenosis and radiculopathy. *Pain Physician.* 2004;7(3):311–317.

43. Asgarzadie F, Khoo LT. Minimally invasive operative management for lumbar spinal stenosis: overview of early and long-term outcomes. *Orthop Clin North Am.* 2007;38(3): 387–399.

44. Weinstein JN, Tosteson TD, Lurie JD, et al. Surgical versus nonsurgical therapy for lumbar spinal stenosis. *N Engl J Med.* 2008;358(8):794–810.

45. Malmivaara A, Slatis P, Heliovaara M, et al. Surgical or nonoperative treatment for lumbar spinal stenosis A randomized controlled trial. *Spine.* 2007;32(1):1–8.

46. Weinstein JN, Tosteson TD, Lurie JD, et al. Surgical versus nonoperative treatment for lumbar spinal stenosis four-year results of the Spine Patient Outcomes Research Trial. *Spine.* 2010;35(14):1329–1338.

47. Slatis P, Malmivaara A, Heliovaara M, et al. Long-term results of surgery for lumbar spinal stenosis: a randomized controlled trial. *Eur Spine J.* 2011;20(7):1174–1181.

48. Atlas SJ, Keller RB, Wu YA, Deyo RA, Singer DE. Long-term outcomes of surgical and nonsurgical management of lumbar spinal stenosis: 8 to 10 year results from the Maine Lumbar Spine Study. *Spine.* 2005;30(8):936–943.

49. Tallarico RA, Madom IA, Palumbo MA. Spondylolysis and spondylolisthesis in the athlete. *Sports Med Arthrosc.* 2008;16(1):32–38.

50. Metz LN, Deviren V. Low-grade spondylolisthesis. *Neurosurg Clin N Am.* 2007;18(2):237–248.

51. Ruiz-Cotorro A, Balius-Matas R, Estruch-Massana AE, Vilaró Angulo J. Spondylolysis in young tennis players. *Br J Sports Med.* 2006;40(5):441–446.

52. Hu SS, Tribus CB, Diab M, Ghanayem AJ. Spondylolisthesis and spondylolysis. *J Bone Joint Surg Am.* 2008;90(3):656–671.

53. Kim HJ. Green DW. Spondylolysis in the adolescent athlete. *Curr Opin Pediatr.* 2011;23(1):68–72.

54. Standaert CJ, Herring SA. Spondylolysis: a critical review. *Br J Sports Med.* 2000;34(6):415–422.

55. Millard L. The Scotty dog and his collar. *J Ark Med Soc.* 1976;72(8):339–340.

56. Butt S, Saifuddin A. The imaging of lumbar spondylolisthesis. *Clin Radiol.* 2005;60(5):533–546.

57. Szypryt EP, Twining P, Mulholland RC, Worthington BS. The prevalence of disc degeneration associated with neural arch defects of the lumbar spine assessed by magnetic resonance imaging. *Spine.* 1989;14(9):977–981.

58. Birch JG, Herring JA, Maravilla KR. Splitting of the intervertebral disc in spondylolisthesis: a magnetic resonance imaging finding in two cases. *J Pediatr Orthop.* 1986;6(5): 609–611.

59. Wood KB, Fritzell P, Dettori JR, Hashimoto R, Lund T, Shaffrey C. Effectiveness of spinal fusion versus structured

rehabilitation in chronic low back pain patients with and without isthmic spondylolisthesis: a systematic review. *Spine*. 2011; 36(21 suppl):S110–S119.

60. Tsirikos AI, Garrido EG. Spondylolysis and spondylolisthesis in children and adolescents. *J Bone Joint Surg Br*. 2010; 92(6):751–759.

61. Miller SF, Congeni J, Swanson K. Long-term functional and anatomical follow-up of early detected spondylolysis in young athletes. *Am J Sports Med*. 2004;32(4):928–933.

62. Watters WC III, Bono CM, Gilbert TJ. An evidence-based clinical guideline for the diagnosis and treatment of degenerative lumbar spondylolisthesis. *Spine J*. 2009;9(7): 609–614.

63. Kalichman L, Hunter DJ. Diagnosis and conservative management of degenerative lumbar spondylolisthesis. *Eur Spine J*. 2008;17(3):327–335.

64. Gibson JN, Waddell G. Surgery for degenerative lumbar spondylosis: updated Cochrane Review. *Spine*. 2005;30(20): 2312–2320.

65. Darouiche RO. Spinal epidural abscess. *N Engl J Med*. 2006; 355(19):2012–2020.

66. Pilkington SA, Jackson SA, Gillett GR. Spinal epidural empyema. *Br J Neurosurg*. 2003;17(2):196–200.

67. Chao D, Nanda A. Spinal epidural abscess: a diagnostic challenge. *Am Fam Physician*. 2002;65(7):1341–1346.

68. Reihsaus E, Waldbaur H, Seeling W. Spinal epidural abscess: a meta-analysis of 915 patients. *Neurosurg Rev*. 2000;23(4): 175–204.

69. Grewal S, Hocking G, Wildsmith JA. Epidural abscesses. *Br J Anaesth*. 2006;96(3):292–302.

70. Davis DP, Salazar A, Chan TC, et al. Prospective evaluation of a clinical decision guideline to diagnose spinal epidural abscess in patients who present to the emergency department with spine pain. *J Neurosurg Spine*. 2011;15:765–770.

71. O'Phelan KH, Bunney EB, Weingart SD, Smith WS. Emergency neurological life support: spinal cord compression (SCC). *Neurocrit Care*. 2012;17(suppl 1):S96–S101.

72. An HS, Seldomridge JA. Spinal infections: diagnostic tests and imaging studies. *Clin Orthop Relat Res*. 2006;444: 27–33.

73. Winters ME, Kluetz P, Zilberstein J. Back pain emergencies. *Med Clin North Am*. 2006;90(3):505–523.

74. Tunkel AR, Pradhan SK. Central nervous system infections in injection drug users. *Infect Dis Clin North Am*. 2002; 16(3):589–605.

75. Tompkins M, Panuncialman I, Lucas P, Palumbo M. Spinal epidural abscess. *J Emerg Med*. 2010;39(3):384–90.

76. Zimmerli W. Clinical practice. Vertebral osteomyelitis. *N Engl J Med*. 2010;362(11):1022–1029.

77. Diehn FE. Imaging of spine infection. *Radiol Clin North Am*. 2012;50(4):777–798.

78. DeSanto J, Ross JS. Spine infection/inflammation. *Radiol Clin North Am*. 2011;49(1):105–127.

79. McHenry MC, Duchesneau PM, Keys TF, Rehm SJ, Boumphrey FR. Vertebral osteomyelitis presenting as spinal compression fracture. six patients with underlying osteoporosis. *Arch Intern Med*. 1988;148(2):417–423.

80. Swift PS. Radiation for spinal metastatic tumors. *Orthop Clin North Am*. 2009;40(1):133–144.

81. Abrahm JL, Banffy MB, Harris MB. Spinal cord compression in patients with advanced metastatic cancer: "All I care about is walking and living my life". *JAMA*. 2008;299(8): 937–946.

82. Levack P, Graham J, Collie D, et al. Don't wait for a sensory level—listen to the symptoms: a prospective audit of the delays in diagnosis of malignant cord compression. *Clin Oncol (R Coll Radiol)*. 2002;14(6):472–480.

83. Prasad D, Schiff D. Malignant spinal-cord compression. *Lancet Oncol*. 2005;6(1):15–24.

84. Kienstra GE, Terwee CB, Dekker FW, et al. Prediction of spinal epidural metastases. *Arch Neurol*. 2000;57(5): 690–695.

85. Walcott BP, Jaglowski JR, Curry WT Jr. Spinal epidural metastasis. *Arch Neurol*. 2010;67(3):358–359.

86. Aslan S, Cetin B, Akinci M, Cetin M, Yucekule N, Cetin A. Computed tomography in detecting bone metastases of breast carcinoma. Is it better than plain x-ray? *Saudi Med J*. 2006;27(9):1326–1328.

87. Gabriel K, Schiff D. Metastatic spinal cord compression by solid tumors. *Semin Neurol*. 2004;24(4):375–383.

88. Abdi S, Adams CI, Foweraker KL, O'Connor A. Metastatic spinal cord syndromes: imaging appearances and treatment planning. *Clin Radiol*. 2005;60(6):637–647.

89. Loughrey GJ, Collins CD, Todd SM, Brown NM, Johnson RJ. Magnetic resonance imaging in the management of suspected spinal canal disease in patients with known malignancy. *Clin Radiol*. 2000;55(11):849–855.

90. Colletti PM, Siegel HJ, Woo MY, Young HY, Terk MR. The impact on treatment planning of MRI of the spine in patients suspected of vertebral metastasis: an efficacy study. *Comput Med Imaging Graph*. 1996;20(3):159–162.

91. Zaidat OO, Ruff RL. Treatment of spinal epidural metastasis improves patient survival and functional state. *Neurology*. 2002;58(9):1360–1366.

92. Heimdal K, Hirschberg H, Slettebo H, Watne K, Nome O. High incidence of serious side effects of high-dose dexamethasone treatment in patients with epidural spinal cord compression. *J Neurooncol*. 1992;12(2):141–144.

93. Sorensen S, Helweg-Larsen S, Mouridsen H, Hansen HH. Effect of high-dose dexamethasone in carcinomatous metastatic spinal cord compression treated with radiotherapy: a randomised trial. *Eur J Cancer*. 1994;30A(1):22–27.

94. Higdon ML, Higdon JA. Treatment of oncologic emergencies. *Am Fam Physician*. 2006;74(11):1873–1880.

95. van der Linden YM, Dijkstra SP, Vonk EJ, Marijnen CA, Leer JW; Dutch Bone Metastasis Study Group. Prediction of survival in patients with metastases in the spinal column: results based on a randomized trial of radiotherapy. *Cancer*. 2005;103(2):320–328.

96. Patchell RA, Tibbs PA, Regine WF, et al. Direct decompressive surgical resection in the treatment of spinal cord compression caused by metastatic cancer: a randomised trial. *Lancet*. 2005;366(9486):643–648.

97. Waters JD, Peran EM, Ciacci J. Malignancies of the spinal cord. *Adv Exp Med Biol*. 2012;760:101–113.

98. Wang VY, Chou D, Chin C. Spine and spinal cord emergencies: vascular and infectious causes. *Neuroimaging Clin N Am*. 2010;20(4):639–650.

99. Liu WH, Hsieh CT, Chiang YH, Chen GJ. Spontaneous spinal epidural hematoma of thoracic spine: a rare case report and review of literature. *Am J Emerg Med*. 2008; 26(3):384.e1-384.e12.

100. Kubota T, Miyajima Y. Spinal extradural haematoma due to haemophilia A. *Arch Dis Child*. 2007;92(6):498.

101. Herd AM. A major pain in the neck. Spinal epidural hematoma. *Can Fam Physician*. 2005;51:497–506.

102. Ain RJ, Vance MB. Epidural hematoma after epidural steroid injection in a patient withholding enoxaparin per guidelines. *Anesthesiology*. 2005;102(3):701–703.

103. Chen JC, Chen Y, Lin SM, Yang HJ, Su CF, Tseng SH. Acute spinal epidural hematoma after acupuncture. *J Trauma*. 2006;60(2):414–416.

104. Litz RJ, Gottschlich B, Stehr SN. Spinal epidural hematoma after spinal anesthesia in a patient treated with clopidogrel and enoxaparin. *Anesthesiology*. 2004;101(6): 1467–1470.

105. Kirazli Y, Akkoc Y, Kanyilmaz S. Spinal epidural hematoma associated with oral anticoagulation therapy. *Am J Phys Med Rehabil*. 2004;83(3):220–223.

106. Gilbert A, Owens BD, Mulroy MF. Epidural hematoma after outpatient epidural anesthesia. *Anesth Analg*. 2002;94(1):77–78.

107. Henderson RD, Pittock SJ, Piepgras DG, Wijdicks EF. Acute spontaneous spinal epidural hematoma. *Arch Neurol*. 2001; 58(7):1145–1146.

108. Lin IY. Diagnostic pitfall: nontraumatic spinal epidural hematoma mimicking a brainstem stroke. *Ann Emerg Med*. 2004;44(2):183–184.

109. Hsieh CT, Chang CF, Lin EY, Tsai TH, Chiang YH, Ju DT. Spontaneous spinal epidural hematomas of cervical spine: report of 4 cases and literature review. *Am J Emerg Med*. 2006; 24(6):736–740.

110. Hammerstedt HS, Edlow JA, Cusick S. Emergency department presentations of transverse myelitis: two case reports. *Ann Emerg Med*. 2005;46(3):256–259.

111. Borchers AT, Gershwin ME. Transverse myelitis. *Autoimmun Rev*. 2012;11(3):231–248.

CHAPTER 9
Cervical Spine Trauma

Michael E. Nelson, MD

INTRODUCTION

The prompt diagnosis of a cervical spine (C-spine) injury is imperative to provide early treatment and prevent secondary spinal cord injury. Since 2010, motor vehicle collisions (MVCs) account for the majority of spinal cord injuries (38%), followed by falls (30.5%), acts of violence (i.e., gunshot wounds, 13.5%), and sporting injuries (9%). Cervical spine injuries are found in 2% to 4% of blunt trauma patients that undergo imaging. The cervical spine is the most common location in the spine to be injured, accounting for upward of 50% to 60% of spinal injuries. Unfortunately, a delay in diagnosis occurs in one-quarter of cases. Spinal cord injuries lead to significant reductions in life expectancy as well as high individual lifetime costs for care, ranging from $2.1 to $4.7 million based on age at the time of injury.

The upper cervical spine, consisting of the occiput, C1 (atlas), and C2 (axis), is unique from the remainder of the cervical spine. It is designed to allow for rotation of the head. The C1 vertebra is a ring structure that articulates with the occiput. The C2 vertebra is composed of a body with a bony projection (dens) that goes through the anterior portion of the ring of C1. The dens is stabilized by both the transverse and the alar ligaments (Fig. 9–1). The transverse ligament is located along the posterior surface of the dens, attaching on either side of C1.

Injury to this ligament may be catastrophic to the patient in the form of atlantoaxial instability and a high cervical cord lesion.

The lower cervical spine can be divided into two columns, where disruption of an entire column is required to alter stability. The anterior column consists of the anterior and posterior longitudinal ligaments and the vertebral body. The posterior column comprises the pedicle, lamina, articular facet joints, and ligamentum flavum.

Spinal Immobilization

Immobilization of the cervical spine has been a long-standing practice after traumatic events in the prehospital setting on the premise that it will prevent further neurologic deterioration. Patients are typically placed in a rigid collar and transported to the emergency department (ED) for evaluation. Evidence demonstrates risks associated with routine immobilization, including skin ischemia; pressure sores; and increased respiratory effort, pain, intracranial pressure, and aspiration risk. Cervical immobilization also increases extraction time and compromises the ability to maintain a safe airway. No studies have confirmed the benefits of spinal immobilization, or demonstrated improved patient outcomes or prevention of neurologic deterioration. Thus, clearance of the cervical spine and removal of the cervical collar in a timely manner in patients that do not require immobilization is paramount.

Imaging

Not all patients with a traumatic source of neck pain will require imaging. Two groups have attempted to safely reduce the rate of cervical spine imaging in the setting of trauma based on the absence of high-risk criteria. The National Emergency X-Radiography Utilization Study (NEXUS) group, consisting of 34,069 patients, identified five criteria that were 99.6% sensitive in excluding a clinically significant cervical spine injury (Table 9–1). The Canadian C-Spine

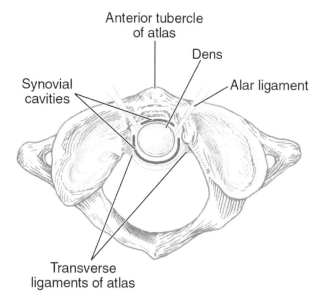

Figure 9–1. The transverse and alar ligaments and their importance in stabilizing the C1 and C2 vertebrae.

▶ TABLE 9–1. **NEXUS CRITERIA TO CLINICALLY EXCLUDE CERVICAL SPINE FRACTURE**

- No midline tenderness
- No focal neurologic deficit
- Normal alertness
- No intoxication
- No painful distracting injury

If all five criteria are met, imaging is not performed.

▶ TABLE 9–2. **CANADIAN C-SPINE RULE**

GCS 15
Stable condition
Age older than 16 y
Not pregnant
No prior cervical spine surgeries or vertebral disease
Absence of high-risk features
- Age older than 65 y
- Paresthesias in extremities
- Dangerous mechanism (fall ≥ 3 ft or five stairs, axial load, rollover/ejection, MVC > 100 km/h [~ 62 mph])

Presence of low-risk features to assess for range of motion
- Simple rear-end MVC
- Sitting in the emergency department
- Ambulatory at any time
- Delayed onset of neck pain
- No midline cervical spine tenderness

Able to rotate neck 45 degrees left and right

GCS, Glasgow Coma Scale; MVC, motor vehicle collision.
If all these criteria are met, imaging is not performed.

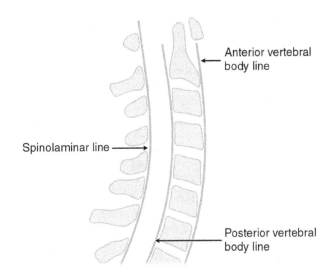

Figure 9–2. Loss of alignment of the anterior and posterior vertebral body line or the spinolaminar line suggests an unstable injury.

Rule (CCR) detected 100% of 151 clinically significant C-spine injuries in 8924 patients. In this rule, to be considered for exclusion from needing C-spine radiographs, patients must have a Glasgow Coma Scale of 15 and no high-risk features (age older than 65, dangerous mechanism, or extremity paresthesias). Next, low risk factors are assessed. In patients with a low risk factor (simple rear-end MVCs, sitting in ED, ambulatory at any time, delayed onset of neck pain, or absence of midline C-spine tenderness), neck rotation is tested. If patients are able to actively rotate the neck 45 degrees to both the left and the right, no radiographs are needed (Table 9–2).[11]

When NEXUS criteria were applied to the CCR data set, the sensitivity of NEXUS criteria was 92.7%.[12] In a prospective cohort study (in Canadian EDs), the CCR had higher sensitivity (99.4% vs. 90.7%) and specificity (45.1% vs. 36.8%) versus the NEXUS criteria and would have led to a reduction in radiography rates, although patient populations were different between the two studies.[13]

Plain radiographs have historically been used as a screening test for cervical spine injury. The typical trauma series includes an anteroposterior (AP), an open-mouth (odontoid), and a lateral view. The plain radiographs detect approximately 65% to 75% of injuries and should include the C7-T1 junction because a high number of injuries occur at C7.[14–16] In the multitrauma unconscious patient, the sensitivity and adequacy of plain films is reduced and has little role, making computed tomography (CT) the imaging test of choice.[16] Flexion-extension radiographs are controversial and not performed routinely, especially when CT and magnetic resonance imaging (MRI) are available.

The interpretation of plain radiographs is addressed in this chapter when discussing each injury; however, the clinician should have a systematic approach to avoid missing important injuries. Before beginning, assess the adequacy of the films, specifically whether the open-mouth view allows visualization of the dens and lateral masses and whether the lateral view demonstrates all cervical vertebrae and the top of T1. Next, consider the alignment of the vertebrae on the lateral view (Fig. 9–2). Look closely for any fractures of the vertebral bodies or posterior bony structures. Loss of height of a vertebral body suggests a compression fracture. An abnormal angle between vertebral bodies suggests an unstable fracture. Finally, evaluate the prevertebral soft tissues and the predental space (Fig. 9–3).

Because plain radiographs are less sensitive and frequently inadequate at demonstrating the entirety of the cervical spine, CT scan of the cervical spine is the more common initial

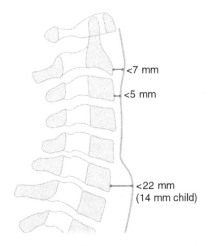

Figure 9–3. In adults, the prevertebral soft tissues should be <7 mm at C2, <5 mm at C3, and <22 mm at C6. In children, 14 mm is the acceptable limit at C6.

imaging study of choice in trauma patients. In addition, when a fracture is seen on plain radiographs, CT is useful to further define the traumatic injury. The sensitivity for detecting injuries is 97% to 100%, and the specificity is 99.5%. A negative CT scan that includes sagittal reconstructions has been shown to exclude both fracture and clinically significant ligamentous injury, even in patients with persistent neck pain. Cervical spine immobilization can often be discontinued with a normal CT at the discretion of the physician. In fact, recent practice management guidelines from the Eastern Association for the Surgery of Trauma recommend discontinuation of cervical collar immobilization after a negative high-quality C-spine CT alone in the obtunded blunt trauma patient. Additional studies support clearance of the cervical spine in intoxicated patients after blunt trauma with no gross motor deficits after a normal CT. MRI is useful for soft tissue, ligamentous, disk, or spinal cord injuries but poor for detecting osseous injuries. Disadvantages of MRI include a high false-positive rate in trauma and obvious time and patient access constraints in the emergency setting. In patients with neurologic deficits, despite a negative high-resolution CT, an MRI should be considered for spinal cord injury such as central cord syndrome. Isolated, clinically significant cervical spine or ligamentous injury with a negative CT and a normal motor examination, however, is extremely rare. Vertebral artery injury can also occur, particularly with complete spinal cord injury, fractures through the foramen transversarium, vertebral subluxation, or cervical spinal facet dislocations. Obtain vascular imaging in these circumstances or if patients are demonstrating lateralizing neurologic deficits not explained by a CT of the head.

Spinal Cord Injury

Neurogenic shock occurs most commonly after cervical spine injury (19% of patients), followed by thoracic (7%) and lumbar (3%) injuries. Vital signs demonstrate a low systolic blood pressure (<100 mm Hg) and bradycardia (<60–80 beats/min). These abnormalities usually occur several hours after cord injury. The pathogenesis is related to loss of sympathetic tone and decreased peripheral vascular resistance. Bradycardia is present because of the disruption of sympathetic activity to

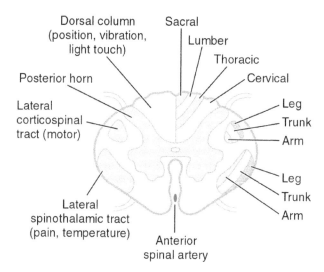

Figure 9–4. The anatomy of a cross-section of cervical spinal cord.

the heart resulting in unopposed vagal activity. Neurogenic shock should be distinguished from the term "spinal shock," which refers to an initial loss with a gradual recovery of some neurologic function after a spinal cord injury.

Knowledge of the location of nerve tracts within the spinal cord will help the clinician understand the syndromes that occur after injury (Fig. 9–4). A patient with a complete cord syndrome will present early with flaccid paralysis and loss of sensation below the injury. Reflexes are absent, and there will be no response to the Babinski test. Priapism may appear and generally lasts for a day. Within 1 to 3 days, hyperactive reflexes, a positive Babinski, and spasticity develop, reflecting the upper motor neuron injury.

Incomplete cord injury is usually more challenging to diagnose. Several classic variants exist, but there is significant disparity in presentation. The *anterior cord syndrome* occurs in most cases from hyperflexion of the cervical spine. The anterior two-thirds of the cord are affected, but the dorsal columns—controlling light touch, proprioception, and vibratory sense—are spared to a variable degree (Fig. 9–5). *Central cord syndrome* is due to hyperextension injury and

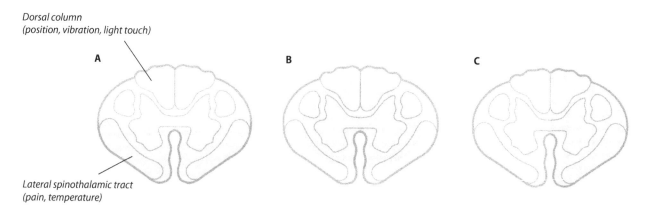

Figure 9–5. Incomplete spinal cord syndromes. **A.** Anterior cord. **B.** Central. **C.** Brown-Séquard.

occurs frequently in patients with preexisting cervical degenerative joint disease. In this setting, the central portion of the cord is compressed between the ligamentum flavum and bony osteophytes. Clinically, the patient will exhibit motor impairment that is greatest in the upper extremities with variable amounts of sensory loss and bladder dysfunction (Fig. 9–5B). Finally, the *Brown-Séquard syndrome* is a rare condition due to unilateral loss of cord function from hemisection of the spinal cord (Fig. 9–5C). The patient will exhibit paralysis with loss of proprioception, vibration, and light touch on the side of the damage and loss of pain and temperature sensation on the contralateral side.

Treatment

Neurogenic shock should be considered in the patient with hypotension, bradycardia, and traumatic spinal cord injury once other causes of shock have been excluded. No consensus on the optimal treatment of neurogenic shock exists. Crystalloid fluid infusion and cervical stabilization may be all that is necessary in mild cases. Vasopressors and inotropes are indicated if vascular instability persists.

In patients with blunt traumatic spinal cord injury, high-dose steroids were considered as a treatment option early post injury.[27,28] Even within the recommended 8-hour window, steroids carry an increased incidence of complications such as sepsis, gastrointestinal bleeding, and pneumonia. In addition, the evidence for the efficacy of steroids to produce a small gain in the total motor and sensory score was seen only in a post-hoc analysis and does not provide long-term benefit. This fact increases the likelihood that a statistical difference will be found when one does not exist and generally precludes the results from being used to change clinical practice.[29] Therefore, without compelling evidence for the efficacy of a high-dose steroid regimen, steroids should be used with caution or not at all.[30,31] Several medical societies have stated that this treatment is not a "standard of care," and recent literature recommends not using steroids in spinal cord injury as the risk of harm outweighs the potential benefit.[32–35]

Other treatment options such as GM-1 ganglioside, naloxone, thyrotropin-releasing hormone, and tirilazad have failed to demonstrate any meaningful effect in neurologic function. Small studies demonstrated a trend toward clinical improvement with therapeutic hypothermia, but routine use cannot be advocated.[36,37]

Classification

The cervical spine is divided into two segments for the purposes of this chapter. High cervical spine injuries are those that involve the occiput, C1, and C2. The remainder of the chapter focuses on injuries to the third through seventh cervical vertebrae. This discussion categorizes injuries based on the mechanism of injury. Clinical stability of each injury is discussed. Loss of stability refers to the inability of the spine to maintain relationships under normal physiologic loads. With instability comes the inherent risk of secondary spinal cord injury.

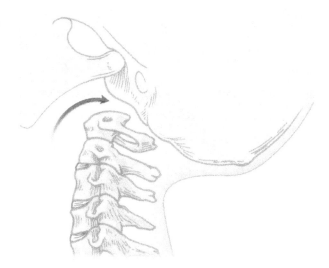

Figure 9–6. Atlanto-occipital dislocation.

HIGH CERVICAL INJURIES

Atlanto-occipital Dissociation

Atlanto-occipital dissociation (also known as internal decapitation) involves a disruption of all of the ligamentous connections between the occiput and the atlas (Fig. 9–6). The skull may be anterior, posterior, or distracted from the cervical spine. Due to the significant force applied to the head and neck, this injury is frequently fatal. Radiographs demonstrate displacement of the occipital condyles from the superior articulating facets of the atlas. The distance between the tip of the clivus (i.e., basion) and a line extending from the posterior cortex of C2 (basion–axial interval) should be less than 12 mm. A second measurement between the basion and the superior surface of the dens (basion–dental interval) should also be less than 12 mm.[38] Immediate neurosurgical referral is indicated, and any type of axial traction is to be avoided as it may increase the displacement of this highly unstable injury.

Atlantoaxial Dislocation

The most common atlantoaxial dislocation is anterior with either transverse ligament rupture or odontoid fracture. Posterior and rotatory injuries are less common. A pure transverse ligament rupture is more common in elderly individuals, but can also occur in younger patients following trauma, such as a MVC.[39]

The clinical presentation is variable, with death common from high-level cord compression between the odontoid and posterior arch of the atlas. Radiographs reveal an abnormal relationship between the atlas and axis. In the anterior dislocation, there is an increased distance (>3 mm) between the posterior aspect of the anterior arch of the atlas and the odontoid process. A distance between 3 and 5 mm suggests transverse ligament disruption, whereas a distance

Normal

Less than 3 mm

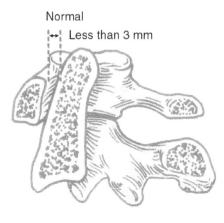

Abnormal

3–5 mm

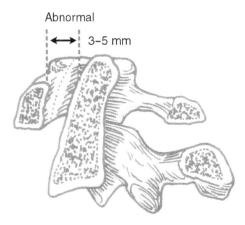

Figure 9–7. A widened predental space is evidence of transverse and alar ligaments' rupture.

greater than 5 mm is consistent with rupture of both the transverse and alar ligaments (Fig. 9–7). Open-mouth plain radiographic views or, preferably, CT scan will demonstrate an odontoid fracture. Consult a spine surgeon for stabilization and reduction.

C1 Burst Fracture (Jefferson Fracture)

The Jefferson burst fracture is due to axial loading when the spine is neither flexed nor extended. This results in fractures of the anterior and posterior arches of C1 on the left and right (Fig. 9–8A). On plain films, prevertebral soft-tissue swelling is usually evident on the lateral view, but the fractures themselves can be difficult to appreciate. The open-mouth view demonstrates displacement of the lateral masses of the atlas (Fig. 9–8B). CT scan is necessary to fully appreciate the fracture pattern (Fig. 9–8C).

Fractures of the ring of the atlas can be stable or unstable based on the integrity of its ligamentous support, specifically the transverse and alar ligaments. Displacement of the lateral masses of the atlas by a distance of 7 mm or more, seen commonly on the open-mouth view, is evidence of a ruptured transverse ligament (Fig. 9–8D). This constitutes an unstable injury in which the odontoid process can compress the spinal cord.

Jefferson burst fractures are associated with additional cervical spine fractures, with an incidence of 50%. Definitive treatment generally consists of immobilization with a rigid collar or halo traction (Fig. 9–9). Fractures associated with transverse atlantal ligament disruption can be treated with rigid immobilization or surgical stabilization.

C1 Arch Fractures

In addition to the axial loading (i.e., Jefferson burst fracture), other mechanisms can cause fractures of the C1 arch. Hyperextension can cause avulsion of the anterior tubercle of the atlas (Fig. 9–10). This injury will be seen on the lateral radiograph or CT scan, and there is frequently associated soft-tissue swelling. If the avulsion consists of the entire anterior arch, then this injury may be unstable.

Hyperextension with compression can direct a force across the posterior arch of the atlas that will cause fracture at the junction of the posterior arch and the lateral mass. The lateral radiograph best demonstrates this fracture and is seen as a vertical fracture with little or no displacement and no prevertebral swelling. There will be no lateral displacement of the C1 articular masses on the open-mouth view, as seen in a burst fracture. This fracture is frequently associated with other cervical spine fractures, particularly the dens. If isolated, this fracture may be stable.

Consultation with a spine surgeon is recommended for any fracture of the C1 arch, and the patient should be kept immobilized.

Odontoid Fractures

Odontoid fractures consist of three main types (Fig. 9–11). Type I is an avulsion of the tip of the dens at the site of attachment of the alar ligament, which is an uncommon injury and is stable as long as the transverse ligament remains intact. If the patient complains of any neurologic symptoms, then suspect another injury or a ruptured transverse ligament. Type I dens fractures may be associated with atlanto-occipital dissociation.

Type II fractures are transverse at the base of the odontoid and are unstable. Type III fractures occur through the body of the axis, often involving an articulating facet. If this fracture is displaced, it is usually unstable.

One-quarter of these patients will present with neurologic deficits, whereas the majority will report a severe high cervical pain with muscle spasm made worse with any attempts at movement.

Radiographically, these injuries are best seen on CT scan, although the open-mouth view is the best plain film method to make the diagnosis (Fig. 9–12). Flexion-extension views are contraindicated, as displacement may be potentially fatal. Type II and III fractures require immediate referral for stabilization.

Hangman's Fracture

The hangman's fracture, also referred to as traumatic spondylolisthesis of the axis, is a hyperextension injury of the high cervical spine that produces a fracture at the pedicles

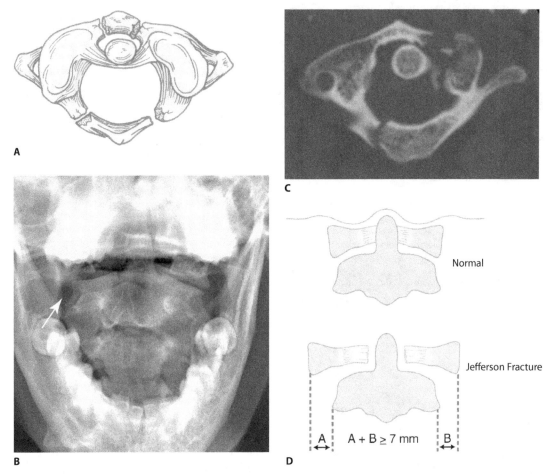

A

B

C

D

Normal

Jefferson Fracture

A   A + B ≥ 7 mm   B

Figure 9–8. Jefferson fracture. **A.** Schematic of a C1 Jefferson fracture with an intact transverse ligament. **B.** Abnormal widening on the open-mouth view (*arrow*). **C.** CT scan. **D.** On the open-mouth view, displacement of the lateral masses of C2 is seen in an unstable Jefferson fracture.

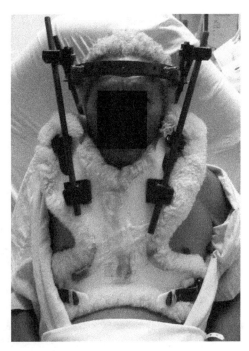

Figure 9–9. A halo device for cervical spine stability.

of C2 with anterior displacement of C2 on C3 (Fig. 9–13). This fracture was seen in judicial hangings but is now more common following MCVs and diving accidents. Although this injury is highly unstable, the patient may present without significant neurologic dysfunction because of the large diameter of the spinal canal at this level. Many patients are treated effectively with external immobilization.

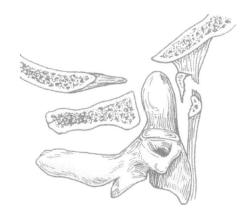

Figure 9–10. Avulsion fracture of the anterior mass of C1.

Type I

Type II

Type III

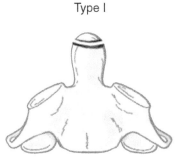
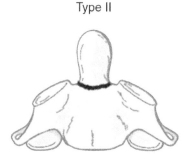
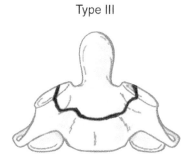

Figure 9–11. Odontoid fractures.

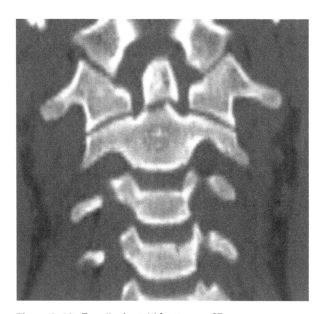

Figure 9–12. Type II odontoid fracture on CT scan.

C3-C7 INJURIES

The forces that lead to injuries of the lower cervical spine can be used for classification and aid in the understanding of the ligamentous and bony injuries present. Flexion, flexion-rotation, extension-rotation, extension, and vertical compression all produce distinct injury patterns that are discussed in this section.

Flexion

Flexion Teardrop Fracture

The flexion teardrop fracture is an extremely unstable injury produced by severe hyperflexion and compressive forces as might occur with diving into the shallow end of a pool. Complete ligamentous disruption occurs with facet joint disruption and a comminuted fracture of the vertebral body that frequently pushes fragments into the spinal canal (Fig. 9–14). The resultant forces create a large triangular

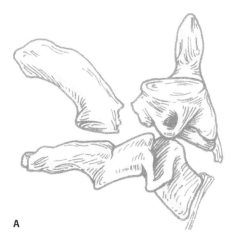

A

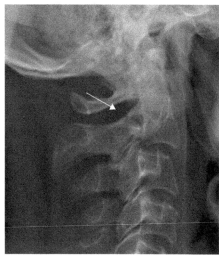

B

Figure 9–13. Hangman's fracture.
A. Schematic. **B.** Lateral radiograph.

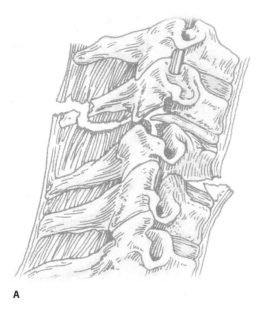

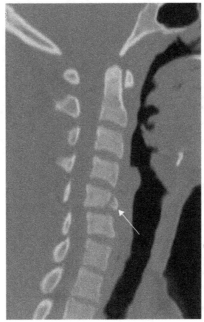

Figure 9–14. Flexion teardrop fracture. **A.** Schematic. **B.** C5 flexion teardrop fracture on CT.

fragment off the anterior portion of the vertebral body in the shape of a teardrop. Neurologic deficit is common, either in the form of a complete cord injury or an anterior cord syndrome. Radiographically, the anterior inferior corner fracture of the vertebral body is evident on the lateral view. The upper cervical spine is flexed, and the involved vertebra is displaced and rotated anteriorly.

When this injury occurs at the C3-C5 levels, apnea can occur from respiratory muscle paralysis. Intubation will be necessary in this circumstance, and the patient will require continuous immobilization. Consult with a spine surgeon for definitive care.

Clay Shoveler's Fracture

Clay shoveler's fracture occurs when the head and the upper cervical vertebrae are forced into flexion against the action of the supraspinatus ligament and erector muscles, resulting in an avulsion fracture of one or more of the spinous processes of C7, C6, and T1, in that order of frequency (Fig. 9–15). This fracture is named due to its association with Australian

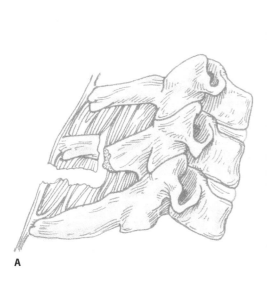

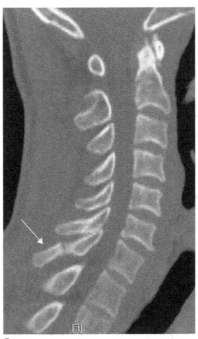

Figure 9–15. Clay shoveler's fracture. **A.** Schematic. **B.** Lateral radiograph.

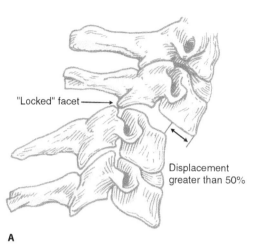

"Locked" facet

Displacement greater than 50%

A

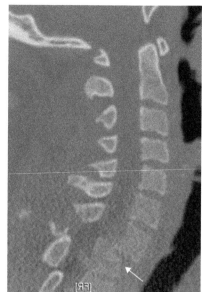

B

Figure 9–16. Bilateral facet dislocation. **A.** Schematic. **B.** Lateral radiograph with more than 50% subluxation of C7 on T1.

clay miners in the 1930s. It more commonly occurs today after direct trauma to the spinous process or after decelerating MVCs. Patients will complain of point tenderness over the involved area. This is a stable injury and requires analgesics and early referral.

Bilateral Facet Dislocation

Severe hyperflexion results in the rupture of the posterior ligamentous complex, which allows the superior facets to pass up and over the inferior facets, where they rest in the intervertebral foramina creating a very unstable injury. The majority of these injuries occur between C5 and C7. Patients will present with neck pain and the inability to move the head from a midline position. On examination, there is often prominence of the spinous process of the inferior vertebrae. Cord or nerve root compression can lead to neurologic deficits. Radiographs are characterized by an anterior displacement of the superior vertebral body of at least 50% of its width (Fig. 9–16). The term *perched facets* refers to an incomplete bilateral dislocation where the inferior aspect of the superior facets rests on the superior aspect of the inferior facets. Emergent reduction can result in significant recovery of neurologic deficits.

Wedge Compression Fracture

Wedge compression fractures occur from forceful flexion with some axial compressive forces that impact the vertebral body (Fig. 9–17). The anterior portion of the superior endplate of the vertebral body fractures. Posterior structures remain intact in most cases, but their involvement makes this fracture unstable. Loss of the anterior vertebral height by more than half or multiple adjacent wedge fractures may also make this injury unstable. For this reason, these fractures should be considered unstable until proven otherwise.

Hyperflexion Sprain

A hyperflexion sprain is also referred to as an anterior subluxation. Hyperflexion causes the posterior ligamentous structures to rupture without associated fractures (Fig. 9–18). On radiographs, there may be a widening of the spinous processes at the level of the ligamentous rupture. Angulation of two vertebrae by more than 11 degrees and more than 3.5 mm horizontal displacement of adjacent cervical segments on lateral films are abnormal, suggest instability, and are consistent with this injury (Fig. 9–19).

Flexion-Rotation

Unilateral Facet Dislocation

Unilateral facet dislocation occurs from a combination of flexion and rotation. The joint opposite the side of rotation

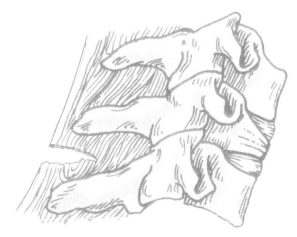

Figure 9–17. Wedge compression fracture. Posterior ligamentous injury may make this fracture unstable.

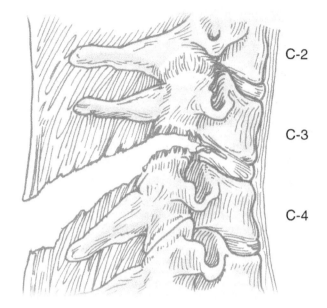

Figure 9–18. Hyperflexion sprain.

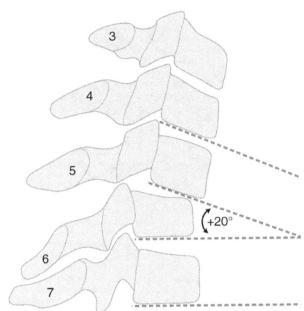

Figure 9–19. More than 11 degrees of angulation of two cervical vertebrae suggest an unstable injury.

becomes dislocated as the superior facet moves anteriorly and superiorly above the inferior facet. In the absence of concomitant fractures, stability remains because the contralateral joint remains intact. Clinically, neck pain usually localizes to the affected side, and the head is rotated away from the lesion. Nerve root impingement is frequent, but the spinal cord is rarely involved. The lateral radiograph

shows the vertebral body anteriorly displaced by a distance of approximately 25% of the diameter of the vertebral body (Fig. 9–20). Treatment of this condition frequently requires open reduction and internal fixation as this injury can be very difficult to reduce by traction and may have varying degrees of ligamentous injury.[44]

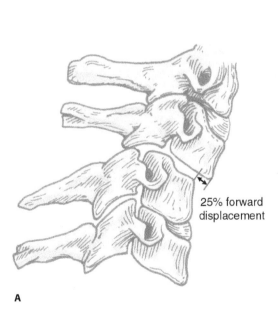

25% forward displacement

A

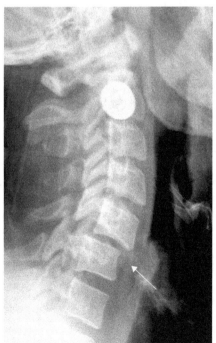

B

Figure 9–20. Unilateral facet dislocation. **A.** Schematic. **B.** Lateral radiograph.

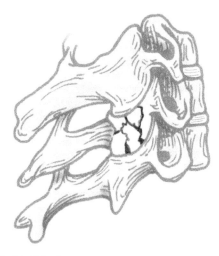

Figure 9–21. Pillar fracture.

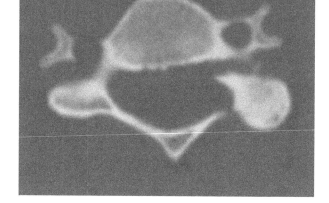

Figure 9–22. Pedicolaminar fracture on CT scan.

Extension-Rotation

Pillar Fracture

This fracture of the pillar of the facet joint is caused by a hyperextension and rotation mechanism (Fig. 9–21). Hyperextension brings the facet bones together, and as the head rotates, a force is directed toward a single pillar that causes it to fracture. Radiographically, the AP projection will demonstrate an abnormality of the lateral column. The fracture line is usually vertical. On the lateral view, the injury is difficult to identify. A "double-outline" sign occurs when the fracture is displaced posteriorly and causes two radiographic shadows.   A tear in the anterior longitudinal ligament may also occur with this fracture. A pillar fracture is considered stable.

Pedicolaminar Fracture Separation

This injury involves unilateral fractures of the pedicle and lamina with varying degrees of displacement and disruption of the anterior longitudinal ligament and disk. The term "separation" refers to the fact that with a fracture to both the pedicle and laminae on one side, the articular pillar (i.e., facet) becomes a free-floating fragment. If the disk above and below the fractured vertebra is involved, then this becomes an unstable injury. On the AP view, there is disruption of the lateral column similar to the appearance of a pillar fracture. On the lateral radiograph, these injuries resemble a laminar or pillar fracture. Occasionally, there is anterolisthesis of the involved vertebra by approximately 3 mm. CT is useful to determine the full extent of the injury (Fig. 9–22).

Extension

Hyperextension Sprain

Hyperextension sprains occur from a blow to the face or forehead, or after a rear-end MVC. The posterior structures act as a fulcrum, and the anterior longitudinal ligament and

intervertebral disk rupture (Fig. 9–23). With significant ligamentous disruption, the superior vertebra can move posteriorly and compress the spinal cord. If the posterior ligamentous complex is also disrupted, dislocation may occur. On examination, there is usually pain and tenderness over the anterior muscles (i.e., sternocleidomastoid and scalenes). There may be dysphagia and hoarseness secondary to injury of the throat and esophagus. Posterior cord injury with motor loss distal to the lesion is most common. Radiographs will exhibit soft-tissue swelling and an anteriorly widened disk space may also be apparent. If this injury is suspected, CT or MRI should be used to confirm ligamentous disruption. Patients with a normal neurologic examination and negative imaging studies can be treated with analgesics and early referral. Others require immediate consultation with a spine surgeon.

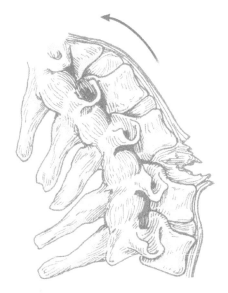

Figure 9–23. Hyperextension sprain.

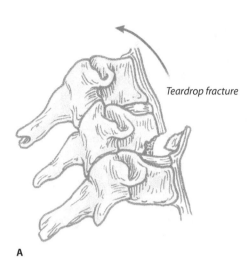

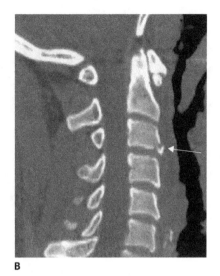

Figure 9–24. Extension teardrop fracture. **A.** Schematic. **B.** CT scan.

Extension Teardrop Fracture

The extension teardrop fracture is similar to a hyperextension sprain, but the anterior longitudinal ligament avulses the inferior portion of the anterior vertebral body (Fig. 9–24). The triangular-shaped fragment's height is usually higher than its width. Extension teardrop fractures are usually more common in elderly patients with osteoporosis. It is an unstable injury, and central cord syndrome is seen in up to 80% of patients with this injury.[45] Advanced imaging (CT, MRI) is required to evaluate the spinal canal. Consult a spine surgeon and maintain cervical immobilization.

Laminar Fracture

Isolated laminar fractures are uncommon but occur most frequently in older patients with cervical stenosis. With hyperextension and compression, the lamina can fracture (Fig. 9–25). More commonly, however, the lamina will fracture as part of a burst fracture, a flexion teardrop fracture, or pedicolaminar fracture-separation.[45] On the lateral radiograph, a vertical fracture line may be seen, but CT is more sensitive. Isolated laminar fractures are stable, but fragments can enter the spinal canal and cause neurologic findings. This injury requires cervical immobilization and referral.

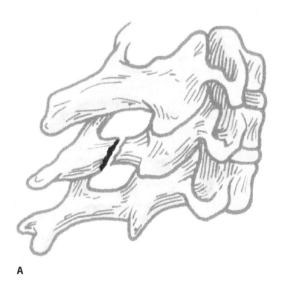

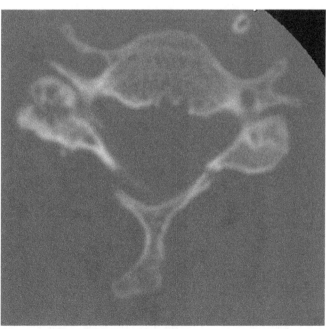

Figure 9–25. Laminar fracture. **A.** Schematic. **B.** CT scan demonstrating bilateral laminar fractures.

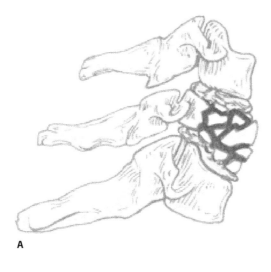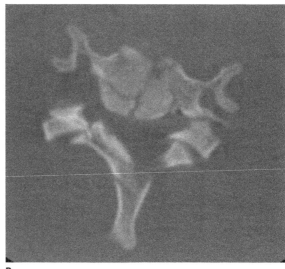

Figure 9–26. Burst fracture. **A.** Schematic. **B.** CT scan.

Vertical Compression

Burst Fracture

Burst fractures are due to an axial load that causes a comminuted fracture of the vertebral body (Fig. 9–26) and are most common at the C5 level. Frequently, fragments displace into the spinal canal. The posterior ligament complex remains intact, but a fracture of the posterior arch is frequently present. The burst fracture appears similar to the flexion teardrop, but the anterior fragment of the body is usually larger. Immediate consultation with a spine surgeon is indicated for this potentially unstable fracture.

SUMMARY

Cervical spine injuries represent a potentially devastating injury to the patient and a financial burden to society. Early recognition and proper stabilization of cervical injuries is paramount. CT is the initial imaging test of choice for the cervical spine in trauma patients and useful for osseous injuries. Fracture and injury pattern recognition aides in determining appropriate early consultation or referral for definitive management.

REFERENCES

1. National Spinal Cord Injury Statistical Center (NSCISC). Facts and figures at a glance. Birmingham: University of Alabama at Birmingham; 2017. https://www.nscisc.uab.edu/Public/Facts%20and%20Figures%20-%202017.pdf. Accessed December 14, 2017.
2. Chen Y, Tang Y, Vogel LC, DeVivo MJ. Causes of spinal cord injury. *Top Spinal Cord Inj Rehabil.* 2013;19(1):1–8. doi:10.1310/sci1901-1.
3. Lowery DW, Wald MM, Browne BJ, et al. Epidemiology of cervical spine injury victims. *Ann Emerg Med.* 2001;38(1):12–16.
4. Badhiwala JH, Lai CK, Alhazzani W, et al. Cervical spine clearance in obtunded patients after blunt traumatic injury. *Ann Intern Med.* 2015;162(6):429–437.
5. Oteir AO, Smith K, Stoelwinder JU, et al. Should suspected cervical spinal cord injury be immobilised?: a systematic review. *Injury.* 2015;46:528–535.
6. Hood N, Considine J. Spinal immobilisation in pre-hospital and emergency care: a systematic review of the literature. *Australas Emerg Nurs J.* 2015;18:118–137.
7. Abram S, Bulstrode C. Routine spinal immobilization in trauma patients: what are the advantages and disadvantages? *Surgeon.* 2010;8(4):218–222. doi:10.1016/j.surge.2010.01.002.
8. Purvis TA, Carlin B, Driscoll P. The definite risks and questionable benefits of liberal pre-hospital spinal immobilisation. *Am J Emerg Med.* 2017;35(6):860–866. doi:10.1016/j.ajem.2017.01.045.
9. Kwan I, Bunn F, Roberts I. Spinal immobilisation for trauma patients. *Cochrane Database Syst Rev.* 2001;(2):CD002803.
10. Hoffman JR, Mower WR, Wolfson AB, Todd KH, Zucker MI. Validity of a set of clinical criteria to rule out injury to the cervical spine in patients with blunt trauma. National Emergency X-Radiography Utilization Study Group. *N Engl J Med.* 2000;343(2):94–99.
11. Stiell IG, Wells GA, Vandemheen KL, et al. The Canadian C-Spine Rule for radiography in alert and stable trauma patients. *JAMA.* 2001;286(15):1841–1848.
12. Dickinson G, Stiell IG, Schull M, et al. Retrospective application of the NEXUS low-risk criteria for cervical spine radiography in Canadian emergency departments. *Ann Emerg Med.* 2004;43(4):507–514.
13. Stiell IG, Clement CM, McKnight RD, et al. The Canadian C-Spine Rule versus the NEXUS low-risk criteria in patients with trauma. *N Engl J Med.* 2003;349(26):2510–2518.
14. Goldberg W, Mueller C, Panacek E, et al. Distribution and patterns of blunt traumatic cervical spine injury. *Ann Emerg Med.* 2001;38(1):17–21.

15. Mower WR, Hoffman JR, Pollack CV Jr, et al. Use of plain radiography to screen for cervical spine injuries. *Ann Emerg Med.* 2001;38(1):1–7.

16. Blackham J, Benger J. "Clearing" the cervical spine in the unconscious trauma patient. *Trauma.* 2011;13:65–79.

17. Schenarts PJ, Diaz J, Kaiser C, Eddy V, Morris JA Jr. Prospective comparison of admission computed tomographic scan and plain films of the upper cervical spine in trauma patients with altered mental status. *J Trauma.* 2001;51(4):663–668.

18. Mathen R, Inaba K, Munera F, et al. Prospective evaluation of multislice computed tomography versus plain radiographic cervical spine clearance in trauma patients. *J Trauma.* 2007;62(6):1427–1431.

19. Bailitz J, Starr F, Beecroft M, et al. CT should replace three-view radiographs as the initial screening test in patients at high, moderate, and low risk for blunt cervical spine injury: a prospective comparison. *J Trauma.* 2009;66(6):1605–1609.

20. Como JJ, Diaz JJ, Dunham M, et al. Practice management guidelines for identification of cervical spine injuries following trauma: update from the eastern association for the surgery of trauma practice management guidelines committee. *J Trauma.* 2009;67(3):651–659.

21. Ryken TC, Hadley MN, Walters BC, et al. Radiographic assessment. *Neurosurgery.* 2013;72(suppl 2):54–72.

22. Schuster R, Waxman K, Sanchez B, et al. Magnetic resonance imaging is not needed to clear cervical spines in blunt trauma patients with normal computed tomographic results and no motor deficits. *Arch Surg.* 2005;140(8):762–766.

23. Patel MB, Humble SS, Cullinane DC, et al. Cervical spine collar clearance in the obtunded adult blunt trauma patient: a systematic review and practice management guideline from the Eastern Association for the Surgery of Trauma. *J Trauma Acute Care Surg.* 2015;78:430–41.

24. Bush L, Brookshire R, Roche B, et al. Evaluation of cervical spine clearance by computed tomographic scan alone in intoxicated patients with blunt trauma. *JAMA Surg.* 2016;151(9):807–813.

25. Inaba K, Byerly S, Bush LD, et al. Cervical spinal clearance: a prospective Western Trauma Association multi-institutional trial. *J Trauma Acute Care Surg.* 2016;81(6):1122–1130.

26. Harrigan MR, Hadley MN, Dhall SS, et al. Management of vertebral artery injuries following non-penetrating cervical trauma. *Neurosurgery.* 2013;72(suppl 2):234–243

27. Bracken MB. Steroids for acute spinal cord injury. *Cochrane Database Syst Rev.* 2012;(1):CD001046.

28. Bracken MB. Methylprednisolone and acute spinal cord injury: an update of the randomized evidence. *Spine.* 2001;26(suppl 24):S47–S54.

29. Spencer MT, Bazarian JJ. Evidence-based emergency medicine/systematic review abstract. Are corticosteroids effective in traumatic spinal cord injury? *Ann Emerg Med.* 2003;41(3):410–413.

30. Short DJ, El Masry WS, Jones PW. High dose methylprednisolone in the management of acute spinal cord injury—a systematic review from a clinical perspective. *Spinal Cord.* 2000;38(5):273–286.

31. Hugenholtz H, Cass DE, Dvorak MF, et al. High-dose methylprednisolone for acute closed spinal cord injury—only a treatment option. *Can J Neurol Sci.* 2002;29(3):227–235.

32. Hugenholtz H. Methylprednisolone for acute spinal cord injury: not a standard of care. *CMAJ.* 2003;168(9):1145–1146.

33. Hurlbert RJ, Hadley MN, Walters BC, et al. Pharmacological therapy for acute spinal cord injury. *Neurosurgery.* 2013;72(suppl 2):93–105.

34. Evaniew N, Belley-Cote EP, Fallah N, et al. Methylprednisolone for the treatment of patients with acute spinal cord injuries. A systematic review and meta-analysis. *J Neurotrauma.* 2016;33:468–481.

35. Rogers WK, Todd M. Acute spinal cord injury. *Best Practice Res Clin Anaesthesiol.* 2016;30:27–39.

36. Levi AD, Casella G, Green BA, et al. Clinical outcomes using modest intravascular hypothermia after acute cervical spinal cord injury. *Neurosurgery.* 2010;66(4):670–677.

37. Dididze M, Green BA, Dietrich WD, et al. Systemic hypothermia in acute cervical spinal cord injury: a case-controlled study. *Spinal Cord.* 2013;51(5):395–400.

38. Theodore N, Aarabi B, Dhall SS, et al. The diagnosis and management of traumatic atlanto-occipital dislocation injuries. *Neurosurgery.* 2013;72(suppl 2):114–126.

39. Naim-ur-Rahman, Jamjoom ZA, Jamjoom A. Ruptured transverse ligament: an injury that is often forgotten. *Br J Neurosurg.* 2000;14(4):375–377.

40. Harris J Jr. The cervicocranium: its radiographic assessment. *Radiology.* 2001;218(2):337–351.

41. Ryken TC, Aarabi B, Dhall SS, et al. Management of isolated fractures of the atlas in adults. *Neurosurgery.* 2013;72(suppl 2):127–131.

42. Ryken TC, Hadley MN, Aarabi B, et al. Management of isolated fractures of the axis in adults. *Neurosurgery.* 2013;72(suppl 2):132–150. doi:10.1227/NEU.0b013e318276ee40.

43. Laporte C, Laville C, Lazennec JY, et al. Severe hyperflexion sprains of the lower cervical spine in adults. *Clin Orthop Relat Res.* 1999;363:126–134.

44. Gelb DE, Aarabi B, Dhall SS, et al. Treatment of subaxial cervical spine injuries. *Neurosurgery.* 2013;72(suppl 2):187–194.

45. Rao SK, Wasyliw C, Nunez DB Jr. Spectrum of imaging findings in hyperextension injuries of the neck. *Radiographics.* 2005;25(5):1239–1254.

CHAPTER 10

Thoracolumbar Spine Trauma

Sean Dyer, MD

INTRODUCTION

This chapter addresses traumatic fractures and dislocations to the thoracolumbar (TL) spinal column. With the exception of vertebral compression fractures, TL spine injuries are uncommon, and when present, are frequently overlooked. This is likely due to the fact that other more significant injuries in the traumatized patient distract the clinician and because signs and symptoms of the vertebral injury are often subtle. Early diagnosis and treatment of these injuries improves neurologic outcome.

Imaging

In victims of blunt trauma receiving thoracic and/or lumbar spine radiographs, approximately 6% will have a fracture. Imaging is recommended in the setting of one of the following :

- Back pain or midline back tenderness
- Abnormal neurologic examination
- Any other spine fracture
- Glasgow Coma Scale <15
- Major distracting injury
- Alcohol or drug intoxication
- High-energy mechanism (fall >10 ft, high-speed motor vehicle collision [MVC])
- Cervical spine fracture

The imaging modality is controversial, but computed tomography (CT) scan is more sensitive than plain films for detecting fractures. Multidetector CT of the abdomen and chest with reconstructions of the spine is as accurate for detecting TL spine fractures as dedicated spinal CT. This technique also saves time and cost.

Patients that have a normal mental status, no signs of intoxication, a normal physical and neurologic exam, no suspicion for a high-energy mechanism, and no complaint of TL spine pain can be reliably excluded from a TL spine injury with no need for radiologic evaluation.

Classification

Fractures of the TL spine are most common at the junction of the rigidly fixed thoracic spine and the flexible lumbar spine. Approximately 50% of all fractures of the TL region occur between T11 and L3. However, because the spinal canal is wider in this location than in the cervical spine, complete cord lesions are less common.

Several classification schemes exist that attempt to predict both the bony and neurologic stability of the injury. In 2005, the Thoracolumbar Injury Classification and Severity Score (TLICS) was developed that used the fracture morphology (compression, rotational/translation, or distraction), patient's neurologic status, and the integrity of the posterior ligamentous complex, as seen on advanced imaging, to predict stability and the need for operative intervention.

The three-column classification system developed by Denis, divides the spinal column into three sections: anterior, middle, and posterior (Fig. 10–1). The anterior column consists of the anterior longitudinal ligament and the anterior half of the vertebral bodies and discs. The middle column is made up of the posterior longitudinal ligament and the posterior half of the vertebral bodies and discs. Finally, the posterior column consists of the supraspinous and interspinous ligaments and facet joints. Mechanical stability is present if two or three columns are intact. Although this scheme is simple to understand, several studies have demonstrated that nonoperative treatment of two-column injuries may achieve a satisfactory outcome.

Due to the complexity of these injuries and the frequent need for diagnostic imaging and expert consultation, no one classification system should be relied on by the emergency provider and thoracolumbar fractures should be considered unstable until proven otherwise.

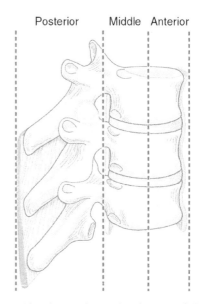

Posterior   Middle   Anterior

Figure 10–1. The three-column classification of the thoracolumbar spine.

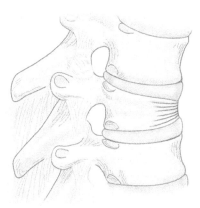

Figure 10–2. An anterior wedge compression fracture is a stable fracture because it involves only the anterior column.

COMPRESSION INJURIES

Compression Fractures

The vertebral compression fracture (VCF) is a common injury in the elderly osteoporotic population, making it the most common fracture in the thoracic and lumbar spine (Fig. 10–2). VCFs affect half of all individuals by the age of 80. These fractures are due to an axial force and flexion, often from a fall. However, in the osteoporotic patient, a VCF may occur after any type of trauma, even as trivial as a sneeze. VCFs are also associated with the muscle contraction that comes with an epileptic seizure and have been reported in patients riding in vehicles that have gone over a speed bump.[16,17]

In awake patients, pain and tenderness are present at the site of the fracture, most commonly, the midthoracic or upper lumbar region. Neurologic injury is not associated with this fracture, and therefore, neurologic complaints or findings on examination should prompt the clinician to consider other more serious injuries. In addition, young, healthy patients generally do not sustain this type of fracture, so careful consideration of another more serious injury should be undertaken. This is especially true after a high-energy traumatic mechanism.[14]

This fracture is best seen on the lateral radiograph, where the vertebral body takes on a wedge shape (Fig. 10–3). The vertebral body is compressed anteriorly and the posterior cortex of the vertebral body is normal, differentiating these fractures from a burst fracture. CT scan is recommended whenever the integrity of the posterior vertebral body and posterior column structures are questionable, as plain radiographs do not adequately evaluate the posterior vertebral body cortex.[18] The patient should be considered to have an unstable fracture until it is clear that the anterior vertebral body is all that is involved.

If the middle and posterior columns are determined to remain intact, a VCF is a stable injury without risk of causing spinal cord injury.[10]

The treatment of a simple wedge-shaped vertebral compression fracture is pain relief and early mobilization with increasing activity as the pain subsides. Physical therapy

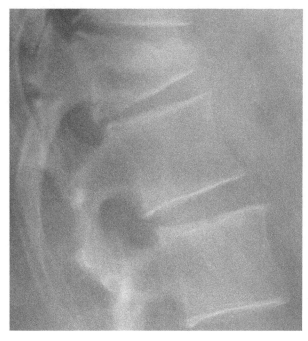

Figure 10–3. Anterior wedge compression fracture of T12.

may be appropriate, and activity is rarely restricted by 3 to 4 months following the injury.

Long-term instability of the spine can occur with severe compression fractures (>50% loss of the body height) or when multiple adjacent wedge fractures are present.

Burst Fractures

A burst fracture is a comminuted fracture of the vertebral body due to axial compression (Fig. 10–4). In some cases, the posterior column is disrupted as well. A burst fracture is distinguished from a simple osteoporotic compression fracture because the posterior vertebral body cortex is fractured.

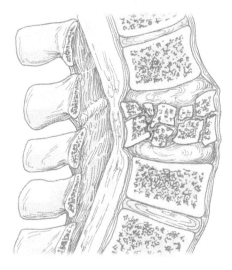

Figure 10–4. Sagittal view of a burst fracture. This comminuted fracture is due to axial compression.

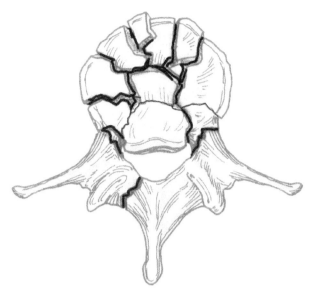

Figure 10–5. Transverse view of a burst fracture showing retropulsion of bony fragments into the spinal canal.

Posterior vertebral body fractures provide an additional risk to the spinal cord because there is frequently retropulsion of bony fragments into the spinal canal (Fig. 10–5).

Burst fractures are most common from a fall, but MVCs also account for a high number of these injuries. They have been reported after an atraumatic seizure. The majority of burst fractures occur in the T12 or L3 region. In 10% of cases, there is more than one burst fracture. They account for approximately 15% of vertebral fractures. Examination of the spine reveals tenderness at the level of the fracture, but the interspinous distance is unchanged. Neurologic deficits are present in approximately half of patients. Complete loss of motor function is present in one-third of patients.

On plain radiographs, there is loss of height of both the anterior and posterior cortex of the vertebral body. These findings are most apparent on the lateral radiographic view. The spine remains well aligned. Posterior element fractures are present in two-thirds of cases, although they are difficult to visualize on plain films.

The loss of height of the posterior cortex of the vertebral body is often difficult to appreciate on plain films, causing this injury to be misdiagnosed as a simple compression fracture. In one study, plain films improperly misdiagnosed burst fractures 25% of the time.

CT adequately details the degree of retropulsion and the presence of fractures in the posterior column and also impacts the treatment plan. Patients with a 50% reduction in the midsagittal diameter of the spinal canal are at an increased risk of progressive neurologic dysfunction.

These fractures are at risk for being unstable if there is suspicion for a ligamentous injury. Special attention should be given to the space between the spinous processes, as any indication of widening is suggestive of an unstable fracture.

In addition, there can be subtle vertebral body translation suggesting disruption of multiple spinal columns and a fracture-dislocation.

The patient should be managed with strict spinal immobilization, and consultation with an orthopedic or neurosurgical spine specialist should be obtained. Frequent neurologic reevaluations are warranted to detect changes in status. Patients with simple compression or stable burst fractures and no neurologic deficits can be treated with a brace that allows early mobilization. Prior to discharge, repeat upright radiographs should be taken with the brace in place as sometimes there can be some degree of "settling" and return to the postinjury alignment.

Flexion-Distraction Injuries

This injury results from rotation about a fulcrum that is located within the vertebral body. The anterior column fails due to a compressive mechanism, and the middle and posterior columns are disrupted by a distraction/tension force (Fig. 10–6). Radiographic findings include anterior impaction of the vertebral body and posterior distraction with fanning of the spinous processes. If the injury is only through the bony elements, it is usually treated with a hyperextension cast or brace, but more severe fractures and those with intra-abdominal injuries may require surgical intervention. The Chance fracture, described next, is a unique morphology of the flexion-distraction injuries and is known to be unstable. Consultation with a spine specialist should be obtained for all these types of fractures.

Chance Fractures

The Chance fracture, first described by G.Q. Chance in 1948, occurs after flexion of the spinal column about an axis that is anterior to the anterior longitudinal ligament and involves all three spinal columns failing under tension. It involves a horizontal splitting of the vertebra through all three columns and is therefore an unstable injury

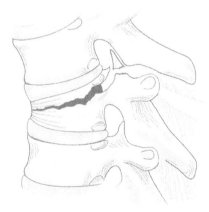

Figure 10–6. Chance fracture.

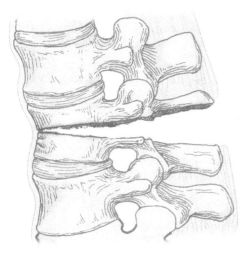

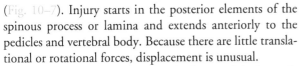

Figure 10–7. Flexion-distraction injury.

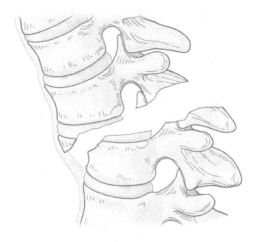

Figure 10–8. Fracture-dislocation (translational) injury due to a shearing force.

(Fig. 10–7). Injury starts in the posterior elements of the spinous process or lamina and extends anteriorly to the pedicles and vertebral body. Because there are little translational or rotational forces, displacement is unusual.

This injury was most common in the era of the lap-only seatbelt, where sudden deceleration forces caused severe hyperflexion and distraction of the spine. Today, most Chance fractures occur after falls or crush injuries. Tenderness is present over the involved vertebrae, most commonly, T12, L1, or L2. Chance fractures are associated with significant intra-abdominal injuries, with an incidence approaching 50%.

On the anteroposterior view, disruption of the pedicles, loss of vertebral height, or transverse process fracture may be noted. The lateral view demonstrates fractures through the spinous process, laminae, or pedicles. More subtle findings include an increase in the distance of adjacent spinous processes or an increase in the height of the posterior vertebral body.

A CT scan should be ordered to determine the extent of injury and the involvement of the spinal canal, as well as to diagnose intra-abdominal injuries. Because the disruption is oriented on a horizontal plane, this injury could be missed on CT if axial images are not supplemented by sagittal reformatted images.

Since these injuries are unstable, the spine should be kept immobilized and consultation with an orthopedic or neurosurgical spine specialist should be obtained.

Fracture-Dislocation Injuries

Fracture-dislocation or translational injuries occur after a shearing mechanism. They are rare, accounting for less than 2% of thoracic-lumbar-sacral (TLS) spine fractures. All three columns fail and the alignment of the spinal canal is affected in the transverse plane (Fig. 10–8). Because both the bony and ligamentous elements are disrupted, this is

inherently an unstable injury, and there is almost always an associated neurologic and/or musculoskeletal injury. Most commonly, the shear force is directed in a posterior to anterior direction and is the result of direct trauma to the back.

Plain radiographs can demonstrate this injury, and several variations may be seen. When translational injuries occur in the thoracic region, the lateral radiograph will demonstrate displacement of the superior vertebral body anteriorly. The vertebral bodies remain essentially intact, but the spinous process of the superior vertebra and the articular processes of the inferior segment are fractured. In the lumbar region, the direction of displacement is opposite, with the superior vertebra displaced in a more posterior direction. This dislocation can be somewhat more subtle, with no more than one-third of the width of the vertebral body displaced. The inferior portion of the superior vertebral body may be avulsed, and frequently, there is a facet joint or pedicle fracture. A CT scan is useful for giving more detailed information on the extent of bony injury.

These injuries are unstable, so the spine should be kept immobilized and consultation with an orthopedic or neurosurgical spine specialist should be obtained. Because of the almost universal occurrence of spinal cord injury, an early decision about the use of steroids should be made. Refer to Chapter 9 for a further discussion of steroids in acute traumatic spinal cord injury.

MINOR INJURIES

Transverse process, spinous process, and pars interarticularis fractures were classified by the previously accepted "Denis system" as minor injuries and are all stable in the absence of neurologic deficits. These fractures are caused by direct blows in the majority of cases, although forceful muscle contractions may also be causative. They are more

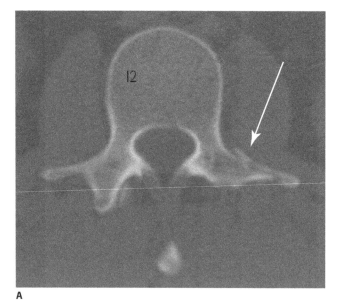
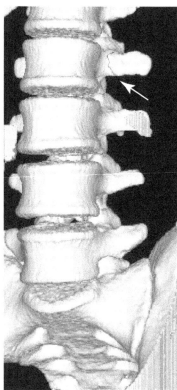

Figure 10–9. Transverse process fracture of L1. **A.** Axial CT image (*arrow*). **B.** CT 3D reconstruction (*arrow*).

common in the lumbar region. Transverse process fractures represent 14% of all TLS spine injuries, whereas the others represent approximately 1%. In patients with a transverse process fracture diagnosed on plain film, a CT scan should be obtained (Fig. 10–9). In one study, 3 of 28 patients (11%) had another spine injury that was only visualized on CT. Neurologic complications are unusual. Management includes rest, pain relief, and referral.

REFERENCES

1. Bernstein M. Easily missed thoracolumbar spine fractures. *Eur J Radiol.* 2010;74(1):6–15.
2. Bellabarba C, Fisher C, Chapman JR, Dettori JR, Norvell DC. Does early fracture fixation of thoracolumbar spine fractures decrease morbidity or mortality? *Spine.* 2010;35(9 suppl): S138–S145.
3. Holmes JF, Miller PQ, Panacek EA, Lin S, Horne NS, Mower WR. Epidemiology of thoracolumbar spine injury in blunt trauma. *Acad Emerg Med.* 2001;8(9):866–872.
4. Hsu JM, Joseph T, Ellis AM. Thoracolumbar fracture in blunt trauma patients: guidelines for diagnosis and imaging. *Injury.* 2003;34(6):426–433.
5. O'Connor E, Walsham J. Review article: indications for thoracolumbar imaging in blunt trauma patients: a review of current literature. *Emerg Med Australas.* 2009;21(2):94–101. doi:10.1111/j.1742-6723.2009.01164.x.
6. Inaba K, DuBose JJ, Barmparas G, et al. Clinical examination is insufficient to rule out thoracolumbar spine injuries. *J Trauma.* 2011;70:174–179.
7. Sixta S, Moore FO, Ditillo MF, et al. Screening for thoracolumbar spinal injuries in blunt trauma: an Eastern Association for the Surgery of Trauma practice management guideline. *J Trauma Acute Care Surg.* 2012;73(5 suppl 4):S326–S332.
8. Gill DS, Mitra B, Reeves F, et al. Can initial clinical assessment exclude thoracolumbar vertebral injury? *Emerg Med J.* 2012; 30:679–682.
9. Chang CH, Holmes JF, Mower WR, Panacek EA. Distracting injuries in patients with vertebral injuries. *Emerg Med.* 2005; 28(2):147–152.
10. Ballock RT, Mackersie R, Abitbol JJ, Cervilla V, Resnick D, Garfin SR. Can burst fractures be predicted from plain radiographs? *J Bone Joint Surg Br.* 1992;74(1):147–150.
11. Roos JE, Hilfiker P, Platz A, et al. MDCT in emergency radiology: is a standardized chest or abdominal protocol sufficient for evaluation of thoracic and lumbar spine trauma? *AJR Am J Roentgenol.* 2004;183(4):959–968.
12. Brandt MM, Wahl WL, Yeom K, Kazerooni E, Wang SC. Computed tomographic scanning reduces cost and time of complete spine evaluation. *Trauma.* 2004;56(5):1022–1026.
13. Vaccaro AR, Lehman RA Jr, Jurlbert RJ, et al. A new classification of thoracolumbar injuries: the importance of injury morphology, the integrity of the posterior ligamentous complex, and neurologic status. *Spine.* 2005;15:2325–2333.
14. Wood KB, Li W, Lebl DR, Ploumis A. Management of thoracolumbar spine fractures. *Spine J.* 2014;1(14):145–164.

15. Mirza SK, Mirza AJ, Chapman JR, Andeson PA. Classifications of thoracic and lumbar fractures: rationale and supporting data. *Am Acad Orthop Surg.* 2002;10(5):364–377.

16. Aslan S, Karcioglu O, Katirci Y, Kandis H, Ezirmik N, Bilir O. Speed bump-induced spinal column injury. *Am J Emerg Med.* 2005;23(4):563–564.

17. Napier RJ, Nolan PC. Diagnosis of vertebral fractures in post-ictal patients. *Emerg Med J.* 2011;28(2):169–170.

18. Campbell SE, Phillips CD, Dubovsky E, Cail WS, Omary RA. The value of CT in determining potential instability of simple wedge-compression fractures of the lumbar spine. *AJNR Am J Neuroradiol.* 1995;16(7):1385–1392.

19. Roohi F, Fox A. Burst fracture of the first lumbar vertebra and conus-cauda syndrome complicating a single convulsive seizure: a challenge of diagnosis in the emergency department. *Emerg Med.* 2006;31(4):381–385.

20. Bensch FV, Koivikko MP, Kiuru MJ, Koskinen SK. The incidence and distribution of burst fractures. *Emerg Radiol.* 2006; 12(3):124–129.

21. DeWald RL. Burst fractures of the thoracic and lumbar spine. *Clin Orthop Relat Res.* 1984;(189):150–161.

22. Dai LY, Wang XY, Jiang LS, Jiang SD, Xu HZ. Plain radiography versus computed tomography scans in the diagnosis and management of thoracolumbar burst fractures. *Spine.* 2008; 33(16):E548–E552.

23. Krueger MA, Green DA, Hoyt D, Garfin SR. Overlooked spine injuries associated with lumbar transverse process fractures. *Clin Orthop Relat Res.* 1996;(327):191–195.

PART III

Upper Extremities

CHAPTER 11

Hand

David E. Manthey, MD and Kim L. Askew, MD

INTRODUCTION

Hand injuries account for up to 15% of all trauma cases seen in the emergency department (ED). Their complex anatomy, ability to perform fine movements, and importance in daily life make missing these injuries potentially devastating.

Terminology

The hand has a *dorsal* and a *volar* surface, and the same terms are used when discussing the digits. In addition, each digit has a *radial* border and an *ulnar* border. The muscle mass at the base of the thumb is the *thenar* eminence, and the muscle mass along the ulnar border of the hand is the *hypothenar* eminence.

The motions of the wrist include radial and ulnar deviation and extension and flexion. Motions of the thumb include flexion and extension, abduction and adduction, and opposition (Fig. 11–1). The digits are named the thumb and the index, long, ring, and little fingers, respectively. The thumb is the first digit, and the little finger is the fifth digit.

History

When a patient presents to the ED with a hand complaint, the physician should first ascertain if there is a history of trauma because the approach to and the differential diagnosis of a traumatized hand are quite different from that of a nontraumatized hand. Important historical points to be elicited in evaluating traumatic hand injuries include:

- Time elapsed since the injury
- Environment in which the injury occurred (contamination)
- Mechanism of injury (crush, laceration, etc.)
- Position of hand during injury (specifically for lacerations)

In the nontraumatized hand, the most important historical questions are:

- When did the symptoms begin?
- What functional impairment has been experienced?
- What activities worsen the symptoms?

Examination

Anatomically, the hand is a group of highly mobile gliding bones connected by tendons and ligaments to a "fixed center." This fixed center consists of the second and third

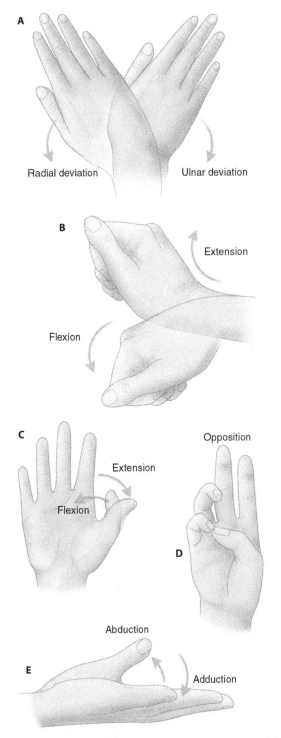

Figure 11–1. Terms used to describe motion of the hand and the digits.

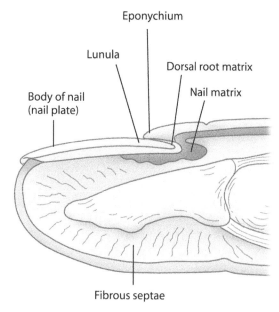

Figure 11–2. Fibrous septa extend from the bone to the skin and serve to stabilize fractures of the distal phalanx.

metacarpal bones. The remainder of the hand is suspended from these two relatively immobile bones. All intrinsic movements of the hand are relative to and dependent on the stability and immobility of these two bones.

The skin of the volar hand and fingers is fixed to the underlying bone by fibrous septa. This helps with grip, limits movement, and does not allow significant swelling. The dorsal hand has looser, thinner skin. This allows a fairly extensive space for swelling from trauma or infection. The venous and lymphatic drainage takes place on the dorsum of the hand. Any condition that causes inflammation and swelling in the hand can lead to lymphatic congestion and nonpitting edema over the dorsal aspect of the hand.

The fingertip is defined as the structures distal to the insertion of the flexor and extensor tendons on the distal phalanx. It comprises the nail (plate), nail bed, pulp, and distal phalanx (Fig. 11–2). The nail complex consists of the eponychium (cuticle or dorsal roof), perionychium (nail edge), hyponychium (where the nail adheres to the nail bed at the tip of the nail), and the nail bed or matrix (under the nail plate). The nail bed comprises a germinal matrix and a sterile matrix. The germinal matrix is proximal, ending at the distal aspect of the lunula, and accounts for approximately 90% of nail growth. The sterile matrix continues from the germinal matrix and makes up the majority of the nail bed, keeping the nail tightly affixed to the finger.

Tendon and Muscle Assessment

The muscles and tendons of the hand are divided into (1) extrinsic flexors, (2) extrinsic extensors, and (3) intrinsic muscles.

There are 12 flexor tendons contained in the volar compartment of the forearm that serve to flex the wrist, hand, and digits, as well as provide radial and ulnar deviation. They are the flexor carpi radialis, flexor carpi ulnaris, palmaris tendon, flexor pollicis longus, four flexor digitorum superficialis (FDS) tendons, and four flexor digitorum profundus (FDP) tendons.

Nine extensor tendons course over the dorsal aspect of the forearm and wrist. The extensor tendons include the extensor carpi radialis longus, extensor carpi radialis brevis, extensor carpi ulnaris, abductor pollicis longus, extensor pollicis longus, extensor pollicis brevis, extensor digitorum communis, extensor digiti minimi, and extensor indicis proprius. The most common site of tendon injury is over the dorsum of the hand where the extensor tendons are more superficial and exposed to injury.

The intrinsics, which lie in the body of the hand, are composed of 20 individual muscles, which are responsible for fine motor movement of the hand and can be divided into four groups: the thenar, hypothenar, interossei (dorsal and palmar), and lumbrical muscles. The thenar muscles, which control the fine movements of the thumb, are comprised of three short muscles located at the base of the thumb. The hypothenar muscles on the opposite side of the palm from the thenar comprise three muscles that control the actions of the little finger.

Tendons function best when they are at an optimal position of stretch. The *extensor carpi radialis brevis* is the most important of the wrist extensors, acting to stretch the flexor tendons to obtain a powerful grasp. To demonstrate this point, compare the power to grasp an object with the wrist in flexion and in approximately 15 degrees of extension.

Hand tendons are quite mobile and are held in place by pulleys that prevent the tendon from dislodging from its normal position. The flexor tendons are also ensheathed by a synovial membrane that acts as a lubricant to permit normal gliding of the tendon. The tendons are almost avascular in the adult and receive their blood supply from the muscles proximally and the site of insertion distally.

Flexor Tendons

Flexor Digitorum Profundus. The four FDP tendons insert on the volar aspect of the distal phalanx of the respective digits and are tested by asking the patient to flex the distal interphalangeal (DIP) joint while the proximal joints are held in an extended position by the physician (Fig. 11–3A).

Flexor Digitorum Superficialis. The four FDS tendons are tested by asking the patient to hold all fingers fully extended and having him/her flex the finger to be tested. If the DIP joint is permitted to relax, then flexion at the proximal phalangeal (PIP) joint is independent of the FDP (Fig. 11–3B).

Flexor Pollicis Longus. This tendon inserts on the volar aspect of the distal phalanx of the thumb. It is tested by having the patient flex the interphalangeal (IP) joint while the

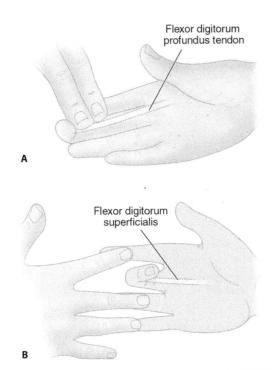

Figure 11–3. **A.** Testing the flexor digitorum profundus (FDP) function. **B.** Testing the flexor digitorum superficialis (FDS) function.

metacarpophalangeal (MCP) joint is held in an extended position by the physician.

Flexor Carpi Radialis. The flexor carpi radialis inserts on the volar aspect of the index metacarpal. This tendon is palpated just radial to the midline with the wrist flexed against resistance.

Flexor Carpi Ulnaris. The flexor carpi ulnaris is palpated under tension when the wrist is flexed against resistance and the thumb and little finger are opposed. It inserts on the pisiform and is easily palpated at this point.

Palmaris Longus. The palmaris longus is palpated by flexing wrist against resistance and opposing the thumb and the little fingers. The tendon lies in the midline, where it attaches to the palmar fascia. This tendon is congenitally absent in one-fifth of the population.

Extensor Tendons

The extensor tendons pass under the extensor retinaculum at the wrist and are divided into six fibro-osseous compartments over the dorsal aspect of the wrist (Fig. 11–4). The dorsal compartments and the retinaculum act to stabilize the extensor tendons and prevent bow stringing. The six fibro-osseous compartments containing the nine extensor tendons are presented next.

Abductor Pollicis Longus and Extensor Pollicis Brevis.
The abductor pollicis longus inserts at the dorsal base of the

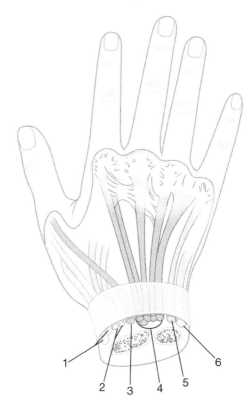

Figure 11–4. The extensor tendons and the six compartments that enclose them at the wrist. 1, abductor pollicis longus and the extensor pollicis brevis; 2, extensor carpi radialis longus and the extensor carpi radialis brevis; 3, adjacent to these is the extensor pollicis longus tendon; 4, extensor digitorum communis and the extensor indicis are contained; 5, extensor digiti minimi is enclosed; 6, extensor carpi ulnaris.

thumb metacarpal and the extensor pollicis brevis inserts at the base of the proximal phalanx of the thumb. These tendons can be tested by asking the patient to forcefully spread the hand. The abductor pollicis longus is palpated just distal to the radial styloid. The extensor pollicis brevis is palpated under tension over the dorsum of the thumb metacarpal.

Extensor Carpi Radialis Longus and Brevis. These tendons insert at the dorsal base of the index and middle metacarpal, respectively. They are evaluated by asking the patient to make a fist and extend the wrist forcibly (Fig. 11–5A). These tendons are of utmost importance to the function and strength of the hand because they are the primary extenders of the wrist.

Extensor Pollicis Longus. The extensor pollicis longus passes around Lister tubercle on the dorsal aspect of the radius and inserts on the distal phalanx of the thumb. It forms the ulnar border of the anatomic snuffbox and can be easily seen by extending the thumb (Fig. 11–5B). Only this tendon can extend the thumb and forcibly hyperextend it at the IP joint. It is tested by asking the patient

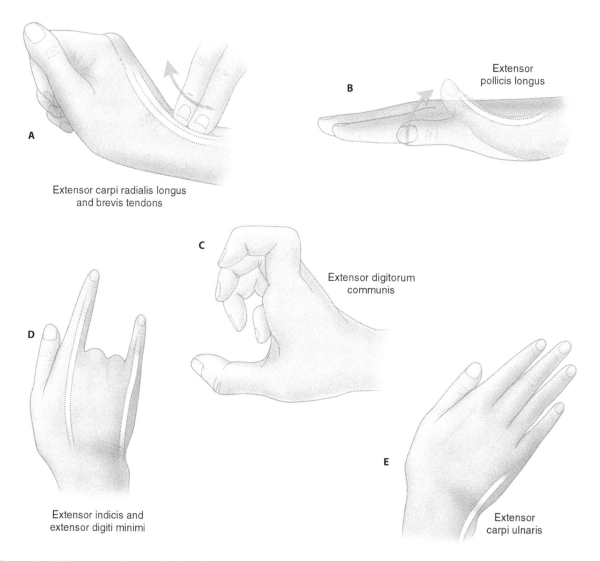

Figure 11–5. Extensor tendon examination. *A.* Extensor carpi radialis longus and brevis tendons. *B.* Extensor pollicis longus, with the hand flat on the table, the thumb extends in the plane of the table. *C.* Extensor digitorum communis, the MCP joints should be held in extension and the IP joints flexed. Compare the strength of extension at the MCP joint to the opposite hand. *D.* Extensor indicis and extensor digiti minimi. Hold the adjacent fingers in a flexed position to eliminate the function tendons of the communis tendons. *E.* Extensor carpi ulnaris.

to hyperextend the distal phalanx of the thumb against resistance.

Extensor Digitorum Communis and Extensor Indicis Proprius.
These tendons are tested by asking the patient to flex the IP joints into a tight claw and actively extend the MCP joint (Fig. 11–5C). This permits the examiner to visualize the extensor digitorum communis. Asking the patient to first make a fist and then extend the index finger, while the other fingers remain flexed, tests the extensor indicis proprius.

Extensor Digiti Minimi.
The extensor digitorum minimi is in the next compartment and can be tested at the same time as the extensor indicis proprius. Ask the patient

to first make a fist, and then extend the index and the little fingers while the long and ring fingers remain flexed (Fig. 11–5D).

Extensor Carpi Ulnaris.
This tendon inserts at the dorsal base of the fifth metacarpal and is evaluated by asking the patient to ulnar deviate the hand while the examiner palpates the taut tendon over the ulnar side of the wrist just distal to the ulnar head (Fig. 11–5E).

Intrinsic Muscles
There are three volar interossei and four dorsal interossei muscles (Fig. 11–6A and B). They originate along the length of the metacarpal bones and insert at the proximal phalanx and extensor expansion (Fig. 11–6C). The dorsal

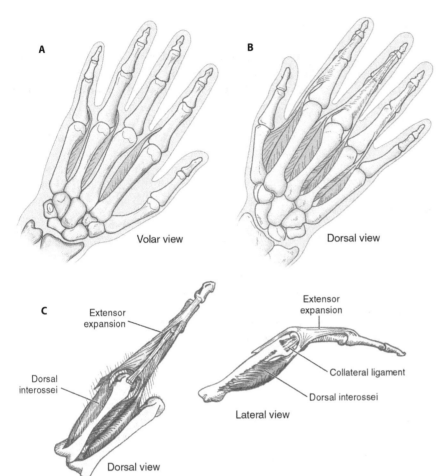

Figure 11–6. **A.** Volar interossei and **(B)** dorsal interossei muscles. **C.** The interossei and their relationship to the extensor expansion.

interossei abduct the fingers and are tested by spreading the hand forcibly against resistance (Fig. 11–7A). The volar interossei adduct the fingers and are tested by placing a piece of paper between the extended fingers and asking the patient to resist withdrawal of the paper from between the fingers (Fig. 11–7B).

The four lumbrical muscles allow flexion at the MCP joints, while maintaining extension at the IP joints. They

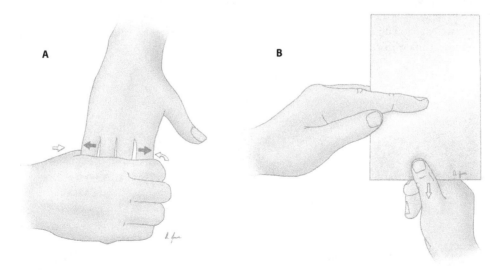

Figure 11–7. **A.** To test the dorsal interossei, spread the fingers forcibly against resistance. **B.** Placing a piece of paper between the fingers and asking the patient to resist withdrawal of the paper tests the volar interossei.

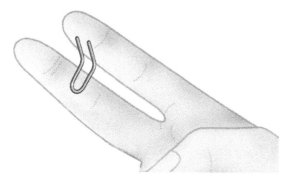

Figure 11–8. Two-point discrimination is the most sensitive indicator of a neurologic deficit involving the sensory branches of the nerves supplying the hand.

originate on the tendons of the flexor digitorum profundus and insert on the lateral band and central slip of the extensor tendons. The interossei muscles also assist in this function (i.e., MCP joint flexion, IP joint extension).

The thenar muscles comprise the abductor pollicis brevis, flexor pollicis brevis, and the opponens pollicis. The hypothenar muscles are comprised of the abductor digiti minimi, the flexor digiti minimi brevis, and the opponens digiti minimi. The thenar and hypothenar muscles are tested by asking the patient to cup the palm and pinch the thumb and little fingertips together forcibly. One can feel the tone of these muscles and compare them with the normal side.

Neurologic Assessment

Two-point discrimination is the most sensitive test for sensory function. This is best performed with a paper clip with its two ends separated by approximately 5 mm (Fig. 11–8). A normal individual is able to distinguish two blunt points that are 2 to 5 mm apart at the fingertips and 7 to 10 mm apart at the base of the palm. The dorsum of the hand is the least sensitive, with a normal threshold of 7 to 12 mm.

Digital nerve assessment should initially begin by examining an uninjured finger to estimate the patient's normal ability. Start at 1 cm, and decrease the distance until two points are no longer felt. It is important to test one digital nerve at a time by placing both points of the paper clip on the same side of the fingertip instead of spanning both sides of the finger, which is in effect checking two separate nerves.

Radial nerve sensation is performed with pinprick and two-point discrimination over the dorsum of the thumb web space. The motor branches of the radial nerve are tested by extension of the wrist and the MCP joint.

Ulnar nerve sensation is best tested over the little finger. There are several tests that can be used to assess motor branches of the ulnar nerve. They are as follows:

- Ask the patient to forcibly spread the fingers and compare the strength to the normal side.
- Have the patient flex the DIP joint of the ring and little fingers against resistance.
- Test the adduction of the thumb by having the patient hold a piece of paper between the thumb and the side of the phalangeal region of the index finger. When the adductor pollicis is weak, the IP joint of the thumb flexes with this maneuver and is called a *positive Froment sign* (Fig. 11–9).
- Have the patient place the ulnar edge of the hand on the examination table, and then have him/her attempt to abduct the index finger against resistance.

Median nerve sensation is tested by evaluating pinprick and two-point discrimination over the distal aspect of the index and long fingers. Motor strength is best assessed by thumb abduction (have the patient raise the thumb toward the ceiling while the dorsal hand is flat on the examination table). This tests the function of the abductor pollicis, which is reliably innervated by the motor nerve branch of the median nerve. Alternatively, the wrist and IP joints of the thumb and index fingers are flexed against resistance. Having the patient bring the small finger and thumb together is commonly used to test median nerve motor function, but can be falsely negative and therefore should not be used.

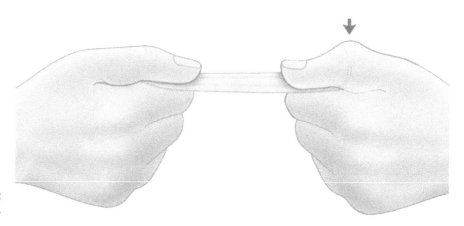

Figure 11–9. A positive Froment sign. Note the flexed IP joint (*arrow*).

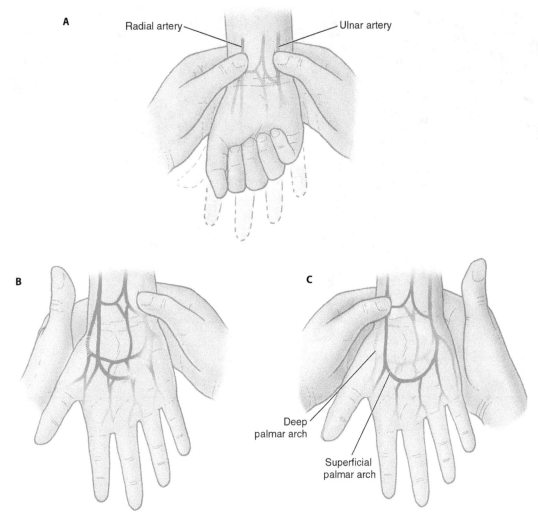

Figure 11–10. Allen test is performed to ascertain the patency of the radial and ulnar arteries. **A.** The patient is asked to make several fists while the examiner compresses the radial and ulnar arteries. The patient then opens the hand and the examiner releases pressure from one of the arteries. **B.** In the patient with a patent vessel, an erythematous flush should be noted in the hand when pressure is released. **C.** The same is done with the vessel on the opposite side.

Vascular Assessment

The vascular supply to the hand is provided by the radial and ulnar arteries, which combine within the hand to form the superficial and deep palmar arches. The integrity of these vessels can best be tested by the *Allen test*. This is performed by compressing the radial and ulnar arteries at the wrist while having the patient make a fist several times to exsanguinate the hand. Next, the radial artery is released; if blood flows to all the digits, then the radial artery is patent and good collateral flow exists into the radial artery system (Fig. 11–10). The same is done to test the ulnar artery. If both vessels are injured, then at least one, usually the ulnar, must be repaired.

Injuries to vascular structures usually do not affect perfusion of the hand because of extensive anastomoses. If initial inspection reveals a dusky or cool finger or hand, prompt intervention is needed. Capillary refill and pulse oximetry waveforms can give some indication of blood flow to injured digits.

Imaging

All significant hand injuries, including those with any degree of swelling, should be evaluated radiographically, even if the likelihood of a fracture seems remote. Chip or avulsion fractures may not be suspected on the basis of clinical examination and yet, if undetected, may result in a significant disability. A minimum of three views should be obtained when a hand fracture is suspected (anteroposterior [AP], lateral, and oblique) (Fig. 11–11). Metacarpal injuries may require special views for adequate radiographic visualization. For example, fractures of the fourth and fifth metacarpals are frequently undetected until a lateral view with 10 degrees of supination is obtained. Second and third metacarpal injuries are often detected on a lateral view with 10 degrees of pronation. Finger injuries require a true lateral view without superimposition of the other digits. One should not accept and subsequently base a diagnosis on inadequate radiographs of the hand.

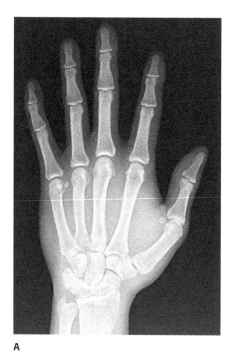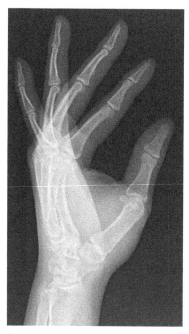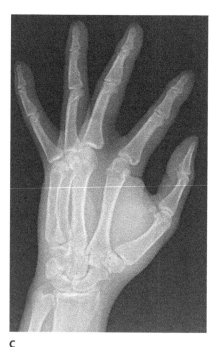

A   B   C

Figure 11–11. Normal radiographs of the hand. **A.** AP. **B.** Lateral. **C.** Oblique views.

HAND FRACTURES

The ED management of hand fractures is not complex but requires an understanding of both bony and soft-tissue anatomy to implement a therapy based on sound medical judgment. Improperly treated, these fractures can result in a crippling disability. For example, a small degree of rotational malalignment with a metacarpal or proximal phalanx fracture will result, if uncorrected, in a partially disabled hand. Only with a thorough understanding of essential hand anatomy can one correctly diagnose hand injuries and initiate appropriate therapy.

TREATMENT

The clinician should be aware that the wounds overlying fractures may communicate with the bony fragments. Although open fractures of long bones (i.e., tibia) generally require operative washout, the available literature suggests some differences in the bones of the hand. Open fractures of the metacarpals and phalanges are classified as clean (without significant contamination) or dirty (grossly contaminated or delay in treatment longer than 24 hours). Small (<1 cm), clean, open fractures without significant soft-tissue injury or fracture comminution of the bones of the hand have a lower incidence of infection (1.5%), and it is often acceptable to thoroughly irrigate them and close the wound in the ED. However, consultation should be obtained and antibiotics should be administered in all cases.

Dirty, open hand fractures have a higher incidence of infection (15%) and therefore will require operative washout.

Mobility is a critical consideration in the management of fractures. Those bones with a high degree of mobility can withstand a greater degree of angulation with the retention of normal function. Those bones with less mobility (second and third metacarpals) require a much more precise reduction to ensure a return to full function.

Another important concept in hand fractures is rotation. For the hand to function smoothly, all of its parts must work together as a unit. When the patient makes a fist, all the fingers normally point in the same direction (Fig. 11–12A). Rotational deformities from fractures of the middle or proximal phalanges or metacarpals interrupt the unit, resulting in malpositioning or overlap (Fig. 11–12B). Another method of diagnosing rotational deformities, which is more useful in the acutely injured hand, is to compare the plane of the fingernails on each hand. In the normal hand, the plane of the nail plate will be similar to the corresponding finger on the other hand. With rotation, there will be a discrepancy between these planes (Fig. 11–13).

> **Axiom:** *Rotational malalignment is never acceptable in fractures of the metacarpals or phalanges. Angulation is acceptable in more mobile bones but is unacceptable in stationary bones (i.e., second and third metacarpals).*

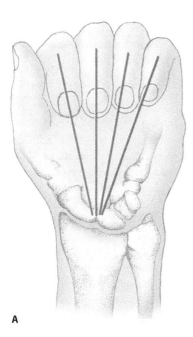
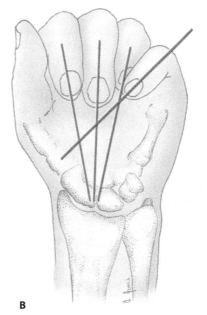

A   **B**

Figure 11–12. **A.** In the normal hand, the fingers will point to the same location in the wrist. **B.** With rotational malalignment of a fracture, the finger of the involved digit points in a different direction.

Hand injuries are best anesthetized by nerve blocks, usually at the wrist. Metacarpal blocks are employed in managing phalangeal fractures. Refer to Chapter 2 for further description of regional nerve blocks of the hand.

Two general principles need to be emphasized when treating hand fractures:

- Never immobilize a finger in full extension. Fingers should be immobilized in the position of function with 50 to 90 degrees of MCP joint flexion and 15 to 20 degrees of IP joint flexion to prevent stiffness and contractures. If stable reduction is only possible in full extension, internal fixation is required prior to immobilization in flexion. In flexion, the collateral ligaments are taut and will aid in maintaining a reduction (Fig. 11–14).⁵ The thumb is typically immobilized, slightly abducted, and neither flexed nor extended (Fig. 11–15).
- Avoid casts or splints beyond the distal palmar crease. If distal plaster immobilization is required, as in proximal and middle phalanx fractures, a gutter splint (radial or ulnar) immobilizing the involved digit, along with the adjacent normal digit (Fig. 11–16 and Appendix A–3), should be used.

Approximately 85% of all hand fractures are treated conservatively with immobilization, as described throughout the chapter. Countertraction (splint) or percutaneous Kirschner wires are frequently employed in unstable hand fractures.

The most frequent complications of hand fractures include *deformities* and *chronic joint stiffness*. Hand fractures

Mild rotational malalignment

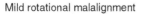
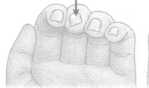
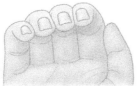

Figure 11–13. With rotational malalignment, the planes of the fingernails are not parallel when one compares the injured nail to the normal fingernails of the opposite hand.

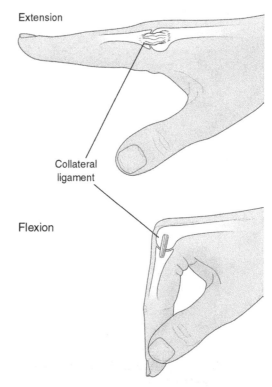

Extension

Collateral ligament

Flexion

Figure 11–14. The collateral ligament is taut in flexion and lax in extension.

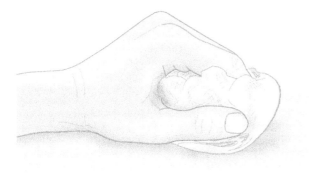

Figure 11–15. Proper position to immobilize the hand. The thumb is immobilized, slightly abducted, and neither flexed nor extended.

have a tendency to develop early lymphatic stasis and edema. The exudate consists of a protein-rich fluid that has a tendency to stimulate the development of adhesions among the tendons, synovial sheaths, and joints. This

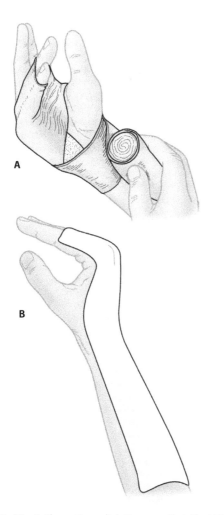

Figure 11–16. **A.** The gutter splint. Once applied, the MCP joint should be 50 to 90 degrees of flexion. **B.** An alternative to the gutter splint is a dorsal splint, with an extension hood extending to the PIP joints.

complication often leads to fibrosis and stiffness. Early elevation with gentle compression and early motion of the hand are helpful in reducing edema.

DISTAL PHALANX FRACTURES

Distal phalanx fractures represent 15% to 30% of all hand fractures. It is important to understand the anatomy of the distal phalanx when diagnosing and treating these injuries. Fibrous septa extend from the distal aspect of the distal phalanx (i.e., tuft) to the skin and serve to stabilize fractures of the distal phalanx. Traumatic hematomas can form between these septa and may elevate pressure within this closed space, causing severe pain.

The flexor and extensor tendons attach to the volar and dorsal aspects of each distal phalanx, respectively. In the second through fifth digits, the *flexor profundus* attaches to the volar aspect, whereas the *terminal slip of the extensor tendon* attaches on the dorsal surface (Fig. 11–17). In the thumb, the flexor pollicis longus inserts on the volar base of the distal phalanx and the extensor pollicis longus on the dorsal base.

These tendons can avulse bone when subjected to excessive stress. Clinically, there will be loss of function, whereas radiographically small avulsion fractures along the base of the phalanx are often seen. These fractures are considered intra-articular.

Distal phalanx fractures are classified as either *extra-articular* or *intra-articular* fractures.

Distal Phalanx Fractures: Extra-Articular

Extra-articular fractures of the distal phalanx may be longitudinal, transverse, comminuted, or transverse with displacement (Fig. 11–18). The most common fracture is a comminuted fracture. When this fracture occurs in the distal aspect of the bone where the fibrous septa attach, it is known as a tuft fracture.

The mechanism of injury is a direct blow to the distal phalanx. The force of the blow will determine the severity of the fracture. Examination typically reveals tenderness and swelling over the distal phalanx, including the pulp. Subungual hematomas are frequently noted,

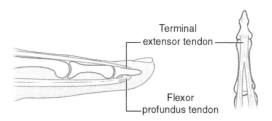

Figure 11–17. The flexor profundus tendon attaches to the volar aspect of the distal phalanx whereas the terminal slip of the extensor tendon attaches to the dorsal surface.

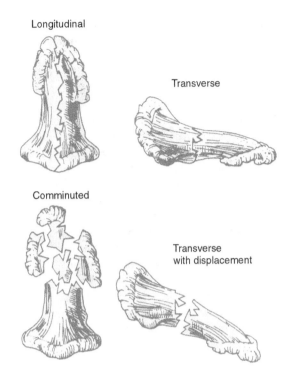

Figure 11–18. Extra-articular phalanx fractures.

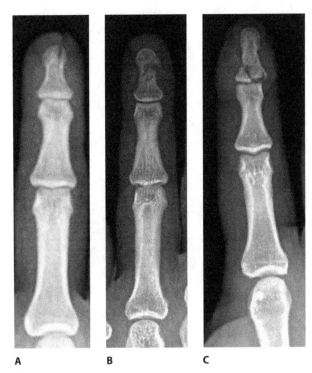

A   B   C

Figure 11–20. Distal phalanx fractures. **A.** Tuft fracture. **B.** Shaft fracture. **C.** Intra-articular fracture.

indicating a nail bed laceration (Fig. 11–19). AP and lateral views are generally adequate in demonstrating the fracture and any displacement (Fig. 11–20). Subungual hematomas with nail bed lacerations are frequently seen associated with injuries. Incomplete avulsion of the nail plate is often associated with transverse distal phalanx fractures.

Treatment

Nondisplaced fractures are managed with a protective splint, elevation, and analgesics. Either the simple volar or hairpin splint (Fig. 11–21 and Appendix A–2) is recommended to accommodate any swelling. These fractures require 3 to

4 weeks of splinting. Comminuted fractures may remain painful for several months thereafter.

Displaced transverse fractures need to be reduced with dorsal traction on the distal fragment followed by immobilization with a volar splint and then repeat radiographs for documentation of position. This may be difficult as soft tissues may be interposed between the fragments. If the fracture is irreducible and left untreated, nonunion of fracture fragments may result; therefore, orthopedic referral is indicated for the placement of a Kirschner wire.[6,7]

An associated subungual hematoma, regardless of the size, does not require that the nail be removed, as long as the nail plate remains intact.[8,9] Trephination, using electrocautery or an 18-gauge needle, is recommended for patient comfort (Fig. 11–22).

Open distal phalanx fractures are associated with disruption and laceration of the nail plate. Unlike other open fractures, these injuries may be treated in the ED using these guidelines (Fig. 11–23):

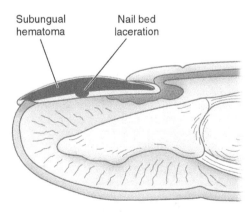

Figure 11–19. Schematic representation of nail bed laceration causing a subungual hematoma.

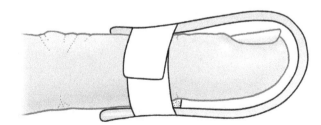

Figure 11–21. Hairpin splint.

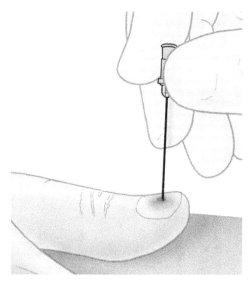

Figure 11–22. The drainage of a subungual hematoma.

1. Regional anesthesia with a digital block is followed by sterile preparation of the hand.
2. Using a pair of fine scissors or hemostat, the nail plate is dissected bluntly from the nail bed, being careful not to further damage the nail bed and dorsal roof matrix.
3. With the nail removed, the nail bed laceration is explored and thoroughly irrigated with normal saline. The nail bed can then be elevated and the fracture reduced.

4. The nail bed is sutured using a minimum number of 5-0 absorbable interrupted sutures. Suturing the nail bed will help support the fracture reduction because the bed is adherent to the dorsal aspect of the distal phalanx. Two prospective trials support the use of tissue adhesives to repair the nail bed.
5. A nonadherent gauze (e.g., Xeroform) or the patient's recently removed nail should be placed back in the nail fold (under the dorsal roof matrix separating it from the nail bed) and secured with tissue adhesive or two simple sutures on either side. Separating the bed from the roof prevents the development of adhesions (synechia) that can result in the regrowth of a deformed nail.
6. The entire digit is dressed with gauze and splinted for protection. The outer dressing can be changed as needed, but the material separating the nail bed from the roof matrix should remain in place for 10 days.
7. Antibiotics are prescribed for 7 to 10 days.
8. Repeat radiographs for documentation of reduction are indicated. If the fracture remains unstable, a pin may be inserted by the orthopedist.

Distal Phalanx Fractures: Intra-Articular, Dorsal Surface (Mallet Finger)

These fractures are classified based on the degree of articular surface involvement and the presence of displacement (Fig. 11–24).

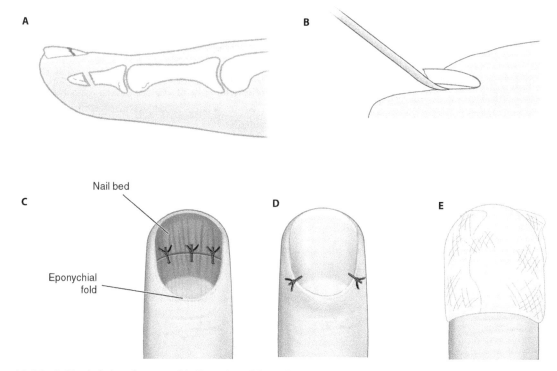

Figure 11–23. **A.** Distal phalanx fracture with disruption of the nail. **B.** The nail is removed. **C.** The nail bed repaired with absorbable suture. **D.** The eponychial fold (i.e., dorsal roof matrix) is identified and the nail is placed back into the fold. **E.** Nonadhesive gauze should be placed over the nail bed.

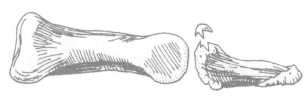

(<25% of articular surface)

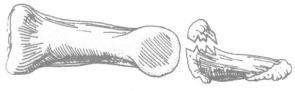

(>25% of articular surface)

Figure 11–24. Intra-articular distal phalanx avulsion fractures—dorsal surface.

Mallet finger is a commonly used term for these injuries. The mechanism is due to forced flexion of the distal phalanx with the finger in taut extension. The fracture is commonly seen in basketball, baseball, and softball players when the ball accidentally hits the tip of the finger causing forced flexion. When this occurs, the tendon may stretch, resulting in a 15- to 20-degree loss of extension; the tendon may rupture, resulting in up to a 45-degree loss of extension (soft-tissue mallet finger); or the tendon may avulse a bone fragment from the distal phalanx, resulting in up to a 45-degree loss of extension (bony mallet finger) (Fig. 11–25).

On examination, there is swelling and tenderness over the dorsal aspect of the joint and loss of active extension at the DIP joint (Fig. 11–26A). A true lateral view is essential for avulsion fractures to determine if the fragment is displaced and if >25% of the articular surface is involved (Fig. 11–26B). These fractures may be associated with nail plate injuries.

Treatment

Management is dependent on three variables: patient reliability, the size of the avulsion fragment, and degree of displacement.

Nondisplaced. In the reliable patient, treatment is conservative, with either a volar or dorsal splint. Dorsal splints provide better fixation as there are fewer soft tissues between the splint and the fracture (Fig. 11–27).

The DIP joint is extended with flexion permitted at the PIP joint. The finger must be maintained in this position for 6 to 8 weeks. Flexion of the DIP at any point during this period may result in a chronic flexion deformity. To stress this point, the patient is instructed to hold the tip of the finger in extension against the top of a table when changing the splint. After 6 to 8 weeks, the splint can be removed during the daytime with the patient cautioned against finger flexion for an additional 4 weeks.

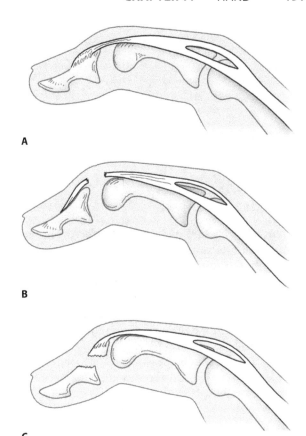

Figure 11–25. Three ways the extensor tendon can be disrupted. ***A.*** A stretch of the tendon without division of the tendon. ***B.*** When the tendon is ruptured from its insertion on the distal phalanx, there is a 40-degree flexion deformity present, and the patient cannot actively extend the tendon at the DIP joint. ***C.*** A fragment of the distal phalanx can be avulsed with the tendon.

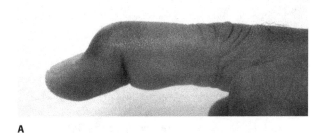

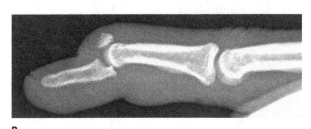

Figure 11–26. ***A.*** Flexion deformity of a "mallet finger." ***B.*** The radiograph reveals a large bony avulsion with subluxation of the joint.

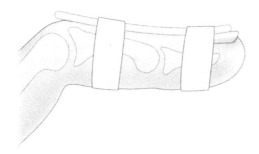

Figure 11-27. A dorsal splint on the DIP joint.

Volar avulsion fracture

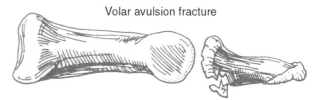

Figure 11-29. Intra-articular distal avulsion fracture—volar surface.

Displaced and >25% of Articular Surface. This fracture is frequently associated with some degree of subluxation of the DIP joint. Management involves dorsal splint immobilization with orthopedic referral (Fig. 11-27). Controversy exists regarding the benefits of continued immobilization versus surgical intervention; however, closed reduction and internal fixation with Kirschner wires is usually necessary.

If the fracture is improperly treated, a hyperextension PIP deformity (swan-neck) may result from an imbalance between the ruptured extensor tendon and the unopposed distal attachment of the flexor tendon (Fig. 11-28).

Distal Phalanx Fractures: Intra-Articular, Volar Surface

The flexor profundus tendon inserts on the base of the distal phalanx. Avulsion injuries due to tension on this tendon are classified as intra-articular fractures (Fig. 11-29).

This is an uncommon injury resulting from forceful hyperextension while the flexor profundus tendon is tightly contracted. The patient will be unable to flex the distal phalanx. Tenderness over the volar aspect of the distal phalanx or palm, secondary to tendon retraction after its rupture, will be present. The lateral view is best for demonstrating this fracture. Associated injuries are rarely seen with this fracture.

> **Axiom:** *Patients with traumatic swelling and tenderness over the volar aspect of the distal phalanx with additional palmar pain have a rupture of the flexor profundus tendon until proven otherwise.*

Treatment

The ED management consists of a volar finger splint (Appendix A–2) and orthopedic referral for early surgical fixation.

MIDDLE PHALANX FRACTURES

Fractures of the middle and proximal phalanges have many similarities in their anatomy, mechanisms of injury, and treatment. Middle phalanx fractures are less common than proximal phalanx fractures. Because the majority of applied axial force is absorbed by the proximal phalanx, there is a higher incidence of proximal phalanx fractures and PIP joint dislocations than middle phalanx fractures. Middle phalanx fractures usually occur at the narrow shaft.

The attachment of the extensor tendon is limited to the proximal dorsal portion of the middle phalanx. The flexor superficialis tendon is divided and broadly inserts along the lateral margins of nearly the entire volar surface of the bone, exerting the predominant deforming force in middle phalanx fractures (Fig. 11-30). As a result, a fracture at the *base* of the middle phalanx will typically result in volar displacement of the distal segment, whereas a distal shaft fracture will usually present with volar displacement of the proximal segment.

A final anatomic point to consider is the cartilaginous volar plate at the base of the middle phalanx. Intra-articular fractures may be complicated by injury of this cartilaginous plate.

Rotational malalignment must be discovered and corrected early (Fig. 11-31). As previously mentioned, rotational deformity is suspected when all fingers of the closed fist do not point to the same point on the wrist or the

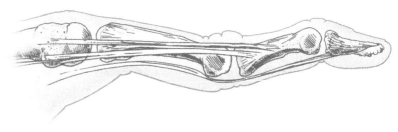

Figure 11-28. If a mallet fracture is treated improperly, a hyperextension deformity will occur at the PIP joint. This is secondary to an imbalance between the ruptured extensor tendon and the unopposed distal flexor tendon.

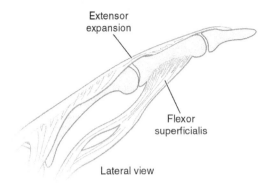

Figure 11–30. The tendons attaching to the middle phalanx.

plane of the nail plates vary.[15] Rotational deformities can be detected radiographically by comparing the diameter of the phalangeal fragments. Asymmetry suggests a rotational deformity (Fig. 11–32).

There are three methods of treating middle phalanx fractures: dynamic splinting, gutter splints, and internal

fixation. The method selected is dependent on the type of fracture, its stability, and the experience of the physician.

Dynamic Splinting: This involves taping the injured digit to the adjacent uninjured one, allowing maximal use of the hand with early mobilization to prevent stiffness. This treatment method is indicated only for nondisplaced, stable fractures that are impacted or transverse (Appendix A–2).[16]

Gutter Splints: The radial and ulnar gutter splints are used in stable fractures with no rotation or angulation (Appendix A–3). The gutter splint offers more immobilization than is possible with dynamic splinting. Radial gutter splints are used for fractures of the second and third digits, while ulnar gutter splints are applied for fourth and fifth digit fractures. The procedure for applying these splints can be found in Chapter 1 and Appendix A–3.

Internal Fixation: Internal fixation, usually with Kirschner wires, is required for unstable fractures or intra-articular avulsion fractures where precise reduction is necessary.

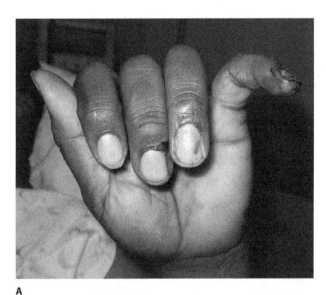

A

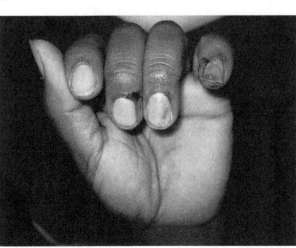

C

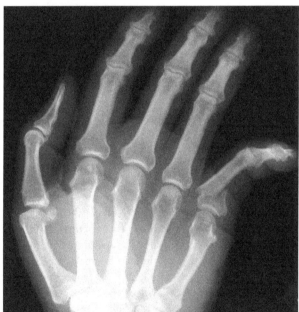

B

Figure 11–31. Patient with an angulated and rotated proximal phalanx fracture on **(A)** clinical examination and **(B)** radiograph. **C.** Reduction should correct malalignment prior to splinting.

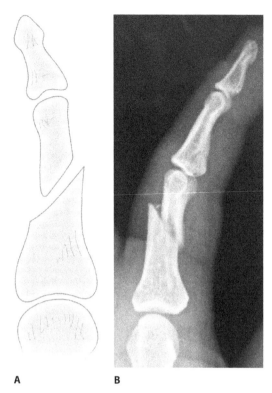

A   **B**

Figure 11–32. With rotational malalignment, there is asymmetry of the diameters of the shaft at the fracture site. **A.** Schematic of rotated middle phalanx fracture. **B.** Radiograph of a rotated proximal phalanx fracture.

Middle Phalanx Fractures: Extra-Articular

The appearance of these fractures is dependent on the pull of the flexor and extensor tendons (Fig. 11–33). The flexor mechanism exerts the predominant force and tends to displace the larger of the fracture fragments in a volar direction.

A direct blow to the middle phalanx is the most commonly encountered mechanism for fractures. Indirect trauma, such as twisting along the longitudinal axis, may result in a spiral fracture of the middle phalanx, although PIP joint dislocation is more common. On examination, pain and swelling will be localized over the fracture area. Clinical and radiographic recognition of rotational deformities should be noted. AP, lateral, and oblique views are essential to identify fracture lines as well as angulation and rotational deformities. Associated injuries include digital neurovascular injuries or tendon rupture (acute or delayed).

Treatment

Nondisplaced Transverse. These fractures may be treated with dynamic immobilization or a gutter splint (Appendices A–2 and A–3) for 10 to 14 days, followed by repeat radiographs to ensure proper healing.

Displaced or Angulated Transverse. These fractures are unstable and may remain so even after reduction. The ED management of these fractures includes

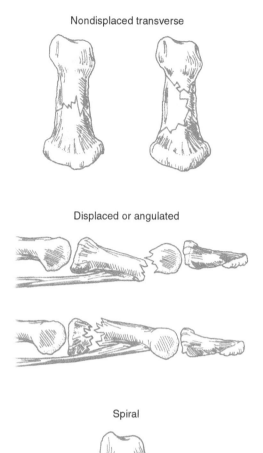

Nondisplaced transverse

Displaced or angulated

Spiral

Figure 11–33. Middle phalanx fractures—extra-articular.

immobilization in a gutter splint (Appendix A–3), ice, elevation, and orthopedic referral. If orthopedic consultation is not available, the emergency physician may attempt to reduce these fractures. The method of reduction includes gentle longitudinal traction in conjunction with flexion and manipulation of the distal fragment. If the fracture is unstable with slight extension, internal fixation will be necessary. If the reduced fracture is stable, use a gutter splint to immobilize for 4 to 6 weeks (Appendix A–3). Postreduction radiographs for documentation of position are recommended, followed by referral to an orthopedist.

Spiral or Oblique. The emergency management of these fractures consists of immobilization in a gutter splint (Appendix A–3), ice, elevation, and orthopedic referral. If

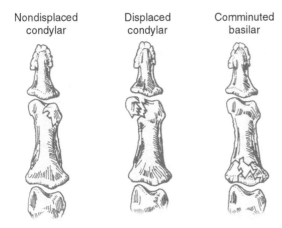

Nondisplaced condylar   Displaced condylar   Comminuted basilar

Figure 11–34. Middle phalanx fractures—intra-articular.

rotational malalignment exists, emergent referral is indicated for early correction to avoid malunion.

Middle Phalanx Fractures: Intra-Articular

These fractures can be divided into three types: (1) nondisplaced condylar fractures, (2) displaced condylar fractures, and (3) comminuted basilar fractures (Fig. 11–34). Intra-articular avulsion fractures are discussed separately because they do not share common therapeutic principles with the preceding three types.

Two mechanisms commonly result in intra-articular middle phalanx fractures. Rarely, direct trauma results in these fractures. The most common mechanism is a longitudinal force transmitted from the distal phalanx. On examination, a fusiform swelling and tenderness are present over the involved joint. AP, lateral, and oblique views are usually adequate in demonstrating these fractures (Fig. 11–35). The most frequent complications include joint stiffness and arthritic degeneration, which may occur despite optimum therapy.

Treatment

Nondisplaced Condylar. Dynamic splinting (Appendix A–2) with early motion exercises is the recommended mode of therapy.

Displaced Condylar. Emergency management includes immobilization in a gutter splint (Appendix A–3), ice, elevation, and referral for operative pinning.

Comminuted Basilar. Emergency management includes immobilization in a gutter splint (Appendix A–3), ice, elevation, and referral for traction splinting.

Middle Phalanx Fractures: Avulsion

These fractures are the result of avulsion by the (1) central slip of the extensor tendon, (2) volar plate (Wilson fracture), and (3) collateral ligaments (Fig. 11–36).

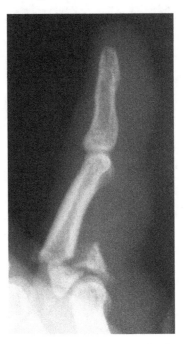

Figure 11–35. A comminuted intra-articular fracture of the middle phalanx.

Avulsion of the extensor tendon's central slip is caused by forced flexion with the finger in extension. Complete tear of the central slip of the extensor tendon without avulsion of bone can occur. Left untreated, these injuries will result in a boutonniere deformity. Hyperextension at the PIP joint will result in volar plate avulsion fractures

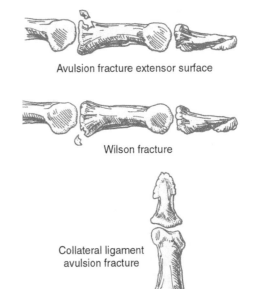

Avulsion fracture extensor surface

Wilson fracture

Collateral ligament avulsion fracture

Figure 11–36. Middle phalanx fractures—avulsion.

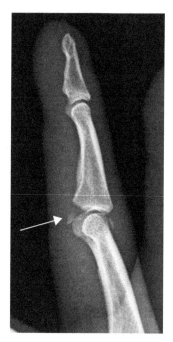

Figure 11–37. Wilson fracture.

(Fig. 11–37). Subluxation or dislocation of the PIP joint is often associated. Extreme medial or lateral stresses of the digit at the proximal IP joint will result in an avulsion of bone caused by the collateral ligaments.

Avulsion fractures are difficult to diagnose clinically without radiographs. Initially, there will be a point of tenderness without swelling or deformity at the PIP joint. Later, there will be fusiform swelling and tenderness of the PIP joint. Early diagnosis can be made by anesthetizing the digit and examining for range of motion and joint stability. Dorsal avulsion fractures will prevent full extension, whereas PIP laxity will accompany collateral ligament injuries. Lateral joint instability is present following a collateral ligament bony avulsion.

Treatment
Avulsion fractures should be immobilized for a brief period of time to reduce the incidence of joint stiffness. Repeat radiographic examinations are indicated to ensure proper positioning during healing, and early referral is needed.

Extensor Tendon Avulsion Fracture. Dorsal surface avulsion fractures require internal fixation; therefore, urgent referral is indicated. Tendon avulsions without fractures can be treated by splinting the PIP joint in full extension for 5 to 6 weeks. The DIP joint should not be splinted and should undergo active and passive range of motion exercises throughout the splinting period.

Volar Plate Avulsion Fracture (Wilson Fracture). If the fragment is <30% of the joint surface, closed treatment is recommended. The PIP joint is splinted in 45 to 50 degrees of flexion for 4 weeks after any dislocation or subluxation has been reduced. This management is controversial, as some hand surgeons will elect internal fixation for all of these fractures to repair the volar plate. A conservative approach for fractures where there is no subluxation of the joint has also been employed. Early orthopedic referral is advised.

Collateral Ligament Avulsion Fracture. Most surgeons recommend surgical fixation. Early consultation is strongly recommended so the appropriate therapeutic program can be selected.

PROXIMAL PHALANX FRACTURES

There are no tendons that attach to the proximal phalanx. However, tendons that lie in close proximity can complicate fracture management. Proximal phalanx fractures tend to have volar angulation secondary to traction from the interosseous muscles and extensor tendons.

As in middle phalanx fractures, recognizing and treating rotational deformities is essential. There are three methods of treating proximal phalanx fractures: dynamic splinting, gutter splints, and internal fixation. The techniques are similar to those described for treating middle phalanx fractures.

Proximal Phalanx Fractures: Extra-Articular
Two mechanisms of injury are commonly associated with extra-articular proximal phalanx fractures. A direct blow to the proximal phalanx can result in a transverse or comminuted fracture (Fig. 11–38). An indirect blow that results in torque applied along the longitudinal axis of the digit frequently causes a spiral fracture. On examination, pain and swelling are localized over the site of the fracture. Longitudinal compression of the digit results in fracture-site pain. Rotational deformities are commonly associated with proximal phalanx fractures. Clinical recognition of rotation of the digit is essential because all rotational deformities are unacceptable. AP, oblique, and true lateral views of the digits are obtained (Fig. 11–39). Rotational deformities are suspected when there is a discrepancy in the diameter of the phalangeal fragments. Associated injuries include digital nerve contusion or transection. Infrequently, acute tendon rupture occurs. If partial tendon rupture occurs, delayed limited motion can result due to adhesions. This complication, commonly seen following displaced and spiral fractures, results in a loss of motion that may require surgical intervention.

Treatment
There is a tendency to underestimate the potential disability encountered with proximal phalanx fractures. A thorough physical examination followed by the correction of

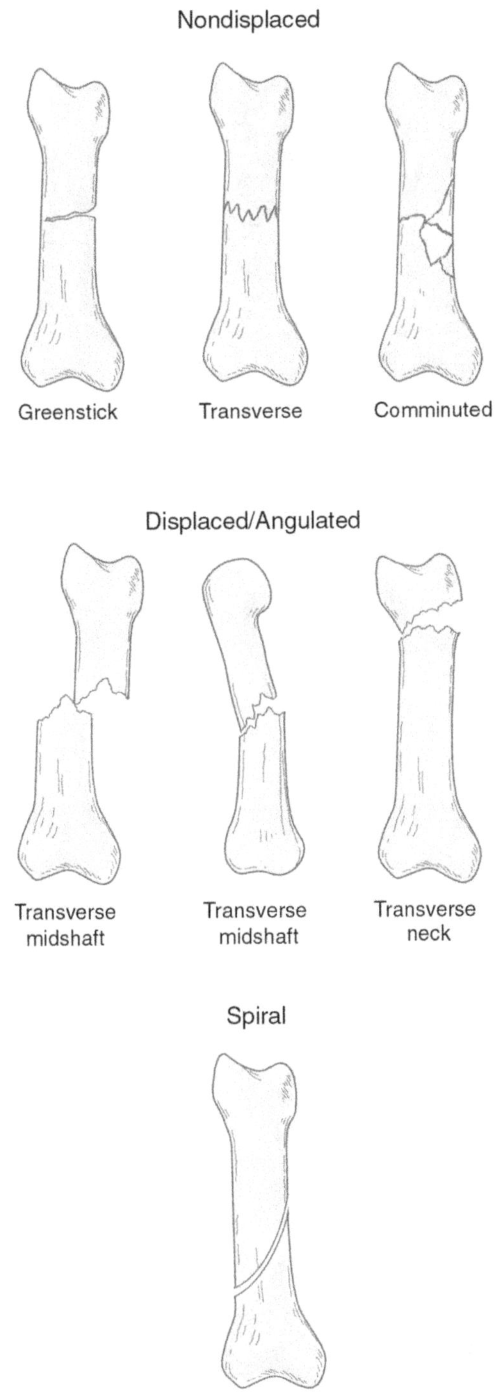

Nondisplaced

Greenstick   Transverse   Comminuted

Displaced/Angulated

Transverse   Transverse   Transverse
midshaft   midshaft   neck

Spiral

Figure 11–38. Proximal phalanx fractures—extra-articular.

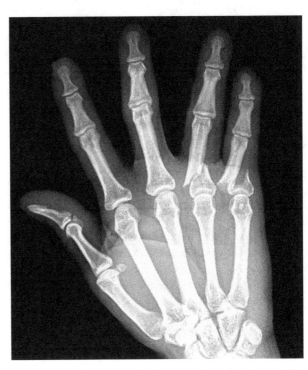

Figure 11–39. Extra-articular fractures of the fourth and fifth proximal phalanges.

angulation and rotation with immobilization will, in most cases, result in a full restoration of function.[17] Rotational deformities may be clinically unapparent unless enhanced by one of the following three tests:

- Convergence test toward the scaphoid
- Comparison of the finger and nail planes
- Measurement of the radiographic diameter of the fracture fragments

Nondisplaced Transverse. Nondisplaced proximal phalanx shaft fractures include greenstick, transverse, and comminuted fractures. The greenstick fracture is a stable fracture with no tendency for displacement or angulation because the periosteum is intact. This fracture should be treated with dynamic splinting followed by early motion exercises (Appendix A–2). A radiographic examination should be repeated in 7 to 10 days to exclude delayed displacement or rotation. Nondisplaced comminuted or transverse fractures can be unstable if the periosteum is not intact. These fractures are treated by one of two methods, depending on stability[17]:

- A gutter splint (Appendix A–3) is our recommendation. In 10 to 14 days, a repeat x-ray is obtained, and if the fragments are properly positioned, a dynamic splint is used.
- A dynamic splint (Appendix A–2) with early motion exercises with a repeat x-ray in 5 to 7 days to ensure proper position.

Displaced or Angulated Transverse. Commonly encountered displaced extra-articular fractures of the proximal phalanx include displaced and angulated transverse shaft or neck fractures. These fractures are unstable, sometimes even following reduction. The emergency management of these fractures includes immobilization in a gutter splint (Appendix A–3), ice, elevation, and orthopedic referral. If orthopedic referral is not available, the emergency physician may reduce these fractures. The method of reducing these fractures is as follows:

1. Anesthesia using either a wrist or metacarpal block.
2. The MCP joint is flexed to 90 degrees to tighten the collateral ligaments and reduce the displacing force of the intrinsic muscles. While flexing the MCP joint, longitudinal traction is applied to gain length.
3. Traction is continued while the PIP is flexed to 90 degrees. The fracture is reduced in this position. If there is loss of reduction with slight extension of the PIP, the fracture is unstable and requires internal fixation. If the fracture cannot be reduced using this method, interposition of tissue should be suspected.
4. If the reduction is stable, a short-arm cast to the palmar crease (with a dorsal extension to the PIP) or a gutter splint with the MCP in flexion is applied. More MCP flexion may be necessary to achieve near-anatomic alignment.[18] Postreduction radiographs for documentation of position are recommended.
5. Referral for orthopedic follow-up.

Spiral or Oblique. The emergency management of spiral fractures consists of immobilization in a gutter splint (Appendix A–2), ice, elevation, and orthopedic referral. In many instances, internal fixation is necessary.

Proximal Phalanx Fractures: Intra-Articular

These intra-articular fractures can be divided into two types: (1) nondisplaced fractures that involve <20% of the articular surface; and (2) displaced, comminuted, or nondisplaced fractures involving >20% of the articular surface (Fig. 11–40). Small, nondisplaced fractures are uncommon and are treated closed, whereas displaced, comminuted, or large fractures are more common and require surgical fixation.

The most frequent mechanism is avulsion secondary to collateral ligament traction. The indirect transmission of a longitudinal force, however, may result in a condylar fracture. On examination, a fusiform swelling and tenderness are present over the involved joint. Joint instability suggests avulsion of the collateral ligament. AP, lateral, and oblique views are usually adequate in demonstrating these fractures (Fig. 11–41). Avulsion fractures may result in detachment of the collateral ligament with subsequent joint instability.

Treatment

Small (<20% Articular Surface) and Nondisplaced.
Intra-articular avulsion fracture of the base of the proximal phalanx of the second through the fifth finger may be treated conservatively if the fragment is stable and involves <20% of the articular surface. Dynamic splinting with active motion exercises and early referral for close monitoring are recommended (Appendix A–2).[12,13,19]

Nondisplaced

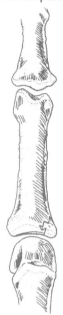

Nondisplaced

Displaced or comminuted

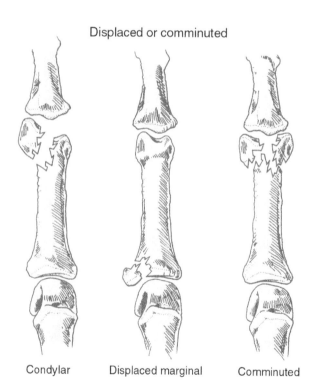

Condylar   Displaced marginal   Comminuted

Figure 11–40. Proximal phalanx fractures—intra-articular.

Large (>20% Articular Surface), Displaced, or Comminuted. Emergency management includes immobilization in a gutter splint (Appendix A–2), ice, elevation, and referral for pin fixation or open reduction and internal fixation.

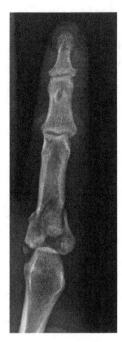

Figure 11–41. Comminuted intra-articular fracture of the base of the proximal phalanx.

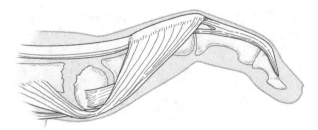

Figure 11–42. A metacarpal fracture that is not properly reduced will develop a compensatory MCP joint hyperextension and PIP joint flexion known as pseudoclawing.

METACARPAL FRACTURES (2 THROUGH 5)

Metacarpal fractures represent as many as one-third of all hand fractures. These fractures are divided into two groups: the first metacarpal and metacarpals 2 through 5. This distinction is based on the fact that the mechanical function of the first metacarpal is distinct from the remaining metacarpals.

Metacarpal fractures 2 through 5 are described on the basis of one of four segments—the *head* (the most distal segment), *neck*, *shaft*, and *base*.

The intermetacarpal ligaments tightly connect the heads of the metacarpals, whereas at the bases, there is a great amount of variation in mobility. The fourth and fifth finger metacarpals have from 15 to 25 degrees of AP motion. The second and third finger metacarpals have virtually no motion at their bases, representing the *fixed center* of the hand from which the remaining bones are suspended. The normal "degree of mobility" is of critical concern when reducing metacarpal fractures. Angulated fractures of the fourth and fifth metacarpals do not require a precise reduction because their normal mobility allows for compensation. Angulated fractures of the second and third metacarpals, however, require a more precise reduction because residual angulation will inhibit normal function.

In addition, the degree of acceptable angulation is wider with more distal fractures. In other words, the more proximal the fracture, the greater is the extent of deformity at the distal portion of the metacarpal. For example, a 30-degree volar deformity of the fifth metacarpal may be acceptable if it occurs at the neck. If it occurs at the

level of the midshaft, however, the same 30-degree volar deformity would be unacceptable because it would create abnormal hyperextension at the MCP joint and flexion of the PIP joint (Fig. 11–42).

Metacarpal Head Fractures

These are uncommon fractures with many disabling complications, even with optimum therapy. These fractures occur distal to the attachment of the collateral ligaments (Fig. 11–43). The most common mechanism is a direct blow or a crushing injury that typically results in a comminuted fracture. On examination, tenderness and swelling are present over the involved MCP joint. Pain is increased and localized over the MCP joint with axial compression of the extended digit.

AP and lateral views are usually adequate for demonstrating this fracture (Fig. 11–44). At times, oblique views may be necessary to adequately visualize the fracture fragments. A 10-degree pronated lateral view is helpful in assessing index and middle finger metacarpal fractures. A 10-degree supinated lateral view is helpful in assessing ring and small finger metacarpal fractures. Collateral ligament avulsions can often be visualized with the Brewerton view taken with the MCP joints flexed 65 degrees with the dorsal surface on the plate and the beam angled 15 degrees radially. Injuries associated with metacarpal head fractures include (1) extensor tendon damage, (2) a crush injury to the interosseous

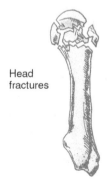

Head fractures

Figure 11–43. Metacarpal fractures—head (2 through 5).

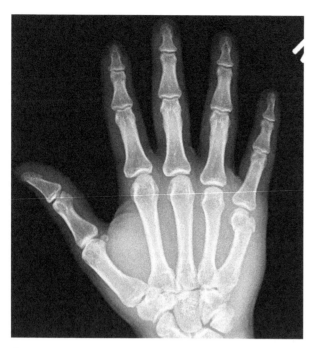

Figure 11–44. Radiograph of a fifth metacarpal head fracture.

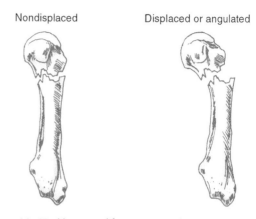

Neck fractures

Nondisplaced   Displaced or angulated

Figure 11–45. Metacarpal fractures—neck (2 through 5).

muscle resulting in fibrosis, and (3) collateral ligament avulsion. Complications include rotational malalignment, chronic arthritis, or extensor tendon injury/fibrosis.

Treatment

Emergency management should include elevation, ice, analgesics, and immobilization of the hand in a soft bulky dressing (Appendix A–5). A gutter splint can be used alternatively.

All metacarpal head fractures require referral. Metacarpal head fractures with large intra-articular defects generally require intraoperative fixation to establish a near-normal joint relationship. For small intra-articular fragments, most consultants will immobilize the hand only for a short time and then begin motion exercises. One study demonstrated that nondisplaced avulsion fractures involving less than 25% of the width of the joint can be treated with early active motion and without pin fixation. Many of these fractures require arthroplasty later.

Fractures associated with adjacent lacerations should be considered open, and emergent orthopedic consultation with operative exploration, irrigation, and repair is recommended.

Metacarpal Neck Fractures

Metacarpal neck fractures are referred to as *boxer's fractures* when they affect the fourth and/or fifth metacarpal. Boxer's fractures are common, accounting for 5% of all upper-extremity fractures and 20% of hand fractures. Neck fractures are almost always unstable and have some degree of volar angulation (Fig. 11–45). Even after reduction, loss of normal alignment in a volar direction is common.

The definition of successful reduction is dependent on the anatomic mobility of the involved metacarpal. In the fifth metacarpal, where the normal excursion is 15 to 25 degrees, up to 40 degrees of angulation is acceptable without limitation of normal function. In the fourth metacarpal, up to 30 degrees of angulation is acceptable. This is in contradistinction to fractures of the second and third metacarpals, where more accurate anatomic reductions (no more than 10 degrees) are essential for the restoration of normal function.

Direct impaction forces, such as a punch with a clenched fist, frequently result in neck fractures. On examination, tenderness and swelling are present over the involved metacarpal joints. Rotational deformities may accompany these fractures and must be diagnosed and corrected early.

AP, lateral, and oblique views are usually adequate in defining the fracture and in determining the amount of angulation and displacement (Fig. 11–46). A 10-degree pronated lateral view is helpful in assessing index- and middle-finger metacarpal fractures. A 10-degree supinated lateral view is helpful in assessing ring- and small-finger metacarpal fractures.

Associated injuries are not commonly seen with these fractures. Occasionally, this fracture will be accompanied by injuries to the digital nerves. Long-term complications of metacarpal neck fractures include collateral ligament injury due to poor fracture alignment, extensor tendon injuries, rotational malalignment, dorsal bony prominence that compromises extensor function, pseudoclawing, or pain with grasp due to a volarly angulated head.

Treatment

Rotational deformities must be diagnosed and treated early. Fractures associated with adjacent lacerations should be considered open, and emergent orthopedic consultation is recommended.

Metacarpal neck fractures are divided into two treatment groups: those involving the fourth and fifth metacarpals, and those involving the second and third metacarpals.

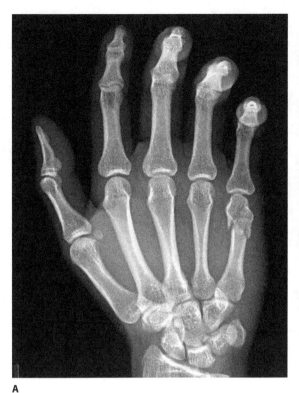
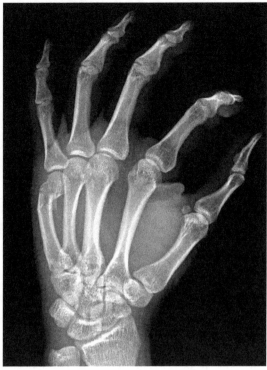

A   **B**

Figure 11–46. Fracture of the fifth metacarpal neck with volar angulation (boxer's fracture). **A.** AP. **B.** Oblique view.

Metacarpal Neck Fractures: Digits 4 or 5

Nondisplaced, Nonangulated. The management includes ice, elevation, and immobilization. An ulnar gutter splint is frequently used temporarily, but likely overimmobilizes in the long term and will result in decreased range of motion. Another option is a volar splint to the palmar crease and a dorsal splint extending to, but not including, the PIP (MCP at 90 degrees). This will allow PIP and DIP motion immediately and is seen as an improvement over the ulnar gutter splint. Protected MCP motion begins in 3 to 4 weeks. However, more recent evidence supports immediate mobilization of single fifth metacarpal neck fractures with only buddy taping (to prevent rotational deformity).[19] This approach may be considered, generally, after orthopedic consultation.

Angulated. This is an area of some controversy. Classically, fifth metacarpal neck fracture angulated >40 degrees and fourth metacarpal neck fractures with angulation of >30 degrees were reduced. Some evidence suggests that angulation up to 70 degrees resulted in adequate healing. Fractures with >70 degrees of angulation are reduced by adhering to the following steps:

1. An ulnar nerve block is used to achieve adequate anesthesia.
2. Finger traps are placed on the involved digits for 10 to 15 minutes to disimpact the fracture.
3. After disimpaction, the MCP and PIP joints are flexed to 90 degrees (Fig. 11–47).

4. The physician applies a volar-directed force over the metacarpal shaft and, simultaneously, dorsally directed pressure over the flexed PIP joint. Reduction is completed with this maneuver (Video 11–1).

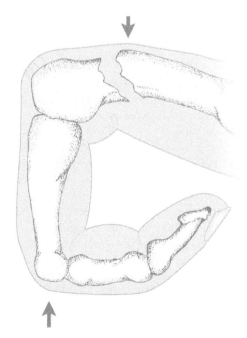

Figure 11–47. The 90-to-90 method of reduction of a fracture of the metacarpal. The proximal phalanx is used to push the metacarpal fracture into a good position.

5. Immobilize with a volar splint to the palmar crease and a dorsal splint extending to, but not including, the PIP, with the wrist extended 30 degrees and the MCP joints flexed 90 degrees. Alternatively, an ulnar gutter splint can be applied.

6. A postreduction radiograph is recommended to ensure maintenance of proper position. The radiograph should be repeated at 1 week to ensure stability of the reduction.

These fractures require close follow-up because they have a tendency to develop recurrent volar angulation despite immobilization. If the reduction is unstable, pin fixation may be necessary, and early referral is indicated.

Metacarpal Neck Fractures: Digits 2 or 3

Nondisplaced, Nonangulated. The recommended therapy for nondisplaced, nonangulated fractures of the neck of metacarpal 2 or 3 includes ice, elevation, and immobilization in a radial gutter splint (Appendix A–3), extending from the distal elbow just proximal to the PIP joint. The wrist should be in 20 degrees of extension, and the metacarpal joint should be in 50 to 60 degrees of flexion. Close follow-up to detect angulation or rotational malalignment is strongly urged. *Caution: Displacement is difficult to correct if detected after 1 week. These fractures require follow-up radiographic examinations at 4 to 5 days post injury to exclude delayed displacement.*

Displaced or Angulated >10 degrees. The emergency management of displaced or angulated second or third digit metacarpal neck fractures >10 degrees includes ice, elevation, and immobilization in a volar or radial gutter splint with referral (Appendix A–3). Accurate reduction of these fractures is imperative and frequently can only be maintained with pinning.

Metacarpal Shaft Fractures

There are four types of metacarpal shaft fractures: nondisplaced transverse, displaced transverse, oblique or spiral, and comminuted (Fig. 11–48). The clinician should be aware that a lesser degree of angulation is acceptable for metacarpal shaft fractures than neck fractures. Each of these fractures is discussed separately in the Treatment section.

There are two mechanisms that result in metacarpal shaft fractures. A direct blow to the hand may result in comminuted, transverse, or short oblique fractures with dorsal angulation secondary to the pull of the interosseous muscles. An indirect blow resulting in a rotational force applied to the digit frequently causes a spiral shaft fracture. Angulation is uncommon with spiral fractures because the deep transverse metacarpal ligament has a tendency to shorten and rotate these fractures.

On examination, tenderness and swelling are present over the dorsal aspect of the hand. The pain is increased

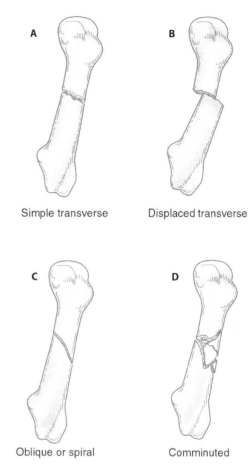

Simple transverse   Displaced transverse

Oblique or spiral   Comminuted

Figure 11–48. Metacarpal fractures—shaft (2 through 5).

with motion, and in most cases, the patient is unable to make a fist. Metacarpal shaft fractures are often associated with rotational malalignment. Rotational deformities can be detected clinically on the basis of the convergence test using the plane of the nail plate or noting the radiographic diameter of the fracture fragments. Rotational deformities must be excluded early in the management of these fractures. For example, just 5 degrees of rotation of the metacarpal shaft can result in 1.5 cm of movement of the fingertip from its normal position.

AP, lateral, and oblique views are often necessary for accurate visualization of the fracture (Fig. 11–49). A 10-degree pronated lateral view is helpful in assessing index- and middle-finger metacarpal fractures. A 10-degree supinated lateral view is helpful in assessing ring- and small-finger metacarpal fractures. With more proximal shaft fractures, the tendency for dorsal angulation becomes greater. Rotational malalignment is suspected when there is either a discrepancy in the shaft diameter or metacarpal shortening.

Long-term complications frequently associated with these fractures include malrotation, dorsal bony prominence with compromise of extensor function, or a painful grip due to volar angulation of the distal bone fragment.

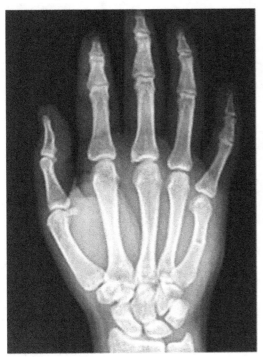

A

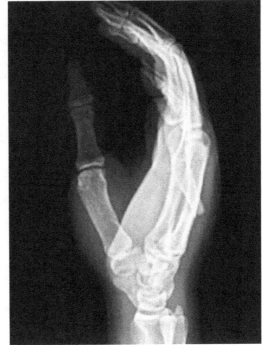

B

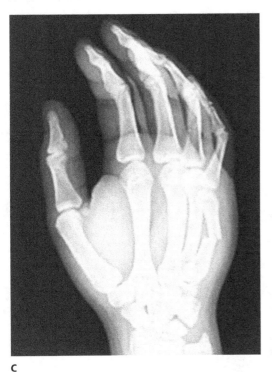

C

Figure 11–49. A. AP, (**B**) lateral, and (**C**) oblique radiographs of a fifth metacarpal shaft fracture with dorsal displacement and approximately 30 degrees of volar angulation.

Treatment

Angulation within the metacarpal shaft is not acceptable in the index and middle metacarpals, whereas up to 10 degrees for the ring metacarpal and 20 degrees in the small metacarpal is acceptable.[2,20]

Nondisplaced Transverse Fractures. Nondisplaced transverse fractures are treated with a gutter splint extending from the proximal forearm to the fingertip (Appendix A–3). The wrist is extended 30 degrees, with the MCP joint in 90 degrees of flexion and the PIP and DIP in extension. Early referral and repeated radiographic examinations are recommended.

Displaced Transverse Fractures. Displaced or angulated transverse fractures require elevation, ice, immobilization, and consultation for reduction and follow-up. Emergency reduction when consultation is unavailable may be accomplished by the following method:

1. A wrist block is used to achieve adequate anesthesia.
2. The fracture fragments are manipulated into position using a volar-directed force over the dorsally angulated fragment while traction is maintained. Rotational deformities must also be corrected at this time.
3. A well-molded dorsal and volar splint, including the entire metacarpal shaft but not the MCP joints, should be applied. The wrist is extended 30 degrees.
4. The patient is referred for follow-up and frequent radiographic examinations, including postreduction views, to ensure proper positioning.

Oblique or Spiral. These fractures require ice, elevation, immobilization in a bulky compressive dressing or gutter splint, and referral for reduction and pinning (Appendix A–5).

Comminuted. The emergency management of comminuted metacarpal shaft fractures includes ice, elevation, and immobilization in a bulky compressive dressing or volar splint with early referral (Appendix A–5).

Metacarpal Base Fractures

Metacarpal base fractures are usually stable injuries (Fig. 11–50). Rotational malalignment of the base will be magnified in its

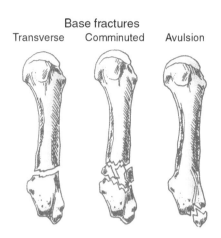

Figure 11–50. Metacarpal fractures—base (2 through 5).

presentation at the tip of the digit. Two mechanisms result in metacarpal base fractures. A direct blow over the base of the metacarpal may result in a fracture. Indirectly, digital torsion is an uncommon fracture mechanism. On examination, tenderness and swelling are present at the base of the metacarpals. Pain is exacerbated with flexion or extension of the wrist or with longitudinal compression.

AP and lateral views are generally adequate in defining these fractures (Fig. 11–51A). Intra-articular base fractures often require a CT scan to fully evaluate the carpometacarpal

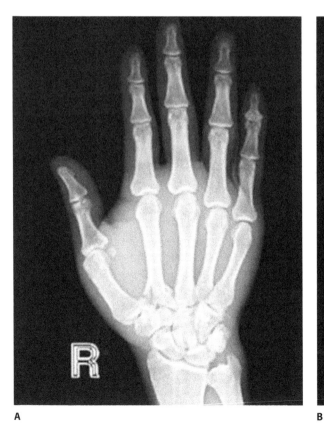

A

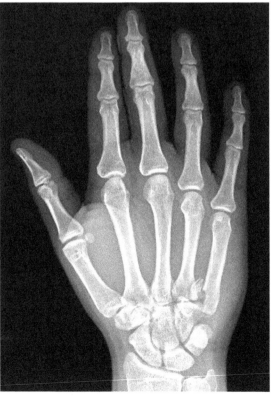

B

Figure 11–51. ***A.*** Fracture of the base of the second metacarpal. ***B.*** Reverse Bennett fracture.

relationship. Always exclude a carpal bone fracture when a metacarpal base fracture is detected.

A unique fracture occurs at the base of the fifth metacarpal when the extensor digit quinti avulses the bone away from a fragment that is held in place by the intermetacarpal ligament. Frequently, an intra-articular step-off is created. Because of the similarity of these injuries, this fracture subluxation is called a *reverse Bennett fracture*. If the fracture is comminuted, the term *reverse Rolando fracture* is used. There will be swelling and tenderness at the fifth carpometacarpal joint. Routine radiographs are diagnostic (Fig. 11–51B).

Fractures at the base of the fourth and fifth metacarpals may cause injury to the motor branch of the ulnar nerve, resulting in paralysis of the intrinsic hand muscles with the exception of the hypothenar muscles. This neural injury is frequently associated with crush injuries. The neural damage may not be apparent initially, secondary to swelling and pain. Metacarpal base fractures may also be associated with tendon injury and chronic carpometacarpal joint stiffness.

Treatment

The emergency management of metacarpal base fractures includes ice, elevation, and immobilization in a bulky compressive dressing with referral (Appendix A–5). Many orthopedic surgeons prefer a volar splint in managing these fractures. Arthroplasty may be necessary if an intra-articular fracture is noted.

Reverse Bennett and Rolando fractures should be treated with an ulnar gutter splint (Appendix A–3). If an intra-articular step-off is present, definitive treatment is pinning.

FIRST METACARPAL FRACTURES

The first metacarpal is biomechanically distinct from the remaining metacarpals because of its high degree of mobility. For this reason, fractures of the first metacarpal are uncommon, and angulation deformities can be accepted without functional impairment.

Fractures of the first metacarpal are classified into three types: extra-articular, intra-articular, and fractures of the sesamoid bones of the thumb.

First Metacarpal Fractures: Extra-Articular

Extra-articular fractures of the first metacarpal are more common than intra-articular fractures. There are three types of extra-articular fractures: transverse; oblique; and, in children, epiphyseal plate fractures (Fig. 11–52).

First metacarpal fractures are usually the result of a direct blow or impaction. Longitudinal torque or distal angular forces typically result in a metacarpal dislocation rather than a fracture. Longitudinal torque associated with a direct blow often results in an oblique fracture. On examination,

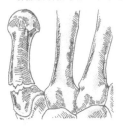

Transverse base fracture

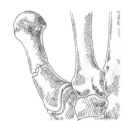

Transverse shaft fracture

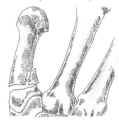

Epiphyseal plate fracture (in children)

Figure 11–52. First metacarpal fractures—extra-articular.

pain and tenderness are present over the fracture site. This is increased with motion.

AP and lateral views are generally adequate for defining shaft fractures. Intra-articular fractures or epiphyseal plate fractures often require oblique views to accurately define the fracture lines and displacement.

Treatment

Because of the normal mobility of the first metacarpal, 30 degrees of angular deformity can be accepted without subsequent functional impairment. The emergency physician should immobilize the extremity in a short-arm thumb spica splint (Appendix A–7) with definitive therapy in a short-arm thumb spica cast (Appendix A–6) for 4 weeks.

Fractures with >30 degrees of angulation require a closed manipulative reduction after regional anesthesia, followed by postreduction radiographs. Oblique fractures may be unstable and complicated by rotational deformities, often requiring percutaneous pinning. Epiphyseal plate injuries require referral for definitive management and follow-up.

First Metacarpal Fractures: Intra-Articular Base

There are two types of intra-articular first metacarpal base fractures (Fig. 11–53). The first type, a *Bennett fracture*, is a fracture with subluxation or dislocation of the metacarpal joint. The other type of intra-articular first metacarpal base fracture is a *Rolando fracture*, which is a comminuted T or Y fracture involving the joint surface.

The most common mechanism is an axial force directed against a partially flexed metacarpal, such as striking a rigid object with a clenched fist. The major indirect deforming forces are supplied by the abductor

Intra-articular base fractures
Bennett fracture—dislocation

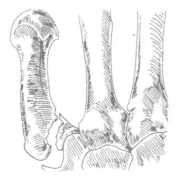

Rolando fracture

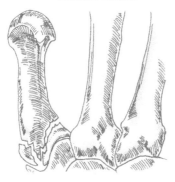

Figure 11-53. First metacarpal fractures—intra-articular.

pollicis longus, which in conjunction with the extrinsic extensors, results in lateral and proximal subluxation of the metacarpal shaft. The anterior oblique ligament (trapezium origin) and the deep ulnar ligament (ulna origin) insert on the base of the first metacarpal and usually hold the proximal fragment in place.

Routine views of the thumb are generally adequate in defining the fracture fragments (Fig. 11-54). Intra-articular base fractures often require CT scans to fully evaluate the carpometacarpal relationship.

The most common complication is the development of traumatic arthritis. In Bennett fracture, this may be secondary to an inadequate reduction; yet, in the Rolando fracture, it may occur despite optimum management.

Treatment

Bennett Fracture—Dislocation. The emergency management of these fractures includes ice, elevation, immobilization in a thumb spica splint (Appendix A-7), and emergent orthopedic consultation or referral. In some instances, after reduction, a very carefully molded plaster cast followed by radiographic confirmation of anatomic positioning will be elected for definitive management. The thumb should be abducted, and the MCP joint should not be hyperextended. Reduction must be stable for this fracture to be treated nonoperatively. Surgery is indicated when >25% of the articular surface is involved and the fracture is more than 1 to 2 mm displaced. In most cases, a satisfactory

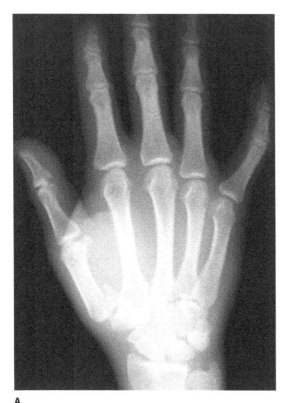

A

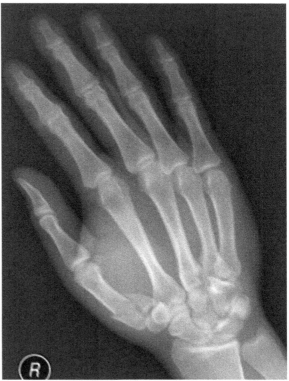

B

Figure 11-54. *A.* Bennett fracture. *B.* Rolando fracture.

reduction cannot be maintained or achieved, and percutaneous wiring is recommended.[6,11,22]

Rolando Fracture. The emergency management of this fracture includes ice, elevation, immobilization in a thumb spica splint (Appendix A–7), and referral. This fracture has a poor prognosis, which is primarily dependent on the degree of comminution. Definitive management of this fracture consists of open reduction and internal fixation or external fixation, depending on the size of the bone fragments.[22]

First Metacarpal Sesamoid Fracture

The thumb has three sesamoids, two at the MCP joint, and a third at the IP joint in 60% to 80% of thumbs (Fig. 11–55).[23] The ulnar sesamoid sits over the ulnar condyle of the distal first metacarpal. The radial sesamoid sits over the narrow radial condyle of the first metacarpal head. The sesamoids of the thumb are embedded in the fibrous plate of the MCP joint. The accessory collateral ligaments insert into the lateral margins of the MCP sesamoids. The tendon of the adductor pollicis inserts on the ulnar sesamoid, and the flexor pollicis brevis inserts on the radial sesamoid.

Sesamoid bone fracture occurs following an MCP hyperextension. On examination, the volar surface of the MCP joint shows tenderness and swelling. The collateral ligaments should be stressed to assess their integrity. Volar plate injuries, evident by hyperextension instability or a hyperextended, locked MCP joint, should be assessed and documented.

Routine views of the hand may demonstrate the fracture. The lateral view is more sensitive than the AP view, which will rarely demonstrate a sesamoid fracture. If doubt exists, radial and ulnar oblique views of the thumb, along with comparison views, may be helpful. A bipartite sesamoid

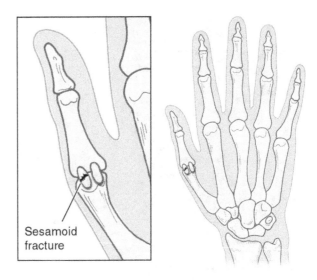

Figure 11–55. Thumb sesamoid fracture.

bone is a rare finding (0.6%) and should be distinguished from a fracture by its smooth borders.[23]

Hyperextension deformity of the thumb MCP joint can complicate unstable volar plate injuries. If chronic post-traumatic arthritis develops, treatment consists of surgical excision of the sesamoid bone.

Treatment

Closed fractures of the sesamoids without hyperextension instability can be treated with a thumb spica splint (Appendix A–7) with the thumb MCP joint in 30 degrees of flexion for 2 to 3 weeks. Consultation for operative repair is recommended when a sesamoid fracture causes the MCP joint to be locked in hyperextension or is associated with clinical MCP joint instability.

HAND SOFT-TISSUE INJURY AND DISLOCATIONS

The following discussion is divided into traumatic and nontraumatic conditions of the hand. Traumatic disorders include soft-tissue wounds, tendon injuries, nerve injuries, vascular injuries, and injuries to the ligaments and joints. Nontraumatic disorders consist of noninfectious inflammatory conditions, constrictive or compressive injuries, and infections of the hand.

TRAUMATIC HAND INJURIES

Rings

The examiner must note the presence of a ring on any finger of a traumatized hand and remove it (Fig. 11–56). Failure to do so may cause an obstruction of venous return, increased swelling, and eventually poor arterial blood flow

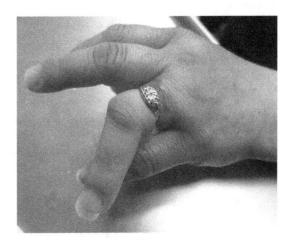

Figure 11–56. The ring noted on this traumatized digit should be removed.

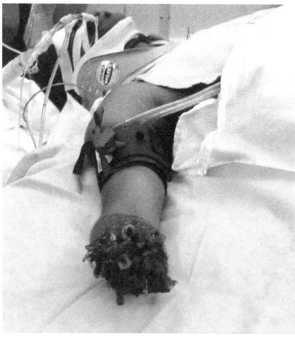

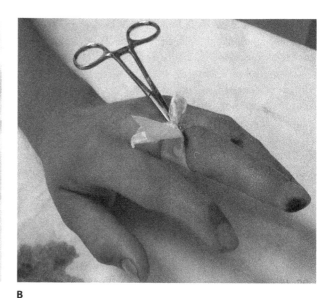

A

B

Figure 11–57. ***A.*** Pneumatic tourniquet used to stop hemorrhage in a patient with a hand amputation. ***B.*** Digital tourniquet using a latex glove and hemostat.

to the digit. Multiple techniques have been described to remove a ring in a swollen digit, but generally, the sooner the ring is removed the better.

Wound Type

It is important to take a thorough history to determine how the injury occurred. The type of wound frequently impacts management decisions. *Incisional wounds* are those caused by a sharp object such as a knife or glass. Although these are usually clean wounds that can be closed primarily, they can be contaminated in certain occupations such as fish handling.

Puncture wounds must be assessed and treated carefully. Foreign bodies are assumed present and the risk of infection considered high, especially when the puncture occurs secondary to a human or animal bite. They are most commonly not closed. Refer to the Fight Bite Injuries (in humans) and Animal Bites sections in this chapter for further details.

Blast wounds are very serious injuries owing to the forceful penetration of foreign objects. Early closure may seal in necrotic tissue as well as foreign material. The first step in treatment is to evaluate nerve and tendon function with careful documentation and local debridement. The hand should be rechecked 36 to 72 hours after injury for final debridement and wound closure in the operating room because there is a latent period before the impact of the concussive force on the circulation is clinically apparent.

Crush injuries, amputations, and high-pressure injection injuries are discussed later.

Control of Bleeding

To assess a wound, one must have control of bleeding. This is usually possible with the application of a sterile pressure dressing. When this is not feasible, however, proximal control is best achieved by the use of a pneumatic tourniquet (Fig. 11–57A). If one is unavailable, a blood pressure cuff placed in the normal position over the arm can be used, but these may deflate during the procedure. Prior to placing the tourniquet, a precursory evaluation of nerve and tendon function is performed. Cast padding is placed under the cuff. The arm can be elevated and compressed with an ace bandage to improve venous drainage of the limb, after which the cuff is rapidly inflated to 250 to 300 mm Hg or 100 mm Hg above systolic pressure. This provides good control of bleeding, can remain in place for 20 to 30 minutes, which permits enough time to clean the wound and ligate bleeding vessels.

If a single digit is injured and hemostasis is required to repair an injury, a sterile glove can be used by cutting off a latex "digit" and wrapping it around the base of the patient's finger. The latex is secured firmly using a hemostat (Fig. 11–57B). Alternatively, have the patient don a surgical glove one full size smaller than his/her hand. Cut off the fingertip of the injured digit and roll the glove down. It will tighten into a tourniquet at the base of the digit while exsanguinating the finger. Finally, commercially available finger tourniquets may be used. The amount of time that the tourniquet is applied should be limited to less than 30 minutes.

Local anesthesia with epinephrine injected into the hand and digits will also decrease bleeding. The use of epinephrine in such a manner has been considered taboo since the 1950s. Recent studies using the typical concentrations included with commercially available local anesthetics (1:100,000) have not uncovered a single case of digital ischemia despite thousands of uses.[25] Based on these data, epinephrine, in the proper concentration, is safe to use in the digit.

Contamination and Wound Closure

Initial care of the wound includes careful assessment and evaluation of the extent of injury, followed by pressure irrigation. An examination of nerve and tendon functions should be performed in addition to direct inspection for tendon or joint involvement (Fig. 11–58). The surrounding skin is cleansed with an antibacterial solution such as povidone-iodine (Betadine) or chlorhexidine. Judicious debridement and removal of foreign material and any non-viable tissue should follow when indicated. The patient's perception of a foreign-body sensation in a digit or the hand suggests that one is present even if not visualized on radiographs.[24]

Whether to close the wound is then decided on the basis of patient factors (e.g., age, diabetes), time since injury, mechanism of injury, and the degree of contamination. A clean wound can be converted to a dirty one by poor care within the ED, and a dirty wound can be converted to a clean one by careful debridement and irrigation. The nature of the offending agent must also be considered; wounds from a knife or glass are generally clean, whereas wounds secondary to bites from animals are not. Crush injuries have macerated tissue and are at a higher risk of infection.

Clean wounds have little contamination and can be closed after irrigation with saline. Dirty wounds are cleansed thoroughly and debrided, and delayed closure is preferred if there is any question about continued contamination. The time interval between the insult and its treatment is ascertained because a delay in seeking care is a risk factor for wound infection.

Prophylactic antibiotics are not recommended in clean soft-tissue wounds of the hands. The infection rate is no different with or without their use.[26,27] The use of antibiotics in a contaminated wound is controversial and the use of antibiotics in an animal bite wound is standard.

Foreign Bodies

Glass, metal, and wood are the most common foreign materials seen in hand wounds (Fig. 11–59). Although some foreign bodies are inert and cause little reaction, others can cause significant problems. On examination, a small laceration or puncture wound with local hemorrhage may be present. The foreign body is usually located within the area of maximal tenderness. All wounds, especially of the hands, should be considered to have a foreign body present until proven otherwise.

The workup begins with a plain radiograph. Fluoroscopy may be of benefit for both foreign-body localization and removal. Ultrasound, computed tomography (CT), and magnetic resonance imaging (MRI) are more advanced techniques for identification. Refer to Chapter 5 for a full discussion.

Glass is radiopaque.[28] Small pieces of glass may not require removal, whereas larger ones tend to migrate and become symptomatic as fibrous reaction envelops them. Metallic particles may remain inert and, if asymptomatic, do not require removal. Symptomatic metal fragments may be allowed to remain until a capsule forms around them, facilitating their removal.

Wood and plastic are radiolucent. Ultrasound and CT may demonstrate these substances. Plastic is perhaps the most difficult substance to detect, often requiring MRI. Wood can

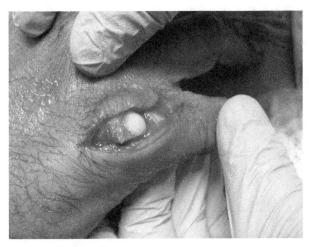

Figure 11–58. Laceration of the hand involving the joint of the MCP.

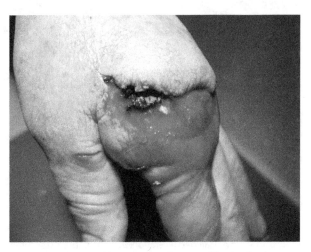

Figure 11–59. Hand laceration with a metal foreign body.

be inert but is frequently stained with toxic dyes or contains oils or resins that induce an inflammatory response.

If the emergency physician is unable to remove the foreign body, the injured hand should be splinted and the patient referred. Often, waiting several days to reexplore the area may prove beneficial as small fragments may encapsulate and gradually migrate to the surface.

Subungual Hematoma and Nail Bed Injuries

The fingertip is defined as the area distal to the insertions of the flexor and extensor tendons on the distal phalanx. Injuries of the fingertip are classified here as subungual hematoma, nail bed injuries, and fingertip amputations. To assess the fingertip after injury, gauze applied by the patient or in triage must first be removed. When a fingertip or nail bed is adherent to gauze, it can be removed easily by soaking the fingertip in a 1% solution of lidocaine for 20 minutes.

A subungual hematoma, regardless of the size, does not require nail removal as long as the nail plate is intact. Trephination of symptomatic subungual hematomas using electrocautery or an 18-gauge needle is recommended (Fig. 11-22).

If the nail plate is lacerated or avulsed, the nail is removed, and any lacerations to the nail bed are repaired (Fig. 11-60). If a distal phalanx fracture is associated with disruption or laceration of the nail plate, it is considered an open fracture but may be treated in the ED.

The technique for repairing nail bed lacerations includes:

1. Regional anesthesia using a digital block. The hand is then prepared and draped in a sterile manner.
2. Using a pair of fine scissors, the nail is dissected bluntly from the nail bed.
3. With the nail removed, the nail bed laceration is explored and thoroughly irrigated with normal saline (Fig. 11-60A). The nail bed is then sutured using a minimum number of 5-0 absorbable interrupted sutures (Fig. 11-60B). Alternatively, a tissue adhesive (e.g., Dermabond) may be used.

4. A nonadherent gauze (e.g., Xeroform) or the patient's recently removed nail is placed back in the nail fold to separate the dorsal roof matrix from the nail bed (Fig. 11-60C). The material is sutured in place with two simple sutures on either side to ensure that it does not dislodge. A tissue adhesive (e.g., Dermabond) has also been used successfully to secure the nail and prevent dislodgement. Separating the bed from the roof prevents the development of adhesions (synechia) that can ultimately result in the regrowth of a deformed nail.
5. The entire digit should be dressed with gauze and splinted for protection. The outer dressing can be changed as needed, but the material separating the nail bed from the roof matrix remains in place for 10 days.
6. Prophylactic antibiotics are recommended when there is an associated distal phalanx fracture or significant wound contamination.

Fingertip Amputation

Fingertip amputations are classified on the basis of whether exposed bone is present. An amputation without exposed bone can be allowed to heal by secondary intention (Fig. 11-61). Management in the ED consists of cleansing the wound and application of a nonadherent (e.g., Xeroform or Vaseline) dressing. When the distal phalanx is exposed, treatment is more complex and may require a Rongeur to trim the bone back. The soft tissue is then sutured so the bone is no longer exposed, a nonadherent dressing is placed, and the wound is allowed to heal by secondary intention. Consultation with a hand surgeon is recommended if the emergency physician is uncomfortable with the procedure. Prophylactic antibiotics are indicated only in grossly contaminated wounds. Nonmicrosurgical reattachment of a clean, sharply amputated distal tip can be employed as a "biologic" dressing, but the patient should be told that the tip will likely not be viable. In children,

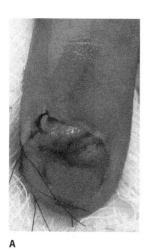 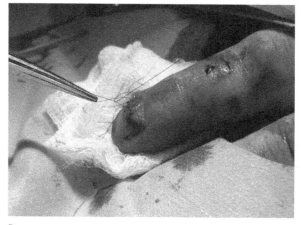 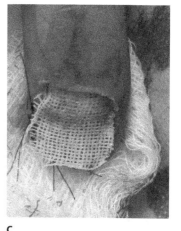

A   **B**   **C**

Figure 11-60. **A.** Nail bed laceration. **B.** Absorbable 5-0 suture is used to approximate the wound edges. **C.** If the nail plate is unavailable, a single layer of nonadhesive gauze is used to keep the eponychium separated from the nail bed.

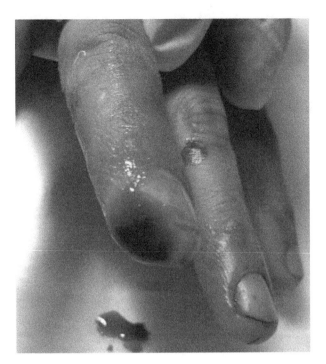

Figure 11–61. Fingertip injury.

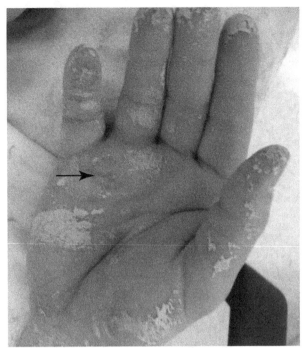

Figure 11–62. High-pressure injection injury to the hand secondary to a paint gun. Note the small entrance wound (*arrow*). This patient required operative debridement.

treatment is similar except that nonmicrosurgical reattachment has greater success than in adults.[29]

Other potential treatments include skin grafts, replantation, and flaps. Replantation is an expensive option requiring a surgeon skilled in microvascular techniques. When successful, however, sensation, length, cosmesis, and range of motion (ROM) are preserved, and the incidence of chronic pain is low. Success rates range from 70% to 90%, and children do especially well. If the amputation is proximal to the lunula, this is the only procedure that will preserve the nail. Because the amputated tip does not possess muscle, the period of ischemia that allows successful replantation is prolonged (8 hours warm; 30 hours cold).[31]

Nonetheless, conservative treatment (i.e., healing by secondary intention) alone yields good results in most cases. The authors of studies supporting this approach cite the natural regenerative properties of the fingertip, simplicity, decreased cost, preservation of length, improved cosmesis, low incidence of painful neuromas and stiffness, and good return of sensation. Disadvantages include higher incidence of nail deformity and the need for frequent dressing changes.[32–41] Areas of greater than 1 to 1.5 cm^2 may require split-thickness skin grafting.

High-Pressure Injection Injuries

These injuries are surgical emergencies and occur to individuals who work with a machine that sprays liquids at high pressure. Examples of such instruments include paint guns, grease guns, concrete injectors, plastic injectors, and diesel fuel jets.[42] The nondominant hand is most often affected

when the patient attempts to clean the nozzle of the gun while it is still operating.

Initially, the patient may have minimal symptoms, and the skin wound is usually small (Fig. 11–62). Despite the trivial wound externally, the emergency physician should be aware that significant tissue injury has occurred below the surface. With time, the extremity becomes swollen, pale, and excruciating pain develops. Severe tenderness to palpation or pain with passive motion is elicited.

Injection injuries may cause extensive loss of tissue, have a high infection rate, and a high rate of amputation. Factors that increase the risk of amputation include the type of material, amount injected, and the pressure of the injection. Oil-based paints appear to be particularly harmful. Injections with *water* under pressure may be observed in the hospital. A pressure >7000 lb/in^2 has been associated with a 100% amputation rate.[43] Also, the time to treatment is significant, with some authors suggesting that patients treated in less than 10 hours after the injury fare better than those with delayed treatment.

A radiograph of the extremity should always be performed as it may help determine the spread of the material and the extent of surgical exploration and debridement necessary. Grease will appear as a lucency.[44] Treatment in the ED consists of administering a prophylactic broad-spectrum antibiotic and, if needed, tetanus immunization. High-pressure injection injuries secondary to water can be treated conservatively without surgical debridement in many cases.[45] High-pressure injections due to organic solvents, however, are a major source of tissue irritation. Not all injuries result in significant injection of foreign material. If there is no tenderness at or around the injection site several hours after the injury, then a significant injection has not occurred and operative intervention is not necessary. Surgery is usually necessary, however, when tenderness is noted proximal and distal to the site of injection. Surgical consultation is required for these cases, and will most often result in irrigation and debridement of necrotic tissue in the operating room.

Crush Injuries

Crush injuries to the hand are common. The underlying tissue is congested and ischemic, whereas the surface wounds often appear quite simple and may mislead the emergency physician regarding the full extent of the injury. If extensive soft-tissue injury is present, primarily closed lacerations have a high rate of infection. Potential occult soft-tissue injuries include closed tendon ruptures and, in the case of a finger, digital artery injury. The hand should be placed in a universal hand dressing (Appendix A–5), elevated, and referred to a hand surgeon.

Mangled Hand Injuries

Mangled hand injuries occur secondary to the use of farming equipment, the use of industrial equipment (e.g., punch press), gunshot wounds, motor vehicle collisions, firecrackers, and the use of household equipment (e.g., lawn mowers) (Fig. 11–63). Treatment of these injuries

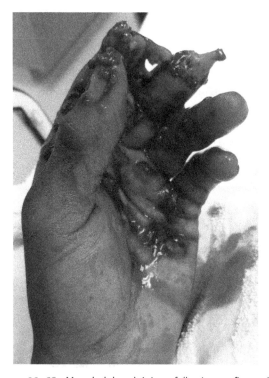

Figure 11–63. Mangled hand injury following a firecracker exploding in the hand.

is difficult. Only a precursory assessment of the extremity circulation and gross neurologic assessment is performed in the ED. Preliminary radiographs should be obtained, and the hand covered with sterile dressings and immobilized while awaiting patient transfer or the consultation of a hand surgeon.

Blind clamping of vascular structures should never be performed. If direct pressure does not work, the hand should be elevated and a blood pressure cuff applied proximal to the zone of injury and inflated to a pressure 100 mm Hg above systolic pressure. Immediate surgery is needed when external hemorrhage cannot be controlled.

Pain control with parenteral narcotics or regional anesthesia is usually warranted. Prophylactic broad-spectrum parenteral antibiotics are indicated. Tetanus prophylaxis is administered as needed. Operative replantation to salvage the amputated portion can be attempted and has become increasingly more successful with the evolution of surgical techniques and instruments.

Hand injuries associated with the use of snow blowers and lawn mowers are generally less severe, but seen more frequently. Injuries occur to the dominant dorsal side of the hand and fingers in almost all cases, with extensive lacerations and contusions. Usually, the long and ring fingers are injured. The majority of these injuries can be managed in the ED, although some require operative intervention for debridement and repair.

A degloving injury occurs when the soft tissue of the hand or digit is separated from the underlying bone. In a "pure" degloving injury, the tendons, bones, and joints remain intact and only the skin is removed. This is often called a *ring injury* because the ring finger is the most commonly involved digit when jewelry becomes hooked and torn from the digit. Treatment includes replantation when the degloved skin is available and the vessels are not damaged. If unsuccessful, secondary reconstruction using a skin flap is required.

Amputation

Amputation of the hand or finger is not common. Care of the stump includes achieving hemostasis first. Point control of a bleeding vessel with a pressure dressing is usually the initial method. The use of proximal tourniquets with patients is discouraged unless being used for temporary control or for life-threatening bleeding. Use for more than 3 hours may lead to irreversible ischemia. Blind ligation or clamping may lead to unnecessary damage to the nerves or vessels. Prophylactic antibiotics and tetanus are indicated.

Care of the amputated part involves gentle cleansing if heavily contaminated, wrapping in saline-soaked gauze, and storage in a sealed plastic bag. The bag is then placed into another bag filled with ice water (Fig. 11–64). Properly maintained digits have approximately 12 hours of viability.

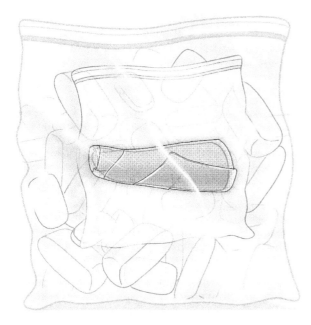

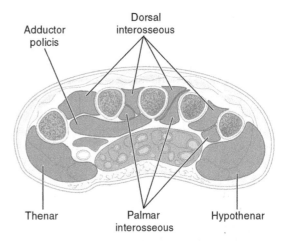

Figure 11–66. Cross section of the palm, through the metatarsal shafts, showing the compartments of the hand.

Figure 11–64. Proper storage of an amputated part requires that the tissue is wrapped in moist gauze, placed in a bag, and then placed in another bag full of ice water.

The classic indications for replantation include amputation between the PIP and DIP joints; amputation of the thumb, multiple digits, and wrist or forearm (Fig. 11–65); amputations in children; and midpalmar amputation. However, all amputated parts proximal to the fingertip should be considered for replantation, and consultation with a hand surgeon should occur. Success is not only related to viability, but also to the restoration of a functional hand. It should always be emphasized that the replanted digit will never function normally and will likely have some sensory problems, as well as chronic stiffness and weakness.

Hand Compartment Syndromes

Acute compartment syndrome of the hand is a relatively rare phenomenon that occurs when the tissue pressure within an enclosed space is elevated to the extent that there is decreased blood flow within the space, decreasing tissue oxygenation. This syndrome is most often a result of a traumatic condition, but nontraumatic entities such as an infectious process may also be causative. The most common causes include fractures, crush injuries, burns, major vascular injury, prolonged hand compression, and iatrogenic injuries such as a cast or compressive dressing.

There are a total of 10 compartments within the hand (Fig. 11–66).[59] The volar and dorsal interosseous muscles are enclosed in fascia between the metacarpals. These compartments constitute 7 of the 10 hand compartments—4 dorsal interosseous and 3 volar interosseous compartments. The remaining three compartments

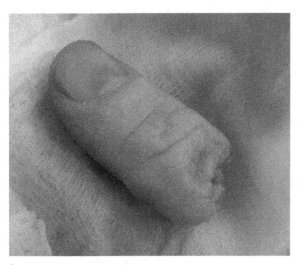

A

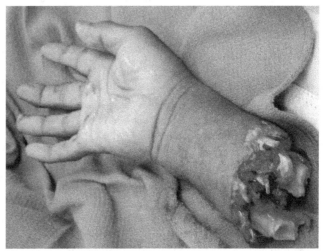

B

Figure 11–65. ***A.*** Thumb amputation between the MCP and IP joints. ***B.*** Hand amputation. Both of these amputations were replanted.

comprise the thenar muscles, hypothenar muscles, and adductor pollicis muscle.

The clinical findings are similar to those of other compartment syndromes in the body—disproportionate pain that is increased on passive muscle stretch and unrelieved by immobilization. The intrinsic interosseous compartments of the hand are tested individually to adequately exclude a limited syndrome. Note that passive stretching of the muscle should occur in the direction opposite to the muscle's normal actions. The volar interosseous muscles are tested by passive *abduction* of the second, fourth, and fifth digits. The dorsal interosseous muscles are tested by passive *adduction* of the second and fourth digits, in addition to medial and lateral movements of the third digit. When testing these interosseous compartments, the MCP joint is placed in full extension and the PIP joint in flexion. The adductor compartment is tested by palmar abduction of the thumb, thereby stretching the adductor pollicis muscle. In a similar manner, the thenar and hypothenar compartments are stretched when the examiner radially abducts the thumb (thenar) and extends and adducts the small finger (hypothenar).

Compartment pressure measurements provide more objective information and are used in conjunction with clinical findings. Measurements can be taken using a Stryker device or the infusion technique. The needle is inserted on the dorsal surface of the hand between the metacarpals to measure the interosseous compartment pressures. For the remaining three compartments, a palmar approach is preferred. Compartment pressure measurements within the hand are difficult and best performed after consultation with a hand surgeon.

Left untreated, compartment syndrome within the hand will result in muscle necrosis and fibrosis. The function of the hand will be severely limited with significant contracture deformities at both the PIP and MCP joints. For more details regarding the diagnosis and treatment of compartment syndromes, refer to Chapter 4.

Tendon Lacerations

Open tendon injuries usually result from a sharp object that lacerates the skin and underlying tendon. The evaluation of a tendon in this setting should include an examination of the tendon's function and a visual inspection of the tendon within the wound. There are many pitfalls to the diagnosis of open tendon injuries.

Functional Examination

The functional assessment of the flexor and extensor tendons is presented at the beginning of this chapter. Further tips to properly diagnose tendon injuries in the face of skin laceration are provided in the following paragraphs.

When examining a tendon, always test both active motion and strength (against resistance). In both partial and complete tendon lacerations, tendon motion may be preserved, and the only clue to the diagnosis is loss of strength. For partial lacerations, a tendon may have 90% of its width transected and still have normal motion. Therefore, to adequately assess a tendon for injury, *one must test motion against resistance.*

In lacerations to the dorsal surface of the hand, several pitfalls exist:

1. Lacerations over the PIP joints and the MCP joints may transect the central slip of the extensor tendon, and the diagnosis is not made until the hood mechanism decompensates and leads to deformity.
2. Disruption of an extensor digitorum communis tendon proximal to the juncturae tendinea may preserve some finger extension due to the function of the other extensor digitorum communis tendons.
3. The index and little fingers each have two extensor tendons. Finger extension may be preserved when there is laceration to only one of the tendons.
4. The intrinsic muscles of the hand can extend the PIP and DIP joints despite an extensor tendon laceration.

In lacerations to the flexor surface of the hand, finger flexion may be preserved despite complete disruption of the flexor digitorum superficialis as long as the flexor digitorum profundus is intact. In this scenario, strength will be limited.

Visual Examination

Control of bleeding and good lighting is required to obtain an adequate examination. When the skin wounds are small, the tendon may be difficult to locate so the skin must be stretched with a hemostat for proper visualization. In larger lacerations, the tendon injury may be overlooked in the face of other more obvious injuries. Lastly, patient cooperation is essential and is often lacking, particularly in the intoxicated patient.

In open wounds, an incomplete injury to the tendon is common and may be difficult to assess. The position of the hand when the injury occurred is important to determine. If the volar aspect of the hand is lacerated while the fingers are held in flexion, then a partial injury to the flexor tendons will be distal to the skin wound if the hand is examined in extension. However, if the hand were in the extended position at the time of injury, the tendon injuries would lie at the wound edges with hand extension. *Therefore, when a tendon is visualized at the base of a laceration, its surface should be inspected while the fingers undergo a full range of motion.*

Axiom: *A negative examination of a patient with a suspected tendon injury should always be reevaluated to be certain of the diagnosis, particularly in the uncooperative patient.*

Treatment

In lacerations to the hand where tendons are transected, the expected outcome is determined to a large extent by how dirty and complex the wound is. Adhesions are accentuated by touching the tendons or even by blood extravasation around the tendon. Therefore, every attempt is made to avoid unnecessary manipulation of the injured tendon.

In general, definitive repair of an open complete tendon injury can be performed primarily, delayed primarily, or secondarily. Since the 1980s, the length of time that a tendon can be repaired primarily has been gradually extended.[61] There is no conclusive evidence that suggests that immediate repair results in better clinical outcome than delayed primary repair (within 7 days of injury).[60,62] A secondary repair is performed after edema has subsided and the scar has softened, usually more than 4 weeks after injury. Secondary tendon repairs result in worse functional outcome.

Delayed primary repairs are performed when other trauma exists and repair of the hand must be deferred or when the wound is not optimal for repair because of infection or swelling. Secondary repairs are performed when associated injuries compromise the patient or wound complications are likely.

Partial Tendon Lacerations. Open partial tendon injuries can be splinted without surgical repair. Controversy exists as to the best treatment of partial tendon injuries, and therefore, consultation with a hand surgeon is recommended.[63] Some hand surgeons repair flexor tendons that have injury to >50% of the tendon surface, although little evidence supports this practice. The perceived benefits include avoiding future entrapment, rupture, or triggering. Even less evidence exists regarding the best treatment of partial extensor tendon injuries; thus, many adopt the same principles as flexor tendons—repair of extensor tendons with >50% of the surface lacerated.[2] There is some evidence that partial tendon lacerations, regardless of the percentage of tendon injury, heal well without sutures, as long as a portion of the tendon is apposed.[64]

For partial extensor tendon injuries, the position to splint the hand is important and contrary to routine practice. With these injuries, the hand is splinted with the MCP joint in full extension to avoid additional strain on the already injured tendon. The digit should remain in this position for 3 to 4 weeks and then be slowly returned to full flexion. Partial flexor tendon injuries are splinted in the position of function with the MCP joint at 50 degrees of flexion and the IP joints at 20 degrees of flexion for 3 to 4 weeks.

Flexor Tendon Lacerations. Flexor tendon injuries have been categorized into five zones to assist in planning treatment (Fig. 11–67).

- *Zone I* extends from the distal insertion of the profundus (FDP) tendon to the site of the superficialis (FDS) insertion. Injuries here generally result in the proximal tendon retracting.

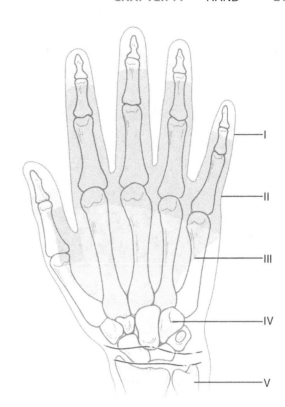

Figure 11–67. Flexor tendon laceration classification.

- *Zone II* injuries are in the area often referred to as "no man's land" because these injuries are very difficult to repair and were previously treated with secondary grafting.[65] Unfortunately, they are the most commonly seen flexor tendon lacerations in emergency medicine and technically the most difficult to repair.[66] The profundus and superficialis tendons interweave closely, and injuries here may injure the vinculum providing the blood supply to the tendons. Repairs in this area are quite complex and should only be attempted by a qualified hand surgeon.
- *Zone III* injuries extend from the distal edge of the carpal tunnel to the proximal edge of the flexor sheath. These injuries generally have a good result with primary repair.
- *Zone IV* injuries include the carpal tunnel and its related structures. Injuries here require careful exploration for associated injuries.
- *Zone V* flexor tendon injuries are those that occur proximal to the carpal tunnel. In zone V injuries, it is essential that the surgeon has adequate exposure and conducts an exhaustive search for any injuries in major structures.

Patients with complete flexor tendon injuries require consultation with a hand surgeon for repair within the operating room (Fig. 11–68). Complete flexor tendon lacerations are usually repaired within 12 to 24 hours, although this time frame can be extended and may depend on your institution or the individual surgeon.[2] Following repair, the hand is splinted with extension blocked.

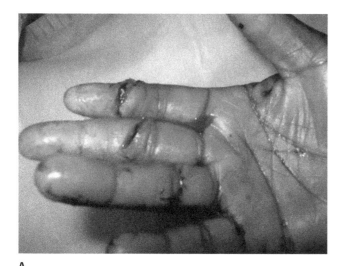

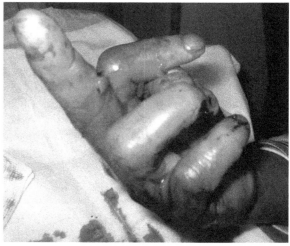

A   **B**

Figure 11–68. **A.** This patient sustained flexor tendon lacerations zone I (2nd digit) and zone II (3rd digit). **B.** When flexion was tested, it was clear he had lacerated the FDP of the 2nd digit (unable to flex at the DIP joint while maintaining PIP flexion) and both the FDP and FDS of the 3rd digit (unable to flex finger at all).

Extensor Tendon Lacerations. A classification system used to divide extensor tendon injuries into eight zones and aid in treatment decisions has been devised by Kleinert and Verdan (Fig. 11–69). The zones of injury are remembered more easily if the physician considers that starting at the DIP joint (zone I), odd-numbered zones are over joints and even-numbered zones are over bones (Fig. 11–70). The thumb is numbered in a similar fashion into five zones.

- *Zone I* injuries are over the distal phalanx. Treatment of open zone I injuries involves repair of the tendon laceration if loss of extension is present at the DIP joint. A dorsal splint is applied to maintain the DIP joint in extension for 6 weeks. During this time, the PIP and MCP joints are allowed to move freely.

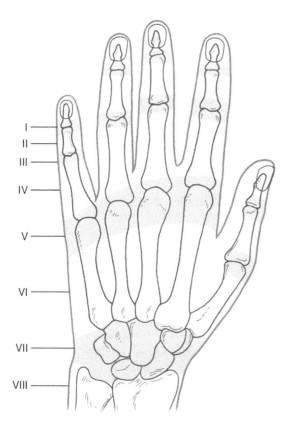

Figure 11–69. Extensor tendon laceration classification.

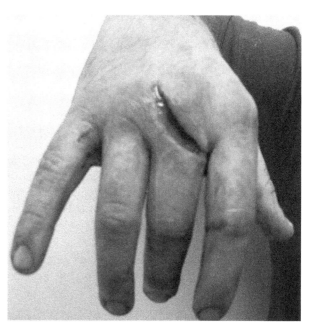

Figure 11–70. This patient sustained a zone V extensor tendon laceration. Note the flexed resting position of the digit compared to the other digits.

- *Zone II* injuries are over the middle phalanx. The treatment here is identical to that for zone I injuries.
- *Zone III* is over the PIP joint. These injuries can be either open or closed, with the central tendon being the most commonly injured structure in both scenarios. This injury frequently leads to a boutonniere deformity if untreated. Open injuries are treated with primary repair and splinted with the wrist in 30 degrees of extension, the MCP at 15 to 30 degrees of flexion, and the PIP in a neutral position. Zone III injuries are associated with a high rate of associated injuries (80%) and generally have a poor outcome.[68] These injuries should undergo primary repair by a hand surgeon.
- *Zone IV* injuries include the area over the proximal phalanx. These injuries are treated with primary or delayed repair with a volar splint for 3 to 6 weeks, as described for zone III injuries. A high rate of complications and associated injuries are noted with zone IV tendon lacerations.[68]
- *Zone V* injuries are over the MCP joint. When from a human bite, the wound must be explored, thoroughly irrigated, and left open. If the joint capsule is not injured and the wound is not secondary to a human bite, it can be repaired with 4-0 or 5-0 absorbable suture. Following repair, the finger should be splinted with the wrist in 45 degrees of extension and the MCP joint in a neutral position.
- *Zone VI* injuries involve the extensor tendons over the dorsum of the hand. The extensor tendons are very superficial in this zone, and even apparently minor wounds may involve the tendons. Following repair, 4 weeks of immobilization is required with the wrist at 30 degrees of extension, the MCP joint in a neutral position, and the DIP and PIP joints free. Tendons at this site tend not to retract because they are connected to adjacent structures and tendons. On the dorsal hand, lacerations causing extensor tendon rupture will often lead to adhesions.[55]
- *Zone VII* injuries occur over the carpal bones and are uncommon. These lacerations often involve the extensor retinaculum and are at risk for developing adhesions after repair. A volar splint is applied with the wrist in 20 degrees of extension and the MCP joint placed in neutral position. These injuries should undergo primary repair by a hand surgeon.[66]
- *Zone VIII* injuries involve the extensor tendon at the level of the distal forearm and are usually a result of deep lacerations. The tendon may retract due to the elasticity of the musculotendinous junction. These injuries should undergo primary repair by a hand surgeon. A volar splint is placed with the wrist in 20 degrees of extension and the MCP joint placed in neutral position.

Most open extensor tendon lacerations are repaired by an experienced hand surgeon. *Successful repair can be accomplished either immediately or after a delay of up to 7 days following the injury.*[68] After 7 days, the tendon ends retract or soften. If the tendon will not be repaired on the day of presentation, the wound should be irrigated and debrided, the skin closed loosely with simple interrupted sutures, and the hand splinted, as previously described. Prophylactic antibiotics are prescribed.

The emergency physician may choose to repair certain extensor tendon lacerations if they have the skill and experience to do so. Zones IV, V, and VI tendon lacerations without joint involvement, bony fracture, or human bite wounds may be sutured using a mattress, figure-of-eight, or modified Kessler or Bunnell stitch. Nonabsorbable 4-0 or 5-0 suture is recommended. Following repair and splinting, the patient is referred to a hand surgeon to initiate a rehabilitation program.

Closed Tendon Injuries

Great forces are required for a closed injury to cause tendon rupture. Closed tendon injuries are the result of either a blunt impact or an opposing force sustained by a contracting muscle-tendon unit. Forces acting against the tendon while it is contracting may avulse the bone at the insertion of the tendon or rupture the tendon without bony injury. Closed tendon injuries are easily missed and, unfortunately, chronic deformities often result if they go untreated.

Jersey Finger

An avulsion injury of the FDP tendon is called a *jersey injury*, named because it often occurs when an athlete grabs an opponent's jersey. The mechanism of injury is forceful extension of a flexed DIP joint. Although rare, this injury is the most common closed flexor tendon injury.[48] The index finger is involved in 75% of cases, but any finger can be affected.[70] On examination, a subtle flexion deformity is noted at the DIP joint, and the patient will be unable to flex the distal phalanx when the PIP joint is extended (Fig. 11–71). If this injury goes untreated, a flexion contracture at the PIP joint

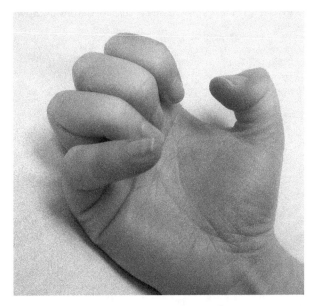

Figure 11–71. Jersey finger. The normal cascade of flexion is disrupted. In this patient, flexion at the DIP joint of the fifth digit is absent.

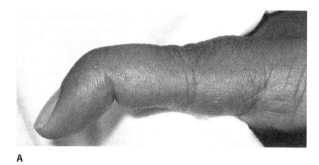

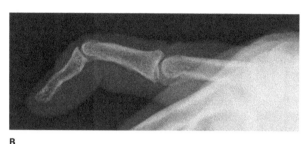

Figure 11–72. A mallet finger deformity **(A)** without associated fracture **(B)**.

may result, or the patient will complain that he/she is unable to make a fist. A radiograph is obtained to assess for an avulsion fracture. In the ED, the patient should be splinted using a dorsal splint with 30 degrees of wrist flexion, 70 degrees of MCP flexion, and 30 degrees of IP flexion. A jersey finger is best treated surgically. Referral to a hand surgeon is needed within 7 to 10 days.

Mallet Finger

A *mallet finger* is a flexion deformity at the DIP joint in which there is incomplete active extension of the DIP joint (Fig. 11–72). This injury is usually sustained from a sudden

blow to the tip of the extended finger. The insertion of the extensor tendon may be avulsed, or there may be an avulsion fracture of the distal phalanx with the tendon still attached. For this reason, a radiograph of the finger should be obtained. Acutely, the patient will have minimal pain and little functional disability. The classic flexion deformity may not be present until several days post injury.

Treatment is to splint the DIP joint in extension (Fig. 11–27). Hyperextension, as has been previously suggested, is avoided. In addition, the patient is allowed to have normal range of motion at the PIP joint. The splint remains in place for 6 weeks. If the splint is removed at any time during this treatment period and the DIP joint is allowed to flex, another 6 weeks of immobilization is warranted. In patients who use the hand a great deal and depend on finger motion at their fingertips, plaster immobilization may be recommended. If left untreated, a flexion deformity of the DIP joint is seen when the PIP is extended and is called a *mallet finger*. Occasionally, a chronic mallet finger will develop into a swan-neck deformity of the digit.

Central Slip Rupture

Disruptions of the *central slip of the extensor tendon* at the dorsal base of the middle phalanx should be identified because failure to do so may result in a boutonniere deformity of the digit (Fig. 11–73). Central slip disruption can be caused by three closed mechanisms: deep contusion of the PIP joint, acute forceful flexion of the extended PIP joint, or palmar dislocation of the PIP joint. Thus, one should suspect this injury whenever one encounters a painful swollen PIP joint with any of the aforementioned mechanisms.

On examination, extension at the PIP joint is tested. A 15- to 25-degree loss of extension with decreased strength against resistance should make one suspect this injury. Tenderness at the PIP joint is maximal over the central slip on

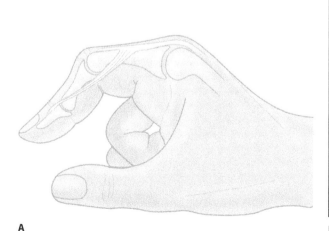

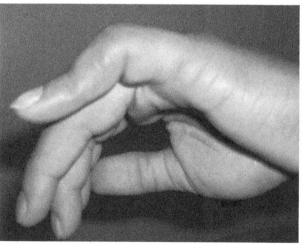

Figure 11–73. The boutonniere deformity. **A.** The lateral bands of the extensor tendon slip volarly and cause PIP flexion and DIP extension. **B.** Clinical photo.

the dorsal aspect of the PIP joint. Elson's test has also been described and modified to test for central slip rupture. In this test, the PIP joint of the injured finger is flexed to 90 degrees and held in position against the middle phalanx of the same finger on the opposite hand. The patient is asked to attempt to extend the PIP against the resistance of the opposite finger. If the central slip is ruptured, the DIP joint will extend and become rigid. This occurs because the lateral bands are stretched more in the setting of a ruptured central slip and do not allow as much mobility at the DIP joint.[73]

The boutonniere deformity (flexion of the PIP joint and hyperextension of the DIP joint) may be present acutely, but usually does not show up for 7 to 14 days following the injury. Gradually, the lateral bands stretch and slip volar to the axis of the PIP joint, and become flexors of the PIP joint.

Ultrasound, performed by experienced providers, has proven useful in diagnosing these injuries.[74]

The treatment is to keep the PIP joint in constant and complete extension, while the DIP and MCP joints are allowed to move freely.[54] Referral to a hand surgeon is indicated as operative repair is required in some cases.

Boxer's Finger

A traumatic blow to the dorsal aspect of the MCP joint may result in *rupture of the extensor hood*.[75,76] This injury is also referred to as "boxer's knuckle" or "boxer's finger" because it is commonly associated with blunt trauma seen with the act of punching. The extensor tendon injury is disruption of the peripherally located sagittal bands that hold the longitudinal central tendon in place. When rupture of these fibrous bands occurs, the result is subluxation of the tendon either ulnarly (common) or radially (Fig. 11–74 and Video 11–2).

On examination, marked swelling, decreased joint mobility, and extensor lag are seen. Subluxation of the extensor tendon is made worse by joint flexion and a palpable defect is noted at the site of the sagittal band rupture.

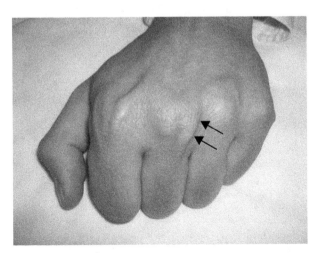

Figure 11–74. Boxer's finger. Note the ulnar position of the extensor tendon as it passes the MCP joint.

The tendon may relocate, causing pain at the MCP joint, as the finger is extended.

Surgery is almost universally successful, but a trial of conservative management with splinting may be attempted. The emergency physician should bring the MCP joint into extension until the tendon relocates, and then the hand is splinted in that position. Other injuries to the MCP joint to be included in the differential diagnosis include contusions, synovitis, collateral ligament ruptures, articular fractures, and capsular tears.[75]

Neurovascular Injuries

Three nerves supply the hand with sensory and muscular branches: radial, ulnar, and median. The sensory innervation of the ulnar nerve is very constant, whereas others vary. Of all the sensory nerves, the significance of the median nerve is the most important to normal hand function, and the radial nerve is the least significant with regard to sensory distribution.

There are varying degrees of nerve injury. In a *neurotmesis*, the nerve is completely disrupted. This is due to penetrating trauma or a fracture fragment. In an *axonotmesis*, there is variable motor and sensory dysfunction. In these patients, the proximal and distal ends of the nerves are separated; however, the Schwann cells are maintained. In a *neurapraxia*, there is no loss of continuity of the nerve and dysfunction is temporary.

Nerve injuries can result from contusions, lacerations, and puncture wounds to the hand. Check for nerve function in every hand injury to avoid delay in diagnosis. Contusions usually result in a neurapraxia with no loss of continuity of the nerve, in which case function is usually regained and treatment is simply observation. Lacerations can result in an axonotmesis or a neurotmesis.[77]

Ulnar Nerve Injury

Lacerations of the ulnar nerve at the distal forearm and wrist result in hypothenar muscle weakness, loss of finger abduction, adduction (interosseus muscles), and flexion, as well as adduction of the thumb. Sensory loss at the tip of the fifth digit is typical of ulnar nerve dysfunction. Laceration of the ulnar nerve in the proximity of MCP joints of the thumb, ring finger, and middle finger will result in loss of finger abduction and adduction, weakness of thumb flexion, and adduction, while the hypothenar muscles and ulnar sensation remain intact. Deep volar hand lacerations of the MCP joints can cause isolated injury to the digital nerves and distal sensory loss with normal motor function.[1]

The specific signs of ulnar nerve injury are as follows:

- Loss of sensation at the tip of the fifth digit
- Deformity of the hand such as Duchenne sign (clawing of the ring and little fingers)
- Inability to actively adduct the little finger
- Hyperflexion of the IP joint of the thumb on a powerful pinch (Froment sign) (Fig. 11–9)

Intrinsic and hypothenar muscle paralysis with muscle wasting and loss of digital abduction and adduction may also occur. Bouvier sign, the inability to actively extend the IP joint on passive flexion of the MCP joint, is also present.

Ulnar neuropathy in bicyclists is a common overuse injury. Patients experience insidious onset of numbness, weakness, and loss of coordination in one or both hands, usually after several days of cycling. The most common sites are the ring and little fingers on the ulnar side. To prevent this problem, cyclists should wear padded gloves and a pad on the handlebars. In addition, the top bar of the handlebar should be level with the top of the saddle. If symptoms continue, these individuals must stop riding.

Radial Nerve Injury

The radial nerve supplies little sensory innervation to the hand, and its motor contribution is primarily wrist extension. Refer to Chapter 8 for further discussion of radial nerve injury.

Median Nerve Injury

Lacerations to the motor branches of the median nerve require repair by a hand surgeon. Median nerve injury commonly occurs at the wrist. Refer to Chapter 8 for further discussion of median nerve injury.

Neuroma

Neuromas are composed of disorganized axons interwoven with scar tissue. They may be quite painful, particularly when they occur over pressure points. Neuromas usually occur after injury to the nerve when the nerve remains intact. Neuromas may follow years after an injury. When the sensory branches of a nerve are involved, neuromas can be very painful and often enlarge insidiously.

The most common sites of neuromas are the sensory branches of the radial nerve at the distal third of the forearm and the wrist. A neuroma in this area may follow trivial trauma that the patient may not recall. Other common sites are the main median nerve, the palmar cutaneous branches at the wrist, and the main ulnar nerve with its dorsal sensory branches to the wrist. The treatment usually depends on how symptomatic the patient is and may include surgical intervention.

Vascular Injuries

Vascular injury is often caused by repetitive trauma. The ulnar artery is susceptible to injury at the segment between the distal margin of the tunnel of Guyon and the palmar aponeurosis, where the superficial palmar arch begins. Repetitive impact among baseball catchers, touring cyclists, and handball players may cause an aneurysm with either thrombosis or vascular spasm. Symptoms of vascular injury include one or more cold digits, pain, intermittent mottling, and stiffness. An aneurysm may present with a mass.

Ligamentous Injuries and Dislocations

Ligamentous injuries to the hand are very common and often missed. The consequence of these injuries is chronic joint stiffness, pain, and swelling.

Collateral Ligament Injury

The collateral ligaments provide support against lateral displacement of the joints of the finger. On examination, one will note ecchymosis or localized tenderness to one or both sides of the IP joint. A vital part of the assessment is to check stability by *lateral stress tests* (Fig. 11–75 and Video 11–3) and active motion at the IP joints and the MCP joints of the hand. Stable joints that are painful on lateral stress testing indicate a partial tear or sprain of the collateral ligaments supporting the joint.

In performing a stress test of the collateral ligaments of the digits, one must always compare the same joint on the opposite hand. Minimal opening of a few millimeters with a good end point indicates that the collateral ligament is ruptured but the volar plate is intact. If one notices wide

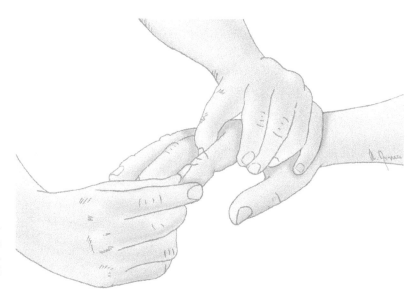

Figure 11–75. The lateral stress test is performed by holding the phalanx on either side of the joint and attempting to open the joint. Minimal opening indicates that the collateral ligament is ruptured on that side.

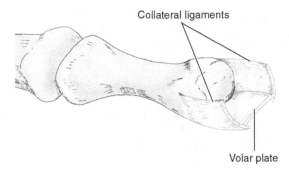

Figure 11–76. The collateral ligaments on either side of the joint and the volar plate form a boxlike support around the joint.

opening on stress testing, the volar plate must be ruptured because of the boxlike nature that the collateral ligaments and volar plate form around the joint (Fig. 11–76). Thus, wide opening indicates that both the collateral ligament and the volar plate are ruptured. Wide opening of the joint should be treated in a gutter splint and referred for assessment by a hand surgeon to determine whether surgical repair is necessary. Functional stability is evaluated by active motion. If the patient cannot perform motion due to pain, or stress testing is limited by pain, a digital block will facilitate the examination. Supplemental stress radiographs may be helpful in difficult cases.

If a partial tear is indicated by appropriate stress testing, as previously described, the treatment is rest with complete immobilization for 10 to 14 days in a malleable finger splint (Appendix A–2). Immobilization should be with the PIP joint splinted at 30 degrees of flexion and the MCP splinted at 45 degrees of flexion. When the thumb MCP is involved, it should be splinted in 30 degrees of flexion. After immobilization of the involved digit, active motion is encouraged for the remainder of the hand.

Capsular thickening and chronic swelling of the involved joint at the end of the immobilization period suggests the initial damage was greater than first believed and more protection is needed. This should be provided by buddy (dynamic) splinting the digit to the adjacent normal one for 5 to 7 days (Appendix A–2). The problem at this point is no longer instability, but stiffness, decrease in range of motion, and pain at the involved joint. Swelling may persist for several weeks after a sprain to the finger joints.

Acute complete ruptures require splinting for 3 to 5 weeks with the joint flexed 35 degrees, followed by guarded active motion with buddy splinting for protection for an additional 3 weeks.[80] Some authors prefer surgical repair of unstable injuries. Consultation with an orthopedist is indicated.

Distal Interphalangeal Joint Injuries

The DIP joint is stabilized by strong collateral accessory ligaments laterally and the fibrous plate volarly. Dorsal support is minimal and includes the extensor mechanism that blends with the dorsal capsule. The collateral ligaments are

thick, rectangular bands that arise laterally from the condyle and pass distally and volarly to insert into the volar lateral articular margin and the volar plate. The volar plate provides support to the distal joint and is square shaped and 2- to 3-mm thick.

Disruption of these ligamentous structures is only clinically important if it produces joint instability, which can be assessed by active motion and lateral stress testing. These tests are most valid under digital anesthesia after the reduction of a dislocation. If reduction is maintained through full range of motion, then adequate ligamentous support can be assumed and only 10 to 14 days of immobilization is needed. If, however, displacement occurs in the last 15 degrees of joint extension, then major disruption must be assumed and immobilization in 30 degrees of flexion for a full 3 weeks is indicated.

Dislocations are most commonly dorsal (Fig. 11–77). Reduction is by simple longitudinal traction and manipulation into its normal position (Video 11–4). Reduction is usually without complication; however, irreducible dislocations due to soft-tissue entrapment have been reported.[81,82]

Proximal Interphalangeal Joint Injuries

The integrity of the PIP joint is maintained by the two collateral ligaments on either side and the volar plate on the volar aspect, which together form a boxlike support around the joint (Fig. 11–76). For instability to occur at the joint, there must be disruption of two of these three supporting structures. The PIP joint is prone to develop stiffness after injury, even with good immobilization, and this complication should be communicated to the patient.

There are three types of injuries that occur at the PIP joint:

- Dislocations: dorsal (common), volar (rare), and lateral
- Volar plate injuries
- Fracture dislocations

PIP Joint Dislocation. Lateral dislocations are classified as collateral ligament injuries (rupture) because spontaneous reduction is the rule here. Dorsal dislocations of the PIP joint are quite common, whereas volar (palmar) dislocations are rare (Fig. 11–78). Volar dislocations are invariably associated with disruption of the central slip of the extensor tendon from its insertion at the base of the middle phalanx.[83]

Dorsal dislocations are caused by hyperextension of the PIP joint such as occurs when the outstretched finger is struck by a ball. For this injury to occur, there must be rupture of the volar plate or collateral ligaments. Lateral dislocations are caused by abduction or adduction stresses to the finger, usually while it is in the extended position. The radial collateral ligament is more commonly injured than the ulnar collateral. Volar dislocations are caused by a combination of (1) varus or valgus forces causing a rupture of the collateral ligament and the volar plate and (2) an anteriorly directed force displacing the base of the middle

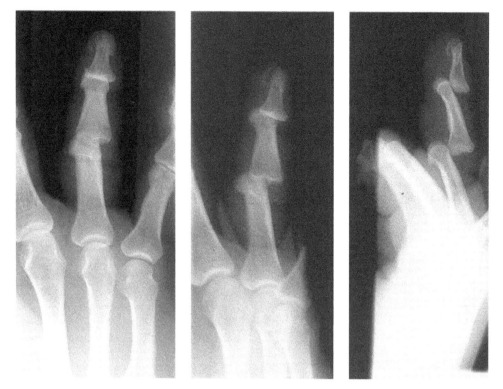

Figure 11–77. Dorsal dislocation of both the PIP and DIP joints.

phalanx forward and rupturing the central slip of the extensor mechanism.

Acute swelling and pain may camouflage a dislocation; however, this is not often the case and the deformity is usually obvious. A radiograph of the digit should be obtained before reduction is performed. Following reduction, the emergency physician should examine the collateral ligaments and the volar plate by stress testing to assess the full extent of the injury.

If there is suspicion of rupture of the collateral ligament or a questionable examination, stress views may be taken and compared with the normal side.

A dorsal dislocations is reduced by longitudinal traction and manipulation back to its normal position (Fig. 11–79 and Video 11–5A and B). This may require some initial hyperextension, which avoids entrapment of the torn volar plate. If the joint is stable, after reduction, then early motion (dynamic splinting) is indicated after an initial period of immobilization. If unstable, then it is splinted for 3 weeks with the PIP joint in 15 degrees of flexion, after which an extension block splint should be used for an additional 3 weeks.

Volar dislocations are usually easily reduced, but are commonly associated with a boutonniere deformity, which results when the central slip ruptures. The volar plate or collateral ligament may also be injured. Because surgical intervention may be needed, referral is indicated.

Irreducible dislocations are uncommon, but may occur with any of the aforementioned dislocations. In most cases, soft tissue or a bony fragment becomes interposed in the joint space and blocks reduction of the dislocation. This is suspected in any case in which one or two attempts at reduction prove unsuccessful. These cases may require open reduction to extract and repair the interposed ligament, tendon, or volar plate.

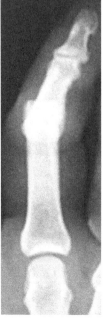

Figure 11–78. Volar dislocation of the PIP joint of the finger.

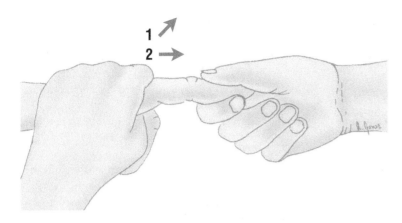

Figure 11–79. Interphalangeal joints are reduced with initial gentle hyperextension (*arrow 1*) and then longitudinal traction (*arrow 2*). Hyperextension will aid in the reduction and help avoid trapping the volar plate.

Open dislocations require antibiotic therapy and thorough debridement (Fig. 11–80). One study of 18 open dislocations of the PIP joint suggested that these injuries are best cared for in the operating room because treatment in the ED is associated with a poorer prognosis.[87] Repair of the collateral ligaments and reattachment of the volar plate are performed as needed.

The complications of PIP joint injuries and dislocations are restricted joint motion, which is a common sequel. The most common complication is *persistent thickening* of the PIP joint. Volar plate and collateral ligament instability are further problems.

PIP Joint Volar Plate Injury. The volar plate of the PIP joint may be ruptured when a blow occurs at the end of the finger, causing a hyperextension force. The volar plate may be torn from its distal attachment at the base of the middle phalanx, and a small piece of bone may be avulsed with it.

Injuries to the volar plate will cause a hyperextension deformity at the PIP joint on extension of the finger, whereas pain and catching or locking is noted with flexion of the digit. If the hyperextension deformity is severe, the patient may have a compensatory flexion deformity of the DIP joint secondary to the action of the FDP tendon (swan-neck deformity). Maximal tenderness is observed over the volar aspect of the finger joint, and pain is increased on passive hyperextension and relieved by passive flexion. In addition, there is loss of the normal end point of finger extension provided by an intact volar plate. To perform an adequate examination, a digital or metacarpal block is usually indicated.

Radiographs in patients with a volar plate avulsion may reveal a small bone fragment avulsed from the base of the middle phalanx.

Volar plate injuries are treated with splinting the PIP joint in 30 degrees of flexion for 3 to 5 weeks.

PIP Joint Fracture Dislocation. Fracture dislocations occur when the extended finger is struck in such a way that longitudinal compression occurs along with hyperextension. The end result is a fracture through the volar lip of the middle phalanx and dorsal displacement of the middle phalanx and distal portion of the finger. This commonly occurs when the extended finger is struck by a ball.[88]

Patients with fracture dislocations are unable to flex the PIP joint and have swelling, pain, and deformity. On radiographs, there is dorsal subluxation of the middle phalanx with a fracture of the volar lip of the middle phalanx that may involve up to one-third of the articular surface.

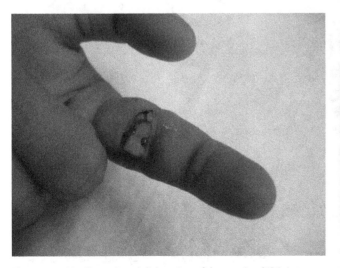
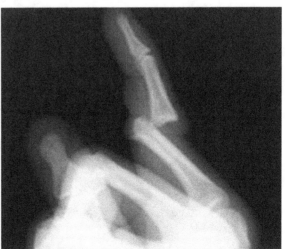

Figure 11–80. Open dorsal dislocation of the proximal IP joint.

Fracture dislocations may be reduced as per the routine method. If the fragment is large or unstable, open reduction and fixation are indicated. All of these injuries should be referred.

Metacarpophalangeal Joint Injuries

The MCP joints are condyloid joints that have, in addition to flexion and extension, as much as 30 degrees of lateral motion while the joint is extended. Because of the shape of this articulation, the joint is more stable in flexion when the collateral ligaments are stretched than in extension.

Collateral ligament and volar plate injuries of the MCP joint usually occur with hyperextension stresses applied to the MCP joint with the finger extended. The patient presents with massive ecchymosis and swelling of the joint. The radiograph is usually negative, but an avulsion fracture may be noted. The treatment of this injury is a gentle compressive dressing with light plaster reinforcement. These patients may require prolonged immobilization depending on the degree of injury and are referred for follow-up care. Nondisplaced fractures due to collateral ligament avulsion can be treated conservatively if the fragment involves less than 25% of the articular surface.

Dislocations. Dislocations at the MCP joint are usually dorsal (Fig. 11–81). The complex anatomy of the MCP joint protects against dislocation, but also leads to a higher incidence of irreducible dislocations. There are two types of dorsal MCP joint dislocations: simple and complex.

Simple dorsal dislocations have a dramatic appearance clinically, with the MCP joint held in 60 to 90 degrees of hyperextension and the finger ulnar-deviated. The index finger is most commonly involved and the metacarpal head is prominent. This dislocation is usually reduced with closed techniques. Reduction is achieved by further hyperextension of the MCP joint, followed by dorsal pressure at the base of the proximal phalanx. Longitudinal traction may convert a simple dislocation into a complex one. After successful reduction, immobilize the MCP joint in 60 degrees of flexion.

Complex dorsal dislocations appear subtle clinically, with the proximal phalanx nearly parallel to the metacarpal. Other findings include a palpable metacarpal head on the volar surface with dimpling of the palmar skin. They are often impossible to reduce with closed techniques due to the interposition of the volar plate and the arrangement of ligaments and lumbrical muscles that actually tighten around the head of the metacarpal as traction is applied.

Subluxation at the MCP joint occurs when the proximal phalanx is locked in hyperextension and the articular surfaces are in partial contact. Reduction is performed by flexion of the digit after longitudinal traction using finger traps with 5 lb of weight applied to disengage the proximal phalanx.

Carpometacarpal Joint Injuries

These rare injuries are caused by forceful dorsiflexion combined with a longitudinal impact. Dorsal dislocation is most common (Figs. 11–82 and 11–83). A high-energy force is required, and this injury is more common in boxers or after motorcycle crashes. Examination reveals considerable swelling in the dorsum of the hand that may cause

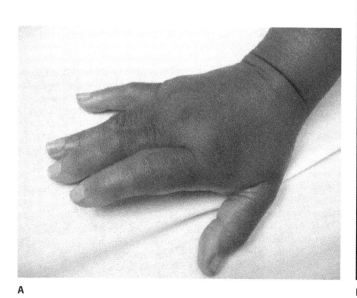

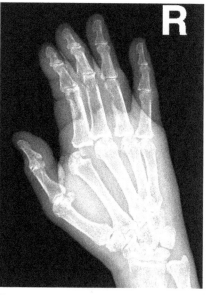

A   **B**

Figure 11–81. Complex MCP joint dislocation of the second digit. This dislocation could not be reduced by closed methods. **A.** Note the subtle appearance of this dislocation. **B.** Radiograph.

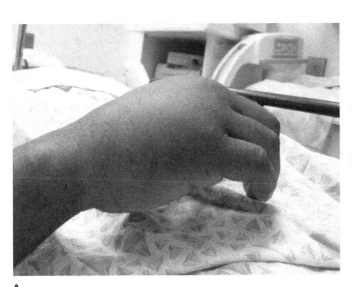

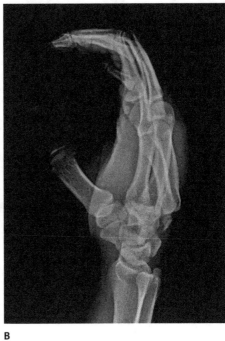

A

B

Figure 11–82. Carpometacarpal dislocation of the fourth and fifth digits. ***A.*** Acutely, swelling obscures the diagnosis of this injury. ***B.*** The lateral radiograph demonstrates this dislocation best.

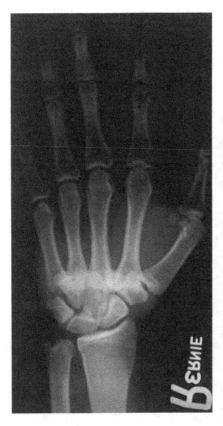

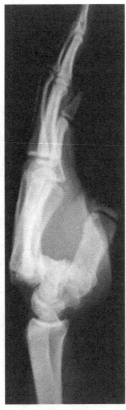

Figure 11–83. A rare posterior dislocation of all of the carpometacarpal joints.

the diagnosis to go undetected. When swelling is not as severe, the proximal metacarpals are palpated dorsally. Treatment includes reduction by traction with manipulation of the proximal metacarpal to its normal position (Video 11–6). The hand is immobilized (Appendix A–11), and the patient is referred. Unsuccessful or unstable closed reductions require open reduction and fixation. Complications include hand compartment syndrome, chronic stiffness, and nerve injury.

Thumb Ligamentous Injuries and Dislocations

IP joint injuries of the thumb are handled similarly to distal IP joint injuries of the fingers. The most common injury is a dorsal dislocation, and these injuries are often open. Reduction is usually simple after a median nerve block. The joint usually remains stable because the volar plate remains attached to the distal phalanx. The joint is immobilized for 3 weeks in slight flexion.

The MCP joint of the thumb is very mobile, and dislocations here are quite common (Fig. 11–84). The collateral ligaments are thick and provide good support for the joint. The volar plate contains two sesamoid bones that serve as the insertions for the flexor pollicis brevis (radial sesamoid) and the adductor pollicis (ulnar sesamoid). Because of the mobility of this joint, dislocations here are far more common than at the digits and are of two types, dorsal and lateral, each with equal frequency.

Dorsal dislocation of the thumb MCP joint occurs with extreme hyperextension or shearing forces, and disruption of the volar-supporting structures almost always occurs.

Displacement varies from a subluxation of the phalanx to complete dislocation with the proximal phalanx resting over the metacarpal head. For the latter to occur, the volar plate and the collaterals must completely tear. When dislocation is associated with this degree of disruption of the supporting structures, reduction is usually easy and proceeds as follows: Flexion of the metacarpal relaxes the muscles, and extension of the IP joint tightens the flexor tendon. Longitudinal traction is then applied until distraction occurs and the MCP joint is flexed. After reduction, the digit is splinted for 3 weeks in flexion. If there is more than 40 degrees of lateral instability, surgical repair may be indicated. The amount of instability must always be assessed after reduction.

Lateral dislocations of the thumb MCP joint present with only local pain and swelling because they frequently have spontaneously reduced. To diagnose this injury, perform stress examinations of the ulnar and radial collateral ligaments of the thumb.

Trapezio-Metacarpal Joint Injuries

Dislocation of the trapezio-metacarpal joint of the thumb is an uncommon injury (Fig. 11–85). The mechanism is usually indirect, where a longitudinal force is directed along the axis of the thumb with the joint in flexion. Associated injuries include carpal and metacarpal fractures. Treatment is immediate reduction followed by immobilization in a short thumb spica splint (Appendix A–7) initially, and then a cast (Appendix A–6) for 6 weeks. Failure to maintain closed reduction or delayed presentation warrants fixation with percutaneous pinning.

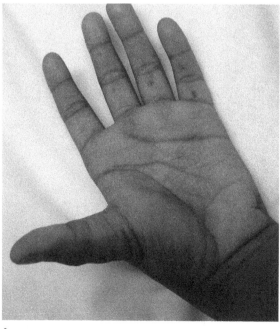
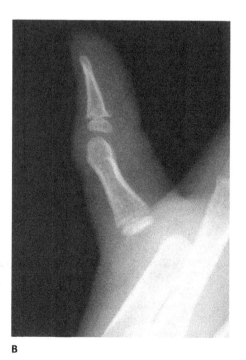

A   B

Figure 11–84. MCP dislocation of the thumb. **A.** Clinical photo. **B.** Radiograph.

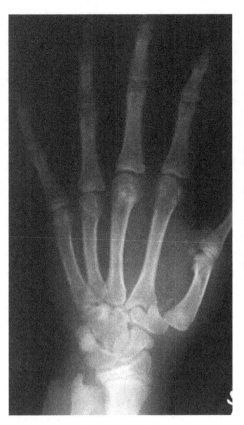
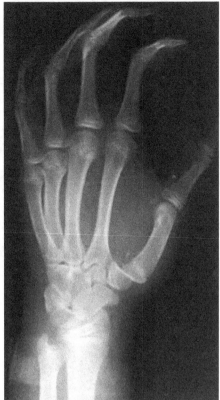

Figure 11–85. Carpometacarpal dislocation of the thumb.

Gamekeeper's Thumb

Ulnar collateral ligament rupture is 10 times more common than injury to the collateral ligament on the radial side. This injury can be very disabling, whereby the patient has a weak pinch and cannot resist an adduction stress. This injury is called gamekeeper's thumb based on a description of ulnar collateral ligament laxity in Scottish gamekeepers due to their method of breaking the necks of wounded hares.[89] It is also seen commonly in skiers (skier's thumb) who have fallen where the ski pole abducts the thumb at the MCP joint. If this injury is missed, it may result in significant disability.

To diagnose ulnar collateral ligament injury, the examiner provides a radial-directed stress with the MCP joint in flexion (Fig. 11–86). Flexion allows the volar plate to relax and makes the test more sensitive. The degree of opening is compared with the normal side. Whether a partial or complete tear is suspected, the patient is placed in a thumb spica splint. A radiograph should be obtained, especially after acute injuries, to exclude an avulsion fracture at the base of the proximal phalanx, "gamekeeper's fracture" (Fig. 11–87).

Definitive treatment depends on the degree of joint opening present. If the joint opens <20 degrees, no surgically correctable instability exists. The thumb should be splinted in the position of function for 3 weeks. If there is >20 degrees of instability, the patient is referred for repair of this ligament. Unfortunately, when >20 degrees of instability exists,

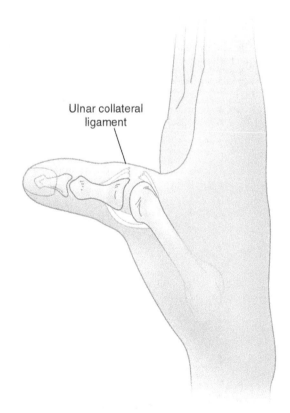

Ulnar collateral
ligament

Figure 11–86. Examining for disruption of the ulnar collateral ligament of the thumb at the MCP joint.

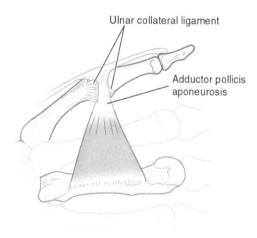

Figure 11–87. Avulsion fracture in a patient with Gamekeeper's thumb.

splinting alone is ineffective in two-thirds of cases because the aponeurosis of the adductor pollicis becomes interposed between the ends of the disrupted ligament and the ligament cannot heal (Fig. 11–88).

Although some surgeons believe that 40 degrees of opening can be treated without surgery, we recommend that all those with >20 degrees of opening at the joint be referred.

Ulnar collateral ligament

Adductor pollicis
aponeurosis

Figure 11–88. If the aponeurosis of the adductor pollicis of the thumb becomes interspersed between the two ruptured ends of the ulnar collateral ligament, healing will not occur.

Patients with gamekeeper's thumb have been successfully treated with a special thumb splint designed to reduce motion simulating the injury. Surgical ligamentous reconstruction has been shown to be effective in achieving painless stability, even if delayed for years after the injury.

OVERUSE INJURIES

Myositis
Muscle soreness in the hand can occur with activity in an unconditioned patient. Treatment generally consists of rest, nonsteroidal anti-inflammatory agents, and future avoidance of similar activity. If the pain and soreness persist, other sources such as strains, sprains, stress fractures, or chronic exertional compartment syndrome are considered.

Tendonitis
Tendonitis is present when active and passive tension of the tendons accentuates the pain. The tenderness is usually well localized over the involved tendon. The condition may occur de novo, but usually presents after repetitive stress of the involved tendon. Swelling and erythema are infrequent with simple tendonitis. When the flexors of the digits are involved, the tenderness is most often over the MCP joint area. The treatment is local injection with a steroid, which affords excellent relief.

Tenosynovitis generally occurs without a recognized precipitating cause; however, a history of excessive stress on the tendon is often obtained. The most common site for this form of tendonitis is the extensor tendon sheath. On examination, the patient has a soft, nontender, diffuse subcutaneous swelling over the base of the hand confined to the area proximal to the extensor retinaculum. In some cases, one may get a dumbbell deformity with swelling seen on either side of the extensor retinaculum. The same condition may be seen with the flexors but is often not recognized due to the fat padding and the thickened skin of the palm. Commonly, the flexor tendons distal to the MCP joint are affected, and this is easily recognized. The treatment for this form is rest and injection with steroids. Steroid injection usually affords prompt relief. A change in any precipitating activity is advisable.

Tendonitis involving the extensor tendons usually affects one of the six extensor tendon compartments. Tendonitis within the first compartment, containing the abductor pollicis longus and extensor pollicis brevis, is referred to as de Quervain tenosynovitis. Further discussion of this condition is provided in Chapter 8. Intersection syndrome is a more proximal tendonitis within the second extensor compartment commonly seen in rowers and weightlifters. Tendonitis within the third compartment affecting the extensor pollicis longus is rare, but when it does occur, it is usually at Lister tubercle. This may occur after a Colles fracture. Patients with tendonitis of the extensor digiti indicis (fourth) or minimi (fifth) present with pain at the wrist that can be reproduced by full passive flexion of the wrist. Patients who present with stenosing tenosynovitis of the extensor carpi ulnaris tendon (sixth) often require surgical release.

Flexor carpi ulnaris tendonitis may be bilateral and may require surgical excision of the pisiform. Flexor carpi radialis tendonitis causes local tenderness just proximal to the thenar eminence and pain with radial wrist deviation.[93] Patients who have flexor tendonitis of the digits present with a stabbing or burning pain proximal to the carpal tunnel that mimics carpal tunnel syndrome.

Bowler's Thumb

This condition is due to perineural fibrosis that is caused by compression of the ulnar digital nerve of the thumb. Classically, this condition results due to adaptive changes in response to chronic insertion and compression of the thumb while grasping a bowling ball. Other activities, such as baseball, and occupational injuries have been implicated. An acute form of bowler's thumb has also been described.[95] Patients complain of tingling and hyperesthesia at the pulp of the thumb. Usually, a tender, palpable lump is present on the ulnar side of the thumb.

Trigger Finger

This condition, also known as stenosing tenosynovitis, is an idiopathic condition that occurs more commonly in middle-aged women. A secondary form occurs in patients with connective tissue disorders. Clinical findings include painful blocking of flexion and extension when a nodule on a flexor tendon catches on the tendon pulley at the MCP joint. At times, the patient complains only about the PIP joint, which is the site of referred pain from the proximal flexor pulley.

The ring and long fingers are the most commonly involved digits, but any digit may be affected, including the thumb. Active closing of the fist reproduces locking or snapping as the tendon slides through the pulley (Fig. 11–89 and Video 11–7). If the swelling is proximal to the pulley, then the digit can flex but not extend easily. However, if the swelling is distal to the pulley, then the digit can passively, but not actively, flex.

Two types of trigger finger occur: diffuse and nodular.[96,97] The distinction is made based on the findings of physical examination. The nodular type is more common and responds to steroid injection with a success rate of 93%.[96,98] For the diffuse type, the success rate of steroid injection is less impressive with only half of patients showing improvement.[97]

Radiographs should not be obtained because they do not change management.[99] Treatment consists of massage, ice, nonsteroidal anti-inflammatory medications, and splinting. If the digit is locked, surgical intervention is often required. For lesser degrees of triggering, an injection of lidocaine (1 mL) and triamcinolone 40 mg/mL (0.5 mL) into the tendon sheath is recommended. Some authors prefer betamethasone because it is water soluble and, therefore, less likely to cause tenosynovitis or leave a residue in the tendon sheath. The

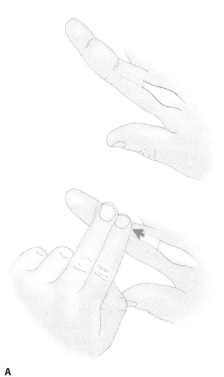

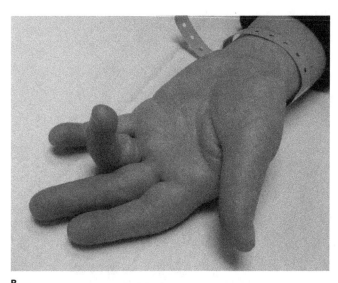

A   **B**

Figure 11–89. **A.** Trigger finger occurs when a fibrous thickening of the tendon does not allow it to slide through the pulley. **B.** Clinical photo of a finger locked in place due to trigger finger.

most common site of injection is over the palpable nodule on the palmar aspect of the palm in the region of the metacarpal head. After inserting a 25-gauge needle, the patient is asked to move the finger. Slight grating of the needle will be felt, but paradoxical motion of the needle and syringe suggests the needle is in the tendon and should be withdrawn. A more proximal palmar approach may also be used, but is believed to be more painful and thus not recommended. Ultrasound-guided injection has proven to be very useful.

Following the injection, extension of the finger is usually possible. The MCP joint should be splinted in extension with free motion of the PIP and DIP joints. This will allow the nodule to rest underneath the flexor tendon pulley. A removable splint is worn for 7 to 10 days (Appendix A–2).

Appropriate follow-up should be arranged because repeat injections and/or surgical release may be required.

PYOGENIC GRANULOMA

This is a benign type of granulomatous vascular tumor that occurs frequently on the volar pulp or periungual area of a digit (Fig. 11–90). It is a solitary, pedunculated or sessile structure that bleeds easily with minimal trauma. It is minimally painful. Pyogenic granulomas often develop over a period of 1 to 3 months at a site where previous injury or foreign-body penetration has occurred. The size of the granuloma may be up to 2 cm in diameter, but is usually approximately 3 to 5 mm. The origin of pyogenic granulomas is unclear, although it is believed they represent a disorder of angiogenesis.

Removal of larger lesions is the treatment of choice. Various methods have been described, including silver nitrate application, electrocautery, avulsion, and surgical excision. One method for removal is described as follows:

1. A digital tourniquet is placed.
2. The lesion is excised flush with the surface of the skin.

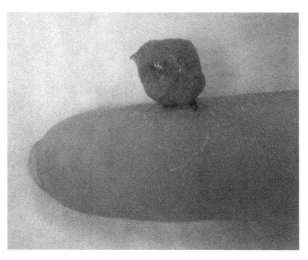

Figure 11–90. Pyogenic granuloma.

3. The base of the lesion is cauterized with silver nitrate applicators.
4. Following removal, the patient is instructed to keep the lesion dry for 2 weeks. The lesion is allowed to heal by secondary intention.

This method had a 85% success rate in one study, but required more than one treatment in most cases.   Recurrence is less likely with complete surgical removal, leaving a margin of normal tissue.

INFECTIONS

Many things favor the development of infections in the hand, including retained foreign bodies, tight dressings around wounds, or congestive states following fractures. *Staphylococcus aureus* is isolated from 50% of all hand infections, followed by β-hemolytic *Streptococcus*, which accounts for 15% (Table 11–1). Other common organisms are *Aerobacter aerogenes*, *Enterococcus*, and *Escherichia coli*. *Eikenella corrodens* is an organism that is isolated from approximately one-third of human bite wounds. *Pasteurella multocida*, a facultative anaerobe, is present in the oral flora of approximately two-thirds of domestic cats and one-half of dogs.   Infection with these organisms is usually rapid and associated with significant cellulitis and lymphangitis. Multiple organisms, however, are isolated from 70% of all hand infections. Rapid inflammation occurring within hours usually indicates that *Streptococcus* is the infecting organism in contrast with *S aureus*, which usually takes several days to develop into an infection. The hallmarks of infection in the hand are warmth, erythema, and pain. Swelling and tenderness are other signs. Infections involving the tendons cause a limitation of motion and tenderness over the involved tendon.

▶ TABLE 11–1. **COMMON PATHOGENS IN HAND INFECTIONS**

Infection	Most Likely Organism
Felon	*Staphylococcus aureus*, oral anaerobes
Flexor tenosynovitis	*S aureus*, *Streptococci*, gram-negative bacteria
Herpetic whitlow	Herpes simplex 1 and 2
Deep space infection	*S aureus*, anaerobes, gram-negative bacteria
Cellulitis	*Streptococcus* spp.
IV drug user	Gram-positive and -negative, anaerobes, *S aureus*
Human bite	*S aureus*, *Eikenella corrodens*, anaerobes
Animal bite	*Pasteurella*, gram-positive cocci, anaerobes

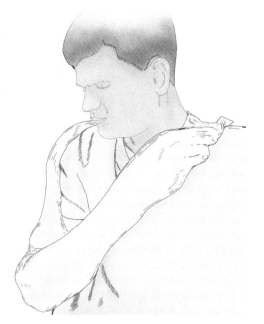

Figure 11–91. A dressing used for elevation of the hand. The stockinette is applied along the entire upper extremity and cut at both ends to form a "Y." The stockinette is fitted onto the upper extremity and the ends are then tied together.

The mainstay of treatment of any hand infection includes splinting and elevation as well as appropriate antibiotics. Antibiotic choices have changed recently with the surge in cases of community-acquired methicillin-resistant *S aureus* (MRSA). Clindamycin or Bactrim (sulfamethoxazole and trimethoprim) are good initial options for patients who will likely be discharged. In more serious infections, vancomycin should be considered. Augmentin remains the antibiotic of choice for both human and animal bites. The clinician should be familiar with bacterial sensitivity patterns within their community and

institution. Wound cultures should be obtained in any ill patient whenever fluid is available.

Elevation of the hand can be accomplished by using a stockinette (Fig. 11–91). This is an inexpensive dressing and works far better than a sling for elevating the hand. Tetanus prophylaxis must be administered when any wound is noted in patients not already immunized. Splinting should be in a position permitting maximal drainage for all hand infections (Appendix A–5).

Furuncle or Carbuncle

Furuncles or carbuncles of the hand are common and occur over hair-bearing regions (Fig. 11–92A). These infections are usually caused by *S aureus* and, when seen early, may be treated with rest, immobilization, elevation, and systemic antibiotics. Once the abscess is well localized, drainage occurs either spontaneously or through a small incision made over the point of maximal fluctuance with an 11-blade scalpel. Applying warm compresses facilitates drainage. If these infections are not treated adequately, they may lead to cellulitis of the hand.

Cellulitis

Cellulitis can occur after an abrasion and/or a puncture, or with any wound of the hand that has been inadequately immobilized or neglected (Fig. 11–92B). This infection is commonly found in intravenous drug users. Cellulitis may develop rapidly or slowly, depending on the offending agent. The hand should be immobilized to control congestion and the limb is elevated. In cases where the cellulitis is progressing rapidly over a period of hours, operative intervention must be considered because of the likelihood of a necrotizing soft-tissue infection. Necrotizing soft-tissue infections require immediate decompression and debridement as well as intravenous antibiotics. Patients with cellulitis of the hand that compromises function should be admitted.

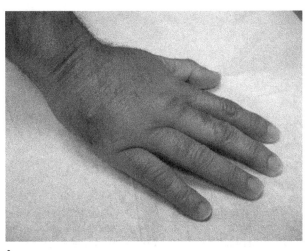

A

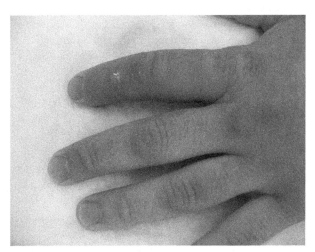

B

Figure 11–92. **A.** Carbuncle on the dorsum of the hand. **B.** Cellulitis of the second digit.

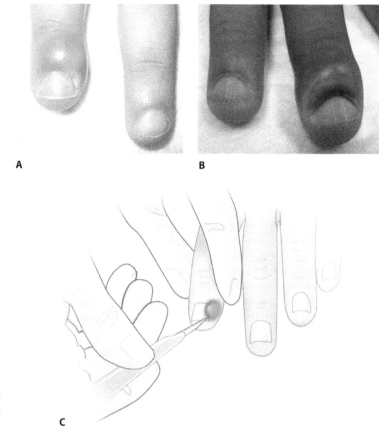

Figure 11–93. **A.** Paronychia. **B.** Eponychia (compare to the normal digit). **C.** Drainage of a paronychia.

Paronychia and Eponychia

A *paronychia* is an infection of the fold of the nail on the radial or ulnar side (Fig. 11–93A). The term *eponychia* is used when there is involvement of the basal fold of the nail (Fig. 11–93B). These may be associated with cellulitis when the infection extends proximally into the tissues around the nail fold. The typical patient comes into the ED with an abscess well localized around the nail fold or at the base of the nail. Most of these are due to staphylococcal infection and are treated by incision and drainage. An 11-blade scalpel is used and the "incision" is carried out by holding the blade against the nail and entering the abscess through the nail fold (Fig. 11–93C and Video 11–8). The nail fold is simply uplifted off the nail and drainage occurs. The patient should be advised to continue warm soaks. If cellulitis is present proximally, the patient is prescribed oral antibiotics.

If this condition is not treated appropriately, a subungual abscess or felon may develop. A subungual abscess floats the fingernail off its bed and is drained by removing the base of the fingernail under digital block anesthesia. The distal nail plate is not usually excised. A tiny loose pack of fine meshed gauze is inserted to separate the matrix from the eponychial fold for a few days.

Felon

A *felon* is a subcutaneous abscess of the pulp space of the distal fingertip (Fig. 11–94A). This infection resides within the vertically oriented fibrous septa that originate on the periosteum and insert on the skin. Left untreated, this infection may spread, infecting the distal phalanx or the flexor tendon sheath. Clinically, there is a rapid onset of throbbing pain and swelling distal to the DIP joint.

Early infection is treated by elevation, oral antibiotics, and warm soaks alone, although most patients present later and require drainage. Incision and drainage should be at the *point of maximum tenderness* in these infections. There is some controversy regarding the best incision to treat a felon. A longitudinal midline incision, which spares the flexion crease (Fig. 11–94B) avoids injury to the vessels and the digital nerves. The scalpel is used to penetrate the dermis only, and a mosquito hemostat is used to gently dissect the soft tissues until the abscess cavity is drained. Controversy remains about the painful scar in the pulp of the finger. A unilateral longitudinal incision ("high lateral") is also acceptable if fluctuance is noted laterally, but care must be taken to avoid injury to the terminal branches of the digital nerves. A rule of thumb is to bend the DIP joint and the upper extent of the flexion fold defines how high the incision should be. Lower than that puts the neurovascular structures at risk. Other incisions for this common problem have been advocated (fish-mouth, through-and-through, transverse palmar, hockey-stick), all of which invoke necrosis and

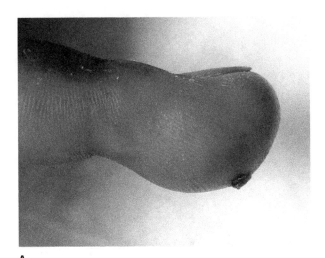

A

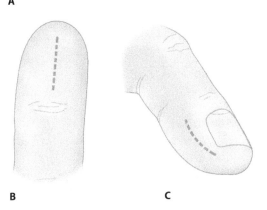

B   C

Figure 11–94. **A.** Felon. **B.** Drainage via the longitudinal incision. **C.** Drainage via a high lateral incision.

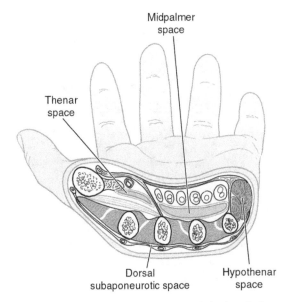

Figure 11–95. Cross-sectional anatomy of the hand, demonstrating the thenar, midpalmar, hypothenar, and dorsal subaponeurotic spaces.

ischemia, lead to anesthesia of the tip of the digit, and produce a more painful scar than the midline incision.

Following drainage, the finger is dressed and splinted, and the patient is started on a course of antibiotics for 10 days. The patient is instructed to elevate the finger for 48 hours. At this time, the dressing is removed, the wound reexamined, and twice-a-day dressing changes with saline soaks are begun. The wound is allowed to heal secondarily.

Deep Space Infections

There are five potential spaces located deep inside the hand that represent potential sites of infection (Fig. 11–95). These infections, referred to as deep subfascial space infections, represent 5% to 15% of all hand infections. The emergency physician should distinguish between infections of the web space, midpalmar space, dorsal aponeurotic space, thenar space, and hypothenar space.

Web Space Infection

Interdigital web space infections present with painful swelling of the web space and distal palmar regions (Fig. 11–96A). Pain and swelling are noted on both the dorsal and the volar surfaces, giving the abscess an hourglass appearance, but are usually more significant on the dorsum. Depending on the degree of swelling, the fingers may be abducted. These infections are also known as a *collar button abscess* and are most often caused by a puncture wound to the web space.

Treatment includes drainage by making an incision on the dorsal and volar aspects of the abscess, ensuring the incision does not cross the web space between the fingers to avoid the development of future dysfunction[110] (Fig. 11–97). Longitudinal incisions on both the volar and the dorsal aspects of the abscess have been described, along with a combination of a longitudinal dorsal incision and an X-shaped volar incision. This infection often leads to stiffness at the MCP joint, unless treated early with incision and drainage, elevation, and antibiotics. Hand consultation for this infection is appropriate.

Midpalmar Space Infection

Infection here is secondary to (1) extension of an infection from the adjacent flexor sheaths or (2) a puncture wound of the palm of the hand. The palmar fascia is under great tension, and maximal edema forms over the dorsum of the hand. However, the point of maximal tenderness is the midpalm. The concavity of the palm is lost. This abscess requires immediate drainage in the operating room.

Dorsal Subaponeurotic Space Infection

The dorsum of the hand is covered by loose, redundant skin that permits significant edema to accumulate from any of the infections occurring elsewhere in the hand. This dorsal edema must be differentiated from infections along the dorsum of the hand, namely the subaponeurotic space that is contained by extensor tendons and the metacarpals. Infection on the dorsum of the hand due to a subcutaneous

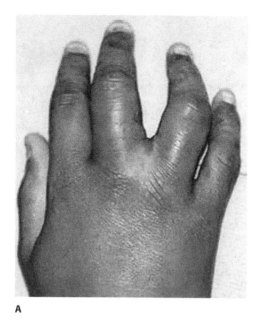
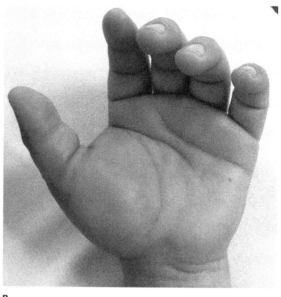

A   **B**

Figure 11–96. **A.** Web space (collar button) abscess (*Used with permission from Kyle Jeray, MD.*) **B.** Thenar space infection.

abscess or a subaponeurotic space infection is accompanied by tenderness, which is not present with simple dorsal edema. These infections usually require drainage through multiple incisions and hand consultation.

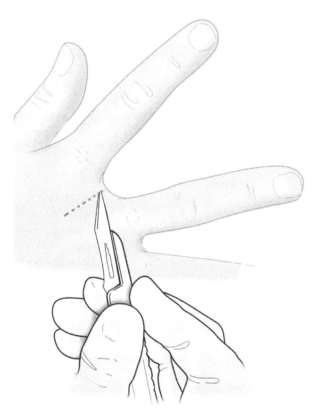

Figure 11–97. A web space infection should be drained by a longitudinal dorsal incision between the fingers.

Thenar Space Infection

This infection is diagnosed by noting considerable thenar and first web space swelling and tenderness (Fig. 11–96B). The patient will abduct the thumb because the volume within the thenar space is greatest in this position. The examiner will also elicit pain with passive adduction or opposition. These infections usually require drainage through multiple incisions and hand consultation.

Hypothenar Space Infection

This infection is extremely rare. Swelling and tenderness are noted at the hypothenar eminence. Treatment involves a longitudinal incision on the ulnar aspect of the palm and is best performed by a consulting hand surgeon.

Flexor Tenosynovitis

The flexor tendons are covered by a closed tendon sheath and bursae that may become infected by puncture wounds or lacerations (Fig. 11–98). The joint creases, where the tendon and its surrounding sheath are in close proximity to the skin, are particularly susceptible. *Streptococcus* and *S aureus* are the most common infecting agents. Disseminated gonorrhea should be considered in sexually active patients without a history of trauma. Because there is no obstruction to spread the infection, usually the entire tendon sheath becomes involved.

Kanavel described four cardinal signs of acute flexor tenosynovitis that are usually present (Fig. 11–99):

- Excessive tenderness over the course of the tendon sheath, limited to the sheath (Video 11–9)
- Symmetric enlargement of the whole finger
- Excruciating pain on passively extending the finger, along the entire sheath
- Flexed resting position of the finger

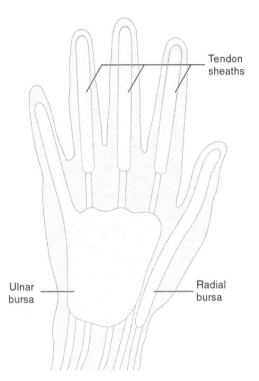

Figure 11–98. Flexor tendon sheaths of the hand. Note that the flexor sheath of the flexor pollicis longus communicates with the radial bursa and the sheath of the little finger communicates with the ulnar bursa.

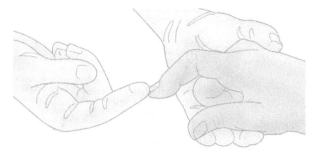

Figure 11–100. Testing for acute suppurative flexor tenosynovitis. Uplifting the nail of the involved digit without palpating the tendon causes exquisite pain.

Passive extension of the finger stretches the involved synovial sac and results in pain. This is best accomplished by avoiding palpation of the finger directly and extending the finger by lifting up on the nail alone (Fig. 11–100).

These patients are splinted and the hand is elevated. Intravenous antibiotics are administered in the ED. Consultation with a hand surgeon is obtained, and the patient is admitted for intravenous antibiotics alone if the infection is early (within 24 hours). If the infection is well established or no improvement is seen with antibiotics, surgical treatment is necessary. Limited incisions and catheter irrigation alone are becoming more common

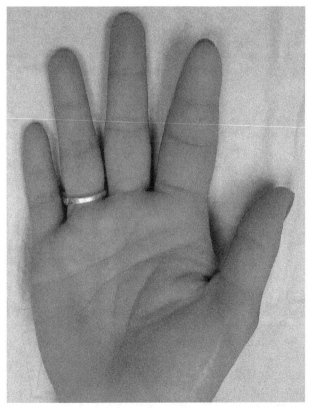

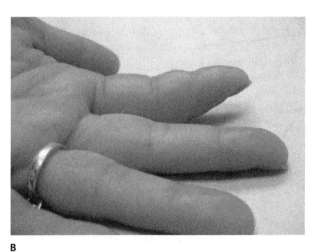

A   **B**

Figure 11–99. Flexor tenosynovitis of the second digit. **A.** Symmetric enlargement of the digit. **B.** Flexed resting position.

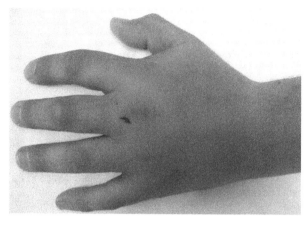

Figure 11–101. Infected fight bite injury over the middle-finger MCP joint.

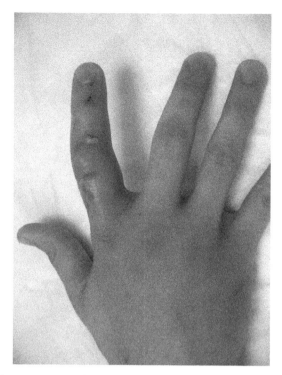

Figure 11–102. Infected finger due to an animal bite.

as a means to avoid more invasive surgery. If improperly treated, these infections may result in chronic tendon scarring or the development of a deep space infection of the hand.

Fight Bite Injuries

A human bite wound is a very serious injury, especially when it occurs over poorly vascularized tissues such as the ligaments, joints, or tendons in the hand. The overall incidence of infection for human bites is 10%. Although a variety of organisms are involved, the prime pathogens are anaerobic *Streptococcus* and *S aureus*.

Injuries to the hand, especially the MCP joint, following a fist fight, are typically referred to as "closed (clenched) fist" or "fight bite" injuries. Fight bites are self-sealing and prone to infection of the soft tissues, joint space, and tendon sheath. The additional challenge to the emergency physician is that the wound is small (3–5 mm) and may appear quite innocuous (Fig. 11–101). These wounds are treated with the utmost expediency and are never closed.

Radiographs are recommended in an effort to search for associated fractures, tooth fragments, or signs of osteomyelitis. Proper treatment of infected fight bite injuries involves debridement thorough irrigation, immobilization (Appendix A–5), elevation, and systemic antibiotics. Antibiotics include a β-lactamase inhibitor (ampicillinsulbactam) or a second-generation cephalosporin (cefoxitin). Admission for hospitalization and operative debridement are indicated if the wound is infected.

If the wound is not infected at the time of presentation, careful exploration of the wound in the ED is indicated. The wound must be carefully extended and explored to exclude tendon injury or joint involvement (Video 11–10). If these injuries are excluded, the patient may be managed conservatively on an outpatient basis. Irrigation is performed, and the wound is allowed to heal by secondary intention. Prophylactic antibiotics are administered and follow-up arranged in the next 1 to 2 days.

Animal Bites

Approximately half of all persons in the United States are bit by an animal at some point in their lifetime (Fig. 11–102). Dog bites are the most common animal-inflicted bite, accounting for 80% of the total and up to 1.5% of all ED visits. Approximately 15% to 20% of dog bite wounds become infected. Infection is more likely with deeper wounds, crush wounds, puncture wounds, and wounds on the hand. *P multocida*, *S aureus*, and anaerobic organisms account for most cases. Augmentin is the antibiotic of choice and is administered prophylactically for 3 to 7 days in high-risk wounds and for 2 weeks if cellulitis is present. Tetanus prophylaxis is administered as with any wound. Hospitalization is recommended in systemically ill patients, those with rapidly spreading cellulitis, or involvement of bone, joint, or tendon.

Domestic cat bites account for only 5% of all animal bites, but 50% will become infected due to cats' thin, sharp teeth that drive bacteria deep into tissues. Irrigation and debridement is recommended, and the wound is not closed primarily. The most common organism in cat bites is *P multocida*, but *Staphylococcus*, *Streptococcus*, and anaerobes are also seen. Augmentin is the antibiotic most commonly used for both prophylaxis and infection.

Rabies vaccination or animal quarantine for rabies evaluation should also be considered in an unprovoked attack.

REFERENCES

1. Hainline B. Nerve injuries. *Med Clin North Am*. 1994;78(2): 327–343.

2. Harrison BP, Hilliard MW. Emergency department evaluation and treatment of hand injuries. *Emerg Med Clin North Am*. 1999;17(4):793–822, v.

3. Swanson TV, Szabo RM, Anderson DD. Open hand fractures: prognosis and classification. *J Hand Surg [Am]*. 1991;16(1): 101–107.

4. McLain RF, Steyers C, Stoddard M. Infections in open fractures of the hand. *J Hand Surg [Am]* 1991;16(1):108–112.

5. Rajesh G, Ip WY, Chow SP, Fung BK. Dynamic treatment for proximal phalangeal fracture of the hand. *J Orthop Surg (Hong Kong)*. 2007;15(2):211–215.

6. Lee SG, Jupiter JB. Phalangeal and metacarpal fractures of the hand. *Hand Clin*. 2000;16(3):323–332, vii.

7. Kozin SH, Thoder JJ, Lieberman G. Operative treatment of metacarpal and phalangeal shaft fractures. *J Am Acad Orthop Surg*. 2000;8(2):111–121.

8. Batrick N, Hashemi K, Freij R. Treatment of uncomplicated subungual haematoma. *Emerg Med J*. 2003;20(1):65.

9. Seaberg DC, Angelos WJ, Paris PM. Treatment of subungual hematomas with nail trephination: a prospective study. *Am J Emerg Med*. 1991;9(3):209–210.

10. Strauss EJ, Weil WM, Jordan C, Paksima N. A prospective, randomized, controlled trial of 2-octylcyanoacrylate versus suture repair for nail bed injuries. *J Hand Surg Am*. 2008;33(2): 250–253.

11. Langlois J, Thevenin-Lemoine C, Rogier A, Elkaim M, Abelin-Genevois K, Vialle R. The use of 2-octylcyanoacrylate (Dermabond®) for the treatment of nail bed injuries in children: results of a prospective series of 30 patients. *J Child Orthop*. 2010;4(1):61–65.

12. Corley FG Jr, Schenck RC Jr. Fractures of the hand. *Clin Plast Surg*. 1996;23(3):447–462.

13. Light TR, Bednar MS. Management of intra-articular fractures of the metacarpophalangeal joint. *Hand Clin*. 1994;10(2): 303–314.

14. Lubahn JD. Mallet finger fractures: a comparison of open and closed technique. *J Hand Surg [Am]*. 1989;14(2 pt 2): 394–396.

15. Bowman SH, Simon RR. Metacarpal and phalangeal fractures. *Emerg Med Clin North Am*. 1993;11(3):671–702.

16. Maitra A, Burdett-Smith P. The conservative management of proximal phalangeal fractures of the hand in an accident and emergency department. *J Hand Surg [Br]*. 1992;17(3): 332–336.

17. McLain RF, Steyers C, Stoddard M. Infections in open fractures of the hand. *J Hand Surg [Am]*. 1991;16(1):108–112.

18. Burkhalter WE. Closed treatment of hand fractures. *J Hand Surg [Am]*. 1989;14(2 pt 2):390–393.

19. Dunn JC, Kusnezov N, Orr JD, Pallis M, Mitchell JS. The boxer's fracture: splint immobilization is not necessary. *Orthopedics*. 2016;39(3):188–192.

20. Ashkenaze DM, Ruby LK. Metacarpal fractures and dislocations. *Orthop Clin North Am*. 1992;23(1):19–33.

21. Sawant N, Kulikov Y, Giddins GE. Outcome following conservative treatment of metacarpophalangeal collateral ligament avulsion fractures of the finger. *J Hand Surg [Eur]*. 2007;32(1): 102–104.

22. Soyer AD. Fractures of the base of the first metacarpal: current treatment options. *J Am Acad Orthop Surg*. 1999;7(6): 403–412.

23. Mohler LR, Trumble TE. Disorders of the thumb sesamoids. *Hand Clin*. 2001;17(2):291–301, x.

24. Daniels JM, Zook EG, Lynch JM. Hand and wrist injuries: part II. Emergent evaluation. *Am Fam Physician*. 2004;69(8): 1949–1956.

25. Lalonde D, Bell M, Benoit P, Sparkes G, Denkler K, Chang P. A multicenter prospective study of 3,110 consecutive cases of elective epinephrine use in the fingers and hand: the Dalhousie project clinical phase. *J Hand Surg [Am]*. 2005;30(5): 1061–1067.

26. Grossman JA, Adams JP, Kunec J. Prophylactic antibiotics in simple hand lacerations. *JAMA*. 1981;245(10): 1055–1056.

27. Haughey RE, Lammers RL, Wagner DK. Use of antibiotics in the initial management of soft tissue hand wounds. *Ann Emerg Med*. 1981;10(4):187–192.

28. Horton LK, Jacobson JA, Powell A, Fessell DP, Hayes CW. Sonography and radiography of soft tissue foreign bodies. *AJR Am J Roentgenol*. 2001;176:1155–1159.

29. Fassler PR. Fingertip injuries: evaluation and treatment. *J Am Acad Orthop Surg*. 1996;4(1):84–92.

30. Hassan MS, Kannan RY, Rehman N, Platt AJ. Difficult adherent nail bed dressings: an escape route. *Emerg Med J*. 2005; 22(4):312.

31. de Alwis W. Fingertip injuries. *Emerg Med Australas*. 2006;18(3):229–237.

32. Illingworth CM. Trapped fingers and amputated finger tips in children. *J Pediatr Surg*. 1974;9(6):853–858.

33. Chow SP, Ho E. Open treatment of fingertip injuries in adults. *J Hand Surg [Am]*. 1982;7(5):470–476.

34. Bossley CJ. Conservative treatment of digit amputations. *N Z Med J*. 1975;82(553):379–380.

35. Holm A, Zachariae L. Fingertip lesions. An evaluation of conservative treatment versus free skin grafting. *Acta Orthop Scand*. 1974;45(3):382–392.

36. Lamon RP, Cicero JJ, Frascone RJ, Hass WF. Open treatment of fingertip amputations. *Ann Emerg Med*. 1983;12(6): 358–360.

37. Louis DS, Palmer AK, Burney RE. Open treatment of digital tip injuries. *JAMA*. 1980;244(7):697–698.

38. Mennen U, Wiese A. Fingertip injuries management with semi-occlusive dressing. *J Hand Surg [Br]*. 1993;18(4): 416–422.

39. Lee LP, Lau PY, Chan CW. A simple and efficient treatment for fingertip injuries. *J Hand Surg [Br]*. 1995;20(1):63–71.

40. Fox JW, Golden GT, Rodeheaver G, Edgerton MT, Edlich RF. Nonoperative management of fingertip pulp amputation by occlusive dressings. *Am J Surg*. 1977;133(2): 255–256.

41. Douglas BS. Conservative management of guillotine amputation of the finger in children. *Aust Paediatr J*. 1972;8(2): 86–89.

42. Schnall SB, Mirzayan R. High-pressure injection injuries to the hand. *Hand Clin*. 1999;15(2):245–248, viii.

43. Schoo MJ, Scott FA, Boswick JA, Jr. High-pressure injection injuries of the hand. *J Trauma*. 1980;20(3):229–238.

44. Proust AF. Special injuries of the hand. *Emerg Med Clin North Am*. 1993;11(3):767–779.

45. Verhoeven N, Hierner R. High-pressure injection injury of the hand: an often underestimated trauma: case report with study of the literature. *Strategies Trauma Limb Reconstr.* 2008;3(1): 27–33.

46. Hogan CJ, Ruland RT. High-pressure injection injuries to the upper extremity: a review of the literature. *J Orthop Trauma.* 2006;20(7):503–511.

47. Reagan DS, Grundberg AB, Reagan JM. Digital artery damage associated with closed crush injuries. *J Hand Surg [Br].* 2002;27(4):374–377.

48. Perron AD, Brady WJ, Keats TE, Hersh RE. Orthopedic pitfalls in the emergency department: closed tendon injuries of the hand. *Am J Emerg Med.* 2001;19(1):76–80.

49. Graham TJ. The exploded hand syndrome: logical evaluation and comprehensive treatment of the severely crushed hand. *J Hand Surg Am.* 2006;31(6):1012–1023.

50. Gupta A, Wolff TW. Management of the mangled hand and forearm. *J Am Acad Orthop Surg.* 1995;3(4):226–236.

51. Wilhelmi BJ, Lee WP, Pagensteert GI, May JW Jr. Replantation in the mutilated hand. *Hand Clin.* 2003;19(1):89–120.

52. Proano L, Partridge R. Descriptive epidemiology of a cluster of hand injuries from snowblowers. *J Emerg Med.* 2002;22(4): 341–344.

53. Dietzel DP, Gorosh J, Burke EF, Singer RM. Snowblower injuries to the hand. *Am J Orthop.* 1997;26(12):863–867.

54. Chin G, Weinzweig N, Weinzweig J, Geldner P, Gonzalez M. Snowblower injuries to the hand. *Ann Plast Surg.* 1998;41(4): 390–396.

55. Blair WF, Steyers CM. Extensor tendon injuries. *Orthop Clin North Am.* 1992;23(1):141–148.

56. Adani R, Castagnetti C, Landi A. Degloving injuries of the hand and fingers. *Clin Orthop Relat Res.* 1995;(314):19–25.

57. Adani R, Busa R, Castagnetti C, Castagnini L, Caroli A. Replantation of degloved skin of the hand. *Plast Reconstr Surg.* 1998;101(6):1544–1551.

58. Schlenker JD, Koulis CP. Amputations and replantations. *Emerg Med Clin North Am.* 1993;11(3):739–753.

59. Ortiz JA Jr, Berger RA. Compartment syndrome of the hand and wrist. *Hand Clin.* 1998;14(3):405–418.

60. Dellaero DT, Levin LS. Compartment syndrome of the hand. Etiology, diagnosis, and treatment. *Am J Orthop.* 1996;25(6): 404–408.

61. Steinberg DR. Acute flexor tendon injuries. *Orthop Clin North Am.* 1992;23(1):125–140.

62. Gelberman RH, Siegel DB, Woo SL, Amiel D, Takai S, Lee D. Healing of digital flexor tendons: importance of the interval from injury to repair. A biomechanical, biochemical, and morphological study in dogs. *J Bone Joint Surg Am.* 1991;73(1): 66–75.

63. Hariharan JS, Diao E, Soejima O, Lotz JC. Partial lacerations of human digital flexor tendons: a biomechanical analysis. *J Hand Surg [Am].* 1997;22(6):1011–1015.

64. Wray RC Jr, Weeks PM. Treatment of partial tendon lacerations. *Hand.* 1980;12(2):163–166.

65. Strickland JW. Flexor tendon injuries: I. foundations of treatment. *J Am Acad Orthop Surg.* 1995;3(1):44–54.

66. Hart RG, Uehara DT, Kutz JE. Extensor tendon injuries of the hand. *Emerg Med Clin North Am.* 1993;11(3):637–649.

67. Kleinert HE, Verdan C. Report of the committee on tendon injuries (international federation of societies for surgery of the hand). *J Hand Surg [Am].* 1983;8(5 pt 2):794–798.

68. Newport ML. Extensor tendon injuries in the hand. *J Am Acad Orthop Surg.* 1997;5(2):59–66.

69. Carl HD, Forst R, Schaller P. Results of primary extensor tendon repair in relation to the zone of injury and pre-operative outcome estimation. *Arch Orthop Trauma Surg.* 2007;127(2): 115–119.

70. Hankin FM, Peel SM. Sport-related fractures and dislocations in the hand. *Hand Clin.* 1990;6(3):429–453.

71. Hoffman DF, Schaffer TC. Management of common finger injuries. *Am Fam Physician.* 1991;43(5):1594–1607.

72. Brzezienski MA, Schneider LH. Extensor tendon injuries at the distal interphalangeal joint. *Hand Clin.* 1995;11(3):373–386.

73. Schreuders T, Soeters J, Hovius S, Stam H. A Modification of Elson's test for the diagnosis of an acute extensor central slip injury. *British J of Hand Therapy.* 2006;11(4):112–113.

74. Westerheide E, Failla JM, van Holsbeeck M, Ceulemans R. Ultrasound visualization of central slip injuries of the finger extensor mechanism. *J Hand Surg [Am].* 2003;28(6): 1009–1013.

75. Hame SL, Melone CP Jr. Boxer's knuckle. Traumatic disruption of the extensor hood. *Hand Clin.* 2000;16(3): 375–380, viii.

76. Arai K, Toh S, Nakahara K, Nishikawa S, Harata S. Treatment of soft tissue injuries to the dorsum of the metacarpophalangeal joint (boxer's knuckle). *J Hand Surg [Br].* 2002;27(1):90–95.

77. Chan RK. Splinting for peripheral nerve injury in upper limb. *Hand Surg.* 2002;7(2):251–259.

78. Gupta A, Kleinert HE. Evaluating the injured hand. *Hand Clin.* 1993;9(2):195–212.

79. Morgan RL, Linder MM. Common wrist injuries. *Am Fam Physician.* 1997;55(3):857–868.

80. Adams KM, Thompson ST. Continuous passive motion use in hand therapy. *Hand Clin.* 1996;12(1):109–127.

81. Murakami Y. Irreducible dislocation of the distal interphalangeal joint. *J Hand Surg [Br].* 1985;10(2):231–232.

82. Inoue G, Maeda N. Irreducible palmar dislocation of the proximal interphalangeal joint of the finger. *J Hand Surg [Am].* 1990;15(2):301–304.

83. Spinner M, Choi BY. Anterior dislocation of the proximal interphalangeal joint. A cause of rupture of the central slip of the extensor mechanism. *J Bone Joint Surg Am.* 1970;52(7): 1329–1336.

84. Peimer CA, Sullivan DJ, Wild DR. Palmar dislocation of the proximal interphalangeal joint. *J Hand Surg [Am].* 1984; 9A(1):39–48.

85. Itadera E. Irreducible palmar dislocation of the proximal interphalangeal joint caused by a fracture fragment: a case report. *J Orthop Sci.* 2003;8(6):872–874.

86. Ostrowski DM, Neimkin RJ. Irreducible palmar dislocation of the proximal interphalangeal joint. A case report. *Orthopedics.* 1985;8(1):84–86.

87. Stern PJ, Lee AF. Open dorsal dislocations of the proximal interphalangeal joint. *J Hand Surg [Am].* 1985;10(3):364–370.

88. Glickel SZ, Barron OA. Proximal interphalangeal joint fracture dislocations. *Hand Clin.* 2000;16(3):333–344.

89. Newland CC. Gamekeeper's thumb. *Orthop Clin North Am.* 1992;23(1):41–48.

90. Pichora DR, McMurtry RY, Bell MJ. Gamekeepers thumb: a prospective study of functional bracing. *J Hand Surg [Am].* 1989;14(3):567–573.

91. Fairhurst M, Hansen L. Treatment of "Gamekeeper's Thumb" by reconstruction of the ulnar collateral ligament. *J Hand Surg [Br]*. 2002;27(6):542–545.

92. Botte MJ, Fronek J, Pedowitz RA, Hoenecke HR Jr, Abrams RA, Hamer ML. Exertional compartment syndrome of the upper extremity. *Hand Clin*. 1998;14(3):477–482, x.

93. Thorson E, Szabo RM. Common tendinitis problems in the hand and forearm. *Orthop Clin North Am*. 1992;23(1):65–74.

94. Stern PJ. Tendinitis, overuse syndromes, and tendon injuries. *Hand Clin*. 1990;6(3):467–476.

95. Ostrovskiy D, Wilbourn A. Acute bowler's thumb. *Neurology*. 2004;63(5):938.

96. Saldana MJ. Trigger digits: diagnosis and treatment. *J Am Acad Orthop Surg*. 2001;9(4):246–252.

97. Freiberg A, Mulholland RS, Levine R. Nonoperative treatment of trigger fingers and thumbs. *J Hand Surg [Am]*. 1989;14(3):553–558.

98. Newport ML, Lane LB, Stuchin SA. Treatment of trigger finger by steroid injection. *J Hand Surg [Am]*. 1990;15(5):748–750.

99. Katzman BM, Steinberg DR, Bozentka DJ, Cain E, Caligiuri DA, Geller J. Utility of obtaining radiographs in patients with trigger finger. *Am J Orthop*. 1999;28(12):703–705.

100. Fleisch SB, Spindler KP, Lee DH. Corticosteroid injections in the treatment of trigger finger: a level I and II systematic review. *J Am Acad Orthop Surg*. 2007;15(3):166–171.

101. Tallia AF, Cardone DA. Diagnostic and therapeutic injection of the wrist and hand region. *Am Fam Physician*. 2003;67(4):745–750.

102. Godey SK, Bhatti WA, Watson JS, Bayat A. A technique for accurate and safe injection of steroid in trigger digits using ultrasound guidance. *Acta Orthop Belg*. 2006;72(5):633–634.

103. Fleming AN, Smith PJ. Vascular cell tumors of the hand in children. *Hand Clin*. 2000;16(4):609–624.

104. Walsh JJ, Eady JL. Vascular tumors. *Hand Clin*. 2004;20(3):261–262, vi.

105. Quitkin HM, Rosenwasser MP, Strauch RJ. The efficacy of silver nitrate cauterization for pyogenic granuloma of the hand. *J Hand Surg [Am]*. 2003;28(3):435–438.

106. Witthaut J, Steffens K, Koob E. Reliable treatment of pyogenic granuloma of the hand. *J Hand Surg [Br]*. 1994;19(6):791–793.

107. Allieu Y, Chammas M, Hixson ML. External fixation for treatment of hand infections. *Hand Clin*. 1993;9(4): 675–682.

108. Jebson PJ. Infections of the fingertip. Paronychias and felons. *Hand Clin*. 1998;14(4):547–555, viii.

109. Clark DC. Common acute hand infections. *Am Fam Physician*. 2003;68(11):2167–2176.

110. Jebson PJ. Deep subfascial space infections. *Hand Clin*. 1998;14(4):557–566, viii.

111. Abrams RA, Botte MJ. Hand infections: treatment recommendations for specific types. *J Am Acad Orthop Surg*. 1996;4(4):219–230.

112. Burkhalter WE. Deep space infections. *Hand Clin*. 1989;5(4):553–559.

113. Perron AD, Miller MD, Brady WJ. Orthopedic pitfalls in the ED: fight bite. *Am J Emerg Med*. 2002;20(2):114–117.

114. Taplitz RA. Managing bite wounds. Currently recommended antibiotics for treatment and prophylaxis. *Postgrad Med*. 2004;116(2):49–52, 55–56, 59.

115. Overall KL, Love M. Dog bites to humans—demography, epidemiology, injury, and risk. *J Am Vet Med Assoc*. 2001;218(12):1923–1934.

116. Presutti RJ. Prevention and treatment of dog bites. *Am Fam Physician*. 2001;63(8):1567–1572.

117. Kravetz JD, Federman DG. Cat-associated zoonoses. *Arch Intern Med*. 2002;162(17):1945–1952.

CHAPTER 12

Wrist

Andrea L. Blome, MD and Megan E. Healy, MD

INTRODUCTION

The wrist comprises eight carpal bones that articulate with the radius proximally and the metacarpals distally. Motions include flexion, extension, radial deviation, and ulnar deviation. The carpal bones are divided into a proximal row of four bones and a distal row of four bones (Fig. 12-1). The proximal row, from radial to ulnar surfaces, includes the scaphoid, lunate, and triquetrum. The distal row, from radial to ulnar surfaces, includes the trapezium, trapezoid, capitate, and hamate. The pisiform, a sesamoid bone enclosed in the sheath of the flexor carpi ulnaris tendon, lies adjacent to the volar surface of the triquetrum and does not articulate with the forearm bones or with any of the remaining carpal bones.

Of the forearm bones, only the radius articulates with the carpal bones. The ulna has a nonosseous fibrocartilaginous union with the triquetrum and the radius, known as the triangular fibrocartilage complex (TFCC). The ulna articulates with the radius at the distal radioulnar joint (DRUJ). An interosseous membrane, dorsal and palmar radioulnar ligaments, and the TFCC stabilize this joint. Injury to the

bones or ligaments of the DRUJ may significantly affect wrist mechanics, leading to subluxation or dislocation. If not treated properly, an injury to these structures may result in long-term limitation of movement, arthritis, or painful range of motion.

The ligaments of the wrist are considered extrinsic if they join the carpal bones to the radius, ulna, or metacarpals, and intrinsic when they link the carpal bones to one another. The ligaments of the wrist are also classified as dorsal, volar, or interosseous. The volar ligaments are stronger than their dorsal counterparts and provide the greatest stability. Injury to these ligaments results in carpal instability and is discussed later in this chapter.

Many important neurovascular structures pass through Guyon canal formed by the pisiform and the hook of the hamate (Fig. 12-2). The deep branch of the ulnar nerve and artery supply the three hypothenar muscles, the interossei, the two ulnar lumbricals, and the adductor pollicis. A fracture to either the hamate or the capitate may result in neurovascular bundle damage and

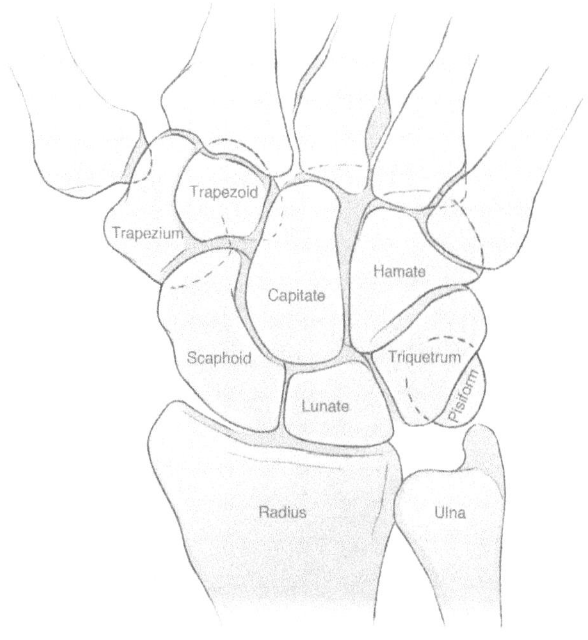

Figure 12-1. The bony anatomy of the wrist.

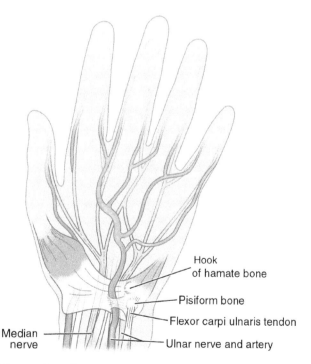

Figure 12-2. There are several important neurovascular structures of the wrist. The ulnar nerve and artery are confined within the Guyon canal.

subsequent impairment of normal function. The median nerve lies in close proximity to the volar surfaces of the lunate and the capitate and may be injured following a fracture or dislocation.

It is essential to understand the relationship between the tendons and the carpal bones. The tendon of the flexor carpi ulnaris virtually engulfs the pisiform in its attachment. The close proximity of the flexor carpi radialis to the tubercle of the trapezium is also noteworthy. Trapezium fractures may result in tendon damage with subsequent pain during normal motion.

Examination

A meticulous examination combined with an in-depth knowledge of wrist anatomy will aid in the accurate diagnosis of wrist injuries. Localized tenderness of a bone or joint usually indicates the involved structure.

The radial portion of the wrist has several significant palpable bony structures. With the hand held palm side down and deviated slightly in a radial direction and the thumb extended, the anatomic snuffbox becomes prominent (Fig. 12–3). The dorsal aspect is made up of the extensor pollicis longus, whereas the tendons of the extensor pollicis brevis and the abductor pollicis longus form the palmar border of the snuffbox. The proximal border of the box is the radial styloid, followed by the scaphoid at the proximal base and the trapezium at the distal base. If the thumb is now flexed, the first carpometacarpal joint is palpated distal to the trapezium (Fig. 12–4).

As the examiner moves over the dorsum of the wrist, Lister tubercle of the distal radius can be palpated (Fig. 12–5). This tubercle serves as a landmark in locating the lunate and the capitate. With the hand held in a neutral position, there is a small indentation in the skin corresponding to the capitate (Fig. 12–6A). With the hand in flexion, the lunate becomes easily palpable just distal to

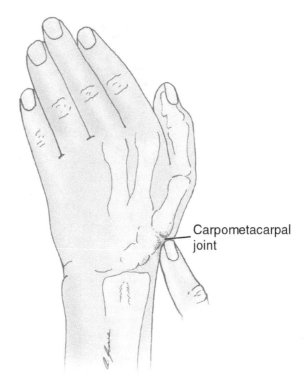

Figure 12–4. With the thumb flexed, the first carpometacarpal joint can be visualized and palpated.

Lister tubercle (Fig. 12–6B). Lister tubercle and the capitate form a straight line that transects the third metacarpal (Fig. 12–7). The triquetrum can be palpated just distal to the ulnar styloid (Fig. 12–8).

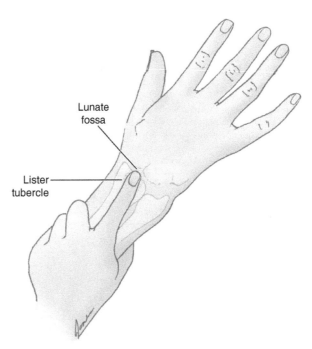

Figure 12–5. Lister tubercle can be palpated over the dorsal aspect of the radius.

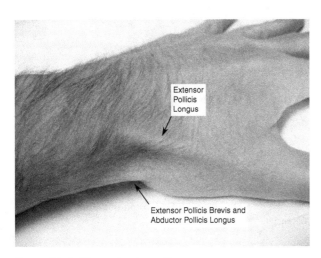

Figure 12–3. The anatomic snuffbox.

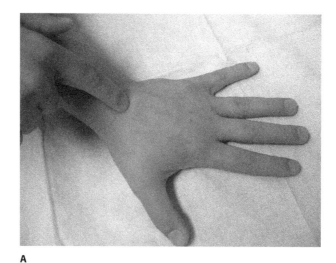

A

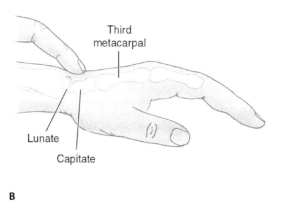

B

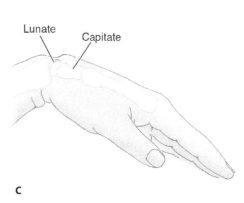

C

Figure 12–6. The lunate fossa. **A.** Palpation. **B.** With the hand in the neutral position, a small indentation is noted that corresponds to the capitate. **C.** With the hand held in flexion, the lunate becomes easily palpated distal to Lister tubercle.

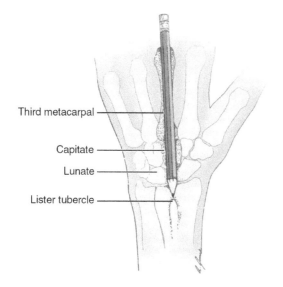

Figure 12–7. Lister tubercle and the capitate form a straight line that transects the third metacarpal.

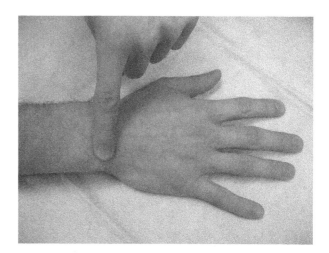

Figure 12–8. The dorsal surface of the triquetrum is palpated just distal to the ulnar styloid.

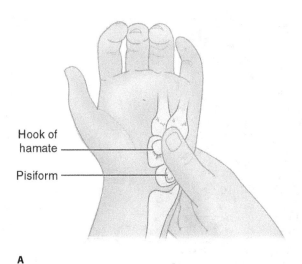
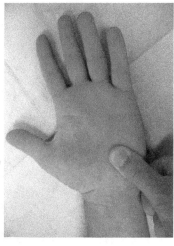

Figure 12–9. ***A.*** The pisiform is easily palpated at the base of the hypothenar eminence on the volar aspect of the hand. ***B.*** The hook of hamate can be palpated with deep palpation, under the tip of the examiner's finger.

The pisiform is easily palpated at the base of the hypothenar eminence on the volar surface of the wrist (Fig. 12–9A). The flexor carpi ulnaris tendon inserts into the pisiform and is best examined with the fist clenched and the wrist flexed. The hook of the hamate can be palpated by placing the interphalangeal (IP) joint of one's thumb over the pisiform, with the distal phalanx directed toward the web space between the thumb and index fingers. With deep palpation, the hook of the hamate can be felt under the tip of the examiner's thumb (Fig. 12–9B).

Lastly, the volar and radial structures include the tuberosity of the scaphoid and the tubercle of the trapezium. With the wrist radial deviated, the tuberosity of the scaphoid is the most prominent structure palpated. The trapezial ridge is found by palpating just distal to the scaphoid in the line in the same axes of the index finger.

Imaging

Standard plain radiographs are the first-line modality in the diagnosis of suspected wrist injuries. The minimum number of radiographic views includes posteroanterior (PA), lateral, and oblique views with the wrist in a neutral position (Fig. 12–10). Other views may be indicated depending on the suspected site of fracture.

The carpal bones are visualized best in the PA view. The three carpal arcs should be identified (Fig. 12–11A). The first arc is outlined by the proximal joint surface of the scaphoid, lunate, and triquetrum. The second arc is made up of the distal joint surfaces of the proximal row. The third arc consists of the proximal articular surface of the lunate and hamate.[12] Any disruption of these arcs suggests injury—fracture, dislocation, or both. In addition, the spacing between the carpal bones is normally constant, independent of wrist positioning. A variation in spacing is abnormal and may reflect subluxation, arthritis, or an old fracture. The normal width between the scaphoid and the lunate is 1 to 2 mm in the PA projection. A distance ≥3 mm between the scaphoid and the lunate are abnormal and suggest carpal instability (scapholunate dissociation).

The oblique view is useful as it demonstrates the radial structures better. This radiograph is obtained with the wrist in 45 degrees of pronation. In this view, the distal scaphoid, trapezium, trapezoid, and first and second carpometacarpal joints can be seen more clearly than in the PA view.

The lateral view is first assessed for adequacy. The ulna should not project >2 mm dorsal to the radius. Once the lateral view is determined to be adequate, the clinician should note the dorsal aspect of the triquetrum. The ulnar styloid points to the dorsal aspect of the triquetrum on the lateral view. A dorsal avulsion fracture of the triquetrum will be identified only on the lateral view.

Carpal alignment is also assessed on the lateral view. Abnormalities in carpal alignment are a clue to carpal instability due to ligamentous injury. The clinician should first note that the radius, lunate, and capitate make up a straight line. It may be helpful to view the lateral wrist radiograph for this purpose in the horizontal plane. The scaphoid is projected over the lunate at its proximal portion, and as it extends more distally, it is positioned volarly. A line drawn through the center of the lunate and the center of the scaphoid should make an angle between 30 and 60 degrees. This angle is known as the scapholunate angle (Fig. 12–11B). The capitolunate angle is measured in a similar manner by drawing a line through the center of the capitate and lunate. The angle that these lines make should be less than 30 degrees (Fig. 12–11C).[5]

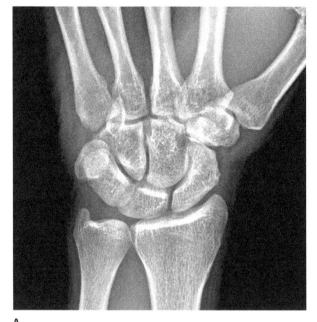

A

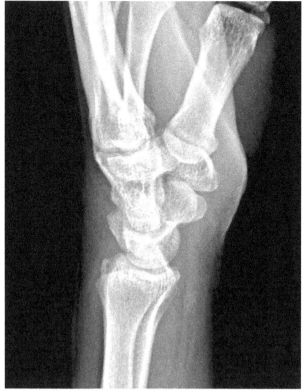

B

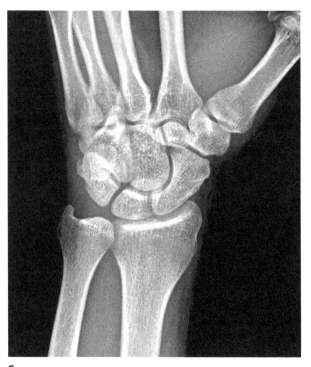

C

Figure 12–10. Normal radiographs of the wrist. *A.* AP. *B.* Lateral. *C.* Oblique views.

Additional views may be obtained to better visualize suspected fractures. A PA view with maximum ulnar deviation of the wrist (scaphoid view) will allow better visualization of the scaphoid. The carpal tunnel view is used to detect fractures of the hook of the hamate and pisiform. This radiograph is obtained with the wrist hyperextended and the beam directed across the volar aspect of the wrist. An additional oblique film with the hand supinated 45 degrees will better demonstrate the pisiform and the palmar aspects of the triquetrum and hamate.

Ninety percent of all wrist fractures will be visualized with the standard plain radiographic views. Compression

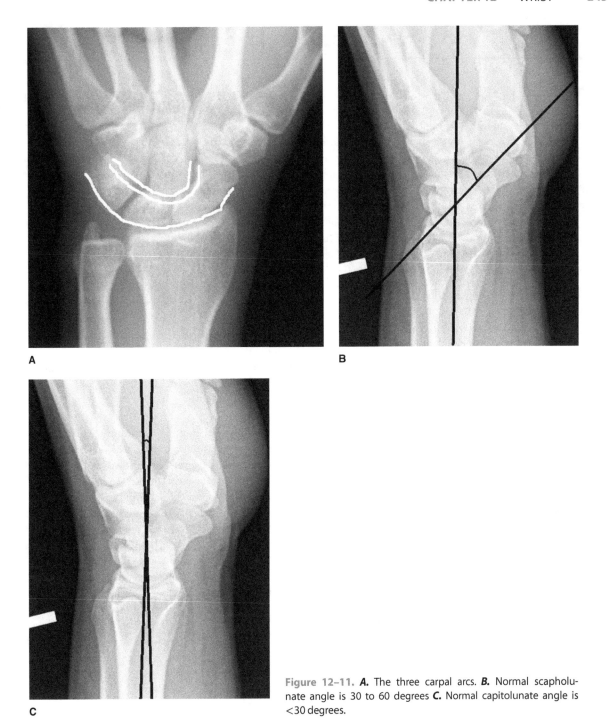

Figure 12–11. **A.** The three carpal arcs. **B.** Normal scapholunate angle is 30 to 60 degrees **C.** Normal capitolunate angle is <30 degrees.

fractures or minimally displaced carpal fractures may not be readily apparent on plain radiographs. Other imaging techniques, including computed tomography (CT), bone scans, and magnetic resonance imaging (MRI), may be necessary but are not routinely used on the initial visit. Careful assessment of bone surfaces with ultrasound may identify fractures not visualized on initial plain radiographs. Among other fractures, ultrasound has been used to detect occult fractures of the waist of the scaphoid and fractures of the hook of the hamate. Once a fracture is detected on ultrasound, CT imaging should be performed to more precisely define the type of fracture.

WRIST FRACTURES

CARPAL FRACTURES

The carpals are a complex set of bones that form multiple articulations. Because radiographs often reveal significant bony overlap, a careful history and clinical examination are necessary to accurately diagnose these fractures. The scaphoid is not only the most frequently fractured carpal bone, but it is also one of the most frequently missed carpal bone fractures. The triquetrum is the second most commonly fractured carpal bone, and the lunate is the third most frequently fractured. Carpal fractures are associated with several common complications.

- *Other injuries.* Patients often suffer a second fracture or ligamentous injury.
- *Nerve injury.* Many carpal fractures are associated with at least a transient median nerve neuropathy. Fractures of the hook of the hamate or pisiform may be complicated by ulnar nerve compromise.
- *Poor healing.* Carpal fractures and especially scaphoid fractures may suffer the sequelae of nonunion or avascular necrosis (AVN). In many patients, this is secondary to inadequate immobilization.

Scaphoid Fractures

The scaphoid is the most commonly fractured carpal bone, accounting for 60% to 70% of carpal injuries.   The high incidence of fractures relates to the size and the position of the scaphoid. The scaphoid is classified as a proximal carpal bone. Anatomically, however, it extends well into the area of the distal carpal bones. Radial deviation or dorsiflexion of the hand is normally limited by impingement of the radius on the scaphoid. With stress, fractures frequently result.

The blood supply to the scaphoid penetrates the cortex on the dorsal surface near the tubercle waist area. Therefore, there is no direct blood supply to the proximal portion of the bone. Because of this tenuous blood supply, scaphoid fractures have a tendency to develop delayed union or AVN.

Axiom: *The more proximal the scaphoid fracture, the greater the likelihood that the bone will develop AVN.*

It is imperative for the clinician to realize that a patient presenting with a "sprained wrist" may have an occult scaphoid fracture. This injury can often be excluded acutely on the basis of physical examination. As is discussed later in this chapter, normal radiographs do not exclude this fracture.

Axiom: *Patients presenting with symptoms of a sprained wrist must have the diagnosis of an acute scaphoid fracture ruled out.*

Scaphoid fractures are divided into four types—middle-third (waist), proximal-third, distal-third, and tubercle fractures (Fig. 12–12). This classification lists scaphoid fractures in order of decreasing frequency. Fractures of the scaphoid waist represent >50% of all scaphoid fractures. The more proximal the fracture line, the higher the incidence of complications (proximal > waist > distal > tubercle). Scaphoid stress fractures have also been reported.

Mechanism of Injury
Scaphoid fractures commonly result from forceful hyperextension of the wrist. Simple falls from a standing height and sports injuries are the most common mechanisms of injury. The particular type of fracture is dependent on the position of the hand and forearm at the time of injury. Middle-third fractures occur secondary to radial deviation, with hyperextension resulting in impingement of the scaphoid waist by the radial styloid process.

Examination
On examination, there is maximum tenderness over the floor of the anatomic snuffbox. Tenderness within the anatomic snuffbox has been shown to be 90% sensitive for detecting scaphoid fractures and has a specificity of 40%. Palpation of the scaphoid tubercle for tenderness has a similar sensitivity (87%) with an improved specificity (57%). This test is performed by radially deviating the wrist and palpating over the palmar aspect of the scaphoid. Axial compression of the thumb in the line with the first metacarpal and supination against resistance may also elicit pain from a scaphoid fracture. The most accurate examination for detecting the presence of an *occult* scaphoid fracture was shown to be the reproduction of pain when the patient pinched the tips of his/her thumb and index finger together or when he/she pronated his/her forearm. In addition, ulnar deviation of the pronated wrist has been shown to produce pain in the anatomic snuffbox in patients with a scaphoid fracture, and in one small study, the absence of this finding had a negative predictive value of 100%.

Imaging
Routine plain radiographs of the wrist, including PA, lateral, and oblique views, may demonstrate the fracture (Fig. 12–13). If a scaphoid fracture is suspected clinically, an ulnar-deviated scaphoid view should be obtained. Despite this additional film, up to 30% of scaphoid fractures may not be demonstrated on initial plain radiographs. In addition, these fractures can take up to 1 to 2 weeks to become evident on plain films. An indirect sign of an acute scaphoid fracture is displacement of the

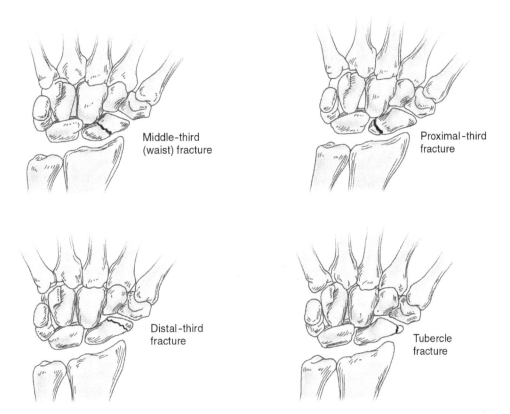

Figure 12–12. Scaphoid fractures.

scaphoid fat stripe.[16] This finding, however, was present in only 50% of radiographically occult scaphoid fractures in one study.[17] In some instances, a comparison view of the uninjured wrist may also be helpful.

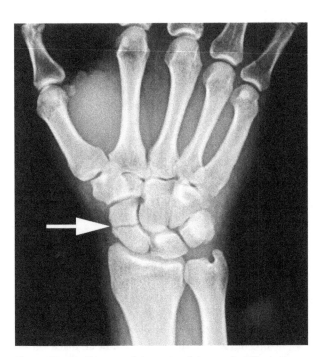

Figure 12–13. Fracture of the waist of the scaphoid (*arrow*).

Although plain radiography remains the standard initial imaging technique, other imaging modalities should be considered. CT scan is the preferred modality to assess the intricacies of a scaphoid fracture, including fracture location and deformity. MRI is excellent in the detection of clinically suspected scaphoid fractures if initial radiographs are negative. Limited MRI of the wrist has been shown in multiple studies to be 100% sensitive for detecting scaphoid fractures, even in the acute setting.[18] On ultrasound, scaphoid cortical interruption and an effusion in the radiocarpal joint are considered diagnostic of a scaphoid fracture.[19]

If a fracture is identified, displacement between the fracture fragments or an unexplained variation in position between the fragments on different views indicates an unstable fracture. Fracture dislocation usually implies dorsal displacement of the distal fragment and carpal bones. The proximal fragment and lunate generally maintain their normal relationship with the radius.

Scaphoid fractures are sometimes confused with a bipartite scaphoid. This is a rare congenital anomaly (incidence <0.5%) that may be mistaken for a scaphoid waist fracture.[20] The presence of a normal smooth bony margin is indicative of this normal variant.

An old scaphoid fracture that has not healed properly should not be confused with an acute injury. Radiographically, nonunion will be associated with sclerotic fragment margins. In addition, the radiolucent distance separating

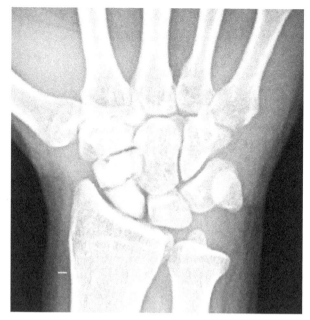

Figure 12–14. Nonunion of a scaphoid fracture. Note the sclerotic fragment margins and the elongated radiolucent distance separating the fragments.

the fragments will be similar to the distance between other carpal bones (Fig. 12–14).

Associated Injuries

The majority (90%) of scaphoid fractures have no associated injuries. Injuries associated with scaphoid fractures include the following:

- Radiocarpal joint dislocation
- Proximal and distal carpal row dislocation
- Distal radial fracture
- Bennett fracture of the thumb
- Lunate fracture or dislocation
- Scapholunate dissociation

Treatment

The treatment of scaphoid fractures is controversial and fraught with complications. In general, distal fractures and transverse fractures heal with fewer complications when compared with proximal or oblique fractures. Immobilization is recommended; however, the best method remains unclear. The appropriate length of the thumb spica splint—short arm versus long arm—has been debated. In one prospective, randomized study, the time to union was longer (12.7 vs. 9.5 weeks), and the rate of nonunion was greater in patients treated with short-arm thumb spica immobilization. A more recent systematic review of randomized trials reported that nonunion rates and functional outcomes did not differ based on the cast type. Another randomized study of

292 patients demonstrated no benefit for immobilization of the thumb. Despite this study, many orthopedists still prefer the thumb be immobilized.

As with other fractures, ice and elevation are important adjuncts in the initial management of scaphoid fractures. The management of scaphoid fractures is divided into (1) patients with clinically suspected scaphoid fractures without radiographic evidence, (2) nondisplaced scaphoid fractures, and (3) displaced scaphoid fractures.

Clinically Suspected Scaphoid Fractures without Radiographic Evidence.

Up to 30% of patients with clinically suspected scaphoid fractures who do not have plain radiographic evidence of such an injury will ultimately be diagnosed with a scaphoid fracture. Therefore, it is our view that such patients should be treated as having a nondisplaced scaphoid fracture, and the wrist and forearm immobilized in a thumb spica splint. The thumb should be in a position as if the patient was holding a wine glass. The wrist should be splinted in slight flexion with neither ulnar nor radial deviation (Appendix A–7).

After 7 to 10 days, a repeat physical examination and radiographic examination should be performed. If a fracture is identified, a long-arm thumb spica cast should be applied for an additional 4 to 5 weeks (total of 6 weeks). This should be followed by a short-arm thumb spica cast until clinical and radiographic signs of union are clearly seen. If a fracture is not identified, but the examination remains clinically suspicious, the splint should be reapplied and the patient reexamined at 7- to 10-day intervals.

Alternative methods for the early detection of an occult fracture include bone scan, CT, and MRI. Bone scanning 4 days post injury is sensitive for the detection of occult scaphoid fractures, but has a high number of false-positive results. CT scan is readily available to most emergency physicians, has an improved sensitivity over plain films, and is more sensitive and specific than bone scanning. A false-negative CT scan may still occur. MRI is very sensitive for the detection of occult scaphoid fractures; however, it is not readily available. In one study of patients with clinical suspicion of scaphoid fracture and negative plain films, MRI within the first 2 weeks of injury detected occult scaphoid fractures in 20% of patients, and in another 20%, a fracture of the distal radius or another carpal bone was found. Another noted advantage of MRI evaluation of the scaphoid is the demonstration of viability of the fracture fragments.

Nondisplaced Scaphoid Fractures.

A thumb spica splint (Appendix A–7) should be applied. If a nondisplaced distal fracture is noted, a short-arm thumb spica splint can be used. If a nondisplaced midbody or proximal scaphoid fracture is noted, a long-arm spica splint should be applied. Follow-up with a hand surgeon should be arranged within 5 to 7 days for definitive treatment.

Most fractures are evaluated with CT to precisely define the location, pattern, and displacement, as these factors are not always apparent on plain radiographs.[26] If the CT scan confirms that the fracture is truly nondisplaced, then a long-arm thumb spica cast is applied. After 6 weeks, a short-arm thumb spica cast is applied for the remaining duration of immobilization, totaling 8 to 12 weeks. At this time, clinical and radiographic signs of union are usually present and casting is discontinued. Due to their higher rate of complications, proximal-third fractures are immobilized for a greater duration (12–16 weeks) than middle or distal-third fractures (8–12 weeks).

Casting of nondisplaced scaphoid fractures has long been the standard practice but more recently early surgical intervention is being offered as an option to patients who want to return to full function more rapidly. Surgery may allow earlier discontinuation of a cast and subsequent return to work or sports. The risk of surgery must be weighed against the more than 95% expected union rate with casting. Several authors also recommend primary operative management for proximal scaphoid fractures even if they appear nondisplaced due to their higher rate of nonunion.[21]

Displaced Scaphoid Fractures. Displaced fractures have a nonunion rate of 50% to 55% (compared to 5%–15% in fully immobilized nondisplaced fractures) and therefore require more aggressive initial management.[33,34] With significant displacement, angulation, or comminution, consultation with a hand surgeon should be obtained. The patient should be placed in a thumb spica splint and referred to a hand surgeon for open reduction and internal fixation.[22,26] Absolute indications for internal fixation include displacement of 1 mm or 15 degrees of angulation.[35,36]

Complications

The following complications of scaphoid fractures may occur despite optimum treatment.

- AVN is associated with proximal-third fractures, displaced fractures, comminuted fractures, or fractures that are inadequately immobilized. AVN will occur approximately 30% of the time, with proximal fractures having the highest incidence.[1,26]
- Delayed union, malunion, or nonunion may be encountered. Nonunion may occur in as many as 5% to 10% of all cases. Risk factors associated with nonunion include proximal fractures, fracture instability, and delay in care.[37]
- Radiocarpal arthritis with subsequent wrist pain and/or stiffness.[38]

Triquetrum Fractures

Triquetrum fractures are the second most common carpal bone fracture, representing 3% to 5% of all carpal fractures.[39] Triquetrum fractures can be divided into two types—dorsal chip (avulsion) fractures and transverse fractures (Fig. 12–15). The dorsal chip fractures are much more common, accounting for up to 93% of all triquetrum fractures.[39]

Mechanism of Injury

Dorsal chip fractures are usually secondary to a hyperextension injury with the wrist in ulnar deviation. In this position, the hamate forces the triquetrum against the dorsal lip of the radius, resulting in fragment shearing. If the wrist is held in flexion during a fall, an avulsion

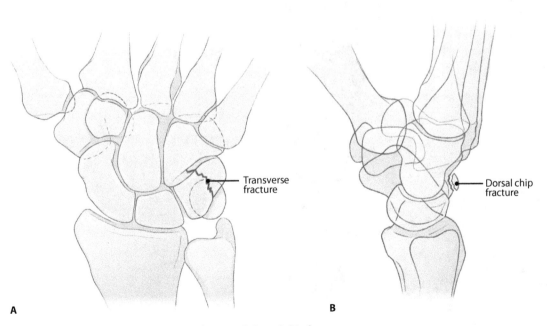

Figure 12–15. Triquetrum fractures. ***A.*** Transverse fracture. ***B.*** Dorsal chip fracture.

fracture at the attachment of the strong dorsal ligaments may also occur.

Transverse fractures are secondary to a direct blow to the dorsum of the hand and are frequently associated with perilunate dislocations.

Examination

There will be dorsal swelling and tenderness localized over the area of the triquetrum (just distal to the ulnar styloid). Wrist extension may reproduce or exacerbate the pain.

Imaging

Dorsal chip fractures are visualized on the lateral radiograph (Fig. 12–16). In this view, the ulnar styloid usually "points" to the dorsal aspect of the triquetrum. Transverse fractures are best visualized on PA and oblique radiographs.

Associated Injuries

Triquetrum injuries are frequently associated with scaphoid fractures, scapholunate instability, distal radius and ulnar styloid fractures, and ulnar nerve injuries. The deep branch (motor) of the ulnar nerve lies in close proximity to the triquetrum and may be compromised.

Treatment

Dorsal Chip (Avulsion) Fracture. The wrist should be immobilized by applying a volar splint with the wrist in slight extension. This provides protection while allowing for icing and elevation. A short-arm cast can be placed in 3 to 4 days after the swelling has subsided. Chip fractures are generally of little consequence as most go on to an asymptomatic

fibrous union, but they do indicate underlying soft-tissue injury that must be allowed to heal with 4 to 6 weeks of cast immobilization.

Transverse Fracture. Guidelines for treating triquetrum body fractures are less clear. Displacement and other carpal injuries must be excluded radiographically before treatment. Nondisplaced body fractures can be immobilized with a short-arm cast for 4 to 6 weeks. If there is >1 mm of displacement or other associated intercarpal ligamentous injuries, operative repair should be considered.

Complications

As mentioned previously, damage to the deep branch of the ulnar nerve with subsequent motor impairment may accompany this fracture. The triquetrum possesses a rich vascular supply, and therefore, neither dorsal chip fractures nor transverse fractures are associated with AVN.

Lunate Fractures

Fractures of the lunate are rare and only make up approximately 0.5% to 6.5% of all carpal bone fractures. These fractures usually result from high-energy trauma and are typically associated with other carpal and ligamentous injuries. The most common lunate fractures are lunate body fractures (Fig. 12–17) and dorsal avulsion fractures. Lunate body fractures may occur in any plane with varying degrees of comminution. As with scaphoid fractures, the clinical suspicion of a fracture mandates treatment to prevent the development of osteonecrosis of the lunate, also known as Kienböck's disease.

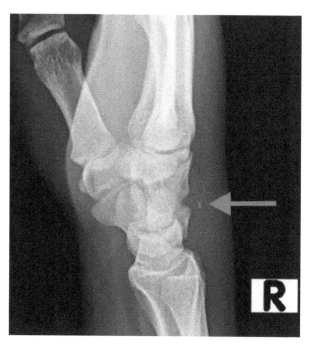

Figure 12–16. Triquetrum fracture. The dorsal chip fracture is only visualized on the lateral radiograph (*arrow*).

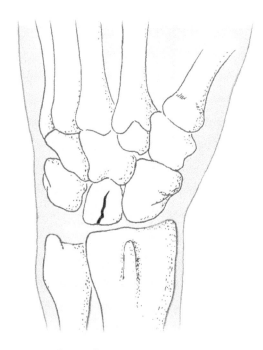

Figure 12–17. Lunate fracture.

Mechanism of Injury

Lunate fractures generally result from an indirect mechanism such as hyperextension (dorsal avulsion fracture). Fractures of the body of the lunate occur from direct axial compression. Although 75% of patients with Kienböck's disease have a prior history of significant wrist trauma, chronic repetitive trauma can also lead to this condition.[45]

Examination

Pain and tenderness will be present dorsally over the area of the lunate (just distal to Lister tubercle). In addition, axial compression of the third metacarpal will exacerbate the pain. Swelling may be minimal because of the intracapsular location of the lunate.

Imaging

A fracture line is often difficult to detect on routine wrist films. If a fracture is suspected clinically, CT scan and MRI are often necessary to make the diagnosis.[35] Both are more sensitive than plain radiographs for the detection of lunate fractures. Kienböck's disease presents in four distinct radiographic stages. In stage I, the plain radiographs are generally normal. In stage II, lunate sclerosis is noted, whereas in stage III, lunate collapse becomes apparent (Fig. 12–18). Finally, in stage IV, severe lunate collapse is present with intra-articular degenerative changes in the surrounding joints.[45] MRI performed early may detect diminished blood flow to the lunate and early signs of Kienböck's disease.

Associated Injuries

Other carpal fractures and carpal instability frequently accompany lunate fractures, and it is important to exclude these injuries.

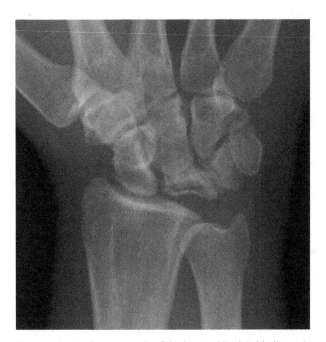

Figure 12–18. Osteonecrosis of the lunate (Kienböck's disease).

Treatment

As with scaphoid fractures, treatment should be initiated on the basis of clinical or radiographic evidence of a fracture.[46] It is generally recommended that the patient be immobilized in a long-arm thumb spica splint (Appendix A–7) with the MCP joints flexed to relieve the compressive forces across the lunate. Orthopedic referral after initial immobilization is strongly recommended. Definitive management includes cast immobilization for a total of 6 to 8 weeks in patients with nondisplaced fractures. Displaced (>1 mm) or unstable fractures require operative repair. Options for operative repair include Kirschner wires, cannulated screws, or suture anchors into the bone. The treatment of Kienböck's disease is not standardized and is beyond the scope of this chapter.

Complications

Inadequately treated lunate fractures tend to develop osteonecrosis of the proximal fragment. With time, there will be compression and collapse of this fragment; however, osteonecrosis may develop despite adequate treatment.

Capitate Fractures

The capitate is the largest of the eight carpal bones. It articulates with the scaphoid and the lunate proximally; the trapezoid and the hamate along its lateral surfaces; and the second, third, and fourth metacarpals distally. Isolated capitate fractures are extremely rare, accounting for only 1.3% of all carpal bone fractures.[47] Capitate fractures are usually transverse and most often nondisplaced due to the stability offered by the intercarpal ligaments (Fig. 12–19).

Mechanism of Injury

Two mechanisms of injury result in fractures of the capitate. A direct blow or crushing force over the dorsal aspect of the wrist may result in a fracture. Indirectly, a fall on the outstretched hand may also result in a fracture. The capitate is well protected in the center of the wrist, so a high-energy force is required to result in a fracture.

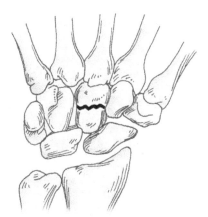

Figure 12–19. Capitate fracture.

Examination

Tenderness and swelling over the dorsal aspect of the hand in the area of the capitate will be present. Axial compression or movement of the third metacarpal exacerbates the pain.

Imaging

In patients with nondisplaced fractures, the initial radiographs are often nondiagnostic. In one study, 57% of initial radiographs failed to show the fracture or were read as normal. If the initial radiographs are nondiagnostic but the clinical suspicion of a fracture remains high, CT or MRI should be considered.

Associated Injuries

Most capitate fractures are associated with additional wrist injuries, including scaphoid fractures, distal radius fractures, lunate dislocations or subluxations, and carpometacarpal dislocations. An entity known as scaphocapitate syndrome is a unique injury that causes a scaphoid waist fracture and proximal capitate fracture.

Treatment

The extremity should be immobilized in a short-arm thumb spica splint (Appendix A–) with the wrist in slight dorsiflexion and the thumb immobilized to the IP joint in the wine glass position. Definitive management requires casting for 8 weeks for nondisplaced fractures.

If significant displacement is present, open reduction and internal fixation are indicated with early mobilization following surgery.

Complications

Capitate fractures may be associated with several complications:

- Malunion or AVN
- Posttraumatic arthritis, especially after comminuted capitate fractures
- Median nerve neuropathy or carpal tunnel syndrome

Hamate Fractures

The body of the hamate articulates distally with the bases of the fourth and fifth metacarpals, radially with the capitate, and proximally with the triquetrum and lunate. The hook of the hamate is the distal border of Guyon canal that contains the ulnar artery and nerve. Hamate fractures account for 1% to 4% of all carpal fractures. These fractures can be divided into four types on the basis of location, with fractures of the hook of the hamate being the most common type (Fig. 12–20):

- Distal articular surface
- Hook of the hamate
- Comminuted body
- Proximal pole articular surface

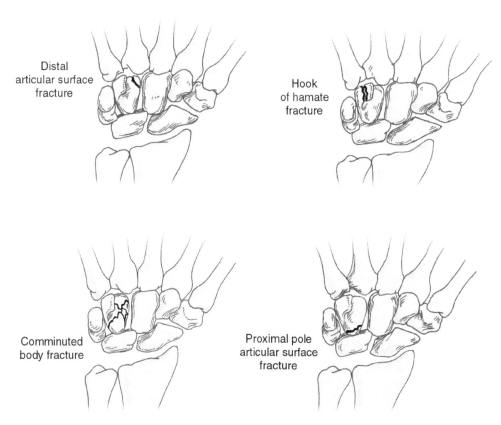

Distal articular surface fracture

Hook of hamate fracture

Comminuted body fracture

Proximal pole articular surface fracture

Figure 12–20. Hamate fractures.

Mechanism of Injury

Each type of hamate fracture generally results from a particular mechanism of injury. Distal articular surface fractures typically result from a fall or blow to the flexed and ulnar-deviated fifth metacarpal shaft. Fractures of the hook of the hamate are common in athletes involved in racket sports. During a forceful swing, the base of the racket (golf club, bat, etc.) compresses the hook, resulting in a fracture. Alternatively, a fall on the outstretched dorsiflexed hand can also result in these fractures. Direct crushing forces produce comminuted body fractures. Proximal pole or osteochondral fractures are impaction injuries that generally occur with the hand dorsiflexed and in ulnar deviation.

Examination

Tenderness is usually localized over the hypothenar eminence. Swelling will be minimal or absent. Distal articular fractures will exhibit increased pain with axial compression of the fifth metacarpal. Hook fractures exhibit tenderness over the palm of the hand in the area of the hamate hook (2 cm distal and radial to the pisiform) (Fig. 12–9). Pain is reproduced when the fourth and fifth digits are extended against resistance while the wrist is held in slight ulnar deviation. With this maneuver, known as "the hook of the hamate pull test," the flexor tendons become taut against the fractured hook and cause pain. Fractures of the body and proximal articular surface demonstrate increased pain with wrist motion.

Imaging

Routine radiographs, including oblique views, may not be adequate in demonstrating hamate fractures.[49]

Hamate body fractures may be visualized with standard wrist views (Fig. 12–21). The hook of the hamate is best visualized with a carpal tunnel view or CT scan (Fig. 12–22).[50] CT scanning has a sensitivity of 100% and a specificity of 94% for detecting fractures of the hook of the hamate.[51]

Of note, the hook of the hamate develops from a different ossification center and, in some adults, may persist as a separate small round ossicle (os hamulus proprium). This normal variant can be misinterpreted as a hamate fracture.

Associated Injuries

Ulnar nerve or arterial injuries frequently accompany hamate fractures. In addition, rupture of the flexor tendons (flexor digitorum profundus) has been reported.

Treatment

Nondisplaced hamate fractures are treated with an ulnar gutter splint for wrist immobilization (Appendix A–3) followed by a short-arm cast for a period of 6 to 8 weeks. All displaced fractures of the body and hook fractures where the patient cannot tolerate prolonged immobilization should be referred for operative intervention after the extremity has been splinted. Displaced or nonunited hamate hook fractures are treated with excision.

Complications

Fractures of the hamate, particularly the hook, can injure branches of the ulnar artery and nerve; thus, it is important

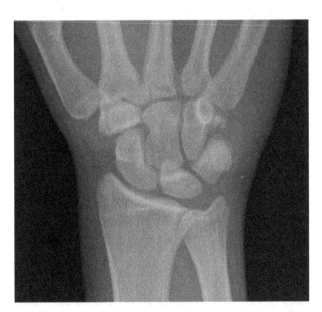

Figure 12–21. Fracture of the body of the hamate extending into the distal articular surface.

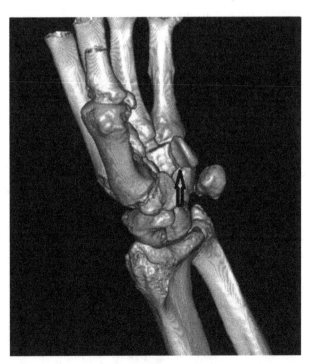

Figure 12–22. Hook of the hamate fracture on CT scan (*arrow*). Plain radiographs were negative.

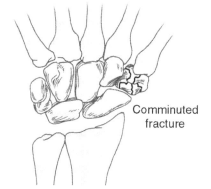
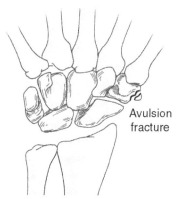

Figure 12–23. Trapezium fractures.

to ensure blood flow and sensation is intact to the fourth and fifth digits. Ulnar nerve injuries may result in interosseous atrophy with possible loss of grip strength. In addition, hamate fractures may lead to arthritis at the fifth carpometacarpal joint.

Trapezium Fractures

Trapezium fractures represent 1% to 5% of all carpal fractures. Isolated fractures are rare. These fractures usually occur in association with other injuries, such as fracture/dislocations of the first metacarpal, scaphoid fractures, and distal radius fractures. Trapezium fractures may be classified into three types (Fig. 12–23).

- Vertical fractures
- Comminuted fractures
- Avulsion fractures (trapezial ridge fracture)

Mechanism of Injury

Trapezium fractures are generally the result of one of three mechanisms. Vertical and comminuted fractures occur when the adducted thumb is driven forcefully into the articular surface of the trapezium. The bone is crushed between the radial styloid process and the first metacarpal. The trapezial ridge is a longitudinal palmar projection off the trapezium that serves as the radial attachment for the transverse carpal ligament. The trapezial ridge is fractured after direct trauma, such as a fall on an outstretched hand, or when the transverse carpal ligament causes an avulsion fracture.

Examination

The patient with a trapezium fracture will note pain at the base of the thenar eminence. They typically present with minimal swelling but may have significant discomfort (more than expected from other carpal bone fractures). In addition, the pain will be increased with thumb motion or axial compression of the thumb. In particular, there may be pain and weakness with pinching (e.g., making the "OK" sign or touching the thumb to the tip of the fifth digit).

Imaging

Trapezium fractures can be difficult to visualize on standard radiographic views. Routine studies may be adequate in demonstrating vertical and comminuted fractures (Fig. 12–24A). A carpal tunnel view or CT scan may reveal a fracture of the trapezial ridge (Fig. 12–24B).

Associated Injuries

Trapezium fractures may be associated with radial artery injury, first metacarpal fractures, distal radial fractures, and first metacarpal dislocations. The flexor carpi radialis courses along the base of the trapezial ridge and is therefore frequently injured following a fracture.

Treatment

The emergency management of these fractures includes elevation and ice. Immobilization with a short-arm thumb spica splint is recommended (Appendix A–7). Nondisplaced fractures and avulsion fractures can be managed with cast immobilization, whereas displaced fractures (>1 mm) require operative repair.

Complications

Trapezium fractures may be complicated by the development of arthritis involving the first metacarpal joint, tendonitis, or rupture of the flexor carpi radialis.

Pisiform Fractures

The pisiform is a sesamoid bone that lies on the volar surface of the wrist. It is unique in that it articulates only with one bone, the triquetrum. The pisiform is rarely fractured and accounts for only 1% of all carpal bone fractures. Anatomically, it is important to recall that the deep branch of the ulnar nerve and artery pass in close proximity to the radial surface of the bone within Guyon canal. In addition, the tendon of the flexor carpi ulnaris attaches to the volar surface of the pisiform.

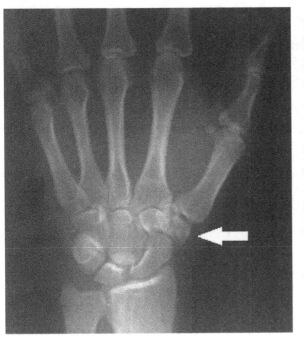
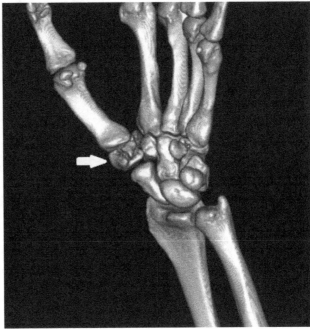

A   **B**

Figure 12–24. **A.** Comminuted fracture of the trapezium (*arrow*). **B.** Trapezial ridge fracture seen on CT scan.

Pisiform fractures are classified as follows (Fig. 12–25):

* Avulsion fractures
* Transverse body fractures
* Comminuted fractures

Mechanism of Injury

There are two common mechanisms resulting in pisiform fractures. A direct blow or fall on the outstretched hand can result in a transverse or comminuted body fracture. Indirectly, a fall on the outstretched hand with tension on the flexor carpi ulnaris may result in an avulsion fracture.

Examination

Tenderness will be present over the area of the pisiform (base of the hypothenar eminence). Ulnar-sided wrist pain will be elicited with resisted wrist flexion. It is important to always examine and record the function of the motor branch of the ulnar nerve when a pisiform fracture is suspected.

Imaging

Diagnosis of a pisiform fracture is difficult on standard views because the adjacent and overlying bones prevent an unobstructed view. If not seen on standard radiographs, the pisiform may be visualized with a carpal tunnel view or an oblique film with the wrist supinated 30 to 45 degrees. Alternatively, a CT scan will usually delineate a fracture.

Associated Injuries

Pisiform fractures may be associated with the following:

* Damage to the motor branch of the ulnar nerve
* Triquetrum fractures
* Hamate fractures
* Distal radial fractures

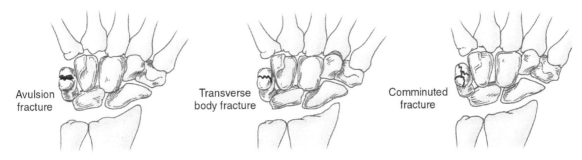

Avulsion fracture   Transverse body fracture   Comminuted fracture

Figure 12–25. Pisiform fractures.

Treatment

Initial treatment includes immobilization with an ulnar gutter splint (Appendix A-3). Definitive management consists of a short-arm cast for 6 weeks, followed by active movement of the flexor carpi ulnaris. Excision of the pisiform is necessary in cases of nonunion.

Complications

Complications related to a missed pisiform fracture include pisotriquetral chondromalacia or subluxation, loose fragments in the joint space, and degenerative arthritis. Pisiform fractures may be complicated by an impairment of the deep branch of the ulnar nerve. However, most ulnar nerve palsies that are present at initial presentation will resolve in 8 to 12 weeks and require only close observation.

Trapezoid Fractures

Trapezoid fractures are exceedingly rare (<1% of carpal fractures) due to the strong ligamentous attachments to the adjacent carpal bones (Fig. 12-26). Its keystone shape and position afford protection. Consequently, dorsal dislocation is much more common than fracture.

Mechanism of Injury

Fractures are most often due to a crush injury (direct dorsal trauma) or a high-energy axial force that pushes the second metacarpal into the trapezoid.

Examination

Point tenderness over the dorsal aspect of the wrist proximal to the base of the second metacarpal is noted. Concomitant injuries may obscure this finding. Gentle motion of the second metacarpal may elicit pain.

Imaging

Trapezoid fractures are difficult to visualize on standard wrist views. With several structures overlapping on these views, CT scan is the best imaging modality if the index of suspicion is high for fracture. Dislocations are best seen on the AP view as evidenced by a loss of the normal linear relationship with the proximal joint surface of the second metacarpal.

Associated Injuries

A fracture of the trapezoid rarely occurs in isolation. Fractures or dislocations of the adjacent metacarpal bases are frequently associated. Dorsal dislocation of the trapezoid can occur. It is reduced using longitudinal traction followed by palmar flexion of the wrist and dorsal pressure on the trapezoid.

Treatment

Initial management consists of ice and elevation. Immobilization with a thumb spica splint (Appendix A—) should be provided. Definitive management consists of cast immobilization or operative repair, depending on the degree of stability.

Complications

These fractures have a high incidence of nonunion and AVN. Because the trapezoid receives 70% of its interosseous blood supply through dorsal branches, dorsal fracture/dislocations often disrupt the blood supply and increase the risk of AVN.

DISTAL RADIUS FRACTURES

Distal radius fractures are among the most common long bone fractures encountered in the emergency department (ED). It has been noted that there is a bimodal distribution of these injuries primarily affecting children/adolescents and the elderly. These fractures include extension-type fractures (Colles), flexion-type fractures (Smith), and push-off fractures (Hutchinson and Barton). These types of distal radius fractures are considered separately after a brief review of the essential anatomy. The classification systems for distal radius fractures are complex. We discuss one of these classification systems and provide practical guidance to the emergency physician treating these injuries.

Essential Anatomy

The emergency physician should be aware of the essential anatomy of the distal radius to assess three important measurements that can be identified on a radiograph of the wrist: volar tilt, radial tilt, and radial length. Restoration of normal anatomy accomplished by either closed reduction and/or operative fixation will be necessary to ensure a good functional outcome. Failure to correct deformities may lead to abnormal wrist biomechanics and motion, as well as the development of traumatic arthritis.

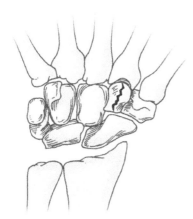

Figure 12-26. Trapezoid fracture.

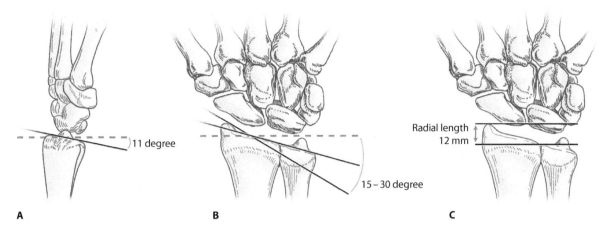

Figure 12–27. A. The normal radiocarpal joint is at an angle of 11 degrees in the volar direction, as shown in the lateral view. **B.** The normal angulation of the ulna in relation to the radiocarpal joint is 15 to 30 degrees. **C.** The normal radial length is 12 mm.

Volar Tilt. The normal radiocarpal joint angle is measured on the lateral view and ranges from 1 to 23 degrees (average of 11 degrees) in a volar direction (volar tilt) (Fig. 12–27A). Fractures associated with volar angulation generally result in good functional recovery, whereas fractures associated with dorsal angulation of the radiocarpal joint will have a poor functional recovery if adequate reduction is not accomplished.

Radial Tilt. The normal angulation of the radioulnar joint seen on the PA view of the wrist is 15 to 30 degrees (radial tilt) (Fig. 12–27B). The evaluation of this angle is essential when treating fractures of the distal radius because inadequate reduction resulting in loss of this angle will lead to an inhibition of ulnar hand motion.

Radial Length. This measurement is also viewed on the PA view of the wrist. It is the distance between two lines: one line perpendicular to the long axis of the radius passing through the distal tip of the radial styloid, and a second line intersecting the distal articular surface of the ulnar head (Fig. 12–27C). Normal radial length is 12 mm. If restoration of radial length cannot be restored after closed reduction, operative fixation may be necessary. In a study of displaced intra-articular radius fractures, restoration of radial length by operative intervention was more strongly correlated with improved functional status than restoration of radial or volar tilt.[58]

Classification

Many classification systems have been described for fractures of the distal radius.[55,57,59] Ideally, a classification system would allow the treating physician to initiate treatment with an understanding of the expected outcome. However, because of the large number of variables, no single classification system is optimal, with some being more clinically applicable than others.

More recently, Fernández proposed a classification system based on mechanism of injury with the added benefit of offering guidelines for treatment.[60] This system is as follows:

- *Type I*: Extra-articular metaphyseal bending fractures
  Colles (dorsal angulation) and Smith (volar angulation)
- *Type II*: Intra-articular shearing fractures
  Barton (dorsal and volar)
- *Type III*: Intra-articular compression fractures
  Complex articular and radial pilon fractures
- *Type IV*: Avulsion fractures
  Radiocarpal fracture dislocations
- *Type V*: High-velocity mechanism with extensive injury

Type I fractures can be reduced by the emergency physician. Types II through V fractures may undergo initial closed reduction in the ED; however, due to a high rate of complications, it is recommended that these patients have close orthopedic follow-up, as many of these cases will require operative intervention.

Most type I distal radius fractures can be managed nonoperatively after successful closed reduction (for displaced fractures). In most cases, types II through V fractures will ultimately require operative management due to their unstable nature.

Unstable fractures that are at high risk for secondary displacement even when properly casted after initial reduction include fractures of the distal radius that show more than 20 degrees of dorsal or volar angulation on initial radiographs, displacement more than two-thirds the width of the shaft in any direction, metaphyseal comminution, more than 5 mm of shortening, an intra-articular component, an associated ulna fracture, or advanced osteoporosis.[61]

A major limitation of most classification systems for distal radius fractures is that the radiographic appearance of the fracture does not clearly delineate a particular treatment method. Many other factors, including patient's age and functional status, occupation, bone density, surrounding soft-tissue injury, and the stability of closed reduction, are important to the orthopedic surgeon when considering the need for operative fixation. Osteopenia increases the need for operative fixation, as adequate closed reduction is difficult to maintain.

Associated Ulna Fractures

Fractures of the distal ulna are frequently associated with distal radius fractures and may contribute to the need for operative intervention. Approximately 60% of distal radius extension-type fractures are associated with fractures of the ulnar styloid, and 60% of ulnar styloid fractures are associated with fractures of the ulnar head or neck. Ulnar styloid fractures signify avulsion by the ulna collateral ligament complex. However, this injury is rarely significant, and appropriate treatment of the distal radius fracture is all that is necessary. Ulnar head or neck fractures may create an unstable DRUJ, and therefore, these fractures should be referred to an orthopedic surgeon for follow-up.

Extension-Type (Colles) Fracture

The distal radius is one of the most frequently fractured long bones, and the extension-type or Colles fracture is the most common wrist fracture seen in adults (Fig. 12–28).

Mechanism of Injury

Most distal radius fractures occur as a result of a fall on an outstretched hand. The amount of comminution and location of the fracture line depends on the force of the fall and the brittleness (age) of the bone. A supinating force often results in an associated ulnar fracture.

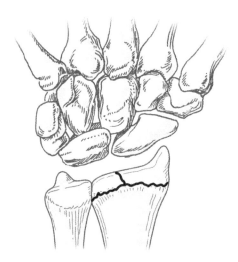

Figure 12–28. Distal radius fracture with intra-articular involvement.

Examination

Examination typically reveals pain, swelling, and tenderness of the distal forearm. The displaced angulated fracture typically resembles a dinner fork (Fig. 12–29). Documentation of the neurologic status with special emphasis on median nerve function should be stressed. Elbow or proximal forearm tenderness may be indicative of proximal radial head subluxation or dislocation.

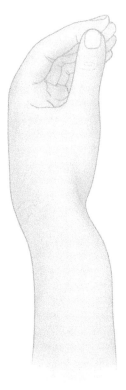

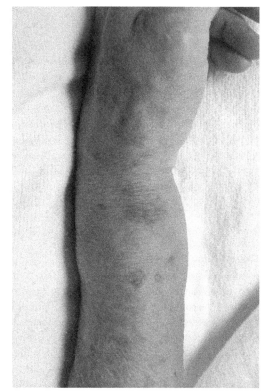

Figure 12–29. The dinner fork deformity described at the distal radius in a Colles fracture. *A.* Schematic. *B.* Clinical image.   A

B

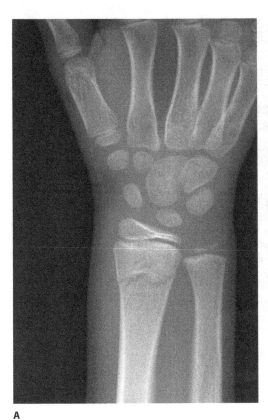
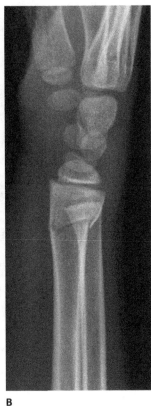

A   **B**

Figure 12–30. Extension-type (Colles) fracture. **A.** PA view. **B.** Lateral view.

Imaging

A PA and lateral view of the wrist is usually sufficient for demonstrating the fracture[63] (Fig. 12–30). Colles fractures are characterized by dorsal displacement or angulation of the distal radius (Fig. 12–31). Impaction of the dorsal cortex is frequently noted. With more substantial forces, comminution of the distal cortex of bone and intra-articular extension is seen.

When evaluating these fractures, the physician should address the following questions:

- *Is there an associated ulnar styloid or neck fracture (Fig. 12–32)?* These fractures may create an unstable DRUJ and require more urgent orthopedic referral.
- *Does the fracture involve the radioulnar or radiocarpal joint?* The more intra-articular involvement, especially if a step-off is present, the more likely traumatic arthritis will develop. CT or MRI may be helpful in delineating the extent of radiocarpal or radioulnar involvement; however, these tests may be performed on an outpatient basis.
- *What are the measurements of the volar tilt (lateral), radial tilt (PA), and radial length (PA)?* Loss of the normal anatomy increases the risk of complications.
- *Is there evidence of distal radioulnar subluxation on the lateral radiograph?* The ulna should not project more than 2 mm dorsal to the radius on a true lateral radiograph. Distances greater than 2 mm suggest distal radioulnar subluxation.

Associated Injuries

Extension-type fractures of the distal radius can be associated with several significant injuries, including ulnar styloid and neck fractures, carpal bone fractures, distal radioulnar subluxation, ligamentous injuries, flexor tendon injuries, and median and ulnar nerve injury.

Treatment

Colles fractures, which are nondisplaced and nonangulated with near-normal radial tilt, volar tilt, and radial length, can be immobilized in a volar or sugar-tong splint (Appendix A–11).[61,64] Other nondisplaced distal radius fractures are managed the same way. For displaced or angulated fractures with loss of normal anatomic alignment, closed reduction is performed either by a consulting orthopedist or the emergency physician if they are comfortable with the procedure.

Closed reduction of Colles fractures are carried out in the following manner (Fig. 12–33 and Video 12–1):

1. Adequate anesthesia should be provided with a hematoma block or procedural sedation (see Chapter 2 and Video 12–2).
2. *Distraction*: The fingers should be placed in finger traps and the elbow in 90 degrees of flexion. Tape placed around the fingers will protect the skin and prevent the fingers from slipping out. Approximately 5 to 10 lb of weight is suspended from the elbow for a period of

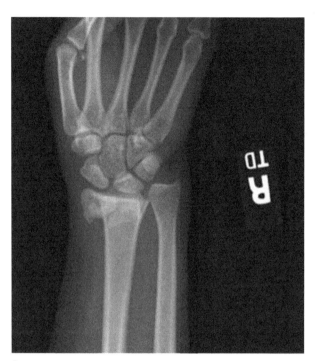

A

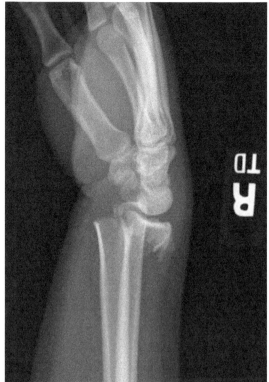

B

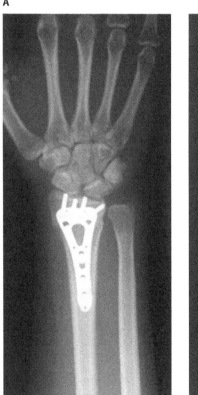

C

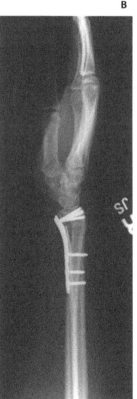

D

Figure 12–31. Extension-type (Colles) fracture with dorsal displacement. **A.** PA view. **B.** Lateral view. **C.** PA view after repair. **D.** Lateral view after repair.

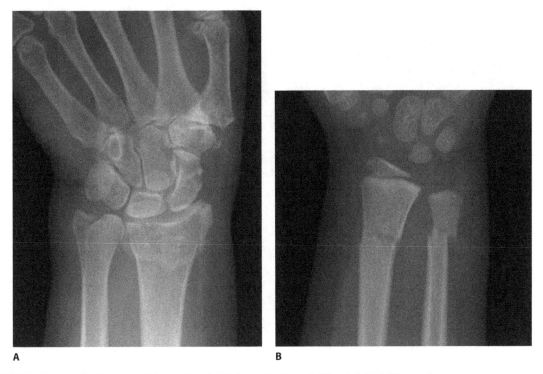

Figure 12–32. Distal radius fractures with associated distal ulna fractures. **A.** Ulna styloid. **B.** Ulna neck.

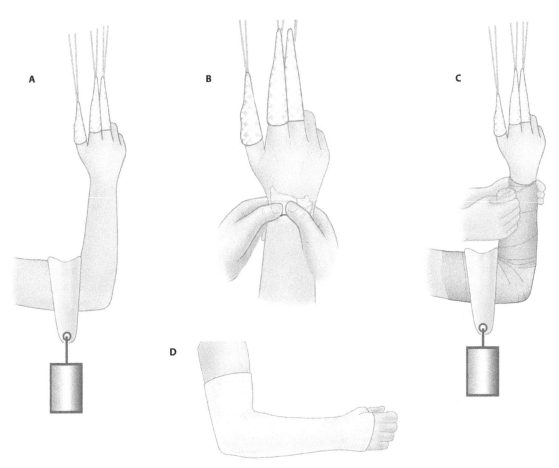

Figure 12–33. The reduction of a Colles fracture. **A.** Distraction with a 10-lb weight and finger traps for 10 minutes. **B.** Disengagement and reapposition with the thumbs over the distal fragment and fingers around the forearm. **C.** The arm is wrapped with padding material and the splint is applied. **D.** The final position of the forearm is neutral with the wrist slightly flexed and ulnar deviated.

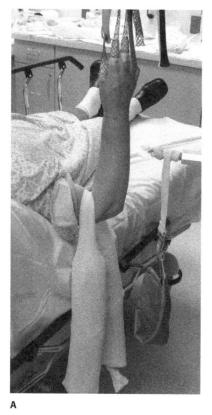
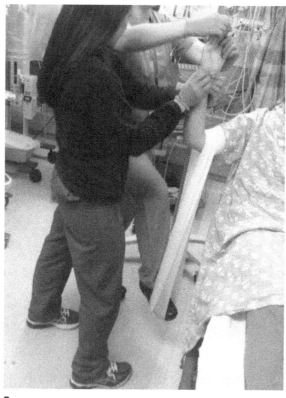

A   **B**

Figure 12–34. *A.* Disengagement of a Colles fracture with finger traps and four bags of saline in stockinette. *B.* Alternatively, a gauze bandage is tied in a circle and wrapped around the patient's arm. The clinician's foot is used to create the distracting force.

5 to 15 minutes or until the fragments disimpact. Four bags of saline in a sling or stockinette weigh almost 9 lb and can be used as an alternative to traditional weights (Fig. 12–34). Alternatively, traction–countertraction can be used to distract the fragments (Video 12–3).

3. *Disengagement*: With the thumbs on the dorsal aspect of the distal fragment and the fingers grasping around the wrist, the force of the injury is re-created by slight extension of the distal fragment to disengage the fracture fragments.

4. *Reapposition*: While maintaining traction, pressure is applied over the distal fragment in a volar direction with the thumbs, and dorsally directed pressure over the proximal segment with the fingers.

5. *Release*: When proper positioning has been achieved, the traction weight is removed. If fluoroscopy is available, the success of the reduction can be evaluated immediately.

When reduction is complete, the forearm is immobilized, and median nerve function is retested and documented. Preparation of the splint materials before the reduction attempt will allow more rapid immobilization once the fracture is reduced. The forearm is wrapped in a thin layer of padding, followed by the application of a sugar-tong splint (Appendix A–11). Excessive padding or the use of commercially available fiberglass splint material is not recommended because the reduction is less likely to

be maintained. Colles fractures are typically immobilized in slight pronation (25 degrees), with the wrist in 15 degrees of palmer flexion and 10 to 15 degrees of ulnar deviation. Postreduction radiographs are obtained to ensure proper reduction. After reduction, the arm should remain elevated for 72 hours to keep swelling at a minimum. Finger and shoulder exercises should begin immediately.

In reducing distal radius fractures, several principles must be remembered. First, patients who present in a delayed fashion (i.e., days later) are more difficult to reduce, and performing a hematoma block alone will often not provide effective pain management. Second, dorsal angulation (tilt) is not acceptable, and volar tilt is difficult to maintain because the extensors of the hand tend to exert dorsal traction. In addition, restoration of normal radial tilt is easily achieved with reduction but frequently difficult to maintain during the healing phase. Radiographs to document that proper reduction is maintained should be obtained at 3 days and 2 weeks post injury. If the reduction cannot be maintained, internal fixation might be required. Guidelines for adequate reduction have been described and include[ ]:

- Radial inclination: 15 degrees or greater on PA view
- Radial length: 5 mm or less shortening on PA view
- Radial tilt: Less than 15-degree dorsal or 20-degree volar tilt on lateral view
- Articular incongruity: 2 mm or less of step-off

Colles fractures, even when managed appropriately, can result in long-term complications.[65,66] For this reason, follow-up with an orthopedist is recommended within 1 week, especially when a fracture is reduced in the ED. Nondisplaced fractures should remain immobilized for 4 to 6 weeks, whereas displaced fractures that are adequately reduced require 6 to 12 weeks of immobilization.

Unstable fractures may require percutaneous pinning, internal fixation, or external fixation.[67,68] Other indications for surgery include open fractures, severely comminuted or displaced (>2 mm) intra-articular fractures, and fractures with more than 3 mm of dorsal displacement or 10 degrees of dorsal angulation after an attempt at closed reduction. Delay beyond 2 to 3 weeks makes operative intervention more difficult because the fracture fragments cannot be manipulated.

Complications

Complications associated with Colles fractures are commonly reported in the literature.[69–71] These complications include neuropathies, degenerative arthritis, malunion, tendon injury, compartment syndrome, and reflex sympathetic dystrophy. Limitation of wrist function after these fractures has been reported to be as high as 90%.[72] Early adequate reduction of the fracture is the most important early aspect of care to reduce complications. Complications of these fractures are typically described as immediate, early (<6 weeks), and late (>6 weeks).[69]

Immediate complications include nerve injury with the median nerve being most commonly affected. Acute carpal tunnel syndrome is more common in patients with severe comminuted fractures and those requiring multiple closed reduction attempts. Other immediate injuries include skin injury during manipulation or as a result of an open fracture, compartment syndrome (rare), or missed associated injuries.

Early complications include median nerve dysfunction, tendon injury, ulnar nerve injury, compartment syndrome, and fracture fragment displacement. The patient with median nerve compression will usually complain of pain and paresthesias over the distribution of the median nerve. If casted, the cast and padding should be split and the arm elevated for 48 to 72 hours. If the symptoms persist, carpal tunnel syndrome should be suspected. *Caution:* The function of the median nerve in distal forearm fractures should always be documented. Persistent pain should be regarded as secondary to median nerve compression until proven otherwise. Another early complication is infection as a result of an open fracture or operative fixation (percutaneous pinning or internal plate fixation).

Late complications include stiffness of the fingers, shoulder, or radiocarpal joint; reflex sympathetic dystrophy; cosmetic defects resulting from displaced fractures; rupture of the extensor pollicis longus; malunion or nonunion; flexor tendon adhesions; and chronic pain over the radioulnar joint with supination.

Flexion-Type (Smith) Fracture

This fracture has often been described as a reverse Colles fracture. It is an uncommon fracture, outnumbered compared to Colles fractures by a factor of 10:1. A Smith fracture rarely involves the DRUJ. The classification system, developed by Thomas, has both therapeutic and prognostic implications.[73]

Mechanism of Injury

Several mechanisms can result in these types of distal forearm flexion fractures, including a fall on a supinated forearm with the hand in dorsiflexion, a punch with the fist clenched and the wrist slightly flexed, or a direct blow to the dorsum of the wrist or distal radius with the hand flexed and the forearm in pronation.

Examination

Pain and swelling will be apparent over the volar aspect of the wrist. The clinical appearance of this fracture is described as a garden spade deformity (Fig. 12-35A). The presence and function of the radial artery and median nerve should be examined and documented.

Imaging

Routine PA and lateral views are adequate for demonstrating this fracture (Fig. 12–35B). Smith fractures are characterized by volar displacement and volar angulation of the distal radius.

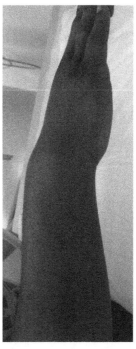
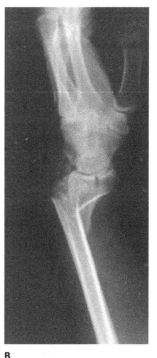

A   B

Figure 12–35. ***A.*** Clinical photo of a Smith fracture. ***B.*** Displaced Smith fracture on lateral radiograph.

Associated Injuries

Carpal fractures or dislocations are uncommonly associated with these fractures.

Treatment

These fractures require emergent orthopedic referral for reduction. If orthopedic referral is unavailable, the fracture may be reduced as follows. Traction is applied using finger traps with 8 to 10 lb of weight at the flexed elbow. The wrist is then flexed until the fragments are disimpacted. With the thumbs against the distal fragment, dorsal pressure is applied until the fragments are properly positioned. The forearm should be immobilized in a sugar-tong splint (Appendix A-11). Postreduction radiographs for documentation of reduction should be obtained. If the reduction remains stable, this fracture can be definitively treated with casting, although these fractures more frequently require surgery. Unstable fractures require pin or plate fixation. Patients with intra-articular involvement require urgent referral for pinning of the bony fragment.

Complications

Complications seen with these fractures include tendon damage, nerve compression, and development of osteoarthritis.

Dorsal and Volar Rim (Barton) Fracture

These fractures are intra-articular and involve the dorsal or volar rim of the distal radius (Fig. 12–36). Using the

classification scheme described by Fernández, Barton fracture is described as a type II shearing mechanism fracture. These fractures require operative repair if the fracture fragment is large or unstable. Barton fractures most commonly involve the dorsal rim of the distal radius (classic Barton fracture), and typically a triangular fragment of bone is noted on a lateral radiograph of the wrist.

Mechanism of Injury

Extreme dorsiflexion of the wrist accompanied by a pronating force may result in a dorsal rim fracture.

Examination

The distal dorsal radius will be tender and swollen. Occasionally, radial nerve sensory branches may be compromised and present as paresthesias in the area of distribution.

Imaging

Lateral radiographs adequately demonstrate the fracture fragment and the degree of displacement (Fig. 12–37).

Associated Injuries

Carpal bone injury or dislocations, along with damage to the sensory branches of the radial nerve, may occur.

Treatment

Management depends on the size of the fracture fragment and the degree of displacement. Nondisplaced Barton fractures should be placed in a sugar-tong splint (Appendix A-11) with the forearm in a neutral position. A large displaced fragment with subluxation or dislocation of the carpal bones requires procedural sedation followed by a closed reduction. If the fracture is stable and in a good position, a sugar-tong splint (Appendix A-11) with the forearm in a neutral position is recommended. If the fracture is unstable or reduced inadequately, open reduction with internal fixation is indicated. A small fragment may be reduced and fixed by the placement of a percutaneous pin.

Complications

Frequent complications include arthritis secondary to intra-articular involvement as well as those complications associated with Colles fractures.

Radial Styloid (Hutchinson) Fracture

This fracture is also known as a chauffeur's or backfire fracture. The term originated in the era of hand-cranked automobiles. The injury historically occurred as a result of recoil of the crank[52] (Fig. 12–38).

Mechanism of Injury

The mechanism involved is similar to that seen in a scaphoid fracture. Here, the force is transmitted from the scaphoid to the styloid.

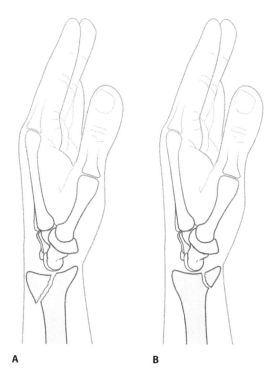

Figure 12–36. Barton fracture. **A.** Dorsal. **B.** Volar.

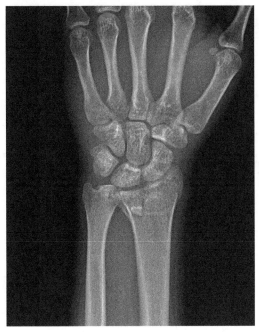 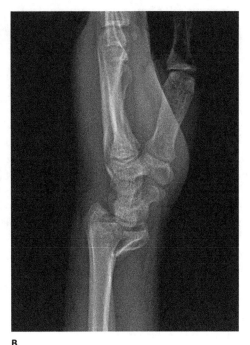

A   **B**

Figure 12–37. Barton fracture. ***A.*** PA. ***B.*** Lateral view demonstrating a fracture of the volar rim of the radius with subluxation of the carpal bones.

Examination

Pain, tenderness, and swelling are noted over the radial styloid.

Imaging

A PA radiograph of the wrist best demonstrates this fracture (Fig. 12–39).

Associated Injuries

Both fractures of the scaphoid and scapholunate dissociation may be associated with these fractures.[67] Up to 70% of radial styloid fractures have extension of injury into the scapholunate ligaments.

Treatment

The forearm should be immobilized in a sugar-tong splint (Appendix A–11) with ice and elevation. These patients require urgent orthopedic referral as percutaneous fixation is indicated for unstable fractures.

Complications

Complications of these fractures include scapholunate ligament disruption and degenerative arthritis.

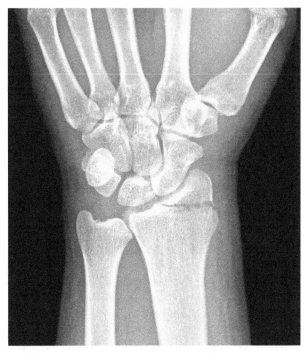

Figure 12–39. Radiograph of a radial styloid fracture (Hutchinson fracture).

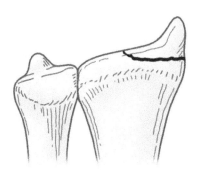

Figure 12–38. Radial styloid fracture (Hutchinson fracture).

WRIST SOFT-TISSUE INJURY AND DISLOCATIONS

LIGAMENTOUS INJURY

Carpal stability is maintained by a complex array of ligaments connecting the bones of the wrist. Ligaments are located on the volar and dorsal sides of the wrist as well as within the intraosseous spaces. The volar ligaments are stronger than the dorsal ligaments with the exception of the space of Poirier, an area on the volar aspect between the lunate and capitate that is often the site of carpal dislocation. Injury to the carpal ligaments can result in loss of the normal alignments of the carpal bones, carpal dislocation, or a combination of the two. With enough force, an associated fracture may occur (scaphoid, capitate, triquetrum, radial, or ulnar styloid). The most common mechanism for these types of injuries is a fall on an outstretched hand; however, a direct blow, distraction, and torquing motions can also produce these injuries.

Carpal instability and associated carpal bone dislocation may be difficult to adequately assess, and radiographic findings may be subtle. Radiographic abnormality may only be noted after stress (e.g., clenched fist), termed *dynamic instability*. Dynamic instability can be seen with partial ligamentous disruption, which frequently progresses to a complete injury over time. Inadequate evaluation during the initial examination or misdiagnosis may lead to progressive loss of range of motion, degenerative arthritis, chronic pain, and disability.

For an overall understanding of ligamentous injuries of the wrist, we briefly review Mayfield's stages of injury. Specific injury patterns are mentioned and covered in greater detail below.

Mayfield described four stages of progressive carpal bone. He found that ligamentous injuries occurred in a sequential and additive fashion. Stage I injuries are associated with a tear of the scapholunate interosseous ligament and the radioscapholunate ligament. When these ligaments are torn, scapholunate dissociation or dorsal intercalated segment instability (DISI) can occur. Stage II injuries occur when there is an additional injury to the volar capitolunate ligament. This results in instability of the scaphoid and capitate. Stage III includes injury to the lunotriquetral interosseous ligament and volar lunotriquetral ligament. When these ligaments are ruptured, there is instability of the scaphoid, capitate, and triquetrum with respect to the lunate. It is at this stage that a dorsal perilunate dislocation occurs. In stage IV injuries, the dorsal radiolunate ligament is ruptured and a lunate dislocation or volar intercalated segment instability (VISI) can occur. In this case, the lunate more frequently displaces anteriorly because the volar radiolunate ligament remains intact.

Intercalated Segment Instability

This condition can be thought of as midcarpal joint collapse. The normal upright position of the lunate on the lateral radiograph is a result of the ligamentous attachments of the adjacent carpal bones. The scaphoid, by way of the scapholunate ligament, pulls the lunate into flexion, while the triquetrum, by way of the lunotriquetral ligament, pulls the lunate into extension. When the scapholunate ligament is disrupted, the unopposed force of the lunotriquetral ligament causes the lunate to tip dorsally, a condition known as DISI. On the lateral radiograph, the distal articular surface of the lunate tilts dorsally, and the scaphoid bone tilts more volarly (Fig. 12–40). The end result is an increase in the capitolunate angle (>30 degrees) and scapholunate angle (>60 degrees). DISI is the most common type of intercalated segment instability and may be seen with scapholunate dissociation or scaphoid fractures.

VISI is present when the lunotriquetral ligament is disrupted. The distal articular surface of the lunate now tilts volarly, creating an increased capitolunate angle (>30 degrees) and a decreased scapholunate angle (<30 degrees). On examination, there is tenderness over the lunotriquetral joint.

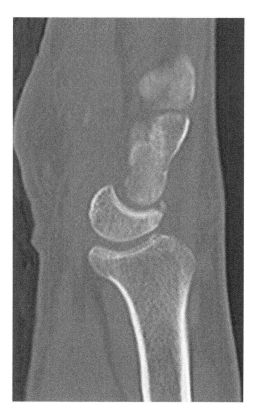

Figure 12–40. Dorsal intercalated segment instability. Note the dorsal tilt of the lunate.

The presence of intercalated segment instability suggests ligamentous disruption that is best treated with reapproximation and operative repair. When this is not possible, another procedure will be required to prevent degenerative arthritis from uneven loads to the carpal joints that occur over time. In the case of disruption of the scapholunate ligament, scapholunate advanced collapse refers to the degenerative condition that follows.

Scapholunate Dissociation

This injury is characterized by the displacement of the scaphoid to a more vertical position in the proximal row of carpal bones. When the scapholunate ligament is ruptured, a gap between the lunate and the proximal pole of the scaphoid is produced. Rupture of the radioscapholunate ligament allows for the volar rotation of the scaphoid and is sometimes termed *rotary subluxation of the scaphoid.*[75] In one study, scapholunate dissociation occurred in 5% of ED patients who did not have a fracture noted on wrist radiographs.[76] This diagnosis can also be challenging in the setting of a concurrent distal radius or carpal bone fracture because of the associated pain and swelling.

Mechanism of Injury

Scapholunate dissociation often occurs as a result of forceful extension of the wrist from a fall on an outstretched hand.

Examination

Patients usually present with wrist pain and swelling. Wrist pain is accentuated at the extremes of motion. The patient may also note crepitus or a snapping sound with wrist motion. A scaphoid shift maneuver known as "Watson's sign" provides a qualitative assessment of the stability of the scaphoid.[77] This maneuver should always be compared to the contralateral side. The scaphoid shift may be subtle or more dramatic. As thumb pressure is withdrawn, the scaphoid returns abruptly to its normal position, sometimes with a resounding "thunk" or "click"[78] (Fig. 12–41). Pain on performance of this test is a more reliable sign of instability than the "click."

Imaging

Scapholunate dissociation is noted radiographically on the PA view as a widening of the *scapholunate joint space.* This joint space should always be noted in any patient with trauma to the wrist. A measurement of ≥3 mm is abnormal and is at times referred to as the "Terry Thomas sign" or "David Letterman sign." A clenched fist PA view forces the capitate head into the scapholunate joint and exposes the ligamentous laxity, making this radiograph a more sensitive means of diagnosis. When rotary subluxation of the scaphoid occurs, an additional radiographic finding on a PA view may be seen, the cortical ring sign (or signet sign). This finding represents the rotation of the normally elongated scaphoid causing the distal pole to be viewed on end. On the lateral view, the scapholunate angle is noted to be >60 degrees due to the volar rotation of the scaphoid (Fig. 12–42).[79,80]

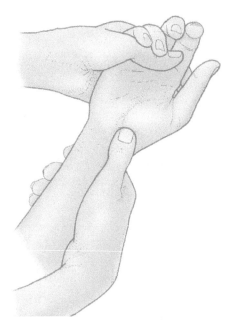

Figure 12–41. The scaphoid shift maneuver to assess for scaphoid stability. The patient's forearm is slightly pronated. The examiner grasps the patient's wrist from the radial side, placing the thumb on the prominence of the scaphoid and wrapping the fingers around the distal forearm. The thumb should put pressure on the scaphoid while the examiner's fingers provide counterpressure. The examiner's other hand grasps the patient's hand at the level of the metacarpal heads. The examiner ulnar deviates and slightly extends the patient's hand, and then moves the patient's wrist radially and into slight flexion while maintaining thumb pressure on the scaphoid. This maneuver is positive if the scaphoid shifts dorsally.

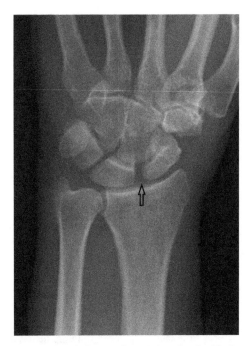

Figure 12–42. Scapholunate dissociation. On the PA view, note the increased distance (≥3 mm) between the scaphoid and lunate, the Terry Thomas sign (*arrow*).

Associated Injuries

Scapholunate dissociation can occur in association with perilunate or lunate dislocation, or it may occur as an isolated injury or in conjunction with a scaphoid fracture or distal radius fracture.

Treatment

All patients with a suspected scapholunate dissociation should be placed in a thumb spica splint (Appendix A-2) and referred to a hand surgeon for close follow-up. Treatment often involves either arthroscopic or open repair of the disrupted ligament.

Complications

Degenerative arthritis with associated limited range of motion and chronic pain can be seen with scapholunate dissociation.

Perilunate and Lunate Dislocations

Perilunate (Stage III) and lunate dislocations (Stage IV) are often considered together, although they represent a progressive degree of injury, as outlined previously. The normal articulation of the radius, lunate, capitate, and third metacarpal makes up a straight line, which is best visualized on the lateral view of the wrist (Fig. 12–43). In a perilunate dislocation, the capitate is dislocated, usually dorsally, in relation to the lunate. With a lunate dislocation, the lunate is dislocated in the volar direction (most commonly) in

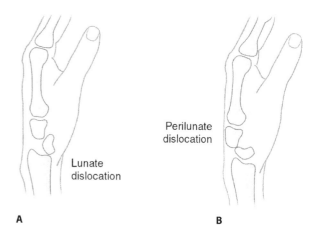

Figure 12–44. A. Volar lunate dislocation **B.** Dorsal perilunate dislocation.

relation to the distal radius and the capitate, which appears in a normal position (Fig. 12–44).

Mechanism of Injury

The mechanism of injury includes excessive hyperextension, ulnar deviation, and intercarpal supination.

Examination

On physical examination, there is dorsal wrist swelling and decreased wrist motion, especially on flexion. A palpable fullness may be noted on the dorsal side of the wrist after a dorsal perilunate dislocation and on the volar surface with a volar lunate dislocation. The median nerve may be compressed in the carpal canal by the lunate. If this occurs, the patient may display signs of an acute median nerve injury.

Imaging

Radiographic abnormalities will be seen on both PA and lateral wrist films. When reading the lateral view of the wrist, an imaginary line should be drawn down the center of the distal radius. This line should bisect directly through the midportion of the lunate and the capitate. The lateral wrist radiograph is the single most important view from which to determine correct alignment of the carpal bones. It is helpful to rotate the image so that the wrist is viewed in the horizontal plane.

In a perilunate dislocation, the PA view reveals a capitate and lunate that overlap. The carpal arcs are disrupted at the scapholunate and triquetrolunate joint. On the lateral film, the capitate is dislocated in relation to the lunate (Fig. 12–45). With a lunate dislocation, the PA film reveals the lunate to have a *triangular appearance*. The lunate is displaced and tilted volarly on the lateral view, the so-called "spilled teacup sign" (Fig. 12–46). The term *midcarpal dislocation* can be used when there is dislocation of the lunate and capitate. In this case, neither bone is aligned over the

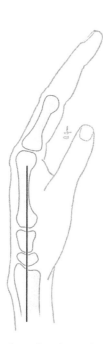

Figure 12–43. Note that a line drawn through the midpoint of the radius and the capitate on the lateral view of the wrist traverses the midpoint of the lunate. If the lunate is dislocated or subluxated, the line will traverse only a fragment of the bone or miss it entirely.

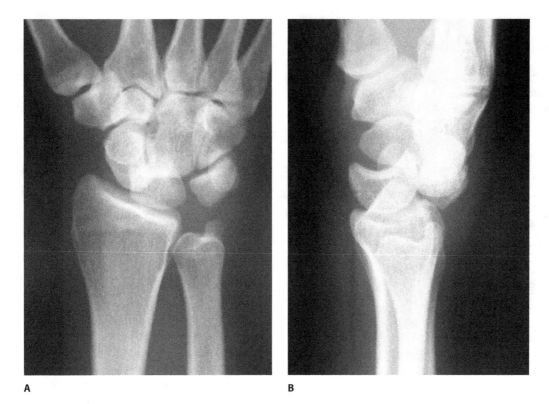

Figure 12–45. Dorsal perilunate dislocation. **A.** On the PA view, note the overlap of the carpal bones. **B.** The lateral view reveals the dorsal location of the capitate and other carpal bones with the lunate articulating normally with the radius.

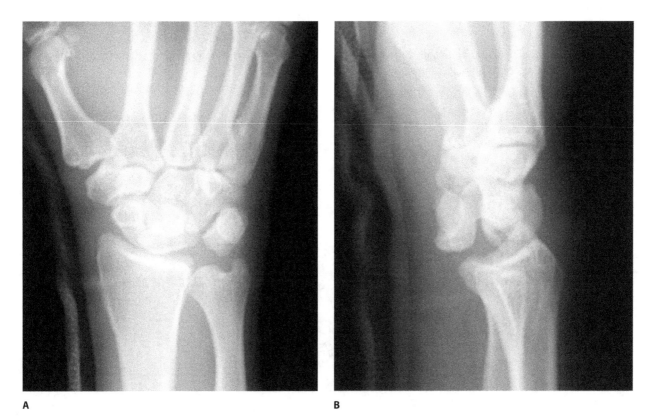

Figure 12–46. Volar lunate dislocation. **A.** PA. **B.** Lateral.

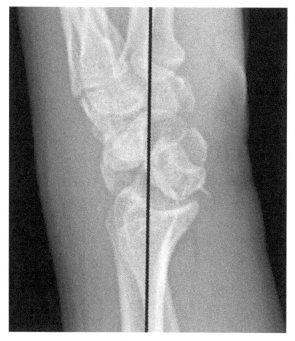

Figure 12–47. Midcarpal dislocation. Note that both the lunate and capitate do not bisect a line drawn through the center of the radius.

center of the distal radius (Fig. 12–47). When a carpal bone fracture is also present, the prefix "trans-" is applied to the name of the bone that is fractured, followed by the site of dislocation (Fig. 12–48).

Associated Injuries

Perilunate and lunate dislocation injuries are associated with scaphoid fractures and, less commonly, capitate fractures.

Treatment

All lunate and perilunate dislocations should be immobilized with the wrist in neutral position in a volar splint and referred immediately for reduction and definitive care.

Closed reduction of lunate and perilunate dislocations requires the use of either a wrist block or procedural sedation to obtain good muscle relaxation and pain control. Finger traps are used with approximately 10 lb of weight for at least 10 minutes prior to reduction. Some authors prefer surgical reduction for complex perilunate dislocations.

Closed or open reduction with percutaneous fixation is indicated for an acute injury. Both perilunate and lunate dislocations usually involve either a scaphoid fracture or rotary subluxation of the scaphoid.

Triangular Fibrocartilage Complex Tear

The term *triangular fibrocartilage complex* (TFCC) is used to describe the major ligamentous stabilizers of the DRUJ and ulnar carpal bones. Injury to this structure often occurs due to a fall but can be seen from repetitive trauma or overuse. Tenderness is localized by palpating in the hollow between the pisiform and the ulnar styloid on the ulnar border of the wrist. Dorsal tears can be diagnosed by the "supination lift test" in which the patient is asked to attempt to lift the examination table with the palm flat on the underside of the table. Eliciting pain or weakness confirms the diagnosis. Treatment is initially conservative with immobilization in slight flexion and ulnar deviation, followed by physical therapy. Arthroscopic repair may be required, so orthopedic referral is recommended whenever this injury is suspected.

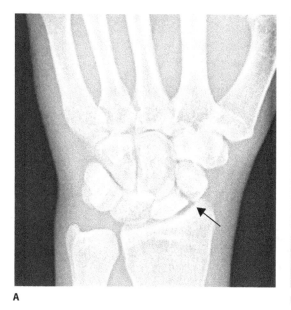
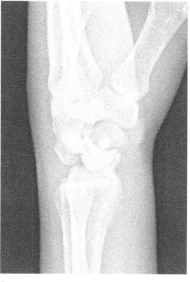

A   B

Figure 12–48. Transcaphoid dorsal perilunate dislocation on (*A*) PA and (*B*) lateral radiographs (*arrow,* scaphoid fracture).

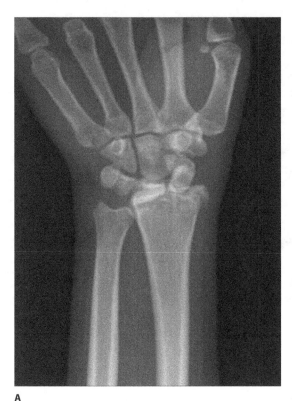
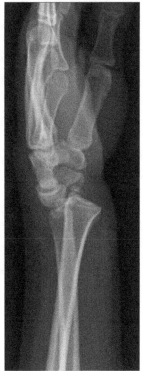

Figure 12–49. Radiocarpal dislocation. *A.* PA view. *B.* Lateral view. In addition, a comminuted intra-articular radius fracture is noted.

Radiocarpal Dislocation

It is estimated that radiocarpal dislocations represent 0.2% of all dislocations (Fig. 12–49).[86] Dorsal dislocation is more common than volar. These injuries often result from high-energy shear and rotational forces; therefore, many associated injuries can be seen, including open and closed fractures, carpal instability, tendon ruptures, and neurovascular compromise. The mechanism is typically forced hyperextension, pronation, and radial inclination. This injury should be differentiated from marginal or rim fractures of the distal radius (Barton fracture) which are viewed as compression injuries.[86] A radiocarpal dislocation is a rare entity in the absence of an intra-articular fracture of the radius.[85,87]

Prompt orthopedic consultation is recommended for radiocarpal dislocation. After closed reduction, a dorsal dislocation should be immobilized with some wrist extension, whereas a volar dislocation is immobilized in wrist flexion. Radiocarpal dislocations have been treated successfully with closed reduction, but most cases require operative intervention.

NERVE COMPRESSION

Carpal Tunnel Syndrome (Median)

Carpal tunnel syndrome (CTS) is the most common compressive neuropathy involving the upper extremities. The carpal tunnel is a confined space located between the carpal

bones and the transverse carpal ligament (Fig. 12–50). Acute CTS can be seen following a distal radius or carpal bone fracture/dislocation or may develop chronically from repetitive strain at the wrist, leading to compression of the median nerve in the carpal tunnel. In addition, several atraumatic conditions have been associated with the development of CTS, including thyroid disorders, pregnancy, diabetes, amyloid, lupus, Lyme disease, and multiple myeloma.[62,88–90]

Classically, a patient will complain of a gradual onset of numbness or tingling along with pain in the thumb, index, and long finger. Often these complaints are bilateral and will be worse at night or with strenuous activities of the hand. At times, the intense paresthesias are described as pain. Symptoms may radiate proximally to the forearm, elbow, or even shoulder but spares the little finger. Sometimes, patients will notice these complaints on awakening.

The earliest objective sensory finding in CTS is diminished vibratory sensation, tested with a tuning fork. More severe median nerve involvement results in abnormal two-point sensory discrimination.[91]

Classic physical examination findings include the Tinel sign and Phalen tests. A Tinel sign is elicited by tapping the volar aspect of the wrist. A positive sign is reported when the patient experiences paresthesias in the distribution of the median nerve (Fig. 12–51A). A Phalen test is performed by having the patient flex his/her wrist for 1 minute. If paresthesias are noted in the hand over the median nerve

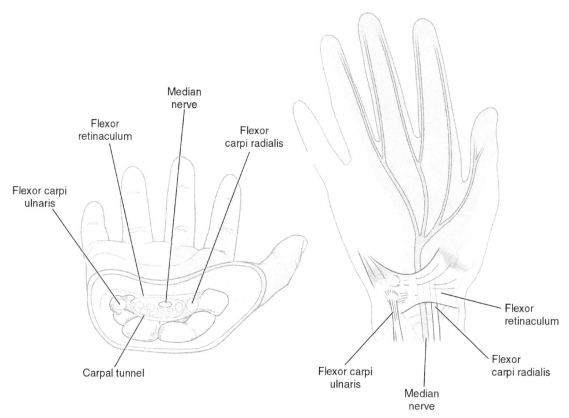

Figure 12–50. The carpal tunnel with the median nerve under the transverse carpal ligament.

distribution, the test is positive (Fig. 12–51B). A blood pressure cuff inflated to 200 mm Hg pressure for 2 minutes may also produce paresthesias in the hand and is reported as a positive tourniquet test. The flick sign is present when patients report that shaking of the hand relieves the paresthesia. Often these tests are helpful in the bedside evaluation of the patient with suspected CTS. However, none is sensitive enough to identify all cases. Currently, electrodiagnostic studies are the recognized standard for the diagnosis of CTS.

Conservative therapy includes avoidance of repetitive wrist and hand motions, wrist splinting, nonsteroidal anti-inflammatory drugs (NSAIDs), and oral or local corticosteroid injection. Oral corticosteroids have been

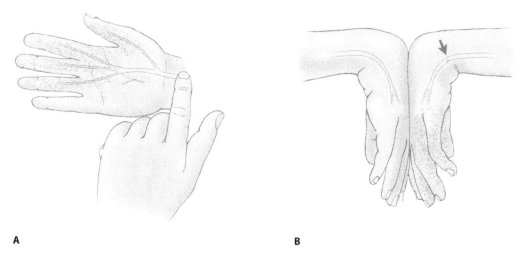

A   B

Figure 12–51. Tests for carpal tunnel syndrome. **A.** The Tinel test is performed by tapping the volar surface of the wrist over the median nerve. **B.** Phalen test is performed by compressing the opposing dorsal surfaces of the hand with the wrist flexed together, as shown. This causes tingling over the median nerve distribution.

shown to be more effective than NSAIDs, and current dose recommendations include prednisone 20 mg per day for 2 weeks.[90] The majority of patients respond to conservative measures, although 80% recur at 1 year.[90] If a positive response is not noted, surgical decompression may be required.

Combined injection of corticosteroid (methylprednisolone 40 mg) and a local anesthetic agent can be both diagnostic and therapeutic. The best site for injection is proximal to the transverse carpal ligament, as this lowers the risk of median nerve damage. The needle is introduced at a 20-degree angle to the skin between the palmaris longus tendon and the flexor carpi radialis, approximately 4 cm proximal to the wrist crease.[93] After inserting the needle beneath the transverse carpal ligament, the steroid-anesthetic solution is injected. To be certain that the needle is positioned appropriately, the provider should elicit paresthesias in the median nerve distribution. At that time, the needle is withdrawn 1 to 2 mm and the contents of the syringe are injected.

Ulnar Nerve Compression

Ulnar tunnel syndrome is compression of the ulnar nerve at the level of the wrist that occurs as the nerve enters the ulnar tunnel or as the deep branch curves around the hook of the hamate in the palm. This may occur in association with repetitive trauma, arthritis, or compression from a ganglion cyst or another benign tumor, as the predominant mechanism is direct compression. This condition occurs in cyclists and others who experience repetitive compression in this area. The ulnar nerve can also be subjected to external compression at the elbow (cubital tunnel syndrome). Refer to Chapter 14 for further discussion of cubital tunnel syndrome.

Patients with an ulnar nerve problem at the wrist will experience an ulnar neuropathy similar to lesions at the elbow, with the exception of the dorsal surface of the hand. Because the cutaneous branch to this region arises proximal to the wrist, dorsal fifth digit sensation will be preserved when the ulnar nerve is compressed at the wrist.

Conservative treatment is initially recommended, which involves proper splinting of the involved extremity and avoidance of the inciting activity. If no improvement is noted after a period of 3 to 4 months, surgery is indicated.

Radial Nerve Compression

Radial nerve compression is less common than neuropathies involving either the median or ulnar nerves.[88] Patients with radial nerve dysfunction can present with complaints of inability to extend the wrist. The most common site for compression of the radial nerve is in the axilla, usually after the incorrect use of crutches, and at the radial tunnel in the elbow. When compression occurs in the spiral groove of the humerus, it is called "Saturday night palsy" because it is seen in intoxicated patients who sleep with their arms resting over the back of a chair. The resulting deficit is primarily motor, with weakness in thumb abduction (abductor pollicis longus), index finger extension (extensor indicis proprius), and wrist extension. Most of these deficits resolve spontaneously as they are secondary to a compressive neuropraxia. Treatment is a cock-up splint worn to prevent wrist drop. Radial neuropathy is further discussed in Chapter 14.

GANGLION CYST

A ganglion cyst, the most common tumor of the hand/wrist, is a synovial cyst that originates from either a joint or the synovial lining of a tendon that has herniated (Fig. 12–52). It contains a jelly-like fluid that may become completely sealed off within the cyst or remain connected to the synovial cavity. The three most common ganglia are the dorsal wrist ganglion, volar wrist ganglion, and the flexor tendon sheath ganglion.[93] The dorsal wrist ganglion, which arises from the scapholunate joint makes up 60% to 70% of all soft-tissue tumors of the wrist.[94] These ganglia can be difficult to detect on clinical examination if small and may only be palpable with the wrist in extreme flexion. Occult dorsal wrist ganglia can produce chronic wrist pain in some patients.

A specific traumatic event to the wrist will be elicited from only 15% of patients. Often, a history of chronic repetitive stress is reported instead. Patients complain of a dull ache or mild pain that is noted over the ganglion. Larger ganglia are less painful than smaller ones, and the pain decreases after rupture. The onset is almost always insidious, although some patients give a history of noting the "bump" over a period of a few days. A history of changing cyst size is often obtained because of the filling and emptying into the parent synovial space. On examination, a firm, nontender, cystic lesion that feels like a bead

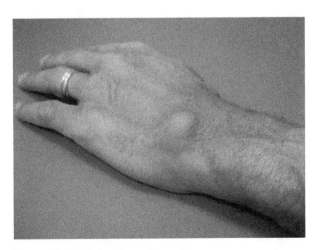

Figure 12–52. A dorsal ganglion cyst.

underneath the skin is noted. Aspiration will show a jelly-like material and confirm the diagnosis. A similar lesion to be aware of is the carpal boss (or carpometacarpal bossing) that is seen over the base of the metacarpals of the index and long fingers.

Most ganglia resolve spontaneously and do not require treatment unless pain is present. Treatment in the ED consists of aspiration with a large-bore needle when the patient complains of symptoms. Initial treatment should include steroid injection of the dorsal capsule followed by immobilization. However, the recurrence rate is very high with this method of treatment, and the patient should be informed of this. In approximately 65% of cases, cure was achieved after injection with a corticosteroid and/or rupture.

When conservative therapy fails, operative treatment with excision of the cyst is indicated. Excision of the dorsal ganglion with a portion of the capsule at the joint is the recommended treatment of choice. In 94% of cases, a cure was achieved after operation. Patients can be advised of this alternative and referred.

DE QUERVAIN TENOSYNOVITIS

De Quervain stenosing tenosynovitis involves the abductor pollicis longus and extensor pollicis brevis in the first dorsal wrist compartment (Fig. 12–53). Patients complain of pain

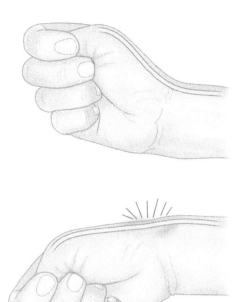

Figure 12–54. Finkelstein test for examining a patient with suspected de Quervain tenosynovitis. The patient will complain of pain over the tendon when the thumb is grasped in the hand (as shown) and the wrist is deviated in the ulnar direction.

over the radial aspect of the wrist with radiation both proximally and distally. There is localized tenderness over the radial styloid where the pulley may look and feel thickened. On examination, the pain is reproduced when the thumb is grasped in the hand and the wrist is deviated in the ulna direction by the examiner. This is commonly referred to as a positive Finkelstein test (Fig. 12–54 and Video 12–4). Although this test is sensitive and considered pathognomonic for de Quervain tenosynovitis, the accuracy of the test can be limited as pain may be elicited in patients with underlying arthritis of the wrist. In the literature, there is some confusion as the above test is sometimes referred to as the Eichoff maneuver. Another description of the Finkelstein test is to have the examiner grasp the patient's thumb and pull it in a longitudinal direction while applying ulnar deviation. The examiner's other hand stabilizes the patient's distal forearm on the ulnar side.

De Quervain tenosynovitis is due to overuse or can be associated with other conditions such as rheumatoid arthritis or pregnancy. Women are more commonly affected than men at a ratio of 10:1. Conservative treatment includes ice application to the radial styloid, NSAIDs, and restriction of thumb and wrist movement with a thumb splint (Appendix A–7). Local injection of steroids has been shown to be effective (Fig. 12–55 and Video 12–5). During the injection, a visible swelling is seen proximal to the extensor retinaculum; this is a guide that the needle is in the tendon sheath. Ultrasound-guided injection has been shown to improve results by

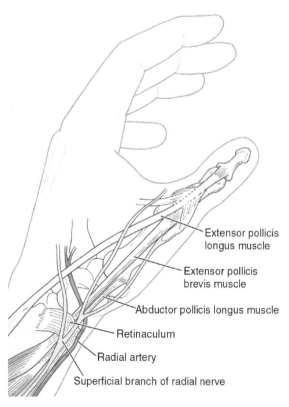

Extensor pollicis
longus muscle

Extensor pollicis
brevis muscle

Abductor pollicis longus muscle

Retinaculum

Radial artery

Superficial branch of radial nerve

Figure 12–53. Anatomy of the first dorsal wrist compartment.

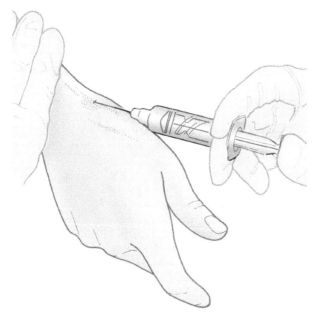

Figure 12–55. Injection for de Quervain stenosing tenosynovitis. The needle is inserted between the tendon and the sheath. If the needle is inserted properly, a sausage-like swelling will be noted in the first compartment as the fluid is injected.

confirming injection of both the sheath of the abductor pollicis longus and the extensor pollicis brevis.[100–102] After injection, the patient should be placed in a simple thumb splint extending from the tip of the thumb to two-thirds of the way down the radial forearm. The splint should remain in place for 10 days.

Surgery is recommended if symptoms recur or persist after two injections in the course of 1 year. In the majority of cases, injection therapy, followed by the administration of a NSAID and splinting of the thumb for a period of 7 to 10 days, is all that is needed.

REFERENCES

1. Abraham MK, Scott S. The emergent evaluation and treatment of hand and wrist injuries. *Emerg Med Clin North Am.* 2010;28(4):789–809.
2. Plancher KD. Methods of imaging the scaphoid. *Hand Clin.* 2001;17(4):703–721.
3. Rosner JL, Zlatkin MB, Clifford P, Ouellette EA, Awh MH. Imaging of athletic wrist and hand injuries. *Semin Musculoskelet Radiol.* 2004;8(1):57–79.
4. Celi J, de Gautard G, Della Santa JD, Bianchi S. Sonographic evidence of a radiographically undiagnosed hook of the hamate fracture. *J Ultrasound Med.* 2008;27(8):1235–1239.
5. Perron AD, Brady WJ, Keats TE, Hersh RE. Orthopedic pitfalls in the ED: scaphoid fracture. *Am J Emerg Med.* 2001;19(4):310–316.
6. Duckworth AD, Jenkins PJ, Aitken SA, Clement ND, Court-Brown CM, McQueen MM. Scaphoid fracture epidemiology. *J Trauma Acute Care Surg.* 2012;72(2):41–45.
7. Pidemunt G, Torres-Claramunt R, Gines A, de Zabala S, Cebamanos J. Bilateral stress fractures of the scaphoid: report in a child and review of the literature. *Clin J Sport Med.* 2012;22(6):511–513.
8. Phillips TG, Reibach AM, Slomiany WP. Diagnosis and management of scaphoid fractures. *Am Fam Physician.* 2004;70(5):879–884.
9. Freeland P. Scaphoid tubercle tenderness: a better indicator of scaphoid fractures? *Arch Emerg Med.* 1989;6(1):46–50.
10. Chen SC. The scaphoid compression test. *J Hand Surg [Br].* 1989;14(3):323–325.
11. Waeckerle JF. A prospective study identifying the sensitivity of radiographic findings and the efficacy of clinical findings in carpal navicular fractures. *Ann Emerg Med.* 1987;16(7):733–737.
12. Unay K, Gokcen B, Oskan K, Poyanli O, Eceviz E. Examination tests predictive of bone injury in patients with clinically suspected occult scaphoid fracture. *Injury.* 2009;40:1265–1268.
13. Powell JM, Lloyd GJ, Rintoul RF. New clinical test for fracture of the scaphoid. *Can J Surg.* 1988;31(4):237–238.
14. Rubin DA, Dalinka RH, Daffner RH, et al. *Acute Hand and Wrist Trauma* (online publication). Reston, VA: American College of Radiology; 2005.
15. Breederveld RS, Tuinebreijer WE. Investigation of computed tomographic scan concurrent criterion validity in doubtful scaphoid fracture of the wrist. *J Trauma.* 2004;57(4):851–854.
16. Terry DW Jr, Ramin JE. The navicular fat stripe: a useful roentgen feature for evaluating wrist trauma. *Am J Roentgenol Radium Ther Nucl Med.* 1975;124(1):25–28.
17. Annamalai G, Raby N. Scaphoid and pronator fat stripes are unreliable soft tissue signs in the detection of radiographically occult fractures. *Clin Radiol.* 2003;58(10):798–800.
18. Smith M, Bain GI, Turner PC, Watts AC. Review of imaging of scaphoid fractures. *ANZ J Surg.* 2010;80(1-2):82–90.
19. Fusetti C, Poletti PA, Pradel PH, et al. Diagnosis of occult scaphoid fracture with high-spatial resolution sonography: a prospective blind study. *J Trauma.* 2005;59:677–681.
20. Doman AN, Marcus NW. Congenital bipartite scaphoid fracture. *J Hand Surg.* 1990;15A:869–873.
21. Burge P. Closed cast treatment of scaphoid fractures. *Hand Clin.* 2001;17(4):541–552.
22. Rettig AC. Management of acute scaphoid fractures. *Hand Clin.* 2000;16(3):381–395.
23. Gellman H, Caputo RJ, Carter V, Aboulafia A, McKay M. Comparison of short and long thumb-spica casts for nondisplaced fractures of the carpal scaphoid. *J Bone Joint Surg Am.* 1989;71(3):354–357.
24. Doornberg JN, Buijze GA, Ham SJ, Ring D, Bhandari M, Poolman RW. Nonoperative treatment for acute scaphoid fractures: a systematic review and meta-analysis of randomized controlled trials. *J Trauma.* 2011;71:1073–1081.
25. Clay NR, Dias JJ, Costigan PS, Gregg PJ, Barton NJ. Need the thumb be immobilised in scaphoid fractures? A randomised prospective trial. *J Bone Joint Surg Br.* 1991;73(5):828–832.
26. Ring D, Jupiter JB, Herndon JH. Acute fractures of the scaphoid. *J Am Acad Orthop Surg.* 2000;8(4):225–231.
27. Murphy D, Eisenhauer M. The utility of a bone scan in the diagnosis of clinical scaphoid fracture. *J Emerg Med.* 1994;12(5):709–712.

28. Brydie A, Raby N. Early MRI in the management of clinical scaphoid fracture. *Br J Radiol*. 2003;76(905): 296–300.

29. Gelberman RH, Wolock BS, Siegel DB. Fractures and non-unions of the carpal scaphoid. *J Bone Joint Surg Am*. 1989; 71(10):1560–1565.

30. Murphy DG, Eisenhauer MA, Powe J, Pavlofsky W. Can a day 4 bone scan accurately determine the presence or absence of scaphoid fracture? *Ann Emerg Med*. 1995; 26(4):434–438.

31. Trumble TE. Avascular necrosis after scaphoid fracture: a correlation of magnetic resonance imaging and histology. *J Hand Surg [Am]*. 1990;15(4):557–564.

32. Barton NJ. Twenty questions about scaphoid fractures. *J Hand Surg [Br]*. 1992;17(3):289–310.

33. Ingari JV. The adult wrist. In: DeLee JC, Drez D, Miller MD, eds. *DeLee & Drez's Orthopaedic Sports Medicine: Principles and Practice*. 3rd ed. Philadelphia, PA: Saunders; 2010.

34. Slade JF III, Jaskwhich D. Percutaneous fixation of scaphoid fractures. *Hand Clin*. 2001;17(4):553–574.

35. Seitz WH Jr, Papandrea RF. Fractures and dislocations of the wrist. In: Bucholz RW, Heckman JD, eds. *Rockwood and Green's Fractures in Adults*. 5th ed. Philadelphia, PA: Lippincott Williams & Wilkins; 2002.

36. Canale ST. *Campbell's Operative Orthopedics*. 10th ed. St. Louis, MO: Mosby, 2003.

37. Adams JE, Steinmann SP. Acute scaphoid fractures. *Orthop Clin North Am*. 2007;38(2):229–235.

38. Berdia S, Wolfe SW. Effects of scaphoid fractures on the biomechanics of the wrist. *Hand Clin*. 2001;17(4):533–540, vii–viii.

39. Marchessault J, Conti M, Baratz ME. Carpal fractures in athletes excluding the scaphoid. *Hand Clin*. 2009;25: 371–388.

40. Papp S. Carpal bone fractures. *Orthop Clin North Am*. 2007; 38:251–260.

41. Hocker K, Menschik A. Chip fractures of the triquetrum. Mechanism, classification and results. *J Hand Surg [Br]*. 1994;19(5):584–588.

42. Teisen H, Hjarbaek J. Classification of fresh fractures of the lunate. *J Hand Surg [Br]*. 1988;13(4):458–462.

43. Brach P, Goitz R. An update on the management of carpal fractures. *J Hand Ther*. 2003;16(2):152–160.

44. Hsu AR, Hsu PA. Unusual case of isolated lunate fracture without ligamentous injury. *Orthopedics*. 2011;34(11): e785–e789.

45. Allan CH, Joshi A, Lichtman DM. Kienbock's disease: diagnosis and treatment. *J Am Acad Orthop Surg*. 2001; 9(2):128–136.

46. Cetti R, Christensen SE, Reuther K. Fracture of the lunate bone. *Hand*. 1982;14(1):80–84.

47. Palumbo DM. An uncommon isolated fracture of the capitate bone. *JAAPA*. 2007;20(12):33–35.

48. De Schrijver F, De Smet L. Isolated fracture of the capitate: the value of MRI in the diagnosis and follow up. *Acta Orthop Belg*. 2002;68(3):310–315.

49. Walsh JJ, Bishop AT. Diagnosis and management of hamate hook fractures. *Hand Clin*. 2000;16(3):397–403, viii.

50. De Schrijver F, De Smet L. Fracture of the hook of the hamate, often misdiagnosed as "wrist sprain". *J Emerg Med*. 2001;20(1):47–51.

51. Steinberg B. Acute wrist injuries in the athlete. *Orthop Clin North Am*. 2002;33(3):535–545, vi.

52. Geissler WB. Carpal fractures in athletes. *Clin Sports Med*. 2001;20:167.

53. Cohen MS. Fractures of the carpal bones. *Hand Clin*. 1997; 13(4):587–599.

54. Jeong GK, Kram D, Lester B. Isolated fracture of the trapezoid. *Am J Orthop*. 2001;30(3):228–230.

55. Ilyas AM, Jupiter JB. Distal radius fractures—classification of treatment and indications for surgery. *Orthop Clin N Am*. 2007;38:167–173.

56. Nellans KW, Kowalski E, Chung KC. The epidemiology of distal radius fractures. *Hand Clin*. 2012;28:113–125.

57. Blakeney WG. Stabilization and treatment of Colles' fractures in elderly patients. *Clin Interv Aging*. 2010;5:337–344.

58. Trumble TE, Schmitt SR, Vedder NB. Factors affecting functional outcome of displaced intra-articular distal radius fractures. *J Hand Surg [Am]*. 1994;19(2):325–340.

59. Jupiter JB, Fernández DL. Comparative classification for fractures of the distal end of the radius. *J Hand Surg*. 1997; 22A:563–571.

60. Fernández DL. Fractures of the distal radius: operative treatment. *Instr Course Lect*. 1993;42:73–88.

61. Fernández DL. Closed manipulation and casting of distal radius fractures. *Hand Clin*. 2005;21(3):307–316.

62. Woolfrey KGH, Woolfrey MR, Eisenhauer MA. Wrist and forearm. In: Marx JA, Hockenberger RS, Walls RM, eds. *Rosen's Emergency Medicine Concepts and Clinical Practice*. 7th ed. USA: Elsevier; 2010.

63. Goldfarb CA, Yin Y, Gilula LA, Fisher AJ, Boyer MI. Wrist fractures: what the clinician wants to know. *Radiology*. 2001; 219:11–28.

64. Black WS, Becker JA. Common forearm fractures in adults. *Am Fam Physician*. 2009;80(10):1096–1102.

65. Cooney WP. Management of Colles' fractures. *J Hand Surg [Br]*. 1989;14(2):137–139.

66. Cooney WP III, Dobyns JH, Linscheid RL. Complications of Colles' fractures. *J Bone Joint Surg Am*. 1980;62(4): 613–619.

67. Szabo RM. Comminuted distal radius fractures. *Orthop Clin North Am*. 1992;23(1):1–6.

68. Hanel DP, Jones MD, Trumble TE. Wrist fractures. *Orthop Clin North Am*. 2002;33:35–57.

69. Turner RG, Faber KJ, Athwal GS. Complications of distal radius fractures. *Orthop Clin N Am*. 2007;38:217–228.

70. Davis DI, Baratz M. Soft tissue complications of distal radius fractures. *Hand Clin*. 2010;26:229–235.

71. McKay SD, MacDermid JC, Roth JH, Roth JH, Richards RS. Assessment of complications of distal radius fractures and development of a complication checklist. *J Hand Surg*. 2001;26:916–922.

72. Bacorn RW, Kurtzke JF. Colles' fracture: a study of two thousand cases from the New York State Workmen's Compensation Board. *J Bone Joint Surg Am*. 1953;35-A(3):643–658.

73. Thomas FB. Reduction of Smith's fracture. *J Bone Joint Surg Br*. 1957;39:463–470.

74. Mayfield JK, Johnson RP, Kilcoyne RK. Carpal dislocations: pathomechanics and progressive perilunar instability. *J Hand Surg [Am]*. 1980;5:226–241.

75. Meldon SW, Hargarten SW. Ligamentous injuries of the wrist. *J Emerg Med*. 1995;13:217–225.

76. Jones WA. Beware the sprained wrist. The incidence and diagnosis of scapholunate instability. *J Bone Joint Surg Br.* 1988;70:293–297.

77. Rettig AC. Athletic injuries of the wrist and hand. Part I: traumatic injuries of the wrist. *Am J Sports Med.* 2003;31:1038–1048.

78. Watson HK, Weinzweig J, Zeppieri J. The natural progression of scaphoid instability. *Hand Clin.* 1997;13:39–49.

79. Vitello W, Gordon DA. Obvious radiographic scapholunate dissociation: x-ray the other wrist. *Am J Orthop.* 2005;34:347–351.

80. Frankel VH. The Terry-Thomas sign. *Clin Orthop.* 1977;(129):321–322.

81. Leversedge FJ, Srinivasan RC. Management of soft-tissue injuries in distal radius fractures. *Hand Clin.* 2012;28:225–233.

82. Grabow RJ, Catalano L III. Carpal dislocations. *Hand Clin.* 2006;22(4):485–500.

83. Martinage A, Balaguer T, Chignon-Sicard B, Monteil MC, Dréant N, Lebreton E. [Perilunate dislocations and fracture-dislocations of the wrist, a review of 14 cases.] *Chir Main.* 2008;27(1):31–39. doi:10.1016/j.main.2007.10.006. Epub 2007 Nov 20.

84. McAdams TR, Swan J, Yao J. Arthroscopic treatment of triangular fibrocartilage wrist injuries in the athlete. *Am J Sports Med.* 2009;37:291–297.

85. Reiter A, Wolf MB, Schmid U, et al. Arthroscopic repair of Palmer 1B triangular fibrocartilage complex tears. *Arthroscopy.* 2008;24(11):1244–1250. doi:10.1016/j.arthro.2008.06.022. Epub 2008 Sep 19.

86. Ilyas AM, Mudgal CS. Radiocarpal fracture-dislocations. *J Am Acad Orthop Surg.* 2008;16:647–655.

87. Dumontier C, Meyer zu Reckendorf G, Sautet A, et al. Radiocarpal dislocations: classification and proposal for treatment. A review of twenty-seven cases. *J Bone Joint Surg Am.* 2001;83-A(2):212–218.

88. Corwin HM. Compression neuropathies of the upper extremity. *Clin Occup Environ Med.* 2006;5:333–352.

89. Tosti R, Ilyas AM. Acute carpal tunnel syndrome. *Orthop Clin N Am.* 2012;43:459–465.

90. Viera AJ. Management of carpal tunnel syndrome. *Am Fam Physician.* 2003;68:265–272.

91. Verdon ME. Overuse syndromes of the hand and wrist. *Prim Care.* 1996;23:305–319.

92. McCabe SJ, Uebele AL, Pihur V, Rosales RS, Atroshi I. Epidemiologic associations of carpal tunnel syndrome and sleep position: is there a case for causation? *Hand (N Y).* 2007;2(3):127–134. doi:10.1007/s11552-007-9035-5.

93. Tallia AF, Cardone DA. Diagnostic and therapeutic injection of the wrist and hand region. *Am Fam Physician.* 2003;67:745–750.

94. Limpaphayom N, Wilairatana V. Randomized controlled trial between surgery and aspiration combined with methylprednisolone acetate injection plus wrist immobilization in the treatment of dorsal carpal ganglion. *J Med Assoc Thai.* 2004;87:1513–1517.

95. Halikis MN, Taleisnik J. Soft-tissue injuries of the wrist. *Clin Sports Med.* 1996;15:235–259.

96. Crop JA, Bunt CW. Doctor, my thumb hurts. *J Fam Prac.* 2011;60:329–332.

97. Ilyas AM, Ast M, Schaffer AA, Thoder J. de Quervain tenosynovitis of the wrist. *J Am Acad Orthop Surg.* 2007;15:757–764.

98. Wasseem M, Khan M, Hussain N, Giannoudis PV, Fischer J, Smith RM. Eponyms: errors in clinical practice and scientific writing. *Acta Orthop Belg.* 2005;71:1–8.

99. Goubau JF, Goubau L, Van Tongel A, Van Hoonacker P, Kerckhove D, Berghs B. The wrist hyperflexion and abduction of the thumb (WHAT) test: a more specific and sensitive test to diagnose de Quervain tenosynovitis than the Eichhoff's Test. *J Hand Surg Eur Vol.* 2013;39(3):286–292. doi:10.1177/1753193412475043. Epub 2013 Jan 22.

100. Rettig AC. Athletic injuries of the wrist and hand: part II: overuse injuries of the wrist and traumatic injuries to the hand. *Am J Sports Med.* 2004;32(1):262–273. doi:10.1177/0363546503261422.

101. Sawaizumi T, Nanno M, Ito H. De Quervain's disease: efficacy of intra-sheath triamcinolone injection. *Int Orthop.* 2007;31(2):265–268. doi:10.1007/s00264-006-0165-0. Epub 2006 Jun 8.

102. Kamel M, Moghazy K, Eid H, Mansour R. Ultrasonographic diagnosis of de Quervain's tenosynovitis. *Ann Rheum Dis.* 2002;61(11):1034–1035.

CHAPTER 13

Forearm

Eric Toth, DO and James Webley, MD

INTRODUCTION

The radius and the ulna lie parallel to each other and are invested at their proximal ends with a relatively large muscle mass. Because of their close proximity, injury forces typically disrupt both bones and their ligamentous attachments. They can be thought of conceptually as two cones lying next to each other pointing in opposite directions (Fig. 13-1).

> **Axiom:** *A fracture of one of the paired forearm bones, especially when angulated or displaced, is usually accompanied by a fracture or dislocation of its "partner."*

The bones of the forearm are bound by several essential ligamentous structures (Fig. 13-2). On either end, the joint capsules of the elbow and wrist hold the radius and ulna together. Anterior and posterior radioulnar ligaments further strengthen these attachments proximally. The distal radioulnar joint contains a fibrocartilaginous articular disk that acts as an energy absorber with compressive forces. The third important ligamentous attachment is the interosseous membrane, which provides both longitudinal stability and load transference between the two bones.

Muscle attachments to the forearm bones are important because of their penchant for displacing fracture fragments. Simply speaking, the shafts of the radius and the ulna are surrounded by four primary muscle groups whose pull frequently results in fracture displacement or

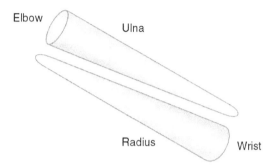

Figure 13-1. The radius and the ulna can be conceptualized as two cones that come together at the ends, thus permitting supination and pronation as the radius "rolls" around the ulna.

nullification of an adequate reduction (Fig. 13-3). These groups are as follows:

- *Proximal*: The biceps and the supinator insert on the proximal radius and exert a supinating force.
- *Midshaft*: The pronator teres inserts on the radial shaft and exerts a pronating force.
- *Distal*: Two groups of muscles insert on the distal radius. The pronator quadratus exerts a pronating force. The brachioradialis and abductor pollicis also produce deforming forces, depending on the location of the fracture. Of these, the brachioradialis exerts the predominant displacing force.

Consider that the ulna is a fixed straight bone around which the radius rotates. The radius, in contradistinction, has a *lateral bow* that must be preserved to allow full pronation

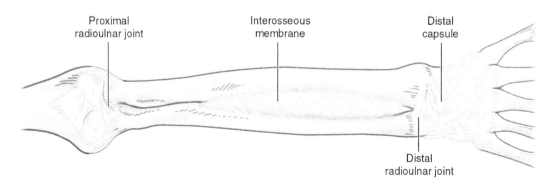

Figure 13-2. The radius and the ulna are joined together by the capsules at either end of the wrist and elbow joints. The interosseous membrane joins the two bones together throughout the shafts.

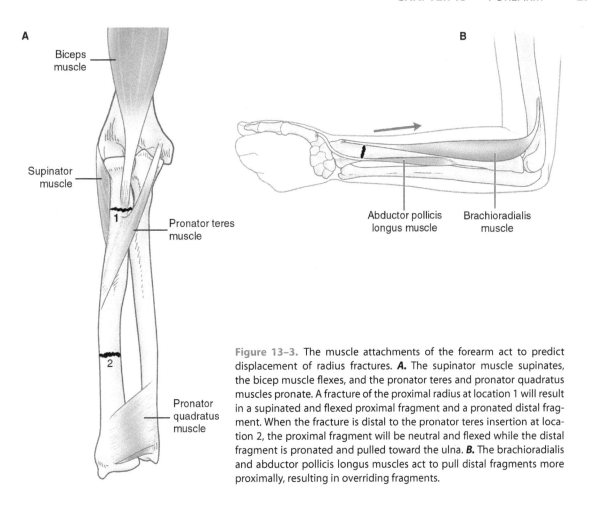

A

Biceps muscle

Supinator muscle

1

Pronator teres muscle

2

Pronator quadratus muscle

B

Abductor pollicis longus muscle

Brachioradialis muscle

Figure 13–3. The muscle attachments of the forearm act to predict displacement of radius fractures. **A.** The supinator muscle supinates, the bicep muscle flexes, and the pronator teres and pronator quadratus muscles pronate. A fracture of the proximal radius at location 1 will result in a supinated and flexed proximal fragment and a pronated distal fragment. When the fracture is distal to the pronator teres insertion at location 2, the proximal fragment will be neutral and flexed while the distal fragment is pronated and pulled toward the ulna. **B.** The brachioradialis and abductor pollicis longus muscles act to pull distal fragments more proximally, resulting in overriding fragments.

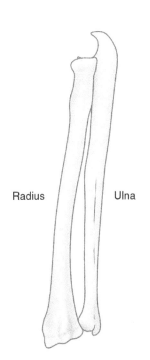

Radius   Ulna

Figure 13–4. The lateral bow of the radius must be preserved to allow full pronation and supination to occur.

and supination after healing (Fig. 13–4). Forearms play an important part in the activities of daily living, and the best patient outcomes often result from careful attention to maintenance of their length and alignment.

Classification

In this chapter, fractures of the radius and ulnar shafts are considered. The shafts of the radius and ulna are defined as the diaphyses of the long bones not encompassed by joint capsules or ligaments. The reader is referred to Chapter 12 for a discussion of distal radius fractures, and Chapter 14 for a discussion of fractures of proximal structures such as the radial head, olecranon, and coronoid process. The classification system used in this chapter for radial and ulnar shaft fractures is based on anatomic as well as therapeutic considerations.

Fractures can occur anywhere along the shaft of the radius or ulna. These fractures are divided into three groups: (1) radial shaft fractures, (2) ulnar shaft fractures, and (3) combined radius and ulna fractures. The Monteggia (ulna fracture with radial head dislocation) and Galeazzi (radius fracture with distal radioulnar dislocation) fractures are classified under their respective single bone fractures but are paid special attention.

FOREARM FRACTURES

RADIAL SHAFT FRACTURES

Radial shaft fractures can be divided into proximal, mid-shaft, and distal fractures (Fig. 13-5). Isolated fractures of the proximal two-thirds of the shaft of the radius are uncommon in adults because this area is well protected by the forearm musculature. A force powerful enough to break the radius is usually sufficient to also break the ulna.

Galeazzi fracture dislocation includes a fracture of the distal radius (usually between 5 and 7.5 cm from the distal articulation) that is obvious both clinically and radiologically. Coupled with the radius fracture is a dislocation of the distal radioulnar joint (DRUJ), which is more subtle.

These are somewhat frequent injuries of the forearm, with up to 3% of children and up to 7% of adult forearm fractures being Galeazzi fractures.

Mechanism of Injury

The usual adult, isolated, radial shaft fracture injury mechanism is a direct blow distally. It is here that the radius is least enshrouded by muscle and therefore more exposed to direct trauma.

Galeazzi fracture dislocations are commonly caused by axial loading (falls) and direct blows (especially motor vehicle accidents).

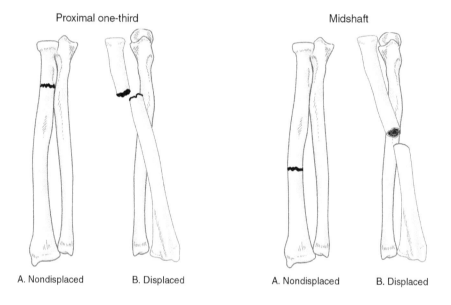

Proximal one-third

A. Nondisplaced   B. Displaced

Midshaft

A. Nondisplaced   B. Displaced

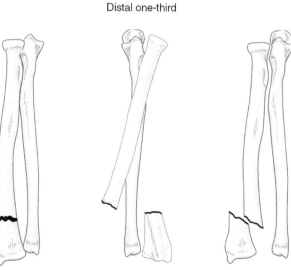

Distal one-third

A. Nondisplaced   B. Displaced   C. Galeazzi fracture

Figure 13-5. Radial shaft fractures.

Examination

Tenderness is present at the fracture site and can be elicited with direct palpation or longitudinal compression of the injured bone.

Galeazzi fracture dislocations demonstrate tenderness over the obvious fracture of the radius as well as in the DRUJ. Displacement of the ulnar head either dorsally or ventrally is commonly felt.[6-8]

Imaging

Routine anteroposterior (AP) and lateral views of the forearm are obtained. Radial shaft fractures are frequently associated with serious but often missed elbow and wrist injuries, so both joints should be seen on radiographs. Isolated, angulated, or displaced radius fractures of the distal shaft suggest that a DRUJ subluxation or dislocation is present.

There are several radiographic signs that suggest an unstable injury of the DRUJ (Figs. 13–6 and 13–7).

- Fracture of the base of the ulnar styloid[1]
- AP view: Widening of the distal radial ulnar joint space
- Lateral view: Dislocation of the distal radius relative to the ulna
- Shortening of the radius by more than 5 mm[9]
- Fracture of the radius more than 7.5 cm from the wrist[5]

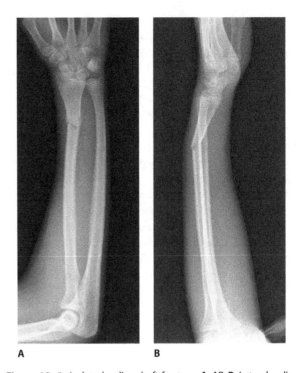

A   **B**

Figure 13–6. Isolated radius shaft fracture. **A.** AP. **B.** Lateral radiograph. This type of angulated fracture of the distal third of the radius should raise suspicion for fracture dislocation; however, radiographic and clinical evidence did not support this diagnosis. This fracture underwent closed reduction and healed well in the cast.

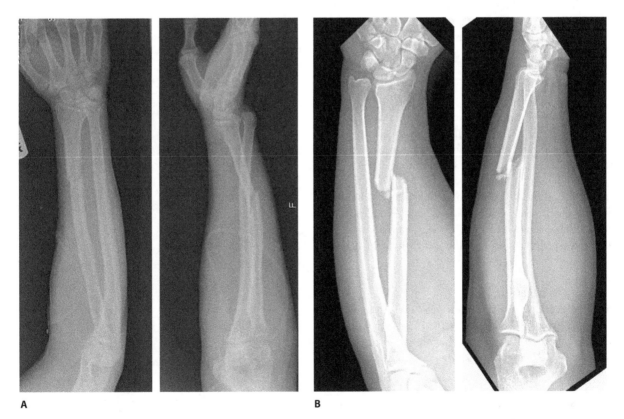

A   **B**

Figure 13–7. Galeazzi fracture dislocations. **A.** Angulated radius fracture. Note the dislocation of the distal radioulnar joint on the lateral view and the shortening of the radius on the AP. **B.** Displaced radius fracture. Note the widening of the radioulnar joint and shortening of the radius of the AP view.

Associated Injuries

A distal radial shaft fracture is frequently associated with a distal radioulnar joint dislocation (*Galeazzi fracture dislocation*). High-energy mechanisms with extensive soft-tissue injury may be associated with acute compartment syndrome.

Treatment

Radius—Proximal One-Third

Nondisplaced. Emergency department (ED) management should include the application of AP splints (Appendix A–10). The elbow should be in 90 degrees of flexion with the forearm in supination. Supination of the forearm is required to prevent the supinating forces of the supinator and biceps muscles that insert on the proximal portion of the radius from causing displacement. Follow-up radiographs to detect displacement are essential. These fractures are rare, and urgent orthopedic referral is appropriate.

Displaced. ED management should include immobilization in a long-arm posterior splint (Appendix A–9) with the forearm in supination and the elbow in 90 degrees of flexion. Discussion with an orthopedist may be prudent as the treatment of choice usually includes open reduction and internal fixation.

If the radius fracture involves the proximal one-fifth of the bone, treatment is controversial. Because of the small size of the proximal fragment, internal fixation is difficult. Most patients are treated with a manipulative reduction and immobilization in AP splints (Appendix A–10). The elbow should be in 90 degrees of flexion and the forearm in supination.

Radius—Midshaft

Nondisplaced. Referral is indicated after immobilization in AP splints (Appendix A–10). The elbow should be in 90 degrees of flexion and the forearm in moderate supination. Follow-up radiographs are strongly encouraged.

Displaced. Discussion with an orthopedist may be prudent as the treatment of choice usually includes open reduction and internal fixation. Initially, immobilize with 90 degrees of elbow flexion and moderate forearm supination (Appendix A–10).

Radius—Distal One-Third

Nondisplaced. Referral is indicated after immobilization in AP splints (Appendix A–10). The elbow should be in 90 degrees of flexion and the forearm in pronation. *An angulated, nondisplaced fracture may be associated with subluxation of the DRUJ.*

Displaced. The treatment of Galeazzi fracture dislocation varies with age. Adults invariably have poor outcomes if they are treated with reduction and casting. Thus, Galeazzi injury was termed "the fracture of necessity" by authors who believed only surgical intervention would allow good patient outcomes. Operative reduction and internal fixation remain the treatments of choice.

Children, as is so often the case in orthopedics, have very good results with conservative treatment. They are frequently treated with reduction and long-arm casting.

Regardless of the patient's age, it seems prudent to involve the orthopedic surgeon early in treatment decisions involving displacement of the distal radial diaphysis.

Complications

Radial shaft fractures are associated with several complicating factors:

- Nondisplaced fractures may undergo delayed displacement due to muscular traction with subsequent poor functional outcomes. Follow-up radiographs to ensure proper positioning are essential.
- Malunion or nonunion may be secondary to inadequate reduction or immobilization.
- Rotational deformities must be detected and treated early.
- DRUJ subluxation or dislocation (Galeazzi fracture) may be unrecognized, and the patient may end up with a poor functional outcome.
- Neurovascular injuries can occur but are uncommon.

ULNAR SHAFT FRACTURES

Ulnar shaft fractures can be classified into three groups: (1) nondisplaced, (2) displaced (>5 mm), and (3) Monteggia fracture dislocations (Fig. 13–8). The midshaft of the ulna is the most frequent location of a fracture (Fig. 13–9).

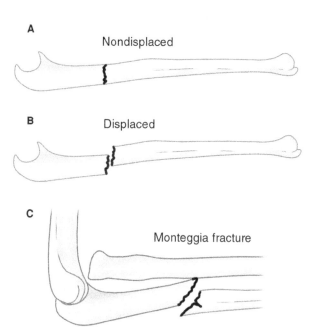

A Nondisplaced

B Displaced

C Monteggia fracture

Figure 13–8. Ulnar shaft fractures.

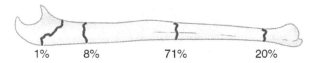

Figure 13–9. The midshaft of the ulna is the most common site for a fracture, often occurring due to a "nightstick"-type injury mechanism.

Monteggia fracture dislocations are displaced fractures of the proximal one-third of the ulnar shaft combined with a radial head dislocation. Radial head dislocations can occur only if there is complete rupture of the annular ligament. Monteggia fracture dislocations account for 1% to 2% of all forearm fractures.[10] Bado's classification system is frequently used and is delineated below with the frequency of the type of injury shown in parentheses[11]:

- *Type I*: Ulnar shaft fracture with anterior dislocation of the radial head (60%). This is the most frequent type in children and young adults.
- *Type II*: Ulnar shaft fracture with posterior or posterolateral dislocation of the radial head (15%). In some studies, this is the most common presentation in adults.[10,12,13]
- *Type III*: Ulnar metaphyseal fractures with lateral or anterolateral dislocation of the radial head (20%). This is a common childhood fracture resulting from a direct blow to the inner elbow.
- *Type IV*: Ulnar and radial shaft fracture (proximal one-third) and anterior dislocation of the radial head (5%).[14]

Mechanism of Injury

A direct blow to the ulna is the most common mechanism, and the resulting fracture is often referred to as a "nightstick fracture," as if the individual was holding up his/her arm to protect the face from the downward strike of a nineteenth-century policeman's nightstick. With the arm up in this manner, the ulna is exposed and not well protected by soft tissues. This mechanism is common in automobile accidents or fights. Excessive pronation or supination can also result in ulnar shaft fractures.

Monteggia fracture dislocation has a number of mechanisms of injury postulated as would be expected by the varying directions of radial head dislocation. Falls on the outstretched hand, falls on the elbow, and direct blows to the ulna are among the suggested mechanisms of injury.[10] Posterior dislocations (Bado, type II) are frequently associated with fractures of the radial head or coronoid process and are most frequent in middle-aged or elderly patients. These patients are believed to have the same mechanism as patients who have dislocated their elbow but osteoporosis allowed a fracture instead.

Examination

Swelling and tenderness with palpation are evident over the fracture site. Palpation of the ulna will elicit pain localized to the fracture site.

Monteggia fracture dislocations are characterized by shortening of the forearm due to angulation. The radial head may be palpable in the antecubital fossa following anterior dislocations. Pain and tenderness will be present over the proximal ulna and are exacerbated by any motion. Crepitus is often felt in the joint if motion is allowed.

Monteggia fracture dislocations characteristically have more pain with pronation and supination than isolated ulnar shaft fractures.

Imaging

AP and lateral views will generally demonstrate the injury (Figs. 13–10 and 13–11). If there is significant displacement, elbow and wrist views should be added to exclude articular injury, subluxation, or dislocation. In any fracture of the ulna, especially proximal fractures, the emergency physician should evaluate the *radiocapitellar line* on the lateral radiograph. A line drawn down the center of the neck and head of the radius should intersect the middle of the capitellum. If this intersection does not occur, the proximal radioulnar joint is disrupted. See Chapter 6 for further details.

Associated Injuries

Fractures of the distal two-thirds of the ulnar shaft are rarely accompanied by joint injuries. However, a fracture to the proximal one-third of the ulna should be evaluated for radial head dislocation.[2] Problems with detection of this injury occur when the radial head is just subluxed or the ulnar injury is a plastic deformation fracture, which is not necessarily appreciated without an entire view of the ulna.[15]

> **Axiom:** *Displaced ulnar fractures are frequently associated with radial fractures or dislocations of the radial head.*

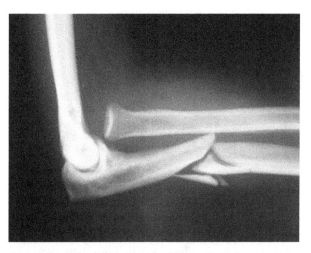

Figure 13–10. Monteggia fracture dislocation with anterior displacement of the radial head. A line drawn through the shaft of the neck of the radius (radiocapitellar line) does not transect the center of the capitellum.

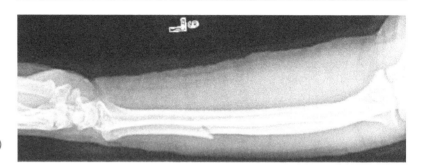

Figure 13–11. Minimally displaced (<5 mm) fracture of the ulna (nightstick fracture).

Infrequently, paralysis of the deep branch of the radial nerve can occur; however, function usually returns without treatment. High-energy mechanisms with extensive soft-tissue injuries may be associated with acute compartment syndrome.

Treatment

Nondisplaced. Nondisplaced or minimally displaced (<5 mm) fractures of the ulnar shaft can typically be treated with a long-arm splint (Appendix A–9). Orthopedic referral is recommended.

Displaced (>5 mm). Cadaver studies have confirmed that displacement of the ulna by 50% of its width causes significant disruption of the interosseous membrane. Proximal one-third fractures of the ulna that are displaced are more likely to have associated injury to the ligamentous structures of the radial head.

Referral after immobilization with a long-arm splint (Appendix A–9) is indicated. A 2012 Cochrane Review was unable to distinguish whether better patient outcomes were associated with surgery. Thus, management remains the surgeon's dilemma. Most orthopedic surgeons prefer open reduction with internal fixation in the management of these fractures, especially if the injury has a high-energy mechanism. Low-energy mechanisms in the elderly might be treated with functional bracing.

Monteggia Fracture Dislocation. In adults, the extremity should be immobilized in a long-arm posterior splint (Appendix A–9). Surgical reduction and repair is the common treatment.

In children, emergency management includes immobilization in a posterior long-arm splint (Appendix A–9). Closed reduction of the injury is typically carried out under general anesthesia.

Regardless of the patient's age, it seems prudent to involve the orthopedic surgeon early in treatment decisions.

Complications

- Paralysis of the deep branch of the radial nerve, which is usually secondary to a contusion and typically heals without treatment
- Nonunion due to an inadequate reduction or immobilization
- Delayed discovery of the radial head dislocation leading to poorer patient outcomes

COMBINED RADIUS AND ULNA FRACTURES

Fractures of the radius and ulna, also known as both bone forearm fractures, are most common in children, and account for 45% of all fractures in childhood. Combined forearm fractures also occur in adults, although the management is very different. In adults, nondisplaced fracture of both forearm bones is rare because a force with enough energy to break both bones typically causes displacement.

The classification of combined radius and ulna fractures is based on displacement and angulation (Fig. 13–12). Plastic deformation and greenstick fractures, incomplete fractures that do not involve both cortices of the bone, are

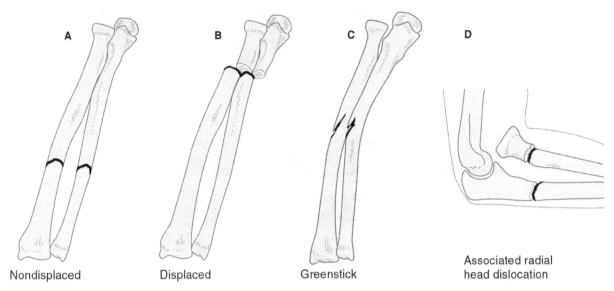

Figure 13–12. Classification of combination fractures of the shafts of the radius and ulna.

also considered. For further discussion of these fractures in children, the reader is referred to Chapter 6.

Mechanism of Injury

Two mechanisms result in fractures of the forearm shaft. In adults, a direct blow, as during a vehicular collision, is the most common mechanism encountered.[20] In children, the most common mechanism is a fall on an outstretched arm.[21]

Examination

Pain, swelling, and loss of function of the hand and forearm are usually encountered. Examination of the elbow and wrist is important to detect possible injury to the proximal or distal ligamentous structures. Deformity of the forearm may be quite obvious (Fig. 13–13). Deficits of the radial, median, and ulnar nerves are not commonly seen but must be excluded.

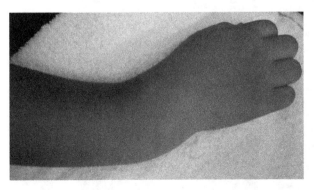

Figure 13–13. Gross deformity of the forearm after a fracture to the radius and ulna.

Imaging

AP and lateral views are adequate for defining the fracture fragments (Figs. 13–14 and 13–15). Wrist and elbow views may also be obtained and evaluated for fracture, dislocation, or subluxation. Subtle subluxation of the DRUJ may only be evident on computed tomography (CT). A line drawn through the radial neck and head should pass through the center of the capitellum (radiocapitellar line). If it does not, injury to the proximal radioulnar joint should be suspected.

Associated Injury

Fracture of the radial and ulnar shaft may be associated with injury to the proximal and DRUJs. Neurovascular involvement is uncommon in closed injuries to the forearm. High-energy mechanisms with extensive soft-tissue injuries may be associated with acute compartment syndrome.

Treatment

Nondisplaced. This is an uncommon injury because a force great enough to break both forearm bones usually causes displacement. Nonetheless, if the bones are neither displaced nor angulated, the patient can be treated with AP splints, with the elbow in 90 degrees of flexion and the forearm in neutral position (Appendix A–10).[20] Definitive management includes a well-molded long-arm cast. *Caution:* Repeat radiographs are required as delayed displacement is common. Prompt orthopedic follow-up is indicated in all cases.

Displaced. In adults, closed reduction generally fails to achieve and maintain proper alignment, and poor patient outcomes ensue.[20] ED management includes long-arm immobilization and a discussion with the orthopedic

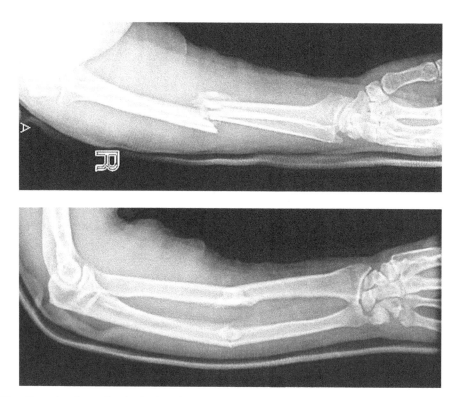

Figure 13–14. AP and lateral radiographs of a displaced combined radius and ulna fracture in an adult. This fracture requires operative fixation.

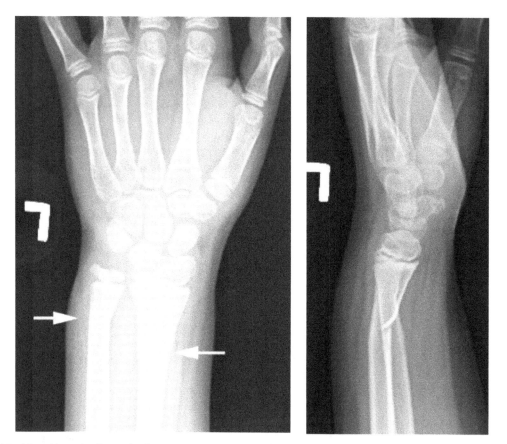

Figure 13–15. AP and lateral radiographs demonstrating a greenstick fracture of the distal radius and a torus fracture of the ulna in a child (*arrows*).

surgeon about operative reduction and internal fixation (Fig. 13–16). Open fractures require prompt operative intervention as outlined in Chapter 1.

In young children, displaced both bone forearm fractures are usually treated with closed reduction and long-arm immobilization. Good results occur in 85% of these patients.[19] Commonly accepted indications for surgery include an unacceptable reduction, loss of an acceptable reduction during follow-up, open fractures, and patients with less than 1 year of growth remaining.[21] Nevertheless, children within a few years of puberty are increasingly receiving surgery to fix these fractures, which are believed to require very accurate reductions much like in adults. The orthopedic surgeon often carries out the reduction and immobilization because these procedures have quite a few nuances. Sedation of the child for reduction is common either in the operating room or as procedural sedation in the ED. A method of closed reduction is described in Figure 13–17.

Combined Proximal One-Third Fractures with Radial Head Dislocation.

These fractures are a variation of the Monteggia fracture (Bado, type IV, as discussed previously) and require open reduction and internal fixation.

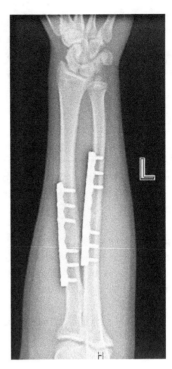

Figure 13–16. Compression plating of the radius and ulna after a displaced fracture in an adult.

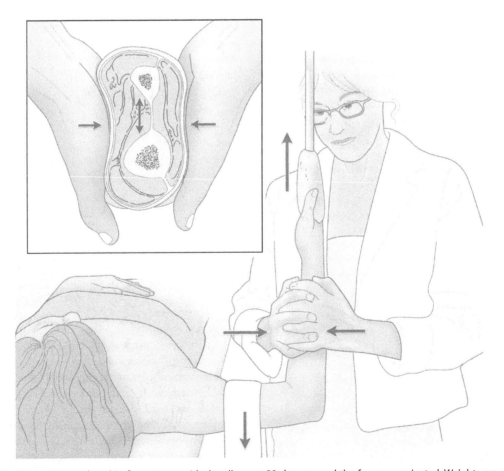

Figure 13–17. The patient is placed in finger traps with the elbow at 90 degrees and the forearm supinated. Weights are added for a period of 5 to 10 minutes to lengthen the bones and help to correct any angular deformity. Under procedural sedation, compression of the volar and dorsal muscle masses forces the radius and ulna apart and puts the interosseous ligament at maximum tension. This act helps to support the fracture fragments. The forearm can be rotated slightly to correct any rotational deformities.

> **Axiom:** *Combined shaft fractures of the proximal one-third of the radius and the ulna are commonly associated with an anterior dislocation of the radial head.*

Acute Plastic Deformation Fracture

This relatively rare injury, usually of the forearm, most frequently occurs in young children because their bones are pliable. It occurs when a longitudinal deforming force causes microfractures without completely breaking the bony cortex.   The microfractured bone remains permanently curved (bowed) after the deforming force has been removed.

Acute plastic deformation fracture (APDF) may include any combination of overt fracture of the radius with APDF of the ulna, overt fracture of the ulna with APDF of the radius, or APDF of both bones simultaneously.

Classically, plastic deformation fracture occurs in a young child with a fall on the outstretched hand injury. There is tenderness over the deformity of the obvious fracture and more diffuse tenderness along the plastically deformed bone due to the extensive microfractures of the cortex. Pronation and supination are limited by the curvature.

Lack of a cortical defect and subtle curvature of the long bone makes discovery of this injury difficult. Nevertheless, as the axiom suggests, when there is a displaced fracture of one bone in the forearm one should be looking for its partner. APDF may be the "partner" to an otherwise obviously displaced fracture in the forearm.

Good AP and lateral x-rays help to discover this injury. If there is doubt about how the films should be interpreted, comparison views of the opposite extremity may be helpful (Fig. 13–18).

Complications of this injury are well known. Natural remodeling may not be adequate to correct the deformity in older children. Bowing of a forearm bone causes abnormalities of the interosseous space, resulting in problems pronating and supinating the forearm, and its consequent poorer patient outcomes. Reduction of the obvious fracture may not be possible without reducing the plastic deformation.

Treatment includes long-arm immobilization with the elbow in 90-degree flexion and the forearm in supination as well as prompt referral to orthopedics. Usually, reduction under anesthesia is performed.

Adult plastic deformity fractures have been described with increasing frequency.   Tianhao described 29 out of 30 injuries resulting from patients having their arm caught in the rollers of a machine. One-third of these patients had a disruption of either the proximal or distal radioulnar joint. In keeping with the concept that APDF occurs in young bones, the 30 patients were between 17 and 24 years of age.

Greenstick Fractures. These represent the commonly occurring middle ground between complete bony fracture and plastic deformation of the bone. One cortex is overtly

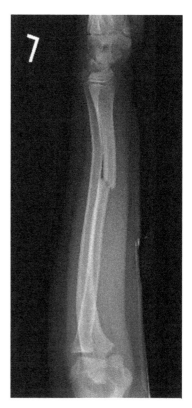

Figure 13–18. Displaced fracture of the radius with plastic deformity of the ulna.

fractured, but the other is plastically deformed (Fig. 13–15). Hence, greenstick fractures only occur in the supple bones of children.

They are initially treated with immobilization in a long-arm splint (Appendix A–9). Referral to an orthopedic surgeon is often appropriate. Reduction of a greenstick fracture may be necessary when angulation is excessive.

Complications

Combined shaft fractures of the radius and the ulna are associated with numerous complications:

- Nerve injury is uncommon in closed injuries but is frequently seen with open fractures. There is an equal frequency of involvement between the radial, ulnar, and median nerves.
- Vascular compromise is an uncommon complication because of the presence of arterial collaterals.
- Nonunion or malunion may ensue.
- Compartment syndromes can occur following combined shaft fractures. It is important to recognize that distal pulses will remain intact despite elevated compartment pressures and compromised capillary flow. The treatment is emergent referral for evaluation and possible *fasciotomy*.
- Synostosis (bone fusion) of the radius and ulna may complicate the management of combined shaft fractures.
- Pronation and supination may be permanently impaired.

FOREARM SOFT-TISSUE INJURY

CONTUSIONS

The tendons of the lower forearm are close to the skin, and *traumatic tenosynovitis* can occur after a direct blow. The treatment for this condition is simple immobilization. Nonsteroidal anti-inflammatory agents are useful for pain. Contusions of the upper forearm are treated the same as contusions elsewhere.

STRAINS

The muscles of the forearm are closely interconnected in the same sheath, and a strain of one muscle often causes discomfort with motion of other nearby muscles. This makes it difficult to isolate individual strains. The mechanism of injury is most often overuse. On examination, the patient will demonstrate swelling and inflammation of the tendon and muscle, which is painful to stress and tender to palpation. The treatment consists of ice compresses followed by local heat and immobilization. Nonsteroidal anti-inflammatory agents are also appropriate.

FOREARM COMPARTMENT SYNDROMES

Acute compartment syndrome is a condition that results from increased fluid pressure within an enclosed fascial space. The increasing compartmental pressure inhibits blood flow through the venules and the capillary bed, resulting in intra-compartmental muscle and nerve ischemia. Time-dependent (6–12 hours) necrosis may result in muscle dysfunction and contracture.[25] The forearm is the most common site for compartment syndrome to develop in the upper extremity.[26] Because the misdiagnosis, or even delay in diagnosis, of this condition may lead to permanent muscle dysfunction and contracture, it is important that emergency physicians be knowledgeable about this condition.

The forearm has three major compartments. The volar compartment is most commonly affected, but compartment syndrome may develop in the dorsal compartment or the lateral compartment, known as the "mobile wad." The lateral mobile wad contains the brachioradialis and the extensor carpi radialis longus and brevis.

Forearm compartment syndrome occurs most commonly after fractures. Nevertheless, isolated soft-tissue injuries account for approximately 25% of occurrences.[25,27] Despite the historical association of supracondylar fractures with compartment syndrome (Volkmann contracture), distal radius fractures are consistently the most common cause of the problem in the forearm.[27,28] Other less common causes include iatrogenic events such as CT-contrast infiltration of an intravenous line, improper use of a pneumatic tourniquet, and complications from thrombolytics.[29]

Clinical Presentation

The clinical presentation of compartment syndrome encompasses the following general sequence, and for further information, the reader is referred to Chapter 4:

* Severe pain is the first and most important symptom to occur. The pain usually seems out of proportion to the severity of the injury.
* As compartment pressure rises, a palpably tense compartment is the most reliable physical finding.[25]
* Increased pain with passive stretch of the enclosed muscles. This is often difficult to distinguish from the underlying pain with movement of the injury.
* Paresis and paresthesias develop later in the syndrome. By this time, some element of muscle necrosis may have begun.
* Pulse may be reduced or absent. This is an ominous finding that occurs only after extensive, irreparable damage has been done. (Do not wait for this finding.)

Although the diagnosis of compartment syndrome is a clinical one, measurement of compartment pressures may assist in making the diagnosis. Compartment pressures should be measured in each compartment of the forearm using a commercially available device.[26] A more detailed discussion of compartment syndrome, can be found in Chapter 4.

To measure the volar compartment, the needle is inserted 1.5 cm medial to a vertical line drawn through the middle of the forearm (Fig. 13–19).[30] Multiple measurements should be taken as the pressures at different sites within the same compartment may be significantly different. The dorsal compartment is measured 1.5 cm lateral to the posterior aspect of the ulna. The mobile wad is measured by inserting the needle within the muscles lateral to the radius. In each case, the needle is inserted to a depth of approximately 1.5 cm.[31]

The normal compartment pressure is between 0 and 8 mm Hg. There is a great deal of literature devoted to what is the dangerous intracompartmental pressure. There is some consensus that the difference between the diastolic blood pressure and the compartment pressure is the most important measurement (ΔP) (this represents the capillary bed perfusion pressure).[25,32] Most authors agree that the diagnosis of acute compartment syndrome is made clinically with pressure measurements used to augment decision making when necessary. Pressure measurements may be most useful when the patient is unable to give a history; that is, if the patient is on a ventilator, in surgery, or a young child, or a host of other possible scenarios. Some

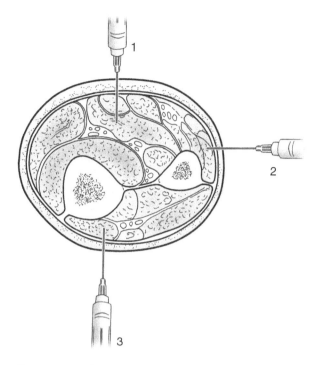

Figure 13–19. Cross-sectional view of the three major compartments of the forearm. 1, volar; 2, lateral (mobile wad); 3, dorsal. (Modified with permission from Reichman EF: *Emergency Medicine Procedures*, 2nd ed. New York: McGraw-Hill; 2013.)

recent evidence suggests that continuous intracompartmental pressure monitoring is a tool that orthopedic surgeons may employ to assist them in evaluating patients with possible or potential acute compartment syndrome.

Treatment

The extremities should not be elevated but rather placed at heart level to optimize arterial pressure and venous drainage. Patients presenting with compartment syndrome symptoms and wearing a cast may have the symptoms relieved by the simple maneuver of removing or splitting the cast and padding. The removal of a constrictive cast and padding can reduce the compartment pressure by 85%.

If symptoms persist after the removal of constrictive casts or bandages, surgical intervention with fasciotomy is often indicated. Orthopedic consultation should be obtained as soon as this condition is strongly suspected. Timely intervention may prevent irreversible damage to the muscles and nerves of the affected compartment. This is one of the few orthopedic problems where emergency intervention is necessary. Fasciotomy is the intervention of choice.

REFERENCES

1. LaStayo PC, Lee MJ. The forearm complex: anatomy, biomechanics and clinical considerations. *J Hand Therapy*. 2006; 19(2):137–144.

2. Reilly TJ. Isolated and combined fractures of the diaphysis of the radius and ulna. *Hand Clin*. 2002;18(1):179–194.

3. Carlsen BT, Dennison DG, Moran SL. Acute dislocations of the distal radioulnar joint and distal ulna fractures. *Hand Clin*. 2010;26:503–516.

4. Eberl R, Singer G, Schalamon J, Petnehazy T, Hoelwarth ME. Galeazzi lesions in children and adolescents: treatment and outcome. *Clin Orthop Relat Res*. 2008;466:1705–1709.

5. Tsismenakis T, Tornetta P III. Galeazzi fractures: is DRUJ instability predicted by current guidelines? *Injury*. 2016;47(7): 1472–1477. doi:10.1016/j.injury.2016.04.003. Epub 2016 Apr 20.

6. Aulicino PL, Siegel JL. Acute injuries of the distal radioulnar joint. *Hand Clin*. 1991;7(2):283–293.

7. Atesok KI, Jupiter JB, Weiss AP. Galeazzi fracture. *J Am Acad Orthop Surg*. 2011;19:623–633.

8. Mikic ZD. Galeazzi fracture-dislocations. *J Am Acad Orthop Surg*. 1975;57-A:1071–1080.

9. Moore TM, Klein JP, Patzakis MJ, Harvey JP Jr. Results of compression-plating of closed Galeazzi fractures. *J Bone Joint Surg Am*. 1985;67(7):1015–1021.

10. Eathiraju S, Mudgal CS, Jupiter JB. Monteggia fracture-dislocations. *Hand Clin*. 2007;23:165–177.

11. Bado JL. The Monteggia lesion. *Clin Orthop*. 1967;50:71–86.

12. Beutel BG. Monteggia fractures in adult and pediatric populations. *Orthopedics*. 2012;35:138–144.

13. Ring D. Monteggia fractures. *Orthop Clin N Am*. 2013;44: 59–66.

14. Morgan WJ, Breen TF. Complex fractures of the forearm. *Hand Clin*. 1994;10(3):375–390.

15. Kozin SH, Abzug JM, Safier S, Herman MJ. Complications of pediatric elbow dislocations and Monteggia fracture-dislocations. *Instr Course Lec*. 2015;64:493–498.

16. Szabo RM, Skinner M. Isolated ulnar shaft fractures. Retrospective study of 46 cases. *Acta Orthop Scand*. 1990;61(4): 350–352.

17. Dymond IW. The treatment of isolated fractures of the distal ulna. *J Bone Joint Surg Br*. 1984;66(3):408–410.

18. Handoll HH, Pearce P. Interventions for treating isolated diaphyseal fractures of the ulna in adults. *Cochrane Database Syst Rev*. 2012;6:CD000523.

19. Rodriguez-Merchan EC. Pediatric fractures of the forearm. *Clin Orthop Relat Res*. 2005;(432):65–72.

20. Schulte LH, Meals CG, Neviaser RJ. Management of adult diaphyseal both-bone forearm fractures. *J Am Acad Orthop Surg*. 2014;22:437–446.

21. Pace JL. Pediatric and adolescent forearm fractures: current controversies and treatment recommendations. *J Am Acad Orthop Surg*. 2016;24(11):780–788. doi:10.5435/jaaos-d-15-00151.

22. Aponte JE Jr, Ghiatas A. Acute plastic bowing deformity: a review of the literature. *J Emerg Med*. 1989;7:181–184.

23. Mabrey JD, Fitch RD. Plastic deformity in pediatric fractures: mechanism and treatment. *J Pediatr Orthop*. 1989;9:310–314.

24. Tianhao W, Yueju L, Yingze Z, Xirui W. Plastic deformation of the forearm in adults: an analysis of 30 cases. *J Orthop Surg Res*. 2014;9:117. doi:10.1186/s13018-014-0117-0.

25. Duckworth AD, Mitchell SE, Molyneux SG, White TO, Court-Brown CM, McQueen MM. Acute compartment syndrome of the forearm. *J Bone Joint Surg Am*. 2012;94(10):e63.

26. Whitesides TE, Heckman MM. Acute compartment syndrome: update on diagnosis and treatment. *J Am Acad Orthop Surg.* 1996;4(4):209–218.

27. Kalyani BS, Fisher BE, Roberts CS, Giannoudis PV. Compartment syndrome of the forearm: a systematic review. *J Hand Surg Am.* 2011;36(3):535–543. doi:10.1016/j.jhsa.2010.12.007.

28. McQueen MM, Gaston P, Court-Brown CM. Acute compartment syndrome. Who is at risk? *J Bone Joint Surg Br.* 2000; 82(2):200–203.

29. Yamaguchi S, Viegas SF. Causes of upper extremity compartment syndrome. *Hand Clin.* 1998;14(3):365–370.

30. Joseph B, Varghese RA, Mulpuri K, Paravatty S, Kamath S, Nagaraja N. Measurement of tissue hardness: can this be a method of diagnosing compartment syndrome noninvasively in children? *J Pediatr Orthop B.* 2006;15(6): 443–448.

31. Reichman EF, Simon RR. *Emergency Medicine Procedures.* New York, NY: McGraw-Hill; 2004.

32. McQueen MM. Acute compartment syndrome in tibial fractures. *Curr Orthop.* 1999;13:113–119.

33. McQueen MM, Duckworth AD, Aitken SA, Court-Brown CM. The estimated sensitivity and specificity of compartment pressure monitoring for acute compartment syndrome. *J Bone Joint Surg Am.* 2013;95:673–677.

34. Friedrich JB, Shin AY. Management of forearm compartment syndrome. *Hand Clin.* 2007;23:245–254.

35. Botte MJ, Gelberman RH. Acute compartment syndrome of the forearm. *Hand Clin.* 1998;14(3):391–403.

CHAPTER 14

Elbow

Carl A. Germann, MD and Brook M. Goddard, MD

INTRODUCTION

The elbow is a hinge joint composed of three articulations: humeroulnar, radiohumeral, and radioulnar. These articulations provide a high degree of inherent stability to the elbow and are supported by several ligamentous structures—the radial collateral, ulnar collateral, annular ligaments, and anterior capsule (Fig. 14–1). The biceps, triceps, brachialis, brachioradialis, and anconeus provide muscular dynamic stability.

Elbow injuries are caused by a direct blow, valgus stress, or axial compression. Acute traumatic injuries may result in fractures to the radius and ulna or the distal humerus. With repetitive valgus stress, such as throwing, patients may develop chondromalacia, loose bodies in the posterior or lateral compartments, injury to the ulnar collateral ligament, injury of the flexor pronator muscle group, osteochondritis dissecans, or ulnar neuritis.

The distal humerus is divided into two condyles (Fig. 14–2). The coronoid fossa is the area of very thin bone that serves as the surface of contact with the coronoid process of the olecranon when the elbow goes into full flexion. The articular surface of the medial condyle is called the trochlea. It serves as the articulating surface of the ulnar olecranon. The lateral articular surface of the distal humerus is the capitellum, which articulates with the radial head.

The nonarticular portions of the condyles are called epicondyles, and serve as points of attachment for the muscles of the forearm—pronator-flexors attach to the medial epicondyle, whereas supinator-extensors attach to the lateral epicondyle. Just proximal to either epicondyle are the supracondylar ridges that also serve as points of attachment for the forearm muscles. The muscles surrounding the elbow impact fracture alignment (Figs. 14–3 and 14–4). With a fracture, continual traction by these muscles results in displacement of the fragments, and on occasion, nullification of an adequate reduction.

Three bursae around the elbow are of clinical significance: one between the olecranon and the triceps; another between the radius and the insertion of the biceps tendon; and, finally, the olecranon bursa, which lies between the skin and the olecranon process. Bursitis about the elbow most commonly involves the olecranon bursa (Fig. 14–5).

Examination

Examination of the elbow reveals several palpable bony landmarks. Laterally, three bony prominences make up a

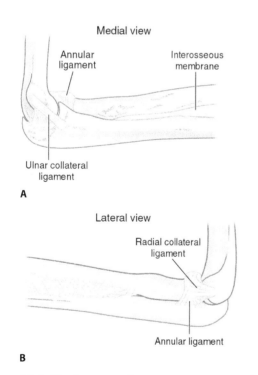

Figure 14–1. The important ligamentous structures of the elbow. The annular ligament holds the radial head in position. The radial collateral ligament is broader and blends with the annular ligament. **A.** Medial view. **B.** Lateral view.

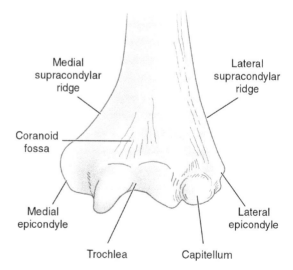

Figure 14–2. The important landmarks of the distal humerus. The bone between the condyles is very thin.

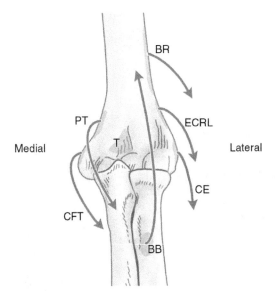

Figure 14–3. The muscles surrounding the elbow. These muscles act to displace fractures occurring at their attachments. BR, brachioradialis; ECRL, extensor carpi radialis longus; CE, common extensor tendon; PT, pronator teres; CFT, common flexor tendon; BB, biceps brachia; T, triceps.

triangle and correspond to the olecranon, radial head, and lateral epicondyle. An effusion of the elbow is indicated by swelling and tenderness between the lateral epicondyle and olecranon.

The neurovascular structures of the elbow include the brachial artery and the radial, ulnar, and median nerves (Fig. 14–6). The ulnar nerve is palpated on the medial surface of the elbow as it runs through the cubital tunnel. Assessment of the neurovascular structures is of critical importance when evaluating and treating elbow fractures. The examination should be repeated after manipulation or splinting and at regular intervals because edema from a fracture may result in neurovascular compromise.

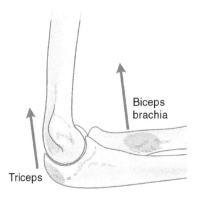

Figure 14–4. The triceps and the biceps act to pull the radius and the ulna proximally and thus cause displacement of elbow fractures.

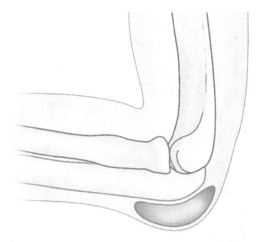

Figure 14–5. The olecranon bursa may become inflamed secondary to infectious or noninfectious causes.

Imaging

The radiographic examination of the elbow should consist of a minimum of an anteroposterior (AP) and lateral radiograph (Fig. 14–7). Oblique views will aid in the diagnosis of some elbow fractures. In most cases, the involved joint should not be extensively manipulated until radiographs have been obtained to exclude apparent fracture and dislocation.

Anteroposterior View

A diagnostic aid in evaluating radiographs of suspected supracondylar fractures in children is the carrying angle. The intersection of a line drawn through the midshaft of the humerus and a line through the midshaft of the ulna

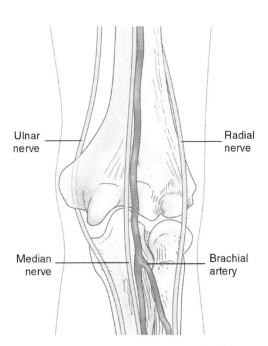

Figure 14–6. The neurovascular structures at the elbow.

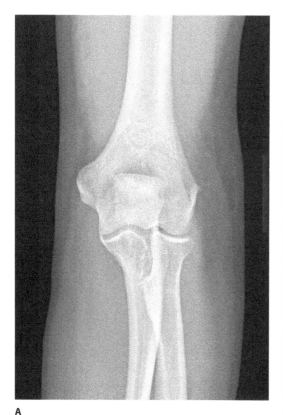

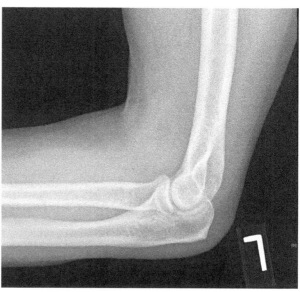

A

B

Figure 14–7. The normal radiographic appearance of bony articulations of the elbow. **A.** AP view. **B.** Lateral view.

on an AP extension view determines the carrying angle (Fig. 14–8). Normally, the carrying angle is between 0 and 12 degrees. Traumatic or asymmetric carrying angles of >12 degrees are often associated with fractures.

Lateral View

The lateral view at 90-degree flexion is the most important view as it allows the physician to note the radiocapitellar and anterior humeral line as well as evaluate the fat pads.

Radiocapitellar Line. A line drawn through the midportion of the radius normally passes through the center of the capitellum on the lateral view of the elbow. In a fracture at the epiphysis of the radial head in children, this line will be displaced away from the center of the capitellum. This may be the only finding suggesting a fracture in a child. In adults, displacement of the radial head, as seen in the Monteggia fracture, will also reveal an abnormal radiocapitellar line (Fig. 14–9).

Anterior Humeral Line. The anterior humeral line is a line drawn on a lateral radiograph along the anterior surface of the humerus through the elbow (Fig. 14–10). Normally, this line transects the middle third of the capitellum. With a supracondylar extension fracture, this line will either transect the anterior third of the capitellum or pass entirely anterior to it.

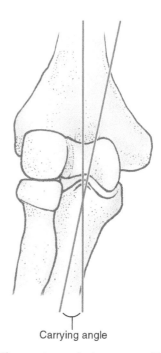

Carrying angle

Figure 14–8. The carrying angle demonstrated by a line drawn through the midshaft of the ulna and another line through the midshaft of the humerus. The normal carrying angle is between 0 and 12 degrees. A carrying angle of >12 degrees is often associated with fractures of the distal humerus.

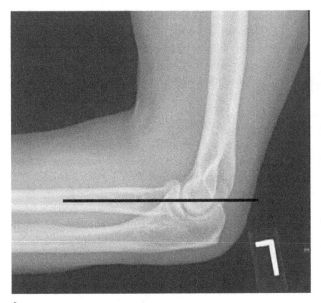
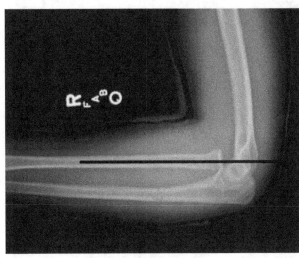

A   B

Figure 14–9. The radiocapitellar line. **A.** A line drawn on the lateral radiograph through the radius normally bisects the capitellum. **B.** An abnormal radiocapitellar line that does not bisect the capitellum indicates a dislocation of the radius (Monteggia fracture dislocation).

Fat Pads. The presence of a bulging anterior fat pad (sail sign) or a posterior fat pad sign is indicative of joint capsule distension (Fig. 14–11). The anterior fat pad is located over the coronoid fossa and is occasionally seen as a thin radiolucent line just anterior to the fossa in many normal radiographs. With a fracture, the joint capsule may be distended with blood, and the anterior fat pad will be displaced anteriorly away from the coronoid fossa. The posterior fat pad lies over the olecranon fossa. Because the olecranon fossa is much deeper, the posterior fat pad is rarely visualized on normal radiographs with the elbow flexed at 90 degrees. Only with joint capsule distension, as with an intra-articular fracture with a capsular hematoma, will the posterior fat pad be visualized. In a child, because cartilaginous growth

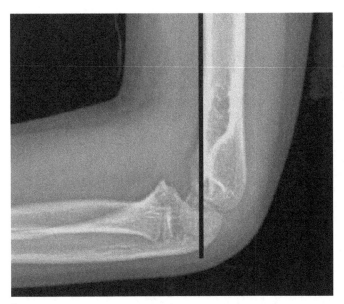
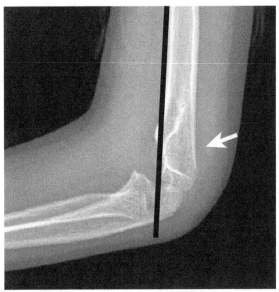

A   B

Figure 14–10. The anterior humeral line. **A.** A line drawn on the lateral radiograph along the anterior surface of the humerus normally transects the middle of the capitellum. **B.** With an extension fracture of the supracondylar region, this line will either transect the anterior third of the capitellum or pass entirely anterior to it. This is especially useful in pediatric physis injuries. The *arrow* indicates a posterior fat pad. (Reproduced with permission from the Sherman SC. Supracondylar fractures, *J Emerg Med* 2011 Feb;40(2):e35–e37.)

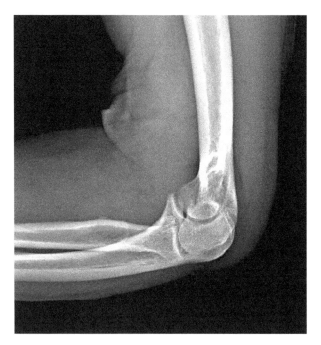

Figure 14–11. Elevation of the anterior and posterior fat pads is seen, suggesting a hemarthrosis. Visualization of a posterior fat pad is always considered abnormal. Careful examination of the radiograph also reveals a marginal radial head fracture.

and various centers of ossification make fracture identification difficult, the detection of a posterior fat pad should be regarded as an intra-articular fracture until proven otherwise.

Although plain films radiographs are usually readily available in the emergency department (ED), point-of-care ultrasound has also been shown to indirectly detect the presence of occult elbow fractures with the presence of a sonographic fat pad sign. The presence of a sonographic fat pad sign has been shown to have a sensitivity of 98% and specificity of 70% for detection of elbow fractures and should prompt reevaluation of the plain-film radiograph, immobilization, and follow-up with orthopedics.

The incidence of a visible radiographic fat pad in elbow fractures without other evidence of fracture ranges widely from 6% to 76%. When magnetic resonance imaging (MRI) was performed on this patient population, occult fractures were discovered in 75% of cases. Fractures of the radial head were most common, accounting for 87% of the occult fractures. Fractures of the olecranon and lateral epicondyle accounted for an equal number of the remaining fractures. Recognition of the fracture did not change management in any of the 20 patients studied.

Axiom: *In a traumatized elbow where a fracture is not seen radiographically, the presence of a posterior fat pad sign strongly suggests an occult fracture.*

ELBOW FRACTURES

OLECRANON FRACTURES

All fractures of the olecranon should be considered intra-articular (Fig. 14–12). It is essential that near-perfect anatomic reduction be achieved to ensure full range of motion.

Mechanism of Injury

Olecranon fractures are usually the result of one of two mechanisms. A fall or direct blow to the olecranon may result in a comminuted fracture. The amount of triceps tone and the integrity of the triceps aponeurosis determine if the fracture will be displaced.

Indirectly, a fall on the outstretched hand with the elbow flexed and the triceps contracted may result in a transverse or oblique fracture. The amount of displacement is contingent on the tone of the triceps, the integrity of the triceps aponeurosis, and the integrity of the periosteum.

Axiom: *All displaced olecranon fractures have either a rupture of the triceps aponeurosis or the periosteum.*

Examination

Patients with olecranon fractures will present with a painful swelling over the olecranon and a hemorrhagic effusion. The patient will be unable to actively extend the forearm against gravity or resistance due to the inadequacy of the triceps mechanism. It is not uncommon for comminuted fractures to result in compromise of ulnar nerve function. It is of critical importance that the initial examination includes documentation of ulnar nerve function.

Imaging

Radiographically, a lateral view with the elbow in 90 degrees of flexion is best for demonstrating olecranon fractures and displacement (Fig. 14–13). Absence of displacement on extension views is not considered definite proof of a non-displaced fracture because the fragments may displace only with elbow flexion. Separation of the fragments or articular incongruity by more than 2 mm is considered sufficient to classify the fracture as displaced.

In children, the olecranon epiphysis ossifies at 10 years of age and fuses by age 16. Interpretation of fractures in children may be difficult, and comparison views should be used whenever doubt exists. In addition, the presence of

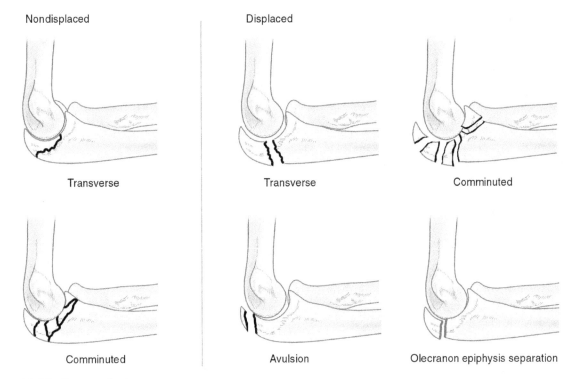

Nondisplaced   Displaced

Transverse   Transverse   Comminuted

Comminuted   Avulsion   Olecranon epiphysis separation

Figure 14–12. Olecranon fractures.

a posterior fat pad or a bulging anterior fat pad should be regarded as indicative of a fracture.

Associated Injuries

Olecranon fractures are frequently associated with ulnar nerve injury; elbow dislocation; anterior dislocation of the radioulnar joint; or concomitant fractures of the radial head, radial shaft, and distal humerus.

Treatment

Nondisplaced. Fractures with <2 mm of separation or articular incongruity are considered nondisplaced. Treatment begins with immobilization in a long-arm splint (Appendix A–9) with the elbow flexed only 50 to 90 degrees and the forearm in a neutral position. This position decreases the pull from the triceps muscle. A cast is used for definitive management, and should be well molded

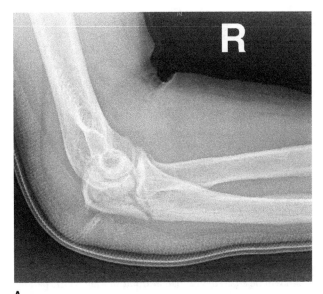

A

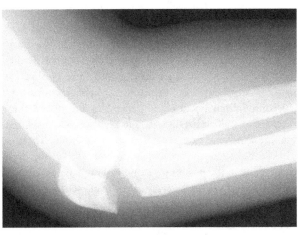

B

Figure 14–13. Olecranon fractures. ***A.*** Nondisplaced. ***B.*** Displaced. Any fracture with >2 mm of separation should be considered displaced and will require surgery.

posteriorly and supported with a collar and cuff. Finger and shoulder range of motion exercises should be started as soon as possible, with repeat radiographs obtained in 5 to 7 days to exclude displacement. Union is complete in 6 to 8 weeks, but the cast may be removed by the orthopedist as early as 1 week in adults to avoid chronic stiffness.

An alternative approach used by some orthopedists in stable fractures is to apply a posterior long-arm splint with the elbow in 90 degrees of flexion (Appendix A–9) and not proceed to casting. Supination and pronation exercises can be initiated in 3 to 5 days, with flexion–extension exercises at 1 to 2 weeks. The protective splint is used until healing is complete (usually 6 weeks).

Displaced. Initial ED management includes splinting in 50 to 90 degrees of flexion with the administration of ice, analgesics, and elevation. Because olecranon fractures are intra-articular, they necessitate anatomic reduction through operative fixation. Displaced fractures of the olecranon include those with displacement of a transverse fracture, a comminuted fracture, an avulsion fracture, or an epiphyseal fracture. These fractures are intra-articular and necessitate anatomic reduction through operative fixation. Therefore, emergent orthopedic referral is indicated.

Complications
The most common complication is the development of shoulder arthritis and inhibition of shoulder mobility. There is a small incidence (5%) of nonunion.

RADIAL HEAD AND NECK FRACTURES

Radial head and neck fractures are relatively common in adults, accounting for one-third of all elbow fractures (Fig. 14–14). Smooth motion of the radial head is essential for full and painless pronation and supination. With fragmentation or displacement, arthritis with restricted motion may result. Therapeutic programs must focus on the restoration and retention of full motion. The classification system that follows is therapeutically oriented. Radial head and neck fractures are divided into three groups: (1) marginal (intra-articular) fractures, (2) neck fractures, and (3) comminuted fractures. In general, nondisplaced fractures are treated closed (at least initially), whereas displaced fractures, in most cases, require open reduction. There is some controversy in the management of these fractures, particularly in the postinjury mobilization phase. As in previous chapters, we make every effort to present both positions where legitimate controversy exists.

Mechanism of Injury
The most common mechanism is a fall on the outstretched hand (indirect). With the elbow in extension,

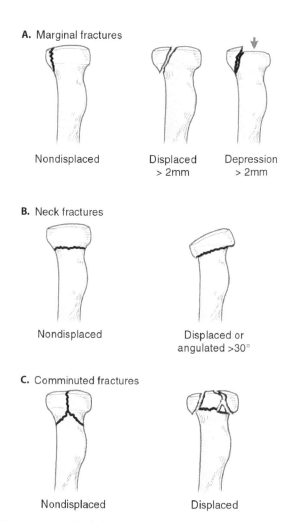

Figure 14–14. Radial head and neck fractures. **A.** Marginal fractures. **B.** Neck fractures. **C.** Comminuted fractures.

the force drives the radius against the capitellum, resulting in a marginal or radial neck fracture (Fig. 14–15). As the force increases, comminution, dislocation, or displaced fragments occur. The fracture pattern in adults and children is variable due to differences in the strength of the proximal radius. In adults, marginal or comminuted fractures of the radial head or neck with articular involvement are common. In children, displacement of the radial epiphysis is common, whereas articular involvement is rare.

Examination
Tenderness will be present over the radial head with swelling secondary to a hemarthrosis. Pain is exacerbated by supination and associated with reduced mobility. Children with epiphyseal injuries may have very little swelling, but pain will be elicited with palpation or motion. If the patient has associated wrist pain, disruption of the distal radioulnar joint should be suspected, and urgent orthopedic referral is recommended.

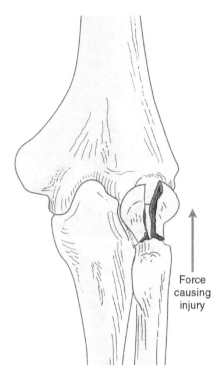

Figure 14–15. Radial head fracture secondary to a fall on an outstretched arm.

> **Axiom:** *Wrist pain associated with a fracture of the radial head suggests disruption of the distal radioulnar joint and the radioulnar interosseous membrane (Essex–Lopresti fracture dislocation).*

Imaging

Visualization of radial head and neck fractures often requires oblique views (Figs. 14–16 and 14–17). Impact fractures of the neck are best seen on the lateral projection. If a radial head fracture is suspected, but not seen, additional views in varying degrees of radial rotation should be obtained. An enlarged anterior fat pad or the presence of a posterior fat pad suggests a joint effusion and strongly suggests an occult fracture, most commonly of the radial head. In addition, the radiocapitellar line should be evaluated in attempting to diagnose pediatric epiphyseal fractures or radial head dislocations.

Associated Injuries

Fracture of the capitellum should be suspected in all proximal radius fractures. This structure must be closely examined, looking for any evidence of fracture.

A valgus strain often results in medial collateral ligament sprain or rupture. In addition, avulsion of the medial epicondyle is frequently seen in both children and adults.

Disruption of the interosseous membrane between the radius and ulna and injury to the distal radioulnar joint ligaments may also occur. An Essex–Lopresti injury should be recognized early as internal fixation is often indicated.

Treatment

For further discussion of epiphyseal fractures, the reader is referred to Chapter 6. In general, radial head epiphyseal fractures with angulation of <15 degrees are best treated with immobilization for 2 weeks in a long-arm posterior splint (Appendix A–9) followed by a sling. Remodeling will generally correct this degree of angulation. With >15 degrees, an orthopedic surgeon should be consulted because reduction is required. Angulation >60 degrees often requires open reduction.

The remainder of the discussion regarding the treatment of radial head and neck fractures applies to adults.

Marginal (Intra-Articular)

Nondisplaced. Marginal radial head fractures with displacement of <2 mm (marginal fractures or minimal depression fractures) are treated with a sling or a long-arm posterior splint (Appendix A–9). If splinted, the splint should remain in place for no more than 3 to 4 days. Early motion exercises are recommended if they can be tolerated (pain).

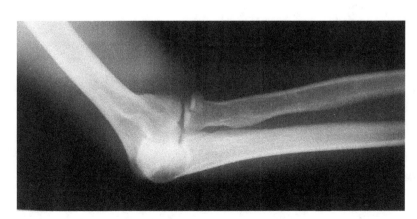

Figure 14–16. A displaced marginal fracture of the radial head.

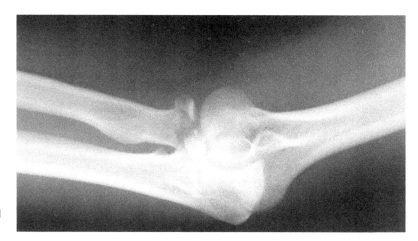

Figure 14–17. Displaced comminuted fractures of the radial head and neck.

Displaced. When there is displacement or depression of >2 mm with more than one-third of the articular surface involved, operative treatment is required. Initial ED management includes aspiration of the hematoma for pain relief and placement of a long-arm posterior splint with the elbow in 90 degrees of flexion and the forearm neutral (Appendix A–9). Displaced fractures with less than one-third of the articular surface involved are reduced and followed by early motion.

Early referral is indicated for all these fractures. Surgical excision of displaced radial head fractures is no longer recommended in young active patients. Better operative techniques and implant placement often make radial head arthroplasty the treatment of choice and has resulted in better outcomes when compared to patients who received open reduction and internal fixation.

Neck

Nondisplaced. Neck fractures without displacement and angulation of <30 degrees are treated with immobilization in a sling or a long-arm posterior splint and urgent orthopedic referral (Appendix A–9). Definitive therapy is controversial.

Displaced. These patients should be placed in a long-arm posterior splint (Appendix A–9). With angulation >30 degrees or significant displacement, operative fixation is recommended.

Comminuted

Nondisplaced. These fractures can be treated conservatively with a long-arm posterior splint (Appendix A–9). Early motion exercises are recommended.

Displaced. These patients should be placed in a long-arm posterior splint (Appendix A–9). With severe comminution of the head, excision of fragments or a prosthetic head replacement is the recommended therapy.

In addition to the treatments outlined in this section, early aspiration of the joint should be considered for radial head and neck fractures, as this serves to reduce pain and facilitate early mobilization. This technique is as follows:

1. The skin of the lateral elbow should be prepped using sterile technique.
2. An imaginary triangle should be constructed over the lateral elbow connecting the radial head, the lateral epicondyle, and the olecranon (Fig. 14–18). Only skin and the anconeus muscle cover the joint capsule in this area, and there are no significant neurovascular structures in the area.
3. The skin should be anesthetized with lidocaine.
4. Using a 20-mL syringe and an 18-gauge needle, the joint capsule is penetrated by directing the needle medially and perpendicularly to the skin. When the capsule is entered, blood is aspirated (usually 2–4 mL).

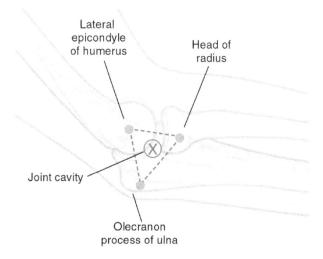

Figure 14–18. The safest place to aspirate the elbow is in the center of a triangle produced by connecting the lateral epicondyle of the humerus, the olecranon, and the radial head. Aspiration should be performed by inserting the needle through the center of this triangle.

Complications

The large majority of patients with nondisplaced fractures of the radial head or neck have excellent outcomes although complications can occur.[16] The most common complication from radial head and neck fractures is decreased elbow range of motion. Early, active range-of-motion exercise in simple, nondisplaced radial head fractures has been shown to reduce the incidence of complications.[17]

CORONOID PROCESS FRACTURES

Coronoid process fractures are classified as (1) nondisplaced, (2) displaced, and (3) displaced with posterior elbow dislocation (Fig. 14–19). These fractures are rarely seen as isolated injuries and are noted more commonly with posterior dislocations of the elbow.[18]

A. Nondisplaced

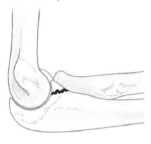

B. Displaced

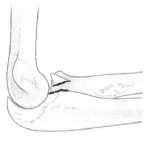

C. Posterior dislocation

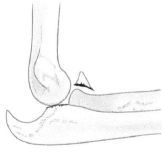

Figure 14–19. Coronoid process fractures. **A.** Nondisplaced. **B.** Displaced. **C.** Posterior dislocation.

Mechanism of Injury

Isolated coronoid process fractures are believed to be due to hyperextension with joint capsule tension and subsequent avulsion. When coronoid fractures are associated with posterior dislocations, the mechanism is a "push-off" injury by the distal humerus.

Examination

Tenderness and swelling over the antecubital fossa is noted frequently.

Imaging

The coronoid fragment is best visualized on a lateral radiograph, although oblique views may be necessary. The fragment may be displaced, as with an avulsion fracture, or impacted against the trochlea, as is frequently noted with fracture dislocations. Nondisplaced coronoid fractures may be missed on radiographs and computed tomography (CT) so MRI should be considered to rule out small fractures.[19]

Treatment

This fracture is commonly associated with elbow dislocations, and a more detailed discussion of treatment can be found in the Elbow Dislocations section of this chapter.

Nondisplaced. Isolated nondisplaced fractures are treated with a long-arm posterior splint (Appendix A–9). The elbow should be in more than 90 degrees of flexion and the forearm in supination. This should be followed by active exercises with sling support. The treatment of these fractures is controversial and early referral is strongly urged.

Displaced. Displaced fractures require emergent orthopedic referral, especially if they are greater than 50% of the size of the coronoid process or the elbow joint is unstable. In both cases, fragment fixation is recommended. If the fracture fragment is small, treatment in a long-arm posterior splint (Appendix A–9), as for nondisplaced coronoid fractures, is appropriate. Small, displaced fracture fragments are managed nonoperatively.[8]

Displaced with Posterior Dislocation. Fracture dislocations are discussed in the Elbow Dislocations section of this chapter. Reduction of the dislocation will frequently result in coronoid fracture reduction.

Complications

Coronoid process fractures are infrequently associated with the development of osteoarthritis.

SUPRACONDYLAR FRACTURES

A supracondylar fracture is a transverse fracture of the distal humerus above the joint capsule in which the diaphysis

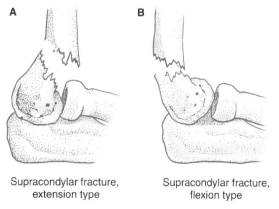

Supracondylar fracture, extension type

Supracondylar fracture, flexion type

Figure 14–20. Supracondylar fractures. **A.** Extension type. **B.** Flexion type.

of the humerus dissociates from the condyles. In children, approximately 60% of all elbow fractures are supracondylar.   The incidence is highest between the ages of 3 and 11 years. They occur more frequently in children because the surrounding ligaments are stronger than the bone. As ligament laxity increases with age, ligament tears without fracture are more common in adults. Distal humerus fractures comprise only 0.5% of all fractures in adults and are most common in osteopenic adults older than 50. In the older age group, these fractures are often comminuted. Supracondylar fractures are covered in further detail in Chapter 6.

Supracondylar fractures are subdivided based on the position of the distal humeral segment into (1) extension-type (posterior angulation or displacement) or (2) flexion-type (anterior angulation or displacement) fractures (Fig. 14–20). The vast majority (95%) of displaced supracondylar fractures are of the extension type.

The most common classification used for extension supracondylar fractures was proposed by Gartland in 1959, who divided them into three types. Type I fractures are nondisplaced. Type II fractures are displaced, but the bony fragments are still partially apposed. Type II fractures were subsequently divided into type IIA (angulated extension fracture with an intact posterior cortex) and type IIB (displaced fracture with partial posterior translation) injuries. Type III fractures include those with complete displacement of the fracture fragments. The diagnosis and management of these fractures varies, depending on the type of fracture that exists.

Mechanism of Injury

Two mechanisms result in fractures of the distal humerus. With the elbow in flexion, a direct blow can result in a fracture. The position of the fragments depends on the magnitude and direction of force, the initial position of the elbow and the forearm (e.g., flexion, supination), and the muscular tone.

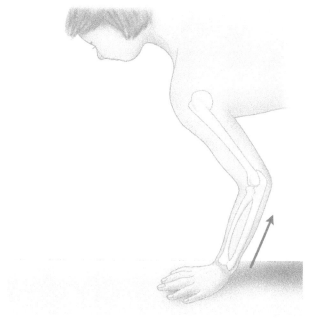

Figure 14–21. The indirect mechanism of producing a supracondylar fracture involves a fall on the outstretched hand.

The indirect mechanism involves a fall on the outstretched hand (Fig. 14–21). As before, the magnitude and direction of force, as well as the position of the elbow and the muscular tone, determine the position of the fracture fragments. More than 90% of supracondylar fractures result from the indirect mechanism. Typically, the fracture is an extension fracture, where the distal fragment is displaced posteriorly.

Flexion fractures, where the distal humeral fragment is displaced anteriorly, account for only 10%. They are usually the result of a direct blow against the posterior aspect of the flexed elbow (Fig. 14–22). The indirect mechanism uncommonly results in a flexion fracture.

Examination

The emergency physician must complete a careful physical examination, with special attention to the brachial, radial,

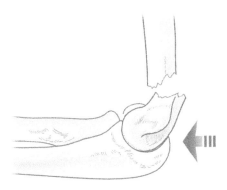

Figure 14–22. With the elbow in flexion, a direct blow to the olecranon can result in a distal humeral fracture.

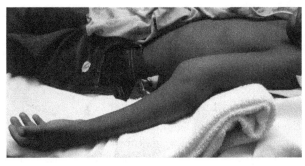

Figure 14–23. Clinical picture of a child with a displaced supracondylar fracture. (Reproduced with permission from the Sherman SC. Supracondylar fractures, *J Emerg Med* 2011 Feb;40(2): e35–e37.)

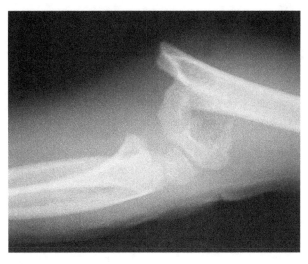

Figure 14–24. Radiograph of the same child in Fig. 14–23 confirms a type III (complete displacement) supracondylar fracture. (Reproduced with permission from the Sherman SC. Supracondylar fractures, *J Emerg Med* 2011 Feb;40(2):e35–e37.)

and ulnar pulses along with the median, radial, and ulnar nerves. Comparison with the uninjured extremity should be a routine part of each examination. Frequently, supracondylar fractures are associated with extensive hemorrhage and swelling, which, in some instances, may result in compartment syndrome.

Recent injuries may demonstrate little swelling with severe pain. The displaced distal humeral fragment can often be palpated posteriorly and superiorly because of the pull of the triceps muscle. As swelling increases, extension supracondylar fractures can be confused with a posterior dislocation of the elbow resulting from the prominence of the olecranon and the presence of a posterior concavity (Fig. 14–23). In addition, the involved forearm may appear shorter when compared with the uninvolved side. In patients with flexion supracondylar fractures, the elbow is usually carried in flexion, and there is a loss of the olecranon prominence.

Imaging

The initial radiographic examination should include AP and lateral views (Fig. 14–24). On the AP film, the forearm should be supinated and the elbow placed in as much extension as possible. The lateral film should be taken with the elbow in 90 degrees of flexion. Additional oblique views with the elbow in extension may be helpful in diagnosing occult fractures.

The distal segment may be displaced, angulated, or rotated with respect to the proximal bone, resulting in various deformities. Approximately 25% of supracondylar fractures are nondisplaced. Radiographic diagnosis in these cases may be exceedingly difficult. Subtle changes, such as the presence of a posterior fat pad, an abnormal anterior humeral line, or an abnormal carrying angle may be the only radiographic clues to the presence of a fracture.

Associated Injuries

Supracondylar fractures are frequently associated with neurovascular complications, especially in the presence of displacement.

The extremity of all patients with supracondylar fractures should be assessed for pulses, color, temperature, and capillary refill. Type III supracondylar fractures present with vascular compromise in approximately 5% to 10% of cases due to impingement by fracture fragments, swelling, or arterial laceration. Document the presence and strength of the radial, ulnar, and brachial pulses. Absent pulses with adequate perfusion are well documented in displaced supracondylar fractures and are made possible by good collateral circulation. Management of a pulseless, well-perfused extremity following adequate reduction varies from observation to operative exploration. Arteriography is not usually necessary.

In patients with intact pulses, a pulse oximeter can be applied to monitor the pulse rate as well as the hemoglobin saturation. The presence of a pulse, however, does not exclude a significant arterial injury.

Function of the radial, median, and ulnar nerves should be tested as deficits can occur with displaced supracondylar fractures. The incidence of nerve injury following type III fractures is 10% to 15%. In those fractures that are posteromedially displaced, neural compromise is more likely to occur.[22] These injuries are common because the nerves are tethered at the elbow and displacement leads to stretching.

The most common nerve injury is to the anterior interosseous nerve. This nerve does not have sensory innervations, and when a deficit is present, only subtle motor findings are seen, making this injury easily missed. The anterior interosseous nerve innervates the flexor digitorum profundus of the index finger (flexion of DIP joint) and the flexor pollicis longus (flexion of IP joint). A deficit is detected by having the patient make an "OK" sign and noting weakened flexion at these two joints. Testing nerve function is important because iatrogenic injuries can occur after multiple attempts at closed reduction or following operative repair. Most nerve injuries are neuropraxias, and function returns without interventions in 3 to 6 months.

Treatment

Extension Supracondylar Fracture. *Type I.* Supra-condylar fractures that are not displaced or angulated are immobilized in a posterior long-arm splint, extending from the axilla to a point just proximal to the metacarpal heads (Appendix A–9). The splint should encircle approximately three-fourths of the circumference of the extremity. The forearm is kept in a neutral position, and the elbow is flexed from 80 to 90 degrees. The distal pulses should be checked, and, if absent, the elbow is extended 5 to 15 degrees or until the pulses return. A sling is used for support, and ice is applied to reduce swelling.

These fractures are stable and require 3 weeks of immobilization followed by early motion. Complications frequently seen following type II and III fractures, such as neurovascular injury and compartment syndrome, are rare after type I injuries. Some authors recommend brief periods (6 hours) of observation in the ED, but in the absence of significant swelling, pain, or pulse deficits, discharge with orthopedic follow-up and return to ED precautions is acceptable.

> **Axiom:** *A cast should never be applied initially on a supra-condylar fracture.*

Types II and III. With an intact neurovascular status, reduction of these fractures should be attempted by an experienced orthopedic surgeon. Emergent reduction by the emergency specialist is indicated only when the displaced fracture is associated with vascular compromise, which immediately threatens the viability of the extremity, where emergent orthopedic consultation is not available (Fig. 14–25):

1. The initial step is to prepare for and administer procedural sedation, as outlined in Chapter 2.
2. While an assistant immobilizes the arm proximal to the fracture site, the physician holds the forearm at the wrist, exerting longitudinal traction until the length is near normal (Fig. 14–25A).
3. The physician now slightly hyperextends the elbow to unlock the fracture fragments while he or she applies pressure in an anterior direction against the distal humeral segment (Fig. 14–25B). At this point, medial and lateral angulation should be corrected. The assistant simultaneously exerts a gentle posteriorly directed force against the proximal humeral segment.

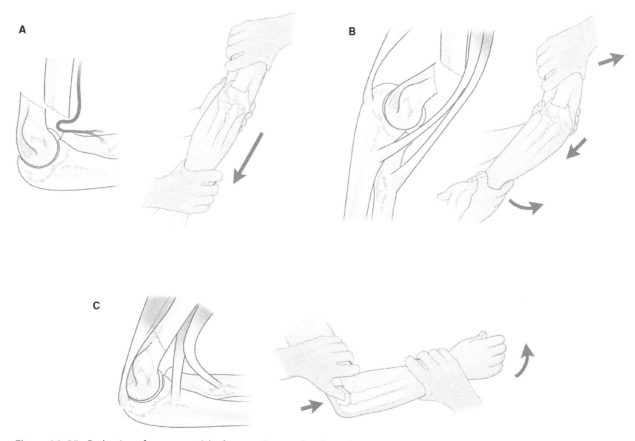

Figure 14–25. Reduction of a supracondylar fracture. See text for discussion.

4. To complete reduction, the elbow is flexed to maintain the proper alignment, and posterior pressure is applied to the distal fragment (Fig. 14–25C). The elbow should be flexed to the point where the pulse diminishes and then extended 5 to 15 degrees and the pulses rechecked and documented.

> **Caution:** *Only one attempt should be made at a manipulative reduction due to the proximity of neurovascular structures and the likelihood of injury with repeated attempts.*

The extremity is immobilized in a long-arm posterior splint (Appendix A–9). Controversy exists about the position of the forearm. In the child, if there is medial displacement of the distal fragment, the forearm should be immobilized in pronation. With lateral displacement, the forearm should be immobilized in supination. Adults are generally immobilized in a neutral position or in slight pronation. A sling should be supplied for support and ice applied to reduce swelling. Postreduction radiographs for documentation of position are essential. Hospital admission for close follow-up of neurovascular status is mandatory. Delayed swelling with subsequent compartment syndrome and neurovascular compromise is common following these fractures.

Definitive treatment of displaced supracondylar fractures is operative pinning after closed reduction. Open reduction is required in a minority of cases. The most common cause of compartment syndrome in children is the displaced supracondylar fracture, and for that reason, emergent (<8 hours) or urgent (within 24 hours) reduction to reduce swelling and improve venous return is required. Fortunately, prompt anatomic reduction and bony stabilization have reduced the incidence of forearm compartment syndrome even in the most severe cases.

Some authors manage type II fractures with closed reduction and casting with close follow-up. Excessive swelling may prohibit a stable closed reduction, however, and approximately 25% will ultimately require pinning due to displacement while in the cast.

Flexion Supracondylar Fracture. Displaced flexion supracondylar fractures also require orthopedic consultation for reduction. Pinning of the fracture is a frequently used treatment modality.[23,24] Where there is limb-threatening neurovascular compromise and emergent orthopedic consultation is not available, an experienced emergency medicine specialist may carry out reduction. With the elbow held in flexion, longitudinal traction–countertraction is applied. The physician then exerts a gentle posteriorly directed pressure over the distal fragment. When the fragment is in position, the elbow is extended and maintained in extension. The extremity is immobilized with a long-arm posterior splint (Appendix A–9). It is our preference to position the elbow at 35 degrees short of full extension to avoid the development of delayed elbow stiffness. Some authors recommend splinting with the elbow in full extension. The patient should be hospitalized and treated with elevation, ice, and analgesics. Operative reduction of supracondylar flexion fractures is indicated when there is a failure of one attempt at manipulative reduction or there are unstable fracture fragments.

Complications

Supracondylar fractures are associated with several complications:

- Neurovascular injuries may present acutely or with delayed symptoms. In all cases where vascular injury is suspected, the consideration of urgent arteriography should be discussed with the consulting orthopedic surgeon. Vascular injury and swelling can lead to compartment syndrome within 12 to 24 hours. If compartment syndrome is not treated in a timely manner, the associated ischemia and infarction may progress to Volkmann ischemic contracture.[25] If compartment syndrome is suspected, urgent surgical consultation should be obtained to assess need for fasciotomy. Ulnar nerve palsy is a delayed complication.
- Cubitus varus and valgus deformities are commonly seen in children. Malposition of the distal humeral fragment after reduction is the most frequent cause.
- Stiffness and loss of elbow motion are common complications in adults secondary to prolonged immobilization. After a stable reduction, pronation and supination exercises should be initiated in 2 to 3 days. Within 2 to 3 weeks, the posterior splint may be removed for flexion–extension exercises.

TRANSCONDYLAR FRACTURES

This transverse fracture transects both condyles, but unlike the supracondylar fracture, this fracture lies within the joint capsule (Fig. 14–26). Transcondylar fractures are most often seen in patients older than 50 with osteopenia. The distal humeral segment may be positioned anterior (flexion) or posterior (extension) to the proximal humeral segment. Therefore, the mechanisms, radiographs, and treatment are identical to those of the supracondylar extension or flexion fractures. This fracture frequently results in the deposition of callus within the olecranon and coronoid fossas with subsequent diminished range of motion. All transcondylar fractures require an urgent consultation with an orthopedic surgeon and are best managed initially in an inpatient setting.

An example of a flexion-type transcondylar fracture is the *Posadas fracture*. This fracture results in anterior displacement of the distal condylar segment (Fig. 14–27). The most common mechanism is a direct blow with the elbow in flexion that displaces the condylar fragments

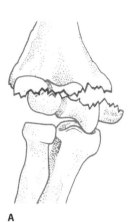

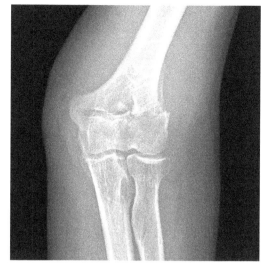

A   **B**

Figure 14–26. Transcondylar fracture. **A.** Schematic. **B.** Radiograph.

anteriorly. In addition to pain and swelling, there is loss of the olecranon prominence with fullness in the antecubital fossa.

The Posadas fracture is associated with a posterior dislocation of the radius or the ulna. Nondisplaced fractures of the transcondylar type are more common than displaced fractures.

The ED management is to splint the fracture in a long-arm posterior splint (Appendix A–9) *without repositioning the arm* because flexion or extension of the joint may result in serious limb-threatening vascular compromise. These fractures are difficult to treat, and an emergent orthopedic consult should be obtained. If there is vascular compromise initially, traction with an olecranon pin is the treatment of choice.

Posadas fractures are associated with several complications, including acute or delayed neurovascular compromise. Diminished range of motion may be secondary to inadequate reduction or callus formation within the joint.

INTERCONDYLAR FRACTURES

Intercondylar fractures generally occur in patients older than 50. This is actually a supracondylar fracture with a vertical component (Fig. 14–28). The terms *T* and *Y* indicate the direction of the fracture line. T fractures have a single transverse line, whereas Y fractures present with two oblique fracture lines through the supracondylar humeral column. Classification is based on the amount of separation between the fracture fragments and is broadly divided into (1) nondisplaced fractures and (2) displaced, rotated, or comminuted fractures.

A nondisplaced fracture has no separation between the capitellum and the trochlea. A displaced fracture exists when

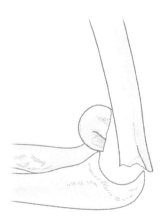

Figure 14–27. Posadas fracture.

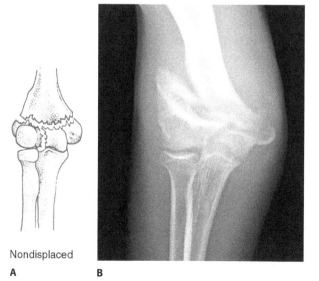

Nondisplaced

A   **B**

Figure 14–28. Intercondylar fractures. **A.** Schematic. **B.** Radiograph.

there is separation between the capitellum and the trochlea without rotation in the frontal plane. This indicates that the capsular ligaments are intact and holding the fragments in their normal position. Displacement with rotation exists when there is separation between the capitellum and the trochlea combined with rotation of the fragments. Rotation is secondary to the pull of the muscles inserting on the epicondyles. Severe comminution of the articular surface and wide separation of the humeral condyles may also occur.

Mechanism of Injury
The most common mechanism is a direct blow driving the olecranon into the distal humerus at the trochlea. The position of the elbow at the time of impact determines whether there will be extension or flexion displacement of the fragments. Extension or posterior displacement of the fragments is more commonly seen. Rotation frequently accompanies these fractures because of the pull of the muscles inserting on the epicondyles. The condyles may separate from each other and from the humeral shaft. The degree of separation depends on the direction and force of injury along with the muscular tone. Generally, larger condylar displacements are associated with greater offending forces.

Examination
On examination, there is shortening of the forearm. With extension fractures, there is a concavity of the posterior arm with prominence of the olecranon.

Imaging
AP and lateral views may demonstrate comminution, and overlapping bony edges may make interpretation difficult. In comminuted fractures difficult to visualize on plain films, CT is often helpful to the surgeon planning operative therapy.

Associated Injuries
Neurovascular injuries are infrequently associated with these fractures.

Treatment
Nondisplaced. This is a stable fracture and can be initially treated with a long-arm posterior splint with the forearm in a neutral position (Appendix A–9). Sling and elevation with ice packs should be used early. Active motion exercises can be started within 2 to 3 weeks.

Displaced, Rotated, or Comminuted. These fractures are uncommonly seen, difficult to treat, and require an emergent orthopedic consultation. Operative treatment of these fractures, which was once considered treacherous, is now the treatment of choice. In patients with contraindications to surgery, other means of treatment such as

olecranon pinning with traction may be used. The therapeutic approach selected depends on the type of fracture, the activity level of the patient, and the judgment and past experiences of the consulting orthopedic surgeon. ED care involves splinting the fracture in the position of presentation and applying ice. Surgical fixation and traction are the two most commonly selected therapeutic modalities. In older patients with severely comminuted fractures, elbow replacement may be considered.

Complications
Intercondylar fractures of the distal humerus may be associated with several complications:

- Loss of elbow joint function (most common)
- Posttraumatic arthritis
- Neurovascular complications (rare)
- Malunion and nonunion (uncommon)

CONDYLAR FRACTURES

The humeral condyle includes an articular portion and a nonarticular epicondylar portion. Condylar fractures, therefore, incorporate both portions of the condyle into the fracture fragment. Fractures may involve either the medial (trochlea and medial epicondyle) or lateral (capitellum and lateral epicondyle) condyle.

The fracture fragment of a condylar fracture may include the lateral trochlear ridge, or it may remain attached to the proximal humeral segment. This distinction is important because fractures in which the lateral trochlear ridge is incorporated into the distal humeral segment demonstrate medial and lateral instability of the elbow, radius, and ulna.

Lateral Condylar Fractures
The lateral condyle is anatomically more exposed, and thus more likely to fracture (Fig. 14–29).

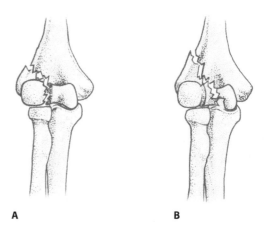

Figure 14–29. Lateral condylar fractures. **A.** Lateral trochlear ridge not included. **B.** Lateral trochlear ridge included.

Mechanism of Injury

Two mechanisms result in lateral condylar fractures. First, with the elbow in flexion a direct force applied to its posterior aspect may result in a fracture. Second, with the elbow in extension, a force causing adduction and hyperextension may result in a fracture. In children, rotation of the fracture fragment is secondary to the pull of the extensor muscles. Fragment rotation is uncommon in adults.

Examination

Physical examination typically reveals tenderness and swelling over the involved condyle.

Imaging

AP and lateral views typically reveal widening of the intercondylar distance. The fractured segment may be displaced proximally, but generally it will be seen posterior and inferior to its normal position. When the lateral trochlear ridge stays with the fragment, translocation of the ulna may occur. In children in whom ossification is incomplete, comparison views should be obtained.

Associated Injuries

No associated injuries are commonly seen.

Treatment

Because of the high rate of complications, all lateral condylar fractures require urgent orthopedic evaluation and follow-up.

Lateral Trochlear Ridge Not Included. When non-displaced, the arm should be immobilized in a long-arm posterior splint with the elbow in flexion, the forearm in supination, and the wrist in extension to minimize distraction by the pull of the extensor muscles (Appendix A–9). The arm should be elevated with a sling and radiographs repeated in 2 days to ensure proper positioning. A long-arm cast can be applied when the swelling is reduced. For displaced fractures, emergent orthopedic consultation should be obtained. The preferred treatment is open reduction with internal fixation. A long-arm posterior splint (Appendix A–9) is placed in the interim.

Lateral Trochlear Ridge Included. Because this fracture is more unstable, initial therapy includes the application of anterior and posterior long-arm splints (Appendix A–10). The elbow should be in more than 90 degrees of flexion with the forearm supinated and the wrist extended. Radiographs should be repeated in 2 or 3 days to ensure proper positioning and a long-arm cast applied. Displaced fractures should be referred immediately to an experienced orthopedic surgeon. These fractures are best treated with open reduction and internal fixation. Closed manipulative reductions often result in cubitus valgus deformities.

Complications

Lateral condylar fractures may result in several complications.

* Cubitus valgus deformity
* Lateral transposition of the forearm
* Arthritis due to joint capsule and articular disruption
* Delayed ulnar nerve palsy
* Overgrowth with subsequent cubitus varus deformity in children

Medial Condylar Fractures

These fractures are less common than lateral condylar fractures (Fig. 14–30).

Mechanism of Injury

Two mechanisms result in medial condylar fractures: (1) a direct force applied through the olecranon in a medial direction and (2) abduction with the forearm in extension.

Examination

Tenderness over the medial condyle with painful flexion of the wrist against resistance is frequently noted.

Imaging

Similar findings as with the lateral condylar fractures are noted, except the distal fragment tends to be pulled anteriorly and inferiorly by the flexor muscles.

Associated Injuries

No associated injuries are commonly seen.

Treatment

Lateral Trochlear Ridge Not Included. A long-arm posterior splint is applied with the elbow flexed, the forearm in pronation, and the wrist in flexion (Appendix A–9). Orthopedic follow-up with repeated radiographs to exclude delayed displacement is strongly urged. Displaced fractures

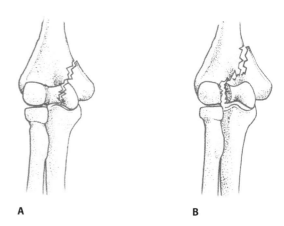

Figure 14–30. Medial condylar fractures. **A.** Lateral trochlear ridge not included. **B.** Lateral trochlear ridge included.

require immobilization, ice, and elevation with emergent referral for surgical fixation.

Lateral Trochlear Ridge Included. Because this fracture is more unstable, initial therapy includes the application of anterior and posterior long-arm splints (Appendix A–10). The elbow should be in more than 90 degrees of flexion with the forearm pronated and the wrist flexed. Radiographs should be repeated in 2 or 3 days to ensure proper positioning and a long-arm cast applied. ED management of displaced fractures includes immobilization, ice, elevation, and emergent referral for surgical fixation.

Complications
Medial condylar fractures are associated with the following complications:

- Posttraumatic arthritis
- Malunion with subsequent cubitus varus deformity
- Ulnar nerve palsy

Capitellum Fractures
Articular surface fractures include the capitellum and trochlea and are very uncommon as isolated injuries, but they may be seen in conjunction with posterior dislocations of the elbow (Fig. 14–31). Trochlear fractures are extremely rare and require emergent orthopedic evaluation and treatment. Capitellum fractures constitute only 0.5% to 1% of all elbow injuries, and 6% of distal humerus fractures.[30]

Mechanism of Injury
The fracture mechanism is usually the result of a blow inflicted on the outstretched hand. The force is transmitted up the radius to the capitellum. The capitellum has no muscular attachments, and, consequently, the fragment may be displaced. In some circumstances, secondary displacement occurs from elbow motion.

Examination
Initially, there may be a silent interval where there is an absence of signs and symptoms. Later, as blood distends the joint capsule, pain and swelling may become quite severe. Anterior displacement of the fracture fragment into the radial fossa may result in incomplete painful flexion. With posterior displacement, the range of motion is complete; however, there is increased pain with flexion.

Imaging
The lateral view usually demonstrates the fragment lying anterior and proximal to the main portion of the capitellum.

Associated Injuries
Radial head fractures are common. Capitellum fractures are associated with a high incidence of ulnar collateral ligament rupture.[31,32]

Treatment
Surgical excision of a small capitellar fragment (articular cartilage and subchondral bone) has been the traditional treatment of choice, but as operative techniques improve, operative fixation is becoming more commonly performed.[14,30] ED management consists of immobilization in a posterior splint, ice, elevation, and analgesics. If a large fragment is present, or a piece of the trochlea is involved, emergent orthopedic consultation for operative reduction is indicated. Both closed and open techniques have been described.[14] An accurate reduction is imperative to ensure normal motion of the radiohumeral joint.

Complications
Capitellum fractures are associated with the following complications:

- Posttraumatic arthritis
- Avascular necrosis of the fracture fragment
- Restricted range of motion

EPICONDYLE FRACTURES

Epicondyle fractures are most commonly seen in children (Fig. 14–32).

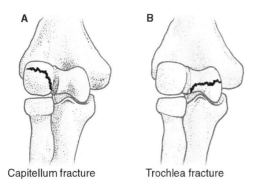

Figure 14–31. Articular surface fractures. **A.** Capitellum fracture. **B.** Trochlea fracture.

Capitellum fracture   Trochlea fracture

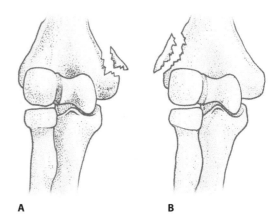

Figure 14–32. Epicondylar fractures. **A.** Medial epicondyle. **B.** Lateral epicondyle.

Medial Epicondyle Fracture

Medial epicondyle fractures are much more common than lateral (Fig. 14–32A). The ossification center for the medial epicondyle appears by ages 5 to 7 years and fuses to the distal humerus by approximately age 20. Medial epicondyle displacement, as an isolated injury, is uncommon. More commonly seen is the palpable avulsion fracture associated with a posterior dislocation of the elbow.

Mechanism of Injury

Three mechanisms are commonly associated with fractures of the medial epicondyle:

* The more common avulsion fracture is associated with childhood or adolescent posterior dislocations. This fracture is rarely associated with posterior dislocations in patients older than 20.
* The flexor pronator tendon is attached to the medial epicondylar ossification center. Repeated valgus stress on the elbow may result in a fracture with fragment displacement distally. This is commonly seen in adolescent baseball players and is called "little league elbow."
* Isolated medial epicondylar fractures in adults are usually due to a direct blow.

Examination

If this fracture is associated with a posterior dislocation, the elbow will be in flexion, and there will be a prominence of the olecranon. Isolated fractures produce localized pain over the medial epicondyle. Pain is increased with flexion of the elbow and the wrist or with pronation of the forearm.

Caution: *When assessing this fracture, examine and document ulnar nerve function before initiating therapy.*

Imaging

Comparison views are essential in children and adolescents. Displaced fragments may migrate and become intra-articular.

Caution: *If the fragment has migrated to the joint line, it should be considered intra-articular.*

The age at which the epicondyles ossify and fuse should be considered before diagnosing a fracture (Fig. 14–33). The medial epicondyle appears at ages 5 to 7 and fuses at ages 18 to 20. The lateral epicondyle appears at ages 9 to 13 and fuses at ages 14 to 16. For further information, the reader is referred to Chapter 6.

Associated Injuries

The most common associated injury is posterior dislocation of the elbow.

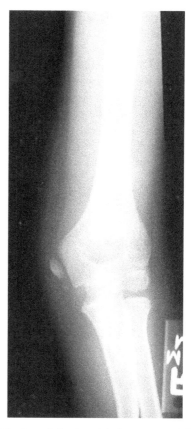

Figure 14–33. A medial epicondyle fracture in a child.

Treatment

Fragments that are displaced <4 mm, as determined by measuring the clear space between the fracture fragment and the humerus, can be immobilized in a long-arm posterior splint (Appendix A–9). The elbow and the wrist should be flexed with the forearm pronated.

If the fracture is associated with an elbow dislocation, the dislocation is reduced first (refer to the Elbow Dislocations section), and the fracture fragments are then assessed. If the epicondyle is within the joint, open reduction is indicated.

Complications

Medial epicondylar fractures are associated with ulnar nerve bony entrapment if persistent displacement is present. Other complications are related to posterior elbow dislocation, and the reader is referred to that section for further details.

Lateral Epicondyle Fracture

This is an exceedingly rare injury that is usually the result of a direct blow. It is much more common for the condyle to fracture than the epicondyle. Most fractures are nondisplaced and can be treated in a similar manner to lateral condylar fractures (Fig. 14–32B).

ELBOW SOFT-TISSUE INJURY AND DISLOCATIONS

ELBOW DISLOCATIONS

Elbow dislocations are among the most commonly seen dislocations in the body, second in frequency only to dislocations of the shoulder and the fingers. The most common elbow dislocation is a posterior dislocation, which accounts for 90% of cases (Fig. 14–34).[33,34] Anterior, medial, and lateral dislocations make up the remainder of the cases. Lateral and medial dislocations can occur in isolation, but they are more often seen in combination with either posterior or anterior dislocations or with fractures. Anterior dislocation of the elbow is almost always associated with fractures.

Posterior Dislocation

Posterior dislocations, in which the olecranon is displaced posteriorly in relation to the distal humerus, account for the majority of dislocations seen at the elbow (Fig. 14–34A).[35] Elbow dislocations are classified as simple or complex, depending on whether there is a fracture in addition to the dislocation. Simple dislocations are more common than complex.

Mechanism of Injury

The mechanism of injury is a fall on the extended and abducted arm. A combination of valgus, supination, and axial forces acts to tear ligamentous attachments and allows the joint to become dislocated.

Examination

Patients with posterior dislocations present to the ED with the limb held in flexion at 45 degrees. The olecranon is prominent posteriorly, and there is usually moderate swelling and deformity at the joint (Figs. 14–35 and 14–36). The peripheral nerves and the distal pulses should be examined.

Significant swelling may make the diagnosis difficult as this may occur with dislocation or supracondylar fracture.

If one palpates the two epicondyles and the tip of the olecranon in patients with a supracondylar fracture, they will be in the same plane, whereas, with dislocations, the olecranon will be displaced from the plane of the epicondyles on palpation.

Imaging

Plain radiographs are diagnostic and reveal an empty olecranon fossa posterior to the distal humerus (Fig. 14–37). Radiographs should be obtained both before and after reduction. Associated fractures include the coronoid process; radial head; and, occasionally, the humeral epicondyles or capitellum (Fig. 14–38). Small fractures of the coronoid are common and should not impact management.[31] When both the coronoid and radial head are fractured in a posterior elbow dislocation, the injury is referred to as the "terrible triad."[36] Fractures are present on 12% to 60% of plain radiographs.[34]

Associated Injuries

Commonly associated injuries are to the peripheral nerves, especially the ulnar nerve, and function should be checked before and after reduction.[37] Ulnar nerve injury occurs in 8% to 21% of patients with posterior elbow dislocations, but the injury usually resolves spontaneously with conservative management.[34] Injury to the brachial artery is rare with posterior dislocations of the elbow.[34,37] Median nerve entrapment may also occur in patients with posterior dislocations.[35]

Complex elbow dislocations are those that occur with a large intra-articular fracture. The radial head and coronoid are the most commonly associated fractures, occurring with an incidence ranging from 12% to 60%. During operative exploration, osteochondral injuries are seen in most cases of acute elbow dislocations. In patients with the "terrible triad" (elbow dislocation with radial head and coronoid process fractures), significant disability frequently occurs.

A fractured medial epicondyle can sometimes become entrapped in the joint, necessitating open reduction. Fractures of the coronoid process are commonly associated

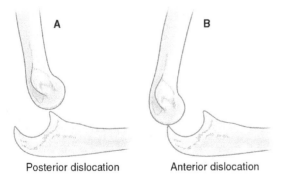

Figure 14–34. **A.** Posterior dislocation of the elbow. **B.** Anterior dislocation of the elbow.

Posterior dislocation   Anterior dislocation

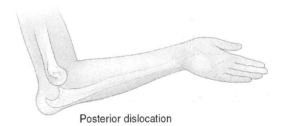

Posterior dislocation

Figure 14–35. The posterior protuberance of the olecranon in a posterior dislocation.

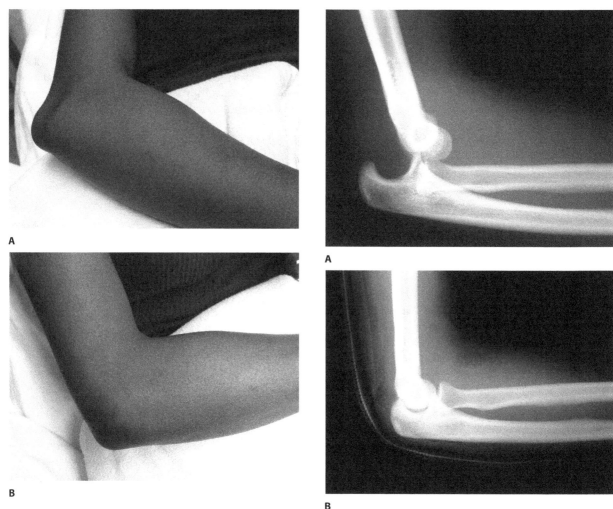

A

B

Figure 14–36. *A.* Posterior elbow dislocation. *B.* The same patient postreduction.

A

B

Figure 14–37. Radiographic appearance of a simple posterior elbow dislocation. *A.* Prereduction. *B.* Postreduction.

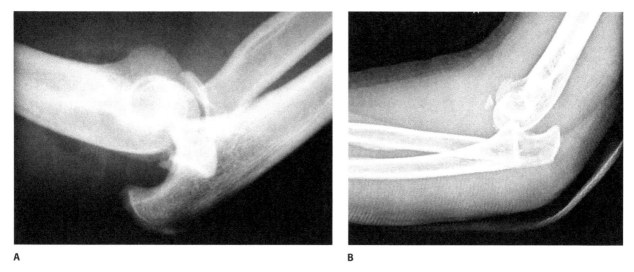

A

B

Figure 14–38. Complex posterior elbow dislocations. *A.* Associated with radial head fracture. *B.* Associated with coronoid process fracture.

injuries and will usually come into near-normal opposition once reduction occurs. Large fragments that are displaced may require operative fixation.

All elbow dislocations not associated with concomitant elbow fractures will demonstrate rupture of the medial and lateral ligaments.[13] Although these ligaments are primary stabilizers of the elbow, surgical repair is rarely needed because the flexor and extensor muscles act as a strong secondary stabilizer that resists redislocation. Recurrent instability in a simple elbow dislocation is seen in only 1% to 2% of cases.[34]

The wrist and shoulder must be examined thoroughly because additional upper-extremity injuries occur in 10% to 15% of cases.[34,38]

Treatment

Early reduction is advocated as delay may damage the articular cartilage or result in excessive swelling or circulatory compromise. If the elbow remains unreduced for more than 7 days, the utility of closed reduction is minimal. Reduction is best accomplished after administering procedural sedation, as described in Chapter 2. Intra-articular local anesthetic is also an option to aid in the reduction. Several reduction techniques have been described to reduce a posterior dislocation. The techniques below apply to posterior dislocation without a medial or lateral component. The Stimson technique is the preferred method because it causes the least amount of discomfort and associated injuries. Whatever technique is employed, it is recommended that slow, continuous, and gentle forces be applied to limit additional soft-tissue injury.

Traction–Countertraction Technique. The forearm is supinated and the elbow is left in slight flexion (approximately 30 degrees). Supination is used to minimize further trauma to the coronoid process. The physician stabilizes the distal humerus with the nondominant hand and distracts the forearm with the dominant hand. A slow, continuous, gentle, longitudinal traction with gradual flexion will reduce the elbow (Fig. 14–39A). If an assistant is available, he/she can grasp the distal humerus while the physician uses both hands to provide traction. Reduction can also be assisted by pressure applied over the olecranon. Hyperextension is contraindicated during reduction because it can lead to neurovascular injury (i.e., median nerve entrapment or brachial artery injury), increase the risk of developing myositis ossificans by damaging muscle, or injure articular surfaces.

Leverage Technique. While supine, the patient's elbow is flexed, forearm supinated, and shoulder abducted. The physician places his/her elbow onto the patient's distal biceps and uses his/her hand to interlock the patient's fingers or grab the wrist. The patient's elbow is gradually flexed while the physician's elbow provides countertraction (Fig. 14–39B and Video 14–1). The end result is a lever with a sufficient longitudinal force to reduce the elbow.[49]

Stimson Technique. This is a modification of the Stimson technique used in shoulder reductions (Fig. 14–39C). The patient should be placed in the prone position with the dislocated elbow hanging perpendicular to the table. A small pillow or folded sheet should support the humerus just proximal to the elbow joint. Weights are then suspended from the wrist with the elbow flexed approximately 30 degrees from the extended position. Over a period of several minutes, the patient's elbow dislocation will reduce. We prefer beginning with approximately 5 lb of weight, which can be increased if needed. This technique is preferred by many because it is least likely to produce forceful manipulation that can result in myositis ossificans.

Kumar Technique. This method involves gentle disengagement of the coronoid process without excessive traction and hyperextension that can lead to soft-tissue damage when the olecranon impinges on the lower humerus.[40] To perform this reduction, the emergency physician stands on the contralateral side of the patient's injured elbow. With one hand, the patient's forearm is grasped (Fig. 14–39D and Video 14–2). With the other hand, the elbow is grasped such that the thumb is placed over the patient's olecranon and the fingers are over the forearm. Gentle traction is applied while the patient's elbow is gradually flexed to disengage the coronoid process from the lower humerus. At the same time, the olecranon is pushed into position with the thumb. This procedure takes about 5 minutes to complete and has a 95% success rate.[40]

Successful reduction is frequently heralded by a "clunking" sound as the articular surfaces return to their normal position. After reduction, the elbow can be checked for stability by putting it through range of motion. If redislocation occurs in extension, the joint is potentially unstable. The lateral and medial ligaments can also be stress tested. If the elbow remains reduced, it is stable and is immobilized at 90 degrees in a long-arm posterior splint[36] (Appendix A–9). If there is significant swelling, a position slightly less than 90 degrees is used. If there is any concern for potential vascular injury or compartment syndrome, the patient should be admitted after appropriate orthopedic consultation.

For patients with stable reductions who will be discharged, the length of immobilization is approximately 5 to 7 days, so follow-up should occur within this time frame. At that time, full range-of-motion exercises should begin with interval use of a splint or sling for comfort and support. Immobilization for >3 weeks is associated with diminished range of motion.[34]

Surgery is indicated in cases in which closed reduction is unsuccessful, redislocation occurs with 50 to 60 degrees of flexion, or unstable fractures are present around the joint.[34,41] Small coronoid fractures do not require further management. Radial head fractures and large coronoid fractures (involving at least 50% of the coronoid process) will usually require operative repair following closed reduction.[36]

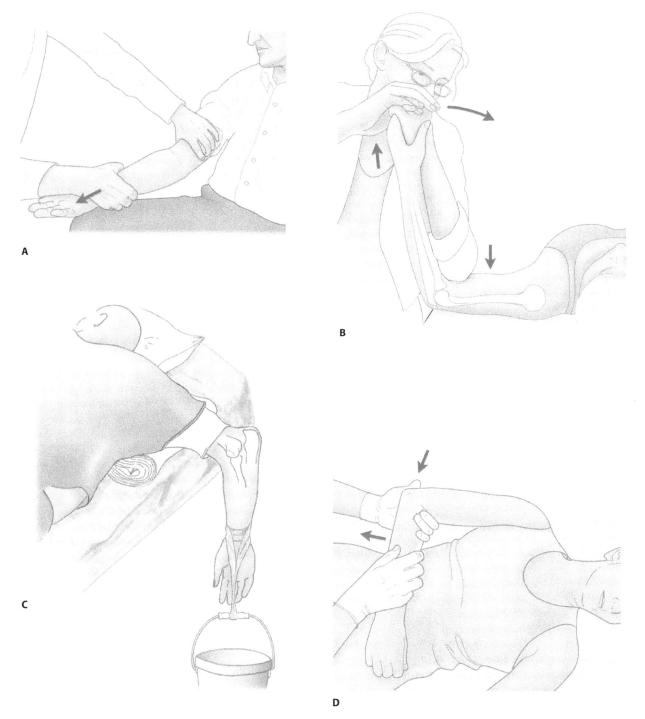

Figure 14–39. Techniques for reduction of a posterior elbow dislocation. **A.** Traction–countertraction. **B.** Leverage. **C.** Stimson. **D.** Kumar.

Complications
- Nerve injuries in up to 20%. The most common are the ulnar and median nerves, but the radial and anterior interosseous nerves can also be affected. They usually resolve with conservative management.
- Posttraumatic joint stiffness. Loss of the terminal 15 degrees of elbow extension after dislocation is common.

- Heterotopic ossification. This is common after posterior elbow dislocation (>75% of patients), but only limits motion in <5%.
- Chronic instability.

Anterior Dislocations
Anterior dislocations are far less common, occurring from a blow to the flexed elbow that drives the olecranon forward.

Associated injuries to bones, vessels, and nerves around the joint are much more common with anterior dislocations, making this dislocation potentially more problematic.

On examination, the arm appears shortened and the forearm is elongated and held in supination. The elbow is usually held in full extension. The olecranon fossa is often palpable anteriorly.

These patients should be splinted, and the vascular and neurologic status assessed. Consultation with an orthopedic surgeon should be obtained for immediate reduction. Many of these dislocations are open, and vascular damage is quite common. Complete avulsion of the triceps mechanism is another commonly associated soft-tissue injury.

Olecranon Bursitis

Olecranon bursitis is the most common form of elbow bursitis seen in the ED. It is secondary to trauma, overuse, crystal disease, autoimmune disease, or infection.[43,44]

One-third of the cases are infectious (septic), and it should be noted that trauma may cause both septic and nonseptic bursitis.[43,45-47] Of more than 150 bursae in the human body, the olecranon bursa is the most commonly infected.[44,45] *Staphylococcus aureus* is responsible for approximately 80% to 90% of cases.[48-50] Other risk factors for septic olecranon bursitis include alcoholism, immunocompromised states, and preexisting bursal disease.[45,50] Approximately one-third of patients with septic olecranon bursitis have a history of a previous episode of olecranon bursitis.[47]

Examination

On examination of the patient with olecranon bursitis, the examiner will note swelling in the posterior aspect of the elbow with slight restriction of flexion due to the inflamed bursa (Fig. 14–40).[49] The bursa will be tender to palpation. Erythema may be present in patients with both septic

and nonseptic bursitis.[47] Patients with septic bursitis usually seek medical attention earlier and are more likely to have fever.[45,47] In patients with bursitis caused by gout or infectious processes, there will be surrounding inflammatory reaction and pain with motion of the elbow. Warmth may be present in both septic and nonseptic bursitis, but the surface temperature between the involved bursa and the unaffected side is significantly greater when infection is the underlying cause.[44]

Diagnosis

Early recognition of septic bursitis is critical to prevent severe sequelae.[43] For this reason, aspiration is recommended in all cases, and fluid is sent for analysis for crystals, cell count, Gram stain, and culture. A purulent aspirate is helpful in diagnosing septic bursitis, but serosanguineous fluid may be septic or nonseptic. The cell count in patients with septic bursitis is usually >1000 WBC/mm^3 with a predominance of neutrophils.[44,45,48] Gram stain will be positive in more than half of the cases of septic bursitis.[47] Frequently, septic olecranon bursitis cannot be ruled out definitively after aspiration, and presumptive antibiotic treatment must be started until the results of the cultures have returned.[51]

Treatment

Noninfectious olecranon bursitis is treated by aspiration and application of a compressive dressing, with local heat and preventive measures directed at the inciting cause. Nonsteroidal anti-inflammatory drugs (NSAIDs) may hasten resolution. Intrabursal injection of methylprednisolone acetate may alleviate symptoms by reducing inflammation but has been recently shown to be associated with increased complications such as higher rate of infection and skin atrophy.[43,52] It should be noted that steroids should be avoided in any patient suspected of having septic bursitis.

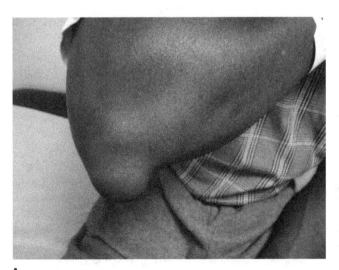
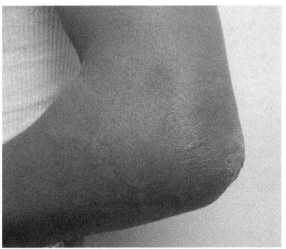

A   **B**

Figure 14–40. Olecranon bursitis. **A.** Noninfectious. **B.** The significant swelling and erythema suggested an infectious etiology.

If conservative management fails, operative treatment may be necessary, but olecranon bursectomy is associated with wound healing problems and should be reserved only for truly chronic cases of olecranon bursitis that interfere with function.[53,54]

In cases of suspected septic bursitis, patients should have the bursa aspirated, and they should be given antibiotics. Given the prevalence of septic bursitis caused by penicillinase producing *S aureus*, empiric antibiotic therapy should be penicillinase resistant.[55] Selective outpatient management with oral antibiotics is successful in most cases.[56] Treatment failures typically include those with extensive infection or those who are immunocompromised.[57] If oral antibiotic therapy fails, aspiration may need to be repeated, and occasionally, incision and drainage in the operating room is required. Percutaneous tube placement for suction irrigation has been attempted and may be beneficial for those with severe septic bursitis.[45,46] Admission for intravenous antibiotics effective against penicillinase producing *S aureus* may be required for severe cases.[47,48,49]

OVERUSE ELBOW INJURIES

The majority of elbow injuries occur from chronic use, particularly in athletes.[50] One helpful way to evaluate a patient with elbow pain is to consider the location of the pain as indicative of potential causes. This information, combined with a thorough history regarding the mechanism of injury and physical examination findings is frequently diagnostic.

Anterior elbow pain is a common presenting problem, particularly in the young athlete. It is usually caused by a stretch or tear of the anterior capsule, distal biceps, or brachialis tendons. This injury can be caused by hyperextension from fall onto the extended elbow. "Climber's elbow" is a strain of the brachialis tendon.

Ectopic bone may deposit after a traumatic blow to the anterior arm. This usually occurs within the brachialis muscle 3 weeks after the injury. Prevention with NSAIDs and early range of motion is of paramount importance. Anterior elbow pain may also result from median nerve entrapment such as with the pronator syndrome.

Medial elbow pain may result from a variety of conditions and is much more common. A medial epicondyle fracture or stress fracture can occur. Medial epicondylitis is due to tendonitis of the flexor or pronator muscle group. An unusual condition called "snapping elbow syndrome" occurs when the ulnar nerve snaps out of the cubital tunnel. Medial elbow pain may result from instability caused by acute or chronic ulnar collateral ligament disruption. Ulnar neuritis is a common cause of medial elbow pain in athletes because of the ulnar nerve's superficial location at the cubital tunnel and its unfavorable response to valgus stresses. Compression can occur proximal to the cubital tunnel because of a tight intramuscular septum. The earliest symptom is medial joint line pain; clumsiness; or heaviness of the hand, fingers, or both.

This is associated with or exacerbated by throwing or overhead activity and may manifest as numbness and tingling in the little and ring fingers.[58]

Posterior elbow pain is less common than medial or lateral elbow pain but more common than anterior pain. Abnormal stresses may cause pain at the attachment of the triceps or olecranon apophysis, which may present in a similar fashion to Osgood–Schlatter disease.[59] Triceps tendonitis is an uncommon cause of posterior elbow pain and is treated with rest. Triceps tendon rupture is very uncommon. A stress fracture of the olecranon is also an uncommon cause of elbow pain that occurs in athletes who throw. Olecranon bursitis is by far the most common condition in this group.

Lateral elbow pain is the most common location of elbow pain in the general population. Lateral epicondylitis, discussed subsequently, is the most common cause. Radial nerve entrapment at the elbow can occur alone or in conjunction with lateral epicondylitis.

EPICONDYLITIS (TENNIS ELBOW)

Epicondylitis can occur on the lateral or medial side of the distal humerus at the site of tendinous insertion of the muscles of the forearm. Both injuries are usually the result of chronic overuse secondary to both recreational and occupational pursuits that require a repeated rotary motion.[60]

Lateral epicondylitis most often occurs in the fourth and fifth decades. It is usually referred to as "tennis elbow" because 10% to 50% of tennis players will develop this condition.[61] Many entities have been implicated, including arthritis of the radiohumeral joint, radiohumeral bursitis, traumatic synovitis of the radiohumeral joint, and periostitis of the lateral epicondyle. At present, none of these can be considered the sole cause of this condition.[60-63] The underlying feature is the presence of tears in the aponeurosis of the extensor tendons.[32] Many patients with tennis elbow have microavulsion fractures of the lateral epicondyle in addition to microscopic tears in the tendon proper.

The patient usually presents with a history of a gradual onset of a dull ache along the outer aspect of the elbow referred to the forearm. The pain increases with grasping and twisting motions.[64] Tenderness is localized over the lateral epicondyle. A reliable test for tennis elbow is elicited by asking the patient to actively extend the wrist and supinate the forearm against resistance (Fig. 14–41). In patients with tennis elbow, this maneuver intensifies the discomfort.[65] The neurologic examination should be normal. MRI is helpful in identifying areas of inflammation suggestive of lateral epicondylitis. Ultrasound also may be useful in making the diagnosis.[66]

Traditionally, treatment of this condition has been to splint the elbow in a flexed position with the forearm supinated and the wrist extended, although counterforce bracing or "tennis elbow bands" has been shown to be

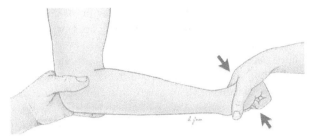

Figure 14–41. Tennis elbow can be diagnosed when pain over the lateral epicondyle is exacerbated by the patient extending the wrist and elbow and supinating the forearm against resistance.

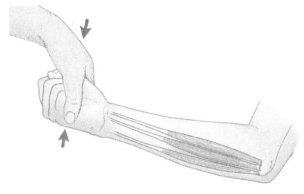

Figure 14–43. A test for medial epicondylitis. Forced flexion of the wrist will cause pain over the medial epicondyle.

quite effective in reducing the symptoms and allowing the individual to continue normal activity (Fig. 14–42).[67,68] Patients with epicondylitis who are treated with splints have higher rates of limited duty, more medical visits, and longer duration of treatment than those managed without splints.[69] The patient should be advised to apply heat to the elbow and rest. NSAIDs such as ibuprofen are of value.

Corticosteroid injections have been shown to be safe and beneficial, with their effects lasting 2 to 6 weeks. The technique for injection requires the elbow to be flexed to 45 degrees. The area of greatest tenderness is identified; the needle is inserted at 90 degrees down to the bone, and then pulled back 1 to 2 mm before injecting.[70]

Treatment with shock therapy, ultrasound, and laser have proven of no value, and in fact, simple stretches and strengthening exercises are the most useful adjuncts as the patient improves.[71-73] Surgical intervention may prove beneficial in refractory cases.[73]

GOLFER'S ELBOW

Medial epicondylitis ("golfer's elbow") is inflammation at the origin of the wrist flexors. It is characterized by pain over the medial epicondyle and medial pain on forced flexion of the wrist (Fig. 14–43). Although seen in golfers, this injury occurs more frequently in individuals who routinely perform household chores, manual labor, or other tasks involving repetitive movements. The treatment of medial epicondylitis is similar to that of lateral epicondylitis. Because of the close proximity of the ulnar nerve, local anesthetic used with the corticosteroid injection may cause a temporary paralysis of the ulnar nerve.

Conservative management is curative in most cases but may take many months. As a last resort, surgical intervention may be necessary.[58]

OSTEOCHONDRITIS DISSECANS

Osteochondritis dissecans refers to a condition in which focal subchondral bone necrosis leads to the disruption of articular cartilage and displacement of a bony fragment into the joint space.[74-76] The condition is rare and most commonly occurs within the femoral condyles at the knee (75% of cases). Other sites include the talar dome and the capitellum of the humerus. Within the elbow, the condition most commonly affects adolescent (ages 12–20) athletes who overload and hyperextend the joint.[77] An adult form has been identified, although it is unclear whether these patients were merely undiagnosed as children.[75]

Gymnasts, due to the nature of their sport, are particularly susceptible to this condition. The symptoms include locking, "giving way," and crepitus on range of motion. Radiographs may reveal a loose body within the joint or demonstrable osteochondritis dissecans. MRI is often helpful in suspicious cases where the radiographs are negative.[77-79]

Treatment is conservative unless there are loose bodies within the joint that require removal. The athlete must refrain from competitive sports for 6 to 8 weeks.

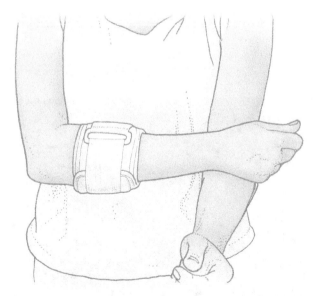

Figure 14–42. Placement of a tennis elbow band. The proximal edge of the band should be placed 2 to 3 cm distal to the lateral epicondyle, over the bulk of the extensor muscles.

Conservative treatment for acute exacerbations consists of splinting the elbow for 3 to 4 days, NSAIDs, and the application of heat. If mechanical symptoms occur and persist, arthroscopic intervention to remove loose bodies is necessary.

For more information, the reader is referred to Chapter 6.

LIGAMENTOUS INJURIES

Sprains involving the ulnar and radial collateral ligaments of the elbow follow acute injuries or chronic overuse. These injuries are diagnosed by appropriate stress testing of the involved ligaments (Fig. 14-44). When there is opening of the joint on a stress examination, one must always assess the neurologic status to exclude associated deficits. Treatment with immobilization of the elbow in a flexed position is the appropriate ED management in most cases.

Ulnar Collateral Ligament Injury

Ulnar collateral ligament injury is a common problem in overhead throwers. The ligament complex comprises three portions—an anterior bundle, a posterior bundle, and an oblique bundle. A sprain or rupture of this ligament compromises medial and valgus stability in the elbow joint. Thus, an accurate diagnosis, indicating the degree of tear, is important to determine appropriate treatment.

The history and examination are crucial to diagnosing ulnar collateral ligament insufficiency, in that there is usually tenderness medially over the ligament. Point tenderness inferior and distal to the medial epicondyle is elicited. Posterior medial joint line tenderness is also present, and one must examine the ulnar nerve within the ulnar groove because this may sometimes be involved in the injury. Routine radiographs may show calcification within the ligament or chronic traction spurs from repetitive stresses.

Rest, ice, and NSAIDs are the mainstay of therapy. The treatment of any patient with significant opening should include a posterior mold with the elbow in 90 degrees of flexion. Because the elbow is a hinge joint, opening indicates a significant disruption of the joint capsule. When medial joint opening occurs, there may be an associated injury (stretch) of the brachial artery, and therefore, pulses should always be documented. In severe cases, surgical intervention may be necessary to reestablish stability. Arthroscopy is performed initially. Reconstruction, often called "Tommy John surgery," may be needed in athletes as this may be a career-ending injury.

NEUROPATHIES

Compressive neuropathies can be subtle and are often overlooked in the upper extremity. These nerve injuries are classified into three types—neurapraxia, axonotmesis, and neurotmesis—as described in Chapter 1. Few of the lesions ever fit exclusively into one category.

Neurapraxia is the mildest form, which is characterized by reduced function but anatomic continuity within the nerve. This injury is caused by loss of axon excitability or segmental demyelination. This is the most common nerve injury. In axonotmesis, there is axonal injury and distal degeneration, with the connective tissue supporting the nerve structure remaining intact. In neurotmesis, there is complete disruption of the nerve.

Radial Neuropathy

Radial neuropathy that occurs at or distal to the radial groove of the humerus will retain motor strength to the triceps muscle. However, motor deficits will include paralysis of the brachioradialis, supinator, and extensors of the wrist, which can be identified by wrist drop on examination (Fig. 14-45). Sensory deficits include loss of sensation to the dorsal web space between the thumb and index fingers.

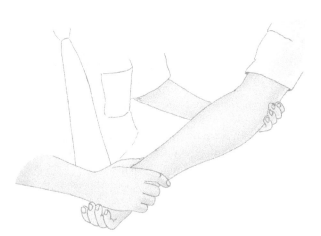

Figure 14-44. Stress test of the collateral ligaments of the elbow.

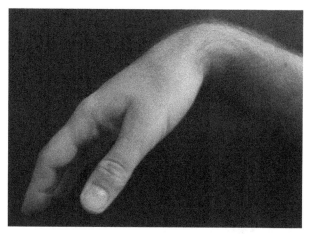

Figure 14-45. Wrist drop seen in a radial neuropathy.

High Radial Nerve Palsy

Injury to the radial nerve above the elbow is unusual and usually secondary to trauma such as crutch use or tourniquets. This injury is differentiated from other forms of radial nerve injury because the triceps muscle will be involved.

When compression occurs as the radial nerve spirals around the humerus, the injury is sometimes referred to as "Saturday night palsy." This condition can occur after humerus fractures or after compression (i.e., intoxicated patients who fall asleep with their arm resting on the back of a chair).

Nerve injury in the spiral groove may also be seen in injuries from gymnastics or wrestling. Compression may occur at the fibrous area around the origin of the lateral head of the triceps or at the intermuscular septum. In this compressive injury, a mixed-motor and sensory involvement occurs.

Conservative treatment using a volar splint with the wrist in 20 degrees of extension will often result in complete recovery, although the time required varies.[91] Surgical exploration of the radial nerve is indicated only when symptoms persist or there is evidence of degeneration.

Radial Tunnel Syndrome

The radial tunnel is defined by the anatomic structures from the elbow to the distal extent of the supinator muscle.[92] This is the most common site for a compressive neuropathy of the radial nerve. Compression is usually due to a fibrous band of tissue and may occur at many sites within the radial tunnel.[93–95] Patients complain of soreness and aching just distal to the lateral epicondyle over the extensor muscle mass. This condition can often be confused with lateral epicondylitis, but on examination, maximal tenderness will be elicited over the anterior radial neck. There is a chronic deep ache that is common at night that is unlike the sharp, knifelike pain of lateral epicondylitis.[92,96–98] There is no true sensory involvement because the sensory branch of the radial nerve is more superficial and does not pass through the radial tunnel. Motor weakness is uncommon.[99] The patient with radial tunnel syndrome often exhibits pain with resisted supination of the extended forearm, which is made worse with wrist flexion.

Treatment consists of rest, NSAIDs, and wrist splinting for 3 to 6 months. If there is no improvement, surgical decompression may be indicated.

Median Neuropathy

Injury to the median nerve proximal to the elbow results in loss of sensation of the palmar surface of the thumb and the index and middle fingers.[94] Motor deficits include loss of forearm pronation, wrist and digit flexion, and thumb abduction. Chronic deficits result in thenar muscle atrophy.

There are a number of median nerve syndromes that occur in the elbow and forearm, only a few of which are discussed here.

Pronator Syndrome

Pronator syndrome is a compression neuropathy of the median nerve at any one of several sites at the elbow and proximal forearm. Sites adjacent to the pronator teres muscle include (1) beneath the bicipital aponeurosis and (2) as the nerve passes between the humeral and ulnar heads.[91,94,100] This syndrome is seen in athletes whose sports require repetitive forceful pronation and gripping.

Several clinical indicators help confirm the diagnosis of a pronator syndrome. Pain with resisted pronation when the elbow is extended and the wrist flexed suggests localization of compression within the pronator teres. One of the most sensitive tests for pronator syndrome is when deep, direct palpation of the proximal forearm over the pronator teres reproduces symptoms.

This condition may be confused with carpal tunnel syndrome as both will cause numbness, paresthesias, and muscle weakness in the median nerve distribution.[101] Some noted differences include a lack of nocturnal symptoms in pronator syndrome and a negative Tinel sign.

The workup should include radiographs and electrodiagnostic studies. Initial management is rest, NSAIDs, and occasional splinting. Surgical treatment is only necessary when the symptoms are refractory for 6 months or more.[102]

Anterior Interosseous Nerve Syndrome

Anterior interosseous nerve syndrome is uncommon and may present clinically with vague forearm pain or pain with activity.[100] The anterior interosseous nerve is a branch of the median nerve. In contrast to pronator syndrome, pain is elicited with resisted flexion of the long finger. Muscle atrophy without sensory deficits is found late. Motor weakness usually begins within a day after the pain is noted.

Carpal tunnel syndrome, the most common site of median nerve compression, is discussed in Chapter 12.

Ulnar Neuropathy

Ulnar neuropathy results in impaired adduction or abduction of the digits due to loss of motor strength to the interosseous muscles. Sensory deficits include loss of sensation to the small finger. Fixed deficits are rare, but the characteristic lesion is that of a "claw hand" with hyperextension at the metacarpophalangeal joint of the ring and small fingers with flexion at the proximal interphalangeal and distal interphalangeal joints (Fig. 14–46).

Cubital Tunnel Syndrome

Cubital tunnel syndrome is an ulnar nerve entrapment syndrome near the elbow and is the second most common compressive neuropathy in the upper extremity.[94,103] The nerve descends down the arm without branching and passes through the groove between the medial epicondyle and the olecranon. This is a potential site of compression or traction. However, the most common site of compression is 1 to 2 cm distal to the ulnar groove. At this location, the

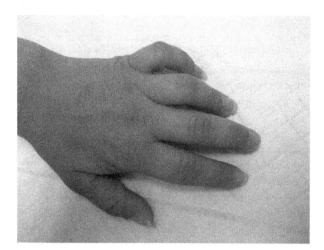

Figure 14–46. "Claw hand" occurring secondary to an ulnar nerve palsy. This patient was diagnosed with cubital tunnel syndrome.

nerve passes into the cubital tunnel and between the two heads of the flexor carpi ulnaris.

The act of throwing is often responsible for ulnar nerve traction at the elbow in the athlete. Holding a tool in a position repetitively can lead to this entrapment, and in some cases, a ganglion cyst causes compression of the nerve.

Patients classically present with medial elbow and forearm pain and paresthesias radiating into the ring and little fingers. Motor findings are subtle and ulnar neuropathy at the elbow is difficult to differentiate from neuropathy caused elsewhere. The elbow flexion test, in which pain is elicited with elbow flexion, may be useful.

Nonoperative treatment consists of rest, ice, NSAIDs, and night splinting with the elbow at 45 degrees of flexion and the forearm in the neutral position. An elbow pad can prevent injury to the nerve in athletes. The natural history of this disorder is spontaneous resolution in as many as half the cases. If this treatment regimen is unsuccessful or testing demonstrates a significant neuropathy, surgery may be indicated.

REFERENCES

1. Dugas AJ, Cain EL. Elbow injuries in sports. *Orthop Sports Med*. 2005;1(4):1–12.
2. Rabiner JE, Khine H, Avner JR, Friedman LM, Tsung JW. Accuracy of point-of-care ultrasonography for diagnosis of elbow fractures in children. *Ann Emerg Med* 2013;61(3):9–17. doi:10.1016/j.annemergmed.2012.07.112. Epub 2012 Nov 9.
3. Blumberg SM, Kunkiv S, Crain EF, Goldman HS. The predictive value of a normal radiograph anterior fat pad sign following elbow trauma in children. *Pediatr Emerg Care*. 2011;27:596–600.
4. Goswami GK. The fat pad sign. *Radiology*. 2002;222:419–420.
5. O'Dwyer H, O'Sullivan P, Fitzgerald D, Lee MJ, McGrath F, Logan PM. The fat pad sign following elbow trauma in adults: its usefulness and reliability in suspecting occult fracture. *J Comput Assist Tomogr*. 2004;28(4):562–565.
6. Major NM, Crawford ST. Elbow effusions in trauma in adults and children: is there an occult fracture? *AJR Am J Roentgenol*. 2002;178(2):413–418.
7. Nork SE, Jones CB, Henley MB. Surgical treatment of olecranon fractures. *Am J Orthop*. 2001;30(7):577–586.
8. McKay PL, Katarincic JA. Fractures of the proximal ulna olecranon and coronoid fractures. *Hand Clin*. 2002;18(1):43–53.
9. Hak DJ, Golladay GJ. Olecranon fractures: treatment options. *J Am Acad Orthop Surg*. 2000;8(4):266–275.
10. Rettig AC. Traumatic elbow injuries in the athlete. *Orthop Clin North Am*. 2002;33(3):509–522, v.
11. Rosenblatt Y, Athwal GS, Faber KJ. Current recommendations for the treatment of radial head fractures. *Orthop Clin N Am*. 2008;39:173–185.
12. Sun H, Duan J, Li F. Comparison between radial head arthoplasty and open reduction and internal fixation in patients with radial head fractures (modified Mason type III and IV): a meta-analysis. *Eur J Orthop Surg Traumatol*. 2016;26(3):283–291.
13. Phillips CS, Segalman KA. Diagnosis and treatment of post-traumatic medial and lateral elbow ligament incompetence. *Hand Clin*. 2002;18(1):149–159.
14. Rizzo M, Nunley JA. Fractures of the elbow's lateral column radial head and capitellum. *Hand Clin*. 2002;18(1):21–42.
15. Pike JM, Athwal GS, Faber KJ, King GJ. Radial head fractures—an update. *J Hand Surg Am*. 2009;34:557–565.
16. Duckworth AD, Wickramasinghe NR, Clement ND, Court-Brown CM, McQueen MM. Long-term outcomes of stable radial head fractures. *J Bone Joint Surg Am*. 2014;96(20):1716–1723. doi:10.2106/JBJS.M.01354.
17. Paschos NK, Mitsionis GI, Vasiliadis HS, Georgoulis AD. Comparison of early mobilization protocols in radial head fractures. *J Orthop Trauma*. 2013;27(3):134–139. doi:10.1097/BOT.0b013e31825cf765.
18. Doornberg JN, Ring D. Coronoid fracture patterns. *J Hand Surg Am*. 2006;31:45–52.
19. McGinley JC, Roach N, Hopgood BC, Kozin SH. Nondisplaced elbow fractures: a commonly occurring and difficult diagnosis. *Am J Emerg Med*. 2006;24:560–566.
20. Goodwin RC, Kuivila TE. Pediatric elbow and forearm fractures requiring surgical treatment. *Hand Clin*. 2002;18(1):135–148.
21. Wu J, Perron AD, Miller MD, Powell SM, Brady WJ. Orthopedic pitfalls in the ED: pediatric supracondylar humerus fractures. *Am J Emerg Med*. 2002;20(6):544–550.
22. Lyons ST, Quinn M, Stanitski CL. Neurovascular injuries in type III humeral supracondylar fractures in children. *Clin Orthop Relat Res*. 2000;(376):62–67.
23. Lee S, Park MS, Chung CY, et al. Consensus and different perspectives on treatment of supracondylar fractures of the humerus in children. *Clin Orthop Surg*. 2012;4:91–97.
24. Shrader MW. Pediatric supracondylar fractures and pediatric physeal elbow fractures. *Orthop Clin North Am*. 2008;39:163–171.
25. Wu J, Perron AD, Miller MD, Powell SM, Brady WJ. Orthopedic pitfalls in the ED: pediatric supracondylar humerus fractures. *Am J Emerg Med*. 2002;20(6):554–550.
26. Ring D, Jupiter JB. Fractures of the distal humerus. *Orthop Clin North Am*. 2000;31(1):103–113.

27. Morrey BF. Fractures of the distal humerus: role of elbow replacement. *Orthop Clin North Am.* 2000;31(1):145–154.

28. Miller AN, Beingessner DM. Intra-articular distal humerus fractures. *Orthop Clin N Am.* 2013;44(1):35–45.

29. Ring D, Jupiter JB, Gulotta L. Articular fractures of the distal part of the humerus. *J Bone Joint Surg Am.* 2003;85:232–238.

30. Mehdian H, McKee MD. Fractures of capitellum and trochlea. *Orthop Clin North Am.* 2000;31(1):115–127.

31. Rosenberg ZS, Blutreich SI, Schweitzer ME, Zember JS, Fillmore K. MRI features of posterior capitellar impaction injuries. *AJR Am J Roentgenol.* 2008;190(2):435–441.

32. Guitton TG, Doornberg JN, Raaymakers EL, Ring D, Kloen P. Fractures of the capitellum and trochlea. *J Bone Joint Surg Am.* 2009;91:390–397.

33. Hobgood ER, Khan SO, Field LD. Acute dislocations of the adult elbow. *Hand Clin.* 2008;24:1–7.

34. Cohen MS, Hastings H II. Acute elbow dislocations: evaluation and management. *J Am Acad Orthop Surg.* 1998;6(1):15–23.

35. Kuhn MA, Ross G. Acute elbow dislocations. *Orthop Clin North Am.* 2008;39:155–161.

36. Ring D, Jupiter JB. Fracture-dislocation of the elbow. *Hand Clin.* 2002;18(1):55–63.

37. Martin BD, Johansen JA, Edwards SG. Complication related to simple dislocations of the elbow. *Hand Clin.* 2008;24:9–25.

38. Hildebrand KA, Patterson SD, King GJ. Acute elbow dislocations: simple and complex. *Orthop Clin North Am.* 1999;30(1):63–79.

39. Hankin FM. Posterior dislocation of the elbow. A simplified method of closed reduction. *Clin Orthop Relat Res.* 1984;(190):254–256.

40. Kumar A, Ahmed M. Closed reduction of posterior dislocation of the elbow: a simple technique. *J Orthop Trauma.* 1999;13(1):58–59.

41. Mehta S, Sud A, Tiwari A, Kapoor SK. Open reduction for late-presenting posterior dislocation of the elbow. *J Orthop Surg (Hong Kong).* 2007;15(1):15–21.

42. Hodge DK, Safran MR. Sideline management of common dislocations. *Curr Sports Med Rep.* 2002;1(3):149–155.

43. Del Buono A, Franceschi F, Palumbo A, Denaro V, Maffulli N. Diagnosis and management of olecranon bursitis. *Surgeon.* 2012;10(5):297–300.

44. Aaron DL, Patel A, Kayiaros S, Calfee R. Four common types of bursitis: diagnosis and management. *J Am Acad Orthop Surg.* 2011;19:359–367.

45. Small LN, Ross JJ. Suppurative tenosynovitis and septic bursitis. *Infect Dis Clin North Am.* 2005;19:991–1005.

46. Valeriano-Marcet J, Carter JD, Vasey FB. Soft tissue disease. *Rheum Dis Clin North Am.* 2003;29(1):77–88.

47. Stell IM. Septic and non-septic olecranon bursitis in the accident and emergency department—an approach to management. *J Accid Emerg Med.* 1996;13(5):351–353.

48. Wasserman AR, Melville LD, Birkhahn RH. Septic bursitis: a case report and primer for the emergency clinician. *J Emerg Med.* 2009;37(3):269–272.

49. Laupland KB, Davies HD, Calgary Home Parenteral Therapy Program Study Group. Olecranon septic bursitis managed in an ambulatory setting. *Clin Invest Med.* 2001;24(4):171–178.

50. Cea-Pereiro JC, Garcia-Meijide J, Mera-Varela A, Gomez-Reino JJ. A comparison between septic bursitis caused by Staphylococcus aureus and those caused by other organisms. *Clin Rheumatol.* 2001;20(1):10–14.

51. Choudhery V. The role of diagnostic needle aspiration in olecranon bursitis. *J Accid Emerg Med.* 1999;16(4):282–283.

52. Sayegh ET, Strauch RJ. Treatment of olecranon bursitis: a systematic review. *Arch Orthop Trauma Surg.* 2014;134(11):1517–1536. doi:10.1007/s00402-014-2088-3. Epub 2014 Sep 19.

53. Reilly D, Kamineni S. Olecranon bursitis. *J Shoulder Elbow Surg.* 2016;25(1):158–167. doi:http://dx.doi.org/10.1016/j.jse.2015.08.032

54. Degreef I, De Smet L. Complications following resection of the olecranon bursa. *Acta Orthop Belg.* 2006;72:400–403.

55. Laupand KB, Davies HD. Olecranon septic bursitis managed in an ambulatory setting. *Clin Invest Med.* 2001;24:171–178.

56. Stell IM. Management of acute bursitis: outcome study of a structured approach. *J R Soc Med.* 1999;92(10):516–521.

57. Chumbley EM, O'Connor FG, Nirschl RP. Evaluation of overuse elbow injuries. *Am Fam Physician.* 2000;61(3):691–700.

58. Ciccotti MC, Schwartz MA, Ciccotti MG. Diagnosis and treatment of medial epicondylitis of the elbow. *Clin Sports Med.* 2004;23:693–705.

59. Rudzki JR, Paletta GA. Juvenile and adolescent elbow injuries in sports. *Clin Sports Med.* 2004;23:581–608.

60. Whaley AL, Baker CL. Lateral epicondylitis. *Clin Sports Med.* 2004;23:677–691.

61. Walz DM, Newman JS, Konin GP, Ross G. Epicondylitis: pathogenesis, imaging, and treatment. *Radiographics.* 2010;30:167–184.

62. Zhu J, Hu B, Xing C, Li J. Ultrasound-guided, minimally invasive, percutaneous needle puncture treatment for tennis elbow. *Adv Ther.* 2008;25(10):1031–1036.

63. Altan L, Kanat E. Conservative treatment of lateral epicondylitis: comparison of two different orthotic devices. *Clin Rheumatol.* 2008;27(8):1015–1019.

64. Greiwe RM, Saifi C, Ahmad CS. Pediatric sports elbow injuries. *Clin Sports Med.* 2010;29:677–703.

65. Tosti R, Jennings J, Sewards JM. Lateral epicondylitis of the elbow. *Am J Med.* 2013;126:357e1–357e6.

66. Tran N, Chow K. Ultrasonography of the elbow. *Semin Musculoskelet Radiol.* 2007;11(2):105–116.

67. Assendelft W, Green S, Buchbinder R, Struijs P, Smidt N. Tennis elbow. *Clin Evid.* 2004;(11):1633–1644.

68. Walther M, Kirschner S, Koenig A, Barthel T, Gohlke F. Biomechanical evaluation of braces used for the treatment of epicondylitis. *J Shoulder Elbow Surg.* 2002;11:265–270.

69. Derebery VJ, Davenport JN, Giang GM, Fogarty WT. The effects of splinting on outcomes for epicondylitis. *Arch Phys Med Rehabil.* 2005;86(6):1081–1088. doi:10.1016/j.apmr.2004.11.029

70. Cardone DA, Tallia AF. Diagnostic and therapeutic injection of the elbow region. *Am Fam Physician.* 2002;66(11):2097–2100.

71. Van Hofwegen C, Baker CL III, Baker CL Jr. Epicondylitis in the athlete's elbow. *Clin Sports Med.* 2010;29:577–597.

72. American Academy of Family Physicians. Information from your family doctor. Exercises for tennis elbow. *Am Fam Physician.* 2007;76(6):849–850.

73. Johnson GW, Cadwallader K, Scheffel SB, Epperly TD. Treatment of lateral epicondylitis. *Am Fam Physician*. 2007; 76(6):843–848.

74. Nobuta S, Ogawa K, Sato K, Nakagawa T, Hatori M, Itoi E. Clinical outcome of fragment fixation for osteochondritis dissecans of the elbow. *Ups J Med Sci*. 2008;113(2):201–208.

75. Hixon AL, Gibbs LM. Osteochondritis dissecans: a diagnosis not to miss. *Am Fam Physician*. 2000;61(1):151–156, 158.

76. Debeer P, Brys P. Osteochondritis dissecans of the humeral head: clinical and radiological findings. *Acta Orthop Belg*. 2005;71(4):484–488.

77. Yadao MA, Field LD, Savoie FH 3rd. Osteochondritis dissecans of the elbow. *Instr Course Lect*. 2004;53:599–606.

78. Kijowski R, De Smet AA. MRI findings of osteochondritis dissecans of the capitellum with surgical correlation. *AJR Am J Roentgenol*. 2005;185(6):1453–1459.

79. Baker CL 3rd, Romeo AA, Baker CL Jr. Osteochondritis dissecans of the capitellum. *Am J Sports Med*. 2010; 38(9):1917–1928.

80. Rahusen FT, Brinkman JM, Eygendaal D. Results of arthroscopic debridement for osteochondritis dissecans of the elbow. *Br J Sports Med*. 2006;40(12):966–969.

81. Field LD, Altchek DW. Elbow injuries. *Clin Sports Med*. 1995;14(1):59–78.

82. Chen FS, Rokito AS, Jobe FW. Medial elbow problems in the overhead-throwing athlete. *J Am Acad Orthop Surg*. 2001; 9(2):99–113.

83. Hariri S, Safran MR. Ulnar collateral ligament injury in the overhead athlete. *Clin Sport Med*. 2010;29:619–644.

84. Nassab PF, Schickendantz MS. Evaluation and treatment of medial ulnar collateral ligament injuries in the throwing athlete. *Sports Med Athros*. 2006;14:221–231.

85. Meyes A, Palmer B, Baratz ME. Ulnar collateral ligament reconstruction. *Hand Clin*. 2008;24:53–67.

86. O'Holleran JD, Altchek DW. The thrower's elbow: arthroscopic treatment of valgus extension overload syndrome. *HSS J*. 2006;2(1):83–93.

87. Dines JS, Elattrache NS, Conway JE, Smith W, Ahmad CS. Clinical outcomes of the DANE TJ technique to treat ulnar collateral ligament insufficiency of the elbow. *Am J Sports Med*. 2007;35(12):2039–2044.

88. Vitale MA, Ahmad CS. The outcome of elbow ulnar collateral ligament reconstruction in overhead athletes: a systematic review. *Am J Sports Med*. 2008;36(6):1193–1205.

89. Koh JL, Schafer MF, Keuter G, Hsu JE. Ulnar collateral ligament reconstruction in elite throwing athletes. *Arthroscopy*. 2006;22(11):1187–1191.

90. Bencardino JT, Rosenberg ZS. Entrapment neuropathies of the shoulder and elbow in the athlete. *Clin Sports Med*. 2006; 25:465–487.

91. Plancher KD, Peterson RK, Steichen JB. Compressive neuropathies and tendinopathies in the athletic elbow and wrist. *Clin Sports Med*. 1996;15(2):331–371.

92. Loh YC, Lam WL, Stanley JK, Soames RW. A new clinical test for radial tunnel syndrome—the rule-of-nine test: a

cadaveric study. *J Orthop Surg (Hong Kong)*. 2004;12(1): 83–86.

93. Stanley J. Radial tunnel syndrome: a surgeon's perspective. *J Hand Ther*. 2006;19(2):180–184.

94. Andreisek G, Crook DW, Burg D, Marincek B, Weishaupt D. Peripheral neuropathies of the median, radial, and ulnar nerves: MR imaging features. *Radiographics*. 2006;26(5): 1267–1287.

95. Popinchalk SP, Schaffer AA. Physical examination of upper extremity compressive neuropathies. *Orthop Clin North Am*. 2012;43:417–430.

96. Lo YL, Fook-Chong S, Leoh TH, et al. Rapid ultrasonographic diagnosis of radial entrapment neuropathy at the spiral groove. *J Neurol Sci*. 2008;271(1-2):75–79. doi:10.1016/j.jns.2008.03.014. Epub 2008 May 12.

97. Shao YC, Harwood P, Grotz MR, Limb D, Giannoudis PV. Radial nerve palsy associated with fractures of the shaft of the humerus: a systematic review. *J Bone Joint Surg Br*. 2005; 87(12):1647–1652.

98. Neal SL, Fields KB. Peripheral nerve entrapment and injury in the upper extremity. *Am Fam Physician*. 2010;81: 147–155.

99. Matsubara Y, Miyasaka Y, Nobuta S, Hasegawa K. Radial nerve palsy at the elbow. *Ups J Med Sci*. 2006;111(3): 315–320.

100. Lee MJ, LaStayo PC. Pronator syndrome and other nerve compressions that mimic carpal tunnel syndrome. *J Orthop Sports Phys Ther*. 2004;34(10):601–609.

101. Rehak DC. Pronator syndrome. *Clin Sports Med*. 2001; 20:531–540.

102. Sellards R, Kuebrich C. The elbow: diagnosis and treatment of common injuries. *Prim Care*. 2005;32:1–16.

103. Gellman H. Compression of the ulnar nerve at the elbow: cubital tunnel syndrome. *Instr Course Lect*. 2008;57: 187–197.

104. Kroonen LT. Cubital tunnel syndrome. *Orthop Clin N Am*. 2012;43:475–486.

105. Boursinos LA, Dimitriou CG. Ulnar nerve compression in the cubital tunnel by an epineural ganglion: a case report. *Hand (N Y)*. 2007;2(1):12–15. doi:10.1007/s11552-006-9013-3.

106. Descatha A, Leclerc A, Chastang JF, Roquelaure Y, Study Group on Repetitive Work. Incidence of ulnar nerve entrapment at the elbow in repetitive work. *Scand J Work Environ Health*. 2004;30(3):234–240.

107. Wiesler ER, Chloros GD, Cartwright MS, Shin HW, Walker FO. Ultrasound in the diagnosis of ulnar neuropathy at the cubital tunnel. *J Hand Surg Am*. 2006;31(7):1088–1093.

108. Ochi K, Horiuchi Y, Tanabe A, Waseda M, Kaneko Y, Koyanagi T. Shoulder internal rotation elbow flexion test for diagnosing cubital tunnel syndrome. *J Shoulder Elbow Surg*. 2012;21:777–781.

109. Szabo RM, Kwak C. Natural history and conservative management of cubital tunnel syndrome. *Hand Clin*. 2007; 23(3):311–318, vi.

CHAPTER 15

Upper Arm

Casey Glass, MD

UPPER ARM FRACTURES

HUMERAL SHAFT FRACTURES

Fractures of the humerus are classified as proximal, midshaft, and distal. In this chapter, we discuss concerns related to midshaft fractures and disorders of the muscles of the upper arm. Proximal humerus fractures are discussed in Chapter 16, and distal fractures are discussed in Chapter 14. Humeral shaft fractures are relatively uncommon, representing only 3% of all fractures.[1] Humerus fractures are responsible for 370,000 emergency visits yearly, of which humeral shaft fractures represent about 13%.[2,3] The incidence of humeral shaft fractures is bimodal with peaks around age 10 and age 80.[4] Most humeral shaft fractures occur in children at a rate of ~290 per 100,000 population as compared to 63 to 69 per 100,000 population in the population as a whole.[3-5] Among the elderly, humeral shaft fracture disproportionately affects women at a rate of ~2:1. In developing nations, limited data suggest a peak incidence during middle age with motor vehicle accidents as a primary cause.[6]

The humeral shaft extends from the insertion of the pectoralis major to the supracondylar ridges. Humeral shaft fractures can be described based on the number of fracture lines and relative position of fracture fragments using the AO fracture classification system. This information is useful to the orthopedic consultant as the classification of the fracture correlates with the need for surgical repair. Simple fractures (AO Type A) have one fracture line and may be spiral, oblique, or transverse. Wedge fractures (AO Type B) have multiple fracture lines and a wedge-shaped defect from the humeral shaft. The proximal and distal parts of the humerus remain in close contact. Complex fractures (AO Type C) usually include multiple fracture lines, and the proximal and distal portions of the humerus are no longer in close contact (Fig. 15–1).

Essential Anatomy

The extensive musculature surrounding the humeral shaft may result in distraction and displacement of the bony fragments after a fracture. The deltoid inserts along the anterolateral humeral shaft, whereas the pectoralis major inserts on the medial intertubercular groove (Fig. 15–2). The supraspinatus inserts into the greater tuberosity of the humeral head, resulting in abduction and external rotation.

The biceps and the triceps insert distally and tend to displace the distal fragment proximally.

A fracture proximal to the pectoralis major insertion may be accompanied by abduction and external rotation of the humeral head because of the action of the supraspinatus (Fig. 15–2A). A fracture between the insertion of the pectoralis major and the deltoid will usually result in adduction of the proximal fragment secondary to the pull of the pectoralis major (Fig. 15–2B). Fractures distal to the deltoid insertion usually result in abduction of the proximal fragment secondary to the pull of the deltoid muscle (Fig. 15–2C).

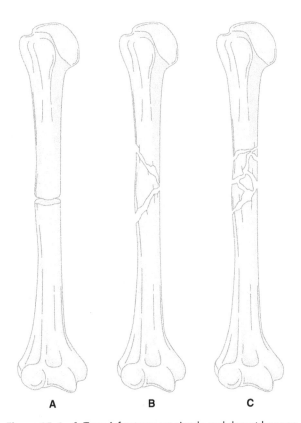

A   **B**   **C**

Figure 15–1. **A.** Type A fractures are simple and do not have an associated fracture fragment. They can be transverse, oblique, or spiral. **B.** Type B fractures have a free wedge-shaped fragment. The humeral shaft ends remain in close proximity. **C.** Type C fractures are complex (comminuted) fractures, where there is increased distance between the fractured ends of the humerus with interposed fracture fragments.

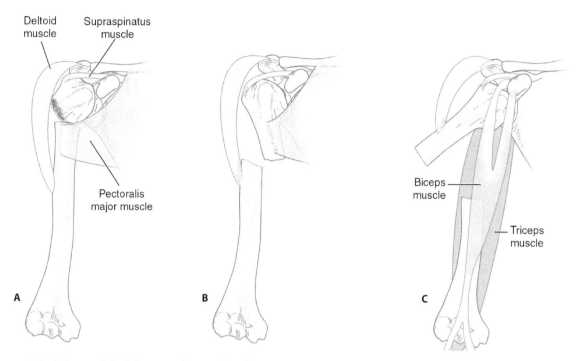

Figure 15–2. In humeral shaft fractures, the muscles of the proximal humerus cause displacement of the fracture fragments. Five muscles play a major role in displacing fractures in this region: the deltoid, supraspinatus, pectoralis major, biceps, and triceps. ***A.*** In fractures between the rotator cuff and the pectoralis major, abduction and rotation of the proximal fragment occur. ***B.*** Fractures occurring between the pectoralis major insertion and the deltoid insertion are associated with adduction deformity of the proximal fragment. ***C.*** Fractures occurring below the deltoid insertion are associated with abduction of the proximal fragment.

The neurovascular bundle of the upper extremity extends along the medial border of the humeral shaft. Although any of these structures may be injured with a fracture, the most commonly injured structure is the radial nerve. The radial nerve lies in close proximity to the humeral shaft at the junction of its middle and distal thirds, and fractures in this area are most often associated with radial nerve involvement (Fig. 15–3).

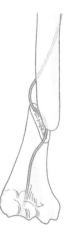

Figure 15–3. The radial nerve courses in the lateral intermuscular septum along the lateral aspect of the humerus and can be involved in fractures of the shaft.

Mechanism of Injury

Several mechanisms cause humeral shaft fractures. The most common mechanism of injury is direct or indirect trauma to the arm from a fall.   Direct force to the humerus typically results in a transverse fracture, and an indirect mechanism results in a spiral fracture. In addition, a violent contraction in an area of pathologically weakened bone may result in a fracture.

Examination

The patient will present with pain and swelling over the area of the humeral shaft. On examination, shortening, obvious deformity, or abnormal mobility with crepitation may be detected (Fig. 15–4). It is imperative that a thorough neurovascular examination accompanies the initial assessment of all humeral shaft fractures.

The examiner should give particular emphasis to the radial nerve function and document the time at which radial nerve injury is first detected. This information is important because of the following reasons:

- Damage at the time of injury is most often a transient neurapraxia due to nerve compression.
- Damage detected after manipulation or immobilization may lead to axonotmesis if the pressure is not relieved.
- Damage detected during healing is typically due to a slowly progressive axonotmesis.

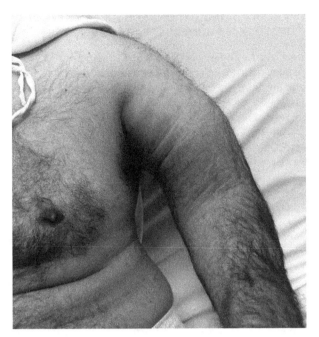

Figure 15–4. A patient with deformity due to a humeral shaft fracture.

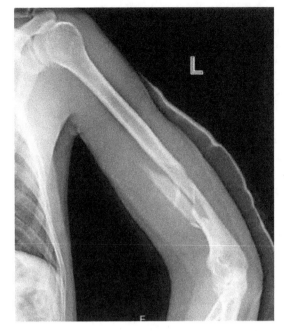

Figure 15–5. Comminuted fracture of the distal one-third humeral shaft.

Radial nerve examination should include assessment of sensation over the lateral upper arm and deltoid, triceps strength, supination strength, and active wrist extension. The examiner should not rely on extension of the digits as evidence of radial nerve function because the intrinsic muscles of the hand can accomplish this movement.

Imaging

Anteroposterior and lateral views of the entire humerus are essential (Fig. 15–5).

Associated Injuries

Humeral shaft fractures may be associated with several significant injuries, including brachial artery injury, nerve injury, or additional fractures to the shoulder or distal humerus. Radial nerve injury is present in 2% to 17% of humeral shaft fractures.[8,9] Fractures in the middle third and middle–distal portions of the bone and transverse or spiral fracture patterns are more often associated with radial nerve injury.[8] The injury may be partial or complete and may involve motor or sensory fibers. The majority of cases of radial nerve dysfunction occur at the time of injury, but injury can occur after closed reduction or operative repair. The injured extremity should be reexamined for nerve function after manipulation or splinting because movement of the fracture may cause a radial nerve injury.[10]

Treatment

Emergent operative intervention is indicated for open fractures and fractures associated with vascular injury. In the absence of these situations, management of humeral shaft fractures includes ice, analgesics, and application of a coaptation splint. Downward traction before or during splint application may aid in reduction (Fig. 15–6 and

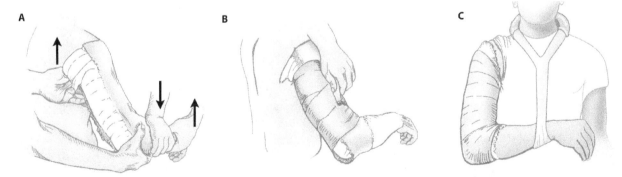

Figure 15–6. ***A, B.*** A U-shaped coaptation splint, sometimes referred to as a "sugar-tong" splint, is applied to fractures of the humeral shaft to maintain reduction. ***C.*** The arm is then suspended at the wrist from the neck in a collar and cuff apparatus.

Appendix A–12). A collar and cuff (or sling and swathe support) is then applied (Appendix A–13). A collar and cuff permits the splint itself to deliver inline traction to the fracture via gravity as the elbow is unsupported.

The urgency of orthopedic follow-up is contingent on the underlying alignment of the fracture. Type A fractures that remain displaced or angulated after reduction and splinting, as well as Type B and C fractures require urgent follow-up as these fractures are more likely to require surgical intervention. Nondisplaced Type A fractures with near anatomic alignment (less than 15 degrees of angulation in any plane) require less urgent follow-up.

Indications for the operative management of humeral shaft fractures are listed in Table 15–1. Approximately 60% of humeral shaft fractures are treated surgically, with younger patients and patients with open fractures more likely to receive a surgery. Operative repair of humeral shaft fractures may be accomplished with open or minimally invasive plate fixation or intramedullary nail placement.

Nonoperative management may be accomplished through the continued use of the coaptation splint or via a functional brace with a fitted plastic orthesis (Sarmiento brace). These methods provide dependency traction and stabilization of the fracture through the compressive forces of the surrounding soft tissues. Functional bracing has the advantage of allowing motion at the elbow and shoulder during healing that improves functional outcome. Functional bracing is associated with acceptable clinical outcomes greater than 90% of the time. The patient should begin hand exercises immediately, with shoulder circumduction exercises started as soon as pain permits.

Humeral shaft fractures generally take 10 to 12 weeks to heal. Spiral fractures heal faster than transverse fractures because of their larger surface area. Fractures close to the elbow or the shoulder are associated with longer healing periods and higher rates of nonunion.

Patients with associated radial nerve injury should be urgently referred to an orthopedist, especially if it occurs

▶ **TABLE 15–1. INDICATIONS FOR SURGICAL REPAIR OF MIDSHAFT HUMERUS FRACTURES**

Brachial artery injury or open fracture (emergent)
Inability to maintain alignment of less than 15-degree angulation
Associated ipsilateral forearm fractures
Segmental fracture, pathologic fracture, or bilateral humeral shaft fractures
Associated fractures that require early mobilization
Interposed soft tissues that do not allow proper alignment
Brachial plexus injury (soft-tissue sleeve surrounding the humerus will lose its stability)
Additional injuries that require a prolonged recumbent position (i.e., no dependency traction)
Noncompliance with nonoperative techniques

following reduction attempts. Although operative exploration was historically indicated, recent literature suggests that conservative management is appropriate for most patients. However, operative intervention may be considered for open fractures or high-energy injuries such as those secondary to gunshot wounds because these injuries have an increased association with nerve transection. When managed conservatively, function begins to return after ~10 weeks, with significant improvement at ~26 weeks. Up to 70% of patients treated conservatively will recover.

Complications
Humeral shaft fractures can be associated with several significant complications.

• Delayed development of radial nerve palsies
• Nonunion or delayed union
• Shoulder adhesive capsulitis (may be prevented by early circumduction exercises)
• Myositis ossificans of the elbow (may be avoided by using active routine exercises)
• Compartment syndrome (rare)

UPPER ARM SOFT-TISSUE INJURY AND DISLOCATIONS

BICEPS TENDON RUPTURE

The biceps brachii muscle is a flexor and supinator of the forearm. The muscle has two proximal attachments with the short head originating on the coracoid process and the long head just above the glenoid. The distal attachment is on the tuberosity of the radius (Fig. 15–7). Disruption of this muscle unit is not uncommon because, similar to the gastrocnemius and hamstring muscles, it has exposure to greater potential forces because it crosses two joints. Disruption can occur at the long head of the biceps tendon,

the musculotendinous portion, muscle belly, or the distal attachment. Rupture of the long head of the biceps tendon is most common, whereas muscle disruption is least common. The presentation, whether proximal or distal disruption is present, is that of a "Popeye"-shaped upper arm (Fig. 15–8).

Long Head of the Biceps Tendon Rupture
Rupture of the long head of the biceps can occur anywhere along its route. The condition often occurs in men during their sixth or seventh decade of life following a chronic

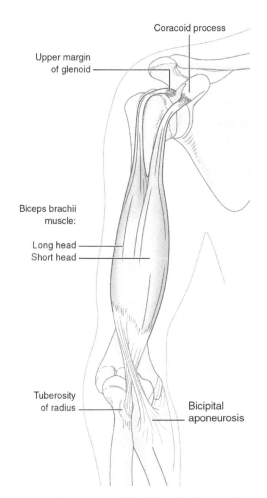

Coracoid process

Upper margin
of glenoid

Biceps brachii
muscle:

Long head
Short head

Tuberosity
of radius

Bicipital
aponeurosis

Figure 15–7. The anatomy of the biceps brachii muscle.

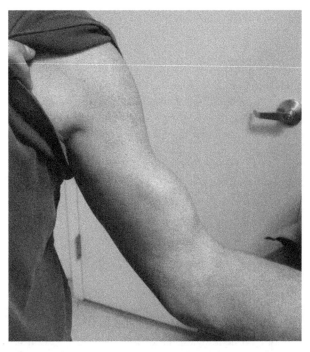

Figure 15–8. A patient with rupture of the biceps tendon. Note the "Popeye" appearance of the muscle.

bicipital tenosynovitis that has left the tendon weakened. In younger patients, it may occur more suddenly, following forceful contraction of the biceps during lifting an object or during athletic activity.[20–23]

The patient usually notices an immediate sharp pain in the region of the bicipital groove, and the biceps is noted to bulge within the arm. There is tenderness to palpation within the bicipital groove. The diagnosis can be confirmed by asking the patient to contract the biceps with the arm abducted and externally rotated to 90 degrees, at which point attempted flexion at the elbow will cause the biceps to move away from the shoulder.[24]

For definitive treatment, surgical reattachment to the bicipital groove is recommended in most active patients. In elderly patients with the condition, repair may not be indicated. If the decision is made not to repair the tendon, negatives include the cosmetic appearance of the arm and a loss of elbow flexion strength of approximately 10% to 20%, which is usually well tolerated.[24,25] Surgical repair usually results in excellent resolution of deformity and permits return to function in about 90% of patients.[25,26,27]

Patients with an acute rupture of the biceps muscle belly are treated conservatively in a Velpeau bandage with the elbow flexed to 90 degrees (Appendix A–13).

Distal Biceps Tendon Rupture

Distal biceps tendon injuries occur at a rate of 2.5 per 100,000 people in the United States, and the average age of affected patients is 43 years. Men are affected more often than women, and injury usually involves the dominant arm.[28] Usually, the injury occurs as a result of a sudden eccentric load on the forearm while the elbow is flexed.[29,30] This injury is less common than proximal disruption, accounting for 3% of biceps tendon injuries, although it seems to be becoming more common, possibly due to an increase in the activity level of patients in their fifth and sixth decades.[31,32]

Patients often describe a tearing sensation accompanied by pain in the region of the antecubital fossa. Similar to patients with long head of the biceps rupture, these patients will present with a visible deformity of the muscle belly and weakness to flexion and supination. Partial tears, which may not present with the same muscle retraction and deformity, are difficult to diagnose. Distal biceps tendon integrity can be assessed with the "hook test," where the examiner hooks his/her index finger under the lateral aspect of the distal biceps tendon (Video 15–1).[33] The squeeze test is analogous to the Thompson test for Achilles tendon rupture. With the forearm slightly pronated and resting on the patient's leg, the examiner squeezes the biceps and should note the slight supination of the forearm if the distal biceps tendon is intact (Video 15–2). The supination mechanism of the biceps can also be evaluated by use of the Supination-Pronation test. The examiner observes the movement of the biceps muscle belly while the patient supinates and

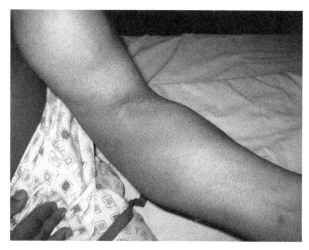

Figure 15–9. Distal biceps tendon rupture. Note the increased distance from the antecubital crease to the distal edge of the biceps muscle in the abnormal extremity.

pronates the forearm. An intact muscle will move toward the shoulder with supination and toward the elbow with pronation. The biceps crease interval, the distance between the antecubital crease and the distal biceps muscle, can also be measured. More than 6 cm or a 20% increase in the affected arm is abnormal (Fig. 15–9). If the diagnosis is unclear, ultrasonography or magnetic resonance imaging (MRI) may be useful.

Acute complete rupture of the distal tendon of the biceps is treated with early surgical reattachment to maintain strength. Partial tears are initially treated conservatively with immobilization; surgical repair is reserved for refractory dysfunction.

TRICEPS TENDON RUPTURE

The triceps brachii muscle consists of three muscle groups that collectively insert on the olecranon process to extend the elbow and, to a lesser extent, adduct the arm. The long head of the triceps originates on the infra-glenoid tubercle of the scapula. The medial head originates from the posterior humerus and radial groove. The lateral head originates on the posterior humerus lateral to the radial groove (Fig. 15–10).

Triceps tendon rupture is very rare, representing less than 1% of tendon injuries. The mechanism is usually a fall against an outstretched arm while the triceps is contracted, with or without a blow to the posterior elbow. Hyperparathyroidism secondary to renal failure, olecranon bursitis, anabolic steroid use, or weight lifting may be contributing factors.

The tendon is usually disrupted at the insertion into the olecranon, and the injury can be associated with an avulsion fracture of the olecranon, which may be visible as a bony "flake" on lateral plain films of the elbow. The patient presents with posterior elbow swelling and tenderness, with

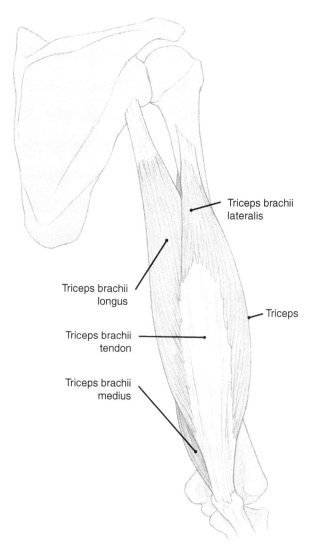

Figure 15–10. The anatomy of the triceps brachii muscle.

a limited ability to extend the elbow against gravity. These injuries may be missed pain in the posterior elbow limits motion at the time of injury and swelling prevents palpation of the gap caused by withdrawal of the tendon.

Treatment involves splinting at 30 degrees of elbow flexion and urgent orthopedic consultation. Most patients require surgical repair.

ARM COMPARTMENT SYNDROME

There are three compartments of the upper arm. The anterior flexor compartment contains the biceps and brachialis muscles, whereas the posterior extensor compartment contains the triceps. The deltoid muscle is surrounded by its own fascia and is the third compartment.

Compartment syndrome of the upper arm is unusual and much less common than in the forearm and leg. There are several explanations for the infrequent incidence of this condition. The fascia of the upper arm musculature is thinner and more distensible. In addition, the muscles of the arm communicate with the shoulder.[41]

Nonetheless, upper arm compartment syndrome has been reported after muscle contusion, humerus fracture, subcutaneous injection, shoulder dislocation, tendon rupture, steroid use, exercise, blood pressure monitoring after thrombolytic therapy, as a complication of dialysis access, secondary to anticoagulant use, and tourniquet use.[42–53]

The only reliable finding is severe pain, and as a result, the condition is easily missed.[54] When the anterior compartment is involved, the elbow may be held in mild flexion.[50] Diagnostic measures and treatment are similar to compartment syndrome in other locations, and the reader is referred to the discussion in Chapter 4 for further information.

ARM CONTUSIONS

Contusions of the muscles of the upper arm are common, but not disabling, injuries with no major complications. The treatment of these injuries is a sling for protection. Ice in the first 24 hours is recommended, followed by heat.

The physician should rule out an underlying fracture and test for injury to the radial nerve from a contusion to the lateral aspect of the distal arm. Contusion of the radial nerve as it courses in close approximation to the humerus along the spiral groove is an infrequent injury. As the nerve courses further, it goes laterally above the lateral epicondylar ridge and is subject to contusions by a direct blow. The patient complains of a tingling sensation extending down the forearm and into the hand over the distribution of the nerve. The treatment is symptomatic.

Patients with repeated contusions to the arm may develop ectopic bone deposition. *Anterior lateral humeral exostosis*, also called *blocker's exostosis* because of its association with American football lineman, is an abnormal deposition of bone at the attachment of the deltoid muscle onto the humerus. The injury is initiated by a direct blow in this region that produces a contusion and periostitis at the insertion of the deltoid tendon. Later, a potentially painful and irritative exostosis develops at the site of injury. When significant discomfort occurs, the patient should be referred for consideration of excision.

REFERENCES

1. Ekholm R, Adami J, Tidermark J, Hansson K, Törnkvist H, Ponzer S. Fractures of the shaft of the humerus. An epidemiological study of 401 fractures. *J Bone Joint Surg Br*. 2006;88(11): 1469–1473.
2. Kim SH, Szabo RM, Marder RA. Epidemiology of humerus fractures in the United States: nationwide emergency department sample, 2008. *Arthritis Care Res*. 2012;64(3):407–414.
3. Bergdahl C, Ekholm C, Wennergren D, Nilsson F, Möller M. Epidemiology and patho-anatomical pattern of 2,011 humeral fractures: data from the Swedish Fracture Register. *BMC Musculoskelet Disord*. 2016;17:159.
4. Holloway KL, Bucki-Smith G, Morse AG, Brennan-Olsen SL, Kotowicz MA, et al. Humeral fractures in South-Eastern Australia: epidemiology and risk factors. *Calcif Tissue Int*. 2015;97(5):453–465. doi:10.1007/s00223-015-0039-9. Epub 2015 Jul 14.
5. Beerekamp MSH, de Muinck Keizer RJO, Schep NWL, Ubbink DT, Panneman MJM, Goslings JC. Epidemiology of extremity fractures in the Netherlands. *Injury*. 2017; 48(7):1355–1363. doi:10.1016/j.injury.2017.04.047. Epub 2017 Apr 24.
6. Ezeuko VC, Ehimigbai AR, Esechie EL. Assessment of some demographic risk factors associated with diaphyseal humeral fractures among Nigerians. *Burns Trauma*. 2015;3:3.
7. Kellam JF, Audigé L. Fracture classification. In: Rüedi TP, Buckley RE, Moran CG, eds. *AO Principles of Fracture Management*, Vol 1, 2nd ed. AO Publishing; 2007. www2.aofoundation.org. Accessed May 31, 2017.
8. Shao YC, Harwood P, Grotz MR, Limb D, Giannoudis PV. Radial nerve palsy associated with fractures of the shaft of the humerus: a systematic review. *J Bone Joint Surg Br*. 2005; 87(12):1647–6452.
9. Bumbasirevic M, Palibrk T, Lesic A, Atkinson H. Radial nerve palsy. *EFORT Open Rev*. 2016;1(8):286–294.
10. Jones M, Kang HW, O'Neill C, Maginn P. Iatrogenic radial nerve palsy following closed reduction of a simple diaphyseal humeral fracture: beware the perfect x-ray. *Case Rep Emerg Med*. 2016;2016:2636450. http://dx.doi.org/10.1155/2016/2636450. Accessed January 11, 2018.
11. Schoch BS, Padegimas EM, Maltenfort M, Krieg J, Namdari S. Humeral shaft fractures: national trends in management. *J Orthop Traumatol*. 2017;18(3):259–263. doi:10.1007/s10195-017-0459-6. Epub 2017 May 8.
12. Heineman DJ, Poolman RW, Nork SE, Ponsen KJ, Bhandari M. Plate fixation or intramedullary fixation of humeral shaft fractures. *Acta Orthop*. 2010;81(2):216–223.
13. Heineman DJ, Bhandari M, Poolman RW. Plate fixation or intramedullary fixation of humeral shaft fractures—an update. *Acta Orthop*. 2012;83(3):317–318.
14. Sarmiento A, Zagorski JB, Zych GA, Latta LL, Capps CA. Functional bracing for the treatment of fractures of the humeral diaphysis. *J Bone Joint Surg Am*. 2000;82(4):478–486.
15. Kapil Mani KC, Gopal Sagar DC, Rijal L, Govinda KC, Shrestha BL. Study on outcome of fracture shaft of the humerus treated non-operatively with a functional brace. *Eur J Orthop Surg Traumatol*. 2013;23(3):323–328.
16. Papasoulis E, Drosos GI, Ververidis AN, Verettas DA. Functional bracing of humeral shaft fractures. A review of clinical studies. *Injury*. 2010;41(7):e21–e27. doi:10.1016/j.injury.2009.05.004. Epub 2009 Jun 11.
17. Mahabier KC, Vogels LM, Punt BJ, Roukema GR, Patka P, Van Lieshout EM. Humeral shaft fractures: retrospective results of non-operative and operative treatment of 186 patients. *Injury*. 2013;44(4):427–430.
18. Kapil Mani KC, Gopal Sagar DC, Rijal L, Govinda KC, Shrestha BL. Study on outcome of fracture shaft of the humerus treated non-operatively with a functional brace. *Eur J Orthop Surg Traumatol*. 2013;23(3):323–328.

19. Lang NW, Ostermann RC, Arthold C, Joestl J, Platzer P. Retrospective case series with one year follow-up after radial nerve palsy associated with humeral fractures. *Int Orthop.* 2017; 41(1):191–196. doi:10.1007/s00264-016-3186-3. Epub 2016 Apr 14.

20. Cope MR, Ali A, Bayliss NC. Biceps rupture in body builders: three case reports of rupture of the long head of the biceps at the tendon-labrum junction. *J Shoulder Elbow Surg.* 2004;13(5):580–582.

21. Ferry AT, Lee GH, Murphy R, Romeo AA, Verma NN. A long-head of biceps tendon rupture in a fast pitch softball player: a case report. *J Shoulder Elbow Surg.* 2009;18(1):e14–e17.

22. Carmichael KD, Foster L, Kearney JP. Biceps muscle rupture in a water skier. *Orthopedics.* 2005;28(1):35–37.

23. Tangari M, Carbone S, Gallo M, Campi A. Long head of the biceps tendon rupture in professional wrestlers: treatment with a mini-open tenodesis. *J Shoulder Elbow Surg.* 2011; 20(3):409–413.

24. Ejnisman B, Monteiro GC, Andreoli CV, de Castro Pochini A. Disorder of the long head of the biceps tendon. *Br J Sports Med.* 2010;44(5):347–354.

25. Elser F, Braun S, Dewing CB, Giphart JE, Millett PJ. Anatomy, function, injuries, and treatment of the long head of the biceps brachii tendon. *Arthroscopy.* 2011;27(4):581–592.

26. Anthony SG, McCormick F, Gross DJ, Golijanin P, Provencher MT. Biceps tenodesis for long head of the biceps after auto-rupture or failed surgical tenotomy: results in an active population. *J Shoulder Elbow Surg.* 2015;24(2):e36–e40.

27. McMahon PJ, Speziali A. Outcomes of tenodesis of the long head of the biceps tendon more than three months after rupture. *World J Orthop.* 2016;7(3):188–194.

28. Kelly MP, Perkinson SG, Ablove RH, Tueting JL. Distal biceps tendon ruptures: an epidemiological analysis using a large population database. *Am J Sports Med.* 2015;43(8):2012–2017.

29. Miyamoto RG, Elser F, Millett PJ. Distal biceps tendon injuries. *J Bone Joint Surg Am.* 2010;92(11):2128–2138.

30. Sarda P, Qaddori A, Nauschutz F, Boulton L, Nanda R, Bayliss N. Distal biceps tendon rupture: current concepts. *Injury.* 2013;44(4):417–420.

31. Alberta FG, Elattrache NS. Diagnosis and treatment of distal biceps and anterior elbow pain in throwing athletes. *Sports Med Arthrosc.* 2008;16(3):118–123.

32. Turkel G, Lomasney LM, Demos T, Marra G. What is your diagnosis? Biceps tendon rupture at the radial tuberosity. *Orthopedics.* 2007;30(11):974–977.

33. O'Driscoll SW, Goncalves LB, Dietz P. The hook test for distal biceps tendon avulsion. *Am J Sports Med.* 2007; 35(11):1865–1869.

34. Metzman LS, Tivener KA. The supination-pronation test for distal biceps tendon rupture. *Am J Orthop.* 2015;44(10): E361–E364.

35. Bain GI, Johnson LJ, Turner PC. Treatment of partial distal biceps tendon tears. *Sports Med Arthrosc.* 2008;16(3):154–161.

36. Yeh PC, Dodds SD, Smart LR, Mazzocca AD, Sethi PM. Distal triceps rupture. *J Am Acad Orthop Surg.* 2010;18(1):31–40.

37. Gharanizadeh K, Mazhar FN, Molavy N, Bagherifard A, Shariatzadeh H. Avulsions of triceps brachii: associated injuries and surgical treatment; a case series. *Acta Orthop Belg.* 2016;82(2):197–202.

38. Foulk DM, Galloway MT. Partial triceps disruption: a case report. *Sports Health.* 2011;3(2):175–178.

39. Desai B, Slish J, Allen B. Bilateral and simultaneous rupture of the triceps tendon in a patient without predisposing factors. *Case Rep Emerg Med.* 2012;2012:920685. doi:10.1155/2012/920685.

40. Naito K, Homma Y, Morita M, Mogami A, Obayashi O. Triceps tendon avulsion: a case report and discussion about the olecranon ossification nucleus. *Eur J Orthop Surg Traumatol.* 2013;(2):S193–S196.

41. Leversedge FJ, Moore TJ, Peterson BC, Seiler JG III. Compartment syndrome of the upper extremity. *J Hand Surg Am.* 2011; 36(3):544–559.

42. Alford JW, Palumbo MA, Barnum MJ. Compartment syndrome of the arm: a complication of noninvasive blood pressure monitoring during thrombolytic therapy for myocardial infarction. *J Clin Monit Comput.* 2002;17(3–4):163–166.

43. Knapke DM, Truumees E. Posterior arm and deltoid compartment syndrome after vitamin B12 injection. *Orthopedics.* 2004;27(5):520–521.

44. Kim KC, Rhee KJ, Shin HD. Recurrent dorsal compartment syndrome of the upper arm after blunt trauma. *J Trauma.* 2008; 65(6):1543–1546.

45. Fung DA, Frey S, Grossman RB. Rare case of upper arm compartment syndrome following biceps tendon rupture. *Orthopedics.* 2008;31(5):494.

46. Lee WY, Hsu HH, Yen TH, Wang LJ, Lee SY. Acute left-arm compartment syndrome due to cephalic arch stenosis in a dialysis patient. *Ann Vasc Surg.* 2013;27(1):111.e1–111.e3. doi:10.1016/j.avsg.2012.04.016. Epub 2012 Sep 12.

47. Zimmerman DC, Kapoor T, Elfond M, Scott P. Spontaneous compartment syndrome of the upper arm in a patient receiving anticoagulation therapy. *J Emerg Med.* 2013;44(1): e53–e56.

48. Erturan G, Davies N, Williams H, Deo S. Bilateral simultaneous traumatic upper arm compartment syndromes associated with anabolic steroids. *J Emerg Med.* 2013;44(1):89–91.

49. Oh JY, Laidler M, Fiala SC, Hedberg K. Acute exertional rhabdomyolysis and triceps compartment syndrome during a high school football camp. *Sports Health.* 2012;4(1):57–62.

50. Aynardi MC, Jones CM. Bilateral upper arm compartment syndrome after a vigorous cross-training workout. *J Shoulder Elbow Surg.* 2016;25(3):e65–e67.

51. Tuna S, Duymus TM, Mutlu S, Ketenci IE, Ulusoy A. Upper extremity acute compartment syndrome during tissue plasminogen activator therapy for pulmonary embolism in a morbidly obese patient. *Int J Surg Case Rep.* 2015;8C:175–178.

52. Titolo P, Milani P, Panero B, Ciclamini D, Colzani G, Artiaco S. Acute compartment syndrome of the arm after minor trauma in a patient with optimal range of oral anticoagulant therapy: a case report. *Case Rep Orthop.* 2014:(2014):980940. doi:10.1155/2014/980940. Epub 2014 Jan 6.

53. Brownlee WJ, Wu TY, Van Dijck SA, Snow BJ. Upper limb compartment syndrome: an unusual complication of stroke thrombolysis. *J Clin Neurosci.* 2014;21(5):880–882.

54. von Keudell AG, Weaver MJ, Appleton PT, et al. Diagnosis and treatment of acute extremity compartment syndrome. *Lancet.* 2015;386(10000):1299–1310. doi:10.1016/S0140-6736(15)00277-9.

CHAPTER 16

Shoulder

Adnan Hussain, MD and Sanjeev Malik, MD

INTRODUCTION

The shoulder is composed of the proximal humerus, clavicle, and scapula. The joints of the shoulder include the sternoclavicular (SC), the acromioclavicular (AC), and the glenohumeral. There is also an articulation between the scapula and the thorax. Figures 16–1 to 16–3 provide the essential anatomy, both osseous and ligamentous, that must be understood to comprehend the disorders involving the shoulder. Superficial to the ligaments are the muscles that support the shoulder and provide for its global range of motion. The rotator cuff surrounds the glenohumeral joint and is composed of the supraspinatus, infraspinatus and teres minor muscles (insert on the greater tuberosity), and the subscapularis muscle (inserts on the lesser tuberosity) (Fig. 16–4). Superficial to these muscles is the deltoid, which functions as an abductor of the shoulder.

The clavicle is an oblong bone, the middle portion of which is tubular and the distal portion, flattened. It is anchored to the scapula laterally by the *AC* and the *coracoclavicular (CC)* ligaments. The *SC* and the *costoclavicular* ligaments anchor the clavicle medially (Fig. 16–3). The clavicle serves as points of attachment for both the sternocleidomastoid and the subclavius muscles. The ligaments and the muscles act in conjunction to anchor the clavicle and, thus, maintain the width of the shoulder and serve as the attachment point of the shoulder to the axial skeleton.

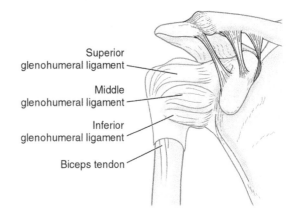

Figure 16–2. The ligaments around the shoulder.

The scapula consists of the body, spine, glenoid, acromion, and coracoid process. The bone is covered with thick muscles over its entire body and spine. On the posterior surface, the supraspinatus muscle covers the fossa superior to the spine, whereas the infraspinatus and teres minor muscles cover the fossa below the spine. The anterior surface of the scapula is separated from the rib cage by the subscapularis muscle. These muscles offer protection and support for the scapula. The scapula is connected to the axial skeleton only by way of the AC joint. The remainder of the scapular support is from the thick investing musculature surrounding its surface.

Examination

When examining the shoulder, start by assessing neurovascular structures. Neurovascular injuries frequently

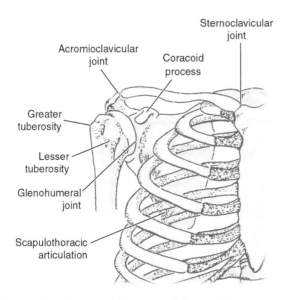

Figure 16–1. The essential anatomy of the shoulder.

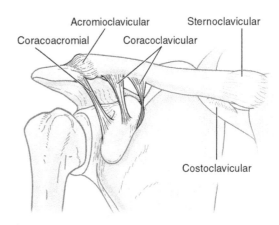

Figure 16–3. The ligamentous attachments of the clavicle to the sternum medially and the acromion laterally.

Anterior view

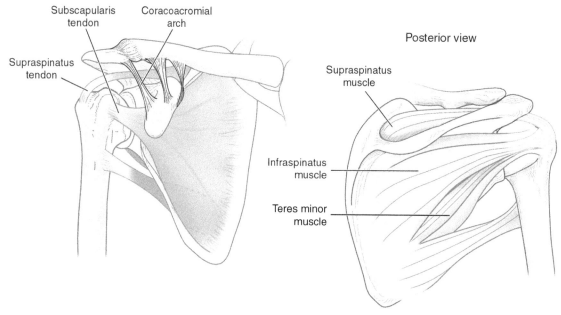

Figure 16–4. The rotator cuff.

accompany traumatic shoulder injuries. The structures in closest proximity to the shoulder include the brachial plexus, axillary nerve, and axillary artery (Fig. 16–5).

The range of motion of the shoulder can be assessed by testing internal and external rotation, as well as abduction

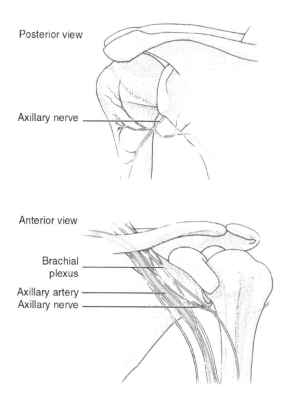

Figure 16–5. The course of the important neurovascular structures surrounding the shoulder.

(Fig. 16–6). With the arm abducted to 90 degrees, an individual can typically rotate to 90 degrees each of internal and external rotation. Throwing athletes may have developed a greater extent of external rotation with more limited internal rotation. In addition, internal rotation can be measured by having the patient put his/her hand on his/her back and gradually walk up the spine. Expected internal rotation allows the patient to reach the base of the scapula. Normal shoulder abduction and forward flexion is to 180 degrees.

The glenohumeral joint and scapulothoracic articulation function as a unit in abducting the humerus. The ratio of scapular to glenohumeral movement is 1:2; therefore, for every 30 degrees of abduction of the arm, the scapula moves 10 degrees and the glenohumeral joint moves 20 degrees (Fig. 16–7). If the glenohumeral joint is completely immobilized, the scapulothoracic articulation is capable of providing 65 degrees of abduction on its own. This "shrugging" mechanism is important for the physician to be aware of in assessing the movements at the shoulder joint that are hampered by certain pathologic entities.

At the SC joint, the clavicle is elevated 4 degrees for every 10 degrees of shoulder abduction. This elevation continues until 90 degrees of abduction have been obtained. The range of motion at the AC joint is approximately 20 degrees. This motion occurs during the first 30 degrees and after 100 degrees of abduction.

A number of structures can be palpated around the shoulder that are common sites of pathology. Palpation of the shoulder begins at the suprasternal notch. Find the SC joint just lateral to the notch. The clavicle is slightly superior to the manubrium, and one is actually palpating the

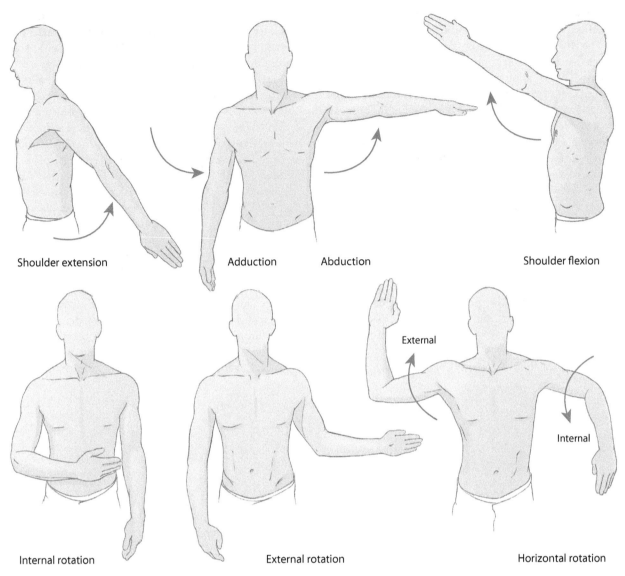

Shoulder extension   Adduction   Abduction   Shoulder flexion

Internal rotation   External rotation   Horizontal rotation

Figure 16–6. The movements of the shoulder.

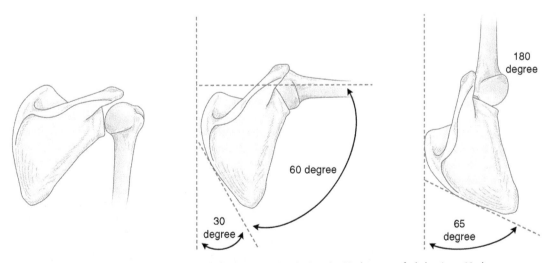

Figure 16–7. The ratio of glenohumeral to scapulothoracic motion is 2:1. At 90 degrees of abduction, 60 degrees occurs at the glenohumeral joint and 30 degrees at the scapulothoracic articulation. With the shrugging mechanism, one can abduct the shoulder 65 degrees because of scapulothoracic movement even though there is no motion at the glenohumeral joint.

proximal end of the clavicle at this point. The clavicle is superficial in its entire course and can be palpated easily.

The *AC joint* is palpated by identifying the lateral border of the clavicle as it approaches the flattened acromion process. The AC joint is more easily palpated if the patient is asked to move the shoulder several times while the examiner palpates the joint. The *greater tuberosity* of the humerus lies lateral to the acromion process and can be palpated by following the acromion process to its lateral edge and then sliding the fingers inferiorly. A small step-off exists between the lateral acromion border and the greater tuberosity.

The *bicipital groove* is bordered laterally by the greater tuberosity and medially by the lesser tuberosity. This structure can be palpated easily if the arm is rotated externally. External rotation places the groove in a more exposed position for palpation and permits the examiner to palpate the greater tuberosity first, then the bicipital groove, and finally the *lesser tuberosity* by moving from a lateral to medial position. The tendon of the biceps lies within this groove.

The *coracoid process* can be palpated by placing the patient in a relaxed position, noting the deepest portion of the clavicular concavity that lies along its lateral third and placing the fingers inferiorly approximately 2 to 3 cm

from the anterior edge of the clavicle. This region is the deltopectoral triangle, and by pressing into this triangle, one will also feel the coracoid process. The *scapula* can be seen posteriorly and covers ribs two through seven.

The *rotator cuff*, although not easily palpable, must be recognized, as it is a common site of pathologic processes. The muscles of the rotator cuff can be tested by assessing strength (Fig. 16-8). The supraspinatus muscle abducts the humeral head. To isolate this muscle, perform the *empty can test*. The affected arm is held upright in the plane of the scapula with the thumb down as if pouring out a can (90 degrees of abduction with 30 degrees of forward flexion and full internal rotation). The patient elevates the arm against resistance. Both the infraspinatus and teres minor externally rotate the arm, although the infraspinatus is responsible for 90% of external rotation strength. To assess the strength of the infraspinatus and teres minor, the *external rotation* test can be performed by having the patient hold the arm adducted to his/her side with the elbow flexed at 90 degrees. Have the patient attempt to externally rotate his/her forearm against resistance. The subscapularis muscle is responsible for internal rotation of the shoulder and can be assessed with the *lift-off test*. Have the patient hold

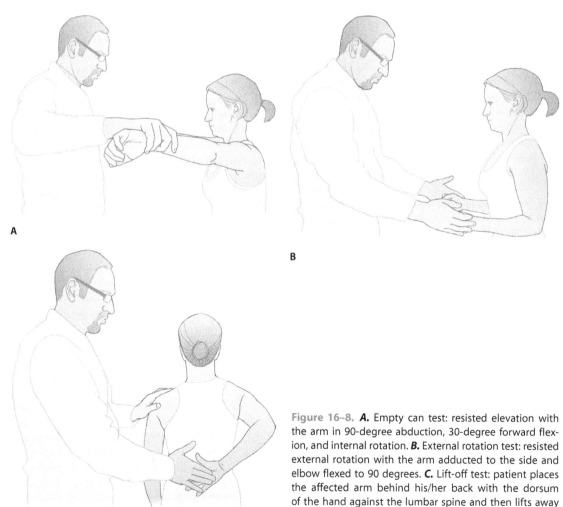

A

B

C

Figure 16–8. *A.* Empty can test: resisted elevation with the arm in 90-degree abduction, 30-degree forward flexion, and internal rotation. ***B.*** External rotation test: resisted external rotation with the arm adducted to the side and elbow flexed to 90 degrees. ***C.*** Lift-off test: patient places the affected arm behind his/her back with the dorsum of the hand against the lumbar spine and then lifts away from the back against resistance.

his/her hand behind his/her back at waist level and lift it away from the body against resistance.

Five bursae exist around the shoulder. The most important is the *subacromial (subdeltoid) bursa* because it separates the muscles of the rotator cuff from the deltoid muscle, acromion, and coracoacromial arch (Fig. 16–9). The subcoracoid bursa is located beneath the coracoid process. The subscapularis bursa is located near the tendinous junction of the subscapularis and the lesser tuberosity. The scapular bursae are located at the superior and inferior medial borders of the scapula and are separated from the chest wall.

Imaging

Radiographs of the shoulder include an anteroposterior (AP) view, "true" AP view (Grashey view), scapular Y view, and an axillary view (Fig. 16–10). The AP view is taken in both external and internal rotation. With the humerus in external rotation, the greater tuberosity is best visualized, whereas in

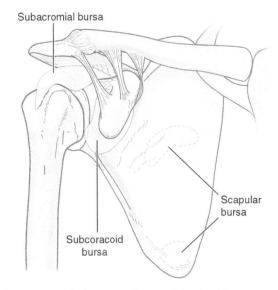

Figure 16–9. The important bursae of the shoulder.

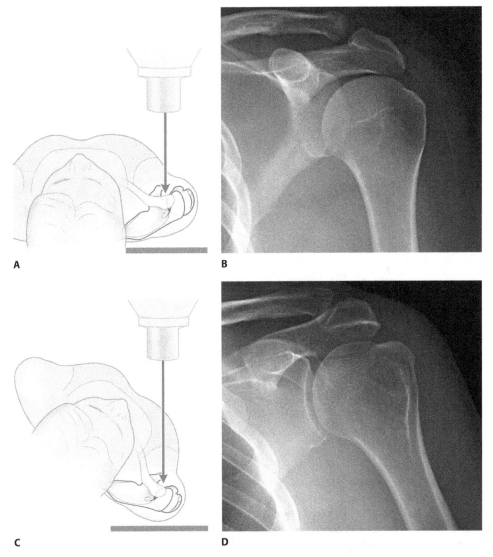

Figure 16–10. Shoulder radiographs. **A.** Anteroposterior (AP) projection. **B.** Normal AP view. **C.** True AP projection (Grashey view). **D.** Normal true AP radiograph. (*continued*)

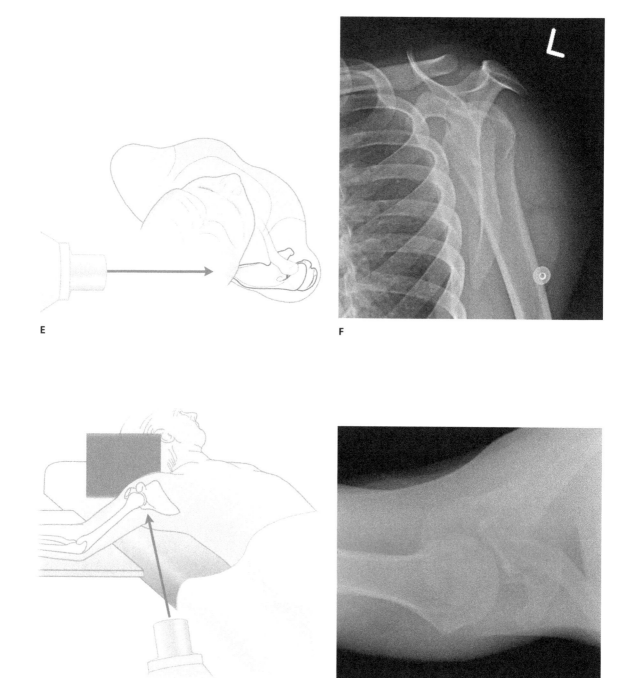

E

F

G

H

Figure 16–10. (*Continued*) *E.* Scapular "Y" projection. *F.* Normal scapular "Y" radiograph. The "Y" is made by the scapular body, spine, and coracoid process. The humeral head is centered at the junction of the "Y." *G.* Axillary projection. *H.* Normal axillary radiograph.

internal rotation, the lesser tuberosity is seen near the glenohumeral joint. A true AP view (Grashey view) is taken with the plate parallel to the scapula and requires the beam to be angled 45 degrees from a medial position to a lateral position toward the shoulder. This view is helpful to confirm a proper articulation of the humeral head with the glenoid.

The scapular Y view and axillary views help to identify glenohumeral dislocations and scapular fractures, as well as proximal humerus fractures. The "Y" is formed by the body, spine, and coracoid process of the scapula. In a normal radiograph, the humeral head is seen at the junction of the "Y." An axillary view, obtained with the arm abducted 90 degrees, is often not tolerated by the patient due to pain. These films may be obtained with the patient supine, standing, or sitting, although we recommend the sitting position.

SHOULDER FRACTURES

PROXIMAL HUMERUS FRACTURES

Proximal humerus fractures account for 3% of upper-extremity fractures and are most commonly seen in the elderly patient.

The proximal humerus is defined as the portion of the humerus proximal to the surgical neck (Fig. 16–11). The surgical neck is the narrowest portion of the proximal humerus. The anatomic neck marks the end of the articular surface of the shoulder joint. The greater and lesser tuberosities are bony prominences located just distal to the anatomic neck.

There are several muscles that insert on and surround the proximal humerus. The supraspinatus, infraspinatus, and teres minor insert on the greater tuberosity and tend to pull fracture fragments in a superior direction with some anterior rotation. The subscapularis muscle inserts on the lesser tuberosity. This muscle tends to pull fracture fragments in a medial direction with posterior rotation. The pectoralis major muscle inserts on the lateral lip of the intertubercular groove, whereas the deltoid muscle inserts on the deltoid tubercle. These muscles tend to exert medial and superior forces, respectively, on the humeral shaft after proximal humerus fractures.

The classification system of proximal humerus fractures was developed by Neer.[13] The proximal humerus is divided into four segments (Fig. 16–12).

- Greater tuberosity
- Lesser tuberosity
- Humeral head
- Humeral shaft

This classification system has both prognostic and therapeutic implications and depends only on the relationship of the bone segments involved and their displacement.

After injury, if all proximal humeral fragments are non-displaced and without angulation, the injury is classified as a *one-part fracture*. If a fragment has greater than 1 cm of displacement or angulation greater than 45 degrees from the remaining intact proximal humerus, the fracture is classified as a *two-part fracture*. If two fragments are individually displaced from the remaining proximal humerus, the fracture is classified as a *three-part fracture*. Finally, if all four fragments are individually displaced, the fracture is a *four-part fracture*. It is important to recall that displacement must be greater than 1 cm or angulation greater than 45 degrees to be considered a separate "part" (Fig. 16–13). Note that three- and four-part fractures are often associated with a dislocation. Articular surface fractures are not included in the Neer system and are discussed separately at the end of the chapter.

Nearly 80% of all proximal humeral fractures are one-part fractures.[1] The humeral fragments are held in place by the periosteum, rotator cuff, and joint capsule. The initial stabilization and management of these fractures should be initiated by the emergency physician. The remaining 20% of proximal humeral fractures (two-, three-, or four-part fractures) require reduction and may remain unstable after reduction.

The treatment of proximal humerus fractures varies depending on the age of the patient and his/her lifestyle. Nondisplaced (i.e., one-part) fractures may be treated with a sling and swathe or a sling alone (Appendix A–13). Early passive exercises are generally recommended (Fig. 16–14). Active exercises are recommended during the later stages of healing. More complex, displaced, or angulated fractures often require operative management and are treated according to the classification system presented later.

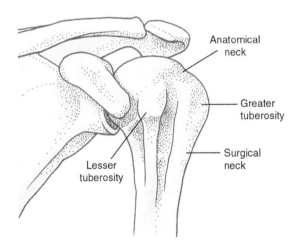

Figure 16–11. Anatomy of the proximal humerus.

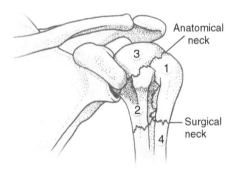

Figure 16–12. The four parts of the proximal humerus referred to in the Neer classification include the (1) greater tuberosity, (2) lesser tuberosity, (3) humeral head, and (4) humeral shaft. Fractures are classified according to displacement of one or more of the "parts" from the remainder. Displacement is defined as separation of greater than 1 cm from the humerus or angulation of the part greater than 45 degrees.

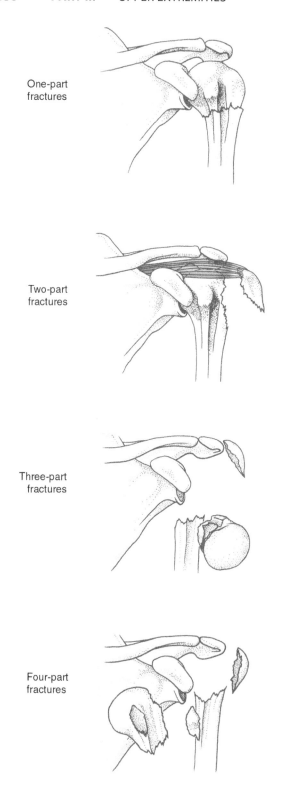

One-part
fractures

Two-part
fractures

Three-part
fractures

Four-part
fractures

Figure 16–13. Examples of one-, two-, three-, and four-part fractures as described by Neer.

Axiom: *Successful treatment of proximal humerus fractures is dependent on early mobility. A compromise in anatomic reduction may be accepted so prolonged immobilization can be avoided.*

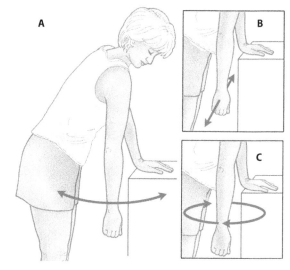

Figure 16–14. Codman exercises. **A.** The exercises begin with the patient's arm suspended and use a back-and-forth swinging movement. **B.** Next, side-to-side movement is performed in a medial–lateral direction. **C.** Finally, clockwise and counterclockwise rotational movements are performed. These three movements are repeated with the arc of movement increased daily as the patient's inflammatory condition improves.

Subsequent discussion of proximal humerus fractures will be divided up into individual fractures and combination fractures as following:

- Surgical neck fractures
- Anatomic neck fractures
- Greater tuberosity fractures
- Lesser tuberosity fractures
- Combination (three- or four-part) fractures
- Articular surface fractures

Surgical Neck Fractures

Surgical neck fractures may alter the angle that the humeral head makes with the shaft. The normal angle between the humeral head and the shaft is 135 degrees (Fig. 16–15). An

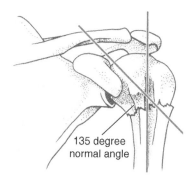

135 degree
normal angle

Figure 16–15. The normal angle between the humeral head and the shaft is 135 degrees. An angle of less than or equal to 90 degrees or greater than 180 degrees is significant and may require reduction, depending on the age and activity of the patient.

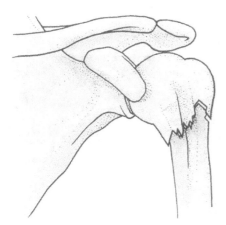

Figure 16–16. Surgical neck fracture.

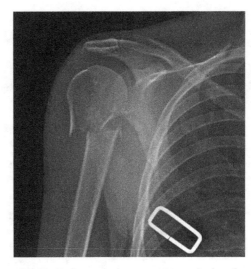

Figure 16–17. Radiograph demonstrating a displaced surgical neck fracture.

angle of less than 90 degrees or greater than 180 degrees may require reduction depending on the age and activity of the patient because healing in this manner can alter the mechanics of the shoulder.

Surgical neck fractures can be divided into three classes—one-part (i.e., nondisplaced and nonangulated), two-part (angulated or displaced), or comminuted fractures. As stated previously, one-part fractures are displaced less than 1 cm and angulated less than 45 degrees from normal (Fig. 16–16).

Mechanism of Injury

Two mechanisms result in surgical neck fractures of the proximal humerus. The most common mechanism is indirect and is due to a fall on the outstretched arm. If the arm was abducted during the fall, the humeral shaft will be displaced laterally. If, however, the arm was adducted during the fall, the humeral shaft will be displaced medially in most cases.

Direct trauma, which is often minimal in the elderly, may result in a surgical neck fracture.

Examination

The patient will present with tenderness and swelling over the upper arm and shoulder. If, on presentation, the arm is held in adduction, the incidence of brachial plexus and axillary arterial injury is low. If the patient presents with the arm abducted, the incidence of neurovascular injury is much more significant. Before the radiographic examination, document the presence of distal pulses and sensory function.

Axiom: *A patient with a suspected surgical neck fracture, who presents with the arm abducted, should have the extremity immobilized in the position of presentation before radiographs. These patients may have a severely displaced fracture, and adduction may result in neurovascular damage.*

Imaging

The trauma series, including an AP view in internal and external rotation, scapular Y view, and axillary view, is usually adequate in demonstrating these fractures (Fig. 16–17). Multidetector computed tomography (CT) is useful for detecting occult fractures not seen on plain radiographs.

Proximal humerus fractures associated with a hemarthrosis may displace the humeral head inferiorly. Radiographically, this is referred to as a *pseudosubluxation*, indicating the presence of an intra-articular fracture (Fig. 16–18). An additional radiographic sign indicating an intra-articular fracture is the presence of a *fat fluid line*.

Associated Injuries

Nondisplaced surgical neck fractures may be associated with a contusion or tear of the axillary nerve, although neurovascular injuries are more common after displaced or comminuted fractures of the surgical neck.

Treatment

A nondisplaced (<1 cm) surgical neck fracture with less than 45-degree angulation is a one-part fracture. A sling is the recommended mode of therapy. Ice and analgesics with hand exercises should be initiated soon after injury. Circumduction exercises should begin as soon as tolerated and be followed by elbow and shoulder passive exercises at 2 to 3 weeks. Shoulder motion exercises can usually be started within 3 to 4 weeks.

In elderly patients with lower physical demands, significant angulation (>45 degrees) can be well tolerated as long as there is some bony contact. However, in young patients, these injuries require reduction. A portion of the periosteum remains intact and will aid in a closed reduction. The emergency department (ED) management consists of immobilization in a sling, analgesics, and urgent referral for reduction.

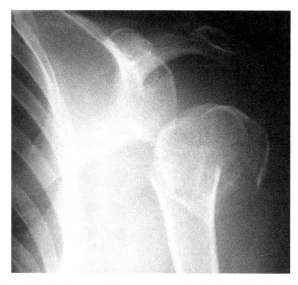
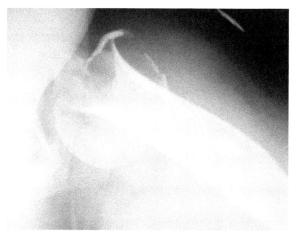

Figure 16–18. Pseudodislocation secondary to hemarthrosis after a proximal humerus fracture. On the AP view, the humeral head appears dislocated, but the axillary view shows proper placement. Despite the fact that both the greater tuberosity and surgical neck are fractured, this injury is classified as a two-part fracture because the greater tuberosity fragment is not displaced.

The emergency management of displaced two-part surgical neck fractures includes sling immobilization, ice, analgesics, and emergent referral. Closed reduction under regional or general anesthesia is preferred followed by immobilization in a sling. If the reduction is unstable, percutaneous pins or open reduction is performed.

If emergent referral is not available in a situation of limb-threatening vascular compromise, reduction using procedural sedation can be carried out using the following methods (Fig. 16–19):

1. With the patient supine or at 45 degrees upright, the physician should apply steady traction to the arm along the long axis of the humerus.

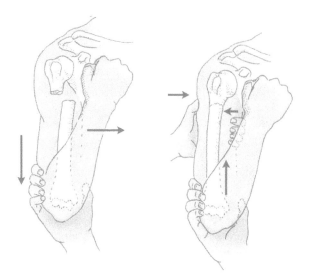

Figure 16–19. The method for reducing a displaced fracture of the proximal humerus. Distraction followed by repositioning of the distal fragment is vital in all reductions.

2. While maintaining traction, the arm is brought across the anterior chest and flexed slightly.
3. While traction is maintained to distract the fragments, the other hand of the physician is placed along the fractured medial border of the humerus. The fragments are manipulated manually back into position, and the traction is gradually released.
4. A complete neurovascular examination must be documented after any attempt at a manipulative reduction. After this, a sling and swathe dressing should be applied.

The emergency management of comminuted surgical neck fractures includes immobilization, ice, analgesics, and urgent referral. Definitive therapeutic alternatives include a hanging cast, internal fixation, or overhead olecranon pin traction.

Complications

Surgical neck fractures are associated with several significant complications.

- Joint stiffness with adhesions can be avoided or minimized with early motion exercises.
- Malunion is common after displaced fractures.
- Myositis ossificans involves calcification at the site of injured adjacent musculature.

Anatomic Neck Fractures

Anatomic neck fractures are through the area of the physis (Fig. 16–20) and can be divided into adult or childhood injuries. Adult injuries are rare and may be classified as nondisplaced or displaced (>1 cm). Childhood injuries are generally limited to 8- to 14-year-olds.

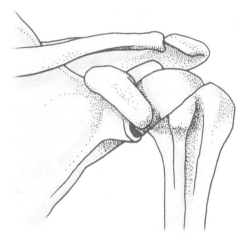

Figure 16–20. Anatomic neck fracture. (Used with permission from the Department of Emergency Medicine, Feinberg School of Medicine, Northwestern University. http://www.feinberg.north western.edu/emergencymed/).

Mechanism of Injury

The usual mechanism is a fall on the outstretched arm.

Examination

Swelling and tenderness to palpation will be apparent in the shoulder area. Pain will be increased with any shoulder motion.

Imaging

Routine radiographic views are generally adequate for demonstrating the fracture. In children, a Salter II injury is most common.

Associated Injuries

Anatomic neck fractures are usually not associated with any serious surrounding injuries.

Treatment

The emergency management of these fractures includes immobilization in a sling and swathe (Appendix A–13), ice, analgesics, and early referral. Both nondisplaced and displaced fractures will require orthopedic referral. Emergent referral is indicated for displaced fractures because they will require open reduction in young patients or early prosthetic replacement in older patients.

Childhood anatomic neck fractures are *proximal humeral epiphyseal* injuries. Ice, sling immobilization, analgesics, and emergent referral are strongly recommended.

Complications

Anatomic neck injuries are often complicated by the development of *avascular necrosis*. It is our recommendation that physicians treating anatomic neck fractures consult with an orthopedic surgeon from the ED before therapy and refer all patients for follow-up.

> **Axiom:** *Anatomic neck fractures are frequently complicated by avascular necrosis. Consult an orthopedic surgeon from the ED for emergent referral.*

Greater Tuberosity Fractures

Greater tuberosity fractures are common and are seen in isolation or in approximately 15% of all shoulder dislocations. These fractures can be nondisplaced or displaced (Fig. 16–21). Displacement is common due to the effect of the rotator cuff muscles. The supraspinatus, the infraspinatus, and the teres minor insert on the greater tuberosity and, when fractured, cause upward displacement of the fragment. The superiorly displaced tuberosity will mechanically block abduction of the shoulder. Displaced fractures of the greater tuberosity are associated with tears of the rotator cuff. Greater tuberosity fractures are an exception to the Neer classification in that only 0.5 cm of displacement is necessary for operative fixation of the fragment.

Mechanism of Injury

Two mechanisms can result in greater tuberosity fractures. Compression fractures are usually the result of a direct blow

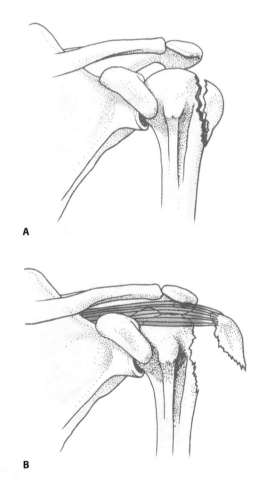

A

B

Figure 16–21. Greater tuberosity fractures. **A.** Nondisplaced. **B.** Displaced (>5 mm).

to the upper humerus, as during a fall. The elderly are particularly susceptible to these injuries due to atrophy and weakening of the surrounding musculature.

Nondisplaced fractures usually result from a fall on the outstretched arm (indirect). Displaced fractures are secondary to a fall on the outstretched arm with rotator cuff contraction resulting in displacement.

Examination

The patient will complain of pain and swelling over the greater tuberosity. The patient will be unable to abduct the arm and will note increased pain with external rotation. Also, external rotation of the shoulder may be inhibited if a posteriorly displaced tuberosity impinges against the posterior glenoid.

Imaging

AP radiographs usually demonstrate these fractures (Fig. 16–22). Although the AP view is able to assess for superior displacement, it often fails to demonstrate precisely the amount of posterior retraction and overlap of the fragment with the articular surface. Axillary radiographs can be used to assess the amount of posterior retraction. If AP radiographs are used alone, the posterior displacement will be underestimated as well as the number of two-part displaced fractures. A nonemergent CT scan will accurately diagnose the degree of displacement if a question remains.

Associated Injuries

Neurovascular injuries are rarely associated with these fractures. Greater tuberosity fractures are commonly associated with anterior shoulder dislocations and rotator cuff tears. Both injuries are more common with displaced fractures.

Treatment

Nondisplaced. The emergency management of nondisplaced fractures of the greater tuberosity consists of ice, analgesics, sling immobilization (Appendix A–13), and early referral because of the high incidence of complications.

Displaced (>0.5 cm). If associated with an anterior shoulder dislocation, reduction of the dislocation often corrects the displacement of the greater tuberosity, and the fracture can then be managed as a nondisplaced fracture.

Management in the ED includes ice, sling immobilization (Appendix A–13), adequate pain control, and early orthopedic referral. If displacement remains or a displaced fracture is present without a shoulder dislocation, the definitive management of these injuries depends on the age and activity of the patient. Young patients require internal fixation of the fragment with repair of the torn rotator cuff. Good bone stock must be present for fixation with screws, and this is frequently lacking in elderly patients. Older patients are usually not candidates for surgical repair and are managed conservatively. Early mobilization in the elderly patient is essential.

Complications

Greater tuberosity fractures may be associated with several complications:

* Compression fractures are often complicated by impingement on the long head of the biceps, resulting in chronic tenosynovitis and eventually tendon rupture.
* Nonunion.
* Myositis ossificans.

Lesser Tuberosity Fractures

Isolated lesser tuberosity fractures are uncommon. They commonly occur in conjunction with posterior shoulder dislocations. Fracture fragments may be small or large (>1 cm) (Fig. 16–23). These injuries are commonly missed on initial presentation.

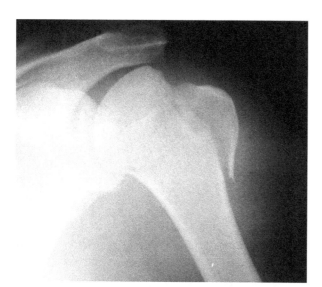

Figure 16–22. Displaced fracture of the greater tuberosity.

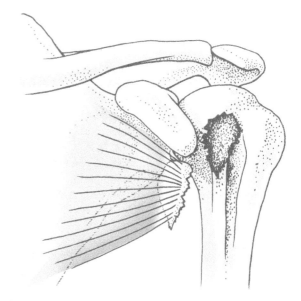

Figure 16–23. Lesser tuberosity fracture.

Mechanism of Injury

Lesser tuberosity fractures are usually associated with an indirect mechanism of injury such as a seizure or a fall on the adducted arm. Both situations result in an intense contraction of the subscapularis muscle to resist the abduction and external rotation force, resulting in an avulsion of the lesser tuberosity.[5]

Examination

Tenderness to palpation will be present over the lesser tuberosity. Pain will be increased with active external rotation or adduction against resistance. In addition, passive external rotation will exacerbate the pain.

Imaging

Routine shoulder views are generally adequate in demonstrating this fracture. An axillary lateral or scapular Y view should be obtained to ensure there is no associated dislocation.

Associated Injuries

Posterior dislocations of the shoulder are commonly associated with these injuries. In addition, nondisplaced surgical neck fractures may be associated with these fractures. Neurovascular injuries are rarely associated with lesser tuberosity fractures.

Treatment

The emergency management of all lesser tuberosity fractures includes ice, analgesics, sling immobilization (Appendix A–13), and early outpatient orthopedic consultation. Nondisplaced fractures may be managed either conservatively or operatively, depending on the preference of the orthopedic surgeon. Due to the rarity of the injury, the medical literature is mixed on which management is preferred with studies supporting both approaches. It is generally agreed that displaced fractures should be managed with open reduction and internal fixation.[6]

Complications

These fractures usually heal without complications because of compensation by the surrounding shoulder musculature. Some surgeons believe that this fracture can lead to a weakening of the anterior capsular support that may predispose to the development of recurrent anterior dislocations. They may also predispose to dislocation of the biceps tendon.[6]

Combination Proximal Humerus Fractures

Combination fractures refer to Neer fractures that are classified as three- or four-part injuries (Figs. 16–24 and 16–25). These fractures are usually the result of severe injury forces and are often associated with dislocations.

Mechanism of Injury

The most common mechanism is a hard fall on the outstretched arm. The segments involved and the amount of

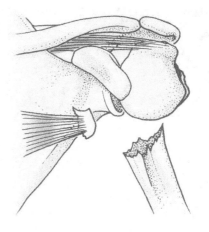

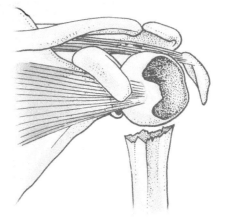

Figure 16–24. Combination fractures—three-part fracture.

displacement are dependent on the force of the fall and the muscular tone at the time of injury.

Examination

Diffuse pain and swelling of the proximal humerus will be apparent and the patient will resist all motion.

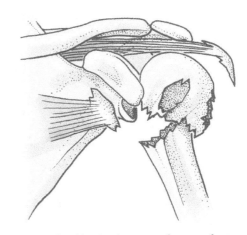

Figure 16–25. Combination fractures—four-part fracture.

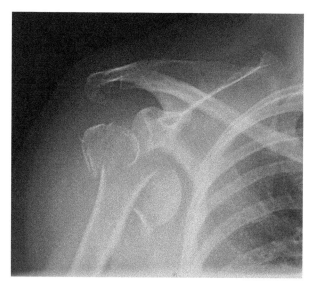

Figure 16–26. Combination fracture of the proximal humerus.

Imaging

AP views and a scapular Y view are generally adequate in delineating these fractures (Fig. 16–26).

Associated Injuries

Combined proximal humerus fractures are associated with several significant injuries:

- Shoulder dislocations
- Rotator cuff injuries
- Injuries to the brachial plexus, the axillary vessels, and the axillary and musculocutaneous nerves

Treatment

Emergency management includes ice, analgesics, sling immobilization, and emergent referral—often necessitating admission. Virtually all combined fractures require surgical repair and, in some instances, the insertion of a prosthesis (four-part fractures).

Complications

As noted previously, neurovascular injuries may complicate the management of these fractures. Four-part fractures are complicated by a high incidence of avascular necrosis of the humeral head secondary to a compromised blood supply.

Articular Surfaces Fractures

Articular surface fractures are referred to as *impression fractures* by some authors (Fig. 16–27). These fractures may be classified as follows: (1) impression fracture with less than 40% involvement, (2) impression fracture with more than 40% involvement, and (3) comminuted articular surface fracture (head splitting).

Mechanism of Injury

Impression fractures are usually secondary to a direct blow to the lateral arm as during a fall. Anterior shoulder dislocations may be associated with an impression fracture on the lateral aspect of the humeral head and are referred to as a Hill–Sachs fracture.

Examination

Impression fractures are associated with only minimal pain with humeral motion. Comminuted articular surface fractures are generally associated with severe pain.

Imaging

Typically, AP views with internal and external rotation are best for visualization of the fracture lines (Fig. 16–28). Impression fractures are often difficult to define, and frequently, secondary signs of fracture are employed in making the correct diagnosis. The presence of a *fat fluid level* on the AP upright film is indicative of an articular surface fracture.

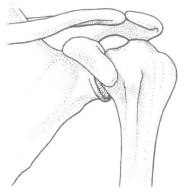

Impression fracture (<40%)

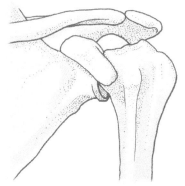

Impression fracture (>40%)

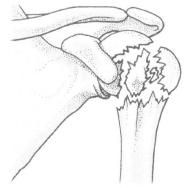

Comminuted articular surface fracture (head splitting)

Figure 16–27. Articular surface fractures.

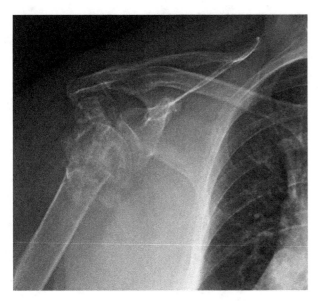

Figure 16–28. Comminuted humeral head fracture.

In addition, inferior pseudosubluxation of the humeral head secondary to a hemarthrosis is often seen in conjunction with impression fractures.

Associated Injuries

Articular surface fractures are often associated with anterior or posterior shoulder dislocations.

Treatment

The emergency management of these fractures includes ice, analgesics, sling immobilization, and early referral. When less than 40% of the articular surface is involved, the arm is immobilized in external rotation. Surgical repair or the insertion of a prosthesis may be indicated for comminuted fractures or impression fractures involving more than 40% of the articular surface. Because elderly patients require early mobility, surgical repair may not be elected.

Complications

Articular surface fractures may be complicated by the following conditions:

* Joint stiffness
* Arthritis
* Avascular necrosis (seen most frequently with comminuted fractures)

CLAVICLE FRACTURES

Clavicle fractures are the most common of all childhood fractures. Overall, clavicle fractures account for 5% of all the fractures seen for all age groups. Clavicle fractures can be divided into three groups in the Allman Classification on

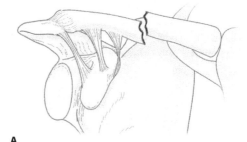

A

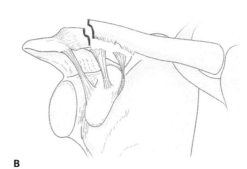

B

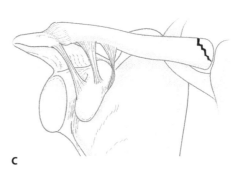

C

Figure 16–29. Clavicle fractures. ***A.*** Middle third. ***B.*** Lateral third. ***C.*** Medial third (involving the sternoclavicular joint).

the basis of anatomy, therapy, and incidence (Fig. 16–29).[7,8] They are distributed as follows:

* Middle third—80%
* Lateral third—15%
* Medial third—5%

The majority of middle-third fractures occur at the junction of the middle and outer thirds of the clavicle, medial to the CC ligaments. They are classified as nondisplaced or displaced. Typically, the proximal fragment is displaced superiorly because of the pull of the sternocleidomastoid. Both the subclavian vessels and the brachial plexus lie in close proximity to the clavicle. Displaced clavicle fractures can be associated with injuries to these vital structures.

Lateral-third fractures occur distal to the CC ligaments. They are divided into three types: (1) nondisplaced, (2) displaced, and (3) articular. Displaced lateral-third fractures are associated with rupture of the CC ligaments. Typically, the proximal clavicular segment will be pulled upward by the sternocleidomastoid. Articular surface fractures involve the AC joint.

Medial-third clavicle fractures are uncommon. Strong forces are required to fracture the medial-third clavicle, and therefore, a diligent search for associated injuries should accompany these fractures.

Mechanism of Injury

Two mechanisms are commonly responsible for clavicle fracture. A direct blow to the clavicle is the first mechanism. A posteriorly directed force may result in a single fracture. If the force is directed inferiorly, the resulting fracture is often comminuted. Neurovascular damage is more likely with inferiorly directed forces.

The indirect mechanism is typified by a fall on the lateral shoulder. The force is transmitted via the acromion to the clavicle. The clavicle usually fractures in the middle-third because the natural "S" shape of the clavicle has a tendency to focus the indirect force at this point.

Lateral-third clavicle fractures are usually the result of a blow from above, directed downward to the lateral third of the clavicle. Articular surface fractures usually result from a blow to the outer aspect of the shoulder (a fall) or a compression force.

Medial-third clavicle fractures can be produced by a direct blow to the medial clavicle, by a force to the lateral shoulder that compresses the clavicle against the sternum, or a fall on the abducted outstretched arm that compresses the clavicle against the sternum.

Examination

The clavicle is subcutaneous over nearly its entire extent, and therefore, fractures can be easily diagnosed on the basis of examination. Patients will have swelling and tenderness over the fracture site (Fig. 16–30). Middle-third clavicle

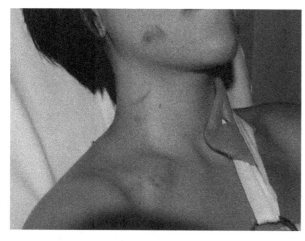

Figure 16–30. Middle-third clavicle fracture with visible soft-tissue swelling. (Used with permission from Northwestern Emergency Medicine teaching file.)

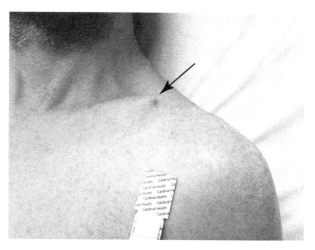

Figure 16–31. Tenting of the skin due to a clavicle fracture (*arrow*).

fractures usually result in a downward and inward slump of the involved shoulder due to loss of support. Patients will usually carry their arm adducted against the chest wall and will resist motion of the extremity. If severe displacement is present that is associated with the tearing of the soft tissues, ecchymosis may be present. All clavicle fractures require examination and documentation of the neurovascular function distal to the injury.

Patients with lateral- or medial-third clavicle fractures will carry the arm in adduction. The pain will be increased with palpation or with attempted abduction. Displaced fractures may have palpable displacement on examination. Despite the subcutaneous nature of the clavicle, open clavicle fractures are uncommon. However, the presence of significant skin tenting should prompt orthopedic consultation for consideration of urgent surgical reduction (Fig. 16–31).

Imaging

The routine clavicle radiograph (apical lordotic, tube-directed, 45-degree cephalad) is generally adequate in defining clavicle fractures (Fig. 16–32).

Articular surface fractures, however, may be difficult to detect radiographically. Tilting the beam 10 to 15 degrees toward the head will avoid superimposing the scapular spine and allow for more subtle detection of injuries. Special techniques such as cone views, lateral views, or weight-bearing (10 lb) films may be helpful for accurate delineation. CT may be necessary when an articular surface fracture is suspected.

Associated Injuries

Subclavian vascular injuries may occur, especially with displaced middle-third clavicle fractures. When a vascular injury is suspected, angiographic studies are strongly recommended. Neurologic damage may involve either contusion or avulsion of the nerve roots. A meticulous neurologic

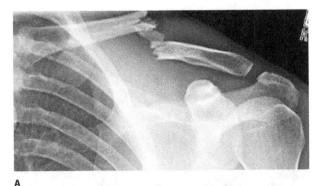

A

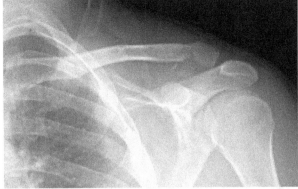

B

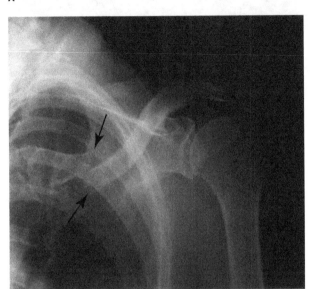

C

Figure 16–32. **A.** Middle-third clavicle fracture. The proximal fragment is displaced superiorly due to the pull of the sterno-cleidomastoid. **B.** Distal-third clavicle fracture. **C.** Medial-third clavicle fracture (*arrow*).

examination of cervical nerve roots 4 through 8 should accompany the diagnosis of any displaced clavicle fracture.

CC ligament damage is associated with lateral-third clavicle fractures.

> **Axiom:** *All displaced lateral-third clavicular fractures are associated with CC ligament rupture and should be treated similar to an AC joint dislocation.*

AC joint subluxation or dislocation may accompany any lateral-third clavicle fracture.

Medial-third clavicle fractures, which usually secondary to severe forces, may be associated with significant underlying organ damage. Intrathoracic injury must be excluded early in the management if the fracture is posteriorly displaced. Sternal fractures or subluxation of the SC joint may be associated with these fractures.

Treatment

Childhood clavicle fractures generally require little treatment because rapid healing with remodeling and full return of function is the usual outcome. Further discussion of clavicle fractures in children is included in Chapter 6. Adult clavicle fractures are associated with more serious complications and, therefore, require a more accurate reduction and closer follow-up to ensure a full return of function.

Middle-Third Clavicle Fractures

Nondisplaced. Nondisplaced fractures have an intact periosteum and, therefore, a sling for support and ice is all that is necessary. Repeat radiographs at 1 week are obtained to ensure proper positioning. Children generally require 3 to 5 weeks of immobilization, whereas adults usually require 6 weeks or more.

Displaced. Attempts at closed reduction in the ED will not improve fracture healing or permanently alter the alignment.[15] Immobilization with a sling is the treatment of choice of the authors. There is no improved outcome when a figure-of-eight clavicle strap is used.[13,14] The figure-of-eight strap does allow patients the ability to use both hands and may allow them to return to activities such as typing

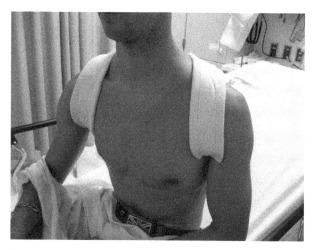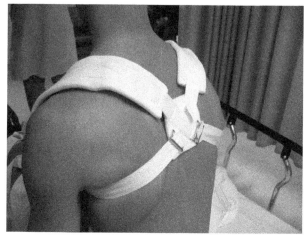

Figure 16–33. Application of figure-of-eight harness for clavicle fractures. Studies have found no major differences in outcomes when compared with a sling.

sooner (Fig. 16-33). In this case, the patient may elect the clavicle strap over a sling. Orthopedic consultation is recommended when there is significant tenting of the skin.

Orthopedic referral for operative consideration is recommended in patients with displaced middle-third clavicle fractures. The incidence of nonunion (15%–20%) and symptomatic malunion (20%–25%) is high. Other factors that are associated with poor outcome include comminution and shortening. Surgical fixation with either a plate or intramedullary nail improves the functional outcome in young active patients with completely displaced midshaft fractures and reduces rates of nonunion and symptomatic malunion (approximately 2%).

Lateral-Third Clavicle Fractures

Nondisplaced. Nondisplaced lateral-third clavicle fractures, which are splinted by the surrounding intact ligaments and muscles, are usually treated symptomatically with ice, analgesics, and early motion.

Displaced. Displaced lateral-third clavicle fractures have a high rate of nonunion (11%). The emergency management of these fractures includes sling immobilization, ice, analgesics, and orthopedic referral for operative consideration. The management of these injuries have been somewhat debatable as nonunion may be relatively asymptomatic, particularly in elderly patients.

Articular Surface Involvement. These patients should be treated symptomatically with ice, analgesics, and a sling for support. Early motion is strongly urged to prevent the development of degenerative arthritis.

Medial-Third Clavicle Fractures

The emergency management includes ice, analgesics, and a sling for support. Displaced medial-third fractures require orthopedic referral for reduction.

Complications

Clavicle fractures may be associated with several complications:

- Malunion is primarily a complication of adult fractures. In children, malunion is uncommon due to the extensive remodeling that normally accompanies these fractures.
- Excessive callus formation may occur, resulting in a cosmetic defect or neurovascular compromise.
- Nonunion.
- Delayed union is frequently associated with displaced lateral-third clavicle fractures treated conservatively.
- Degenerative arthritis may be noted after fractures of the medial or lateral clavicle that extend into the articular surface.

SCAPULAR FRACTURES

Scapular fractures are relatively uncommon injuries that generally occur in patients between 40 and 60 years of age. This type of injury represents only 1% of all fractures and 5% of fractures involving the shoulder. There are a multitude of fracture patterns associated with the scapula. Frequently, scapular fractures, such as a glenoid rim fracture, are associated with glenohumeral dislocations.

Several muscles insert on the scapula and may initiate displacing forces when fractures are encountered. The triceps inserts on the inferior rim of the glenoid fossa, whereas the short head of the biceps, the coracobrachialis, and the pectoralis minor insert on the coracoid process.

Scapular fractures (Fig. 16-34) are classified anatomically into the following:

- Body or spine fractures
- Acromion fractures
- Neck fractures
- Glenoid fractures
- Coracoid process fractures

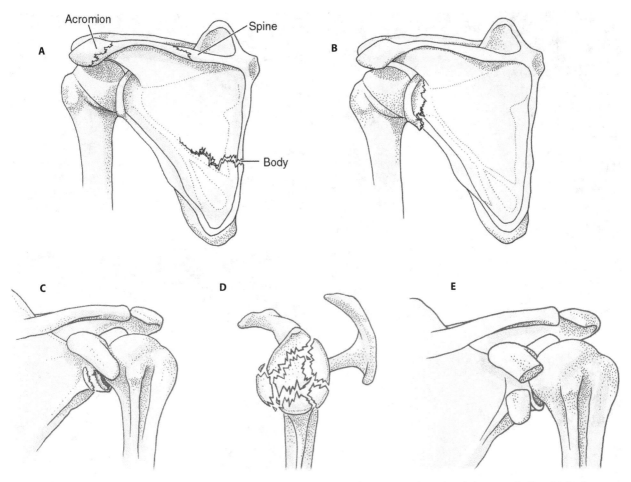

Figure 16–34. Scapula fractures. **A.** Body or spine fractures and acromion fracture. **B.** Glenoid neck fracture. **C.** Glenoid rim fracture. **D.** Comminuted glenoid articular surface fracture. **E.** Coracoid process fracture.

Scapular Body or Spine Fractures

Mechanism of Injury

The mechanism involved is usually a direct blow over the involved area. A great deal of force is necessary to fracture the body or the spine of the scapula, and associated injuries may complicate or mask these fractures. Typically, there is little displacement due to the support of the investing muscles and the periosteum.

Examination

The patient will present with pain, swelling, and ecchymosis over the involved area. The involved extremity will be held in adduction, and the patient will resist abduction. Abduction past the first 90 degrees is largely the result of scapular motion and, thus, will exacerbate the pain.

Imaging

Routine AP and scapular views (Y view) are generally adequate in defining these fractures (Fig. 16–35A). Tangential oblique views may be helpful in defining small body fractures. CT imaging with 3D reconstruction may provide better visualization (Fig. 16–35B).[20]

Associated Injuries

Scapular fractures involving the body or the spine are usually the result of large blunt forces and may be associated with several life-threatening injuries.[21,22] Classic teaching has suggested that a fractured scapula heralds blunt thoracic aortic injury. One recent study found that in patients with scapular fractures following blunt trauma, only 1% had an associated aortic injury.[21] Other associated injuries to consider include[21,22]:

- Pneumothorax or pulmonary contusion.
- Rib or vertebral compression fractures.
- Both upper- and lower-extremity fractures.
- Injuries to the axillary artery, nerve, or brachial plexus are rare.

Treatment

The emergency management of these fractures includes (1) sling or (2) sling and swathe (Appendix A–13) immobilization

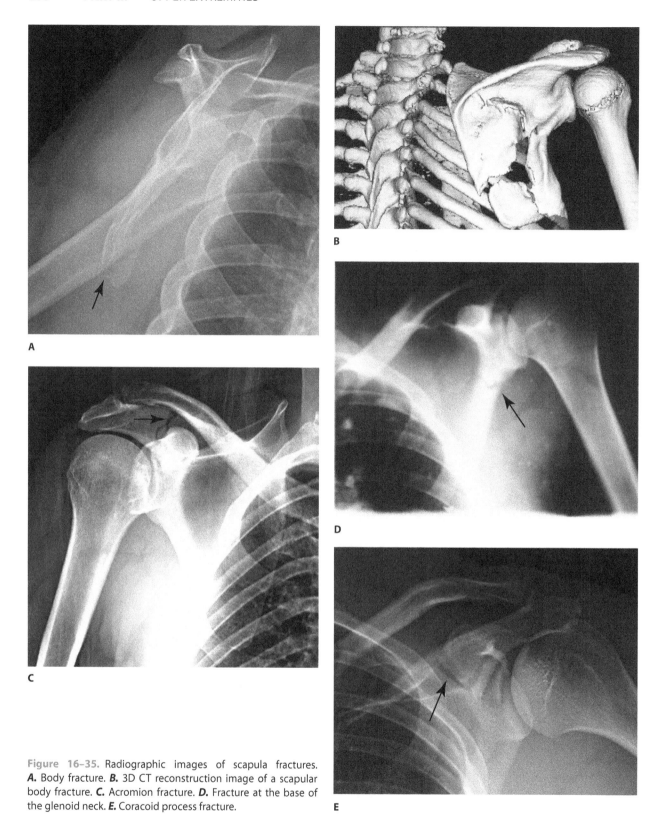

Figure 16–35. Radiographic images of scapula fractures. **A.** Body fracture. **B.** 3D CT reconstruction image of a scapular body fracture. **C.** Acromion fracture. **D.** Fracture at the base of the glenoid neck. **E.** Coracoid process fracture.

with ice and analgesics. *It is essential to exclude the possibility of life- or limb-threatening injuries early when managing these fractures.* After approximately 2 to 3 weeks, limited activity as tolerated is advised. Although absolute surgical indications are debated in the literature, significantly displaced or angulated fractures with functional impairment should be referred urgently for consideration of open reduction and internal fixation.

Complications

Neurovascular or visceral injuries as mentioned previously may complicate the management of these fractures.

Acromion Fractures

Mechanism of Injury

Acromion fractures are usually the result of a direct downward blow to the shoulder. The force required is generally large, and associated injuries often complicate the management of these fractures. Superior dislocation of the shoulder may result in a superiorly displaced fracture of the acromion.

Examination

Tenderness and swelling will be maximal over the acromion process. The pain will be exacerbated with deltoid stressing.

Imaging

Routine scapular radiographs are generally adequate in defining the fracture (Fig. 16–35C). On occasion, CT scanning may be helpful in precisely defining the full extent of the fracture.

Associated Injuries

Acromion process fractures may be associated with the following:

- Brachial plexus injuries
- AC joint injuries or lateral clavicle fractures

Treatment

Nondisplaced fractures can be treated with sling immobilization. Range-of-motion exercises should be started early in the management of these fractures.

Displaced fractures may require internal fixation to avoid compromise of the subacromial space resulting in a restricted range of motion. Internal fixation may be necessary if both the clavicle and scapula are injured together.[20]

Complications

The most frequent complication of acromion fractures is bursitis. Bursitis is most often seen in association with fractures with inferior displacement. Nonunion may also occur.

Glenoid Neck Fractures

Glenoid neck fractures are uncommon injuries that are often associated with humerus fractures (Fig. 16–34B).

Mechanism of Injury

An anterior or posterior force directed against the shoulder is the usual mechanism of injury. In most patients, the glenoid will be impacted. However, if displaced, the fragment will typically be anterior.

Examination

The patient will present with the arm held in adduction and will resist all movement of the shoulder. Medial pressure over the lateral humeral head will exacerbate the patient's pain.

Imaging

AP and tangential views are generally adequate in defining the fracture (Fig. 16–35D). Axillary views may be helpful in delineating displaced fractures. On occasion, CT scanning may be helpful in precisely defining the full extent of the fracture.

Associated Injuries

Proximal humerus fractures or shoulder dislocations are often noted in conjunction with these fractures. Also, an associated fracture of the ipsilateral clavicle may occur. This injury pattern results in a double disruption of the superior suspensory complex (SSC) and results in an unstable shoulder girdle. This is commonly termed the *floating shoulder*.[19]

Treatment

Nondisplaced. The emergency management of these fractures includes sling immobilization, ice, and analgesics. Passive exercise should be started at 48 hours, graduating to active exercise as tolerated.

Displaced. Urgent orthopedic consultation is advised for these patients. Glenoid neck fractures with greater than 40 degrees angulation or 1 to 2 cm of displacement may require operative fixation. Fractures with a second disruption of the SSC are generally managed with operative repair.[23]

Complications

Frequently encountered complications include diminished shoulder mobility or the development of posttraumatic arthritis.

Glenoid Fractures

Fractures of the articular surface of the glenoid are divided into two types: rim fractures and comminuted fractures (Fig. 16–34C and D). Glenoid rim fractures may demonstrate anterior or posterior displacement. In addition, glenoid rim fractures can traverse the rim and the spine. Comminuted fractures involve the entire articular surface of the glenoid.

Mechanism of Injury

Three mechanisms are commonly responsible for glenoid fractures. A direct blow, usually secondary to a fall on the lateral shoulder, may result in a comminuted fracture. A fall on the flexed elbow results in a force that is transmitted up the humerus and to the glenoid rim. This mechanism results in a rim fracture whose displacement is dependent on the direction of force. In addition, violent contraction of the triceps may result in avulsion of the inferior glenoid rim. This mechanism is commonly seen with shoulder dislocations. Approximately 20% of shoulder dislocations are associated with glenoid rim fractures.

Examination

Pain and weakness of the triceps is present with inferior rim fractures. Comminuted articular fractures will present with swelling and pain, which is increased with lateral compression.

Imaging

Routine views as well as an axillary view are generally adequate in defining the fracture. CT scanning is helpful in precisely defining the full extent of the fracture.

Associated Injuries

Shoulder dislocation is commonly associated with glenoid rim fractures.

Treatment

Rim. These patients require orthopedic referral. Intra-articular involvement of >25% of the glenoid surface or more than 5 mm of step-off require operative fixation. If the fracture is managed nonoperatively, sling immobilization, ice, and analgesics are administered. Exercise (pendulum type) should be started as soon as symptoms subside. Displaced fractures associated with dislocations are often reduced simultaneously with the joint reduction.

Comminuted Articular. The emergency management should include sling immobilization, ice, analgesics, and early consultation. Depressed fractures or those with large displaced fragments require operative reduction.

Complications

Glenoid fractures are frequently complicated by the development of arthritis.

Coracoid Process Fractures

The muscles that insert onto the coracoid process include the coracobrachialis, the short head of the biceps, and the pectoralis minor. The ligaments inserting on the coracoid process are the coracoacromial, the CC, and the coracohumeral.

Mechanism of Injury

Two mechanisms commonly result in coracoid process fractures. A direct blow to the superior point of the shoulder may result in a coracoid process fracture. Violent contraction of one of the inserting muscles may result in an avulsion fracture.

Examination

The patient will present with tenderness to palpation anteriorly over the coracoid process. In addition, there will be pain with forced adduction and with flexion at the elbow.

Imaging

Routine radiographs of this fracture should include an axillary lateral view for delineation of any displacement (usually, downward and medially) of the fragment (Fig. 16–35). On occasion, CT scanning may be helpful in precisely defining the full extent of the fracture.

Associated Injuries

Brachial plexus injuries, AC separation, or clavicular fractures are often associated with coracoid fractures.

Treatment

Coracoid process fractures are treated symptomatically. The patient should be given a sling, ice, analgesics, and instructions to begin early motion as tolerated. Associated injuries must be excluded before discharge from the ED. Displaced fractures may be considered for operative repair and early referral is advised.

Complications

No complications are commonly seen after these injuries.

SHOULDER SOFT-TISSUE INJURY AND DISLOCATIONS

ACROMIOCLAVICULAR DISLOCATION

The AC joint functions to allow an increase in elevation and abduction of the arm. Two ligaments provide stability at this joint: the AC and the CC ligaments. The CC ligament is divided into the conoid and the trapezoid ligaments, which function together to anchor the distal clavicle to the coracoid process (Fig. 16–3).

Subluxations and dislocations of the AC joint, "shoulder separation," are common injuries presenting to the ED and account for 10% of all dislocations. These injuries are divided into three types that represent progressive amounts of ligamentous injury—first-degree, second-degree, and third-degree (Fig. 16–36). A first-degree injury to this joint is commonly called a sprain of the AC ligament and involves an incomplete tear of that structure. A second-degree injury involves a subluxation of the AC joint and is always associated with disruption of the AC ligament; however, the CC ligament remains intact. In patients with third-degree AC joint separation, there is disruption of both the AC and CC ligaments, resulting in upward displacement of the clavicle.

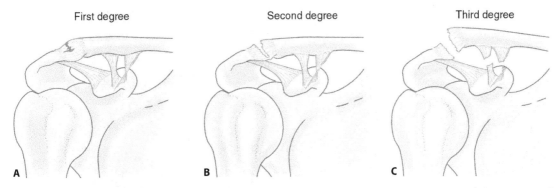

Figure 16–36. Acromioclavicular (AC) separation. **A.** A first-degree "sprain" with intact ligaments. **B.** A second-degree separation with tear of the AC ligament. **C.** A third-degree sprain with tear of both the AC and coracoclavicular (CC) ligaments.

AC separations have been further classified according to the Rockwood Classification based on the direction of displacement of the clavicle (Table 16–1). Type 4 injuries exist when the clavicle is displaced posteriorly into or through the trapezius muscle. Type 5 injuries involve disruption of all ligaments above the joint, and the clavicle is displaced far superiorly toward the base of the neck. In type 6 injuries, the clavicle is displaced inferiorly with the lateral end under the acromion or the coracoid process. This injury is often associated with clavicle fractures, rib fractures, or brachial plexus injuries. Types 4, 5, and 6 AC dislocations are rare. Treatment of these injuries is operative.[25]

Mechanism of Injury

The mechanisms by which these injuries occur are either as a result of a direct force, usually a fall with the arm adducted to the side, or a force from above the acromion that strikes the bony prominence and dislodges it from its attachments to the clavicle. An indirect mechanism by which this injury occurs is a fall on the outstretched arm with the force transmitted

▶ TABLE 16–1. **THE ROCKWOOD CLASSIFICATION FOR ACROMIOCLAVICULAR INJURIES**

Type	Pathology	Clinical Findings	Radiographic Findings	ED Management	Definitive Management
Type I	AC sprain, CC intact	AC tenderness	Normal	Sling 7–10 d, pain control	Conservative
Type II	AC torn, CC sprain	AC tenderness	AC >3 mm	Sling 2–3 wk, pain control	Conservative
Type III	AC torn, CC torn, D and T torn	AC tenderness, deformity	AC >3 mm CCD >13 mm 25%–100% displacement	Sling, pain control	Controversial, nonoperative[a]
Type IV	AC torn, CC torn, D and T torn, posterior displacement of clavicle through trapezius	Prominent acromion	AC >3 mm CCD >13 mm Posterior displacement of clavicle on axillary lateral	Sling, pain control, neurovascular assessment	Surgical
Type V	AC torn, CC torn, D and T torn, severe superior displacement of clavicle	Deformity	AC >3 mm CCD >13 mm 100%–300% displacement	Sling, pain control	Surgical
Type VI	AC torn, CC intact, inferior displacement of clavicle subcoracoid	CCD decreased	Associated trauma AC >3 mm	Sling, pain control	Surgical neurovascular assessment

AC, acromioclavicular; CC, coracoclavicular; D, deltoid attachment at clavicle; T, trapezius attachment at clavicle; CCD, coracoclavicular distance.
[a]Management of Type III injuries is controversial. Nonoperative management is most common but surgical management may be considered in select populations.
Data from Simovitch R, Sanders B, Ozbaydar M, et al. Acromioclavicular joint injuries: diagnosis and management, *J Am Acad Orthop Surg* 2009 Apr;17(4):207-219 and Williams GR, Nguyen VD, Rockwood CR. Classification and radiographic analysis of acromioclavicular dislocations, *Appl Radiol* 1989;18:29–34.

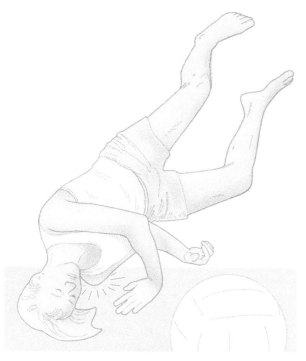

Figure 16–37. A fall onto the shoulder is the most common mechanism for sustaining an AC separation.

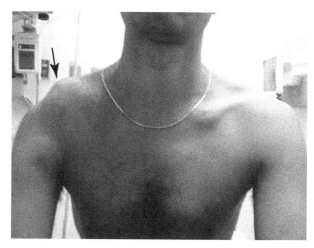

Figure 16–38. AC separation is noted on the right (*arrow*). This deformity represents prominence of the distal clavicle as it separates from the acromion.

to the AC joint. Most injuries of the AC joint are caused by a direct fall onto the point of the shoulder (Fig. 16–37). A more horizontally directed force (i.e., fall to the lateral side of the shoulder) may result in intra-articular damage with no significant injury to the ligaments. This may account for many cases of late degenerative joint disease and pain following a seemingly mild AC sprain.

Examination

The examination of the AC joint starts with inspection. In patients with significant ligamentous disruption (i.e., third-degree injury), a deformity at the top of the shoulder will be apparent in the upright position (Fig. 16–38). This deformity represents a prominence of the distal clavicle, indicating a tear of the AC and CC ligaments. The upward displacement of the clavicle is due to the loss of the suspending CC ligament combined with the downward pull of the shoulder laterally caused by the weight of the arm.

In patients with first-degree injuries, there will be minimal swelling, but pain with palpation of the AC joint or when performing the AC cross-arm adduction test. This test is performed by bringing the arm across the body (Fig. 16–39). Localization of pain to the AC joint confirms that it is the source. The patient with second-degree injury experiences tenderness to mild palpation, and moderate swelling is noted.

The O'Brien test of active compression can also be performed. In this test, the affected arm is brought into 90-degree forward flexion and 10-degree adduction. The arm is resisted from further forward flexion in both full internal rotation (thumb down) and external rotation (thumb up). Pain in internal rotation is suggestive of labral pathology, pain in external rotation is suggestive of AC pathology. It is imperative to match physical examination findings in the context of the clinical picture as the specificity of these tests is limited in isolation.

Imaging

Routine shoulder x-rays in a patient whom one suspects has an AC joint injury should detect significant AC injury

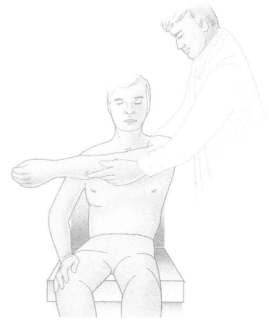

Figure 16–39. Technique for testing for injury or inflammation of the AC joint.

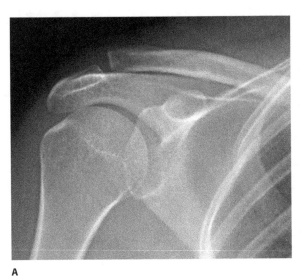
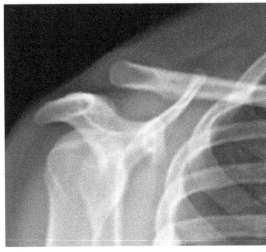

A   **B**

Figure 16–40. AC separation on AP radiograph. **A.** Second-degree injury. **B.** Third-degree injury.

(Fig. 16–40). Simultaneous imaging of both sides on one large cassette is recommended to compare the injured side with the normal side. Tilting the beam 10 to 15 degrees toward the head will avoid superimposing the scapular spine and allow for more subtle detection of injuries.[11] Three measurements should be taken and compared to the opposite side (Fig. 16–41)[25,27]:

- AC joint width (normal is <3 mm)
- Clavicle–coracoid distance (CCD)—the perpendicular distance from the clavicle to the superior portion of the coracoid process (normal is <13 mm)
- Clavicle elevation—the degree of superior displacement of the clavicle compared with the acromion

Patients with first-degree injury will have normal radiographs. The radiographic findings of second-degree injuries are subtle and may be misinterpreted as normal. The AC joint width is increased (≥3 mm or >50% increase when compared with the uninjured side), but the CCD is normal (<13 mm or similar to the opposite side). In addition, the lateral end of the clavicle may be slightly elevated, but the separation from the acromion is no more than one-half its diameter.

In patients with third-degree injury, the inferior border of the distal clavicle is above the midpoint of the acromion. In addition, the CCD is greater than 13 mm. Alternatively, a CCD of 5 mm greater than the CCD on the contralateral normal side is also suggestive of injury.

Stress views may be taken in the AP position with 5 to 10 lb of weight suspended from the arm. Once widely obtained to differentiate second- and third-degree AC separations, the necessity of stress films has been questioned and the authors no longer use them. They can be painful to obtain and of limited accuracy. In one study, stress films provided a significant difference to unmask a third-degree injury in only 4% of cases.[25]

Treatment

The treatment of first-degree injuries is rest, ice, and a sling, with early range of motion.

Second-degree injuries are treated conservatively in a similar fashion to first-degree injuries. The sling should be continued for 2 weeks or until the symptoms resolve, followed by physical therapy and rehabilitation. Early motion will help reduce the development of adhesive capsulitis. Heavy lifting and contact sports are avoided initially while the ligaments heal so as not to convert a partial injury into a complete dislocation. Earlier return to contact sports is acceptable if the joint is covered with a protective pad.

Treatment of third-degree injuries in the acute setting is similar to second-degree injuries with the additional measure of early referral. There is no definitive proof that an AC support (Kenny–Howard harness) makes a difference

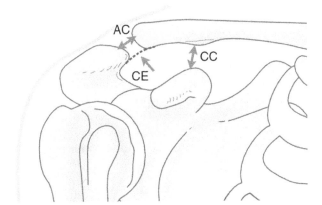

Figure 16–41. Radiographic measurements to determine the degree of AC separation. AC joint width (normal is <3 mm); CC distance (normal is <13 mm); and clavicular elevation (CE) (inferior aspect of the acromion and clavicle should be level).

in terms of long-term function as compared with a sling and ice.

The definitive treatment of third-degree AC joint dislocations is controversial. Although operative intervention has historically been performed for this injury, nonoperative management has been increasingly preferred by orthopedic surgeons. In a 2007 survey of orthopedic surgeons, 81% recommended conservative treatment. Several studies support conservative treatment for third-degree injuries with equivalent rates of functional recovery and pain control. Overhead athletes may be candidates for operative repair. Anatomic fixation may avoid potential complications such as impingement or neurovascular symptomatology. However, surgical intervention is often performed in a delayed time frame.

Complications

Late symptoms of posttraumatic degenerative joint disease may occur after AC joint injury. Persistent pain in the AC joint after first- and second-degree injuries occurs in 8% to 42% of patients. If conservative measures fail, operative management with distal clavicular resection may be necessary.

STERNOCLAVICULAR JOINT DISLOCATION

The SC joint is stabilized by the SC ligament and the costoclavicular ligament (Fig. 16–2). The SC ligament has both anterior and posterior portions. Maximum motion of this joint occurs during internal rotation with the arm elevated above 110 degrees.

A mild sprain of the SC joint involves microscopic, incomplete ligamentous tears of the SC and the costoclavicular ligaments (Fig. 16–42A). A moderate sprain involves subluxation of the clavicle from its manubrial attachment and signifies complete rupture of the SC ligament and partial rupture of the costoclavicular ligament (Fig. 16–42B).

A dislocation of the SC joint involves complete rupture of the SC and costoclavicular ligaments (Fig. 16–42C), permitting the clavicle to be removed from its manubrial attachment. This injury is rare and accounts for less than 1% of all dislocations. Dislocations at this joint are either anterior or posterior. Posterior dislocations are also referred to as retrosternal because the clavicle displaces medially as well as posterior to the sternum. Anterior dislocation of the SC joint is much more common due to the greater strength of the posterior SC ligament. In patients younger than 25 years, the injury is typically a physeal fracture rather than a true dislocation.

Mechanism of Injury

The most common mechanism of injury is a force that thrusts the shoulder forward. It usually involves a tremendous force and most commonly follows a motor vehicle collision (40%), athletics (20%), or falls and other trauma

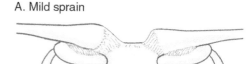

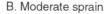

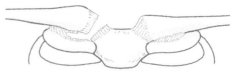

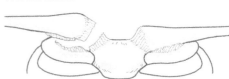

Figure 16–42. Sternoclavicular joint injuries. **A.** Mild sprain occurs when microscopic tears are present in the sternoclavicular and costoclavicular ligaments. **B.** Moderate sprain with tear of the sternoclavicular ligament. **C.** Dislocation with disruption of both the sternoclavicular and costoclavicular ligaments.

(40%). An anterior dislocation occurs indirectly, when a shoulder is laterally compressed (against the ground) and then rolled backward. Conversely, a posterior dislocation is created when a laterally compressed shoulder is rolled forward. A direct anterior force may also produce a posterior dislocation. In the absence of trauma, an infectious process within the SC joint, although rare, should be considered.

Examination

A patient with a mild sprain experiences minimal swelling and complains of tenderness over the joint. Pain is increased by elevation of the arm above 110 degrees. The patient with a moderate sprain experiences pain on abduction of the arm, and swelling is noted over the joint.

A patient with an SC joint dislocation experiences severe pain, which is increased by any motion of the shoulder or when the patient is placed in a supine position. The affected shoulder appears shortened and thrust forward. On inspection, one will note the obvious deformity of an anterior dislocation (Fig. 16–43). Palpation may find that the clavicle is fixed or quite mobile. A patient with a posterior dislocation may present with significant anterior swelling that may mislead the physician into thinking the dislocation is anterior (Fig. 16–44A).

Associated Injuries

Patients with posterior dislocations may constitute a true orthopedic emergency if they present with breathing

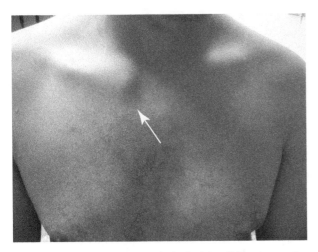

Figure 16–43. Anterior sternoclavicular joint dislocation on the patient's right (*arrow*).

difficulties secondary to tracheal compression, tracheal rupture, or a pneumothorax. Venous congestion may also be seen. These injuries are often associated with fatal injuries to the mediastinum, including the great vessels.[40] Subclavian vein compression may lead to numbness and edema in the extremity. Esophageal compression causes dysphagia. CT angiography can evaluate major vascular injuries.[40,41] These injuries, if present, may necessitate emergency reduction by the physician in the ED.

Although anterior dislocations are not a direct cause of secondary injuries, they may be a marker of significant injuries due to the amount of force required to create them. Greater than two-thirds of patients with anterior dislocations have significant associated injuries that include pneumothorax, hemothorax, pulmonary contusion, and rib fractures.[42]

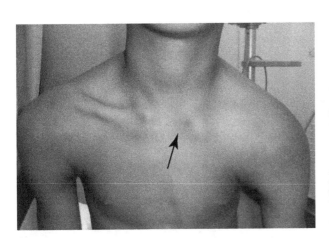

A

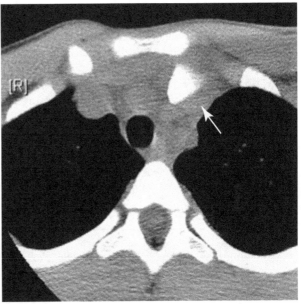

B

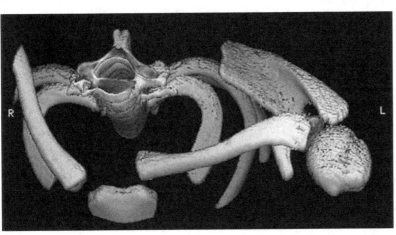

C

Figure 16–44. Posterior sternoclavicular joint dislocation on the left. *A.* Clinical photograph. Swelling is noted over the joint and obscures the diagnosis (*arrow*). *B.* CT demonstrating posterior sternoclavicular joint dislocation with the medial clavicle in proximity to the mediastinal structures (*arrow*). *C.* CT reconstruction in the same patient. (Reproduced with permission from Beecroft M, Sherman SC: Posterior displacement of a proximal epiphyseal clavicle fracture, *J Emerg Med* 2007 Oct;33(3):245-248.)

Imaging

A nonrotated AP radiograph may suggest dislocation if the difference in the height of the medial clavicles is greater than 50% of their width. Lateral views are difficult to interpret due to superimposition of other structures. A Rockwood serendipity view with the beam tilted 40 to 45 degrees cephalad and centered on the sternum is the best plain film for detecting dislocation. A CT scan of the chest is often required to diagnose an SC dislocation and its associated injuries (Fig. 16–44).

Treatment

A mild sprain is treated with ice three to four times daily for a period of 24 hours and a sling for 3 to 4 days. Moderate sprains and subluxations of the joint are treated with a fig-ure-of-eight clavicle strap and a sling to hold the clavicle in its normal position and permit ligamentous healing. This protection should be continued for 6 weeks, and the patient should be advised that problems in the joint that require operative intervention may develop.

In patients with a posterior dislocation with a stable airway and no symptoms of vascular compromise, workup of associated injuries should occur before reduction is attempted because the posteriorly displaced clavicle may be functioning to occlude a vascular injury. Procedural seda-tion is frequently needed to reduce a posterior dislocation of the SC joint. Consultations with an orthopedic surgeon and a thoracic surgeon should be obtained.

> **Axiom:** *In patients with a posterior SC dislocation with a stable airway and no symptoms of vascular compromise, emergent ED reduction is not indicated because the pos-teriorly displaced clavicle may be functioning to occlude a vascular injury*

Dislocations are reduced in the following manner (Fig. 16–45). While the patient is supine, a folded sheet is placed between the shoulders, which serves to separate the clavicle from the manubrium. The arm is abducted, and traction is maintained. In anterior dislocations, the assistant pushes a downward, posterior-directed force on the clavicle toward its normal position. For posterior dislocations, the assistant attempts to pull the clavicle anteriorly. In more difficult posterior dislocations, the clavicle can be grasped with a towel clip (Fig. 16–46).

Anterior dislocations are often unstable. Immediately following reduction of an anterior dislocation, place a pres-sure bandage (e.g., a roll of gauze) over the SC joint to ensure it does not redislocate.

Reduction of a posterior dislocation is usually mechani-cally stable. If it cannot be performed by closed methods, surgical repair is indicated. If reduction of an anterior dislocation is successful, and no other injuries are present, the patient should be placed in a figure-of-eight harness, which should remain for a period of 6 weeks, followed by

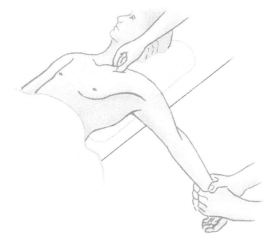

Figure 16–45. Reduction of a displaced sternoclavicular joint injury. The arm is abducted, and traction is applied. With traction maintained, an assistant pushes the clavicle back into its normal position for anterior dislocations or pulls back on the clavicle for posterior dislocations.

protected motion for another 2 weeks. Anterior dislocations are often unstable and may dislocate again. These injuries are not treated operatively because the complications of the procedure outweigh any benefits.

Complications

Although anterior dislocations of the SC joint often remain unstable, they generally do not cause functional impairment. The most common complication of an anterior dislocation is cosmetic, with chronic swelling noted around the joint. Posterior dislocations are less frequent but are fraught with more serious complications, including pneumothorax, lac-eration of the superior vena cava, occlusion of the subclavian

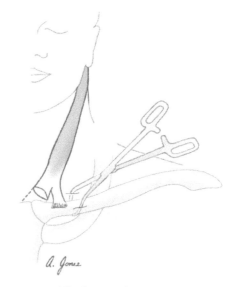

Figure 16–46. In difficult cases of posterior dislocation, the clav-icle can be grasped with a towel clip and replaced.

artery or vein, and rupture or compression of the trachea. Up to 25% of all posterior dislocations of the SC joint are associated with tracheal, esophageal, or great vessel injury, which emphasizes the need for early reduction and consultation.[47]

ANTERIOR SHOULDER DISLOCATION

The shoulder, with its wide range of motion and shallow glenoid, is inherently unstable. As a consequence, shoulder dislocation is a common joint dislocation presenting to the ED, representing approximately 50% of all major dislocations seen by the emergency physician. The most frequent location of a glenohumeral joint dislocation is anterior, accounting for 95% of cases. Approximately 70% of all anterior dislocations of the shoulder occur in patients younger than 30 years.

Posterior dislocations are seen in the remaining 5%, with inferior dislocations (luxatio erecta) being extremely rare.

There are three types of anterior dislocation: *subclavicular*, *subcoracoid*, and *subglenoid* (Fig. 16–47). In 90% of cases, the humeral head is in a subcoracoid location. A subclavicular dislocation is rare. Subclavicular and subglenoid dislocations have either an associated rotator cuff tear or a greater tuberosity fracture. The humeral head can interchange from one position to the next, but it usually remains in one of the three.

Mechanism of Injury
The mechanism by which this injury occurs is usually *abduction* accompanied by *external rotation* of the arm, which disrupts the anterior capsule and the glenohumeral ligaments.[48] Subcoracoid dislocations are often secondary to "hyper" external rotation. Less commonly, they can be seen after convulsions or a direct blow to the posterior

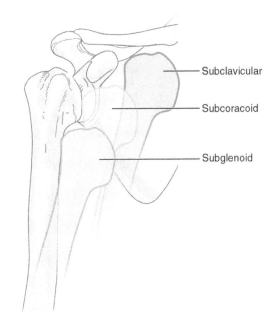

Figure 16–47. The three types of anterior dislocations of the shoulder.

Labels: Subclavicular, Subcoracoid, Subglenoid

aspect of the proximal humerus, displacing it anteriorly. Subglenoid dislocations are usually associated with more abduction than external rotation. A small percentage (4%) of dislocations are atraumatic, occurring while raising an arm or moving during sleep.[48]

Examination
The patient presents with the arms held to the side. In a thin patient, the acromion is prominent, providing the classic "squared off" appearance to the shoulder. The absence of the humeral head can be quite obvious (Fig. 16–48A). In

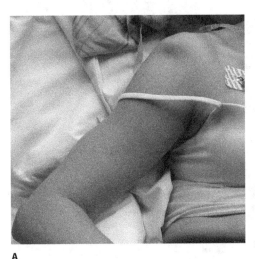
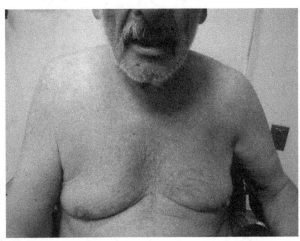

A   **B**

Figure 16–48. Anterior shoulder dislocation. *A.* In a thin individual, absence of the humeral head is straightforward. *B.* In a larger patient, the normal, rounded appearance of the left shoulder compared with a more "squared-off" appearance of the dislocated right shoulder.

other patients, the only finding may be loss of the normal rounded contour of the shoulder (Fig. 16–48B). On palpation, the examiner will note the absence of the humeral head in its usual location while palpating inferior to the acromion. Fullness in the anterior shoulder may be noted, indicating the presence of the humeral head. In most cases, the patient will resist any movement of the arm, only occasionally permitting some abduction and external rotation. Internal rotation and adduction will be quite painful, and therefore, the patient will be unable to use the affected arm to touch the opposite shoulder (Video 16–1).

A full neurovascular examination of the upper extremity should be performed. Associated neurologic injury occurs in 13.5% of anterior glenohumeral dislocations, with the axillary nerve being the most commonly affected. Injury to the axillary nerve can be assessed by testing motor strength and pinprick sensation over the lateral aspect of the arm and comparing it with the other side. Some authors have reported that sensory testing is unreliable and motor weakness (i.e., abduction) is a better indicator of nerve injury. However, testing deltoid muscle strength is impractical to assess during the initial evaluation.

Imaging

Standard shoulder radiographic views (AP and scapular Y views) are typically obtained before reduction is attempted to both confirm the diagnosis and exclude concomitant fractures, which occur in approximately 20% to 25% of cases. Factors associated with a fracture include age over 40, first-time dislocation, presence of humeral ecchymoses, and a traumatic mechanism. When none of these features are present and the clinician is clinically certain of his/her diagnosis, prereduction radiographs can be omitted.

The diagnosis is usually apparent on AP radiographs (Fig. 16–49A). The humeral head will be displaced from the glenoid fossa and fixed in external rotation. In external rotation, the greater tuberosity will be located along the lateral aspect of the humeral head. Any attempt to obtain an internal rotation AP view will be unsuccessful and should be a clue to the diagnosis. Pseudodislocation occurs when a hemarthrosis causes widening of the joint space. This is seen most commonly in patients with proximal humerus fractures (Fig. 16–10).

The scapular Y view will demonstrate anterior dislocation of the humeral head from the glenoid (Fig. 16–49B). Occasionally, a false-negative scapular Y view will occur, so if question still exists, an *axillary view* of the scapula should be obtained. To perform an axillary view, it should be noted that the patient does not need to abduct the arm to 90 degrees as this will be quite impossible in the setting of an anterior dislocation. Approximately 15 degrees of abduction, or just enough to get the x-ray tube between the arm and the body, is usually sufficient. If the patient is ambulatory and has difficulty fully abducting the arm due to pain, a *Velpeau axillary view* will be much easier for the patient and provides similar information (Fig. 16–50). A *true AP (Grashey) view* in which the beam is directed at a 45-degree angle in a medial to lateral direction is also helpful to assess subtle joint incongruity.

In evaluating the radiographs in patients with suspected anterior dislocations of the shoulder, one should look for a defect in the posterior lateral portion of the humeral head. This defect, known as a *Hill–Sachs defect*, is present in up to 40% of cases of anterior shoulder dislocation

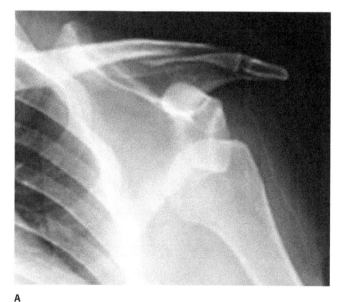
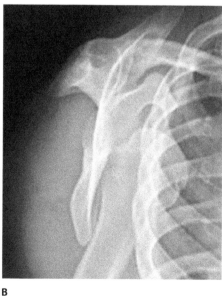

A   **B**

Figure 16–49. Anterior shoulder dislocation. *A.* AP view. *B.* Scapular Y view.

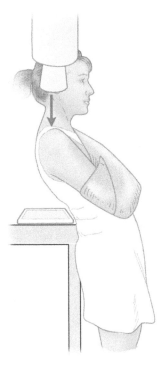

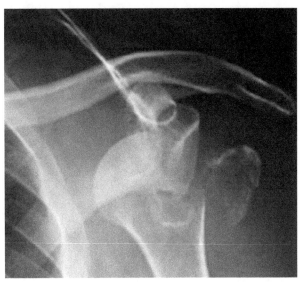

Figure 16–52. Anterior shoulder dislocation with associated fracture of the greater tuberosity.

Figure 16–50. The Velpeau axillary view can be used to diagnose shoulder dislocations in patients who are unable to abduct the arm.

(Fig. 16–51A).[57] It occurs as a result of impaction of the soft base of the humeral head against the anterior glenoid. The longer the humeral head is out of the glenoid fossa, the larger is the defect. This defect commonly occurs with recurrent anterior dislocations. If one suspects a Hill–Sachs deformity, an internal rotation view that will delineate the

defect more clearly can be obtained after the shoulder has been reduced.

Associated Injuries

Associated fractures other than the Hill–Sachs defect include the greater tuberosity and glenoid rim (i.e., Bankart lesion) (Fig. 16–51B). Fractures of the greater tuberosity occur in 15% of patients with anterior shoulder dislocations (Fig. 16–52).[48] In approximately 40% of cases, these fractures occur in patients older than 45 years. Glenoid rim fractures occur in approximately 5% of patients.[48]

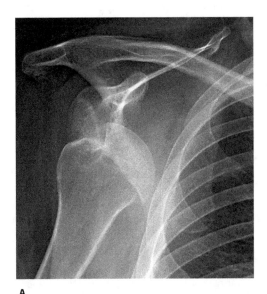

A

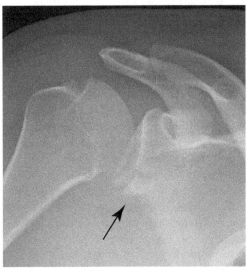

B

Figure 16–51. **A.** Hill–Sachs impaction fracture following an anterior shoulder dislocation. **B.** Glenoid rim (Bankart) fracture (*arrow*).

Soft-tissue injuries also occur. In the young, the common site of capsular tear is between the superior and middle glenohumeral ligaments. In addition to capsular tears, the labrum may be torn from the glenoid by the displacing humeral head. This injury, known as the soft-tissue Bankart lesion, occurs in approximately 90% of patients younger than 30 years who suffer an anterior shoulder dislocation.

Rotator cuff tears occur in 35% to 86% of patients older than 40 years. Inability to abduct the arm following reduction of an anterior shoulder dislocation is a sensitive indicator of a rotator cuff tear. This test is not specific, however, because it may occur in patients with an axillary nerve injury. Rotator cuff tears are important to diagnose early because early surgical repair improves outcome. Biceps tendon injuries may also be seen.

Brachial plexus injury or damage to the axillary nerve occurs in 5% to 14% of cases. An axillary nerve injury is usually a neuropraxia, and full recovery can be expected in most instances.

Treatment

Analgesia

Before performing shoulder reduction, the clinician should consider appropriate analgesia. In cooperative patients with recent, recurrent, and relatively atraumatic dislocations, reduction can often be achieved without procedural sedation. Reduction without analgesia is most effective when reduction techniques that do not require a significant amount of traction are used (e.g., scapular manipulation). If the patient is in significant pain or unable to achieve adequate muscle relaxation, reduction will be difficult. Several options exist to assist in alleviating pain to facilitate a reduction, including intravenous analgesics, procedural sedation, ultrasound (US)-guided nerve blocks, and intra-articular lidocaine. As the use of US in emergency medicine continues to expand, US-guided interscalene nerve or suprascapular nerve blocks have been shown to be effective alternatives with good success rates and short length of stays in the ED setting. Without adequate analgesia and muscle relaxation, anterior shoulder dislocation reduction can be difficult.

A growing body of literature comparing intra-articular lidocaine injection to procedural sedation for shoulder reduction suggests similar success rates but fewer complications, lower cost, and shorter ED length of stays with lidocaine injection (Video 16–2). Lateral and posterior approaches can be taken, although posterior approaches can be guided by ultrasound to ensure injection into the articular space.

With the lateral approach, the site of injection is approximately 1 cm inferior to the lateral edge of the acromion (Fig. 16–53). A 20-g spinal needle is directed medially and inferiorly to a depth of 2.5 to 3 cm. For the posterior

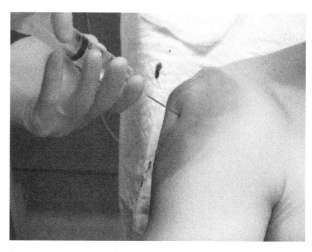

Figure 16–53. Lateral approach to intra-articular injection of lidocaine. A spinal needle is inserted perpendicular to the adducted arm approximately 1 in. below the lateral border of the acromion.

approach, the needle is directed anteromedially through the sulcus between the acromion and humeral head. Intra-articular injection is more effective when the patient presents within 6 hours of dislocation.

Reduction Techniques

Several methods have been described for reducing anterior shoulder dislocations (Table 16–2). No clear evidence supports the superiority of any one technique, and the method used is frequently based on the clinician's experience. The ideal method is quick and simple, requiring the least amount of force. With this goal in mind, we prefer the external rotation, FARES, or the scapular manipulation techniques as the methods of first choice, and in the appropriate setting, reduction is attempted before preparing the patient for procedural sedation.

A description of several techniques for reducing anterior shoulder dislocations are provided as follows.

Cunningham Technique. The patient sits upright with the affected arm adducted and elbow at 90 degrees. The patient is encouraged to relax as much as possible and bring his/her shoulders back. This puts the scapula in the best position to allow reduction. The operator faces the patient, one hand between the patient's forearm and body. This hand applies mild downward traction with the weight of the operator's arm. The operator's other hand massages the trapezius, deltoid, and biceps sequentially with emphasis on kneading the biceps (Fig. 16–54). Relaxation of the muscles results in reduction. The advantages of this technique are that it does not require sedation and can be performed rapidly in a busy emergency department.

▶ TABLE 16–2. **TECHNIQUES FOR REDUCTION OF ANTERIOR SHOULDER DISLOCATION**

Technique	Operators	Position	Description	Disadvantages	Success Rate (%)
Cunningham	One	Seated	Starting position: Patient's arm adducted, elbow at 90 degrees. Operator faces patient. Place one hand between the patient's forearm and body. This hand applies mild downward traction with weight of operator's arm. Other hand massages the trapezius, deltoid, and biceps sequentially, with emphasis on kneading biceps. Relaxation of muscles results in reduction.	None	Unknown (first described in 2003)
Modified Hippocratic (traction–countertraction)	Two	Supine	One operator provides a longitudinal traction force with the arm slightly abducted. Second operator provides countertraction (typically with a bedsheet wrapped around the thorax in the axilla).	Requires significant force	86
FARES	One	Supine	Starting position: Arm adducted with elbow straight and forearm in neutral. Gently apply longitudinal traction while taking the arm into abduction using a vertical oscillatory movement to help with muscle relaxation. Add external rotation after 90-degree abduction and continue abduction, vertical oscillation until reduction achieved.	None	88–95
Kocher	One	Seated	Starting position: Arm should be adducted at the side with elbow flexed. Gently adduct the arm further and externally rotate the elbow. When resistance is felt, the arm is forward flexed upward and then internally rotated.	Higher incidence of fracture	72–100
Milch	One	Supine	Starting position: Arm fully abducted above the head with extended elbow. Apply longitudinal traction and external rotation of arm.	None	70–89
Scapular manipulation	Two	Prone	One operator provides downward traction to arm forward flexed 90 degrees. Second operator attempts to adduct and medially rotate inferior border of scapula.	Difficult to monitor sedation, operator dependent	79–90
External rotation	One	Supine/ seated	Starting position: Arm fully adducted at side with elbow flexed. Perform slow passive external rotation of arm.	None	80–90
Stimson	One	Prone	Arm hangs off stretcher in 90-degree forward flexion and 5- to 10-lb weights attached to affected arm (can combine with scapular).	Equipment, difficult to monitor sedation	91–96
Snowbird	Two	Seated	Starting position: Patient seated in chair with arm adducted and flexed at elbow. Operator applies downward traction by placing foot in a loop of stockinette wrapped around the patient's forearm.	None	97
Spaso	One	Supine	Starting position: Arm forward flexed 90 degrees toward the ceiling. Apply longitudinal traction toward ceiling and passive external rotation.	Operator back discomfort (rare)	67–91

Data from Ufberg JW, Vilke GM, Chan TC, et al. Anterior shoulder dislocations: beyond traction-countertraction, *J Emerg Med* 2004;27(3): 301–6.

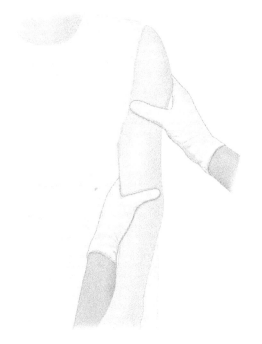

Figure 16-54. The Cunningham technique. The patient is seated with the arm adducted and elbow flexed to 90 degrees as shown. Operator places one hand between the patients forearm and body, applying mild downward traction. The other hand massages the trapezius and deltoid and kneads the biceps resulting in reduction.

Scapular Manipulation Technique. The patient lies prone on the table with the affected arm hanging off of the table, suspended with approximately 5 to 10 lb of weight in a similar fashion to the Stimson technique. The physician then rotates the tip of the scapula medially and the superior aspect of the scapula laterally (Fig. 16-55 and Video 16-3).

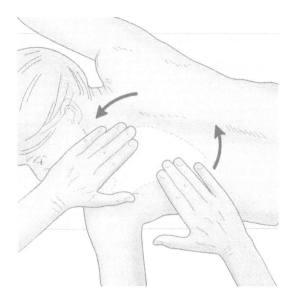

Figure 16-55. Scapular manipulation. The inferior border of the scapula is rotated medially, while the superior border is rotated laterally.

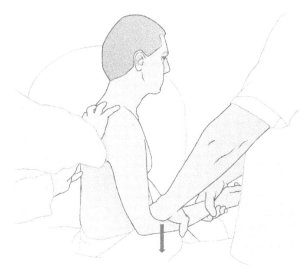

Figure 16-56. In the upright patient leaning the unaffected shoulder against the stretcher, scapular manipulation is performed with gentle downward traction.

This technique is quick, has a high rate of success, and is associated with few complications.   Alternatively, the patient sits upright with the unaffected shoulder leaning up against a stretcher that is placed at 90 degrees. While one person performs scapular manipulation from behind the patient, another individual provides gentle downward traction on the patient's affected, flexed arm (Fig. 16-56 and Video 16-4).

External Rotation Technique. This technique was described by Leidelmeyer and popularized at Hennepin County Emergency Medicine Center.   External rotation of the shoulder acts to overcome internal rotator muscle spasm and unwind the joint capsule, allowing the external rotators of the rotator cuff to pull the humerus back into position. The technique requires little manipulation and permits the shoulder muscles to reduce the dislocation with little or no analgesia. In one case series, 81% of patients were reduced with no sedation. Only one person is required to perform the reduction. Success rates for this maneuver are between 80% and 90%.

To perform the external rotation technique, the patient is supine, upright, or at 45 degrees. The patient's elbow is supported by one hand, and the other hand is used to slowly and gently externally rotate the arm. Gradually, the arm is externally rotated to 90 degrees (Fig. 16-57 and Video 16-5). If the patient experiences any discomfort during external rotation, the examiner should stop and wait a moment until the muscles relax. During this procedure, it is important that the patient be completely relaxed and that the rotation be done gradually and slowly. Reduction is frequently subtle and the "clunk" of the humerus rearticulating with the glenoid is not heard.

Milch Technique. The authors use this technique when external rotation to 90 degrees using the external rotation

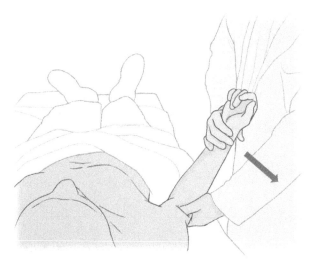

Figure 16–57. External rotation technique (i.e., Hennepin technique) for the reduction of anterior shoulder dislocations.

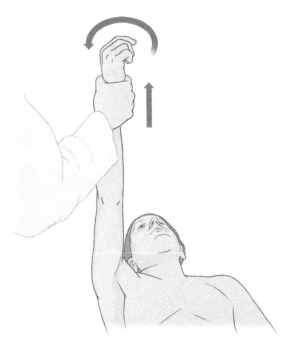

Figure 16–59. Spaso technique for reduction of anterior shoulder dislocations.

technique described previously has not reduced the shoulder spontaneously. The arm is slowly abducted, and the humeral head is lifted into the glenoid if it does not spontaneously reduce on elevation alone (Fig. 16–58 and Video 16–6). Elevation of the arm (i.e., abduction) is believed to aid reduction of the shoulder by eliminating the cross-stresses of the shoulder muscles that normally prevent reduction.[83,84] The modified Milch maneuver incorporates some longitudinal traction if reduction is not successful at 90 degrees abduction and external rotation with 30 degrees forward flexion.[85] Success rates are between 70% and 89%.[60,85,86]

Spaso Technique. The patient is supine and the examiner applies gentle vertical traction and external rotation to reduce the dislocation (Fig. 16–59).[87,88] This technique is rapid, and success is usually achieved within 1 to 2 minutes.

Stimson Technique. The Stimson technique is a safe procedure to reduce an anterior dislocation of the shoulder. The patient is placed in the prone position with the arm dependent over a pillow or folded sheets (Fig. 16–60).

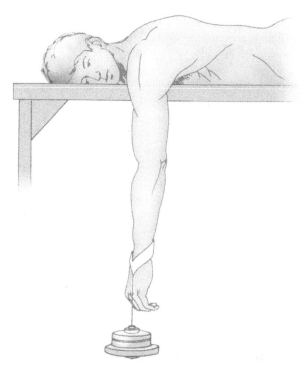

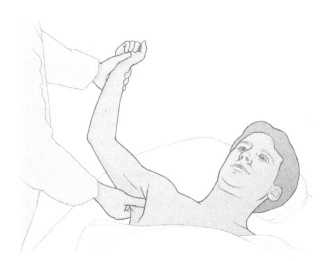

Figure 16–58. Milch technique for reduction of anterior shoulder dislocations.

Figure 16–60. Stimson technique for reduction of anterior shoulder dislocations.

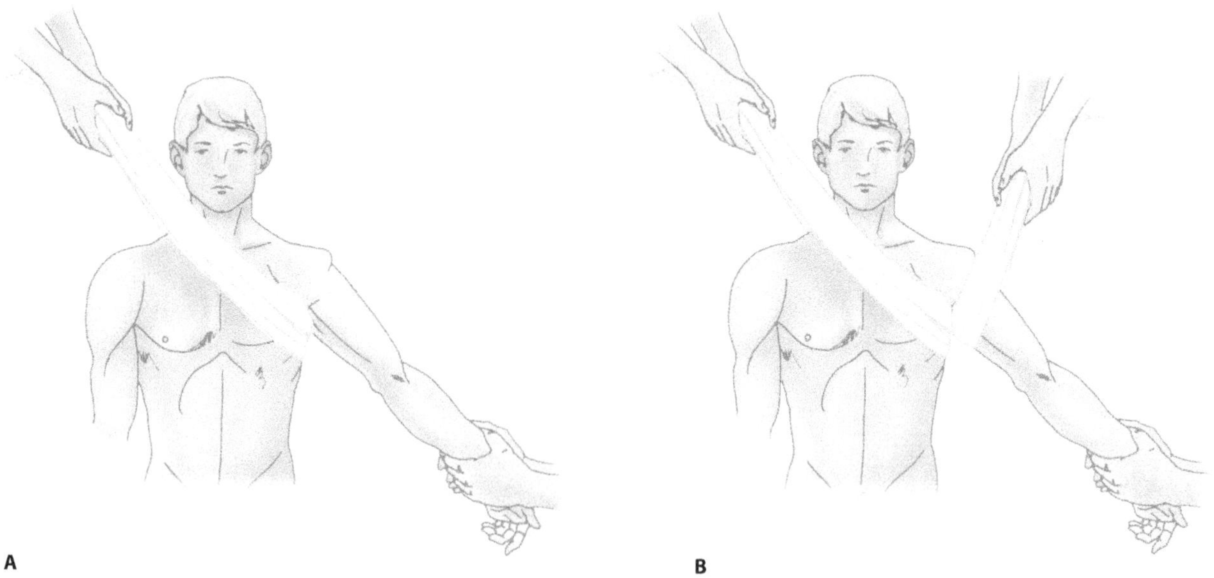

Figure 16–61. ***A.*** Traction–countertraction technique for reducing anterior shoulder dislocations. ***B.*** If a few minutes of traction–countertraction are unsuccessful, gentle lateral traction on the arm may aid the reduction. Using excessive lateral traction should be avoided so as not to produce a proximal humerus fracture.

A strap is added to the wrist or distal forearm, and 10 to 15 lb of weights are applied for a period of 20 to 30 minutes. Procedural sedation is difficult to administer in the prone patient, leaving intra-articular lidocaine as a good alternative anesthetic method. Success rates range from 91% to 96%. If unsuccessful, the examiner may rotate the humerus gently, externally, and then internally with mild force, which usually reduces the dislocation. Alternatively, the examiner may apply scapular manipulation with the patient in the prone position with excellent success rates.

Traction and Countertraction. This method has been advocated for those anterior dislocations that are difficult to reduce by other techniques (Fig. 16–61A). In this method, an assistant applies countertraction with a folded sheet wrapped around the upper chest, and the examiner applies traction to the arm in an inferolateral direction (Video 16–7). This maneuver dislodges the humeral head and will reduce the dislocation. Lateral traction during traction and countertraction can also be employed in patients with good muscle relaxation. Lateral traction involves a perpendicular force to the longitudinal axis of the humerus applied by a second assistant to the proximal humerus in the axilla (Fig. 16–61B and Video 16–8). Lateral traction should be used with some caution. If it is applied before the humeral head is safely below the glenoid rim, fracture to the rim may occur.

FARES Method. The FARES (fast, reliable, safe) method can be done safely with or without analgesia, with successful reduction achieved in 88% to 95% of cases.

To perform this method, the patient should be placed supine on the cart. The examiner uses both hands to grasp the wrist of the affected arm to apply longitudinal traction with the elbow extended and the forearm in neutral position. Slowly abduct the affected arm while using brief 2 to 3 second bursts of a vertical oscillating motion (approximately 5 cm above and below the neutral position) to promote muscle relaxation. Once 90-degree abduction has been achieved, gently externally rotate the arm while maintaining the longitudinal traction and oscillatory movements. Continue abduction until reduction (generally reduced by 120 degrees) (Fig. 16–62 and Video 16–9). This newer method has shown promising results in two small randomized control trials with greater success than external rotation and Kocher and Hippocratic methods.

Several other methods have been described to reduce anterior shoulder dislocations. These include the chair, Eskimo, Kocher, and Hippocratic techniques. The Kocher maneuver, particularly when modified to include traction, is fraught with many complications and should be used with great caution by the emergency physician in reducing anterior dislocations of the shoulder. In our opinion, the Hippocratic technique should never be used under any circumstances in reducing these dislocations.

Successful reduction is frequently signaled by an audible clunk as the humeral head relocates. The shoulder returns to its normal contour, and fullness is felt again below the acromion. The ability to place the hand of the affected extremity on the opposite shoulder further confirms reduction.

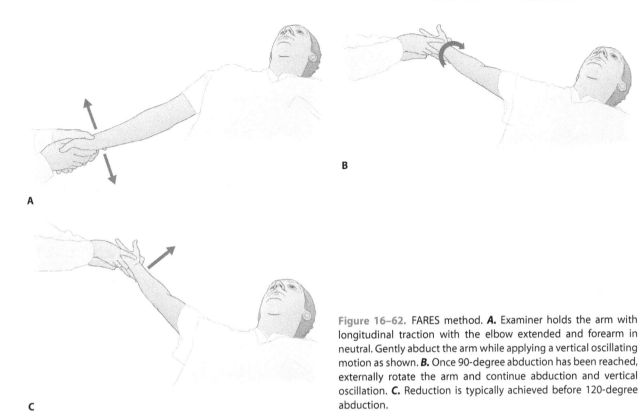

Figure 16–62. FARES method. **A.** Examiner holds the arm with longitudinal traction with the elbow extended and forearm in neutral. Gently abduct the arm while applying a vertical oscillating motion as shown. **B.** Once 90-degree abduction has been reached, externally rotate the arm and continue abduction and vertical oscillation. **C.** Reduction is typically achieved before 120-degree abduction.

A shoulder dislocation is more likely to be irreducible the longer it has been in this position. Should the dislocation be irreducible by the methods listed previously, then general anesthesia is considered and reduction attempted in the operating room. Irreducible dislocations constitute 5% to 10% of cases treated in the ED and are usually due to soft-tissue interposition.

Immobilization and Rehabilitation

Following reduction, the shoulder should be immobilized, and the patient sent for postreduction radiographs. The traditional method of immobilization is adduction and internal rotation, typically with a sling and swathe or a shoulder immobilizer (Appendix A–13). In an effort to reduce the long-term rate of recurrent dislocation, several authors have proposed immobilization in 10 degrees of external rotation.[98–101] This position has been shown in a few studies to reduce redislocation rates.[98,102] In magnetic resonance imaging (MRI) studies, external rotation provides better anatomic reduction of the detached labral lesions.[103–105] The most common method is with a wire-mesh splint covered with sponge that is bent such that half of the splint fits over the anterior trunk and the second half extends forward and is attached to the arm. Commercially available splints are also available to immobilize the shoulder in external rotation. Although seemingly awkward for patients, studies have found this immobilization to be surprisingly well tolerated with good compliance rates.[102]

Recent studies have not shown benefit to external rotation over a typical internal rotation sling.[106,107] Further research is needed to determine the optimal mode of immobilization after primary shoulder dislocation.

The duration of immobilization is also unclear but is generally longer in younger patients due to the higher rates of recurrence. In patients younger than 30 years, 3 weeks of immobilization is advocated. A German study showed equivalent results with 3 weeks of immobilization compared to 5 weeks.[108] After this, gentle active range-of-motion exercises can be instituted; however, the patient should be cautioned against abduction and external rotation. External rotation and abduction should be prohibited for an additional 3 weeks after immobilization has been discontinued. During the time the patient is immobilized, exercises of the wrist, hand, and elbow should be instituted.

In patients older than 30 years, we advocate immobilization for 7 to 10 days, with circumduction (Codman) exercises to begin within 4 to 5 days of injury to reduce stiffness (Fig. 11–13).[109] The patient should avoid abduction and external rotation of the shoulder. Exercise should be performed within a pain-free range of motion following the period of immobilization. Too little movement following a dislocation may result in tightening of the structures around the shoulder and a prolonged time to regain full range of motion.[109]

Following the initial recovery period, strengthening of the subscapularis muscle is advocated to prevent future

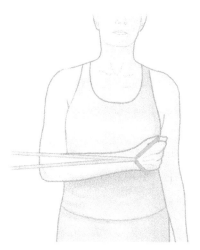

Figure 16–63. Internal rotation exercise using rubber tubing strengthens the subscapularis muscle and helps prevent recurrent dislocations of the shoulder. The elbow is held as close to the chest wall as possible.

redislocation (Fig. 16-63). Exercises can be initiated 2 months after injury. The external rotators can be strengthened by the opposite maneuver. By strengthening these muscles, the capsule, which is a static stabilizer of the joint, is further enhanced by the dynamic muscular stabilizers.

Definitive Treatment

There are several indications for surgery in an acute anterior dislocation of the shoulder besides soft-tissue interposition. In a subglenoid or subclavicular dislocation, complete disruption of the cuff often occurs. Fracture of the greater tuberosity that is displaced more than 5 mm postreduction or a glenoid rim (Bankart) fracture that is displaced more than 5 mm is also an indication for surgery.

Arthroscopic repair of a labral tear (i.e., soft-tissue Bankart lesion) is sometimes recommended in young patients with physically demanding occupations after a first-time dislocation.[98,116-118] Surgery in these patients will significantly reduce the rate of recurrent dislocation.[2] Most agree, however, that unless there is a complication requiring surgery, most patients do not benefit from surgical intervention to stabilize these dislocations.[116-118]

Complications

The most common complication of anterior dislocation is recurrence, which is seen in 60% of patients younger than 30 years and drops off to an incidence of approximately 10% to 15% in patients older than 40 years.[106,119] Operative repair is indicated in patients who have sustained multiple dislocations. Most of the literature demonstrates that patients with recurrent dislocations have extensive capsular tears and at least partial labral detachment resulting in some instability. Bankart lesions have been found at the time of repair in 90% of cases.[120]

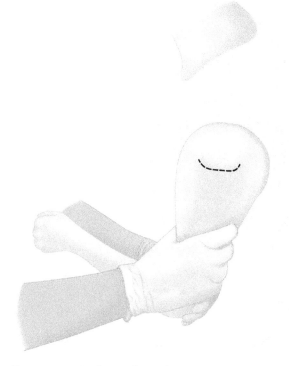

Figure 16–64. Technique for performing the inferior sulcus sign.

Anterior glenohumeral instability may complicate an anterior shoulder dislocation or occur independently in the absence of a previous dislocation. This condition, in which subluxation of the humeral head occurs due to a loss of ligamentous and labral support, is a common, often missed problem in the ED. Subluxation is characterized by sudden sharp pain when the shoulder is forcibly moved into external rotation during abduction. Instability may be suggested by the *inferior sulcus sign.* This can be noted when downward traction on the affected arm results in a visible sulcus below the lateral acromion (Fig. 16-64). In addition, the *shoulder apprehension test* is usually positive. To perform this test, the arm is rotated externally and abducted. Anterior pressure is then applied to the posterior aspect of the humeral head (Fig. 16-65). This causes

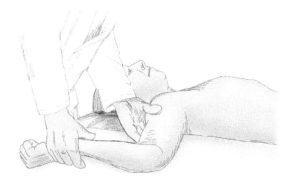

Figure 16–65. Technique for performing shoulder apprehension test.

sudden pain and may cause anterior displacement of the humeral head. When performed 6 to 9 weeks after the initial dislocation, it may be suggestive of an increased risk for recurrent dislocation. However, the exam test cannot be used as a definitive predictor of recurrence alone and has relatively poor sensitivity.[121] When this is a recurrent problem, the patient should be referred for further evaluation as many of these cases require surgical intervention to stabilize the shoulder.

POSTERIOR SHOULDER DISLOCATION

Posterior dislocations are far less common than anterior dislocations, but are the most commonly missed major dislocations of the body. These dislocations are missed in up to 60% to 70% of cases.[122-124] The most frequent cause is suboptimal radiographic evaluation, but they also present with less pain than anterior dislocations and the radiographic findings are subtle. The diagnosis of a posterior shoulder dislocation should be suspected in a patient whose shoulders are blocked to external rotation.

There are three types of posterior dislocations—subacromial, subglenoid, and subspinous—the majority of which are subacromial.

Mechanism of Injury

There are several mechanisms by which this injury occurs. A blow to the anterior aspect of the shoulder and axial loading of the arm when it is adducted and internally rotated are two possible mechanisms. A violent internal rotational force such as would occur during a fall on the forward flexed internally rotated arm is another mechanism. A seizure or an electric shock is a common precursor to posterior shoulder dislocation and occurs because the internal rotators are twice as strong as the external rotator muscles.[125]

Examination

Posterior dislocations are not clinically obvious. The cardinal sign of a posterior dislocation of the shoulder is that the arm is held in adduction and internal rotation. Internal and external rotation of the glenohumeral joint will be very limited. Abduction is severely limited, and external rotation of the shoulder is blocked (Video 16–10). On palpation of the shoulder girdle, the examiner will note a prominence in the posterior aspect of the shoulder accompanied by an anterior flattening of the normal shoulder contour. The coracoid process is usually more obvious than its counterpart on the normal side. *Blocking of external rotation and limitation of abduction occur in all cases of posterior dislocations.* In the subglenoid and subspinous type, the arm is held in 30 degrees of abduction and internally rotated. A subacromial dimple may be present with a posterior dislocation, representing the posteromedial portion of the deltoid.[125]

Imaging

Evidence of a posterior shoulder dislocation on the standard AP view of the shoulder is not always apparent, causing this dislocation to be missed on this view in up to 50% of cases.[126] A lateral projection is essential.

However, there are several radiographic features that will aid the emergency physician in making this diagnosis on a standard AP view.

Rim sign. This is the loss of the normal elliptical pattern produced by overlap of the medial aspect of the humeral head and the anterior glenoid rim (Fig. 16–66). Either superimposition of these two structures or widening of the joint space (>6 mm) suggest a posterior dislocation.

Lightbulb sign. Internal rotation of the humeral head that occurs with a posterior shoulder dislocation results in rotation of the greater tuberosity so it is no longer in its normal lateral position (Fig. 16–67). This is referred to as the "lightbulb" or "ice cream cone" sign because the humeral head appears rounded, as though it sits on top of a cone—the humeral shaft.[127]

Trough line sign. When the humeral head dislocates behind the glenoid, an impaction fracture occurs to its articular surface referred to as the "reverse Hill–Sachs lesion." On the AP radiograph, two parallel lines of cortical bone representing the medial cortex of the humeral head and the base of the impaction fracture on the anterior articular surface are called the trough line sign (Fig. 16–68).[126,128] This was found in 75% of posterior dislocations in one case series.[126]

If a question remains about dislocation, a lateral projection such as a scapular Y or axillary view should be obtained (Fig. 16–69). A CT scan will be diagnostic and also reveals the size of the impaction fracture, aiding the orthopedic surgeon in choosing the best definitive treatment (Fig. 16–70).[123,129]

> **Axiom:** *A scapular Y view or axillary lateral view is essential to exclude a posterior shoulder dislocation, which may be missed in 50% cases.*

Associated Injuries

This dislocation is commonly associated with fractures of the humerus and the posterior aspect of the glenoid rim.[123] An isolated fracture of the lesser tuberosity should lead one to suspect a posterior dislocation until proven otherwise. A reverse Hill–Sachs lesion is an impression defect on the anteromedial part of the humeral head due to compression by the glenoid. It is seen in up to 80% of these patients.[122] Rotator cuff tears are present in up to 20% of cases.[130] Neurovascular complications with this injury are uncommon.

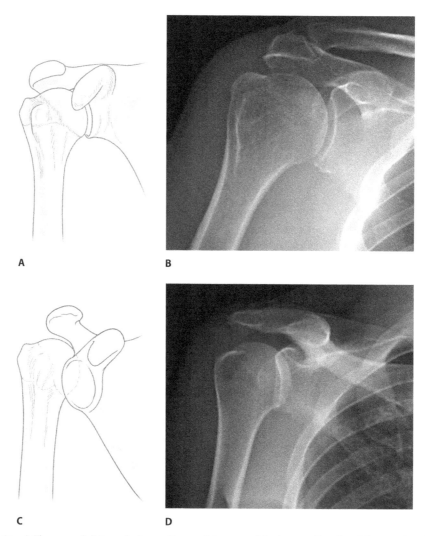

Figure 16–66. Rim sign. **A.** The normal distance between the medial aspect of the humeral head and the anterior glenoid rim. **B.** Normal radiograph. **C.** In the patient with a posterior dislocation, this distance is abnormal. **D.** Superimposition (i.e., Rim sign) seen on a radiograph of a posterior shoulder dislocation.

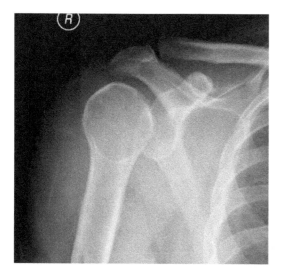

Figure 16–67. Lightbulb sign indicating a posterior shoulder dislocation.

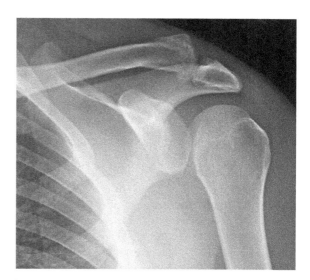

Figure 16–68. Trough sign indicating a posterior shoulder dislocation.

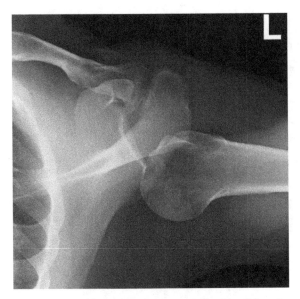

Figure 16-69. Axillary view of a posterior shoulder dislocation.

Axiom: *An isolated fracture of the lesser tuberosity should lead one to suspect posterior dislocation of the shoulder until proven otherwise.*

Treatment

Consultation with an orthopedic surgeon is advised. Closed reduction using axial traction on the flexed and adducted shoulder is usually successful and can be performed in acute dislocations (<3 weeks) when there is a less than 25% articular surface defect.[123] Direct pressure on the posteriorly displaced humeral head may facilitate the reduction. Indications for surgical intervention include significant displacement of the lesser tuberosity that is irreducible on reduction of the dislocation, an articular defect greater than 25%, or a chronic dislocation (>3 weeks).

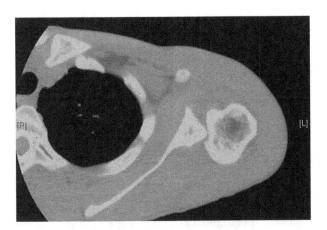

Figure 16-70. CT scan demonstrating a posterior shoulder dislocation. Note the articular impaction fracture.

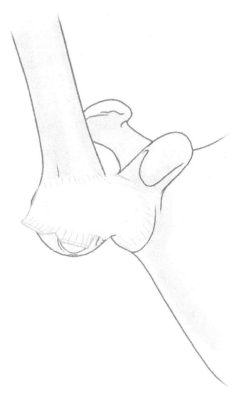

Figure 16-71. Luxatio erecta. The mechanism by which this injury occurs is hyperabduction. This dislocation is always accompanied by both disruption of the rotator cuff and tear through the inferior capsule.

INFERIOR SHOULDER DISLOCATION (LUXATIO ERECTA)

Inferior dislocations of the shoulder are uncommon, accounting for 0.5% of shoulder dislocations (Fig. 16–71). These injuries are more common in men than women and can occur at any age.[131] The term *luxatio erecta* means "to place upward," which refers to the characteristic presentation of the arm in this injury.

Mechanism of Injury

The mechanism by which this injury occurs is forceful hyperabduction.[132]

Examination

This injury is unlikely to be missed because the patient holds the arm elevated 180 degrees and cannot adduct it, as if they are "asking a question" (Fig. 16–72A). These patients usually present with significant pain. The arm appears to be shortened when compared with the normal side. On palpation, the humeral head is felt along the lateral chest wall.

Imaging

Standard shoulder radiographs are diagnostic and reveal the inferior location of the humeral head with the humeral shaft raised upward (Fig. 16–72B).

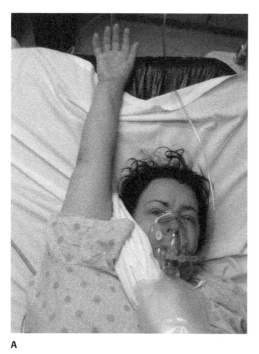
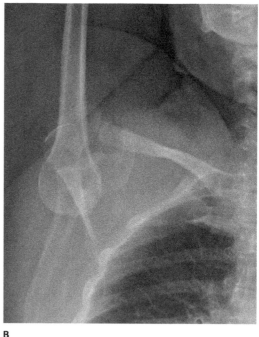

A

B

Figure 16–72. **A.** Patient with an inferior shoulder dislocation (luxatio erecta). **B.** Radiograph.

Associated Injuries

Luxatio erecta may concurrently cause damage to the rotator cuff. In a review of 80 published cases of luxatio erecta, rotator cuff tears were noted in 12% of cases. Patients commonly have neurovascular compression; however, they usually recover function following reduction. The axillary artery and brachial plexus are commonly injured because the humeral head tears through the inferior capsule rather than the anterior capsule as with an anterior dislocation of the shoulder. Vascular injury is not common but occurs more often in luxatio erecta than in any other type of shoulder dislocation. Greater tuberosity fractures are the most common associated fracture. Reduction of the dislocation often reduces the fracture fragment as well.

Treatment

Early reduction is necessary in luxatio erecta to prevent neurovascular sequelae. Reduction is not difficult in most cases, unless the humeral head has torn a small defect in the inferior glenohumeral capsule. In these cases, closed reduction may not be successful, and open reduction may be required. To perform the reduction, the physician applies traction in the longitudinal axis of the humerus while an assistant applies countertraction with a folded sheet wrapped around the supraclavicular region (Fig. 16–73 and Video 16–11). While traction is maintained, the arm is rotated inferiorly in an arch as shown.

Another reduction technique is the two-step closed reduction maneuver in which the inferior dislocation is converted to an anterior location prior to full reduction. To perform this maneuver, the physician should stand on the affected side with the patient in the supine position. One hand (PUSH hand) should be placed on the lateral aspect of the midhumerus with the second hand (PULL hand) positioned over the medial epicondyle. The physician will

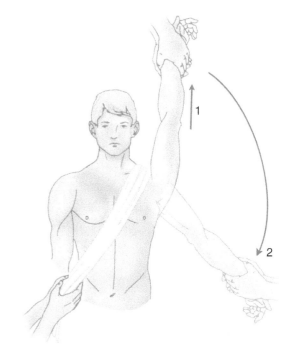

Figure 16–73. Reduction of a luxatio erecta dislocation. Traction is applied by the physician in the longitudinal axis of the humerus while an assistant applies countertraction with a folded sheet. While traction is maintained, the arm is rotated inferiorly in an arc as shown.

provide pressure to the humerus with the push hand while gently pulling at the elbow. This should reduce the humeral head to an anterior location. Ability to adduct the arm against the body confirms the conversion. At this point, the physician may use their preferred technique for reduction of an anterior glenohumeral dislocation.

After reduction, immobilize the shoulder for 2 to 4 weeks. Post injury, the patient must be followed closely for evidence of rotator cuff tears.[131]

IMPINGEMENT SYNDROME

Impingement syndrome involves mechanical compression of the rotator cuff tendons as they pass between the acromion, the rigid coracoacromial ligament, and the head of the humerus (Fig. 16–4).[134] The end result is acute inflammation, edema, and hemorrhage of the rotator cuff tendons. If untreated, fibrosis and tendinosis occur, and eventually the condition progresses to tearing of the rotator cuff tendons. The supraspinatus tendon is most commonly affected because of its proximity to the coracoacromial arch and poorer blood supply.

The condition most commonly affects elderly individuals and young athletes whose sport involves overhead motions (e.g., tennis, swimming). It has also been described in patients with whiplash injury secondary to a seatbelt.[135]

Many anatomic variables contribute to impingement, including a hooked acromion, osteophyte formation, subacromial bursal fibrosis, and coracoacromial ligament thickening. A hook-shaped acromion has been associated with a greater extent of rotator cuff tears.[136,137]

The clinical findings of impingement are characterized by pain that is referred to the lateral aspect of the upper arm in the region of the deltoid and its insertion. Characteristically, the pain is worse at night and is typically exacerbated

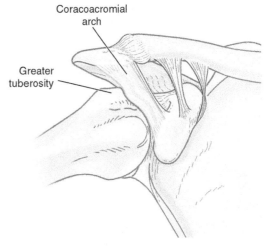

Figure 16–74. In the painful arch syndrome, as the patient elevates and abducts the arm, the tuberosity encroaches on the coracoacromial arch. This causes maximal pain between 60 and 120 degrees.

with overhead activities because the outlet narrows with shoulder abduction (Fig. 16–74). The painful arch is between 60- and 120-degree abduction, which indicates a disorder of a structure in the subacromial region.[138]

Tenderness is maximal below the lateral edge of the acromion. The rotator cuff outlet is further compromised when the shoulder is placed in forward flexion and internal rotation (Fig. 16–75A). Pain may be cleared by external rotation of the humerus during abduction. Pain may also occur with passive forward elevation of the pronated arm to 180 degrees (Fig. 16–75B). High-resolution ultrasonography is useful in diagnosing this condition, as is MRI.[135] In situations where the pain increases at a point beyond 120 degrees of abduction up to full elevation, disorders of the AC joints should be suspected.

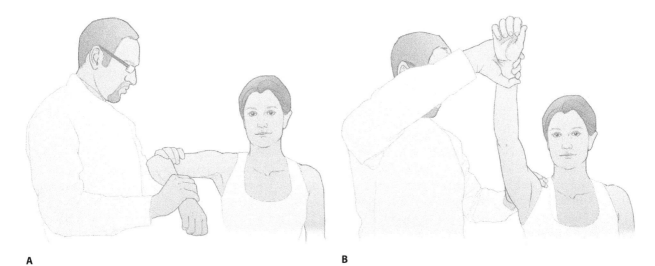

A   **B**

Figure 16–75. **A.** Hawkins sign—internal rotation of the forward-flexed arm with elbow flexion reproduces subacromial impingement. **B.** Neer test—painful forward flexion of the internally rotated arm results in impingement.

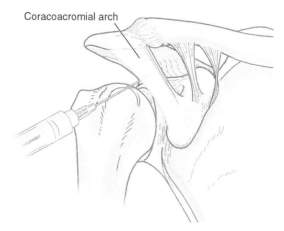

Coracoacromial arch

Figure 16–76. Injection along the coracoacromial arch. Injection should be concentrated under the arch, which is palpable through the needle tip.

Treatment with a local anesthetic and steroid injection may provide immediate relief and support the diagnosis if the pain resolves. Have the patient sit with the arm relaxed at the side. The needle is inserted underneath the anterior edge of the acromion and the coracoacromial ligament at the site of maximal tenderness (Fig. 16–76 and Video 16–12).

SUPRASPINATUS TENDONITIS AND SUBACROMIAL BURSITIS

The pathogenesis, clinical presentation, and treatment of these two conditions are similar, and they will therefore be considered together.

Supraspinatus tendonitis is the most common cause of shoulder pain and is usually caused by degenerative changes in that tendon with advancing age and impingement, as stated previously. Impingement is the cause of approximately three-fourths of the cases, followed by chronic overuse (10%) and acute strains (5%).

The tendons of the supraspinatus, infraspinatus, teres minor, and subscapularis muscles come together and attach on the greater and lesser tuberosities to form the rotator cuff. Tendonitis can occur in any one of these tendons but is much more common where the supraspinatus tendon comes in close proximity with the coracoacromial arch (Fig. 16–77).

The pathogenesis of supraspinatus tendonitis is along a continuum that will ultimately lead to subacromial bursitis. As the supraspinatus tendon traverses under the acromion and the coracoacromial arch, small tears occur. The repair process is associated with inflammatory cells that lead to tendonitis. The patient seen at this stage usually complains of a deep ache in the shoulder with increasing pain on abduction and internal rotation. The inflammatory cells cause significant swelling, and eventually calcium deposits within the tendon.[19] The swelling of the tendon causes worsening impingement on the subacromial bursa that forms the roof of the supraspinatus tendon. At this stage, the tendon becomes an obstacle to pain-free abduction, and the patient

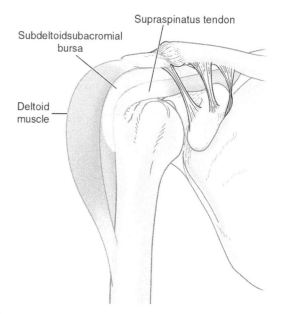

Subdeltoidsubacromial bursa

Supraspinatus tendon

Deltoid muscle

Figure 16–77. The relationship of the supraspinatus tendon and the subdeltoid–subacromial bursa.

complains of increasing pain in the shoulder. Attempts to abduct the arm to 70 degrees cause significant pain.

As the process continues, a severe inflammatory reaction occurs within the bursa, leading to bursitis. As the subacromial bursa swells, partial abduction and adduction are restricted. The arm is held at approximately 30 degrees of abduction. Further adduction or abduction causes increasing pain, and the patient resists any attempt to elevate the arm beyond this point. If the process is allowed to continue, the patient may experience a chronic bursitis leading eventually to adhesive pericapsulitis or bursitis.

This condition usually occurs between the ages of 35 and 50 years. It appears to be more common in sedentary people. Patients usually complain of a deep ache in the shoulder referred to the deltoid region, and the pain may radiate to the entire limb. There is often point tenderness at a "critical point" between the acromion and the greater tuberosity. The pain is increased on abduction and internal rotation of the arm. The onset is usually gradual, but may be acute after overuse of the shoulder, especially in an overhead position. Within 2 to 3 days, the pain becomes increasingly intense at the point of the shoulder.

Radiographic findings include calcification and cystic changes along the greater tuberosity accompanied by sclerosis. These do not occur, however, until the process has become more chronic. Calcification is sometimes seen in asymptomatic patients.

Treatment consists of avoidance of the inciting activity, nonsteroidal anti-inflammatory drugs (NSAIDs), ice, and exercises that prevent muscle atrophy. The patient should be encouraged to initiate range of motion, starting with pendulum (Codman) exercises (Fig. 16–12). Continued motion is essential to reduce the risk of adhesive capsulitis in patients older than 40 years. Physical therapy referral is appropriate.

Treatment with a local anesthetic and steroid injection may provide immediate relief. A lateral approach in which the needle is inserted directly under the acromion is used (Video 16–13). A longer needle directed medially and anteriorly under the acromion provides the best results.[140] Move the needle back and forth through the tendon sheath as this releases the fluid in the bursa and reduces pain. Ultrasound is very useful in both making the diagnosis and aiding in placement of steroid injections.[141] Methylprednisolone (40 mg, 1 mL) and bupivacaine (5–10 mL) are generally effective. The condition may require repeat injections before relief is obtained, so the patient should be referred for follow-up care. Local corticosteroid injections have been commonly performed for this condition with unclear benefit. Some studies have shown a marginal decrease in pain but long-term improvement has not been demonstrated in the limited published literature.[192] In patients with calcific tendonitis/bursitis, which can lead to frozen shoulder syndrome, optimal outpatient treatment includes multiple punctures in the calcific deposits to break up the calcium and treat the condition.[135]

ROTATOR CUFF TEARS

Tears of the rotator cuff are more common in the elderly because of degenerative changes that occur with advancing age, particularly after the fifth decade of life. In patients older than 60 years, full-thickness rotator cuff tears occurred with a reported incidence of 28% in asymptomatic individuals.[134,135] Only 25% of rotator cuff tears are symptomatic.[143]

Disruption of the rotator cuff can occur at any point; however, it is more common in the anterosuperior portion of the cuff near the attachment of the supraspinatus muscle (Fig. 16–78).[144] In this location, the tendon is worn down by impingement occurring between the humeral head and the coracoacromial arch. Other causes include intrinsic degeneration, chronic overuse, or acute overload.[134]

When this injury is seen in the young, it requires a greater degree of trauma. Prior to the fifth decade, rotator cuff tears are more likely to avulse bone.[145] The mechanism by which one disrupts the rotator cuff is usually a sudden powerful elevation of the arm against resistance in an attempt to cushion a fall. It can also occur secondary to heavy lifting or a fall on the shoulder. In a patient older than 50 years, this injury may occur with minimal or no trauma (e.g., during sleep).

The patient presents with complaints of pain aggravated by activity that radiates to the anterior aspect of the arm. There is no relationship between the size of the tear and the level of pain and disability.[146] The most severe pain occurs when one compresses the tendon beneath the coracoacromial arch with passive abduction between 70 and 120 degrees.[147] Abduction is painful and weak. Although no singular examination maneuver is definitive, the rotator cuff can be evaluated in the ED with a comprehensive physical examination, including range of motion, strength testing, and provocative maneuvers as described previously in the section.

Weakness in abduction of greater than 50% compared to the unaffected arm is suggestive of a large or massive tear.[148] Up to 40 degrees of abduction may occur by the "shrugging" mechanism alone in which the patient compensates for glenohumeral motion with scapulothoracic motion. The patient cannot *initiate abduction* if large tears of the supraspinatus occur (Video 16–14). Strength testing of the supraspinatus, infraspinatus, and subscapularis muscles is also helpful in the acute evaluation of rotator cuff tears (Fig. 16–8).

The *drop arm test* is frequently positive in patients with significant tears.[26,149] This test is performed by laterally elevating the arm to the 90-degree position, and asking the patient to hold the arm in this position (Fig. 16–79 and Video 16–15). A slight pressure on the distal forearm or

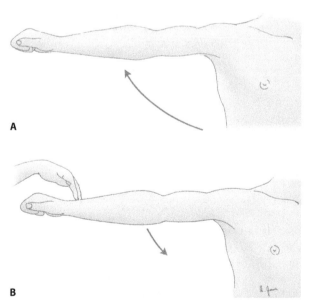

A

B

Figure 16–79. The drop arm test is shown. **A.** The patient or examiner abducts the arm to 90 degrees. **B.** With minimal pressure over the abducted arm, the patient cannot sustain abduction and drops the arm to the side.

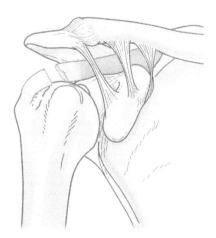

Figure 16–78. A rotator cuff tear is shown. The rotator cuff usually tears along the supraspinatus tendon insertion.

wrist applied by the examiner will cause the patient to suddenly drop the arm. In addition, the patient is unable to bring the arm from the abducted position to the side in a slow fashion, but rather, drops it suddenly. Lidocaine may be infiltrated around the cuff in patients unable to abduct the arm to perform the drop arm test. Injection will also allow the examiner to differentiate a significant tear from tendonitis, as patients with tendonitis will be able to perform better after injection.

All physical examination findings should be interpreted with caution and incorporated into the context of the clinical picture because no singular physical examination maneuver has sufficient predictive value. Multiple studies have shown that physical examination alone has relatively low sensitivity at picking up even moderate tears. However, the combination of age older than 65, night pain, and weakness in external rotation was found to have a specificity of 95% in the diagnosis of rotator cuff tears.

When tears are localized to the posterosuperior aspect of the cuff, pain is elicited on abduction and internal rotation, whereas tears of the anterosuperior cuff cause pain on abduction and external rotation. A defect may be palpable in early cases (i.e., before swelling occurs) of acute rotator cuff rupture below the acromion. Crepitation may be palpated on examination in this region.

Although often not definitive, plain radiographs are the first line in the evaluation of suspected rotator cuff injuries. One may see the acromial morphology and signs of degenerative changes in the rotator cuff, including the following: erosion and periosteal reaction of the greater tuberosity, alterations of the inferior aspect of the acromion, humeral osteophytes, and subchondral erosion in the greater tuberosity. A true AP (Grashey view) is more sensitive than traditional AP views of the shoulder.

The sensitivity of MRI for the diagnosis of full-thickness rotator cuff tears is 100% and the specificity is 95%. MRI is able to differentiate partial cuff tears from intact tendons with a sensitivity of 82% and a specificity of 85%. It is also highly predictive of the size of the full-thickness rotator cuff tear. MR arthrography is an excellent means of detecting the degree of tear. High-resolution, real-time US has been shown to be a good examination technique for rotator cuff tears. Some studies have shown equal accuracy with US and MRI.

Conservative measures remain the mainstay of initial treatment for most rotator cuff tears. Conservative therapy will result in a good outcome in 50% of patients. Passive range-of-motion exercises should be instituted as soon as possible in elderly patients. In the initial period, rest, ice, and NSAIDs should be accompanied by modified activity and physical therapy. With partial-thickness tears, range-of-motion exercises are important to reduce stiffness.

In the young, early surgical repair is indicated for complete tears of the rotator cuff. Arthroscopic rotator cuff repair leads to satisfactory results in more than 90% of cases. In a large study involving more than 400 patients, arthroscopic repairs for moderate tears was the mainstay of treatment with excellent results, and open repair was reserved for massive tears. More recent studies suggest that arthroscopic repair can be considered even in large or massive tears because clinical outcomes are good despite higher incidence of recurrent tear. In the elderly, with more sedentary lifestyles, repair may not be beneficial.

BICIPITAL TENDINOSIS

The long head of the biceps traverses between the greater and lesser tuberosities within the bicipital groove and inserts on the glenoid rim. In this location, it is ensheathed by the capsule of the glenohumeral joint. This position makes the tendon subject to constant trauma and irritation from motions of the shoulder and impingement as described previously. Inflammation around the tendon increases until it moves reluctantly. Bicipital tendinosis rarely occurs in isolation and is commonly a marker for underlying impingement or labral pathology, such as the superior labrum anterior to posterior or SLAP tear.

The patient complains of pain in the biceps region and anterior aspect of the shoulder that radiates down toward the forearm. Abduction and external rotation are the most painful motions, and snap extension of the elbow increases the pain markedly. On examination, there is tenderness to palpation in the bicipital groove (Video 16–10). This irritative process increases with abduction of the shoulder with the elbow fixed in an extended position. A reliable test for diagnosing tenosynovitis of the long head of the biceps is the *Yergason test* (Fig. 16–80). In performing this test, the patient's elbow is held at 90 degrees of flexion. The patient is asked to supinate the forearm as the examiner resists this attempt. This causes pain along the intertubercular groove and is a reliable test to indicate tenosynovitis of the long head of the biceps.

This condition may progress to complete adhesion of the tendon, and either shoulder motion will be restricted or the biceps will rupture proximal to the groove.

The treatment includes immobilization in a sling and injection of the bicipital canal with an anesthetic and

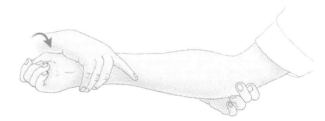

Figure 16–80. The Yergason test. Although this test was originally described for dislocation of the bicipital tendon, it can be used to diagnose tenosynovitis of the long head of the biceps as well. In performing this test, the patient is asked to supinate the forearm against resistance as the elbow is held in flexion.

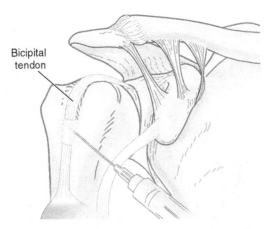

Figure 16–81. Injection of the bicipital tendon sheath along the intertubercular groove.

steroid solution (Fig. 16–81 and Video 16–17).[167] One must be careful not to inject the tendon itself. The injection is usually carried out at several points along the route of the tendon within the bicipital groove. Analgesics and anti-inflammatory agents may be administered as well.

BICIPITAL TENDON SUBLUXATION

The bicipital tendon can subluxate or dislocate out of its groove between the greater and lesser tuberosities (Fig. 16–82). This condition is more likely when there is a congenitally abnormal, shallow bicipital groove. A tear of the subscapularis tendon where it attaches to the lesser tuberosity and extends over the bicipital groove is another predisposing factor. The most common mechanism by which this condition occurs acutely is forced external rotation of the arm with the biceps contracted.

The patient usually complains of a painful snap felt in the anterior aspect of the shoulder during forced external rotation of the arm while the biceps is contracted. With

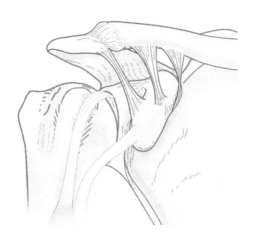

Figure 16–82. Dislocation of the bicipital tendon out of the intertubercular groove.

rotation, the tendon slips back and forth, in and out of the groove. Pain is usually felt in the anterior and lateral aspect of the shoulder and is referred distally and along the anterior aspect of the arm. The pain is typically worse at night; in the acute phase, spasms of the deltoid and subscapularis muscles are common accompanying features. The *Yergason test* should be performed. The stability of the biceps tendon is determined by subluxation of the tendon from its normal position in the intertubercular groove. When supination against resistance is tested, the bicipital tendon will pop out of the groove and the patient will experience pain.

Treatment is usually operative. Both anchoring the tendon to bone (i.e., tenodesis) and releasing the tendon (i.e., tenotomy) are possibilities, and the specific procedure performed depends on a variety of factors, including the age of the patient, activity level, presence of an accompanying rotator cuff tear, and the condition of the tendon itself.[169]

ACUTE TRAUMATIC SYNOVITIS

This is common secondary to sprains of the glenohumeral ligaments or slight tears in the capsule occurring in young athletes. The patient complains of pain over the shoulder joint, and there is tenderness elicited to palpation of the capsule and motion of the shoulder. The anterior/inferior portion of the capsule is the most commonly affected site, usually secondary to abduction–external rotation injuries. The treatment for this condition is immobilization in a sling and the application of warm moist packs. One should begin active range-of-motion exercises as soon as pain will permit.

ADHESIVE CAPSULITIS

Adhesive capsulitis, or "frozen shoulder," usually occurs in women older than 40 years. It may be insidious in onset or occur after an injury.[170] Pain is projected to the anterolateral aspect of the shoulder and to the arm. Nighttime pain is often severe, interfering with sleep.[171] Risk factors include diabetes, trauma, hypertriglyceridemia, and thyroid disease. Diabetes, in particular, is a major risk factor as 20% of diabetics will experience adhesive capsulitis. Furthermore, in a small study, 30% of patients with adhesive capsulitis were diagnosed with diabetes or prediabetes.[172] Due to the strong association, emergency physicians should consider screening patients for diabetes or referring them for diabetic testing when adhesive capsulitis is suspected.

Symptoms typically progress through three traditional phases over the course of several months.[173] The initial "freezing" stage occurs with progressive pain from the synovitis and development of limited range of motion. The middle phase is the "frozen stage" in which the range of motion becomes very limited with a rigid feel. The third phase is the "thawing phase" in which slow improvements in range of motion and pain can occur.

Loss of external rotation is greater than abduction and internal rotation. In most cases, palpation over the bicipital tendon groove elicits pain.   Although the etiology of frozen shoulder in many cases remains unclear, increasingly calcific tendonitis of the rotator cuff and bicipital tendon complexes are being implicated.

Treatment is not the same in all cases and consists of physical therapy, NSAIDs, corticosteroid injections, and surgery. Exercises to improve the range of motion should be done in the painless arc of motion.   Corticosteroids have been shown to improve results but require multiple injections.   Simple excision of the calcified material will initiate a sequence of events leading to recovery in many cases.   Arthroscopically, multiple punctures through these deposits lead to good results.

SCAPULOCOSTAL SYNDROMES AND BURSITIS

The syndromes in this category are a group of conditions with a common course and clinical presentation. They are usually caused by inflammation of the bursae around the scapula or strains of the muscles that insert onto the scapula. Pain in the scapular region is usually secondary to poor posture and occurs more commonly at the end of the day. These conditions can also be seen when the arm has not been used for a protracted length of time because of fractures or other conditions.

The onset of bursitis and muscle strains around the scapula is usually insidious and is characterized by exacerbations and remissions. The most common sites for bursitis to occur in this region are the superior and inferior angles of the scapula. The patient usually experiences pain on any motion of the scapula, and the examiner may elicit crepitation when instructing the patient to bring the arm across the chest. To diagnose this condition, the physician should retract the scapula by asking the patient to place the hand on the opposite shoulder. A trigger point usually at the superior angle or near the base of the spine can be palpated. Lidocaine injection should give the patient relief if the condition is secondary to a bursitis of one of the scapular bursae.

Local injection of a trigger point affords prompt relief and should be attempted in those cases with significant pain. Heat in the form of ultrasound twice a day for 20 minutes each day and diathermy (electrically induced heat treatments) provides good relief for patients with muscle strains. Patients with bursitis in the scapular region can be treated with local injection, heat, and rest.

LONG THORACIC NERVE PALSY

Injury of the long thoracic nerve results in paralysis of the serratus anterior muscle. This nerve is injured due to its length and superficial course. Clinically, this injury is noted by an unusual prominence of the medial and

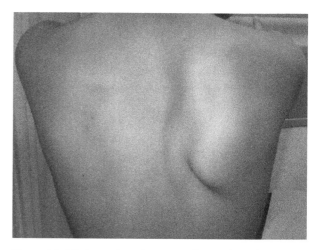

Figure 16–83. Long thoracic nerve palsy on the right creating the classic appearance of the "winged scapula."

inferior borders of the scapula, commonly referred to as the "winged scapula" (Fig. 16–83). The most common cause of this injury is overuse. Other causes include acute trauma, either blunt or penetrating, and the improper use of axillary crutches. The cause is idiopathic in 17% of cases.

Treatment is conservative in most cases, including analgesics and referral for physical therapy. A full range of motion should be encouraged. Recovery may take 12 to 18 months. One-fourth of patients do not recover following conservative management and should be considered for surgical repair.

EXTRINSIC DISORDERS

A number of extrinsic disorders can present as shoulder pain. The astute clinician should consider a referred source of pain when the patient presents with shoulder pain and minimal findings on physical examination. Serious underlying pathology, such as an acute myocardial infarction or an inflammatory process under the diaphragm, may refer pain to the shoulder. Cervical spine disease, brachial plexus neuropathy, neoplastic disease, and thoracic outlet syndrome cause shoulder pain and will be considered subsequently.

Cervical Spine Disease

Cervical spine problems, including disk degeneration, herniation, and osteoarthritis, can cause shoulder pain. The examiner will find restricted range of motion of the neck, and the shoulder pain is often reproduced by neck movement. Neurologic findings, such as a radiculopathy, may be present and can be assessed with the *Spurling test*. This test can be performed by lateral bending of the neck to the affected extremity and applying a downward axial load on the cervical spine. The addition of neck extension with lateral bending may improve the sensitivity.   It is important to examine the cervical spine carefully and order radiographs of the neck if this condition is suspected.

Treatment consists of analgesics and referral. Shoulder pain that radiates beyond the elbow should prompt evaluation of the cervical spine.

Brachial Plexus Neuropathy

This is an uncommon cause of shoulder pain that can present with vague symptoms that are either localized or diffuse throughout the upper extremity. Brachial plexus neuropathy can occur due to allergic conditions, infectious disorders (viral syndromes), or may be idiopathic.

The predominant symptom is pain, which may be localized to the shoulder area or generalized. Within a few weeks, the patient usually develops weakness in the shoulder girdle. This condition usually has a good prognosis.[178]

Neoplastic Disease

Neoplastic disease, particularly of the apical lung, may present with shoulder pain. This may involve the chest wall and brachial plexus producing local pain or radicular pain.

Thoracic Outlet Syndrome

This syndrome includes a number of disorders, including neurologic and vascular compression. In neurologic thoracic outlet syndrome, portions of the brachial plexus can be compressed as the plexus traverses the supraclavicular area and passes through the axilla to the arm. Compression may be due to the scalene muscle, the first rib, the coracoid process, or the tendinous insertion of the pectoralis minor muscle.[178] Patients present with pain noted during certain motions. Thrusting of the shoulders back with the arms dependent at the side while the patient is taking a deep breath may produce pain. The medial trunk of the brachial plexus is the area most commonly affected by compression. Thus, pain may radiate down the forearm along the ulnar nerve distribution, and weakness of grasp may be noted.[179]

The treatment for neurologic thoracic outlet syndrome consists of physical therapy and shoulder muscle strengthening, which provides symptomatic relief. Occasionally, surgery is necessary to relieve the area of compression.[177,179]

Vascular compression may also occur but is less common. Activity-related compression of the venous outflow may result from repetitive shoulder abduction such as performed by overhead athletes. This is commonly referred to as *Paget–Schroetter syndrome* and requires urgent evaluation by a vascular surgery for consideration of thrombolysis.[179]

REFERENCES

1. Neer CS. Displaced proximal humeral fractures. I. Classification and evaluation. *J Bone Joint Surg Am*. 1970;52(6): 1077–1089.
2. Carofino B, Leopold S. Classifications in brief: the Neer classification for proximal humerus fractures. *Clin Orthop Relat Res*. 2013;471(1):39–43.
3. Haapamaki VV, Kiuru MJ, Koskinen SK. Multidetector CT in shoulder fractures. *Emerg Radiol*. 2004;11(2): 89–94.
4. Flatow EL, Cuomo F, Maday MG, Miller SR, McIlveen SJ, Bigliani LU. Open reduction and internal fixation of two-part displaced fractures of the greater tuberosity of the proximal part of the humerus. *J Bone Joint Surg Am*. 1991; 73(8):1213–1218.
5. Geominne S, Debeer P. The natural evolution of neglected lesser tuberosity fractures in skeletally immature patients. *J Shoulder Elbow Surg*. 2012;21(8):e6–e11.
6. Robinson CM, Teoh KH, Baker A, Bell L. Fractures of the lesser tuberosity of the humerus. *J Bone Joint Surg Am*. 2009; 91(3):512–520. doi:10.2106/JBJS.H.00409.
7. Beavis C, Barber A. Clavicle fractures. In: Johnson DH, Amendola A, Barber FA, Field, LD, Richmond JC, Sgaglione NA, eds. *Operative Arthroscopy*. 4th ed. Baltimore: Lippincott Williams & Wilkins; 2012:336–345.
8. Allman FL Jr. Fractures and ligamentous injuries of the clavicle and its articulation. *J Bone Joint Surg Am*. 1967; 49:774–784.
9. Post M. Current concepts in the treatment of fractures of the clavicle. *Clin Orthop Relat Res*. 1989;(245):89–101.
10. Ertl J. Complications of clavicle fractures. In: Archdeacon M, Anglen F, Ostrum R, Herscovici D Jr, eds. *Prevention and Management of Common Fracture Complications*. Thorofare, NJ: SLACK; 2012:77–83.
11. Chalmers PN, VanThiel GS, Ferry ST. Is skin tending secondary to displaced clavicle fracture more than a theoretical risk? A report of 2 adolescent cases. *Am J Orthop*. 2015; 44(10):E414–E416.
12. Zanca P. Shoulder pain: involvement of the acromioclavicular joint (analysis of 1,000 cases). *Am J Roentgenol*. 1971; 112(3):493–506.
13. Lenza M, Buchbinder R, Johnston RV, Belloti J, Faloppa F. Surgical versus conservative interventions for treating broken collarbones in adolescents and adults. *Cochrane Database Syst Rev*. 2013;6:CD009363.
14. Lenza M, Faloppa F. Conservative interventions for treating middle third clavicle fractures in adolescents and adults. *Cochrane Database Syst Rev*. 2016;12:CD007121. doi:10.1002/14651858.CD007121.pub4.
15. Grassi FA, Tajana MS, D'Angelo F. Management of midclavicular fractures: comparison between nonoperative treatment and open intramedullary fixation in 80 patients. *J Trauma*. 2001;50(6):1096–1100.
16. Zlowodzki M, Zelle BA, Cole PA, Jeray K, McKee MD. Evidence-Based Orthopaedic Trauma Working Group. Treatment of acute midshaft clavicle fractures: systematic review of 2144 fractures: on behalf of the Evidence-Based Orthopaedic Trauma Working Group. *J Orthop Trauma*. 2005;19:504–507.
17. Mall N, Foley E, Chalmers P, Cole B, Romeo A, Bach B. Degenerative joint disease of the acromioclavicular joint. *Am J Sports Med*. 2013;41(11):2684–2692.
18. Owens B, Goss T. The floating shoulder. *J Bone Joint Surg Br*. 2006;88(11):1419–1424.
19. Griffith JF, Antonio GE, Yung PS, et al. Prevalence, pattern, and spectrum of glenoid bone loss in anterior shoulder dislocation: CT analysis of 218 patients. *AJR Am J Roentgenol*. 2008;190(5):1247–1254.

20. Cole PA, Gauger EM, Schroder LK. Management of scapular fractures. *J Am Acad Orthop Surg*. 2012;20(3):130–141.

21. Brown CV, Velmahos G, Wang D, Kennedy S, Demetriades D, Rhee P. Association of scapular fractures and blunt thoracic aortic injury: fact or fiction? *Am Surg*. 2005; 71(1):54–57.

22. Veysi VT, Mittal R, Agarwal S, Dosani A, Giannoudis PV. Multiple trauma and scapula fractures: so what? *J Trauma*. 2003;55(6):1145–1147.

23. Lantry JM, Roberts CS, Giannoudis PV. Operative treatment of scapular fractures: a systematic review. *Injury*. 2008; 39(3):271–283.

24. Ferrera PC, Wheeling HM. Sternoclavicular joint injuries. *Am J Emerg Med*. 2000;18(1):58–61.

25. Malik S, Chiampas GC, Leonard H. Emergent evaluation of injuries to the shoulder, humerus and clavicle. *Emerg Med Clin North Am*. 2010;28(4):739–763.

26. Hegedus EJ, Goode AP, Cook CE, et al. Which physical examination tests provided clinicians with the most value when examining the shoulder? Update of a systematic review with meta-analysis of individual tests. *Br J Sports Med*. 2012;46(14):964–978.

27. Bossart PJ, Joyce SM, Manaster BJ, Packer SM. Lack of efficacy of 'weighted' radiographs in diagnosing acute acromioclavicular separation. *Ann Emerg Med*. 1988;17(1):20–24.

28. Weaver JK, Dunn HK. Treatment of acromioclavicular injuries, especially complete acromioclavicular separation. *J Bone Joint Surg Am*. 1972;54(6):1187–1194.

29. Farber AJ, Cascio BM, Wilckens JH. Type III acromioclavicular separation: rationale for anatomical reconstruction. *Am J Orthop*. 2008;37(7):349–355.

30. Tischer T, Salzmann GM, El Azab H, Vogt S, Imhoff AB. Incidence of associated injuries with acute acromioclavicular joint dislocations types III through V. *Am J Sports Med*. 2009; 37(1):136–139.

31. Nissen CW, Chatterjee A. Type III acromioclavicular joint separation: results of a recent survey on its management. *Am J Orthop*. 2007;36(2):89–93.

32. Bjerneld H, Hovelius L, Thorling J. Acromio-clavicular separations treated conservatively. A 5-year follow-up study. *Acta Orthop Scand*. 1983;54(5):743–745.

33. Galpin RD, Hawkins RJ, Grainger RW. A comparative analysis of operative versus nonoperative treatment of grade III acromioclavicular separations. *Clin Orthop Relat Res*. 1985; (193):150–155.

34. Press J, Zuckerman JD, Gallagher M, Cuomo F. Treatment of grade III acromioclavicular separations. Operative versus nonoperative management. *Bull Hosp Jt Dis*. 1997; 56(2):77–83.

35. Spencer EE. Jr. Treatment of grade III acromioclavicular joint injuries: a systematic review. *Clin Orthop Relat Res*. 2007; 455:38–44.

36. Mouhsine E, Garofalo R, Crevoisier X, Farron A. Grade I and II acromioclavicular dislocations: results of conservative treatment. *J Shoulder Elbow Surg*. 2003;12(6):599–602.

37. Wirth MA, Rockwood CA Jr. Acute and chronic traumatic injuries of the sternoclavicular joint. *J Am Acad Orthop Surg*. 1996;4(5):268–278.

38. Song HK, Guy TS, Kaiser LR, Shrager JB. Current presentation and optimal surgical management of sternoclavicular joint infections. *Ann Thorac Surg*. 2002;73(2):427–431.

39. Haddad M, Maziak DE, Shamji FM. Spontaneous sternoclavicular joint infections. *Ann Thorac Surg*. 2002;74(4): 1225–1227.

40. Gove N, Ebraheim NA, Glass E. Posterior sternoclavicular dislocations: a review of management and complications. *Am J Orthop*. 2006;35(3):132–136.

41. Hoekzema N, Torchia M, Adkins M, Cassivi SD. Posterior sternoclavicular joint dislocation. *Can J Surg*. 2008; 51(1):E19–E20.

42. McCulloch P, Henley BM, Linnau KF. Radiographic clues for high-energy trauma: three cases of sternoclavicular dislocation. *AJR Am J Roentgenol*. 2001;176(6):1534.

43. Beecroft M, Sherman SC. Posterior displacement of a proximal epiphyseal clavicle fracture. *J Emerg Med*. 2007; 33(3):245–248.

44. MacDonald PB, Lapointe P. Acromioclavicular and sternoclavicular joint injuries. *Orthop Clin North Am*. 2008;39(4): 535–545.

45. Groh GI, Wirth MA. Management of traumatic sternoclavicular joint injuries. *J Am Acad Orthop Surg*. 2011; 19(1):1–7.

46. Kuzak N, Ishkanian A, Abu-Laban RB. Posterior sternoclavicular joint dislocation: case report and discussion. *CJEM*. 2006;8(5):355–357.

47. Martin SD, Altchek D. Erlanger S. Atraumatic posterior dislocation of the sternoclavicular joint: a case report and literature review. *Clin Orthop Relat Res*. 1993;(292):159–164.

48. Cleeman E, Flatow EL. Shoulder dislocations in the young patient. *Orthop Clin North Am*. 2000;31(2):217–229.

49. Stayner LR, Cummings J, Andersen J, Jobe CM. Shoulder dislocations in patients older than 40 years of age. *Orthop Clin North Am*. 2000;31(2):231–239.

50. Visser CP, Coene LN, Brand R, Tavy DL. The incidence of nerve injury in anterior dislocation of the shoulder and its influence on functional recovery. A prospective clinical and EMG study. *J Bone Joint Surg Br*. 1999;81(4):679–685.

51. Perron AD, Ingerski MS, Brady WJ, Erling BF, Ullman EA. Acute complications associated with shoulder dislocation at an academic emergency department. *J Emerg Med*. 2003;24(2):141–145.

52. Emond M, Le Sage N, Lavoie A, Rochette L. Clinical factors predicting fractures associated with an anterior shoulder dislocation. *Acad Emerg Med*. 2004;11(8):853–858.

53. Hendey GW, Chally MK, Stewart VB. Selective radiography in 100 patients with suspected shoulder dislocation. *J Emerg Med*. 2006;31(1):23–28.

54. Hendey GW. Necessity of radiographs in the emergency department management of shoulder dislocations. *Ann Emerg Med*. 2000;36(2):108–113.

55. Emond M, Le Sage N, Lavoie A, Moore L. Refinement of the Quebec decision rule for radiography in shoulder dislocations. *CEJM*. 2009;11(1):36–43.

56. Goud A, Segal D, Hedayati P, Pan J, Weissman B. Radiographic evaluation of the shoulder. *Eur J Radiol*. 2008; 68(1):2–15.

57. Riebel GD, McCabe JB. Anterior shoulder dislocation: a review of reduction techniques. *Am J Emerg Med*. 1991; 9(2):180–188.

58. Barber FA, Ryu RK, Tauro JC. Should first time anterior shoulder dislocations be surgically stabilized? *Arthroscopy*. 2003;19(3):305–309.

59. Steinmann SP, Moran EA. Axillary nerve injury: diagnosis and treatment. *J Am Acad Orthop Surg.* 2001;9(5):328–335.

60. O'Connor DR, Schwarze D, Fragomen AT, Perdomo M. Painless reduction of acute anterior shoulder dislocations without anesthesia. *Orthopedics.* 2006;29(6):528–532.

61. Blaivas M, Adhikari S, Lander L. A prospective comparison of procedural sedation and ultrasound-guided interscalene nerve block for shoulder reduction in the emergency department. *Acad Emerg Med.* 2011;18(9):922–927.

62. Raeyat Doost E, Heiran MM, Movahedi M, Mirafzal A. Ultrasound guided interscalene nerve block vs procedural sedation by propofol and fentanyl for anterior shoulder dislocations. *Am J Emerg Med.* 2017;35(10):1435–1439. doi:10.1016/j.ajem.2017.04.032. Epub 2017 Apr 14.

63. Tezel O, Kaldirim U, Bilgic S, et al. A comparison of suprascapular nerve block and pro-cedural sedation analgesia in shoulder dislocation reduction. *Am J Emerg Med.* 2014; 32(6):549–552.

64. Fitch RW, Kuhn JE. Intraarticular lidocaine versus intravenous procedural sedation with narcotics and benzodiazepines for reduction of the dislocated shoulder: a systematic review. *Acad Emerg Med.* 2008;15(8):703–708. doi:10.1111/j.1553-2712.2008.00164.x.

65. Kashani P, Asayesh Zarchi F, Hatamabadi HR, et al. Intraarticular lidocaine versus intravenous sedative and analgesic for reduction of anterior shoulder dislocation. *Turk J Emerg Med.* 2016;16(2):60–64.

66. Wakai A, O'Sullivan R, McCabe A. Intraarticular lignocaine versus intravenous analgesia with or without sedation for manual reduction of acute anterior shoulder dislocation in adults. *Cochrane Database Syst Rev.* 2011;(4):CD004919.

67. Miller SL, Cleeman E, Auerbach J, Flatow EL. Comparison of intra-articular lidocaine and intravenous sedation for reduction of shoulder dislocations: a randomized, prospective study. *J Bone Joint Surg Am.* 2002;84-A(12):2135–2139.

68. Tamaoki M, Faloppa F, Wajnsztejn A, Archetti Netto N, Matsumoto MH, Belloti JC. Effectiveness of intra-articular lidocaine injection for reduction of anterior shoulder dislocation: randomized clinical trial. *Sao Paulo Med J.* 2012; 130(6):367–372.

69. Orlinsky M, Shon S, Chiang C, Chan L, Carter P. Comparative study of intra-articular lidocaine and intravenous meperidine/diazepam for shoulder dislocations. *J Emerg Med.* 2002;22(3):241–245.

70. Dhinakharan SR, Ghosh A. Towards evidence based emergency medicine: best BETs from the Manchester Royal Infirmary. Intra-articular lidocaine for acute anterior shoulder dislocation reduction. *Emerg Med J.* 2002;19(2): 142–143.

71. Breslin K, Boniface K, Cohen J. Ultrasound-guided intra-articular lidocaine block for reduction of anterior shoulder dislocation in the pediatric emergency department. *Pediatric Emerg Care.* 2014;30(3):217–220.

72. Kosnik J, Shamsa F, Raphael E, Huang R, Malachias Z, Georgiadis GM. Anesthetic methods for reduction of acute shoulder dislocations: a prospective randomized study comparing intraarticular lidocaine with intravenous analgesia and sedation. *Am J Emerg Med.* 1999;17(6):566–570.

73. Sherman SC, Schaider J. Shoulder dislocation and reduction. UpToDate. n.d. www.uptodate.com. Accessed December 6, 2009.

74. Alkaduhimi H, van der Linde JA, Willigenburg NW, et al. A systematic comparison of the closed shoulder reduction techniques. *Arch Orthop Trauma Surg.* 2017;137(5): 589–599.

75. Cunningham N. A new drug free technique for reducing anterior shoulder dislocations. *Emerg Med.* 2003;15(5–6): 521–524.

76. Baykal B, Sener S, Turkan H. Scapular manipulation technique for reduction of traumatic anterior shoulder dislocations: experiences of an academic emergency department. *Emerg Med J.* 2005;22(5):336–338.

77. Kothari RU, Dronen SC. The scapular manipulation technique for the reduction of acute anterior shoulder dislocations. *J Emerg Med.* 1990;8(5):625–628.

78. Schubert H. Reducing anterior shoulder dislocation. Easy is good. *Can Fam Physician.* 2002;48:469–472.

79. Sagarin MJ. Best of both (BOB) maneuver for rapid reduction of anterior shoulder dislocation. *J Emerg Med.* 2005; 29(3):313–316.

80. Leidelmeyer R. Reduced! A shoulder, subtly and painlessly. *Emerg Med.* 1977;9:233–234.

81. Simon RR. The Hennepin technique. *Ann Emerg Med.* 1984;13(10):981–982.

82. Eachempati KK, Dua A, Malhotra R, Bhan S, Bera JR. The external rotation method for reduction of acute anterior dislocations and fracture-dislocations of the shoulder. *J Bone Joint Surg Am.* 2004;86-A(11):2431–2434.

83. Mattick A, Wyatt JP. From Hippocrates to the Eskimo—a history of techniques used to reduce anterior dislocation of the shoulder. *J R Coll Surg Edinb.* 2000;45(5):312–316.

84. Milch H. Treatment of dislocation of the shoulder. *Surgery.* 1938;3:732–740.

85. Singh S, Yong CK, Mariapan S. Closed reduction techniques in acute anterior shoulder dislocation: modified Milch technique compared with traction-countertraction technique. *J Shoulder Elbow Surg.* 2012;21(12):1706–1711.

86. Amar E. Maman E, Khashan M, Kauffman E, Rath E, Chechik O. Milch versus Stimson technique for nonsedated reduction of anterior shoulder dislocation: a prospective randomized trial and analysis of factors affecting success. *J Shoulder Elbow Surg.* 2012;21(11):1443–1449.

87. Fernández-Valencia JA, Cuñe J, Casulleres JM, Carreño A, Prat S. The Spaso technique: a prospective study of 34 dislocations. *Am J Emerg Med.* 2009;27(4):466–469.

88. Yuen MC, Yap PG, Chan YT, Tung WK. An easy method to reduce anterior shoulder dislocation: the Spaso technique. *Emerg Med J.* 2001;18(5):370–372.

89. Ufberg JW, Vilke GM, Chan TC, Harrigan RA. Anterior shoulder dislocations: beyond traction-countertraction. *J Emerg Med.* 2004;27(3):301–306.

90. Stimson LA. An easy method of reducing dislocations of the shoulder and hip. *Med Rec.* 1900;57:356–357.

91. Sayegh FE, Kenanidis El, Papavasiliou KA, Potoupnis ME, Kirkos JM, Kapetanos GA. Reduction of acute anterior dislocations: a prospective randomized study comparing a new technique with the Hippocratic and Kocher methods. *J Bone Joint Surg Am.* 2009;91(12):2775–2782.

92. Maity A, Roy DS, Mondal BC. A prospective randomised clinical trial comparing FARES method with Eachemapati external rotation method for reduction of acute anterior shoulder dislocation. *Injury.* 2012;43(7):1066–1070.

93. Chung JY, Cheng CH, Graham CA, Rainer TH. The effectiveness of a specially designed shoulder chair for closed reduction of acute shoulder dislocation in the emergency department: a randomised control trial. *Emerg Med J*. 2013; 30(10):795–800.

94. Poulsen SR. Reduction of acute shoulder dislocations using the Eskimo technique: a study of 23 consecutive cases. *J Trauma*. 1988;28(9):1382–1383.

95. Dala-Ali B, Penna M, McConnell J, Vanhegan I, Cobiella C. Management of acute anterior shoulder dislocation. *Br J Sports Med*. 2014;48(16):1209–1215. doi:10.1136/bjsports-2012-091300. Epub 2012 Jul 21.

96. Chitgopkar SD, Khan M. Painless reduction of anterior shoulder dislocation by Kocher's method. *Injury*. 2005; 36(10):1182–1184.

97. Chung CH. Closed reduction techniques for acute anterior shoulder dislocation: from Egyptians to Australians. *Hong Kong J Emerg Med*. 2004;11:178–188.

98. McNeil NJ. Postreduction management of first-time traumatic anterior shoulder dislocations. *Ann Emerg Med*. 2009; 53(6):811–813.

99. Miller BS, Sonnabend DH, Hatrick C, et al. Should acute anterior dislocations of the shoulder be immobilized in external rotation? A cadaveric study. *J Shoulder Elbow Surg*. 2004;13(6):589–592.

100. Funk L, Smith M. Best evidence topic report. how to immobilise after shoulder dislocation? *Emerg Med J*. 2005; 22(11):814–815.

101. Murrell GA. Treatment of shoulder dislocation: is a sling appropriate? *Med J Aust*. 2003;179(7):370–371.

102. Itoi E, Hatakeyama Y, Kido T, et al. A new method of immobilization after traumatic anterior dislocation of the shoulder: a preliminary study. *J Shoulder Elbow Surg*. 2003; 12(5):413–415.

103. Siegler J, Proust J, Marcheix PS, Charissoux JL, Mabit C, Arnaud JP. Is external rotation the correct immobilization for acute shoulder dislocation? An MRI study. *Orthop Traumatol Surg Res*. 2010;96(4):329–333.

104. Seybold D, Schliemann B, Heyer CM, Muhr G, Gekle C. Which labral lesion can be best reduced with external rotation of the shoulder after a first-time traumatic anterior shoulder dislocation? *Arch Orthop Trauma Surg*. 2009;129(3): 299–304.

105. Itoi E, Sashi R, Minagawa H, Wakabayashi I, Sato K. Position of immobilization after dislocation of the glenohumeral joint. A study with the use of magnetic resonance imaging. *J Bone Joint Surg Am*. 2001;83-A(5):661–667.

106. Finestone A. Milgrom C, Radeva-Petrova DR. Bracing in external rotation for traumatic anterior shoulder dislocation of the shoulder. *J Bone Joint Surg Br*. 2009;91(7):918–921.

107. Liavaag S, Brox JI, Pripp AH, Soldal LA, Svenningsen S. Immobilization in external rotation after primary shoulder dislocation did not reduce the risk of recurrence: a randomized control trial. *J Bone Joint Surg Am*. 2011;93(10): 897–904.

108. Schiebel M, Kuke A, Nikulka C, Magosch P, Ziesler O, Schroeder RJ. How long should acute anterior shoulder dislocations of the shoulder be immobilized in external rotation? *Am J Sports Med*. 2009;37(7):1309–1316.

109. Nicholson GG. Rehabilitation of common shoulder injuries. *Clin Sports Med*. 1989;8(4):633–655.

110. Kirkley A, Werstine R, Ratjek A, Griffin S. Prospective randomized clinical trial comparing the effectiveness of immediate arthroscopic stabilization versus immobilization and rehabilitation in first traumatic anterior dislocations of the shoulder: long-term evaluation. *Arthroscopy*. 2005;21(1):55–63.

111. Davy AR, Drew SJ. Management of shoulder dislocation—are we doing enough to reduce the risk of recurrence? *Injury*. 2002;33(9):775–779.

112. Bottoni CR, Wilckens JH, DeBerardino TM, et al. A prospective, randomized evaluation of arthroscopic stabilization versus nonoperative treatment in patients with acute, traumatic, first-time shoulder dislocations. *Am J Sports Med*. 2002;30(4):576–580.

113. Handoll HH, Almaiyah MA, Rangan A. Surgical versus non-surgical treatment for acute anterior shoulder dislocation. *Cochrane Database Syst Rev*. 2004;(1):CD004325.

114. Kralinger FS, Golser K, Wischatta R, Wambacher M, Sperner G. Predicting recurrence after primary anterior shoulder dislocation. *Am J Sports Med*. 2002;30(1):116–120.

115. Chahal J, Marks PH, Macdonald PB, et al. Anatomic Bankart repair compared with nonoperative treatment and/or arthroscopic lavage for first time traumatic shoulder dislocation. *Arthroscopy*. 2012;28(4):565–575.

116. Hovelius L, Olofsson A, Sandstrom B, et al. Nonoperative treatment of primary anterior shoulder dislocation in patients forty years of age and younger. A prospective twenty-five-year follow-up. *J Bone Joint Surg Am*. 2008;90(5): 945–952.

117. Spatschil A, Landsiedl F, Anderl W, et al. Posttraumatic anterior-inferior instability of the shoulder: arthroscopic findings and clinical correlations. *Arch Orthop Trauma Surg*. 2006;126(4):217–222.

118. Chalidis B, Sachinis N, Dimitriou C, Papadopoulos P, Samoladas E, Pournaras J. Has the management of shoulder dislocation changed over time? *Int Orthop*. 2007;31(3):385–389.

119. Cutts S, Prempeh M, Drew S. Anterior shoulder dislocation. *Ann R Coll Surg Engl*. 2009;9(1):2–7.

120. Liu SH, Henry MH. Anterior shoulder instability. Current review. *Clin Orthop Relat Res*. 1996;(323):327–337.

121. Safran O, Milgrom C, Radeva-Petrova DR, Jaber S, Finestone A. Accuracy of the anterior apprehension test as a predictor of risk for redislocation after a first time traumatic shoulder dislocation. *Am J Sports Med*. 2010;38(5):972–975.

122. Kowalsky MS, Levine WN. Traumatic posterior glenohumeral dislocation: classification, pathoanatomy, diagnosis, and treatment. *Orthop Clin North Am*. 2008;39(4):519–533.

123. Cicak N. Posterior dislocation of the shoulder. *J Bone Joint Surg Br*. 2004;86(3):324–332.

124. Feleus A, Bierma-Zeinstra SM, Miedema HS, Verhaar JA, Koes BW. Management in non-traumatic arm, neck and shoulder complaints: differences between diagnostic groups. *Eur Spine J*. 2008;17(9):1218–1229.

125. Von Raebrox A, Campbell B, Ramesh R, Bunker T. The association of subacromial dimples with recurrent posterior dislocation of the shoulder. *J Shoulder Elbow Surg*. 2006; 15(5):591–593.

126. Gor DM. The trough line sign. *Radiology*. 2002;224(2): 485–486.

127. Harris JH, Harris WH. *The Radiology of Emergency Medicine*. 4th ed. Philadelphia, PA: Lippincott Williams & Wilkins; 2000.

128. Cisternino SJ, Rogers LF, Stufflebam BC, Kruglik GD. The trough line: a radiographic sign of posterior shoulder dislocation. *AJR Am J Roentgenol.* 1978;130(5):951–954.

129. Aparicio G, Calvo E, Bonilla L, Espejo L, Box R. Neglected traumatic posterior dislocations of the shoulder: controversies on indications for treatment and new CT scan findings. *J Orthop Sci.* 2000;5(1):37–42.

130. Saupe N, White LM, Bleakney R, et al. Acute traumatic posterior shoulder dislocation: MR findings. *Radiology.* 2008; 248(1):185–193.

131. Groh GL, Wirth MA, Rockwood CA Jr. Results of treatment of luxatio erecta (inferior shoulder dislocation). *J Shoulder Elbow Surg.* 2010;19(3):423–426.

132. Yanturali S, Aksay E, Holliman CJ, Duman O, Ozen YK. Luxatio erecta: clinical presentation and management in the emergency department. *J Emerg Med.* 2005;29(1):85–89.

133. Nho SJ, Dodson CC, Bardzik KF, Brophy RH, Domb BG, MacGillivray JD. The two-step maneuver for closed reduction of inferior glenohumeral dislocation (luxatio erecta to anterior dislocation to reduction). *J Orthop Trauma.* 2006; 20(5):354–357.

134. Morrison DS, Greenbaum BS, Einhorn A. Shoulder impingement. *Orthop Clin North Am.* 2000;31(2):285–293.

135. Shahabpour M, Kichouh M, Laridon E, Gielen JL, De Mey J. The effectiveness of diagnostic imaging methods for the assessment of soft tissue and articular disorders of the shoulder and elbow. *Eur J Radiol.* 2008;65(2):194–200.

136. Hirano M, Ide J, Takagi K. Acromial shapes and extension of rotator cuff tears: magnetic resonance imaging evaluation. *J Shoulder Elbow Surg.* 2002;11(6):576–578.

137. Balke M, Schmidt C, Dedy N, Banerjee M, Bouillon B, Liem D. Correlation of acromial morphology with impingement syndrome and rotator cuff tears. *Acta Orthop.* 2013; 84(2):178–183.

138. Miniaci A, Fowler PJ. Impingement in the athlete. *Clin Sports Med.* 1993;12(1):91–110.

139. Hurt G, Baker CL Jr. Calcific tendinitis of the shoulder. *Orthop Clin North Am.* 2003;34(4):567–575.

140. Sardelli M, Burks RT. Distances to the subacromial bursa from 3 different injection sites as measured arthroscopically. *Arthroscopy.* 2008;24(9):992–996.

141. Awerbuch MS. The clinical utility of ultrasonography for rotator cuff disease, shoulder impingement syndrome and subacromial bursitis. *Med J Aust.* 2008;188(1):50–53.

142. Koester MC, Dunn WR, Kuhn JE, Spindler KP. The efficacy of subacromial corticosteroid injection in the treatment of rotator cuff disease: a systematic review. *J Am Acad Orthop Surg.* 2007;15(1):3–11.

143. Mantone JK, Burkhead WZ Jr, Noonan J Jr. Nonoperative treatment of rotator cuff tears. *Orthop Clin North Am.* 2000; 31(2):295–311.

144. Green A. Chronic massive rotator cuff tears: evaluation and management. *J Am Acad Orthop Surg.* 2003;11(5):321–331.

145. Benson RT, McDonnell SM, Rees JL, Athanasou NA, Carr AJ. The morphological and immunocytochemical features of impingement syndrome and partial-thickness rotator-cuff tear in relation to outcome after subacromial decompression. *J Bone Joint Surg Br.* 2009;91(1):119–123.

146. Krief OP, Huguet D. Shoulder pain and disability: comparison with MR findings. *AJR Am J Roentgenol.* 2006; 186(5):1234–1239.

147. Litaker D, Pioro M, El Bilbeisi H, Brems J. Returning to the bedside: using the history and physical examination to identify rotator cuff tears. *J Am Geriatr Soc.* 2000; 48(12):1633–1637.

148. McCabe RA, Nicholas SJ, Montgomery KD, Finneran JJ, McHugh MP. The effect of rotator cuff tear size on shoulder strength and range of motion. *J Orthop Sports Phys Ther.* 2005; 35(3):130–135.

149. Millstein ES, Snyder SJ. Arthroscopic evaluation and management of rotator cuff tears. *Orthop Clin North Am.* 2003; 34(4):507–520.

150. Hughes PC, Taylor NF, Green RA. Most clinical tests cannot accurately diagnose rotator cuff pathology: a systematic review. *Aust J Physiother.* 2008;54(3):159–170.

151. Koh KH, Han KY, Yoon YC, Lee SW, Yoo JC. True anteroposterior (Grashey) view as a screening radiograph for further imaging study in rotator cuff tear. *J Shoulder Elbow Surg.* 2013;22(7):901–907.

152. Borick JM, Kurzweil PR. Magnetic resonance imaging appearance of the shoulder after subacromial injection with corticosteroids can mimic a rotator cuff tear. *Arthroscopy.* 2008;24(7):846–849.

153. Jesus J, Parker L, Frangos A, Nazarian L. Accuracy of MRI, MR arthrography, and ultrasound in the diagnosis of rotator cuff tears: a meta-analysis. *AJR Am J Roentgenol.* 2009; 192(6):1701–1707.

154. Waldt S, Bruegel M, Mueller D, et al. Rotator cuff tears: assessment with MR arthrography in 275 patients with arthroscopic correlation. *Eur Radiol.* 2007;17(2):491–498.

155. Miller D, Frost A, Hall A, Barton C, Bhoora I, Kathuria V. A 'one-stop clinic' for the diagnosis and management of rotator cuff pathology: getting the right diagnosis first time. *Int J Clin Pract.* 2008;62(5):750–753.

156. Kijima H, Minagawa H, Yamamoto N, et al. Three-dimensional ultrasonography of shoulders with rotator cuff tears. *J Orthop Sci.* 2008;13(6):510–513.

157. Vlychou M, Dailiana Z, Fotiadou A, Papanagiotou M, Fezoulidis IV, Malizos K. Symptomatic partial rotator cuff tears: diagnostic performance of ultrasound and magnetic resonance imaging with surgical correlation. *Acta Radiol.* 2009; 50(1):101–105.

158. Marx RG, Koulouvaris P, Chu SK, Levy BA. Indications for surgery in clinical outcome studies of rotator cuff repair. *Clin Orthop Relat Res.* 2009;467(2):450–456.

159. Matava M, Purcell D, Rudzki J. Partial-thickness rotator cuff tears. *Am J Sports Med.* 2005;33(9):1405–1417.

160. Zumstein MA, Jost B, Hempel J, Hodler J, Gerber C. The clinical and structural long-term results of open repair of massive tears of the rotator cuff. *J Bone Joint Surg Am.* 2008; 90(11):2423–2431.

161. Zingg PO, Jost B, Sukthankar A, Buhler M, Pfirrmann CW, Gerber C. Clinical and structural outcomes of nonoperative management of massive rotator cuff tears. *J Bone Joint Surg Am.* 2007;89(9):1928–1934.

162. Levy O, Venkateswaran B, Even T, Ravenscroft M, Copeland S. Mid-term clinical and sonographic outcome of arthroscopic repair of the rotator cuff. *J Bone Joint Surg Br.* 2008;90(10): 1341–1347.

163. Park MC, Elattrache NS. Treating full-thickness cuff tears in the athlete: advances in arthroscopic techniques. *Clin Sports Med.* 2008;27(4):719–729.

164. Pearsall AW 4th, Ibrahim KA, Madanagopal SG. The results of arthroscopic versus mini-open repair for rotator cuff tears at mid-term follow-up. *J Orthop Surg Res.* 2007; 2:24.

165. Lahteenmaki HE, Hiltunen A, Virolainen P, Nelimarkka O. Repair of full-thickness rotator cuff tears is recommended regardless of tear size and age: a retrospective study of 218 patients. *J Shoulder Elbow Surg.* 2007;16(5): 586–590.

166. Cho NS, Rhee YG. The factors affecting the clinical outcome and integrity of arthroscopically repaired rotator cuff tears of the shoulder. *Clin Orthop Surg.* 2009;1(2):96–104.

167. Churgay CA. Diagnosis and treatment of biceps tendinitis and tendinosis. *Am Fam Physician.* 2009;80(5):470–476.

168. Yergason RM. Supination sign. *J Bone Joint Surg.* 1931; 131:60.

169. Patton WB, McCluskey GM III. Biceps tendinitis and subluxation. *Clin Sports Med.* 2001;20(3):505–529.

170. Shah N, Lewis M. Shoulder adhesive capsulitis: systematic review of randomised trials using multiple corticosteroid injections. *Br J Gen Pract.* 2007;57(541):662–667.

171. Sofka CM, Ciavarra GA, Hannafin JA, Cordasco FA, Potter HG. Magnetic resonance imaging of adhesive capsulitis: correlation with clinical staging. *HSS J.* 2008;4(2):164–169.

172. Tighe CB, Oakley WS Jr. The prevalence of a diabetic condition and adhesive capsulitis of the shoulder. *South Med J.* 2008;101(6):591–595.

173. Manske RC, Prohaska D. Diagnosis and management of adhesive capsulitis. *Curr Rev Musculoskelet Med.* 2008;1(3–4): 180–189.

174. Yoo JC, Ahn JH, Lee YS, Koh KH. Magnetic resonance arthrographic findings of presumed stage-2 adhesive capsulitis: focus on combined rotator cuff pathology. *Orthopedics.* 2009;32(1):22.

175. DePalma AF. The classic. Loss of scapulohumeral motion (frozen shoulder). Ann Surg. 1952;135:193–204. *Clin Orthop Relat Res.* 2008;466(3):552–560. doi:10.1007/s11999-007-0101-7. Epub 2008 Feb 10.

176. Sherman SC, O'Connor M. An unusual cause of shoulder pain: winged scapula. *J Emerg Med.* 2005;28(3):329–331.

177. Anekstein Y, Blecher R, Smorgick Y, Mirovsky Y. What is the best way to apply the Spurling test for cervical radiculopathy? *Clin Orthop Relat Res.* 2012;470(9):2566–2572.

178. Zuckerman JD, Mirabello SC, Newman D, Gallagher M, Cuomo F. The painful shoulder: part I. Extrinsic disorders. *Am Fam Physician.* 1991;43(1):119–128.

179. Nichols AW. Diagnosis and management of thoracic outlet syndrome. *Curr Sports Med Rep.* 2009;8(5):240–249.

PART IV

Lower Extremities

CHAPTER 17

Pelvis

Hany Y. Atallah, MD

INTRODUCTION

Pelvic fractures represent 3% of all skeletal fractures and are exceeded only by skull fractures in their associated complications and mortality.[1] Pelvic fractures range from low-energy stable fractures to high-energy unstable injuries, associated with abdominal injuries, need for major blood transfusion, and even death.[2] The mortality rate for high-energy pelvic fractures ranges from 10% to 20%, but in hemodynamically unstable patients or after open fractures, it increases to 50%.[3,4] Motor vehicle collisions account for approximately two-thirds of all pelvic fractures. Pedestrians struck by automobiles are responsible for 15% of cases. Crush injuries, motorcycle crashes, and falls each account for an additional 5%.[5]

Pubic rami fractures are the most common pelvic fractures with the superior ramus more frequently involved than the inferior ramus. Pubic rami fractures account for more than 70% of all pelvic fractures.[6] The incidence of fractures of the remaining pelvic bones in descending order is the ilium, ischium, and acetabulum. Sacroiliac (SI) fractures are associated with the most significant bleeding. Both the mechanism of injury and the fracture pattern identified on imaging studies are important in predicting associated injuries.

Essential Anatomy

In humans, the pelvic ring serves two important functions: weight support (stability) and protection of the viscera.

There are essentially three bones that combine to form the pelvic ring: two innominate bones (composed of the ischium, ilium, and pubis) and the sacrum (Fig. 17–1). The coccyx is a fourth bone, but it is not incorporated into the pelvic ring. The two innominate bones and the sacrum are united by the formation of three joints (the symphysis pubis and the two SI joints). The ligaments that form the pelvic ring are the strongest in the body.

Weight bearing is transmitted through the bony pelvis along two pathways (Fig. 17–2). When standing, weight is transmitted through the spine to the sacrum and the SI joints and along the arcuate line to the superior dome of the acetabulum and down the femur. In the sitting position, the force is transmitted down the spine to the sacrum and the SI joints and to the ischium by way of the inferior ramus. The bone is very strong in these areas and the anteroposterior (AP) radiograph of the pelvis clearly demonstrates the thick trabecular pattern along these lines of stress. As a result, pelvic fractures more commonly interrupt the ring in areas not involved in weight transmission. A greater force is required to fracture a "weight-bearing" area of the pelvis. In addition, fractures involving the weight-bearing arches are associated with much more pain when stressed than those fractures that do not involve these arches. A good example is the superior ramus fracture. Because this structure is a nonweight-supporting area, it is generally less painful and mechanically stable compared to

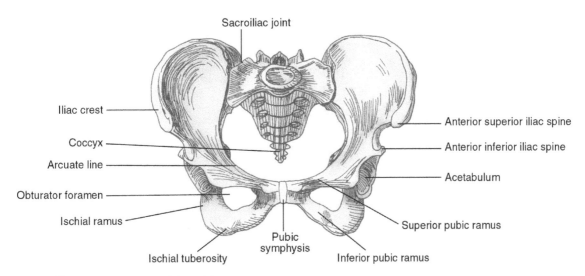

Figure 17–1. The osseous structures of the pelvis.

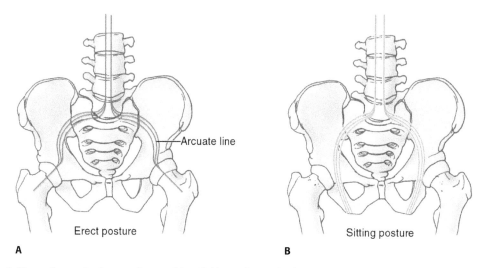

Figure 17–2. *A.* Lines of stress in the standing position. *B.* Lines of stress in the sitting position. Note that in the sitting position the lines go through the ischium.

fractures in weight-supporting portions of the pelvis. A patient with a fracture of the superior pubic ramus may walk into the emergency department (ED), whereas a patient with a fracture through the sacrum will not be able to bear weight without significant pain.

The concept of the pelvis as an anatomic ring also has important implications for fracture detection. The presence of at least two fractures or one fracture and a dislocation is required to cause a displaced fracture in the ring. Therefore, if a displaced pelvic ring fracture is diagnosed, the clinician should search for a second fracture or joint injury. Single breaks in the pelvic ring are unusual and are usually non-displaced and occur near or at a joint (SI joint or symphysis pubis).

> **Axiom:** *A displaced fracture of the pelvic ring indicates that there is at least a second fracture or a fracture plus a joint dislocation, most commonly the SI joint.*

Pelvic stability during ambulation is a combined function of ligaments and bones. Anteriorly, the interpubic ligaments join the two pubic bones forming the symphysis pubis. The anterior pelvic structures (symphysis and rami) are responsible for 40% of pelvic ring stability. Posteriorly, the SI joint is supported by a series of strong ligaments that are the major stabilizers of the pelvic ring (Fig. 17-3). Disruption of the SI ligaments will alter the normal weight-bearing function of the pelvic ring.

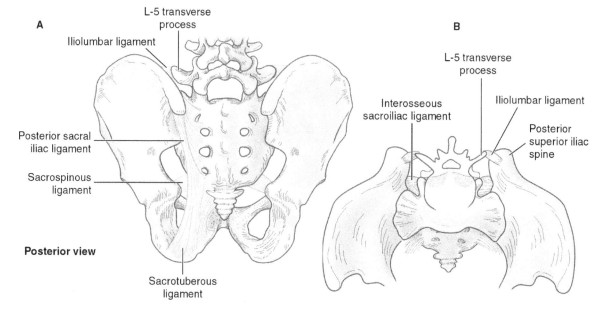

Figure 17–3. The ligaments surrounding the sacroiliac joint are the strongest in the body.

Disruption of the interpubic ligaments may result in diastasis of the pubic symphysis of up to 2.5 cm. The intact ligaments of the SI joint—specifically the sacrospinous, sacrotuberous, and anterior SI ligaments—limit further opening. If these ligaments are sectioned, the pelvis becomes rotationally unstable and will "open like a book." As long as the posterior ligaments of the SI joint (interosseous SI ligament and posterior SI ligament) remain intact, the hemipelvis will remain vertically stable. Additional injury to the posterior SI ligaments results in a pelvis that is unstable both rotationally and vertically.

The muscles attached to the pelvis serve to support the body in the erect position and to provide mobility to the lower limbs. For the purpose of this text, the essential muscular anatomy concerns only those muscles responsible for avulsion fractures:

- The sartorius inserts on the anterior superior iliac spine.
- The rectus femoris inserts on the anterior inferior iliac spine.
- The hamstrings insert on the ischial tuberosity.

The spinal nerves leave the protection of the vertebral column by way of the lumbar intervertebral foramina or the sacral foramina and course along the posterior aspect of the pelvis. Pelvic fractures, particularly those involving the sacrum, may be associated with nerve injury. A thorough neurologic examination of the lower extremities and the sphincters is essential in the assessment of pelvic fractures.

The abdominal aorta descends to the left of the midline and divides at L4 into the two common iliac vessels. At the level of the SI joints, the common iliacs branch to form the external and internal iliacs. The internal iliac artery further divides into anterior and posterior branches. The posterior branch gives rise to the superior gluteal artery, which has an acutely angled base and is exposed to shearing forces with fractures in the area. The anterior branch supplies the viscera of the pelvic cavity. Posterior pelvic (ilium and SI) fractures are associated with more extensive hemorrhage than are anterior pelvic fractures.

The rectum, anus, sigmoid, and descending colon are contained within the bony pelvis. These structures may be damaged with any pelvic fracture but are most commonly injured with fractures associated with penetrating injuries. The genitourinary system is frequently damaged in association with pelvic fractures due to blunt or penetrating trauma. The bladder, lying directly behind the symphysis pubis, is frequently injured following pelvic fractures involving the pubis. Anterior pelvic fractures are also associated with urethral injuries. If the urethra ruptures below the level of the urogenital diaphragm, the extravasation of urine will involve the scrotum, the superficial perineal compartment, and the abdominal wall.

In addition to associated injuries of the pelvic viscera, there is significant risk of injury to the other intra-abdominal organs due primarily to the mechanism of injury. The incidence of abdominal injuries in patients with blunt pelvic fracture in

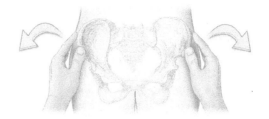

Figure 17–4. Gentle external rotation of the pelvis is used to test for rotational instability.

one study was 16.5%. The most commonly injured organs were the liver (6.1%) and the bladder and urethra (5.8%). In severe pelvic fractures, the incidence of associated abdominal injuries was 30.7%, and the most commonly injured organs were the bladder and urethra (14.6%).

Examination

Patients who present with pelvic pain after a minor trauma and a possible fracture should have a simple six-point examination:

1. External rotation of the pelvis (Fig. 17–4)
2. Internal rotation of the pelvis (Fig. 17–5)
3. Compression of the pubic symphysis
4. Palpation of the anterior superior iliac spine
5. Palpation of the sacrum and coccyx
6. Palpation of the trochanters and ischial tuberosities

The evaluation of a patient with major trauma should begin with a thorough primary survey searching for and treating any immediate life threats. Pelvic fractures may result in exsanguination; therefore, two large bore intravenous lines must be started, and cross-matched blood made available should the need arise. During the secondary survey, an assessment of pelvic injury and stability should take place. All patients with multiple injuries must be suspected of having a pelvic fracture until proven otherwise. Pelvic fractures involving impact from the side tend to compress the pelvis and lead to less bleeding from fractures than AP force pelvic fractures. Therefore, "open book"-type pelvic fractures associated with hypotension should be identified early during the secondary survey.

Following exposure, the examiner should perform a careful inspection of the soft tissues of the pelvis, looking

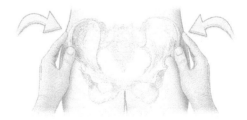

Figure 17–5. Gentle internal rotation of the pelvis may also aid in detecting rotational instability.

specifically for deformity of the pelvis or lower extremities that suggest a pelvic fracture. Examination should continue with a search for lacerations that might indicate an open fracture. This includes visual inspection of the gluteal folds and perineal area, where an injury might be missed otherwise. If there is concern for bone fragments being pushed into the rectum or vagina, the examiner should carefully proceed with a proper exam. Gross blood on rectal or bimanual examination suggests an open pelvic fracture. The risks of missing such an injury are significant and include spread of infection to the soft tissues of the pelvis, thigh, and lower abdomen. The examination of suspected pelvic fractures must include direct palpation of the entire ring, with special emphasis on the pubic symphysis, the SI joints, and the sacrum. Examination of each hip and its range of motion will help exclude an acetabular injury.

Pelvic instability can be detected on physical examination. Rotational instability is present when gentle manual pressure over the anterior superior iliac spines in both external and internal rotation causes significant movement of the pelvis. Bony crepitus may also be noted. Vertical instability can be assessed by noting vertical movement of the pelvis with the examiner's palms palpating the anterior superior iliac spines while a second examiner provides traction and then a vertical load to the lower extremity. Testing for vertical instability is not recommended because, if it is present, the examination will only increase the amount of hemorrhage.

It is of utmost importance to note that only one examination for instability should be permitted because repeated examinations can disrupt hematoma formation and exacerbate or create hemodynamic instability. These patients should be moved or manipulated as little as possible so as not to aggravate hemorrhage or induce further complications.

The genitourinary system is frequently injured with pelvic fractures, and questions relating to hematuria, inability to void, last menses, and vaginal bleeding should be noted on history. During the digital rectal examination, the position of the prostate gland is assessed. Prostate displacement, scrotal ecchymosis, or blood at the urethral meatus indicates possible disruption in the membranous urethra. Unfortunately, physical signs of urethral injury are absent in more than half of patients with these injuries.[8]

A thorough neurologic examination of the lower extremities is important. Particular areas of concern include the L5 and S1 nerve roots. Both motor and sensory functions should be documented. Sacral fractures can injure sacral roots, the obturator nerve, and the L5 nerve roots. The sciatic nerve is commonly injured following acetabular fractures.

Secondary signs of a potential pelvic fracture include the following:

- Destot sign—a superficial hematoma above the inguinal ligament or in the scrotum.
- Roux sign—occurs when the distance measured from the greater trochanter to the pubic spine is diminished

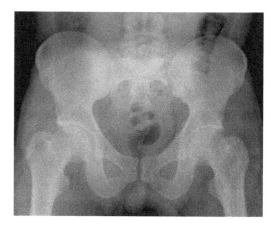

Figure 17–6. Normal pelvis AP radiograph.

on one side, as compared with the other, as might result from an overlapping anterior ring fracture.
- Earle sign—occurs when a large hematoma, an abnormal palpable bony prominence, or a tender fracture line is detected on a rectal examination.

Imaging

An AP radiograph of the pelvis is indicated in the alert trauma patient in the setting of pain or tenderness (Fig. 17–6). This view detects most injuries to the sacral wings, iliac bones, ischium, and pubis. Obvious fracture lines are diagnosed on this film, and suspected fracture areas are the cause for further imaging studies. The initial AP pelvic film allows for classification of the pelvic fracture and guides resuscitation and the need for acute pelvic stabilization in 90% of cases.[ ] If the AP radiograph reveals significant pelvic ring instability, treatment of a hemodynamically unstable patient should be instituted on the basis of this film alone.[ ] Although Advanced Trauma Life Support (ATLS) still recommends performing pelvic radiography in all major blunt trauma patients, more recent evidence suggests that it can be limited to blunt trauma patients who are hemodynamically unstable or have positive pelvic physical examination findings.[ ]

Inlet (AP with x-ray beam angled caudad 45 degrees) and outlet (AP with 45 degrees of cephalic tilt) views may aid in the diagnosis of pelvic ring fractures in hemodynamically stable patients (Fig. 17–7). The inlet view demonstrates the true pelvic inlet. Injuries to the anterior ring are easily identified on this view, whereas posterior injuries may remain subtle. The outlet view is oriented 90 degrees to the anterior sacrum, and therefore, more readily detects fractures of this bone. This projection also detects any bony displacement in the sagittal plane. Both the inlet and outlet views have largely been replaced by computed tomography (CT). Oblique (Judet) views may be useful for diagnosing acetabular fractures, although CT is more sensitive in diagnosing fractures of the acetabulum and sacrum and is therefore the imaging test of choice.[ ]

The CT scan of the pelvis has other advantages. It aids in the evaluation of the integrity of the posterior pelvic

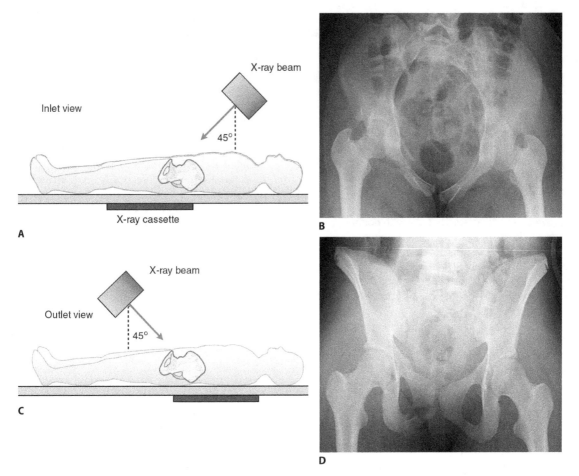

Figure 17–7. Inlet and outlet views of the pelvis. **A.** Technique to obtain inlet view. **B.** Inlet view of the pelvis. The pubic rami are fractured, but the posterior elements (i.e., sacroiliac joints) appear intact. **C.** Technique to obtain on outlet view. **D.** Outlet view of the pelvis. The fracture line extends into the pubic bone.

structures, which facilitates a more accurate assessment of pelvic injury and stability. CT is very helpful in the evaluation of hematoma size and location, as well as in the diagnosis of visceral injuries in patients sustaining pelvic fractures. Visualization of a blush of contrast or a hematoma larger than 10 cm^2 suggests an arterial hemorrhage.[15-17] Three-dimensional CT imaging is being used more frequently and may aid in defining the overall pelvic ring injury.

Elderly osteopenic patients with pelvic pain after a low-energy mechanism of injury who have negative plain films may benefit from a radionuclide scan. A delay of 3 days from the trauma is recommended before scanning.[15,17]

In the setting of high-energy pelvic trauma, additional radiographic studies are often required. In hemodynamically unstable patients, pelvic angiography may be lifesaving if it can occlude arterial bleeding. If a urethral tear is suspected in a male patient, based on the findings of blood at the urethral meatus, hematuria, or a high-riding prostate, a retrograde urethrogram is obtained before placement of a Foley catheter. If this study is normal, a retrograde cystogram is obtained to evaluate the integrity of the bladder. A post void film is imperative to exclude extravasation of dye. A retrograde cystogram should be deferred in a patient who may undergo pelvic angiography because this test will interfere with proper angiographic diagnosis.

PELVIC FRACTURES

There are multiple classification systems for pelvic ring fractures. Pennal and Sutherland were the first to develop a mechanistic classification of pelvic ring injuries.[18] They divided pelvic ring injuries into categories based on the force that caused them—lateral compression (LC), anteroposterior compression (APC), and vertical shear (VS).

Burgess and Young further refined Pennal and Sutherland's system by subdividing the first two categories (LC and APC) into three subcategories (I, II, and III) based on the extent of injury (Table 17–1). With this system, the clinician classifies pelvic fractures by observing both the anterior and posterior injury patterns. The anterior injuries within

▶ **TABLE 17-1. BURGESS AND YOUNG CLASSIFICATION SYSTEM OF PELVIC RING INJURIES**

Lateral Compression (LC)

LC I: Pubic rami fracture (transverse) and ipsilateral sacral compression

LC II: Pubic rami fracture (transverse) and iliac wing fracture

LC III: Pubic rami fracture (transverse) and contralateral open-book injury (i.e., pelvis is run over by an automobile wheel, resulting in the hemipelvis on the side of lateral impact to rotate internally and the contralateral hemipelvis to rotate externally)

Anteroposterior Compression (APC)

APC I: Symphyseal diastasis (1–2 cm) with normal posterior ligaments

APC II: Symphyseal diastasis or pubic rami fracture (vertical) with anterior SI joint disruption

APC III: Symphyseal diastasis or pubic rami fracture (vertical) with complete SI joint disruption

Vertical Shear (VS)

Symphyseal diastasis or pubic rami fracture with complete SI joint disruption, iliac wing, or sacrum (with vertical displacement)

Combined Mechanical (CM)

Combination of other injury patterns (LC/VS or LC/APC)

▶ **TABLE 17-2. TILE CLASSIFICATION SYSTEM OF PELVIC RING INJURIES**

Type A: Stable Pelvic Ring Injury

A1: Fractures not involving the ring; avulsion fractures

A2: Minimal displacement

A3: Transverse fractures of the sacrum or coccyx

Type B: Rotationally Unstable, Vertically Stable Pelvic Ring Injury

B1: External rotation instability; open-book injury

B2: Internal rotation instability; lateral compression injury

Type C: Rotationally and Vertically Unstable Pelvic Ring Injury

C1: Unilateral injury

C2: Bilateral injury (one side rotationally unstable and the other vertically and rotationally unstable)

C3: Bilateral injury (both sides rotationally and vertically unstable)

---

each category (LC and APC) are the same. The degree of posterior injury defines the three subcategories (I, II, and III) in LC and APC mechanisms. These authors also added another category—combined mechanism (CM)—when the fractures noted were a result of a combination of forces (i.e., APC and LC or, more frequently, LC and VS). This system is beneficial to the emergency physician during the initial resuscitation as it helps predict fluid resuscitation requirements; associated skeletal and solid organ injury; the need for acute stabilization of the pelvis; and, ultimately, patient survival. APC III, LC III, and VS injuries are all associated with high-energy mechanisms. APC III injuries are associated with the highest transfusion requirement, highest mortality, and highest rate of neurologic injury.

Tile introduced a modification of the Pennal classification system in 1988, highlighting the importance of the posterior SI complex in maintaining the ability of the pelvis to withstand physiologic force and therefore maintain mechanical stability (Table 17-2). This system combines the mechanism of injury with the potential instability present. In hemodynamically stable patients, Tile's classification aids the orthopedic surgeon and the emergency physician in determining the requirement for surgical stabilization as well as the prognosis.

In this chapter, pelvic fractures are divided into those that do not involve the pelvic ring and those that do (Table 17-3). Fractures that do not disrupt the pelvic ring are mechanically stable fractures and have a low rate of associated injuries.

Pelvic fractures that disrupt the pelvic ring are then further subdivided into nondisplaced mechanically stable fractures and displaced high-energy fractures based on the classification of Burgess and Young.

Mechanically stable fractures generally occur when only one nondisplaced fracture in the pelvic ring is present and the SI joint and symphysis pubis remain intact. Stable, nondisplaced fractures tend to occur near the symphysis pubis or SI joint as the relative mobility of the pelvis in these areas allows a ring transection without additional injury. As mentioned previously, displaced pelvic fractures are usually mechanically unstable and suggest there are two fractures transecting the ring or one fracture and a joint dislocation.

Unstable fractures involve a transection of the pelvic ring in two places with displacement. These fractures represent

---

▶ **TABLE 17-3. PELVIC FRACTURES**

A. No Pelvic Ring Disruption

1. Avulsion
2. Single pubic ramus or ischial ramus
3. Ischial body
4. Iliac wing
5. Horizontal sacral
6. Coccygeal

B. Pelvic Ring Disruption

1. Nondisplaced pelvic ring fractures
   a. Superior and inferior pubic rami
   b. Pubic bone
   c. Ilium body
   d. Vertical sacral fractures
2. Displaced pelvic ring fractures
   a. Straddle injury
   b. Burgess and Young classification
      i. Lateral compression (LC)
      ii. Anteroposterior compression (APC)
      iii. Vertical shear (VS)
      iv. Combined mechanism (CM)

15% of patients with pelvic fractures.[10] The mortality rate for displaced pelvic fractures is high, and life-threatening–associated injuries, including hemorrhage and visceral organ damage, frequently accompany these injuries. These fractures are usually secondary to severe direct forces such as those that occur in a high-speed car collision or after a fall from a significant height.

AVULSION FRACTURES

These fractures generally occur in young athletes and are due to a forceful muscular contraction in an area where the apophyseal centers are not yet fused (Fig. 17–8). They typically fuse at the following ages:

• Anterior superior iliac spine (sartorius insertion) fuses at 16 to 20 years.
• Anterior inferior iliac spine (rectus femoris insertion) fuses at 16 to 20 years.
• Ischial tuberosity (hamstrings insertion) fuses at age 25.

Mean patient age of avulsion fractures is approximately 14 years old, with 75% of patients being male. Most commonly affected are the anterior inferior iliac spine (33.2%), ischial tuberosity (29.7%), anterior superior iliac spine (27.9%), iliac crest (6.7%), lesser trochanter (1.8%), and superior corner of the pubic symphysis (1.2%).[23]

In addition to the preceding injuries, an avulsion at the symphysis pubis by the adductor longus muscle may be seen in young athletes. After the fracture, callus formation is extensive and at times can be mistaken for a neoplasm.

Mechanism of Injury
Each type of avulsion fracture is associated with a different mechanism of injury.

Avulsion of the anterior superior iliac spine is typically seen in young sprinters and is secondary to a forceful contraction of the sartorius. Displacement is usually mild and inhibited by the attachment of the inguinal ligament and fascia lata to this bone. Avulsion of the anterior inferior iliac spine is less frequent and is due to a forceful contraction of the rectus femoris, as can occur during a soccer kick. Avulsion of the ischial tuberosity is typically seen in athletes, such as hurdlers, cheerleaders, and pole vaulters, after a forceful contraction of their hamstrings.

Examination
Patients with an avulsion of the anterior superior iliac spine will have pain and tenderness over the area that is exacerbated with use of the sartorius (flexion or abduction of the thigh). Avulsion of the anterior inferior iliac spine will result in complaints of pain and tenderness in the groin. Active hip flexion using the rectus femoris, as during walking, will be painful. Avulsion of the ischial tuberosity may present with acute or chronic symptoms of pain that worsen with sitting. Tenderness will be elicited with percutaneous and rectal palpation of the ischial tuberosity. Palpation over the sacrotuberous ligament on rectal examination will also greatly exacerbate the pain. In addition, flexion of the thigh with the knee extended is painful, although it is painless with the knee flexed.

Imaging
An AP view is generally adequate in defining the fracture fragment (Fig. 17–9). Nonossified apophyseal centers may confuse the interpretation of these radiographs, and therefore, comparison to the uninjured side is warranted.

Associated Injuries
Avulsion fractures are usually not associated with any other significant injuries.

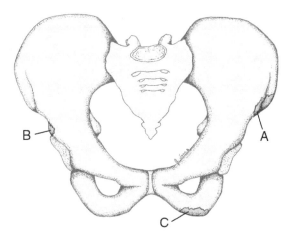

A = Avulsion of the anterior superior iliac spine
B = Avulsion of the anterior inferior iliac spine
C = Avulsion of the ischial tuberosity

Figure 17–8. Avulsion fractures.

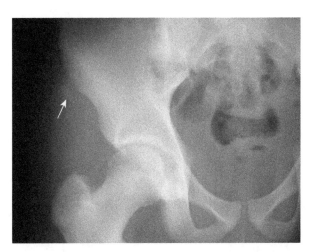

Figure 17–9. Avulsion of the anterior superior iliac spine (*arrow*).

Treatment

The treatment of avulsion pelvic fractures is symptomatic. Referral is indicated for determination of need for surgical intervention. Patients with more than 10 to 15 mm of displacement generally require surgical treatment. With conservative treatment, patients with avulsions of the anterior superior iliac spine should rest in bed for 3 to 4 weeks with the hip in flexion and abduction. The patient may sit as tolerated, although ambulation and vigorous activity should be restricted. Complete recovery takes as long as 8 weeks or more. The treatment of avulsions of the anterior inferior iliac spine is similar, except the hip should be in flexion with no abduction. Patients with avulsions of the ischial tuberosity should be placed on bed rest with the thigh in extension with external rotation and slight abduction. An inflatable ring cushion for sitting is advised.

Surgical treatment may be preferred because it speeds recovery and return to preinjury sport level. The overall success and return to sports rate are higher in patients receiving surgery, especially in patients with fragment displacement greater than 15 mm and high functional demands.

Complications

Avulsion fractures may be followed by the persistence of chronic pain due to the overzealous growth of callus. Surgical excision is occasionally required.

SINGLE PUBIC RAMUS OR ISCHIAL RAMUS FRACTURE

These fractures do not result in complete transection of the pelvic ring (Fig. 17–10). Earlier studies suggested these fractures represented one-third of all pelvic fractures, but recent advances in radiographic techniques have led many clinicians to conclude that they are a rare occurrence and are usually associated with injury to an additional ipsilateral ramus or subtle posterior injury.

Some authors elect to classify these injuries as stress fractures because they are seen in women during the third trimester of pregnancy, in military recruits after a strenuous activity, or in long-distance runners. These fractures are also seen in elderly patients. Most patients with these injuries experience persistent groin discomfort during any activity. All patients recover with an 8- to 12-week rest period, particularly with the avoidance of running.

Mechanism of Injury

In the elderly, the mechanism is generally secondary to a fall. In the young, persistent tension on the adductors and the hamstrings may result in a stress fracture of the inferior ramus.

Examination

The patient will complain of a "deep pain" that is exacerbated with deep palpation or walking. Hamstring stressing will elicit or worsen the pain.

Imaging

An AP pelvic view is obtained first as a general overview of the area. If clinical or radiographic suspicion is high, an outlet view should be obtained. Bone scan may be the only way to demonstrate a stress fracture.

Associated Injuries

These fractures may be accompanied by a hip fracture in elderly patients.

Treatment

Symptomatic treatment is recommended, including analgesics and bed rest, progressing to crutch walking as tolerated.

Complications

Complications are not commonly seen after these fractures.

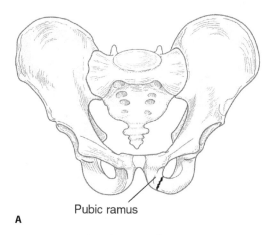
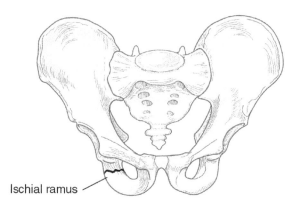

Pubic ramus

Ischial ramus

A   **B**

Figure 17–10. **A.** Single pubic ramus fracture. **B.** Ischial ramus fracture.

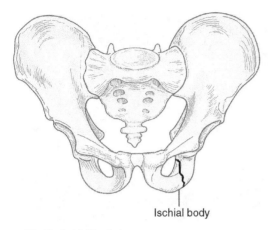

Figure 17–11. Ischial body fracture.

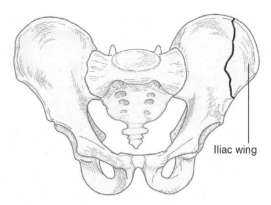

Figure 17–12. Iliac wing fracture (Duverney fracture).

ISCHIAL BODY FRACTURES

Ischial body fractures (Fig. 17–11) are often comminuted and are the least frequent of all pelvic fractures.

Mechanism of Injury
These fractures result from a significant fall landing on the buttocks in the seated position.

Examination
There will be pain and tenderness to deep palpation that is exacerbated with tension on the hamstrings.

Imaging
An AP view of the pelvis is generally adequate in demonstrating this fracture.

Associated Injuries
These fractures usually follow a significant fall, and associated fractures of the lumbar and thoracic spine may accompany these injuries.

Treatment
Symptomatic treatment with 4 to 6 weeks of bed rest is usually adequate. Elderly patients typically require active and passive motion exercises along with earlier mobilization. A pneumatic cushion for sitting is helpful during the later stages of healing.

Complications
Ischial body fractures may be complicated by malunion or excessive callus formation resulting in the development of chronic pain exacerbated by sitting or hamstring stress.

ILIAC WING (DUVERNEY) FRACTURE

Mechanism of Injury
These fractures are usually the result of a medially directed force. A Duverney fracture may be due to a high-energy force and, therefore, may serve to alert the clinician to other injuries. The iliac wing may at times demonstrate medial displacement (Fig. 17–12).

Examination
The patient will complain of tenderness and swelling over the iliac wing. The abductors of the hip insert on the iliac wing, and thus, pain will be exacerbated with walking or stressing of the hip abductors.

Imaging
An AP pelvic view is generally adequate in demonstrating this fracture. Oblique views may be indicated if the fracture is not clearly identified or if displacement is suspected. A CT scan can be obtained in equivocal cases (Fig. 17–13).

Associated Injuries
Although these fractures do not involve the pelvic ring, iliac wing fractures typically follow severe forces and may be accompanied by associated injuries including:

- Acetabular fractures
- Gastrointestinal injuries—uncommon but may be delayed in their presentation
- Solid organ abdominal and thoracic injuries

Treatment
Symptomatic treatment, including bed rest and nonweight bearing until the hip abductors are pain-free, is appropriate. Displaced fractures typically do not require reduction.

Complications
Iliac wing fractures are generally free of long-term complications.

HORIZONTAL SACRAL FRACTURES

Sacral fractures may be either horizontal or vertical. Vertical fractures are secondary to an indirect mechanism; transect

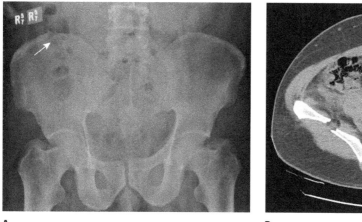

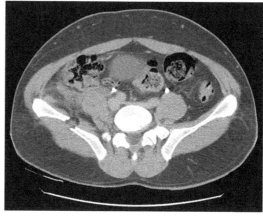

A   **B**

Figure 17–13. Iliac wing fracture on plain radiograph and CT scan. *A.* Plain radiograph. *B.* CT scan.

the pelvic ring; and are commonly associated with an additional, sometimes occult, pelvic ring fracture. The following discussion is limited to horizontal sacral fractures. Isolated horizontal (transverse) sacral fractures account for 2% to 3% of pelvis fractures (Fig. 17–14). Fractures above the level of S2 are less common than fractures below S2.

Mechanism of Injury

A direct blow over the posterior sacrum in an anterior direction is the usual mechanism. These fractures also occur following a fall with landing in the sitting position or a massive crush injury to the pelvis.

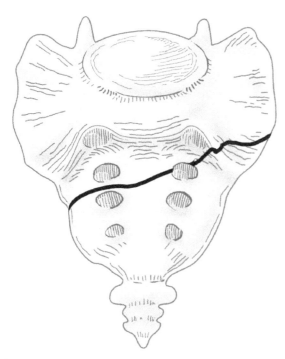

Figure 17–14. Horizontal sacral fracture.

Examination

The patient will complain of tenderness, swelling, and ecchymosis over the sacral prominence. Rectal examination will elicit pain in the sacrum, and displacement can be assessed with a bimanual rectal examination. Blood on the examiner's glove following the digital rectal examination suggests an open fracture. Open fractures require emergent broad-spectrum antibiotics and surgical intervention. Neurologic function of the lower sacral nerves is assessed by noting anal sphincter tone, perineal sensation, and the bladder sphincter.

Imaging

Horizontal sacral fractures may be difficult to detect on routine pelvic radiographs. Horizontal fractures tend to occur distally to the SI joints. A malalignment or buckling of the sacral foramina may be indicative of a displaced sacral fracture. The outlet (AP cephalic) view is better for demonstrating displaced sacral fractures.   A CT scan is very helpful in delineating these fractures when plain films are not definitive.

Associated Injuries

Various series report a 4% to 14% incidence of associated pelvic fractures with horizontal sacral fractures. Fractures above S2 are associated with a greater incidence of neurologic dysfunction than fractures below S2.

Treatment

Nondisplaced horizontal sacral fractures are treated with bed rest for 4 to 5 weeks. An inflated cushion may be used later for sitting. Displaced horizontal fractures require emergent orthopedic referral because of the potential for neurologic injury. It is imperative that the initial examining physician performs a thorough neurologic examination of the patient.

Complications

Horizontal sacral fractures may be complicated by the development of chronic pain or nerve dysfunction secondary to callus formation.

COCCYX FRACTURES

Coccyx fractures tend to be transverse and, because numerous muscle fibers insert here, they are impossible to immobilize (Fig. 17–15). Coccyx fractures are among the easiest fractures to treat and yet the most difficult to cure.

Mechanism of Injury

A fall landing in the sitting position is the most common mechanism of injury. In addition, surgical procedures performed in this area may be complicated by the development of a coccyx fracture.

Examination

The patient will complain of tenderness localized to "one spot." Use of the tensor levator ani or spasm of the anococcygeal muscle, as during sitting or defecation, will exacerbate the pain. Palpation rectally or externally over the coccyx is usually diagnostic. Similar to sacral fractures, rectal examination will elicit pain over the coccyx. Blood on the examiner's glove following the digital rectal examination suggests an open fracture. Open fractures require emergent broad-spectrum antibiotics and surgical intervention.

Imaging

An AP pelvic view, along with a lateral projection with the thighs in flexion, is best for demonstrating these fractures. Coccygeal fractures are often not visualized radiographically.

Associated Injuries

Coccygeal fractures are not commonly associated with any other significant injuries.

Treatment

The treatment is symptomatic with bed rest, inflated cushions, sitz baths, and laxatives to avoid straining. Patients may suffer from debilitating pain that requires narcotic pain medications, nonsteroidal anti-inflammatory drugs (NSAIDs), and laxatives. The patient should be told to expect that the pain may persist for months before recovery. Coccygectomy may be indicated if chronic pain persists despite adequate conservative therapy.

Complications

Chronic pain may persist for several years after coccygeal fractures.

PUBIC RAMI FRACTURES (NONDISPLACED)

This injury is the first of four stable (nondisplaced) fractures of the pelvic ring to be presented. Nondisplaced fractures of the superior and inferior pubic rami are not only very commonly seen, but they are also very stable from an orthopedic standpoint (Fig. 17–16). A common mistake, however, is for the clinician to miss an occult injury to the SI joint in a patient with minimally displaced fractures of the pubic rami.

Mechanism of Injury

This fracture usually results from direct trauma to the area. If the fracture lines run horizontally, a lateral compressive force may be the mechanism of injury. Ipsilateral sacral compression may be present and would classify this fracture as an LC I injury based on the work of Burgess and Young (Table 17–1).[19]

Examination

The patient will present with tenderness, swelling, and ecchymosis over the fracture site. LC of the ring (Patrick test) will exacerbate the patient's pain.

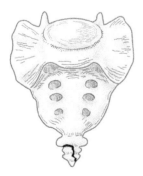 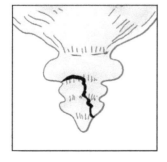

Figure 17–15. Coccyx fracture.

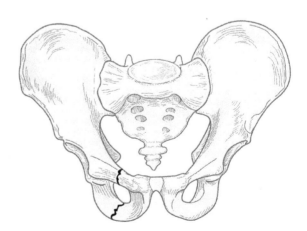

Figure 17–16. Superior and inferior pubic rami fractures (nondisplaced).

Imaging

A routine AP pelvic view is usually adequate in demonstrating the fracture. The ipsilateral SI joint must be inspected carefully for any evidence of disruption. CT scanning is recommended if an SI joint disruption is suspected.

Associated Injuries

Although these fractures are considered mechanically stable, they may still be associated with significant associated injuries. CT scanning is useful in evaluating patients with suspected visceral and/or vascular injuries.

Treatment

Early orthopedic consultation is recommended. These fractures are typically stable and treated symptomatically with bed rest for 3 weeks. Internal fixation of pubic rami fractures is necessary only when a posterior pelvis injury has occurred in combination.

Complications

These fractures may be complicated by the persistence of pain secondary to posttraumatic arthritis.

PUBIC BONE FRACTURE (NONDISPLACED)

This is rare as an isolated injury (Fig. 17–17).

Mechanism of Injury

A direct AP force is the usual mechanism, although indirect forces may add to the displacement.

Examination

The patient will present with tenderness, swelling, or even deformity over the involved area. Pain will be localized and exacerbated with anterior or LC of the pelvis.

Imaging

A routine pelvic view is usually adequate in demonstrating the fracture. Urologic imaging studies are indicated for patients with suspected urinary tract disruption.

Associated Injuries

Damage to the urologic system frequently accompanies these injuries.

Treatment

Although these are typically stable injuries, early orthopedic consultation is recommended. The treatment is symptomatic with bed rest in the lateral position and crutches for ambulation.

Complications

These injuries may be complicated by the development of persistent pain over the involved area.

ILIUM BODY FRACTURE (NONDISPLACED)

Pelvic fractures in this category are isolated, nondisplaced ilium body fractures near the SI joint (Fig. 17–18). These fractures are rare. Typically, posterior pelvic fractures are associated with anterior ring fractures.

Mechanism of Injury

Ilium body fractures near the SI joint are usually the result of a direct force pushing the ilium posteriorly and medially.

Examination

The patient will present with tenderness over the posterior pelvis that is exacerbated with anterior or LC. Straight-leg raise is painful with this type of fracture.

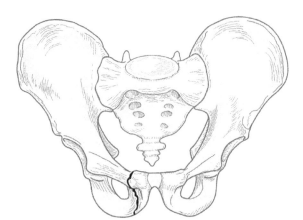

Figure 17–17. Pubic bone fracture (nondisplaced).

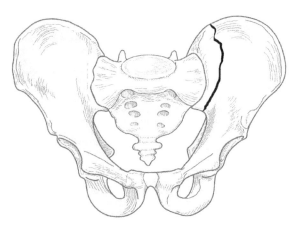

Figure 17–18. Ilium body fracture (nondisplaced).

Imaging

An AP pelvic view is usually adequate for visualizing these injuries. A CT or bone scan is often helpful in delineating these fractures where plain films are not conclusive.[25]

Associated Injuries

These fractures are frequently associated with anterior pelvic fractures.

Treatment

Although these are typically stable fractures and treated symptomatically, early orthopedic consultation is recommended. Bed rest with a pelvic sling or belt is recommended. Ambulation, with crutches initially, should progress as tolerated, with an expected return to normal function within 3 to 4 months.

Complications

These fractures may be complicated by the development of chronic back pain or neurologic compromise.

VERTICAL SACRAL FRACTURES

Vertical sacral fractures usually begin at the weakest point of the bone that is adjacent to the first and second neural foramina (Fig. 17–19).

Mechanism of Injury

Vertical sacral fractures are the result of indirect trauma, as when an anterior force drives the pelvic ring posteriorly.

Examination

The patient will present with tenderness over the posterior pelvis that is exacerbated with anterior or LC. Straight-leg raise is painful with this type of fracture. Patients with this fracture should have a digital rectal examination. Blood on the examiner's glove following the digital rectal examination suggests an open fracture.

Imaging

An AP pelvic view is usually adequate for both of these injuries. Sacral fractures may be better demonstrated on an AP cephalic tilt (outlet) view. A CT scan is helpful in delineating these fractures where plain films are not conclusive (Fig. 17–20).[25]

Associated Injuries

These fractures are frequently associated with anterior pelvic fractures. Vertical sacral fractures have a high incidence of associated neurologic injury.

Denis et al classified sacral fractures by the location of injury.[27] See the Associated Injuries section later in this chapter.

Treatment

Although these are typically stable fractures and treated symptomatically, early orthopedic consultation is recommended. Bed rest with a pelvic sling or belt is advised. These devices are commercially available at orthopedic supply companies. Ambulation with crutches for assistance should progress as tolerated, with an expected return to normal function within 3 to 4 months. Open fractures require emergent broad-spectrum antibiotics and surgical intervention.

Complications

These fractures may be complicated by the development of chronic back pain or neurologic compromise.

STRADDLE INJURY

Straddle fractures are the most common type of displaced pelvic fractures seen (Fig. 17–21). Nearly one-third of these fractures have an associated lower urinary tract injury.

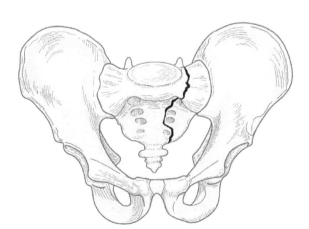

Figure 17–19. Vertical sacral fracture (nondisplaced).

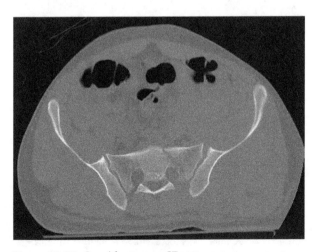

Figure 17–20. Sacral fracture on CT scan.

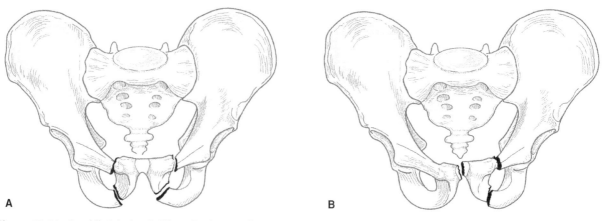

Figure 17–21. Straddle injuries. **A.** Bilateral pubic rami fractures. **B.** Pubic rami fractures and symphysis pubis disruption.

Mechanism of Injury

The most common mechanism is a fall resulting in the straddling of a hard object. LC of the pelvis may result in a similar appearing fracture but without the same incidence of associated GU injuries.

Examination

The patient will present with anterior tenderness, swelling, and ecchymosis. It is important to examine and palpate the perineum, rectum, scrotum, testes, and vagina for lacerations, bony deformities, and hematomas.

Imaging

An AP pelvic view is usually adequate in demonstrating the fracture (Fig. 17-22). CT scanning is valuable in determining the extent of the damage to the underlying tissues and organs as well as the SI joint. Radiographic imaging of the lower urinary tract is also recommended. Ultrasound may

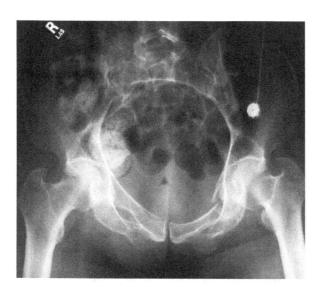

Figure 17–22. Inlet view of a straddle injury with bilateral breaks of both pubic rami.

be needed to evaluate for testicular injury associated with straddle injuries.

Associated Injuries

As mentioned previously, these injuries are associated with a high incidence of vascular and visceral injuries. Up to 33% have an associated lower urinary tract injury, the most common being a urethral rupture. It is therefore imperative that patients with these fractures undergo a radiographic examination of the lower urinary tract, particularly if there is blood at the urethral meatus.

Treatment

Emergent orthopedic consultation is recommended. The emergency management of these fractures includes immobilization and stabilization, including fluid therapy and the exclusion of serious associated injuries. The physician's priority must be directed at the identification and stabilization of associated life-threatening injuries. Operative fixation of the anterior pelvis is necessary after straddle injuries.

Complications

- Posttraumatic arthritis
- Malunion or nonunion
- Pulmonary or fat emboli (early)

BURGESS AND YOUNG

Unstable pelvic ring disruptions are classified on the basis of the system developed by Burgess and Young because the acute management of the patient is best guided by this classification system. As stated previously, this system helps predict fluid resuscitation requirements; associated skeletal and solid organ injury; need for acute stabilization of the pelvis; and, ultimately, patient survival. These fractures are therefore divided by the mechanism of injury into four subtypes: (1) lateral compression (LC), (2) anteroposterior

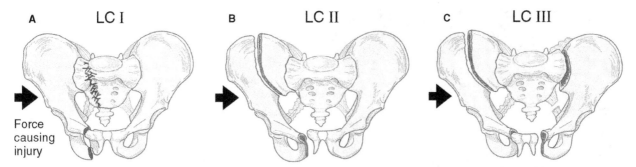

Figure 17–23. Lateral compression injuries. **A.** LC I injury pattern. Note the internally rotated right hemipelvis with transverse pubic rami fractures and sacral impaction fracture. **B.** LC II injury pattern. Lateral impaction of the right hemipelvis results in transverse pubic rami fractures and ilium fracture near the right SI joint. (SI joint disruption may also occur with LC II injuries.) **C.** LC III injury pattern. Lateral compression of the right hemipelvis results in internal rotation of the right hemipelvis (transverse pubic rami fractures and ilium fracture), as well as external rotation of the contralateral hemipelvis (pubic bone fracture and left anterior SI disruption).

compression (APC; open-book injury), (3) vertical shear (VS; Malgaigne fracture), and (4) a combined mechanism (CM) (Table 17–1).[19]

Lateral Compression Mechanism

These injuries are due to an LC force that results in an implosion of the pelvis. The anterior pelvic ligaments (anterior SI, sacrotuberous, and sacrospinous) are shortened in this mechanism rather than stretched. Because these ligaments remain intact, a tamponade effect is created if there is pelvic hemorrhage. Anterior injury is similar in all three subtypes and consists of transverse pubic rami fractures. Pubic rami fractures may occur ipsilaterally (most common), contralaterally, or bilaterally to the applied lateral force. The injury to the posterior structures of the pelvis distinguishes the three subtypes of the LC mechanism (Fig. 17–23).

Lateral Compression I (LC I)

The posterior component of an LC I injury is a sacral impaction fracture (Fig. 17–23A). This fracture is often misdiagnosed as isolated pubic rami fracture unless the posterior components are closely scrutinized (Fig. 17–24A). The posterior elements are demonstrated on an outlet view of the pelvis with close examination of the sacral foramina. CT scan is the most sensitive for detecting an LC I injury (Figs. 17–24B and 17–25). These fractures are generally stable to physical examination and are considered mechanically stable fractures with a low incidence of associated injuries.

Definitive treatment consists of protected weight bearing on the side of injury (crutches for support) and repeat radiographs in 2 to 5 days to ensure that no additional displacement has occurred. External fixation (in the nonacute setting) is required only in patients with debilitating pain due to fracture instability.

Lateral Compression II (LC II)

In the LC II injury, there are transverse pubic rami fractures with either an ipsilateral iliac wing fracture (crescent

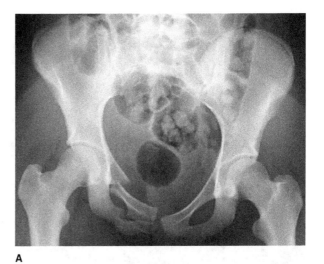

A

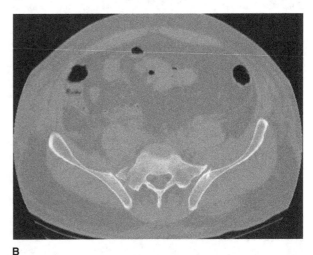

B

Figure 17–24. Lateral compression I injury. **A.** AP view of the pelvis reveals transverse fractures of the right superior and inferior pubic rami consistent with a lateral compression mechanism. Examination of the posterior elements does not identify an obvious fracture. **B.** CT scan of the pelvis of the same patient reveals a sacral ala impaction fracture consistent with an LC I injury.

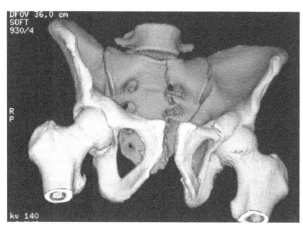

Figure 17–25. Three-dimensional reconstruction of an LC I injury on the patient's left.

fracture) adjacent to the SI joint or ipsilateral SI joint disruption (Figs. 17–23B and 17–26). An LC II injury can be treated with bed rest and delayed open reduction and internal fixation unless hemodynamic instability necessitates the acute application of external fixation. The reader is referred to the Associated Injuries section of this chapter for further discussion.

Definitive treatment consists of both anterior and posterior stabilization. Either an external fixator or open reduction is used anteriorly, whereas open reduction with a plate or screw is required to stabilize the posterior injury.

Lateral Compression III (LC III)

In the LC III injury pattern, LC causes the contralateral hemipelvis to rotate externally (i.e., "open") while the hemipelvis on the side of the impact rotates internally

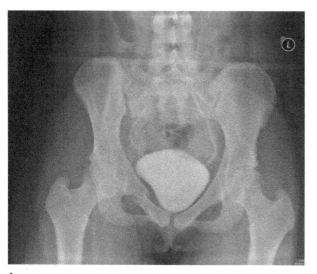

A

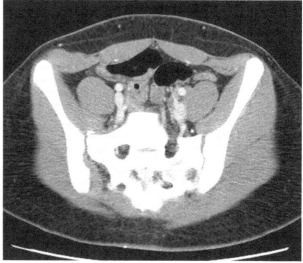

B

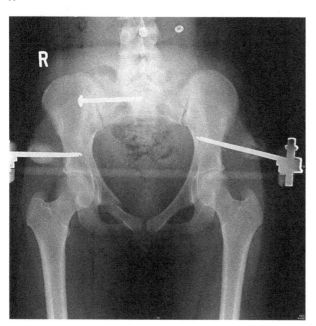

C

Figure 17–26. Lateral compression II injury of an unrestrained passenger involved in an motor vehicle collision (MVC). **A.** AP view of the pelvis reveals fractures of the right pubic rami. In this case, the ilium was not fractured, but the sacroiliac joint was disrupted. **B.** CT scan confirms right SI joint disruption. Note the widening of the posterior portion of the SI joint (arrow). **C.** Operative fixation in this case included an anterior external fixator and a right iliosacral screw.

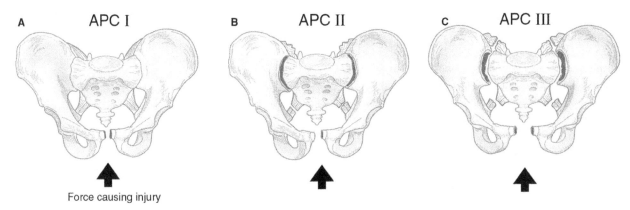

A APC I **B** APC II **C** APC III

Force causing injury

Figure 17–27. Anteroposterior compression injuries. **A.** APC I injury pattern. The ligaments of the pelvic floor and SI joint remain intact while the symphysis pubis ligaments are injured. Separation of the pubic bones >2.5 cm on imaging suggests more significant injury. **B.** APC II injury pattern. Ligaments of the symphysis pubis and anterior SI joint are disrupted. This injury will result in a pelvis that "opens like a book." **C.** APC III injury pattern. In this injury, the pelvis is both rotationally and vertically unstable due to rupture of all the ligaments of the symphysis pubis and SI joint.

(Fig. 17–23C). Pubic rami fractures occur on the side of impact with or without an associated ipsilateral ilium fracture or SI joint disruption. An example of an LC III–type mechanism is a pelvis that is rolled over by an automobile. The initial LC that occurs results in an LC II injury, and as the car wheel hits the contralateral pelvis, it applies an externally rotated force. An LC III injury is mechanically unstable and often necessitates acute application of an external fixator in hemodynamically unstable patients.[19] The reader is referred to the Associated Injuries section later in the chapter for further discussion.

Definitive treatment consists of both anterior and posterior stabilization. Anterior stabilization is similar to LC II injuries. For the posterior injury, the contralateral open-book injury is reduced with percutaneous iliosacral screws. The ipsilateral posterior injury is treated on the basis of the injury present. LC I injury requires no treatment. LC II injury requires plate fixation for ilium fractures and percutaneous iliac screws for displaced sacral fractures.

Anteroposterior Compression Mechanism

These fractures are due to anterior compression of the pelvis. The anterior injury to the pelvis consists of a symphysis pubis diastasis or vertical pubic rami fractures. Anterior force may be due to a directly applied force, as in a crush injury, or indirectly via the lower extremities. The injury to the posterior pelvis defines the subtype (I, II, and III) (Fig. 17–27). APC II and III injuries are also known as open-book injuries or a sprung pelvis.

Anteroposterior Compression I (APC I)

This stable injury occurs following an AP force that results in symphysis pubis diastasis or vertical pubic rami fractures without posterior injury (Fig. 17–27A). This is a rare injury and results from low- to moderate-energy trauma. The anterior ligaments of the SI joint are stretched but not torn. The ligaments of the symphysis pubis normally allow for

0.5 to 1 cm of movement. Any separation beyond 1 cm is considered abnormal (Fig. 17–28A). Subluxation beyond 2.5 cm is associated with posterior ligamentous injury and should be considered unstable (APC II, III). Examination of

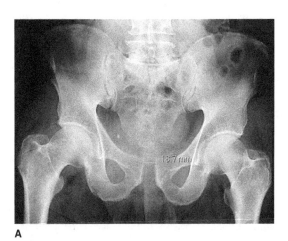

A

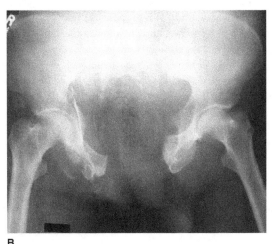

B

Figure 17–28. A. Symphysis pubis diastasis (APC I injury). **B.** "Open-book" injury.

APC I patients will result in little movement to external rotation forces. Third trimester and postpartum patients are susceptible to this injury because the hormonally induced ligamentous laxity allows for more mobility. Patients with APC I injuries suffer from a low incidence of associated injuries.

Definitive treatment is symptomatic with bed rest in the lateral position. Early orthopedic consultation is recommended. These injuries may be complicated by the development of persistent pain over the involved area.

Anteroposterior Compression II (APC II)

In the APC II injury, symphyseal diastasis is accompanied by disruption of the anterior SI ligamentous structures and the ligaments of the pelvic floor (sacrotuberous and sacrospinous) (Fig. 17–27B). The symphysis pubis diastasis is >2.5 cm, and these injuries are considered open-book injuries (sprung pelvis) (Fig. 17–28B). APC II injuries are mechanically unstable to external and internal rotation but do not demonstrate instability to vertical forces due to the intact posterior SI ligaments. APC II injuries are associated with a high rate of hemorrhage and neurologic injury and often require external fixation and arterial embolization in the acute setting. The reader is referred to the Associated Injuries section later in the chapter for further discussion.

Definitive treatment consists of plate fixation of symphysis pubis disruptions and external fixation or open reduction for pubic rami fractures. If external fixation is used, it is left in place for 8 weeks.

Anteroposterior Compression III (APC III)

APC III injuries consist of symphysis pubis dislocation and injury to the anterior and posterior SI ligaments (Fig. 17–27C). These fractures are very unstable because the integrity of the pelvic ring has been abolished. APC III injuries are unstable to both vertical and rotational forces. The ligamentous injuries of the APC III mechanism are similar to VS injuries, except that the hemipelvis is not displaced superiorly. Associated injuries—vascular, visceral, and neurologic—frequently complicate the management of these fractures, resulting in a high morbidity and mortality. It is imperative that the emergency physician aggressively evaluates these patients for the presence of accompanying life-threatening injuries. Like APC II injuries, external fixation is often necessary in the acute setting to control hemorrhage. Patients with this fracture pattern are more likely to require emergent arterial embolization. The reader is referred to the Associated Injuries section later in the chapter for further discussion.

Definitive treatment is similar to APC II injuries anteriorly but also requires stabilization of the posterior injury. Stabilization of the posterior-ring injury is performed with percutaneous iliosacral screws.

Vertical Shear Mechanism

These fractures are distinguished by displacement of the anterior and posterior pelvis vertically and were originally

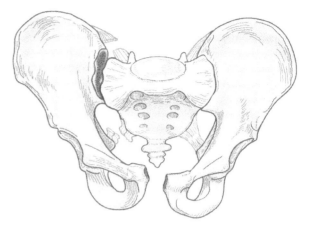

Figure 17–29. Vertical shear injury pattern. Note the right hemipelvis is superior to the left hemipelvis.

described by Malgaigne (Fig. 17–29). Anteriorly, there is usually disruption of the symphysis pubis, although fracture through the pubic rami is a less common presentation. Posteriorly, the injury may occur through the ilium, sacrum, or SI joint. In some cases, there is a small avulsion fragment of the ilium that remains attached to the sacrum.

The classic mechanism for this injury is a fall from a height. If the patient lands on an extended lower extremity, the hemipelvis is displaced vertically upward. In a motor vehicle collision, the patient may suffer from this injury when an extended leg is superiorly displaced into the pelvis by the floor of the car.

The physician will note shortening of the lower extremity on the involved side. Shortening is due to cephalad displacement of the pelvic fragment. Careful measurements from the umbilicus to the anterior superior iliac spine or the medial malleolus will demonstrate shortening on the involved side. Measurements from the anterior superior iliac spine to the malleolus will be the same on both sides, thus excluding a femoral neck fracture. Sacral neurologic deficits may accompany these injuries and must be excluded early on the basis of examination. Visceral injuries frequently accompany these fractures and require a thorough physical and radiographic evaluation.

The emergency management of these fractures includes immobilization along with a rapid and thorough assessment for associated life-threatening injuries. Patients with unstable pelvic fractures with hemodynamic instability despite appropriate fluid therapy should be considered candidates for emergent external fixation. Early external fixation may be a valuable option in reducing blood loss. Patients with VS injuries are more likely to require arterial embolization. The reader is referred to the Associated Injuries section later in the chapter for further discussion.

Definitive treatment depends on the location of the posterior injury. Fractures involving the SI joint or the sacrum require traction for reduction followed by percutaneous iliosacral screw fixation. Anterior stabilization with open

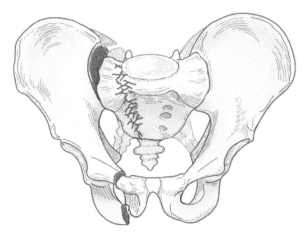

Figure 17–30. Combined mechanisms. Multiple fractures of the pelvis that cannot be classified into any of the other groups.

reduction or external fixation is also required. The external fixator must be left in place for 12 weeks.

Combined Mechanism

These fractures are very unstable as the integrity of the pelvic ring has been abolished (Fig. 17–30). Associated injuries frequently complicate the management of these fractures resulting in a high morbidity and mortality.

Because these injuries are frequently accompanied by other life-threatening injuries, they should be considered within the context of trauma management rather than as isolated fractures of the pelvis. Emergent orthopedic consultation is strongly recommended. The emergency management of these fractures includes immobilization along with a rapid and thorough assessment for associated life-threatening injuries. Patients with unstable pelvic fractures with hemodynamic instability despite appropriate fluid therapy should be considered candidates for emergent external fixation. The reader is referred to the Associated Injuries section for further discussion.

Definitive treatment depends on the types of injury involved and is best guided by an experienced orthopedic surgeon.

Associated Injuries

The mortality rate from pelvic ring disruptions is high (10%–20%) and is a result of the high incidence of multisystem injury.[1,6,28–30] The clinician must consider these injuries in the overall context of the patient. Multiple associated injuries can occur due to the fracture fragments and their effect on adjacent anatomic structures. Early identification of patients with specific pelvic fracture patterns is useful because it predicts the type of associated injury.[21] Pelvic fractures result in associated injuries that affect structures within the vasculature, genitourinary tract, neurologic system, and alimentary tract. Hemorrhage control is the primary concern in the initial stages of management.

Hemorrhage. Up to 4 L of blood can accumulate in the retroperitoneum after a significant pelvic fracture.[10] Half of patients suffering from blunt pelvic fractures admitted to the hospital will require blood transfusions (mean volume 6–8 units).[5,19] With these facts in mind, it is not surprising that hemorrhagic shock is the major cause of death in patients with pelvic fractures. Characteristics of patients who are at risk for death from pelvic fractures include male gender, severe multiple trauma, and major hemorrhage.[31]

However, the emergency physician assessing these patients must also consider other sources of hemorrhage. A large review established that the majority of patients suffering from hemorrhagic fatality after a pelvic fracture did not die as a result of pelvic hemorrhage.[28] Other sources of bleeding, such as the thorax and abdomen, must be evaluated.

The initial pelvic radiograph may be useful to predict significant pelvic hemorrhage. In hemodynamically unstable patients with mechanically stable LC I and APC I fracture patterns, ongoing hypotension was due to intra-abdominal hemorrhage in 85% of cases. In contrast, in patients with mechanically unstable LC II, LC III, APC II, APC III, and VS injuries, significant hemorrhage from the pelvis occurred in 60%.[21] APC injuries have the largest transfusion requirement (15 units), whereas LC injuries required the smallest (4 units).[19] Limitations include the potential difficulty in interpreting these initial films in patients who are often too unstable to undergo CT scanning.[32]

Other radiographic patterns that predict significant hemorrhage include double breaks in the pelvic ring and posterior fracture patterns. Fractures that involve a displaced double-ring break have a twofold increase in the incidence of bleeding requiring transfusion when compared with single-ring fractures. Posterior pelvic fractures are associated with more bleeding than are anterior fractures.

Direct surgical control and repair of bleeding vessels associated with pelvic fractures is not routinely indicated. Bleeding is venous in many cases, and surgical exploration is often futile due to extensive collateral circulation. In addition, loss of a tamponade effect following incision into the retroperitoneum makes this option potentially harmful.[10]

Interventions that have proven useful to control pelvic bleeding include pelvic fixation and angiography. Decisions made regarding the need and appropriate timing of pelvic fixation, angiography, or laparotomy to repair intra-abdominal injury are the source of debate and may be institution dependent; they are also the subject of the following discussion (Table 17–4).

Unstable fractures may be treated with external fixation in an attempt to reduce the intrapelvic volume, tamponade bleeding by opposing bony structures, and prevent clot dislodgement by immobilizing bony fragments.[10,19] Mortality has been shown to decrease with its use.[33,34] In mechanically unstable fractures, acute application of an external fixator should be considered for APC II, APC III, LC III,

▶ **TABLE 17-4.** **DIAGNOSTIC ALGORITHM FOR BLUNT PELVIC TRAUMA**

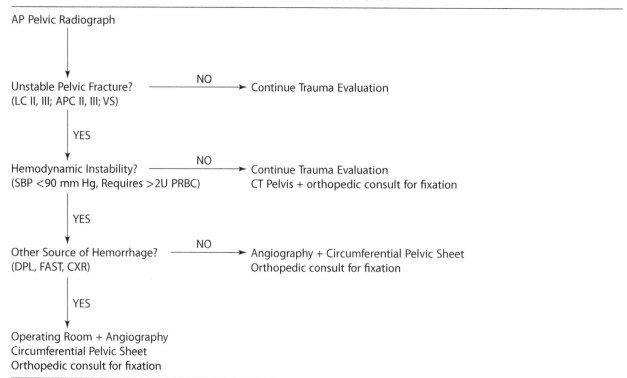

AP Pelvic Radiograph

↓

Unstable Pelvic Fracture? ————NO————→ Continue Trauma Evaluation
(LC II, III; APC II, III; VS)

↓ YES

Hemodynamic Instability? ————NO————→ Continue Trauma Evaluation
(SBP <90 mm Hg, Requires >2U PRBC)   CT Pelvis + orthopedic consult for fixation

↓ YES

Other Source of Hemorrhage? ————NO————→ Angiography + Circumferential Pelvic Sheet
(DPL, FAST, CXR)   Orthopedic consult for fixation

↓ YES

Operating Room + Angiography
Circumferential Pelvic Sheet
Orthopedic consult for fixation

AP, anteroposterior; APC, anteroposterior compression; CT, computed tomography; CXR, chest x-ray; DPL, deep peritoneal lavage; FAST, focused abdominal sonography in trauma; LC, lateral compression; PRBC, packed red blood cells; SBP, systolic blood pressure; VS, vertical shear.

and VS.[10] The type of external fixator and its application should be determined by the orthopedic surgeon based on the specific fracture pattern (Fig. 17–31). Many orthopedists recommend fixator placement before emergency laparotomy whenever possible. Pelvic fixators can be inserted in the ED under local anesthesia with minor skin incisions. Early external fixation of unstable pelvic fractures may be a valuable option in reducing blood loss.

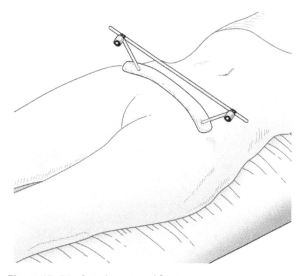

Figure 17-31. Anterior external fixator.

Downsides of external fixator application in the critically injured patient include the time required to place the device, approximately 40 minutes, which may unnecessarily delay other important lifesaving interventions. The other limitation of an external fixator is that it does not provide tremendous support to the posterior pelvis. In addition, some believe that an anteriorly applied external fixator may actually further distract a posterior injury.

Posterior-ring reduction clamps (C-clamps, pelvic clamps, Ganz clamps) are available but are more difficult to apply—generally requiring a skilled orthopedist and fluoroscopy to avoid misplacing the device (Fig. 17–32). These devices are effective in stabilizing the posterior pelvic ring by mechanically compressing the SI joints. Laparotomy is not interfered in a patient with the clamp. Posterior-ring reduction clamps are most common in European centers.

Another simple method for obtaining temporary pelvic stabilization is application of either a commercially available pelvic binder or a sheet wrapped around the pelvis (Fig. 17–33). Advantages of a circumferential pelvic antishock sheet (CPAS) include that it is inexpensive and readily available, and no special training is required for application. Lower extremity and abdominal access is maintained after the sheet is placed. Caution is required in patients with LC pelvic ring injuries or sacral neuroforaminal fractures. Forceful or aggressive CPAS application could worsen visceral injury or sacral nerve root injury in these instances.

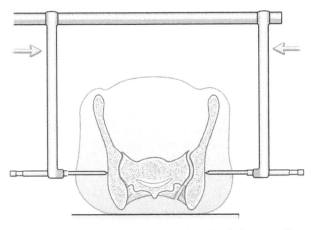

Figure 17–32. Schematic representation of a C-clamp application. This fixator is more difficult to apply but stabilizes the posterior pelvis more than an anterior external fixator.

Angiography with embolization is another important option to halt arterial bleeding from pelvic fractures. Traditional teaching is that pelvic bleeding is due to an arterial source in approximately 10% of cases. However, in patients with pelvic fracture who are hemodynamically unstable and refractory to volume resuscitation, arterial bleeding is more likely than venous bleeding, and up to 80% of these patients will have a significant component of arterial bleeding amenable to embolization.[39–41] For that reason, angiography with arterial embolization is potentially lifesaving in such a patient and should be considered early.[19] Hereto, the fracture pattern may also help indicate which patients might benefit from angiography. Twenty percent of patients with APC II, APC III, and VS injury patterns required embolization in Burgess et al's study,[19] whereas only 2% of patients with an LC injury pattern benefited from embolization.[34]

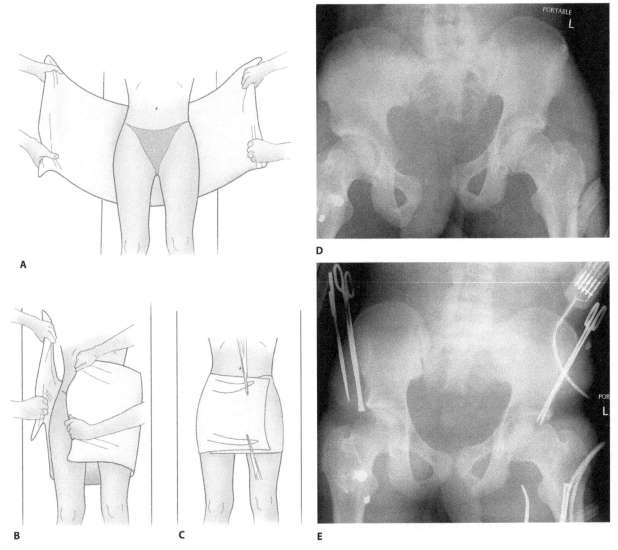

Figure 17–33. Circumferential pelvic antishock sheeting. **A.** A sheet is placed under the pelvis. **B.** The ends are brought together anteriorly. **C.** Hemostats are used to secure the sheet snugly. **D.** An open-book pelvis fracture before pelvic antishock sheeting. **E.** The same patient after pelvic antishock sheeting.

Before angiography, aggressive resuscitation and stabilization with a circumferential sheet or pelvic binder should be performed. If the patient remains hypotensive, and no other source of bleeding is evident (chest, abdomen), then angiography is indicated. In hypotensive patients without other sources of hemorrhage, angiography will reveal an arterial hemorrhage that can be embolized in 73% of patients. In these patients, the emergency physician should not wait for placement of an external fixator if it delays angiography. In hemodynamically unstable patients with evidence of both pelvic and abdominal hemorrhage (positive pelvic radiograph and focused abdominal sonography in trauma examination), the traditional order of laparotomy and then angiography has been questioned. Angiography before laparotomy has potential advantages in being able to embolize abdominal arteries and in avoiding the increase in pelvic volume that comes with opening the abdomen.

Genitourinary. Visceral injuries in conjunction with high-energy pelvic fractures are associated with a high mortality. The most common visceral injury is to the lower urinary tract, specifically the urethra and bladder. Urethral injuries occur with an incidence of 4% to 14% after pelvic ring disruptions, whereas bladder injuries are present in 6% to 11%. Simultaneous bladder and urethral injuries occur in 0.5% to 2.5% of pelvic fractures.

The clinician should consider urinary tract injury after all pelvic fractures. Examination findings such as a difficult-to-palpate prostate ("high riding"), scrotal/perineal swelling, and blood at the urethral meatus are often absent in the early period after injury. For this reason, specific fracture patterns that are associated with a high likelihood of urinary tract injury should be sought. The incidence of lower urologic injury is most common after disruption of the anterior pelvic ring, especially bilateral pubic rami involvement (straddle injury). Urologic injuries occur in 15% of patients with unilateral pubic ramus fractures and increase to 40% in patients after bilateral ramus fractures (straddle injury). Other fracture patterns associated with urinary tract injury include pubic symphysis subluxation (APC I), open-book injuries (APC II, APC III), VS fractures (Malgaigne), and pubic rami fractures with associated SI injury. Urethral injury is uncommon after an isolated posterior injury.

Axiom: *Pelvic fractures are assumed to have an associated urinary tract injury until proven otherwise. Pelvic fractures of the anterior pelvic ring are associated with a higher incidence of injury.*

The urethra is divided into posterior and anterior portions in the male. The posterior portion consists of the prostatic and membranous urethra, whereas the anterior portion consists of the bulbous and penile urethra. The area most susceptible to urethral injury after a pelvic fracture is the bulbomembranous junction. To understand why requires some knowledge of the surrounding anatomy. The prostate is fixed to the pubic bone via the puboprostatic ligaments. The prostate is similarly fixed to the urogenital diaphragm, which attaches to the membranous urethra. When injury to the pelvic ring occurs, the movement of the pubic bone displaces the prostate and creates a shearing force that partially or completely tears the urethra.

Female patients have a smaller incidence of urethral injuries (4.6%) due to the urethra's shorter length and the fact that there is less surrounding structural support. However, a meticulous examination should be performed in a female patient whenever blood is seen at the introitus.

All patients with physical examination findings suggesting a urethral injury should undergo a retrograde urethrogram prior to the passage of a Foley catheter. A Foley catheter inserted prematurely may convert a partial tear into a complete one. Because physical examination findings are unreliable, especially within the first hour after injury, male patients with anterior pelvic ring disruptions should have a retrograde urethrogram considered despite a negative examination.

Using a bulb syringe or a Foley catheter inserted into the fossa navicularis, 30 to 40 cc of water-soluble contrast medium is injected into the urethra while a radiograph is obtained (Fig. 17–34A). If a Foley has been placed prematurely, the urethrogram can be obtained by using an angiocatheter inserted alongside the Foley. A complete tear is diagnosed by extravasation of contrast without filling of the bladder, whereas an incomplete tear is present with extravasation and partial filling of the bladder. Treatment remains controversial, but in general, small anterior urethral tears usually do not require surgical repair as they heal well over an indwelling Foley catheter. A complete tear and posterior urethral injuries are best treated surgically.

Bladder injury can involve an intraperitoneal or extraperitoneal rupture. In 93% of cases of bladder rupture, a pelvic fracture is present concomitantly. Extraperitoneal rupture of the bladder is due to a bony spicule lacerating the anterolateral portion of the bladder in one-third of cases. Another common mechanism of extraperitoneal rupture is compression of an empty bladder. Intraperitoneal rupture occurs through the weakest part of the bladder, the dome, when a force is applied to the full bladder. Gross hematuria will be present in 82% to 97% of patients with a bladder rupture, although this finding does not distinguish between injury of the upper and lower genitourinary tract.

Fractures that disrupt the pelvic ring require a retrograde cystogram following the urethrogram. A retrograde cystogram is performed by instilling 300 cc of water-soluble contrast medium, by gravity alone, into the bladder (Fig. 17–34B). Radiographic views in distention and post voiding should be examined carefully for any evidence of extravasation. False-negative cystograms may result if the bladder is not fully distended or postvoid films are not obtained. Retrograde CT cystograms are also an acceptable alternative for the workup of bladder rupture. Bladder ruptures are treated with operative repair.

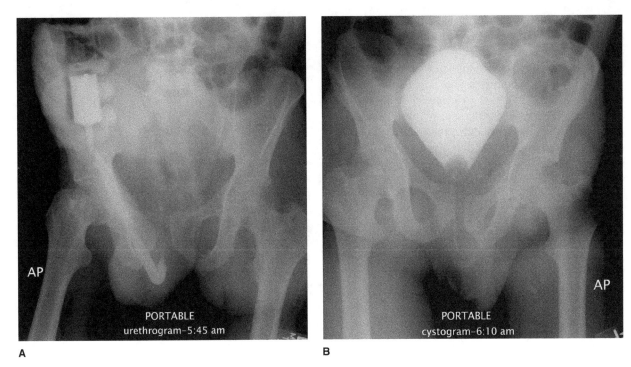

Figure 17–34. Pelvic fractures are frequently associated with genitourinary injury. **A.** Normal urethrogram. **B.** Normal cystogram.

Neurologic. Neurologic injuries are present in 20% of patients with unstable fractures of the pelvic ring. Neurologic injury is more common after SI injury, sacral fractures, or acetabular fractures. Sciatic nerve injury is present in 13% of patients with acetabular fractures.[4]

More than half of patients with neurologic injury due to pelvic fractures will suffer from both sensory and motor deficits. In one study, 50% of patients had a persistent neurologic deficit at 24 months post injury.[46] Following sacral fractures, nerves are damaged due to stretching, small bony fragments, or hematoma formation. These injuries are detected by a thorough neurologic examination, particularly of the L5, S1, and S2 nerve roots.

Denis et al classified sacral fractures by the location of injury (Fig. 17–35).[27] In patients with fractures through the sacral ala (zone I), the incidence of neurologic injury was 6%, with the most likely injury being partial injury to the L5 nerve root. Fractures through the sacral foramina (zone II) had a 28% incidence of neurologic injury. Zone II fractures were most commonly associated with injury to the ventral roots of L5, S1, or S2. Fractures medial to the sacral foramina or horizontal fractures (zone III) had the highest incidence of neurologic injury at 57%. These fractures were the most common and the most devastating as nearly 80% affected bowel, bladder, or sexual function. Horizontal sacral fractures above the S2 level are uncommon but associated with a much higher incidence of neurologic injuries than fractures below S2.[4]

Gastrointestinal. Gastrointestinal injuries associated with fractures are typically seen with penetrating trauma or open fractures. If a lower gastrointestinal injury is suspected, endoscopy should be obtained.

Open Fractures. Open pelvic fractures carry a mortality ranging from 25% to 50%. In the acute phase, death is most often due to hemorrhage, whereas sepsis is the cause of death

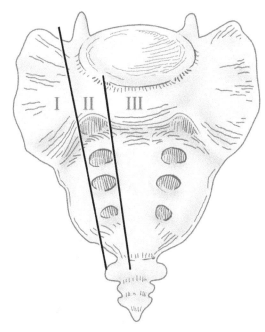

Figure 17–35. Denis classification of sacral fractures. Three zones of injury (I, II, III) exist, with the most medial extension of the fracture fragment used to classify the injury. The more medial the fracture, the higher the incidence of neurologic compromise.

in late cases. High-risk groups include those patients with involvement of the rectum or perineal area. In these patients, a diverting colostomy should be performed early. Rectal involvement is present in one-fourth of patients. One-fourth of women will have an open fracture heralded by a vaginal laceration. Associated injuries are common, with one-third of patients suffering from genitourinary injury. Treatment principles include irrigation and debridement of the open wounds and colostomy when the rectum or perineum are involved. Open pelvic fractures require the early administration of broad-spectrum antibiotics.

Complications

Pelvic fractures may be associated with many long-term complications :

- Chronic SI arthritis presenting as constant low sacral pain may follow SI joint injury.

- Malunion or delayed union.
- Pulmonary and fat emboli (early).
- Sepsis from a ruptured viscus.
- Persistent neurologic deficits, especially following sacral fractures.

ACETABULAR FRACTURES

The acetabulum is divided into four segments—an anterior column and anterior rim (wall) and a posterior column and posterior rim (wall). Fractures of the acetabulum are classified on the basis of their involvement of these structures (Fig. 17–36). The anterior column extends from the iliac crest to the symphysis pubis and includes the anterior rim of the acetabulum. The posterior column starts at the sciatic notch and includes the posterior rim of the acetabulum and ischial tuberosity. The acetabular dome (roof) is

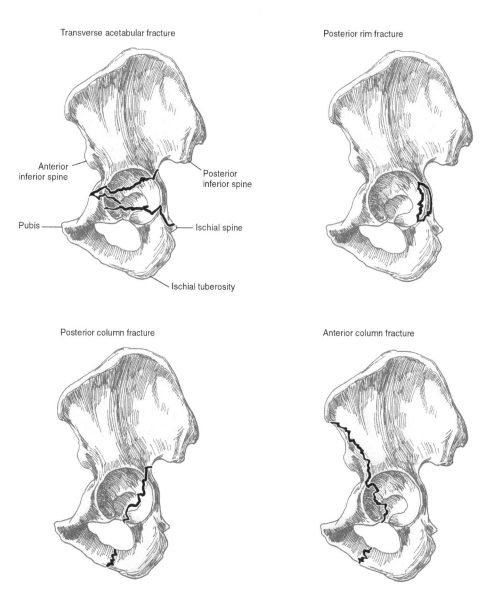

Figure 17–36. Nondisplaced acetabular fractures. Many variant types exist.

the superior weight-bearing area of the acetabulum and includes portions of both the anterior and posterior columns. Transverse fractures of the acetabulum involve portions of the anterior and posterior columns.

The most common fracture pattern involves both columns. Isolated fractures of the posterior column are more common than the anterior column. Posterior rim fractures occur frequently with posterior hip dislocations. Displaced acetabular fractures are referred to as central fracture dislocations when the head of the femur becomes medially displaced into the pelvis (Fig. 17–37).

Acetabular fractures are classified, as described by Letournel and Judet, into simple fracture types and associated fracture types. Simple fracture types include transverse fractures or fractures isolated to a single column or rim. Associated fracture types are more complex and

Acetabular fractures

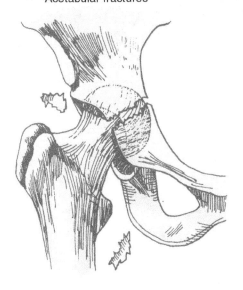

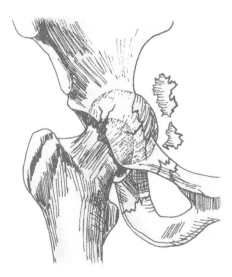

Figure 17–37. Central fracture dislocation.

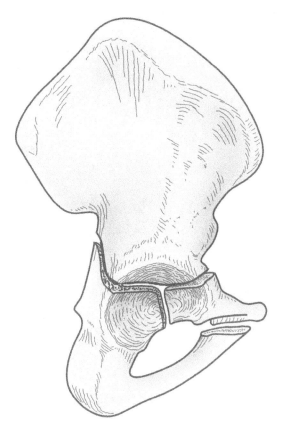

Figure 17–38. T-shaped fracture pattern.

include T- or Y-shaped fractures as well as those fracture patterns that include more than one simple fracture. T-shaped fractures involve both the anterior and posterior columns and have a transverse component (Fig. 17–38). They account for approximately 5% to 10% of acetabular fractures.

Mechanism of Injury

Acetabular fractures are usually the result of high-energy trauma. The most common mechanism of injury is indirect, as with a medially directed blow to the greater trochanter. When this occurs, the femoral head acts as a hammer to fracture the acetabulum. If the femoral head is internally rotated at the time of the injury, a posterior column fracture is produced. Likewise, external rotation of the femoral head causes an anterior column fracture, adduction results in a superior dome fracture, and abduction causes the inferior acetabulum to be injured. This mechanism is commonly seen when a pedestrian is struck by a car.

Another indirect mechanism of injury is by the axial transmission of a force from a blow to the knees transmitted to the femoral head and the acetabulum. This mechanism is encountered frequently in drivers or passengers of cars involved in collisions. The result is often a transverse acetabular fracture or, less commonly, a posterior column fracture.

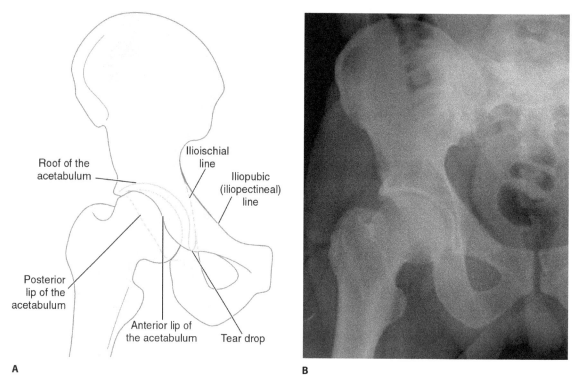

Figure 17–39. AP view of the pelvic acetabulum. These lines should be examined carefully in a patient with suspicion of a fracture. A subtle fracture may displace only one of those lines. *A.* Schematic. *B.* Radiograph.

Examination

The patient will present with pain and tenderness, which increases with attempts at weight bearing. Patients with central acetabular fractures may have ipsilateral leg shortening if associated with displacement or dislocation. Patients with acetabular fractures may have accompanying vascular, visceral, or neurologic injuries. A thorough examination and evaluation for accompanying injuries is strongly recommended.

Imaging

Acetabular fractures may be difficult to detect on the initial AP pelvic radiograph. It is essential that the normal anatomic landmarks surrounding the acetabulum be carefully scrutinized when these injuries are suspected (Fig. 17–39).[40] Disruption of any of these lines suggests a fracture to the corresponding portion of the acetabular bone as follows:

- *Iliopubic (iliopectineal) line.* Fracture of the anterior column.
- *Ilioischial line.* This line represents the medial border of the posterior column with any disruption corresponding to fracture of the posterior column.
- *Posterior lip.* Fracture of the posterior rim. The posterior lip is larger and projects more laterally than the anterior lip.
- *Anterior lip.* This line runs contiguous with the inferior border of the superior pubic rami. Disruption represents fracture of the anterior rim.

- *Teardrop.* This "U"-shaped shadow represents the anterior margin of the acetabular notch. It is contiguous with the ilioischial line, and any separation of these structures represents either rotation of the hemipelvis or a fracture of the posterior column.
- *Roof of the acetabulum.* Fracture of the superior acetabulum.

In some cases, an acetabular fracture will be obvious on the AP radiograph (Fig. 17–40). If an acetabular fracture is suspected, but not evident on AP views of the pelvis or hip, oblique (Judet) views and/or a CT scan should be obtained. The posterior column and the anterior rim are best visualized on a 45-degree external oblique view, whereas the posterior rim and the anterior column are projected best on the 45-degree internal oblique view. Central acetabular fractures are best visualized on a posterior oblique radiograph. Certain pelvic fractures are frequently associated with acetabular fractures that may not be easily visualized radiographically. Eighty percent of intra-articular fragments in the hip joint are not seen on plain film radiography.[14] CT scanning is recommended in all suspected acetabular injuries and has supplanted specialized plain radiographs in most cases. CT scanning, frequently with 3D reconstructions, can be especially helpful in detecting intra-articular bone fragments and for the planning of operative management (Figs. 17–41 and 17–42).

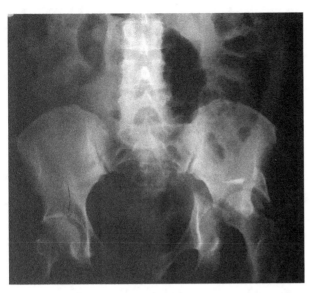

Figure 17–40. Bilateral acetabular fractures. The left acetabulum is severely displaced and disruption of both the iliopubic and ilioischial lines suggests fractures to both the anterior and posterior columns.

Associated Injuries

Acetabular fractures may be associated with the vascular, visceral, and neurologic complications. In addition, acetabular fractures may be associated with fractures of the femur, femoral head, pubic rami, and ipsilateral extremity. Posterior hip dislocations are frequently associated with displaced posterior rim fractures, while anterior hip dislocations are associated with anterior rim fractures. Sciatic nerve injuries occur in 10% to 13% of acetabular fractures.[50]

Treatment

Emergent orthopedic referral is recommended, especially in the setting of a hip dislocation. The emergency management of these fractures includes immobilization of the

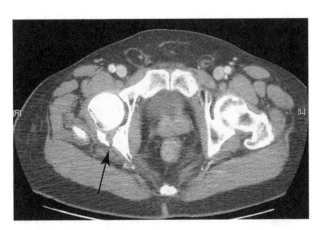

Figure 17–41. CT scan demonstrating a right posterior rim fracture (*arrow*).

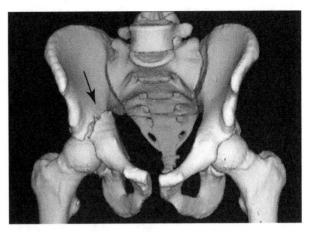

Figure 17–42. Three-dimensional CT reconstruction demonstrating a transverse acetabular fracture (*arrow*).

extremity and a thorough evaluation for accompanying vascular, visceral, or neurologic injuries.

Early normalization of the femoral acetabular relationship is the treatment goal. Surgery is indicated if the femoral head is subluxated out of traction. Open reduction with internal fixation is also recommended for displaced fractures >2 mm.[51] Fractures with impaction of the femoral head are associated with a worse outcome.

Nonoperative treatment of acetabular fractures ranges from traction to full weight-bearing status. For nondisplaced fractures involving the weight-bearing dome, closed treatment with traction to prevent further displacement is required (Fig. 17–43). If the weight-bearing dome is not involved, the patient is allowed to bear weight as tolerated.

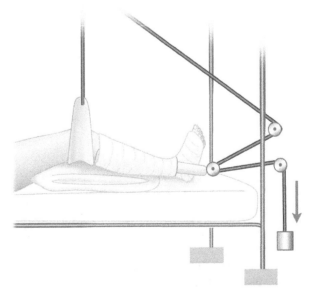

Figure 17–43. Russell traction. The leg is balanced in a suspension apparatus with minimal flexion; 10 to 15 lb of weight will provide good traction.

Complications

The management of acetabular fractures may be complicated by the development of several disorders:

- Osteoarthritis commonly follows even the smallest fractures.
- Traumatic arthritis is commonly noted, especially after displaced central fracture dislocations.
- Avascular necrosis may occur up to a year after the injury. The incidence is dependent on the fracture type and the reduction time. Central acetabular fracture dislocations, which were reduced early, had an avascular necrosis incidence of 15%. If reduction was delayed, there was an incidence of 48%. Other authors report no cases of aseptic necrosis after central acetabular fracture dislocations.
- Sciatic nerve injury may complicate the management of these injuries, especially central displaced fractures.

PELVIC SOFT-TISSUE INJURY

CONTUSIONS

Buttocks

Contusions are a common injury to the buttocks resulting from a direct blow, such as during a fall. The buttocks are protected by a large amount of fatty tissue, and contusion of the gluteus maximus requires a significant force. The patient will complain of pain on sitting and on ambulation, and the examiner will note tenderness to palpation. Other conditions resulting from blunt force to the buttocks include periostitis of the ischial tuberosity, contusion of the ischial tuberosity, and fractures of the tuberosity. These conditions can be differentiated by appropriate x-rays and clinical evaluation. In the patient with periostitis of the ischial tuberosity, the examiner will note exquisite pain over the tuberosity with very little discomfort elsewhere.

The treatment of contusions to the buttocks is symptomatic, with ice packs and rest in a prone position. A pillow or a cushion affords relief from the discomfort until the condition improves. In the patient with periostitis of the ischial tuberosity, injection of the tuberosity with bupivacaine affords good relief. In addition, the patient should be discharged with instructions to use a cushion until the condition clears, as well as appropriate analgesics and ice packs during the first 24 to 48 hours.

Sacrum and the Coccyx

A contusion is a common injury and is due to a direct blow over the sacrum or the coccyx. Owing to the subcutaneous nature of these bones, contusions may be extremely painful, and the patient usually complains of a sharp, localized area of pain that may be quite disabling. On examination, one finds a well-localized area of tenderness over the sacrum or the coccyx with little discomfort elsewhere. Appropriate radiographs should be ordered to exclude fractures.

Although other authors have stated that this condition is not disabling, we have found that it tends to be extremely disabling to the patient. Contusions of the coccyx can lead to a condition called "coccydynia," which has a poor prognosis and for which there is little in the way of adequate treatment. The emergency treatment of contusions of the sacrum and the coccyx includes the early application of cold compresses and the dispensing of a "doughnut" seat and appropriate analgesics, along with referral for follow-up care. Because of the guarded prognosis in contusions of the coccyx, we believe all contusions of this bone should be referred for follow-up care.

Perineum

Contusions of the perineum are uncommon and result from direct blows such as during a fall on a hard object. On examination, the patient will have a painful, ecchymotic, and swollen perineum and may have a painful hematoma. Any patient with a large hematoma in the perineum warrants a urethrogram to exclude urethral injury. The treatment is cold compresses for the first 48 hours followed by warm sitz baths.

Iliac Crest

The most common injury to occur at the iliac crest is a contusion. Contusions of the iliac crest have been called "hip pointers." This diagnosis should not be made without considering an intra-abdominal injury. Periostitis of the iliac crest results from a contusion of the bone and usually poses no problem in diagnosis and treatment. On examination, the patient presents with tenderness localized to any region along the iliac crest from the anterior superior spine to the posterosuperior spine. Treatment of the condition is symptomatic.

SACROILIAC LIGAMENT SPRAIN

This is an uncommon traumatic injury; however, missing its diagnosis in the ED can lead to inappropriate treatment for a herniated disk. The SI articulation, the strongest joint in the body, is rarely injured. When injury does occur, the patient complains of pain localized to the region of the SI joint and referral to the groin and the posterior aspect of the thigh. The mechanism of injury involves wide abduction of the thighs or extremes of hyperextension or hyperflexion.[55,56] The best maneuver to diagnose this condition is to have the patient lie on his/her side and compress downward over the iliac crest. This action compresses the SI joint and will cause pain when there is an SI joint sprain. Alternatively, wide abduction of the supine patient's elevated extended legs will elicit pain over the injured iliosacral or lumbosacral ligaments.

Localized injection of the joint with bupivacaine, analgesics, hot packs, and bed rest are usually all that is needed. If symptoms persist, referral is indicated. For more information about SI joint disease, refer to Chapter 8.

HAMSTRING ATTACHMENT STRAIN

This condition results from forcible flexion of the hip while the knee is extended. In the adolescent, when the epiphysis is not closed, avulsion of the tuberosity with wide separation of the epiphysis can occur. On examination, the patient will present with tenderness over the attachment to the bone with little swelling. A history compatible with the aforementioned mechanism accompanied by pain increased with passive flexion of the hip with the knee extended or active extension of the hip against resistance will help make the diagnosis. X-rays should be obtained to exclude an avulsion fracture.

With incomplete avulsion, treatment consists of splinting the knee in a flexed position to relieve the pressure on the ischial attachment of the tendons. Discharge the patient with crutches for 3 weeks. Active flexion of the thigh should be avoided. In cases where complete avulsion is suspected, the patient should be referred for evaluation of the need for surgical repair.

SCIATIC NERVE COMPRESSION

Sciatica is most commonly believed to be secondary to a herniated nucleus pulposus within the lumbosacral spine. Other causes include posterior facet syndrome, central spinal stenosis, or direct sciatic nerve compression by tumor, aneurysm, or hematoma.[57] This condition is also seen in patients who undergo anesthesia and are recumbent for a prolonged period of time or bedridden. In patients with the piriformis syndrome, trauma to the piriformis muscle results in hematoma formation and subsequent scarring that causes mechanical irritation of the anatomically adjacent sciatic nerve (Fig. 17–44).[58]

Piriformis syndrome accounts for 0.5% to 5% of cases of sciatica.[57] Patients with piriformis syndrome will suffer with the classic symptoms of sciatica, including pain in the buttock and posterior thigh. There is intolerance to sitting and pain with flexion, adduction, and internal rotation of the hip. Tenderness to palpation of the greater sciatic notch is often noted. Functional loss of the piriformis is present, but this does not affect strength because three stronger, short external rotators of the hip exist. The diagnosis of sciatic nerve compression at the level of the piriformis can be confirmed by electrodiagnostic tests.[59]

Conservative therapy includes NSAIDs, physical therapy, ultrasound, or lidocaine injection.[57] Sectioning of the piriformis muscle at its tendinous origin releases the fibrous

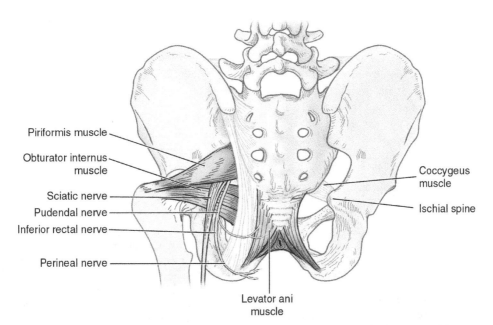

Figure 17–44. Anatomy of the sciatic nerve as it emerges from the posterior pelvis. Note the proximity of the sciatic nerve to the piriformis muscle.

band and is curative if conservative measures fail. Release of the piriformis muscle can be successfully performed through a minimally invasive arthroscopic procedure.

PUDENDAL NERVE PALSY

Pudendal nerve palsy is caused by a compression neuropathy due to forces applied to the perineal region. This is usually a condition that occurs postoperatively following an intramedullary nailing of the femur; however, it can be seen posttraumatically. Numbness of the penis and scrotum, along with erectile dysfunction, are present. The sensory terminal branches of the pudendal nerve are more susceptible to this palsy postoperatively than the motor branches.

GLUTEAL COMPARTMENT SYNDROME

Gluteal compartment syndrome is an extremely rare condition; however, it is one the emergency physician must be aware of because its consequences may be quite serious. The syndrome may result after prolonged immobility, often following drug and alcohol abuse, blunt trauma, or operative positioning. This syndrome has also been reported after bone marrow biopsy and may also be misdiagnosed as deep venous thrombosis.

The gluteal muscles behave as if they were divided into three separate compartments: (1) the tensor fascia lata compartment, (2) the gluteus medius–minimus compartment, and (3) the gluteus maximus compartment. After severe contusions to the buttocks, as would occur during a fall from a height, the patient may present to the ED with tensely swollen buttocks and increasing pain that, over the ensuing 4 to 6 hours, may result in necrosis of the muscles. Patients complain of pain in the buttocks with hip movement, especially in flexion and adduction. In addition, because of the inverse relationship between peripheral nerve conduction block and intracompartmental pressure, the high pressures may cause sciatic neuropathy.

Patients who have a history and examination compatible with this syndrome should be admitted and receive consultation from an orthopedic surgeon. A fasciotomy is performed if the pressure within the compartment is 30 mm Hg or more for a duration of 6 to 8 hours. For further discussion of the compartment syndromes, the reader is referred to Chapter 4.

EXTERNAL OBLIQUE APONEUROSIS RUPTURE

This uncommon condition results from forceful contraction of the abdominal muscles while the trunk is rapidly pushed to the contralateral side. The patient presents with very severe pain over the iliac crest and characteristically

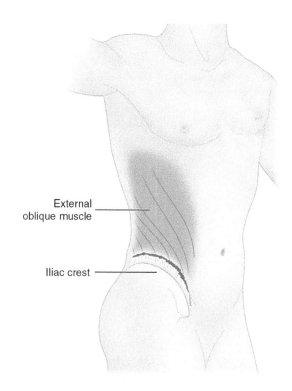

Figure 17–45. Rupture of the external oblique aponeurosis.

walks into the ED in a stooped-over posture from which he/she cannot straighten out due to pain. Examination discloses exquisite tenderness along the entire iliac crest. and in the early stages, one may feel a palpable defect if a large rupture has occurred (Fig. 17–45). In mild cases, only tenderness is noted to palpation. Contraction of the involved muscle elicits significant pain that aids in making the diagnosis and distinguishes it from contusion of the iliac crest. The patient will also complain of pain at the involved iliac crest on flexion to the opposite side.

Treatment for incomplete avulsions of the muscle includes ice for the first 24 to 48 hours, followed by heat, analgesics, and rest. Some physicians have used strapping and taping; however, this has not proved to be entirely beneficial and is not used in the acute stage of this injury. When extensive tears of the aponeurosis exist and a hematoma is present, consultation should be obtained from the orthopedic surgeon.

REFERENCES

1. Peltier LF. Complications associated with fractures of the pelvis. *J Bone Joint Surg Am.* 1965;47:1060–1069.
2. Demetriades D, Karaiskakis M, Toutouzas K, Alo K, Velmahos G, Chan L. Pelvic fractures: epidemiology and predictors of associated abdominal injuries and outcomes. *J Am Coll Surg.* 2002;195(1):1–10.
3. Tile M. Acute pelvic fractures: I. Causation and classification. *J Am Acad Orthop Surg.* 1996;4(3):143–151.

4. Coppola PT, Coppola M. Emergency department evaluation and treatment of pelvic fractures. *Emerg Med Clin North Am.* 2000;18(1):1–27.

5. Poole GV, Ward EF, Muakkassa FF, Hsu HS, Griswold JA, Rhodes RS. Pelvic fracture from major blunt trauma. Outcome is determined by associated injuries. *Ann Surg.* 1991;213(6):532–538.

6. Conolly WB, Hedberg EA. Observations on fractures of the pelvis. *J Trauma.* 1969;9(2):104–111.

7. Cass AS. Bladder trauma in the multiple injured patient. *J Urol.* 1976;115(6):667–669

8. Lowe MA, Mason JT, Luna GK, Maier RV, Copass MK, Berger RE. Risk factors for urethral injuries in men with traumatic pelvic fractures. *J Urol.* 1988;140(3):506–507.

9. Salvino CK, Esposito TJ, Smith D, et al. Routine pelvic x-ray studies in awake blunt trauma patients: a sensible policy? *J Trauma.* 1992;33(3):413–416.

10. Wolinsky PR. Assessment and management of pelvic fracture in the hemodynamically unstable patient. *Orthop Clin North Am.* 1997;28(3):321–329.

11. Fu CY, Wu SC, Chen RJ, et al. Evaluation of pelvic fracture stability and the need for angioembolization: pelvic instabilities on plain film have an increased probability of requiring angioembolization. *Am J Emerg Med.* 2009;27(7):792–796.

12. Paydar S, Ghaffarpasand F, Foroughi M, et al. Role of routing pelvic radiography in initial evaluation of stable, high-energy, blunt trauma patients. *Emerg Med J.* 2012;30(9):724–727.

13. Kricun ME. Fractures of the pelvis. *Orthop Clin North Am.* 1990;21(3):573–590.

14. Resnik CS, Stackhouse DJ, Shanmuganathan K, Young JW. Diagnosis of pelvic fractures in patients with acute pelvic trauma: efficacy of plain radiographs. *AJR Am J Roentgenol.* 1992;158(1):109–112.

15. Sheridan MK, Blackmore CC, Linnau KF, Hoffer EK, Lomoschitz F, Jurkovich GJ. Can CT predict the source of arterial hemorrhage in patients with pelvic fractures? *Emerg Radiol.* 2002;9(4):188–194.

16. Blackmore CC, Jurkovich GJ, Linnau KF, Cummings P, Hoffer EK, Rivara FP. Assessment of volume of hemorrhage and outcome from pelvic fracture. *Arch Surg.* 2003;138(5):504–508.

17. Pereira SJ, O'Brien DP, Luchette FA, et al. Dynamic helical computed tomography scan accurately detects hemorrhage in patients with pelvic fracture. *Surgery.* 2000;128(4):678–685.

18. MacLeod M, Powell JN. Evaluation of pelvic fractures. Clinical and radiologic. *Orthop Clin North Am.* 1997;28(3):299–319.

19. Burgess AR, Eastridge BJ, Young JW, et al. Pelvic ring disruptions: effective classification system and treatment protocols. *J Trauma.* 1990;30(7):848–856.

20. Olson SA, Pollak AN. Assessment of pelvic ring stability after injury. Indications for surgical stabilization. *Clin Orthop.* 1996;(329):15–27.

21. Eastridge BJ, Starr A, Minei JP, O'Keefe GE, Scalea TM. The importance of fracture pattern in guiding therapeutic decision-making in patients with hemorrhagic shock and pelvic ring disruptions. *J Trauma.* 2002;53(3):446–450.

22. Tile M. Pelvic ring fractures: should they be fixed? *J Bone Joint Surg Br.* 1988;70(1):1–12.

23. Eberbach H, Hohloch L, Feucht MJ, Konstantinidis L, Südkamp NP, Zwingmann J. Operative versus conservative treatment of apophyseal avulsion fractures of the pelvis in adolescents: a systematical review with meta-analysis of clinical outcome and return to sports. *BMC Musculoskelet Disord.* 2017;18(1):162. doi:10.1186/s12891-017-1527-z. Published online 2017 Apr 19.

24. Northrop CH, Eto RT, Loop JW. Vertical fracture of the sacral ala. Significance of non-continuity of the anterior superior sacral foraminal line. *Am J Roentgenol Radium Ther Nucl Med.* 1975;124(1):102–106.

25. Newhouse KE, el-Khoury GY, Buckwalter JA. Occult sacral fractures in osteopenic patients. *J Bone Joint Surg Am.* 1992;74(10):1472–1477.

26. Rockwood CA, Green DP, Heckman JD, Bucholz RW, eds. *Rockwood and Green's Fractures in Adults.* 5th ed. Philadelphia, PA: Lippincott Williams & Wilkins; 2001.

27. Denis F, Davis S, Comfort T. Sacral fractures: an important problem. Retrospective analysis of 236 cases. *Clin Orthop.* 1988;227:67–81.

28. Poole GV, Ward EF. Causes of mortality in patients with pelvic fractures. *Orthopedics.* 1994;17(8):691–696.

29. Fox MA, Mangiante EC, Fabian TC, Voeller GR, Kudsk KA. Pelvic fractures: an analysis of factors affecting prehospital triage and patient outcome. *South Med J.* 1990;83(7):785–788.

30. Failinger MS, McGanity PL. Unstable fractures of the pelvic ring. *J Bone Joint Surg Am.* 1992;74(5):781–791.

31. Holstein JH, Culemann U, Pohlemann T, Working Group Mortality in Pelvic Fracture Patients. What are predictors of mortality in patients with pelvic fractures? *Clin Orthop.* 2012;470(8):2090–2097.

32. Hammel J, Legome E. Pelvic fracture. *J Emerg Med.* 2006; 30(1):87–92.

33. Yang AP, Iannacone WM. External fixation for pelvic ring disruptions. *Orthop Clin North Am.* 1997;28(3):331–344.

34. Mirza A, Ellis T. Initial management of pelvic and femoral fractures in the multiply injured patient. *Crit Care Clin.* 2004;20(1):159–170.

35. Tornetta P III, Matta JM. Outcome of operatively treated unstable posterior pelvic ring disruptions. *Clin Orthop.* 1996;(329):186–193.

36. Simonian PT, Routt ML Jr, Harrington RM, et al. Anterior versus posterior provisional fixation in the unstable pelvis. A biomechanical comparison. *Clin Orthop.* 1995;(310):245–251.

37. Heini PF, Witt J, Ganz R. The pelvic C-clamp for the emergency treatment of unstable pelvic ring injuries. A report on clinical experience of 30 cases. *Injury.* 1996;27(suppl 1):S–45.

38. Routt ML Jr, Falicov A, Woodhouse E, Schildhauer TA. Circumferential pelvic antishock sheeting: a temporary resuscitation aid. *J Orthop Trauma.* 2002;16(1):45–48.

39. Miller PR, Moore PS, Mansell E, Meredith JW, Chang MC. External fixation or arteriogram in bleeding pelvic fracture: initial therapy guided by markers of arterial hemorrhage. *J Trauma.* 2003;54(3):437–443.

40. Bassam D, Cephas GA, Ferguson KA, Beard LN, Young JS. A protocol for the initial management of unstable pelvic fractures. *Am Surg.* 1998;64(9):862–867.

41. Cook RE, Keating JF, Gillespie I. The role of angiography in the management of haemorrhage from major fractures of the pelvis. *J Bone Joint Surg Br.* 2002;84(2):178–182.

42. Grimm MR, Vrahas MS, Thomas KA. Pressure-volume characteristics of the intact and disrupted pelvic retroperitoneum. *J Trauma.* 1998;44(3):454–459.

43. Watnik NF, Coburn M, Goldberger M. Urologic injuries in pelvic ring disruptions. *Clin Orthop.* 1996;(329):37–45.

44. Taffet R. Management of pelvic fractures with concomitant urologic injuries. *Orthop Clin North Am.* 1997;28(3):389–396.

45. Clark SS, Prudencio RF. Lower urinary tract injuries associated with pelvic fractures. Diagnosis and management. *Surg Clin North Am.* 1972;52(1):183–201.

46. Reilly MC, Zinar DM, Matta JM. Neurologic injuries in pelvic ring fractures. *Clin Orthop.* 1996;(329):28–36.

47. Hanson PB, Milne JC, Chapman MW. Open fractures of the pelvis. Review of 43 cases. *J Bone Joint Surg Br.* 1991;73(2):325–329.

48. Jones AL, Powell JN, Kellam JF, McCormack RG, Dust W, Wimmer P. Open pelvic fractures. A multicenter retrospective analysis. *Orthop Clin North Am.* 1997;28(3):345–350.

49. Judet R, Judet J, Letournel E. Fractures of the acetabulum: classification and surgical approaches for open reduction. Preliminary report. *J Bone Joint Surg Am.* 1964;46:1615–1646.

50. Oxford CF, Stein A. Complicated crushing injuries of the pelvis. *J Bone Joint Surg Br.* 1967;49(1):24–32.

51. Butler-Manuel PA, James SE, Shepperd JA. Pelvic underpinning: eight years' experience. *J Bone Joint Surg Br.* 1992;74(1):74–77.

52. Gilchrist MR, Peterson DH. Pelvic fracture and associated soft-tissue trauma. *Radiology.* 1967;88(2):278–280.

53. Fanciullo JJ, Bell CL. Stress fractures of the sacrum and lower extremity. *Curr Opin Rheumatol.* 1996;8(2):158–162.

54. Paletta GA Jr, Andrish JT. Injuries about the hip and pelvis in the young athlete. *Clin Sports Med.* 1995;14(3):591–628.

55. Segal NA, Felson DT, Torner JC, et al. Greater trochanteric pain syndrome: epidemiology and associated factors. *Arch Phys Med Rehabil.* 2007;88(8):988–992.

56. DeAngelis NA, Busconi BD. Assessment and differential diagnosis of the painful hip. *Clin Orthop.* 2003;(406):11–18.

57. Parziale JR, Hudgins TH, Fishman LM. The piriformis syndrome. *Am J Orthop.* 1996;25(12):819–823.

58. Benson ER, Schutzer SF. Posttraumatic piriformis syndrome: diagnosis and results of operative treatment. *J Bone Joint Surg Am.* 1999;81(7):941–949.

59. Hughes SS, Goldstein MN, Hicks DG, Pellegrini VD Jr. Extrapelvic compression of the sciatic nerve. An unusual cause of pain about the hip: report of five cases. *J Bone Joint Surg Am.* 1992;74(10):1553–1559.

60. Dezawa A, Kusano S, Miki H. Arthroscopic release of the piriformis muscle under local anesthesia for piriformis syndrome. *Arthroscopy.* 2003;19(5):554–557.

61. Brumback RJ, Ellison TS, Molligan H, Pellegrini VD Jr. Pudendal nerve palsy complicating intramedullary nailing of the femur. *J Bone Joint Surg Am.* 1992;74(10):1450–1455.

62. Owen CA, Woody PR, Mubarak SJ, Hargens AR. Gluteal compartment syndromes: a report of three cases and management utilizing the Wick catheter. *Clin Orthop.* 1978;(132):57–60.

63. Krysa J, Lofthouse R, Kavanagh G. Gluteal compartment syndrome following posterior cruciate ligament repair. *Injury.* 2002;33(9):835–838.

64. Klockgether T, Weller M, Haarmeier T, Kaskas B, Maier G, Dichgans J. Gluteal compartment syndrome due to rhabdomyolysis after heroin abuse. *Neurology.* 1997;48(1):275–276.

65. Bleicher RJ, Sherman HF, Latenser BA. Bilateral gluteal compartment syndrome. *J Trauma.* 1997;42(1):118–122.

66. Roth JS, Newman EC. Gluteal compartment syndrome and sciatica after bone marrow biopsy: a case report and review of the literature. *Am Surg.* 2002;68(9):791–794.

67. Chua HC, Lim T, Lee HC, Lee SW. Gluteal compartment syndrome misdiagnosed as deep vein thrombosis. *Int J Clin Pract.* 2003;57(7):633–634.

68. Kumar V, Saeed K, Panagopoulos A, Parker PJ. Gluteal compartment syndrome following joint arthroplasty under epidural anaesthesia: a report of 4 cases. *J Orthop Surg (Hong Kong).* 2007;15(1):113–117.

69. Heyn J, Ladurner R, Ozimek A, Vogel T, Hallfeldt KK, Mussack T. Gluteal compartment syndrome after prostatectomy caused by incorrect positioning. *Eur J Med Res.* 2006;11(4):170–173.

70. Ryan JB, Wheeler JH, Hopkinson WJ, Arciero RA, Kolakowski KR. Quadriceps contusions. West Point update. *Am J Sports Med.* 1991;19(3):299–304.

71. Schmalzried TP, Neal WC, Eckardt JJ. Gluteal compartment and crush syndromes. Report of three cases and review of the literature. *Clin Orthop.* 1992;(277):161–165.

CHAPTER 18

Hip

Gregory W. Hendey, MD

INTRODUCTION

The hip joint is a ball-and-socket joint composed of the head of the femur and the acetabulum. This articulation has many palpable bony landmarks. The proximal femur consists of a femoral head and neck as well as a greater and lesser trochanter (Fig. 18–1). The anterosuperior iliac spine and the greater trochanter are easily palpated laterally, and the pubic symphysis lies medially. The hip joint is capable of a very wide range of motion.

The joint is enclosed in a capsule that has attachments to the rim of the acetabulum and the femoral neck. Three ligaments are formed by capsular thickenings: the *iliofemoral ligament*, which is located anteriorly; the *pubofemoral ligament*, which is located inferiorly; and the *ischiofemoral ligament*, which is located posteriorly. Additional support is provided by the *labrum acetabulare*, a thick band of cartilage surrounding and extending out from the acetabulum and adding depth to the cavity. A flat, thin-shaped ligament, the *ligamentum teres*, attaches the head of the femur to the acetabulum centrally.

The muscles surrounding the hip joint are large and powerful. They can be divided into three main groups—anterior, medial, and posterior. The anterior muscles include the iliopsoas, tensor fasciae latae, sartorius, and quadriceps femoris. Muscles within the medial compartment adduct the thigh and include the pectineus; gracilis; obturator externus; and adductor magnus, brevis, and longus. Posterior muscles extend the hip and include the semitendinosus, semimembranosus, and biceps femoris.

It is essential that one clearly understands the precarious vascular supply to the proximal femur. The vascular anatomy consists of three main sources, listed in order of importance (Fig. 18–2).

1. Femoral circumflex and retinacular arteries
2. Medullary vasculature
3. Vessel of the ligamentum teres

The femoral circumflex arteries surround the base of the femoral neck and give rise to retinacular arteries that ascend up to supply the femoral head. Disruption of the retinacular blood vessels results in avascular necrosis (AVN) of the femoral head in 84% of cases.[1] In occult, nondisplaced fractures of the femoral neck, the retinacular

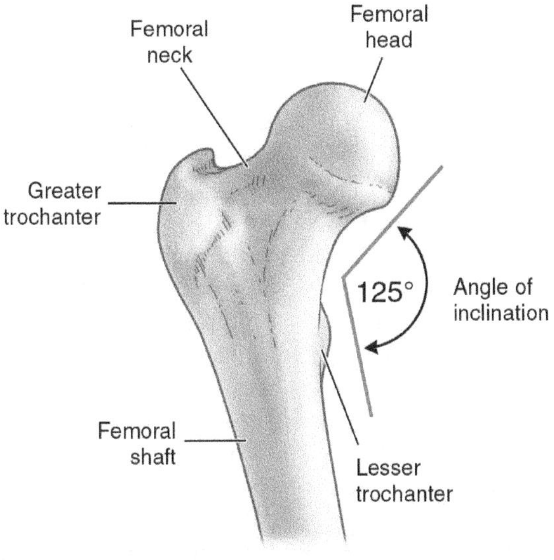

Figure 18–1. The neck-shaft angle should be evaluated in all suspected fractures. Normal angle is 120 to 130 degrees.

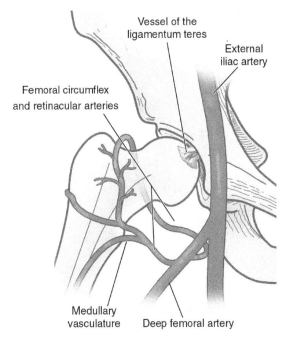

Figure 18–2. The vascular ring around the base of the femoral neck sends intracapsular vessels (retinacular vessels) important in maintaining perfusion to the femoral head.

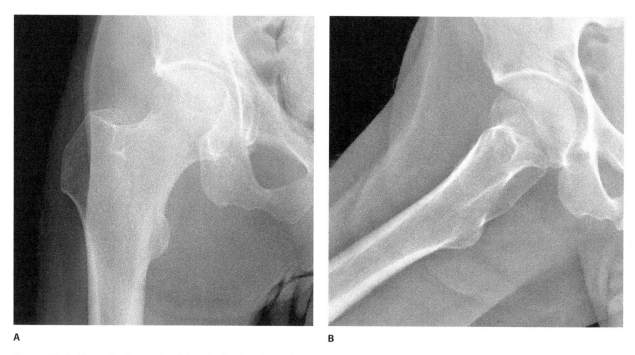

A   **B**

Figure 18–3. Normal radiographs of the hip. **A.** AP radiograph. **B.** External rotational view (i.e., rolled or frog-leg lateral).

vessels are not disrupted, and early diagnosis should prevent complications.

Imaging

Routine radiographs including anteroposterior (AP) and external rotational views (i.e., rolled or frog-leg lateral) are adequate in most cases (Fig. 18–3). A cross-table, lateral view is obtained in a patient with a suspected fracture in place of the external rotational view. This radiograph should be taken perpendicular to the long axis of the femoral neck (Fig. 18–4). Comparison views of the

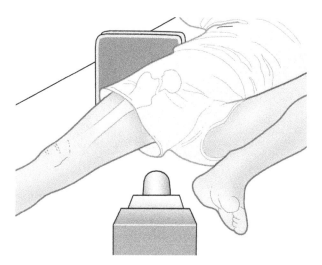

Figure 18–4. A cross-table lateral view of the hip.

hip are often helpful in diagnosing occult fractures, especially in the setting of compression fractures (Fig. 18–5). *Shenton line* should be carefully scrutinized in all patients with a suspected hip injury (Fig. 18–6). In addition, the normal *neck-shaft angle of 120 to 130 degrees* should be evaluated in all suspected fractures. This is obtained by measuring the angle of the intersection of lines drawn down the axis of the femoral shaft and the femoral neck (Fig. 18–1).

Occult Fractures

Occult fractures in elderly osteoporotic patients with hip pain after trauma occur commonly at the femoral neck, intertrochanteric region, or pelvis. Missing an occult femoral neck fracture may result in subsequent displacement, vascular disruption, and eventually AVN. Occult hip fractures are present in 4% to 10% of patients with trauma, hip pain, and negative initial radiographs. Low-energy trauma such as a fall from standing is a common mechanism. Although the clinical examination is useful, some patients with an occult hip fracture are able to bear weight (with pain) and complete examinations such as straight-leg raise, passive rotation, or axial loading.

When the plain films are equivocal in a patient suspected of a hip fracture, magnetic resonance imaging (MRI) is the diagnostic study of choice with a sensitivity and specificity of 100%. MRI will detect fractures as early as 4 to 6 hours following the injury. In patients older than 70 years, MRI is more likely to be positive

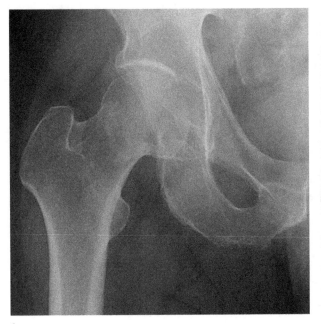
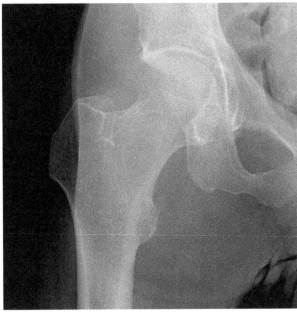

A   **B**

Figure 18–5. *A.* Compression fracture of the femoral neck. Note the hyperdensity and loss of the trabecular pattern of the bone. ***B.*** Normal trabecular appearance of the femoral neck (for comparison).

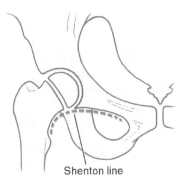

Shenton line

Figure 18–6. Shenton line extends from the inferior border of the femoral neck to the inferior border of the pubic ramus. Interruption of this line suggests a femoral neck fracture.

and require surgical repair. MRI also has the advantage of detecting other pathology not initially detected. In one study, MRI detected pathology in 83% of cases, 23% requiring operative repair. A limited MRI of the hip region only takes approximately 15 minutes. The argument for the cost effectiveness of MRI in this setting is related to avoidance of longer hospitalizations and expensive complications.

Other imaging techniques such as computed tomography (CT) and bone scanning are less sensitive than MRI. CT detects the majority of occult fractures but may miss nondisplaced fractures in osteoporotic trabecular bone. In two studies, CT missed fractures detected by MRI.

HIP FRACTURES

Proximal femur and hip fractures are classified on the basis of anatomy. Intracapsular fractures include fractures of the femoral head and neck. Extracapsular fractures include intertrochanteric, trochanteric, and subtrochanteric fractures.

FEMORAL HEAD FRACTURES

These are uncommon fractures that may present with dislocation or without any significant deformity. Femoral head

fractures are classified into *single* fragment and *comminuted* fractures (Fig. 18–7).

Mechanism of Injury

Fractures with a single fragment are caused by sheer forces that often occur during a dislocation. Anterior dislocations are associated with superior fractures, whereas posterior dislocations are associated with inferior fractures. Comminuted fractures are usually the result of direct trauma and may be associated with severe injuries.

Single fragment

Comminuted

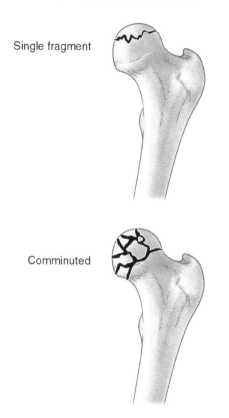

Figure 18–7. Femoral head fractures.

Examination

The patient presents with pain on palpation and rotation. A contusion is often present over the lateral aspect of the thigh, but gross bony deformities are uncommon unless there is an associated dislocation.

Imaging

Routine hip views are usually adequate in demonstrating these fractures. CT or MRI is recommended when plain films are inconclusive.

Associated Injuries

Comminuted fractures may be associated with pelvic or ipsilateral upper-extremity fractures. Posterior fracture dislocations are associated with sciatic nerve injuries, pelvic fractures, and ipsilateral lower-extremity injuries. Anterior fracture dislocations may be associated with arterial injury or venous thrombosis.

Treatment

Single Fragment. The emergency management of these fractures includes immobilization, analgesics, and admission. If associated with a dislocation, reduction followed by immobilization is indicated. Small fragments or superior dome fragments may require operative removal or arthroplasty.

Comminuted. The emergency management of these injuries includes immobilization, analgesics, stabilization of

associated injuries, and admission for arthroplasty as most will undergo AVN if treated conservatively.

FEMORAL NECK FRACTURES

Femoral neck fractures, also referred to as subcaptial fractures, are common. They typically occur in the elderly patient with osteoporosis with a female-to-male ratio of 4:1.[5,13] Femoral neck fractures are rarely seen in young patients unless they are associated with a high-energy mechanism. If this injury is diagnosed in a young patient after minor trauma, a pathologic fracture should be suspected.

Femoral neck fractures may result in long-term disability secondary to disruption of the blood supply, leading to femoral head AVN.

Many systems have been used in the classification of femoral neck fractures based on anatomy and therapeutic results. Garden classifies femoral neck fractures by the degree of displacement on the AP radiograph into four types :

Type I	Incomplete or impacted fractures
Type II	Complete, but nondisplaced
Type III	Partially displaced or angulated fractures
Type IV	Displaced fractures with no contact between the fragments[13]

Because treatment and prognosis are so similar for Garden types I and II (nondisplaced) and Garden types III and IV (displaced), these fractures are often grouped together.[5,13] The classification system used in this text, therefore, defines femoral neck fractures as *nondisplaced* and *displaced* (Fig. 18–8).

Mechanism of Injury

Direct minor trauma, such as a ground-level fall in the elderly, may result in a femoral neck fracture. However, indirect trauma is also a common mechanism in the elderly with osteoporotic bone. Femoral neck stress in combination with a torsion injury may result in a stress, impacted, or partially displaced fracture. The patient then falls, adding displacement or comminution to the injury. Stress fractures are usually initiated along the superior border of the femoral neck.

Examination

Patients with a stress or impacted fracture present with a complaint of minor groin pain or medial thigh or knee pain that is exacerbated with active or passive motion. There may be no history of trauma, and the patient may be ambulatory. There is usually no leg shortening or external rotation, thus making the diagnosis difficult on the basis of examination.

Displaced fractures usually present with severe pain, along with the classic finding of leg shortening and external rotation (Fig. 18–9A).

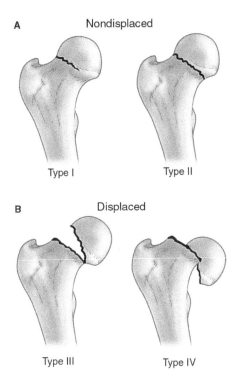

Figure 18–8. Femoral neck fractures.

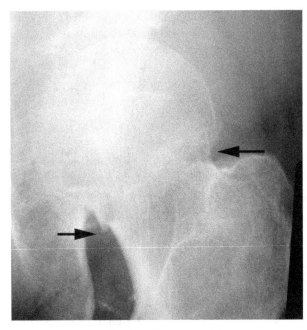

Figure 18–10. A nondisplaced femoral neck fracture.

Imaging

Displaced femoral neck fractures are usually well visualized on the AP and lateral views (Fig. 18–9B). However, nondisplaced fractures may be difficult to visualize radiographically during the acute stage (Fig. 18–10). A distortion of the normal trabecular pattern or a cortical defect may be the only clues to an underlying fracture. An AP view with the lower extremity internally rotated 15 degrees, permitting visualization of the entire femoral neck, is helpful.[15]

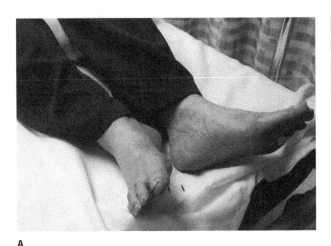

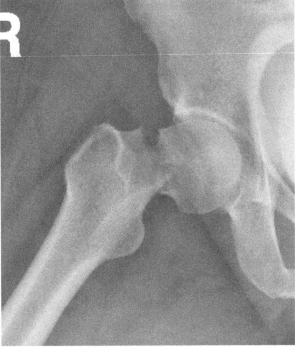

Figure 18–9. Displaced femoral neck fracture on the patient's right. *A.* The leg is shortened and externally rotated. *B.* Radiographic appearance.

Patients with a suspected fracture but normal plain films should undergo CT or MRI. MRI is the gold standard for detecting occult femoral neck fractures.

Associated Injuries

These fractures are usually not associated with other significant injuries.

Treatment

Femoral neck fractures are very painful, and one of the primary responsibilities of the emergency physician is to provide adequate relief. This can be accomplished by intravenous narcotic analgesics or with a femoral nerve block. The technique for blocking this nerve is described in Chapter 2. In addition, the patient will be most comfortable with a pillow placed under the knee to support a mild degree of hip flexion, but traction is not helpful.

Nonoperative management of femoral neck fractures is rarely employed. Surgical fixation is more cost effective and has a lower rate of complications. Operative management is used with nearly all patients, except with those who have significant comorbid illness that precludes surgery or with those who are chronically non-ambulatory.

Nondisplaced. The emergency management of these fractures includes immobilization, analgesics, and emergent orthopedic consultation. Historically, these fractures were treated with bed rest followed by prolonged nonweight-bearing status. Results for nonoperative management are not as good as operative intervention; therefore, repair is the treatment method of choice. Without fixation, 10% to 30% of these fractures will become displaced. Immediate repair also avoids the possibility of future displacement with its deleterious consequences.

The operative method depends on a variety of factors, including the treating orthopedist. The most common surgical repair involves fixation, with the placement of cannulated screws through the lateral aspect of the femur into the femoral head, thus stabilizing the fracture line. Some authors recommend hemiarthroplasty in patients older than 80 because of a lower rate of reoperation.

Displaced. The emergency management of these fractures includes immobilization, analgesics, and emergent orthopedic consultation.

The influence of delay in surgery is controversial, but many consider these fractures an orthopedic emergency because of an increased risk of AVN of the femoral head. Left untreated, 40% will undergo AVN 48 hours post injury, whereas 100% undergo AVN after 1 week.

The definitive treatment of these fractures depends on the patient's age and activity level. In young patients, closed or open reduction and internal fixation with cannulated screws is standard treatment because

it preserves the patient's femoral head. Disadvantages include a higher rate of AVN, nonunion, and reoperation. Hemiarthroplasty is favored in geriatric patients who have less physical demands, as well as patients who present with a delay in diagnosis (>1 week), pathologic fracture, or hip arthritis. Some authors favor total hip replacement over hemiarthroplasty in the elderly population.

Regardless of the operative technique, it remains clear that patients fair better with surgery. There is a 10% mortality rate for those patients treated with internal fixation and a 60% rate for those treated with bed rest. In the elderly, the mortality rate is especially high even after surgery. Within 1 month of injury, death occurs in 21% of women and 37% of men older than 84.

Complications

Femoral neck fractures are associated with several significant complications:

- AVN of the femoral head (up to 35% of patients 3 years after fracture)
- Osteoarthritis
- Operative complications (e.g., osteomyelitis, nail protrusion)
- Nonunion (<5%)

INTERTROCHANTERIC FRACTURES

These fractures represent almost half of all fractures of the proximal femur. Intertrochanteric fractures are extracapsular and involve the cancellous bone between the greater and lesser trochanters. Like femoral neck fractures, they are usually seen in elderly patients with a female-to-male ratio of 4:1 to 6:1. The vascular supply to this region is very good, owing to the large amount of surrounding musculature and the presence of cancellous bone. The internal rotators of the hip remain attached to the proximal fragment, whereas the short external rotators remain attached to the distal segment.

The emergency physician should classify these injuries as stable or unstable (Fig. 18–11). One-half of

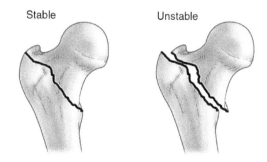

Figure 18–11. Intertrochanteric fractures.

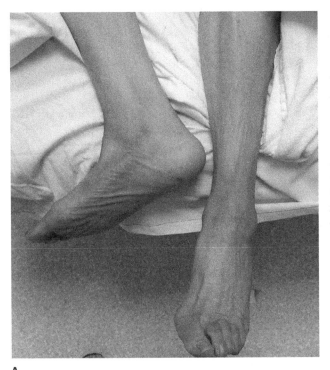
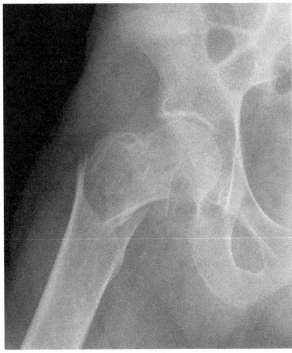

Figure 18–12. An unstable intertrochanteric femur fracture. ***A.*** The leg is externally rotated and shortened. ***B.*** Radiographic appearance.

intertrochanteric fractures are considered unstable.[20] Both classifications of intertrochanteric fractures are described as follows:

- *Stable intertrochanteric fractures.* A single fracture line transects the cortex between the two trochanters, and there is no displacement between the femoral shaft and neck.
- *Unstable intertrochanteric fractures.* There are multiple fracture lines or comminution with associated displacement between the femoral shaft and neck. The fracture line may extend to the subtrochanteric bone or may run in a "reverse oblique direction." An intertrochanteric fracture that runs in a reverse oblique direction has its most superior portion on the medial surface of the femur.

Mechanism of Injury

The majority of these fractures are secondary to direct trauma, such as a fall on the greater trochanter, or transmission of forces along the long axis of the femur. With increasing forces, the greater or lesser trochanters may themselves become fractured. The muscles inserting on the trochanters act to further displace the fragments.

Examination

The patient will present with tenderness, swelling, and ecchymosis over the hip. There is usually significant leg shortening with external rotation secondary to traction by the iliopsoas muscle (Fig. 18–12A).

Imaging

AP and cross-table lateral views are usually adequate in demonstrating these fractures (Figs. 18–12B and 18–13). In a similar manner to femoral neck fractures, the diagnosis of nondisplaced intertrochanteric fractures may be more

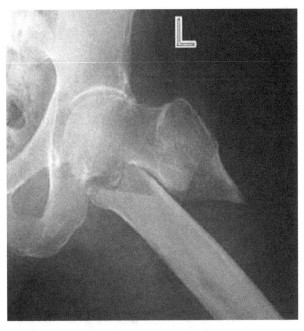

Figure 18–13. Intertrochanteric fracture. Note that the fracture line runs in a reverse oblique direction and into the subtrochanteric bone, making this fracture unstable.

difficult, and occasionally requires advanced radiographic techniques (i.e., MRI, CT).

Associated Injuries

Intertrochanteric fractures may be associated with a significant amount of blood loss secondary to injury of the well-vascularized cancellous bone. Up to three units of blood may be lost after these fractures.

Treatment

The emergency management of these fractures includes immobilization and analgesics. Intravenous narcotics or a femoral nerve block should be administered (see Chapter 2). Skin traction with a 5-lb weight has not demonstrated any benefit and is therefore not recommended.

Definitive treatment is based on the patient's medical condition, bone quality (i.e., osteoarthritis or osteoporosis), and fracture configuration. Surgical fixation is indicated in all patients who are medically stable. Both stable and unstable fractures are treated surgically with internal fixation using a compression hip screw and side plate. Stable fractures can also be treated with intramedullary devices. Early mobilization can be achieved after operative intervention. Patients with a high surgical risk have been successfully treated with external fixation.

Complications

Intertrochanteric fractures are associated with several significant complications:

* Thromboembolism
* Postoperative complications (e.g., osteomyelitis in 5%–8%, nail protrusion)

The mortality rate for these fractures is 10% to 15%. Unlike femoral neck fractures, AVN and nonunion are rarely seen after these injuries, owing to the abundant blood supply.

TROCHANTERIC FRACTURES

Trochanteric fractures are uncommon injuries, usually seen in young patients (Fig. 18-14).

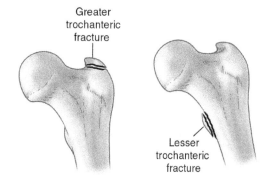

Greater trochanteric fracture

Lesser trochanteric fracture

Figure 18-14. Trochanteric fractures.

Mechanism of Injury

Greater trochanteric fractures are usually secondary to direct trauma as, for example, a fall. A minority of these fractures may be the result of an avulsion injury.

Lesser trochanteric fractures are secondary to avulsion from a forceful contraction of the iliopsoas muscle. They may occur after minimal trauma. Lesser trochanteric fractures are often pathologic in nature.

Examination

Greater trochanteric fractures usually present with pain and tenderness exacerbated with active abduction of the thigh. Lesser trochanteric fractures typically present with pain and tenderness that increase with flexion and rotation of the hip.

Imaging

AP and lateral views are generally adequate in demonstrating this fracture (Fig. 18-15). Internal and external rotation views may be necessary to accurately determine displacement. Nondisplaced fractures may be subtle, and occasionally CT or MRI is necessary to visualize the fracture.

Associated Injuries

There may be significant blood loss at the fracture site. Lesser trochanteric fractures in elderly patients are frequently pathologic and require an appropriate workup as such.

Treatment

Nondisplaced. These fractures are managed symptomatically with ambulation assisted by crutch walking for 3 to 4 weeks. This will decrease the displacing forces on the fragment. Limited weight bearing should be continued until the patient is pain-free. Orthopedic referral for follow-up is recommended.

Displaced. Young patients with greater trochanteric fractures with 1 cm of displacement or lesser trochanteric fractures with 2 cm of displacement require internal fixation. Elderly patients with displaced fractures may be managed symptomatically. In these patients, muscle function returns due to osseous or fibrous union despite the displacement of the fracture fragment.

Complications

The loss of associated muscle function secondary to atrophy is a long-term complication of these fractures.

SUBTROCHANTERIC FRACTURES

Subtrochanteric fractures include those injuries within 5 cm of the lesser trochanter (Fig. 18-16). These fractures usually occur in younger patients and are the result of severe injury forces. The fractures may be spiral, comminuted, displaced, or occur as an extension of an intertrochanteric fracture.

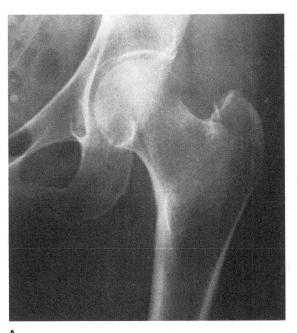

A

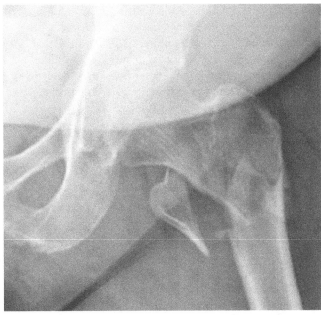

B

Figure 18–15. ***A.*** Greater trochanter fracture without displacement. ***B.*** Lesser trochanter fracture (and subtrochanteric fracture).

Multiple classification systems have been proposed for these fractures. None are universally accepted, however, and they do not impact the emergency management of these fractures.

Mechanism of Injury
In the elderly, the most common mechanism is a fall with a combination of direct and rotational forces. In younger patients, these fractures are more often the result of high-energy trauma.

Examination
The patient will present with pain and swelling in the hip and upper thigh. Deformity may be present if the fracture is displaced. In the setting of a high-energy mechanism, ipsilateral knee injuries or lower-extremity fractures may be seen.

Imaging
The majority of these fractures are diagnosed with plain radiographs only (Fig. 18–17). CT scan may be useful to the surgeon to fully define the operative therapy.

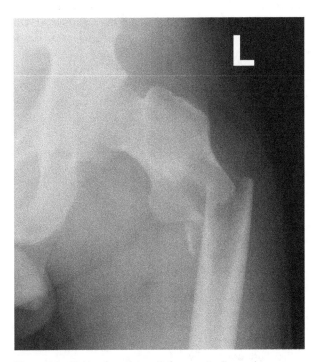

Figure 18–17. A subtrochanteric fracture (radiographic appearance).

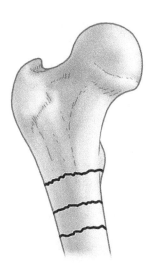

Figure 18–16. Subtrochanteric fractures.

Treatment

The emergency management of these fractures includes immobilization in a Sager splint (see Chapter 1), ice, analgesics, intravenous fluids to correct volume loss, and admission for open reduction and internal fixation. Severely comminuted fractures are best treated with traction, although this treatment is used sparingly.

Complications

Several significant complications are associated with these fractures:

- Venous thromboembolism
- Malunion or nonunion
- Postsurgical complications (e.g., osteomyelitis, mechanical failure of the nail or screw)

HIP SOFT-TISSUE INJURY AND DISLOCATION

AVASCULAR NECROSIS OF THE FEMORAL HEAD

AVN of the femoral head is a result of impaired blood supply, a common complication of many disorders of the hip from infancy to adulthood. In the United States, 10,000 to 20,000 new cases present annually. AVN occurs most often in men between 40 and 50 years of age and is bilateral in 40% to 80% of patients. The chief blood supply to the head comes from branches of the medial and lateral circumflex arteries that enter the capsule distally and pass along the posterior surface of the head. The infarction of the femoral head may be total or incomplete. If incomplete, it is limited to one segment of the femoral head, and the radiographic appearance will be spotty.

Any condition that disrupts the blood supply to the femoral head can cause this disorder (Table 18–1). Trauma to the major blood vessels is the most common cause. Femoral neck fractures that disrupt the retinacular vessels cause AVN. The incidence of AVN after femoral neck fractures is 20% to 30%. AVN is more likely to develop with proximal fractures and those fractures that are improperly reduced, thus permitting greater shearing stresses to occur at the fracture site.

AVN is also commonly seen after hip dislocation at a rate of up to 40%. The pathogenesis is believed to be an ischemic insult to the head while it remains dislocated.

▶ TABLE 18–1. **CONDITIONS ASSOCIATED WITH AVASCULAR NECROSIS OF THE FEMORAL HEAD**

Traumatic
  Femoral neck fracture
  Hip dislocation
Nontraumatic
  Sickle cell disease
  Collagen vascular diseases
  Alcohol abuse
  Exogenous steroid administration
  Cushing disease
  Decompression sickness
  Gaucher disease
  Renal osteodystrophy
  Idiopathic

Reduction results in reperfusion, stressing the importance of early detection and treatment of this condition. In the setting of dislocation, AVN usually becomes clinically apparent within 2 years.

Atraumatic conditions associated with AVN are numerous. Steroid use and alcohol ingestion are associated in as many as 90% of atraumatic cases. Corticosteroid-induced AVN may be either from exogenous administration (common) or Cushing disease (rare). AVN can complicate sickle cell disease due to the impaired circulation of the small vessels that supply the femoral head. Collagen vascular disorders, such as systemic lupus erythematosus and small vessel vasculitis, may also precipitate AVN of the femoral head. Other associated conditions include decompression sickness (Caisson disease), Gaucher disease, and renal osteodystrophy. In 10% to 20% of cases, despite thorough investigation, the cause remains idiopathic.

The articular cartilage covering the necrotic head survives usually because it derives its nutrition from the synovial fluid. If subcondylar bone cortex collapses, the cartilage then undergoes degeneration. The added stress of weight bearing, before bony replacement is complete, can cause collapse and severe degenerative changes.

Clinical Presentation

AVN can be clinically silent, but the most common complaint is pain. The pain is localized to the groin area but may be felt in the buttock or refer to the knee. The onset may be insidious or sudden. On examination, the patient will walk with a limp. Joint motion is decreased and painful. Passive internal rotation will be severely limited. Abduction will also be limited.

The clinical picture will vary, however, depending on the underlying cause and the patient's age. The onset of symptoms does not correlate well with the appearance on radiographs. It is not the death of bone cells that causes hip pain, but rather the collapse and fracture of subchondral bone that heralds the onset of clinical symptoms.

In a child, spasm around the hip appears to be an early sign. A limp or a slight spasm of the hip is often the first clinical manifestation of this disorder. It is followed by pain that is present on weight bearing and often referred to the thigh or knee. A high index of suspicion is needed in the absence of radiographic findings.[46]

Imaging

Radiographs should include AP and "frog-leg" (flexed and externally rotated) lateral views. Multiple systems have been developed for the radiographic classification of AVN of the femoral head. One common system is the Arlet–Ficat staging system that organizes the radiographic appearance into four stages (Fig. 18–18).[35]

Stage	Radiographic Appearance
I	Normal plain radiographs
II	Increased density in femoral head, cystic changes
III	Crescent sign, irregular femoral head
IV	Severe deformity, degenerative changes, collapse

The crescent sign is a curvilinear radiolucent subchondral line along the anterolateral aspect of the proximal femoral head. It is most commonly present on the frog-leg lateral view but may be detected on CT scan.[47]

Early diagnosis of stage I disease can only be established by MRI or bone scan.[19,48,49] Bone scan may show an area of low-uptake representative of the necrotic bone surrounded by an area of increased uptake that corresponds to rapid bone turnover. MRI is highly sensitive for the diagnosis (88%–100% sensitive) and is considered the imaging study of choice for early detection.[35]

Treatment

The emergency physician should keep the patient from bearing weight as pressure may cause the necrotic head to collapse.

The definitive treatment for this condition depends on which stage the AVN has reached. In stage I and early stage II, core decompression is the recommended procedure.[35,44] This involves removing an 8- to 10-mm core of bone from the anterolateral segment of the femoral head through a lateral trochanteric approach. This procedure is highly effective in relieving pain, prevents further changes in the femoral head, and delays the need for total hip arthroplasty.

In the later stages, when collapse and deformation of the femoral head have occurred, reconstruction is necessary. Stage III and stage IV disease require a total hip arthroplasty.[35,50] In young patients, some authors have placed a vascularized fibular graft in the subchondral region of the femoral head that delays the need for hip replacement.[51,52]

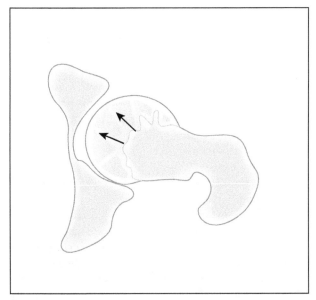

A

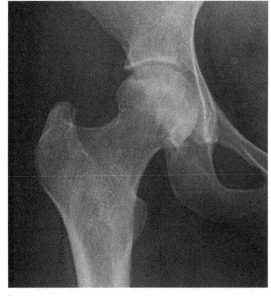

B

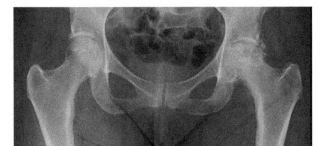

C

Figure 18–18. Avascular necrosis (AVN). **A.** Schematic representation demonstrating subchondral bone collapse, the crescent sign (*arrows*). **B.** Radiograph demonstrating subchondral sclerosis with bone collapse (stage III). **C.** Further joint space narrowing and collapse of the head, heralding stage IV AVN.

SEPTIC ARTHRITIS

Septic arthritis of the hip may occur within the native joint or following hip arthroplasty. When the native joint is affected, 70% of cases occur in patients 4 years of age or younger. The younger the child affected by septic arthritis of the hip, the worse the prognosis.

In children, the infection usually reaches the hip joint from a focus of osteomyelitis within the joint capsule. The osteomyelitis is usually of hematogenous origin and arises in the metaphysis by way of nutrient vessels. From there, it may spread outward and develop as a subperiosteal abscess. The articular cartilage is damaged by the increased intra-articular pressures resulting from the pus produced by the infection. It can withstand these forces for approximately 4 to 5 days before destructive changes occur.

Infection of the native joint is rare in adult patients. In one study of 4 hospitals, only 10 cases occurred over a 10-year period. The majority of cases occur in immuno-compromised patients (including diabetes), in an already diseased hip, following instrumentation, or from contiguous spread of infection. Nonetheless, native joint septic hip arthritis can occur in the absence of these risk factors. In adult patients who undergo total hip arthroplasty, however, the risk of infection is approximately 1%. The increasing number of elderly patients undergoing this procedure makes it likely that the emergency physician will encounter such a patient.

Staphylococcus aureus (*S aureus*) is the most prevalent organism in septic arthritis of the native hip. Methicillin-resistant *S aureus* (MRSA) is common. Adult cases involving prosthetic replacement are caused by gram-positive bacteria in 75% of cases, with the most common bacterium being *Staphylococcus epidermidis* (30%) and *S aureus* (20%). Of gram-negative organisms, *Pseudomonas aeruginosa* is the most common pathogen. Anaerobes, fungi, and mycobacterium may also be involved.

Clinical Presentation

Characteristically, the patient presents to the emergency department (ED) with a fever and severe pain in the affected hip. The onset of symptoms is usually acute, although in patients with underlying rheumatoid arthritis, the onset can be insidious, frequently without fever. In these patients, the diagnosis may be difficult, and the patients may be believed to have an arthritic flare rather than septic arthritis.

On examination, the patient has tenderness anteriorly in the groin and over the hip joint accompanied by grossly restricted motion in all directions and muscle spasm. The patient walks with a limp or does not walk at all. These patients usually do not want any pressure placed on the lower extremity and avoid any movement due to severe pain.

In children, septic arthritis may be confused with transient synovitis. Septic hip is more likely if four of the following are noted: (1) temperature >38.3°C; (2) pain localized to the hip that is worse with gentle passive motion; (3) swelling of the involved joint; (4) systemic symptoms of lethargy, irritability, or toxicity, with no other demonstrable pathologic process; or (5) if a satisfactory response is noted to antibiotic therapy. The hip may be held in the flexed, externally rotated, and abducted position. Unlike transient synovitis in which the patient generally appears well with a mild febrile illness, patients with septic arthritis usually appear toxic. See Chapter 6 for a further discussion of septic arthritis of the hip in children and how it is differentiated from transient synovitis.

Patients who present after total hip arthroplasty will present in one of three stages, depending on the amount of time that has elapsed since their procedure. In stage I infection, purulent drainage is present at the wound site in the days following the procedure. Stage II infections are indolent and present 6 months to 2 years postoperatively. Finally, patients who present later than 2 years after replacement are considered to have stage III infections, which are believed to be due to infection from a hematogenous source.

Laboratory and Imaging

If septic arthritis is suspected, a complete blood count, erythrocyte sedimentation rate (ESR), and C-reactive protein (CRP) may be helpful; however, none of these are diagnostic. The ESR and CRP are sensitive, but they lack specificity. The ESR is elevated in almost all patients with septic arthritis.

Plain radiographs are usually normal initially. Abnormal subluxation of the hip with widening of the joint space is most common. Osteomyelitis of the proximal femur is noted in some.

An ultrasound that demonstrates fluid in the joint suggests septic arthritis. With the patient supine, the knee is slightly flexed and the hip is held in slight internal rotation. The probe is placed below the inguinal ligament and lateral to the neurovascular bundle. It is angled superomedially toward the umbilicus. The acetabulum, femoral head, and femoral neck are easily visualized approximately 3 to 5 cm below the skin. Synovial fluid cannot readily be seen in the normal hip, but if an effusion is present, a hypoechoic area appears, most prominently just anterior to the femoral neck. A comparison view of the other hip may be useful. In some settings, ultrasound-guided arthrocentesis may be accomplished in the ED. In other cases, the procedure may be performed by a radiologist or orthopedic surgeon. Using sterile technique, an 18-gauge spinal needle is introduced in the long axis of the ultrasound probe from the inferior position.

In septic hip arthritis, the synovial white blood cell (WBC) count averages 57,000/mL; however, it can be as low as 10,000/mL or as high as 250,000/mL. Blood cultures are positive in >50% of the cases.

CT scan may also demonstrate an effusion. MRI has demonstrated little usefulness in making this diagnosis and may be difficult to obtain from the ED.[71] However, a gadolinium-enhanced MRI shows a decreased perfusion of the femoral epiphysis and may be useful in making the diagnosis in difficult cases.[72,73]

In adults with a prosthetic replacement, an indium-labeled autologous WBC study is recommended in patients with stage I and II infections.[64] A positive result will be followed by aspiration and arthrography. Radiographs of a patient with stage II disease will reveal a radiolucent line at the bone–cement interface indicative of a loosening prosthesis.

Treatment

Perhaps the most important point for the emergency physician to be aware of is that a delay in diagnosis and treatment is the most important factor affecting the prognosis. The initiation of treatment beyond 3 weeks has been shown to predict the need for hip replacement in adult patients.[74]

In native joint infection, the goals of treatment are to clean the joint to avoid articular cartilage destruction and adhesion formation, as well as to decompress the joint to avoid vascular embarrassment of the epiphysis.[75] Antibiotic coverage should be broad-spectrum until Gram stain and culture results are available.

Definitive therapy includes arthrotomy and early irrigation. More recently, several authors have recommended arthroscopic drainage of the joint.[76–78] Although arthrotomy is considered the standard of care, it may be complicated by AVN or postoperative hip instability. Thus, three-dimensional arthroscopic surgery with large volumes of irrigation fluid is effective and less invasive.[78] Successful treatment requires early and good surgical drainage.[79]

Patients with infected prosthetic hips generally require removal of all the prosthetic components, surgical debridement, and intravenous antibiotics.[64] A one-stage surgical approach in which the hip is reconstructed and antibiotic-infused polymethylmethacrylate beads are implanted locally has been successful in eradicating the infection.

DEGENERATIVE JOINT DISEASE

Degenerative arthritis is very common. For additional information, the reader is referred to Chapter 3.

Degenerative arthritis or osteoarthritis of the hip takes place with advancing age. Among Whites, where osteoarthritis is most common, the prevalence is 3% to 6%.[80] In Asian, Black, and East Indian populations, the prevalence is low.[81] It is accelerated by any incongruity of the articular surface causing abnormal friction. A secondary form occurs after conditions such as AVN, trauma, joint infection, slipped capital femoral epiphysis, congenital hip disease, and rheumatoid arthritis. The primary form is most common, however, and there appears to be a genetic predisposition. Other contributory factors include obesity and occupations that require high physical demands.[80,82–84]

Clinical Presentation

The patient usually complains of an insidious onset of stiffness about the hip. At first, there are repeated attacks of slight pain lasting only a day or two. The pain is exacerbated by prolonged periods of weight bearing. There is often a protective limp due to muscle spasm accompanied by pain and a sense of stiffness that progressively worsens. The pain may be anterior, lateral, or posterior, depending on the site of inflammation. Referral is typically to the anterior and medial aspects of the thigh and the inner aspect of the knee. Characteristically, the pain is worsened with prolonged weight bearing and movement, particularly with *abduction*, *internal rotation*, and *extension*. Patients often complain of worsening pain in cold weather and relief with heat and salicylates.

During an acute exacerbation of osteoarthritis of the hip, there is tenderness over the site of capsular inflammation accompanied by muscle spasm, primarily involving the adductors. The *FABER test* (**F**lexion, **A**bduction, **E**xternal **R**otation) is usually positive. This test is performed by having the patient place the heel of the affected extremity on the dorsum of the normal foot. The patient then "slides" the heel up the leg until the knee is reached. If pain in the groin is elicited, the test is considered positive. This test is not specific but often indicates intra-articular pathology of the hip.

Imaging

In the early stages of this disorder, plain radiographs will be negative. Later, however, one will note an irregular subchondral sclerosis that gradually evolves into joint space narrowing. Additional findings include flattening of the head of the femur at the superior pole, accompanied by cystic changes in this area (Fig. 18–19).

Treatment

Conservative treatment is indicated for acute exacerbations that present to the ED. This includes abstinence from weight bearing, heat, and massage. Nonsteroidal anti-inflammatory medications are an important adjunct in relieving the inflammatory process.

There is no clear consensus regarding the decision to undergo total hip arthroplasty. Many variables are considered, including age, pain severity, functional limitations, bone quality, and surgical risk.[85,86] A survey of orthopedic surgeons found that most surgeons required at least severe daily pain, rest pain several days per week, and destruction of most of the joint space on radiographs before considering surgery.[85] In patients with significant functional limitations, the procedure not only improves quality of life but is cost effective over long-term assisted living.[87]

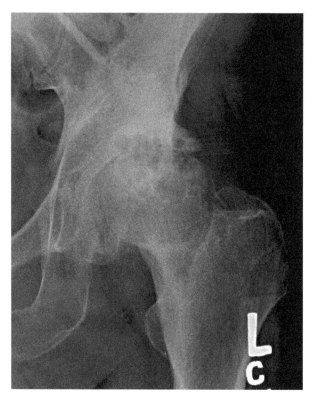

Figure 18–19. Severe degenerative joint disease of the left hip marked by obliteration of the joint space, periarticular sclerotic and cystic changes, and acetabular osteophyte formation.

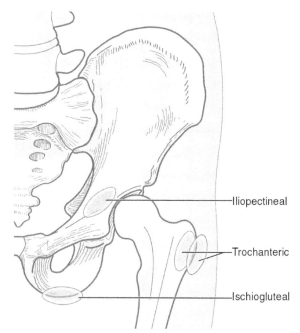

Figure 18–20. The bursae of the hip.

BURSITIS

Many bursae surround the hip, but four are clinically important: the deep trochanteric, superficial trochanteric, iliopsoas (iliopectineal), and ischiogluteal bursa (Fig. 18–20).

The deep trochanteric bursa is located between the tendinous insertion of the gluteus maximus muscle and the posterolateral prominence of the greater trochanter. The superficial trochanteric bursa is located between the greater trochanter and the skin. The iliopsoas bursa is the largest of all the hip bursae. It lies between the iliopsoas muscle anteriorly and the iliopectineal eminence posteriorly along the anterior surface of the hip joint capsule. The ischiogluteal bursa is superficial to the tuberosity of the ischium. The obturator internus bursa has recently been described as a cause of bursitis in some patients.

The usual causes of bursitis include reactive inflammation secondary to overuse or excessive pressure and trauma. Other causes of bursitis are infectious and metabolic conditions, such as gout.

Clinical Presentation

Deep trochanteric bursitis characteristically presents with pain and tenderness localized to the posterior aspect of the greater trochanter, which is increased by *flexion of the hip* and *internal rotation*. Abduction and external rotation of the hip relaxes the gluteus maximus and relieves the pressure on the bursa. Trendelenburg sign is present in three-fourths of patients. This sign is elicited when the patient is asked to stand on the affected leg and the pelvis drops to the unaffected side, indicating inhibition of the gluteus muscles. The pain may radiate down the back of the thigh and any motion may cause discomfort.

Deep trochanteric bursitis is associated with repetitive microtrauma caused by active use of the muscles inserting on the greater trochanter. It is most common between the fourth and sixth decades of life. Degenerative diseases have been associated with this condition, as well as inflammatory arthritis of the hip, obesity, and iliotibial band syndrome.

Calcification around the greater trochanter is evident in many patients with trochanteric bursitis, suggesting concomitant pathology of the gluteus medius muscle (tears) and tendons (tendonitis). Pathologic involvement of several soft-tissue structures has caused some authors to refer to this condition as greater trochanteric pain syndrome.

Superficial trochanteric bursitis presents with tenderness and swelling over the inflamed bursa with accentuation on *extreme adduction* of the thigh.

Iliopsoas bursitis presents with pain and tenderness over the lateral aspect of the femoral triangle (area bound by the inguinal ligament, sartorius, and adductor longus) (Fig. 18–21). Irritation of the adjacent femoral nerve causes pain to be referred along the anterior thigh. This condition is common in sports such as soccer, ballet, or hurling that require extensive use of the hip flexors. The patient usually holds the hip in a position of flexion and abduction with external rotation. Pain is increased by *extension*,

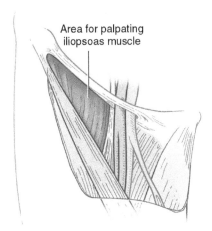

Figure 18–21. Area for palpating the iliopsoas muscle and bursa.

adduction, or *internal rotation* of the hip. This condition must be differentiated from a femoral hernia, psoas abscess, synovitis, or infection of the joint.

Ischiogluteal bursitis is common in patients with occupations requiring prolonged sitting on hard surfaces. Tenderness is elicited over the ischial tuberosity. Pain radiates down the back of the thigh and along the course of the hamstrings, mimicking a herniated disk.

Treatment
The treatment of bursitis is bed rest, heat application, and anti-inflammatory agents. In ischiogluteal bursitis, a cushion or pillow helps relieve the discomfort and prevents recurrence. Sixty percent of the patients with greater trochanteric bursitis treated by injection demonstrated total relief of symptoms from a single injection at 6 months.[93] A rare complication of steroid injection is femoral head necrosis, which has been described due to injection into the joint rather than the bursa.[95] In the event that symptoms are refractory, arthroscopic bursectomy has been successfully employed.[96]

Septic bursitis in one of the bursae about the hip is rare. However, if suspected, this presents a true emergency and must be diagnosed early by the emergency physician. Parenteral antibiotics are indicated. Patients who fail to respond to intravenous antibiotics and percutaneous aspiration of the bursa may require surgical drainage or bursectomy.[97]

CALCIFIC TENDINOPATHY

This condition is comparable to calcific tendinopathy in the shoulder. Amorphous calcium deposits in the tendons of the gluteus medius, lateral to the greater trochanter and superior to the capsule.[98] It is associated with deep trochanteric bursitis, as previously described, and is frequently referred to as greater trochanteric pain syndrome.

Long-distance runners develop tendonitis secondary to the insertion of the iliopsoas tendon on the lesser trochanter.[99]

Clinical Presentation
The patient usually presents with severe pain in the hip. The hip is held in a position of flexion, abduction, and external rotation to relax the involved gluteus medius muscle. Muscle spasm limits motion in all directions. The examiner elicits tenderness over the site of inflammation. If the patient is able to ambulate, a Trendelenburg gait will be noted, in which the pelvis drops to the unaffected side when the patient steps onto the leg of the affected side.

Imaging
The radiograph will often reveal a cloudy opacity in the soft tissues overlying the hip joint.

Treatment
Heat application, rest, and anti-inflammatory agents are usually effective. The calcium depositions are more readily absorbed when broken up by a needling of the involved tendons under local anesthesia.[100] Endoscopic treatment of this condition is also being used.[101]

SNAPPING HIP SYNDROME

Coxa saltans, or snapping hip syndrome, is now regarded as a common cause of hip pain in runners and is typically caused by sudden maneuvers in the course of running.[102] Pain is present in less than one-third of patients.[94] The condition affects young athletes and is slightly more common in women. Snapping hip syndrome is especially common in ballet dancers.[103] This syndrome should be differentiated from a painless, deep "pop" that occurs with normal hip motion and holds no clinical importance. The pain is characterized by a sharp and burning discomfort exacerbated by activity.[102]

There are several causes of snapping hip syndrome. They are classified as external or internal based on their etiology.

External Snapping Hip
External coxa saltans occurs when the iliotibial band or the gluteus maximus tendon snaps over the greater trochanter (Fig. 18–22).[102] This is the most common cause of snapping hip syndrome. Affected patients state that they experience a snapping sensation over the lateral aspect of their hip.[104] Snapping of the tendon over the greater trochanter is frequently demonstrated while walking or upon hip flexion. Passive internal and external rotation of the abducted limb usually demonstrates the snapping.[105] Pain, if present, is mild unless a bursitis of the greater trochanteric bursa develops. External snapping hip caused by the iliotibial band is common in ballet dancers and is also a complication of total hip replacement.

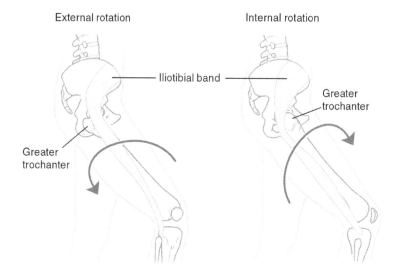

Figure 18–22. In the snapping hip syndrome, the iliotibial band courses over the greater trochanter.

Internal Snapping Hip

An internal cause of snapping hip syndrome is less common but can occur when the iliopsoas tendon snaps over the pelvic brim as it proceeds to its insertion on the lesser tuberosity (Fig. 18–23). Another proposed mechanism is a sudden "flipping" of the iliopsoas tendon over the iliac muscle.

Patients complain of snapping during extension of the flexed hip. It is decreased by internal and increased by external rotation of the hip. Tenderness and pain occur at the anterosuperior spine and medial to the sartorius muscle.

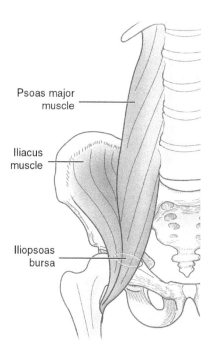

Figure 18–23. Internal snapping hip syndrome occurs when the iliopsoas tendon snaps over the iliopectineal eminence of the pelvic brim as it proceeds to its insertion on the lesser tuberosity.

Psoas major muscle

Iliacus muscle

Iliopsoas bursa

Snapping hip syndrome can also be caused by injuries to intra-articular structures that obstruct the motion of the iliopsoas tendon. Injury to the acetabular labrum, a cartilaginous structure that encircles the acetabulum, or a loose body from an osteochondral injury are two examples. The painful pop or snap is most often anterior but may be posterior and is often accompanied by a sudden weakness of the leg.

Imaging

Plain films of the hip are usually normal in cases of external coxa saltans. Ultrasound has been used to establish the diagnosis, but clinical findings are usually sufficient. If internal causes are suspected, plain radiographs will establish a diagnosis in one-third of patients. If the diagnosis remains unresolved, ultrasound and CT will establish the cause in approximately 90% of patients. MRI is 100% sensitive. MRI demonstrates thickening of the iliotibial band or thickening of the anterior edge of the fascia around the gluteus maximus muscle.

Treatment

Most patients with snapping hip are treated conservatively. The main principle of management is stretching exercises to promote the lengthening of the iliotibial band. Steroid injection is beneficial for eliminating external coxa saltans. If this condition becomes resistant to conservative treatment, surgical lengthening of the band can be performed. This procedure, called a "Z-plasty," has been reported to be highly successful but is rarely necessary. Z-plasty lengthens the tight iliotibial tract and also brings the thickened band anteriorly so it no longer flicks over the greater trochanter during hip flexion. Endoscopic release of the iliotibial band has also been successful in treating this syndrome. Surgery is also indicated for loose bodies. Labral tears are treated with conservative management (nonweight bearing) or arthroscopic debridement.

FEMOROACETABULAR IMPINGEMENT

Femoroacetabular impingement (FAI), also known as hip impingement syndrome, occurs when movement of the femoral head within the acetabulum is limited by excessive bony growth along the femoral neck, acetabular rim, or both.[118] The more common "cam" type of FAI occurs when bony overgrowth along the femoral neck or head comes into contact with the labrum of the acetabulum during hip flexion. In the "pincer" type, excess bone protruding from the acetabular rim contacts the femur during flexion. In both types, range of motion is limited and painful. Over time, the condition may worsen as the bony overgrowth increases and articular cartilage is damaged. Arthritis and destruction of the joint may result.[118]

Clinical Presentation

Although hip impingement may present at any age, it is commonly noted in young, athletic types. The classic symptoms include progressive pain with hip flexion during activity, especially when combined with adduction and internal rotation. Abnormalities may be noted on imaging studies as noted in the next section, but the diagnosis is largely clinical.

Imaging

Plain films are usually obtained early in the diagnostic evaluation, although they neither rule in nor rule out hip impingement syndrome.[119] The primary value of plain films in this setting is to exclude other conditions.

MRI is the best imaging study to evaluate the joint space and is especially valuable in determining whether there is destruction of the cartilage. This becomes important when considering the best treatment options.

Treatment

Conservative treatment may be recommended when there is little joint destruction and little impact on the physical activities of the patient. Rest, restriction of activities, and NSAIDs are often effective in reducing the inflammation and associated pain.

Arthroscopic surgery is recommended for those patients who are more active and more symptomatic with activity.[120] Damaged cartilage may be repaired, and excess bony growth may be shaved to prevent recurrence of hip impingement syndrome. Physical therapy is important in regaining the strength and range of motion that may have been lost over many months of symptoms and recovery.

If left untreated over a prolonged period, damaged cartilage and bone on bone may produce loose bodies that destroy the femoroacetabular joint.[118] Open surgical procedures or total hip replacement may become necessary when the patient has significant joint destruction resulting in severe pain and limitation of daily activities.

HIP DISLOCATION

Hip dislocations constitute 5% of all traumatic joint dislocations and may occur in an anterior or posterior direction.[121,122] Posterior dislocations are more common, accounting for 90% to 95% of all hip dislocations.[1,38,123] Inferior dislocations (luxatio erecta of the hip) have also been reported but are extremely rare.[124]

Posterior Hip Dislocation

The classification of posterior hip dislocations is based on the system developed by Stewart and Milford.[125] In this classification, posterior hip dislocations are graded on the basis of the presence and type of associated fractures.

Grade I   A simple dislocation, without fracture (Fig. 18–24)

Grade II   Dislocation associated with a large acetabular rim fracture that is stabilized after reduction

Grade III Dislocation associated with an unstable or comminuted fracture

Grade IV   Dislocation associated with a femoral head and neck fracture

Mechanism of Injury

Posterior dislocations occur after a blow to the knee while the hip and knee are flexed. In more than 50% of patients, this injury occurs following a high-energy trauma such as automobile accidents where the knee of an unrestrained driver strikes the dashboard (Fig. 18–25).[38,121,122] Fortunately, with the increased use of lap belts, the frequency of

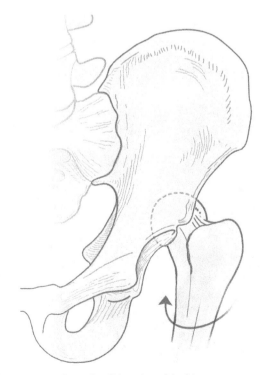

Figure 18–24. Posterior dislocation of the hip.

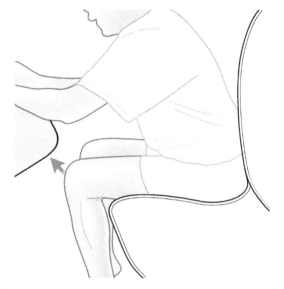

Figure 18–25. Dashboard dislocation.

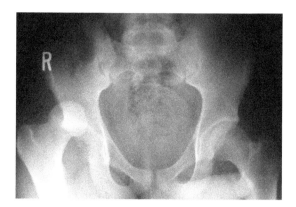

Figure 18–27. Posterior dislocation of the right hip.

these injuries is decreasing. Other high-energy mechanisms include motorcycle collisions, pedestrians struck by automobiles, and sports such as downhill skiing.

Low-energy dislocations are common in children and adults with prosthetic hips. Children younger than 6 years old are especially prone to dislocation after minimal trauma due to general laxity of the surrounding ligamentous structures and the largely cartilaginous acetabulum. Spontaneous dislocations occur in up to 10% of patients after total hip replacement.

Examination

Posterior dislocations present with limb shortening, hip adduction, and internal rotation of the involved extremity (Fig. 18–26). The femoral head may be palpable within the muscle of the buttock. The patient should be carefully evaluated for sciatic nerve injury that may manifest as sensory

and motor deficits. Distal pulses must also be assessed; however, vascular injury is uncommon following a posterior hip dislocation.

Imaging

A single routine AP view of the pelvis is usually adequate in demonstrating these injuries (Figs. 18–27 and 18–28). The femoral head is no longer congruent with the roof of the acetabulum. On a true AP film, the femoral head will appear smaller than the contralateral side due to its posterior displacement. Shenton line should be evaluated whenever a hip injury is suspected (Fig. 18–3). Additional radiographs of the ipsilateral extremity may be indicated on the basis of the physical examination.

Although the dislocation is usually obvious, the radiograph must also be closely inspected for associated fractures. Fractures of the femoral head, neck, and especially the acetabulum

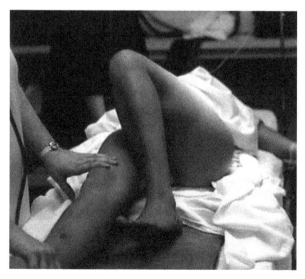

Figure 18–26. Clinical picture of a posterior dislocation of the hip.

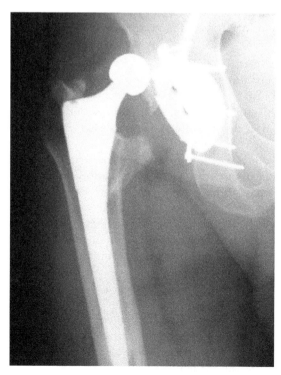

Figure 18–28. Posterior dislocation of a prosthetic hip.

are associated with hip dislocation. If a subtle femoral neck fracture is present, closed reduction of the hip dislocation should not be attempted as it may displace the fracture and increase the likelihood of AVN of the femoral head.

A CT scan of the hip with thin, 2-mm cuts should be obtained in several situations[1,38]:

* Before reduction, if there is suspicion of a femoral neck fracture on plain films
* If closed reduction is unsuccessful, to evaluate for intra-articular bony fragments or loose bodies
* Following reduction, to evaluate the acetabulum for fracture

Associated Injuries

Hip dislocations of a native hip joint may be associated with other significant injuries. In one study, 95% of patients had an associated injury (head, abdomen, chest) severe enough to require hospital admission[130]:

* Acetabular fractures are seen in up to 75% of patients.[127]
* AVN of the femoral head is a consequence of approximately 10% of uncomplicated dislocations.[123] The incidence is 4.8% if the hip is reduced in less than 6 hours, but increases to 50% if reduced after 6 hours.[131] Stewart and Milford grades III and IV were more likely to undergo AVN compared to grades I and II.[131] All hip dislocations must be regarded as true emergencies and reduced promptly to minimize the incidence of AVN of the femoral head.[132]
* Femoral head fractures occur in up to 16% of posterior hip dislocations.[16] Osteochondral fractures due to impaction of the femoral head can cause locking of the dislocated joint.[133]
* Femoral shaft fractures occur in 4% of patients with hip dislocation.[125] Rotation of the shaft after fracture may alter the position of the extremity and confuse the diagnosis.[38]
* Sciatic nerve injury complicates 10% to 13% of posterior hip dislocations.[1,125]
* Ipsilateral knee injuries were present in up to 25% of patients in one series.[125] These injuries vary from ligamentous damage to fractures around the knee.
* Arterial injuries are rare.

Treatment

Posterior hip dislocations are best managed with immobilization and emergent reduction within 6 hours.[131] Delay in reduction increases the rate of AVN of the femoral head and the potential for sciatic nerve injury.[129] Some trauma patients with a hip dislocation have other serious injuries that take precedence, but closed reduction should be accomplished as soon as reasonably possible.

Many closed reduction maneuvers have been described.[126,128,134–136] In all maneuvers, inline traction of the thigh is exerted with countertraction frequently provided by an assistant or sheets tied around the gurney or backboard. Traction should be applied in a steady manner,

as forceful jerky motions will not be successful and may result in femoral neck fractures. If closed reduction under procedural sedation is unsuccessful after two to three attempts, closed or open reduction under general anesthesia should be considered.

Closed reduction should begin by placing the patient on a backboard and administering procedural sedation, as outlined in Chapter 2.

Allis Technique. This method was developed in 1893 by Allis (Fig. 18–29)[128]:

1. The patient should be lowered to the floor while on the backboard, or the physician can stand on the stretcher.
2. An assistant immobilizes the pelvis by holding the iliac crests down.
3. With the hip and knee flexed to 90 degrees, the physician applies traction along the axis of the femur.
4. As traction is maintained, hip rotation, abduction, and adduction may be applied.
5. A second assistant may apply lateral traction to the thigh.

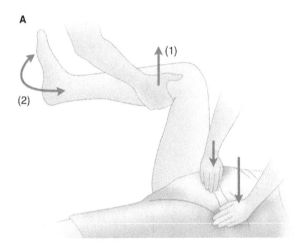

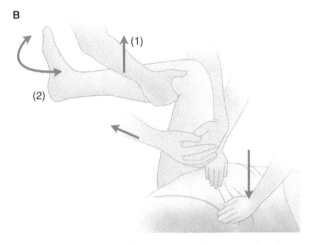

Figure 18-29. *A.* The Allis maneuver. ***B.*** A second assistant applying lateral traction to the thigh may aid in the reduction. (Modified with permission from Reichman EF: *Emergency Medicine Procedures*, 2nd ed. New York: McGraw-Hill; 2013.)

Stimson Technique. Stimson's method of reducing posterior hip dislocations is also safe and effective (Fig. 18–30):

1. The patient is placed prone with the hip flexed over the edge of the stretcher.
2. Traction is applied to the hip by placing pressure over the posterior aspect of the knee by either the physician's hand or knee.
3. External and internal rotation is provided by the hand holding the patient's ankle.
4. An assistant may also apply direct pressure to the femoral head.

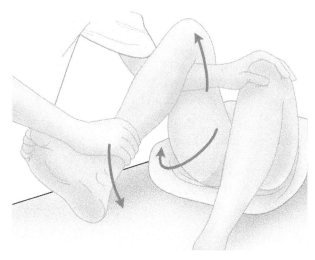

Figure 18–31. The Whistler maneuver.

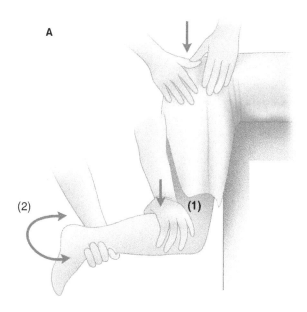

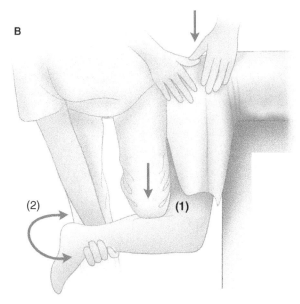

Figure 18–30. ***A.*** The Stimson maneuver. ***B.*** Alternatively, the clinician's knee can be used to reduce the dislocation. (Modified with permission from Reichman EF: *Emergency Medicine Procedures*, 2nd ed. New York: McGraw-Hill; 2013.)

Whistler Technique. Variations of this technique have been described by multiple authors (Fig. 18–31)[136,138,139]:

1. The physician stands on the side of the dislocation and places his/her arm under the knee of the affected leg and onto the unaffected knee.
2. The physician's opposite hand is placed on the anterior aspect of the ankle.
3. The arm under the patient's knee is elevated and traction is applied to the thigh. The palm of the hand on the unaffected knee creates countertraction.
4. The hand on the patient's ankle is used to provide slight internal and external rotation of the hip while also flexing the knee.

Captain Morgan Technique. This technique was developed in Fresno and published in 2011 (Fig. 18–32 and Video 18–1)[139]:

1. The stretcher is lowered as much as possible, and the patient's pelvis is secured to a backboard by a strap.
2. The patient's hip and knee are flexed to 90 degrees.
3. The physician stands on the side of the dislocation and places his/her foot on the backboard with his/her knee under the patient's knee.
4. The physician's hands are used to apply a gentle downward force at the patient's ankle and upward force at the patient's knee. The major force, however, is created by the physician's leg, which applies an upward force by ankle plantarflexion to push off from the backboard.

A careful neurovascular assessment of the extremity should be completed before and after reduction. Successful reduction should be confirmed with a radiograph, and CT scan should be ordered to assess for acetabular fracture (if not already completed). Many patients are admitted with strict nonweight bearing and observation.

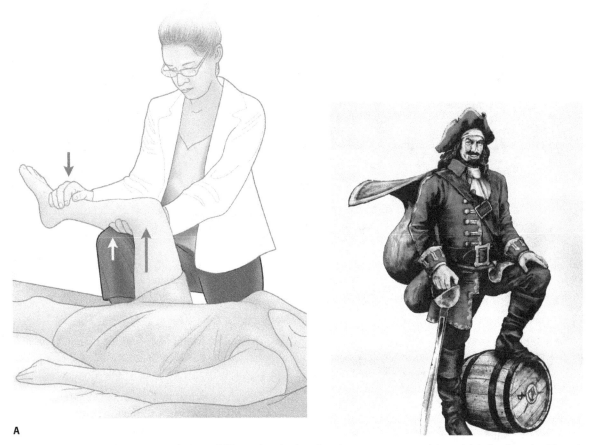

A

Figure 18–32. The *Captain Morgan* technique. **A.** The patient is placed supine on a gurney, and the pelvis is fixed to a backboard with a strap. The patient's hip and knee are flexed to 90 degrees. The physician places one foot on the board, with a knee behind the patient's knee. The physician holds the patient's knee in flexion by holding the ankle down and applies an upward force to the hip by lifting with his or her calf and then gently rotates lower leg. **B.** *Captain Morgan*. (©2018 Diageo. All rights reserved. Used by permission.)

However, select patients without fracture may be discharged with home assistance and good follow-up, particularly those with a recurrent prosthetic hip dislocation. There is no benefit from skeletal traction after reduction.[131]

Operative intervention is necessary in (1) reduced but unstable dislocations, (2) irreducible dislocations, and (3) dislocations associated with proximal femur fractures. In those dislocations complicated by an acetabular fracture, an attempt at closed reduction is indicated. If the reduction is unstable, operative fixation is needed. Closed reduction is unsuccessful in up to 15% of posterior hip dislocations.[38]

Complications

Hip dislocations are associated with several significant complications, including AVN of the femoral head, sciatic nerve injury, and traumatic arthritis.[121,137]

In one study, which followed patients with traumatic posterior dislocations of the hip for an average of 12.5 years, it was found that even with simple dislocations, 24% of the patients had poor results and up to 70%

of the patients had fair-to-poor results.[121] It is clear that even with simple posterior dislocations of the hip treated properly, late osteoarthritis may develop in as many as 20% of cases.

Anterior Hip Dislocation

Anterior dislocations are far less common than posterior dislocations, and many occur in patients with a prosthetic hip. They can be classified as follows (Fig. 18–33):

- Obturator dislocation (most common)
- Iliac dislocation
- Pubic dislocation

Mechanism of Injury

Anterior dislocations are the result of forced abduction resulting in impingement of the femoral neck or trochanter against the superior dome of the acetabulum and a levering of the femoral head through a tear in the anterior capsule.

Obturator dislocations occur when the hip is in flexion at the time of the injury. This type of anterior dislocation

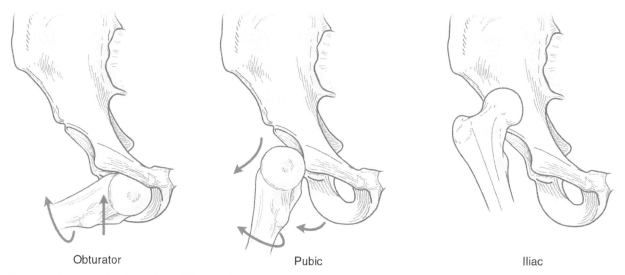

Figure 18–33. Anterior dislocations of the hip. Three types are demonstrated: obturator, pubic, and iliac.

results in a limb fixed in up to 60 degrees of abduction, external rotation, and some flexion.

Injuries to a hip held in extension produces a pubic or iliac dislocation. Pubic dislocations reveal a limb in marked external rotation, full extension, and some abduction. A pubic dislocation can also be the result of severe hyperextension with external rotation, thus forcing the head of the femur anteriorly. Anterior dislocations may be associated with a shear fracture of the femoral head.

Examination

Anterior obturator dislocations usually present with abduction, external rotation, and flexion of the involved extremity. Anterior iliac or pubic dislocations present with the hip in the position of extension, slight abduction, and external rotation. The femoral head is palpable near the anterosuperior iliac spine with iliac dislocations and near the pubis after a pubic dislocation. The neurovascular status of the extremity must be documented in all patients with hip dislocations.

Imaging

Routine hip and pelvic views are usually adequate in demonstrating these injuries (Fig. 18–34). The femoral head will appear larger on the affected side because of its anterior location. Shenton line should be evaluated whenever a hip injury is suspected (Fig. 18–5). Additional radiographs of the ipsilateral extremity may be indicated on the basis of the physical examination.

Associated Injuries

Hip dislocations may be associated with several significant injuries. The associated injuries are similar to a posterior dislocation; however, vascular injury is more common in an anterior dislocation, while sciatic nerve injury is more common after a posterior dislocation.

Treatment

The reduction techniques described previously may be attempted first, but an anterior dislocation of a prosthetic hip may be better treated in the following manner:

1. The patient is placed supine on the gurney and stabilized by an assistant, with the hip and knee straight and the leg in a slightly abducted (20 degrees) and externally rotated position.
2. The physician holds the ankle and applies steady, progressive traction.
3. Further rotation, abduction, and adduction may be added.

As with posterior dislocations, if closed reduction under procedural sedation is unsuccessful, general anesthesia for closed or open reduction is indicated.

Complications

Long-term complications of anterior hip dislocations are similar to posterior dislocations and include AVN of the femoral head and traumatic arthritis.

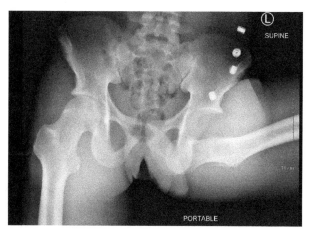

Figure 18–34. Anterior dislocation of the left hip on AP radiograph.

MUSCLE STRAIN AND TENDINOPATHY

Iliopsoas Strain

This is an uncommon injury occurring primarily in dancers and gymnasts. Strain of the iliopsoas may occur at its attachment to the lesser trochanter or at the musculotendinous junction. The usual mechanism of injury is excessive stretch placed on the iliopsoas. On examination, the patient characteristically holds the thigh in a flexed adducted and externally rotated position. Extension and internal rotation of the thigh accentuate pain.

Ice packs and bed rest are the mainstays of management in this injury. The tendon is usually not repaired surgically even if it is completely avulsed or has an incorporated bone fragment.

Gluteus Medius Strain

This is more commonly seen in young athletes; however, even in this group it is an uncommon injury. Strain of the gluteus medius usually occurs as a result of overexertion. Pain is noted on abduction against resistance and is accentuated by having the patient rotate the thigh medially against resistance. The treatment of this injury is the same for any other muscle strain and includes rest, moist heat application, and analgesics.

In young patients with chronic buttocks pain, one should consider gluteus medius tendon tear or even rupture as the cause. In one study, 46% of patients with chronic buttocks pain had this as the etiology. The diagnosis is best made by doing the Trendelenburg test, which is most sensitive for this condition.[139,140]

External Rotator Tendinopathy

This condition can be acute or chronic and commonly involves the external rotators. The external rotators of the thigh include the piriformis, gemellus superior and inferior, obturator internus and externus, quadratus femoris, and gluteus maximus. Tendinopathy of these muscles is characterized by pain and tenderness on active external rotation. Treatment for the condition includes local moist heat application, anti-inflammatory agents, and analgesics. In younger patients with overuse syndromes of the external rotators, treat with cold packs for 20 minutes several times a day as well as ultrasound and ionophoresis.[140]

REFERENCES

1. Rudman N, McIlmail D. Emergency department evaluation and treatment of hip and thigh injuries. *Emerg Med Clin North Am.* 2000;18(1):29–66, v.
2. Caviglia HA, Osorio PQ, Comando D. Classification and diagnosis of intracapsular fractures of the proximal femur. *Clin Orthop.* 2002;(399):17–27.
3. DeLaMora SN, Gilbert M. Introduction of intracapsular hip fractures: anatomy and pathologic features. *Clin Orthop.* 2002;(399):9–16.
4. Cannon J, Silvestri S, Munro M. Imaging choices in occult hip fracture. *J Emerg Med.* 2009;37(2):144–152.
5. Dominguez S, Liu P, Roberts C, Mandell M, Richman PB. Prevalence of traumatic hip and pelvic fractures in patients with suspected hip fracture and negative initial standard radiographs—a study of emergency department patients. *Acad Emerg Med.* 2005;12(4):366–369.
6. Hakkarinen DK, Banh KV, Hendey GW. Magnetic resonance imaging identifies occult hip fractures missed by 64-slice computed tomography. *J Emerg Med.* 2012;43(2):303–307.
7. Hossain M, Barwick C, Sinha AK, Andrew JG. Is magnetic resonance imaging (MRI) necessary to exclude occult hip fracture? *Injury.* 2007;38(10):1204–1208.
8. Perron AD, Miller MD, Brady WJ. Orthopedic pitfalls in the ED: radiographically occult hip fracture. *Am J Emerg Med.* 2002;20(3):234–237.
9. Chana R, Noorani A, Ashwood N, Chatterji U, Healy J, Baird P. The role of MRI in the diagnosis of proximal femoral fractures in the elderly. *Injury.* 2006;37(2):185–189.
10. Sankey RA, Turner J, Lee J, Healy J, Gibbons CE. The use of MRI to detect occult fractures of the proximal femur: a study of 102 consecutive cases over a ten-year period. *J Bone Joint Surg Br.* 2009;91(8):1064–1068.
11. Lubovsky O, Liebergall M, Mattan Y, Weil Y, Mosheiff R. Early diagnosis of occult hip fractures MRI versus CT scan. *Injury.* 2005;36(6):788–792.
12. Hunter GA. Posterior dislocation and fracture-dislocation of the hip. A review of fifty-seven patients. *J Bone Joint Surg Br.* 1969;51(1):38–44.
13. Barnes R, Brown JT, Garden RS, Nicoll EA. Subcapital fractures of the femur. A prospective review. *J Bone Joint Surg Br.* 1976;58(1):2–24.
14. Shah AK, Eissler J, Radomisli T. Algorithms for the treatment of femoral neck fractures. *Clin Orthop.* 2002;(399):28–34.
15. Koval KJ, Zuckerman JD. Hip fractures: I. overview and evaluation and treatment of femoral-neck fractures. *J Am Acad Orthop Surg.* 1994;2(3):141–149.
16. Norris MA, De Smet AA. Fractures and dislocations of the hip and femur. *Semin Roentgenol.* 1994;29(2):100–112.
17. Heim M, Adunski A, Chechick A. Nonoperative treatment of intracapsular fractures of the proximal femur. *Clin Orthop.* 2002;(399):35–41.
18. Hui AC, Anderson GH, Choudhry R, Boyle J, Gregg PJ. Internal fixation or hemiarthroplasty for undisplaced fractures of the femoral neck in octogenarians. *J Bone Joint Surg Br.* 1994;76(6):891–894.
19. Bachiller FG, Caballer AP, Portal LF. Avascular necrosis of the femoral head after femoral neck fracture. *Clin Orthop.* 2002;(399):87–109.
20. Parker MJ. The management of intracapsular fractures of the proximal femur. *J Bone Joint Surg Br.* 2000;82(7):937–941.
21. Bosch U, Schreiber T, Krettek C. Reduction and fixation of displaced intracapsular fractures of the proximal femur. *Clin Orthop.* 2002;(399):59–71.
22. Rodriguez-Merchan EC. Displaced intracapsular hip fractures: hemiarthroplasty or total arthroplasty? *Clin Orthop.* 2002;(399):72–77.
23. Claffey TJ. Avascular necrosis of the femoral head. an anatomical study. *J Bone Joint Surg Br.* 1960;42-B:802–809.

24. Barr JS Jr. Experiences with a sliding nail in femoral neck fractures. *Clin Orthop.* 1973;92:63–68.

25. Koval KJ, Zuckerman JD. Hip fractures: II. Evaluation and treatment of intertrochanteric fractures. *J Am Acad Orthop Surg.* 1994;2(3):150–156.

26. Lindskog DM, Baumgaertner MR. Unstable intertrochanteric hip fractures in the elderly. *J Am Acad Orthop Surg.* 2004;12(3):179–190.

27. Kaplan K, Miyamoto R, Levine BR, Egol EA, Zuckerman JD. Surgical management of hip fractures: an evidence-based review of the literature. II: intertrochanteric fractures. *J Am Acad Orthop Surg.* 2008;16(11):665–673.

28. Larsson S, Friberg S, Hansson LI. Trochanteric fractures. Mobility, complications, and mortality in 607 cases treated with the sliding-screw technique. *Clin Orthop.* 1990;(260):232–241.

29. Dhal A, Varghese M, Bhasin VB. External fixation of intertrochanteric fractures of the femur. *J Bone Joint Surg Br.* 1991;73(6):955–958.

30. Merlino AF, Nixon JE. Isolated fractures of the greater trochanter. Report of twelve cases. *Int Surg.* 1969;52(2):117–124.

31. Gradwohl JR, Mailliard JA. Cough induced avulsion of the lesser trochanter. *Nebr Med J.* 1987;72(8):280–281.

32. Phillips CD, Pope TL Jr, Jones JE, Keats TE, Macmillan RH III. Nontraumatic avulsion of the lesser trochanter: a pathognomonic sign of metastatic disease? *Skeletal Radiol.* 1988;17(2):106–110.

33. Bertin KC, Horstman J, Coleman SS. Isolated fracture of the lesser trochanter in adults: an initial manifestation of metastatic malignant disease. *J Bone Joint Surg Am.* 1984;66(5):770–773.

34. Sims SH. Subtrochanteric femur fractures. *Orthop Clin North Am.* 2002;33(1):113–126, viii.

35. Lavernia CJ, Sierra RJ, Grieco FR. Osteonecrosis of the femoral head. *J Am Acad Orthop Surg.* 1999;7(4):250–261.

36. Ware HE, Brooks AP, Toye R, Berney SI. Sickle cell disease and silent avascular necrosis of the hip. *J Bone Joint Surg Br.* 1991;73(6):947–949.

37. Moran MC. Osteonecrosis of the hip in sickle cell hemoglobinopathy. *Am J Orthop.* 1995;24(1):18–24.

38. Tornetta P III, Mostafavi HR. Hip dislocation: current treatment regimens. *J Am Acad Orthop Surg.* 1997;5(1):27–36.

39. Koch CA, Tsigos C, Patronas NJ, Papanicolau DA. Cushing's disease presenting with avascular necrosis of the hip: an orthopedic emergency. *J Clin Endocrinol Metab.* 1999;84(9):3010–3012.

40. Sadat-Ali M. Avascular necrosis of the femoral head in sickle cell disease. An integrated classification. *Clin Orthop.* 1993;(290):200–205.

41. Tektonidou MG, Moutsopoulos HM. Immunologic factors in the pathogenesis of osteonecrosis. *Orthop Clin North Am.* 2004;35(3):259–263, vii.

42. Itzchaki M, Lebel E, Dweck A, et al. Orthopedic considerations in Gaucher disease since the advent of enzyme replacement therapy. *Acta Orthop Scand.* 2004;75(6):641–653.

43. Mirzai R, Chang C, Greenspan A, Gershwin ME. Avascular necrosis. *Compr Ther.* 1998;24(5):251–255.

44. Hungerford DS, Jones LC. Asymptomatic osteonecrosis: should it be treated? *Clin Orthop.* 2004;(429):124–130.

45. Schroer WC. Current concepts on the pathogenesis of osteonecrosis of the femoral head. *Orthop Rev.* 1994;23(6):487–497.

46. Ohzono K, Saito M, Takaoka K, et al. Natural history of nontraumatic avascular necrosis of the femoral head. *J Bone Joint Surg Br.* 1991;73(1):68–72.

47. Pappas JN. The musculoskeletal crescent sign. *Radiology.* 2000;217(1):213–214.

48. Jackson SM, Major NM. Pathologic conditions mimicking osteonecrosis. *Orthop Clin North Am.* 2004;35(3):315–320, ix.

49. Etienne G, Mont MA, Ragland PS. The diagnosis and treatment of nontraumatic osteonecrosis of the femoral head. *Instr Course Lect.* 2004;53:67–85.

50. Lee SB, Sugano N, Nakata K, Matsui M, Ohzono K. Comparison between bipolar hemiarthroplasty and THA for osteonecrosis of the femoral head. *Clin Orthop.* 2004;(424):161–165.

51. Beaule PE, Amstutz HC. Management of Ficat stage III and IV osteonecrosis of the hip. *J Am Acad Orthop Surg.* 2004;12(2):96–105.

52. Urbaniak JR, Harvey EJ. Revascularization of the femoral head in osteonecrosis. *J Am Acad Orthop Surg.* 1998;6(1):44–54.

53. Griffin PP, Green WT Sr. Hip joint infections in infants and children. *Orthop Clin North Am.* 1978;9(1):123–134.

54. Paterson DC. Acute suppurative arthritis in infancy and childhood. *J Bone Joint Surg Br.* 1970;52(3):474–482.

55. Yeargan SA III, Perry JJ, Kane TJ III, Richardson AB. Hematogenous septic arthritis of the adult hip. *Orthopedics.* 2003;26(8):771–776.

56. Laiho K, Kotilainen P. Septic arthritis due to *Prevotella bivia* after intra-articular hip joint injection. *Joint Bone Spine.* 2001;68(5):443–444.

57. Peravali R, Purohit N, Dutta S, Mohsen Y. Septic arthritis of the hip: a rare complication of fistulizing Crohn's disease. *Colorectal Dis.* 2009;11(3):323–324.

58. Million M, Roux F, Cohen SJ, et al. Septic arthritis of the hip with *Propionibacterium avidum* bacteremia after intraarticular treatment for hip osteoarthritis. *Joint Bone Spine.* 2008;75(3):356–358.

59. Bal BS, Barrett M. Acute sepsis complicating degenerative arthritis of the hip joint: a report of three cases. *J Surg Orthop Adv.* 2005;14(4):190–192.

60. Kumagai K, Ushiyama T, Kawasaki T, Matsusuey Y. Extension of lumbar spine infection into osteoarthritic hip through psoas abscess. *J Orthop Sci.* 2005;10(1):91–94.

61. Freedman KB, Hahn GV, Fitzgerald RH Jr. Unusual case of septic arthritis of the hip: spread from adjacent adductor pyomyositis. *J Arthroplasty.* 1999;14(7):886–891.

62. Edwards SA, Cranfield T, Clarke HJ. A typical presentation of septic arthritis in the immunosuppressed patient. *Orthopedics.* 2002;25(10):1089–1090.

63. Barrett MO, Bal BS. Septic arthritis of the hip in an immune competent adult: the significance of the differential diagnosis. *J Am Board Fam Med.* 2007;20(3):307–309.

64. Fitzgerald RH Jr. Infected total hip arthroplasty: diagnosis and treatment. *J Am Acad Orthop Surg.* 1995;3(5):249–262.

65. Yuan HC, Wu KG, Chen CJ, Tang RB, Hwang BT. Characteristics and outcome of septic arthritis in children. *J Microbiol Immunol Infect.* 2006;39(4):342–347.

66. Frazee BW, Fee C, Lambert L. How common is MRSA in adult septic arthritis? *Ann Emerg Med.* 2009;54(5):695–700.

67. Al Ahaideb A. Septic arthritis in patients with rheumatoid arthritis. *J Orthop Surg.* 2008;3:33.

68. Freeman K, Dewitz A, Baker WE. Ultrasound-guided hip arthrocentesis in the ED. *Am J Emerg Med.* 2007;25(1):80–86.

69. McGillicuddy DC, Shah KH, Friedberg RP, Nathanson LA, Edlow JA. How sensitive is the synovial fluid white blood cell count in diagnosing septic arthritis? *Am J Emerg Med.* 2007;25(7):749–752.

70. Yagupsky P. Differentiation between septic arthritis and transient synovitis of the hip in children. *J Bone Joint Surg Am.* 2005;87(2):459–460.

71. Weishaupt D, Schweitzer ME. MR imaging of septic arthritis and rheumatoid arthritis of the shoulder. *Magn Reson Imaging Clin N Am.* 2004;12(1):111–124, vii.

72. Kwack KS, Cho JH, Lee JH, Cho JH, Oh KK, Kim SY. Septic arthritis versus transient synovitis of the hip: gadolinium-enhanced MRI finding of decreased perfusion at the femoral epiphysis. *AJR Am J Roentgenol.* 2007;189(2):437–445.

73. Yang WJ, Im SA, Lim GY, et al. MR imaging of transient synovitis: differentiation from septic arthritis. *Pediatr Radiol.* 2006;36(11):1154–1158.

74. Matthews PC, Dean BJ, Medagoda K, et al. Native hip joint septic arthritis in 20 adults: delayed presentation beyond three weeks predicts need for excision arthroplasty. *J Infect.* 2008;57(3):185–190.

75. Curtiss PH Jr, Klein L. Destruction of articular cartilage in septic arthritis. II. In vivo studies. *J Bone Joint Surg Am.* 1965;47(8):1595–1604.

76. Mathews CJ, Kingsley G, Field M, et al. Management of septic arthritis: a systematic review. *Postgrad Med J.* 2008;84(991):265–270.

77. Kaminski A, Muhr G, Kutscha-Lissberg F. Modified open arthroscopy in the treatment of septic arthritis of the hip. *Ortop Traumatol Rehabil.* 2007;9(6):599–603.

78. Nusem I, Jabur MK, Playford EG. Arthroscopic treatment of septic arthritis of the hip. *Arthroscopy.* 2006;22(8):902–903.

79. Trampuz A, Zimmerli W. Diagnosis and treatment of implant-associated septic arthritis and osteomyelitis. *Curr Infect Dis Rep.* 2008;10(5):394–403.

80. Hoaglund FT, Steinbach LS. Primary osteoarthritis of the hip: etiology and epidemiology. *J Am Acad Orthop Surg.* 2001;9(5):320–327.

81. Oishi CS, Hoaglund FT, Gordon L, Ross PD. Total hip replacement rates are higher among Caucasians than Asians in Hawaii. *Clin Orthop.* 1998;(353):166–174.

82. Yoshimura N, Sasaki S, Iwasaki K, et al. Occupational lifting is associated with hip osteoarthritis: a Japanese case-control study. *J Rheumatol.* 2000;27(2):434–440.

83. Sturmer T, Gunther KP, Brenner H. Obesity, overweight and patterns of osteoarthritis: the Ulm Osteoarthritis Study. *J Clin Epidemiol.* 2000;53(3):307–313.

84. Marks R, Allegrante JP. Body mass indices in patients with disabling hip osteoarthritis. *Arthritis Res.* 2002;4(2):112–116.

85. Mancuso CA, Ranawat CS, Esdaile JM, Johanson NA, Charlson ME. Indications for total hip and total knee arthroplasties. Results of orthopaedic surveys. *J Arthroplasty.* 1996;11(1):34–46.

86. Quintana JM, Aróstegui I, Azkarate J, et al. Evaluation by explicit criteria of the use of total hip joint replacement. *Rheumatology.* 2000;39(11):1234–1241.

87. Chang RW, Pellisier JM, Hazen GB. A cost-effectiveness analysis of total hip arthroplasty for osteoarthritis of the hip. *JAMA.* 1996;275(11):858–865.

88. Segal NA, Felson DT, Torner JC, et al. Greater trochanteric pain syndrome: epidemiology and associated factors. *Arch Phys Med Rehabil.* 2007;88(8):988–992.

89. DeAngelis NA, Busconi BD. Assessment and differential diagnosis of the painful hip. *Clin Orthop.* 2003;(406):11–18.

90. Butcher JD, Salzman KL, Lillegard WA. Lower extremity bursitis. *Am Fam Physician.* 1996;53(7):2317–2324.

91. Hwang JY, Lee SW, Kim JO. MR imaging features of obturator internus bursa of the hip. *Korean J Radiol.* 2008;9(4):375–378.

92. Bird PA, Oakley SP, Shnier R, Kirkham BW. Prospective evaluation of magnetic resonance imaging and physical examination findings in patients with greater trochanteric pain syndrome. *Arthritis Rheum.* 2001;44(9):2138–2145.

93. Shbeeb MI, Matteson EL. Trochanteric bursitis (greater trochanter pain syndrome). *Mayo Clin Proc.* 1996;71(6):565–569.

94. Morelli V, Smith V. Groin injuries in athletes. *Am Fam Physician.* 2001;64(8):1405–1414.

95. Koudela K Jr, Koudelova J, Koudela K Sr, Kunesova M. [Bursitis iliopectinea]. *Acta Chir Orthop Traumatol Cech.* 2008;75(5):347–354.

96. Fox JL. The role of arthroscopic bursectomy in the treatment of trochanteric bursitis. *Arthroscopy.* 2002;18(7):E34.

97. Zimmermann B III, Mikolich DJ, Ho G Jr. Septic bursitis. *Semin Arthritis Rheum.* 1995;24(6):391–410.

98. Kuroda H, Wada Y, Nishiguchi K, et al. A case of probable hydroxyapatite deposition disease (HADD) of the hip. *Magn Reson Med Sci.* 2004;3(3):141–144.

99. Nguyen JT, Peterson JS, Biswal S, Beaulieu CF, Fredericson M. Stress-related injuries around the lesser trochanter in long-distance runners. *AJR Am J Roentgenol.* 2008;190(6):1616–1620.

100. Holt PD, Keats TE. Calcific tendinitis: a review of the usual and unusual. *Skeletal Radiol.* 1993;22(1):1–9.

101. Kandemir U, Bharam S, Philippon MJ, Fu FH. Endoscopic treatment of calcific tendinitis of gluteus medius and minimus. *Arthroscopy.* 2003;19(1):E4.

102. Paluska SA. An overview of hip injuries in running. *Sports Med.* 2005;35(11):991–1014.

103. Winston P, Awan R, Cassidy JD, Bleakney RK. Clinical examination and ultrasound of self-reported snapping hip syndrome in elite ballet dancers. *Am J Sports Med.* 2007;35(1):118–126.

104. White RA, Hughes MS, Burd T, Hamann J, Allen WC. A new operative approach in the correction of external coxa saltans: the snapping hip. *Am J Sports Med.* 2004;32(6):1504–1508.

105. Brignall CG, Stainsby GD. The snapping hip. Treatment by Z-plasty. *J Bone Joint Surg Br.* 1991;73(2):253–254.

106. Deslandes M, Guillin R, Cardinal E, Hobden R, Bureau NJ. The snapping iliopsoas tendon: new mechanisms using dynamic sonography. *AJR Am J Roentgenol.* 2008;190(3):576–581.

107. Choi YS, Lee SM, Song BY, Paik SH, Yoon YK. Dynamic sonography of external snapping hip syndrome. *J Ultrasound Med.* 2002;21(7):753–758.

108. Wunderbaldinger P, Bremer C, Matuszewski L, Marten K, Turetschek K, Rand T. Efficient radiological assessment of the internal snapping hip syndrome. *Eur Radiol.* 2001; 11(9):1743–1747.

109. Krishnamurthy G, Connolly BL, Narayanan U, Babyn PS. Imaging findings in external snapping hip syndrome. *Pediatr Radiol.* 2007;37(12):1272–1274.

110. Schaberg JE, Harper MC, Allen WC. The snapping hip syndrome. *Am J Sports Med.* 1984;12(5):361–365.

111. Allen WC, Cope R. Coxa saltans: the snapping hip revisited. *J Am Acad Orthop Surg.* 1995;3(5):303–308.

112. Faraj AA, Moulton A, Sirivastava VM. Snapping iliotibial band. Report of ten cases and review of the literature. *Acta Orthop Belg.* 2001;67(1):19–23.

113. Gruen GS, Scioscia TN, Lowenstein JE. The surgical treatment of internal snapping hip. *Am J Sports Med.* 2002; 30(4):607–613.

114. Ilizaliturri VM Jr, Chaidez C, Villegas P, Briseno A, Camacho-Galindo J. Prospective randomized study of 2 different techniques for endoscopic iliopsoas tendon release in the treatment of internal snapping hip syndrome. *Arthroscopy.* 2009; 25(2):159–163.

115. Provencher MT, Hofmeister EP, Muldoon MP. The surgical treatment of external coxa saltans (the snapping hip) by Z-plasty of the iliotibial band. *Am J Sports Med.* 2004; 32(2):470–476.

116. Ilizaliturri VM Jr, Martinez-Escalante FA, Chaidez PA, Camecho-Galindo J. Endoscopic iliotibial band release for external snapping hip syndrome. *Arthroscopy.* 2006;22(5):505–510.

117. Ilizaliturri VM Jr, Villalobos FE Jr, Chaidez PA, Valero FS, Aguilere JM. Internal snapping hip syndrome: treatment by endoscopic release of the iliopsoas tendon. *Arthroscopy.* 2005; 21(11):1375–1380.

118. Volpon JB. Femoroacetabular impingement. *Rev Bras Ortop.* 2016;51(6):621–629. doi:10.1016/j.rboe.2016.10.006.

119. Mascarenhas VV, Rego P, Dantas P, et al. Imaging prevalence of femoroacetabular impingement in symptomatic patients, athletes, and asymptomatic individuals: a systematic review. *Eur J Radiol.* 2016;85(1):73–95. doi:10.1016/j.ejrad.2015.10.016. Epub 2015 Nov 2.

120. Fairley J, Wang Y, Teichtahl AJ, et al. Management options for femoroacetabular impingement: a systematic review of symptom and structural outcomes. *Osteoarthritis Cartilage.* 2016;24(10):1682–1696. doi:10.1016/j.joca.2016.04.014. Epub 2016 Apr 20.

121. Shukla PC, Cooke SE, Pollack CV Jr, Kolb JC. Simultaneous asymmetric bilateral traumatic hip dislocation. *Ann Emerg Med.* 1993;22(11):1768–1771.

122. Sahin V, Karakas ES, Aksu S, Atlihan D, Turk CY, Halici M. Traumatic dislocation and fracture-dislocation of the hip: a long-term follow-up study. *J Trauma.* 2003; 54(3):520–529.

123. Dawson I, Van Rijn AB. Traumatic anterior dislocation of the hip. *Arch Orthop Trauma Surg.* 1989;108(1): 55–57.

124. Ferguson KL, Harris VV. Inferior hip dislocation in an adult: does a rare injury now have a common mechanism? *Am J Emerg Med.* 2000;18(1):117–118.

125. Gillespie WJ. The incidence and pattern of knee injury associated with dislocation of the hip. *J Bone Joint Surg Br.* 1975;57(3):376–378.

126. Walden PD, Hamer JR. Whistler technique used to reduce traumatic dislocation of the hip in the emergency department setting. *J Emerg Med.* 1999;17(3):441–444.

127. Kutty S, Thornes B, Curtin WA, Gilmore MF. Traumatic posterior dislocation of hip in children. *Pediatr Emerg Care.* 2001;17(1):32–35.

128. Nordt WE III. Maneuvers for reducing dislocated hips: a new technique and a literature review. *Clin Orthop.* 1999; (360):260–264.

129. Hillyard RF, Fox J. Sciatic nerve injuries associated with traumatic posterior hip dislocations. *Am J Emerg Med.* 2003; 21(7):545–548.

130. Suraci AJ. Distribution and severity of injuries associated with hip dislocations secondary to motor vehicle accidents. *J Trauma.* 1986;26(5):458–460.

131. Hougaard K, Thomsen PB. Traumatic posterior dislocation of the hip—prognostic factors influencing the incidence of avascular necrosis of the femoral head. *Arch Orthop Trauma Surg.* 1986;106(1):32–35.

132. Rath E, Levy O, Liberman N, Atar D. Bilateral dislocation of the hip during convulsions: a case report. *J Bone Joint Surg Br.* 1997;79(2):304–306.

133. Esenkaya I, Elmali N. [Locked posterior dislocation of the hip: a case report]. *Acta Orthop Traumatol Turc.* 2007;41(2): 155–158.

134. Reichman EF, Simon RR. *Emergency Medicine Procedures.* New York, NY: McGraw-Hill; 2004.

135. Stefanich RJ. Closed reduction of posterior hip dislocation: the Rochester method. *Am J Orthop.* 1999;28(1):64–65.

136. Hendey G, Avila A. The Captain Morgan technique for the reduction of the dislocated hip. *Ann Emerg Med.* 2011; 58(6):536–540.

137. Schlickewei W, Elsasser B, Mullaji AB, Kuner EH. Hip dislocation without fracture: traction or mobilization after reduction? *Injury.* 1993;24(1):27–31.

138. Friedenberg ZB, Baird D. Fracture of the hip: a review of 200 consecutive fractures. *J Trauma.* 1970;10(1):51–56.

139. Bewyer D, Chen J. Gluteus medius tendon rupture as a source for back, buttock and leg pain: case report. *Iowa Orthop J.* 2005;25:187–189.

140. Bewyer DC, Bewyer KJ. Rationale for treatment of hip abductor pain syndrome. *Iowa Orthop J.* 2003;23:57–60.

CHAPTER 19

Thigh

Rachel R. Bengtzen, MD and Alexander P. Skog, MD

INTRODUCTION

The thigh, the largest anatomic portion of any extremity, comprises powerful muscle groups that encase the femoral shaft. The femur is the heaviest and longest bone in the body. It has an excellent blood supply derived from the profunda femoris artery, and its periosteum receives extensive collateral circulation. As a result, the femur is well protected from devascularization and has good healing potential.

The musculature of the thigh is divided into three compartments by intermuscular septa that attach to the linea aspera, a ridge that runs down the posterior aspect of the femur (Fig. 19–1). The anterior compartment contains hip flexors and knee extensors, including the four quadriceps muscles (rectus femoris, vastus medialis, vastus lateralis, and vastus intermedius). The posterior compartment is occupied by the hamstrings, which include the long and short heads of the biceps femoris, as well as the semimembranosus and semitendinosus muscles medially. The medial compartment includes the adductor muscle group, consisting of the adductor longus, brevis, and magnus, as well as the gracilis.

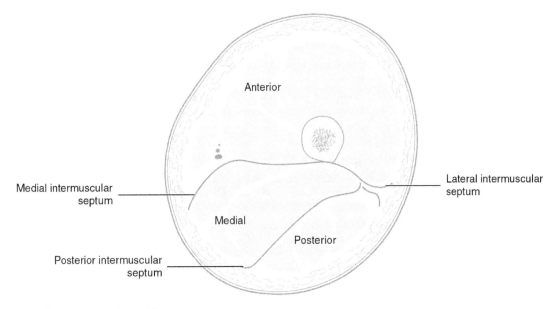

Figure 19–1. Compartments of the thigh.

FEMUR FRACTURES

FEMORAL SHAFT FRACTURES

The femoral shaft in an adult extends from approximately 5 cm distal to the lesser trochanter to a point approximately 5 cm proximal to the adductor tubercle.[1]

Femoral shaft fractures are classified into three types:

- Spiral, transverse, or oblique shaft fractures
- Comminuted femoral shaft fractures
- Open femoral shaft fractures

Distinguishing between spiral, transverse, or oblique fractures does not alter the treatment or prognosis. However, comminuted fractures and open fractures have an overall higher rate of nonunion and longer healing time than simple fractures.[2,3]

Comminuted fractures are further classified by Winquist based on the size of the fracture fragment and the degree of comminution (Fig. 19–2).[1,4] Grade I fractures have minimal or no comminution, and fracture fragments are small (≤25% of the width of the femoral shaft).

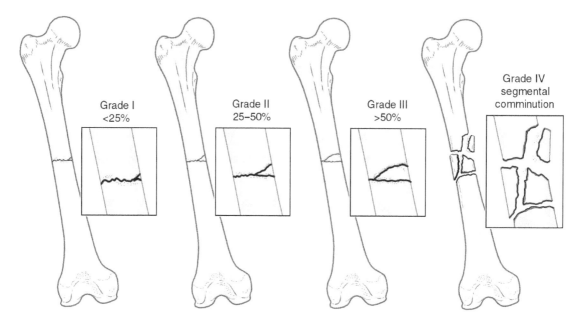

Figure 19–2. Winquist grading of femoral shaft fractures.

Grade II fractures possess a fracture fragment of 25% to 50%, whereas grade III fractures are associated with a large butterfly fragment (>50% of the width of the femoral shaft). Grade IV fractures possess circumferential comminution over an entire segment of bone with complete loss of abutment of the cortices.

Femoral shaft fractures occur with minimal or no trauma and are associated with abnormally brittle bone and increased cortical thickening. These atypical fractures are characterized by a transverse or short oblique morphology and lack of substantial comminution. They most commonly occur in the proximal one-third of the femoral shaft but can be anywhere from an area distal to the lesser trochanter to just proximal to the supracondylar flare of the distal femoral metaphysis. They comprise only 1.1% of all femoral fractures and 3% of all femoral shaft fractures. Although absolute risk remains low, a growing body of evidence suggests that the relative risk of atypical femoral shaft fractures is significantly increased with long-term bisphosphonate use. To mitigate this risk, a drug holiday after 3 to 5 years of treatment is often considered.

Mechanism of Injury

In 49% of cases, femoral shaft fractures are due to a high-energy force. Low-energy mechanisms are more common in children and the elderly. The mechanism of high-energy fractures can be from a direct blow or an indirect force transmitted through the flexed knee. Mechanisms of high-energy force include, most commonly, automobile-related injuries, as well as falls from heights of more than 6 feet and gunshot wounds. Whereas high-energy forces disproportionately affect young males, low-energy fractures are more common in elderly women with ground-level falls. Fracture of the femur following a low-energy

mechanism may suggest a pathologic fracture in adults or nonaccidental trauma (NAT) in pediatrics.

In children, fracture of the femur is the most common musculoskeletal injury requiring hospitalization. Falls and motor vehicle accidents account for approximately three-fourths of these injuries; however, it is estimated that approximately 15% of femoral fractures in children younger than 2 years are due to NAT. The strongest predictors of NAT are age less than 36 months, history or mechanism inconsistent with injury pattern, and physical and/or radiographic evidence of prior trauma. Strongly consider NAT screening for children less than 36 months of age who present with a femoral shaft fracture. Although spiral fractures have been classically associated with NAT, transverse fractures are in fact the most common type of fracture in both accidental and nonaccidental injuries.

Examination

The patient will present with severe pain in the involved extremity and usually will have a visible deformity (Fig. 19–3). The extremity may classically be internally rotated and shortened, as well as exhibit crepitation with movement. The thigh will be swollen and tense secondary to hemorrhage and formation of a hematoma. Signs of compartment syndrome should be noted because femoral fractures cause nearly half of all incidents of thigh compartment syndrome. Neurologic examination should be performed to assess the function of the sciatic nerve. Arterial injuries are rare, but they must be excluded on the initial examination. Arterial injuries associated with a femoral shaft fracture may be suspected in the presence of an expanding hematoma, diminishing or absent distal pulses, or worsening neurologic signs. Neurovascular examination

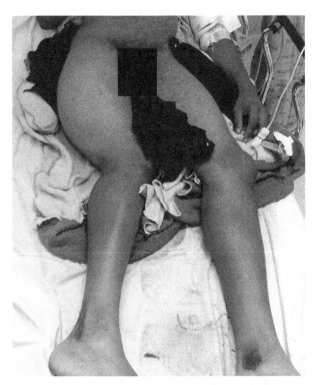

Figure 19–3. Right femur fracture. Note the medial angulation and rotation of the leg. (*Used with permission from Trevonne Thompson, MD.*)

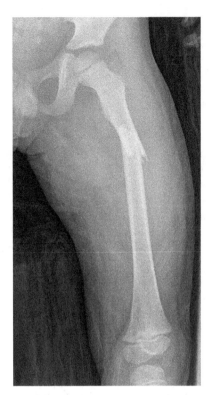

Figure 19–4. Femoral shaft fracture in a child. (*Used with permission from Katharine Hopkins, MD.*)

should be repeated frequently, especially after splinting or other manipulation of the involved extremity.

Imaging

Routine anteroposterior and lateral views are usually adequate in demonstrating the fracture (Figs. 19–4 and 19–5). Pelvis and knee views should be included as there is a significant incidence of associated injury. In addition, stress fractures of the femoral shaft may not be visualized on these routine views, and up to half of associated femoral neck fractures may be missed by plain films.[21]

Associated Injuries

Femoral shaft fractures are frequently associated with additional significant injuries. Associated significant injuries have been shown to occur in up to 80% of bilateral femur fractures and 40% of unilateral femoral shaft fractures.[14] A careful and systematic evaluation should be done on patients with femur fractures to evaluate for potential multiple injuries. Ipsilateral femoral neck fractures are associated with up to 9% of femoral shaft fractures but may be missed in 30% to 50% of cases.[13,21–23] The most common mechanism of injury in these concurrent fractures is an axillary directed force against the knee while sitting, as is commonly seen in motor vehicle collisions when the knee strikes the dashboard.[22]

In pediatric patients where femoral shaft fractures are more common, polytrauma is present in approximately 20% of cases. However, concurrent ipsilateral femoral neck

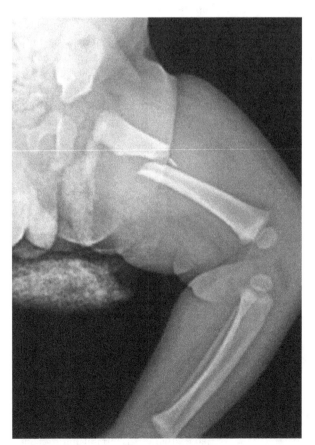

Figure 19–5. Femoral shaft fracture in an infant.

fractures, seen commonly in adults, are much less prevalent, being found in less than 1% of cases. The majority of associated injuries includes other fractures, abdominal injuries, and closed head injuries.

The femoral shaft has a rich blood supply. In adults, fractures are associated with an average blood loss of 25% of blood volume. In children, however, isolated femoral fractures are rarely associated with significant blood loss. Particularly in children, bleeding into the thigh from a closed femoral shaft fracture is not typically enough to cause hypotension.

Associated sciatic nerve injuries are rarely encountered with these fractures secondary to the protective surrounding musculature. The incidence of sciatic or peroneal nerve injury in the setting of a femoral shaft fracture is 2% after a blunt mechanism but increases to 9% after a gunshot wound.

Treatment

The emergency management of this injury begins in the prehospital setting. The extremity should be immobilized in a traction splint or a pneumatic antishock garment. Early application of traction splints provides immobilization, distracts the fracture, reduces incidence of fat embolism, and decreases the potential space for bleeding. The Sager traction splint is illustrated in Chapter 1. In the presence of a sciatic nerve injury, a splint should be placed without traction to avoid further injury to the nerve. Traction splints should not be used in grossly contaminated open fractures, concurrent ipsilateral hip dislocations, or fracture dislocations of the ipsilateral knee or ankle. Pain medications should be provided early, and emergent referral and admission are indicated. Intramedullary nailing is the preferred method for definitive treatment of femoral shaft fractures in adult patients (Fig. 19-6). This treatment has been shown to be superior to other techniques regardless of mechanism of injury and has also been shown to be effective for atypical fractures associated with long-term bisphosphonate use or metastatic disease. Advantages of intramedullary nailing include early patient mobilization, minimally invasive operative technique, reduced delayed bone healing, and low complication rate. This technique can be employed in virtually any fracture along the length of the femoral shaft, including periprosthetic fractures and severely comminuted fractures. However, there are some data suggesting that initial external fixation followed by delayed intramedullary nailing may be preferred in patients with contaminant head, thoracic, or abdominal injury. Retrograde nailing is usually reserved for the treatment of femoral shaft fractures with ipsilateral femoral neck or intertrochanteric fractures, patients with bilateral femur fractures, and the morbidly obese.

The management of open fractures is outlined in Chapter 1. Open fractures of the femoral shaft require emergent operative debridement. Grade I and II open fractures can be treated with immediate closed femoral nailing, with infection as low as 2%. There are conflicting data, and no universal agreement on external fixation versus intramedullary nailing for severe grade IIIB and IIIC open fractures.

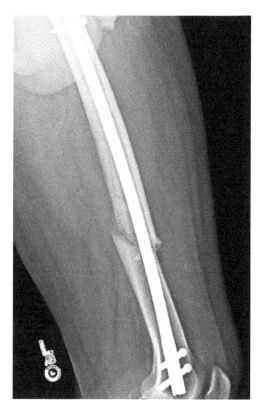

Figure 19–6. Locked intramedullary nailing of a femur fracture.

Management of pediatric femoral shaft fractures is variable, and debate continues as to which fixation methods are most appropriate in different situations. Spica casting is still common in children younger than 5 years, whereas the preferred treatment in children ages 5 to 11 years is flexible intramedullary nails. Locked intramedullary nails are usually reserved for children older than 12 years. Plating is commonly used in unstable fractures, and external fixation is favored in situations involving extensive soft-tissue injury of the thigh. Timing of fracture fixation in patients with multiple injuries remains controversial and an area of continued interest.

Complications

High-energy femoral shaft fractures are often complicated by a variety of other systemic injuries. Both the severity of the fracture itself and the degree of polytrauma are closely associated with mortality. Unilateral fractures associated with head and abdominal injuries have mortality rates as high as 45% and 52%, respectively. Thigh compartment syndrome is a rare complication of femoral shaft fracture.

General complication rates related to the repair of femoral shaft fractures are less than 5%. The most common complications are intraoperative fractures of the femoral neck and postoperative infection requiring surgical revision, each with a rate of 1.4%. Other potential but uncommon complications include delayed union, nonunion, malrotation, and hardware failure.

THIGH SOFT-TISSUE INJURY

THIGH COMPARTMENT SYNDROME

Compartment syndrome of the thigh is a rare clinical entity. It occurs less frequently than compartment syndrome of the calf due to the thigh's ability to accommodate larger volumes of fluid. Of the three compartments within the thigh—anterior, posterior, and medial—the anterior compartment is most commonly affected (Fig. 19–1).[48,49]

Mechanism of Injury

Blunt trauma accounts for approximately 90% of cases of acute thigh compartment syndrome, with motor vehicle collisions being the most common traumatic mechanism.[20] Additionally, many causes of thigh compartment syndrome have been identified, including femoral shaft fractures, muscle contusion or rupture, revascularization injury, external limb compression, and even anticoagulant-induced bleeding into the thigh.[4,20,49-53] In all cases, the underlying pathophysiologic mechanism is similar to that of other compartment syndromes, in which increased pressure within the limited compartmental space exceeds perfusion pressure, leading to circulatory compromise.

Examination

Like other compartment syndromes, the patient will present with severe pain that is exacerbated by passive stretch of the muscles within the involved compartment. The compartment is often swollen, tense, and exquisitely tender to palpation. Late findings may include sensorimotor deficits distal to the thigh. Anesthesia or paresthesia may be an early indication of nerve ischemia, whereas muscle paralysis is often a late sign indicating irreversible muscle and nerve damage.[4,51,54]

Similar mechanisms of injury and clinical symptoms often make compartment syndrome of the thigh difficult to distinguish from severe contusion. Therefore, the diagnosis is often made both clinically and with the aid of intracompartmental pressure measurements.[4,20]

Imaging

Although CT, MRI, and ultrasound have been studied for the diagnosis of compartment syndrome, their use is currently limited and may delay definitive management.[51]

Associated Injuries

The high-energy trauma often involved in thigh compartment syndrome will result in many soft-tissue and musculoskeletal injuries. Femur fractures are associated with up to 44% of cases of thigh compartment syndrome, interestingly with almost one-quarter of these being open fractures. Severe complications, including neurologic deficits, infection, and renal failure are very common. Mortality rates as high as 47% have been reported, most often due to polytrauma and infection.[20]

Treatment

The definitive treatment for thigh compartment syndrome is emergent surgical fasciotomy. The primary cause of poor outcomes from compartment syndrome is a delay of treatment.[51] The generally accepted indication is a difference between diastolic pressure and the measured compartment pressure of less than 30 mm Hg, although this is the subject of continued debate.[4,20,51] Successful outcomes with conservative management involving bed rest, frequent compartment pressure measurements, cooling, and serial clinical examinations have been described in the absence of fracture.[51,55] Nevertheless, early fasciotomy is important to prevent complications of delayed diagnosis, and early surgical consult should be obtained in any patient suspected of having thigh compartment syndrome regardless of compartmental pressures.

QUADRICEPS CONTUSION

Quadriceps contusions, after muscle strains, are the second most common type of quadriceps injury in athletics, comprising approximately 14% of all thigh injuries in high school sports and 19% of all muscle injuries in professional soccer.[54,56,57]

Mechanism of Injury

The usual mechanism of injury is a direct blow to the quadriceps muscles, often from an opponent's knee or sporting equipment.[56,57] This compresses the underlying muscle and soft tissues against the femur, causing myofiber and capillary rupture and the formation of a hematoma.[58]

Examination

The patient will often report a traumatic mechanism and complain of localized pain. The ability to play following injury, as well as the time interval between injury and presentation, are important indicators of injury severity and prognosis.[54] Physical examination will reveal tenderness to palpation, swelling, and often ecchymosis at the site of injury (Fig. 19–7). They may develop difficulty with knee extension.[57] If signs such as pulselessness, paresthesia, or paralysis suggestive of compartment syndrome are found, early surgical consultation should be considered and intracompartmental pressures obtained.

A clinically and prognostically useful classification system grades quadriceps contusions as *mild, moderate,* and *severe.*[57,59] In a mild contusion, the patient has localized tenderness, no alteration of gait, and knee motion without pain up to at least 90 degrees of flexion. In a moderate contusion, the patient displays swelling and a tender muscle mass.

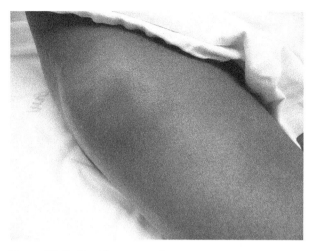

Figure 19–7. Quadriceps contusion.

Knee motion is restricted to <90 degrees, and the patient walks with an antalgic gait. The patient is unable to climb stairs or arise from a chair without considerable discomfort. In patients with severe contusions, the thigh is markedly tender, swollen, and indurated. Knee motion is severely limited (<45 degrees), and there is either a severe limp or the patient is unable to ambulate. Average disability times are progressively longer with increased severity: 13 days for mild, 19 days for moderate, and 21 days for severe.

Imaging

The diagnosis of quadriceps contusions is usually a clinical one. However, imaging may be useful in distinguishing contusions from avulsions and strains, especially when the presentation is subacute. Plain radiographs are usually unremarkable. Ultrasound and MRI are sensitive indicators of soft-tissue injury; however, the availability of ultrasound in the emergency department makes it particularly useful in this circumstance. Hematoma on ultrasound will appear as interruption in the normal architecture of the muscle with localized hypoechogenicity.

Treatment

Treatment of thigh contusions is often approached in a staged manner from the time of injury. The immediate goal is to control propagation of the hematoma by immobilizing the knee of the contused thigh in 120 degrees of flexion for as long as 2 to 48 hours. This can be done by an elastic wrap or an adjustable brace and should be done as soon as possible after the injury occurs. Ice and compression should also be employed during this time, and the patient should ambulate with crutches. In one study involving naval athletes who received immobilization within 10 minutes of injury followed by range-of-motion stretching as described in the following paragraph, the average time from injury to return of unrestricted full athletic activity without disability was 3.5 days.

After the brace is removed, the patient should engage in active, pain-free, range-of-motion stretching of the involved thigh. Once the patient is able to attain full, pain-free range of motion in the ipsilateral knee, functional rehabilitation should begin, and the use of crutches may be discontinued. In athletes, the use of a thigh pad to prevent recurrent injury to the site of the contusion should be encouraged.

The effect of nonsteroidal anti-inflammatory drugs (NSAIDs) on muscle injuries is believed to be paradoxical, with early use leading to improvement but sustained use leading to impairment in functional capacity and histology. There is a theoretical risk of further bleeding risk if given acutely. NSAIDs may diminish pain as well as risk for myositis ossificans. Corticosteroids are not an effective adjunctive therapy for thigh contusions.

Complications

Myositis ossificans occurs as a complication in up to 17% of muscle contusions. It should be suspected if symptoms worsen 2 to 3 weeks after the initial injury. Risk factors for development of myositis ossificans include associated knee effusion, severe injury, and delay in treatment. Compartment syndrome is also a potential complication, especially in contusions with large hematoma formation.

MUSCLE STRAINS AND RUPTURE

Adductor Strains
Mechanism of Injury

Adductor muscle strains are the most common groin injury in athletes. The sports with highest prevalence of this injury include ice hockey and soccer, where strong eccentric contraction of the adductor muscle group is required. This injury is usually caused by forced abduction of the thigh. Decreased adductor strength and range of motion are both risk factors for the development of adductor strains.

Examination

The patient complains of pain that is localized to the groin region. With incomplete rupture, the pain is made worse by passive abduction of the thigh and is accentuated by active adduction against resistance. Ecchymosis may be present (Fig. 19–8). If complete rupture has occurred, the examiner will often see bunching of the muscle along the medial aspect of the thigh near the groin.

Imaging

Imaging is not necessary unless the diagnosis is in question. Ultrasound may be used to diagnose adductor muscle or tendon tears but not strains. MRI can be used to confirm a muscle strain or tear and has prognostic value but is generally not needed for the diagnosis. Pelvis radiographs should be obtained if there is concern for avulsion injury at the origin of the adductor longus.

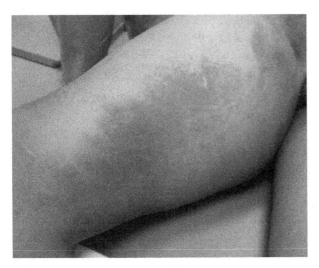

Figure 19–8. Pattern and degree of ecchymosis raises concern for adductor muscle strain or rupture.

Treatment

Adductor strains should be treated with relative rest, ice, and short-term use of NSAIDs, followed by physical therapy. A return to sports is allowed once the patient has regained at least 70% of their former adductor strength and full, pain-free range of motion. This process can take approximately 4 to 8 weeks.

Chronic adductor strains may require up to 6 months of physical therapy. Failure to respond to prolonged physical therapy may be an indication for surgical referral for tenotomy.[65]

Complete rupture of the tendinous insertion of the adductor warrants surgical referral for repair.

Hamstring Strain
Mechanism of Injury

Hamstring strains are common in runners, water skiers, and hurdlers, as well as in other sports such as soccer that involve jumping and kicking. The mechanism is usually a sudden contraction when hamstrings are at maximal length (flexion at hip and extension at the knee). Prior hamstring injury is a major risk factor for hamstring strain. Other potential risk factors include patient age, lack of hamstring flexibility, strength imbalance, fatigued muscles, and increased peak quadriceps torque.[68,69]

Examination

The patient will present with acute onset of posterior thigh pain. There will be pain with weight bearing and an antalgic, stiff-legged gait that usually inhibits athletic activity.

Examination should be performed with the patient in the prone position with the knee flexed. There is usually tenderness to the posterior thigh to palpation. Severe injuries may be accompanied by ecchymosis in the posterior thigh, but this may be absent on acute presentation. The examination should include thorough palpation of the entire muscle belly searching for a defect that represents a tear. Complete tears of the hamstring musculature are rare.[57,70]

Knee flexion should also be tested. If there is less than 30% strength compared to the contralateral uninjured limb and significant posterior thigh or knee ecchymosis, consider an MRI to evaluate for possible proximal hamstring rupture.[68]

Imaging

Usually, the diagnosis of a mild strain is clinical and no imaging is necessary. Plain films are useful in more severe injuries to identify whether avulsion from ischial tuberosity has occurred. In the case of suspected rupture or avulsion, MRI is an important tool that may affect surgical decision making.[68] Some studies have shown that the size of the strain's appearance on MRI may correlate to time lost from sporting activity.[70,71]

Treatment

The acute treatment for noninsertional hamstring strains includes rest and rehabilitation, ice, compression, and elevation, usually for 3 to 7 days. The goal of this treatment is to limit the initial inflammatory response, control hemorrhage and edema, and improve pain.[57,68] NSAIDs are also used during this time. Gradual mobilization as tolerated is made over a period of 2 to 6 weeks, depending on injury severity, and crutches may be used initially until pain-free ambulation is possible.

The risk of hamstring strain recurrence is high, with athletes shown to have 20 times the risk of recurrence in the first 3 weeks back in play compared to their noninjured peers. A progressive agility and trunk stabilization program may reduce the reinjury rate. Stretching has not been definitely shown to improve recurrence rates. To avoid reinjury, the patient should be advised to avoid early return to sports until they are appropriately rehabilitated.[70]

Thigh Muscle Rupture

The rectus femoris, adductors, and hamstrings can rupture anywhere from their origin to their insertion. The patient is often misdiagnosed as having a contusion, so there is a delay in diagnosis. Surgery is more complicated and less effective on chronic ruptures, stressing the importance of timely diagnosis. The telltale signs and symptoms develop with time and may not be present in the acute setting. This emphasizes the need for appropriate instructions to follow up if the mechanism suggests tendon rupture. Recommend close follow-up to patients if they develop a large ecchymosis or a muscle bulge, or if they have weakness. Rupture can occur when a tendon is suddenly eccentrically loaded. For example, hamstring ruptures usually result from sudden flexion at the hip with knee extension. These injuries are more common in water skiers, and they can also occur if a patient slips on an icy surface with his/her leg outstretched.

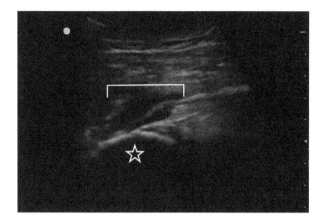

Figure 19–9. Complete hamstring rupture. Curvilinear ultrasound probe, long axis view with gap present between proximal hamstring tendon fibers (*bracket*) and ischial tuberosity (*star*).

Educate patients to look for the development of a large ecchymosis or a mass (suggesting the tendon/muscle is retracted) and weakness.

Examination

The examination should include inspection for ecchymosis or deformity, palpation of bone attachment site, assessment for the presence of an intact tendon bundle, or appreciation of a palpable defect detected during strength testing.

Imaging

For suspected proximal thigh tendon rupture, consider a plain AP radiograph of the pelvis to evaluate for fracture or avulsion fractures. If normal, patients may still have a partial or complete tendon rupture. Consider using ultrasound in the acute and subacute setting to assess for local hematoma, muscle tear, tendon bundle attachment, or complete rupture (Fig. 19–9). MRI in the outpatient setting can confirm the diagnosis.

Treatment

A minimum of 6 weeks is needed for healing when partial rupture involving the muscles of the thigh occurs. Activity is permitted to the tolerance of pain; however, avoid sports or vigorous activity. Ambulation with crutches and a gradual return to activity is advised. Patients with complete ruptures should be made nonweight bearing and subsequently referred to orthopedics. Surgical treatment is indicated for total or near-total hamstring muscle rupture. It is also considered in cases of bony avulsion of the ischial tuberosity when the avulsed fragment is displaced >2 cm. Surgical outcomes are superior when performed in the acute phase (less than 4 weeks from injury).

Fascial Hernia

The muscles of the thigh are invested in fascial sheaths. The fascial sheaths along the anterior and lateral aspects of the thigh are thinner just anterior to the iliotibial band.

The patient may present to the ED with a complaint of a small palpable mass that appears when the quadriceps is contracted and disappears when the muscle is relaxed. Point-of-care musculoskeletal ultrasound may reveal a mushroom-shaped muscle bulging through the fascia. Treatment is usually not necessary; however, if the symptoms warrant, surgical repair may be indicated.

Myositis Ossificans Traumatica

Myositis ossificans traumatica is a common condition in which a non-neoplastic ectopic calcium deposit is found in soft tissue at a site of prior trauma and hematoma. Myositis ossificans occurs as a complication after muscle contusion injuries in 9% to 17% of cases. This condition is commonly seen in the anterior thigh muscles after a moderate or severe contusion. The patient is usually a young athlete playing a contact sport. In most cases of myositis ossificans, the involvement is limited to the middle third of the thigh; however, in some, it extends into the proximal third. Cases of myositis ossificans in the adductor muscles have also been reported. Myositis ossificans can also be congenital, occur after surgery, present as a complication of paraplegia or prolonged immobilization, or be seen in the setting of serious disease such as clotting factor deficiencies. It can also be mistaken for osteosarcoma.

Examination

Myositis ossificans is usually diagnosed 2 to 4 weeks after injury to the thigh. Palpation may reveal a firm and tender mass in the soft tissue. The patient may have limited range of motion due to pain or mass effect.

Imaging

The radiograph usually shows evidence of irregularly shaped heterotopic bone at 2 to 4 weeks post injury (Fig. 19–10). Three forms of myositis ossificans have been described: (1) a type with a stalked connection to the adjacent femur, (2) a periosteal type with continuity between the heterotopic bone and the adjacent femur, and (3) a broad base type with a portion of the ectopic bone projecting into the quadriceps muscle. CT or MRI scans are especially helpful in distinguishing this condition from oncologic causes or in identifying neurovascular entrapments.

Treatment

The emergency physician should be aware of preventive measures to avoid the development of myositis ossificans. The patient with a quadriceps contusion should be cautioned against early active use of the quadriceps and forceful passive flexion of the knee. NSAIDs may decrease incidence by inhibiting mast cell degranulation. Once present, myositis ossificans is usually not severely disabling, although some patients may require surgical excision due to pain once the bone has matured. Once the diagnosis is established, appropriate referral and follow-up are indicated.

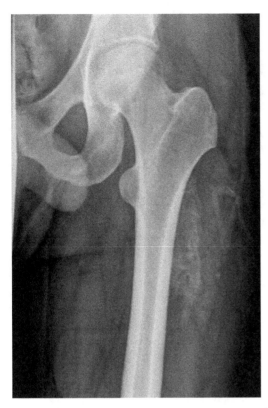

Figure 19–10. Myositis ossificans. (*Used with permission from Erik Foss, MD.*)

REFERENCES

1. Winquist RA, Hansen ST Jr. Comminuted fractures of the femoral shaft treated by intramedullary nailing. *Orthop Clin North Am.* 1980;11(3):633–648.

2. Metsemakers W-J, Roels N, Belmans A, Reynders P, Nijs S. Risk factors for nonunion after intramedullary nailing of femoral shaft fractures: remaining controversies. *Injury.* 2015; 46(8):1601–1607.

3. Bell A, Templeman D, Weinlein JC. Nonunion of the femur and tibia: an update. *Orthop Clin North Am.* 2016;47(2): 365–375.

4. Stein MJ, Kang C, Ball V. Emergency department evaluation and treatment of acute hip and thigh pain. *Emerg Med Clin North Am.* 2015;33(2):327–343.

5. Shane E, Burr D, Abrahamsen B, et al. Atypical subtrochanteric and diaphyseal femoral fractures: second report of a task force of the American Society for Bone and Mineral Research. *J Bone Miner Res.* 2014;29(1):1–23.

6. Abrahamsen B, Einhorn TA. Beyond a reasonable doubt? Bisphosphonates and atypical femur fractures. *Bone.* 2012; 50(5):1196–1200.

7. Donnelly E, Saleh A, Unnanuntana A, Lane JM. Atypical femoral fractures: epidemiology, etiology, and patient management. *Curr Opin Support Palliat Care.* 2012;6(3): 348–354.

8. Lee S, Yin RV, Hirpara H, et al. Increased risk for atypical fractures associated with bisphosphonate use. *Fam Pract.* 2015;32(3):276–281.

9. Giusti A, Hamdy NAT, Dekkers OM, Ramautar SR, Dijkstra S, Papapoulos SE. Atypical fractures and bisphosphonate therapy: a cohort study of patients with femoral fracture with radiographic adjudication of fracture site and features. *Bone.* 2011;48(5):966–971.

10. Schilcher J, Koeppen V, Aspenberg P, Michaëlsson K. Risk of atypical femoral fracture during and after bisphosphonate use. *N Engl J Med.* 2014;371(10):974–976.

11. Adler RA, El-Hajj Fuleihan G, Bauer DC, et al. Managing osteoporosis in patients on long-term bisphosphonate treatment: report of a task force of the American Society for Bone and Mineral Research. *J Bone Miner Res.* 2016;31(1):16–35.

12. Salminen ST, Pihlajamaki HK, Avikainen VJ, Böstman OM. Population based epidemiologic and morphologic study of femoral shaft fractures. *Clin Orthop.* 2000;372:241–249.

13. Enninghorst N, McDougall D, Evans JA, Sisak K, Balogh ZJ. Population-based epidemiology of femur shaft fractures. *J Trauma Acute Care Surg.* 2013;74(6):1516–1520.

14. Willett K, Al-Khateeb H, Kotnis R, Bouamra O, Lecky F. Risk of mortality: the relationship with associated injuries and fracture treatment methods in patients with unilateral or bilateral femoral shaft fractures. *J Trauma.* 2010;69(2):405–410.

15. Loder RT, O'Donnell PW, Feinberg JR. Epidemiology and mechanisms of femur fractures in children. *J Pediatr Orthop.* 2006;26(5):561–566.

16. Blatz AM, Gillespie CW, Katcher A, Matthews A, Oetgen ME. Factors associated with nonaccidental trauma evaluation among patients below 36 months old presenting with femur fractures at a level-1 pediatric trauma center. *J Pediatr Orthop.* 2016.

17. Baldwin K, Pandya NK, Wolfgruber H, Drummond DS, Hosalkar HS. Femur fractures in the pediatric population: abuse or accidental trauma? *Clin Orthop.* 2010;469(3):798–804.

18. Hui C, Joughin E, Goldstein S, et al. Femoral fractures in children younger than three years: the role of nonaccidental injury. *J Pediatr Orthop.* 2008;28(3):297–302.

19. Scherl SA, Miller L, Lively N, Russinoff S, Sullivan CM, Tornetta P III. Accidental and nonaccidental femur fractures in children. *Clin Orthop.* 2000;(376):96–105.

20. Ojike NI, Roberts CS, Giannoudis PV. Compartment syndrome of the thigh: a systematic review. *Injury.* 2010;41(2): 133–136.

21. Boulton CL, Pollak AN. Special topic: ipsilateral femoral neck and shaft fractures—does evidence give us the answer? *Injury.* 2015;46(3):478–483.

22. Hak DJ, Mauffrey C, Hake M, Hammerberg EM, Stahel PF. Ipsilateral femoral neck and shaft fractures: current diagnostic and treatment strategies. *Orthopedics.* 2015;38(4):247–251.

23. Cannada LK, Viehe T, Cates CA, et al. A retrospective review of high-energy femoral neck-shaft fractures. *J Orthop Trauma.* 2009;23(4):254–260.

24. Caldwell L, Chan CM, Sanders JO, Gorczyca JT. Detection of femoral neck fractures in pediatric patients with femoral shaft fractures. *J Pediatr Orthop.* 2016.

25. Song KS, Ramnani K, Cho CH, Bae KC, Lee KJ, Son ES. Ipsilateral femoral neck and shaft fracture in children: a report of two cases and a literature review. *J Orthop Traumatol.* 2013;14(2):147–154.

26. Dodd A, Paolucci EO, Parsons D. Paediatric femoral shaft fractures: what are the concomitant injuries? *Injury.* 2013; 44:1502–1506. doi:10.1016/j.injury.2013.02.012.

27. Chu RS, Browne GJ, Lam LT. Are children with femoral fracture haemodynamically unstable? *Emerg Med*. 2003;15(5–6):453–458.

28. Unal VS, Gulcek M, Unveren Z, Karakuyu A, Ucaner A. Blood loss evaluation in children under the age of 11 with femoral shaft fractures patients with isolated versus multiple injuries. *J Trauma*. 2006;60(1):224–226.

29. Hoppe S, Keel MJB, Rueff N, Rhoma I, Roche S, Maqungo S. Early versus delayed application of Thomas splints in patients with isolated femur shaft fractures: the benefits quantified. *Injury*. 2015;46(12):2410–2412.

30. Lee C, Porter KM. Prehospital management of lower limb fractures. *Emerg Med J*. 2005;22(9):660–663.

31. Wild M, Gehrmann S, Jungbluth P, et al. Treatment strategies for intramedullary nailing of femoral shaft fractures. *Orthopedics*. 2010;33(10):726.

32. Streubel PN, Gardner MJ, Ricci WM. Management of femur shaft fractures in obese patients. *Orthop Clin North Am*. 2011;42(1):21–35.

33. Rhorer AS. Percutaneous/minimally invasive techniques in treatment of femoral shaft fractures with an intramedullary nail. *J Orthop Trauma*. 2009;23(5 suppl):S2–S5. doi:10.1097/BOT.0b013e31819f2569.

34. Lee K-J, Yoo JJ, Oh K-J, et al. Surgical outcome of intramedullary nailing in patients with complete atypical femoral fracture: a multicenter retrospective study. *Injury*. 2017;48(4):941–945.

35. Tanaka T, Imanishi J, Charoenlap C, Choong PFM. Intramedullary nailing has sufficient durability for metastatic femoral fractures. *World J Surg Oncol*. 2016;14:80. doi:10.1186/s12957-016-0836-2.

36. Elmi A, Rohani AR, Tabrizi A, Esmaili S-M. Comparison of outcome of femoral shaft fracture fixation with intramedullary nail in elderly patient and patients younger than 60 years old. *Arch Bone Joint Surg*. 2014;2(2):103–105.

37. Tuttle MS, Smith WR, Williams AE, et al. Safety and efficacy of damage control external fixation versus early definitive stabilization for femoral shaft fractures in the multiple-injured patient. *J Trauma*. 2009;67(3):602–605.

38. Papadokostakis G, Papakostidis C, Dimitriou R, Giannoudis PV. The role and efficacy of retrograding nailing for the treatment of diaphyseal and distal femoral fractures: a systematic review of the literature. *Injury*. 2005;36(7):813–822.

39. Russell, Kregor PJ, Jarrett CA, Zlowodzki M. Complicated femoral shaft fractures. *Orthop Clin North Am*. 2002;33(1):127–142.

40. Mitchell SE, Keating JF, Robinson CM. The treatment of open femoral fractures with bone loss. *J Bone Joint Surg Br*. 2010;92(12):1678–1684.

41. Kovar FM, Jaindl M, Schuster R, Endler G, Platzer P. Incidence and analysis of open fractures of the midshaft and distal femur. *Wien Klin Wochenschr*. 2013;125(13–14):396–401.

42. Madhuri V, Dutt V, Gahukamble AD, Tharyan P. Interventions for treating femoral shaft fractures in children and adolescents. *Cochrane Database Syst Rev*. 2014;29(7):CD009076.

43. Jevsevar DS, Shea KG, Murray JN, Sevarino KS. AAOS Clinical Practice Guideline on the Treatment of Pediatric Diaphyseal Femur Fractures. *J Am Acad Orthop Surg*. 2015;23(12):e101.

44. Li Y, Hedequist DJ. Submuscular plating of pediatric femur fracture. *J Am Acad Orthop Surg*. 2012;20(9):596–603.

45. Kuremsky MA, Frick SL. Advances in the surgical management of pediatric femoral shaft fractures. *Curr Opin Pediatr*. 2007;19(1):51–57.

46. Nahm NJ, Vallier HA. Timing of definitive treatment of femoral shaft fractures in patients with multiple injuries: a systematic review of randomized and nonrandomized trials. *J Trauma Acute Care Surg*. 2012;73(5):1046–1063.

47. Li A-B, Zhang W-J, Guo W-J, Wang X-H, Jin H-M, Zhao Y-M. Reamed versus unreamed intramedullary nailing for the treatment of femoral fractures: a meta-analysis of prospective randomized controlled trials. *Medicine*. 2016;95(29):e4248.

48. Mithofer K, Lhowe DW, Vrahas MS, Altman DT, Altman GT. Clinical spectrum of acute compartment syndrome of the thigh and its relation to associated injuries. *Clin Orthop*. 2004;(425):223–229.

49. King TW, Lerman OZ, Carter JJ, Warren SM. Exertional compartment syndrome of the thigh: a rare diagnosis and literature review. *J Emerg Med*. 2010;39(2):e93–e99.

50. Suzuki T, Moirmura N, Kawai K, Sugiyama M. Arterial injury associated with acute compartment syndrome of the thigh following blunt trauma. *Injury*. 2005;36(1):151–159.

51. McCaffrey DD, Clarke J, Bunn J, McCormack MJ. Acute compartment syndrome of the anterior thigh in the absence of fracture secondary to sporting trauma. *J Trauma*. 2009;66(4):1238–1242.

52. Limberg RM, Dougherty C, Mallon WK. Enoxaparin-induced bleeding resulting in compartment syndrome of the thigh: a case report. *J Emerg Med*. 2011;41(1):e1–e4.

53. Masini BD, Racusin AW, Wenke JC, Gerlinger TL, Hsu JR. Acute compartment syndrome of the thigh in combat casualties. *J Surg Orthop Adv*. 2013;22(01):42–49.

54. Trojian TH. Muscle contusion (thigh). *Clin Sports Med*. 2013;32(2):317–324.

55. Riede U, Schmid MR, Romero J. Conservative treatment of an acute compartment syndrome of the thigh. *Arch Orthop Trauma Surg*. 2006;127(4):269–275.

56. Kary JM. Diagnosis and management of quadriceps strains and contusions. *Curr Rev Musculoskelet Med*. 2010;3(1–4):26–31.

57. Lamplot JD, Matava MJ. Thigh injuries in American football. *Am J Orthop*. 2016;45(6):E308–E318.

58. Hayashi D, Hamilton B, Guermazi A, de Villiers R, Crema MD, Roemer FW. Traumatic injuries of thigh and calf muscles in athletes: role and clinical relevance of MR imaging and ultrasound. *Insights Imaging*. 2012;3(6):591–601.

59. Jackson DW, Feagin JA. Quadriceps contusions in young athletes. Relation of severity of injury to treatment and prognosis. *J Bone Joint Surg Am*. 1973;55(1):95–105.

60. Ryan JB, Wheeler JH, Hopkinson WJ, Arciero RA, Kolakowski KR. Quadriceps contusions. West Point update. *Am J Sports Med*. 1991;19(3):299–304.

61. Pasta G, Nanni G, Molini L, Bianchi S. Sonography of the quadriceps muscle: examination technique, normal anatomy, and traumatic lesions. *J Ultrasound*. 2010;13(2):76–84.

62. Aronen JG, Garrick JG, Chronister RD, McDevitt ER. Quadriceps contusions: clinical results of immediate immobilization in 120 degrees of knee flexion. *Clin J Sport Med*. 2006;16(5):383–387.

63. Prisk V, Huard J. Muscle injuries and repair: the role of prostaglandins and inflammation. *Histol Histopathol.* 2003; 18(4):1243–1256.

64. Joglekar SB, Rehman S. Delayed onset thigh compartment syndrome secondary to contusion. *Orthopedics.* 2009;32(8): 610–612.

65. Morelli V, Weaver V. Groin injuries and groin pain in athletes: part 1. *Primary Care.* 2005;32(1):163–183.

66. Tyler TF, Silvers HJ, Gerhardt MB, Nicholas SJ. Groin injuries in sports medicine. *Sports Health.* 2010;2(3): 231–236.

67. Serner A, Tol JL, Jomaah N, et al. Diagnosis of acute groin injuries: a prospective study of 110 athletes. *Am J Sports Med.* 2015;43(8):1857–1864.

68. Ali K, Leland JM. Hamstring strains and tears in the athlete. *Clin Sports Med.* 2012;31(2):263–272.

69. Ahmad CS, Redler LH, Ciccotti MG, Maffulli N, Longo UG, Bradley J. Evaluation and management of hamstring injuries. *Am J Sports Med.* 2013;41(12):2933–2947.

70. Sherry M. Examination and treatment of hamstring related injuries. *Sports Health.* 2011;4(2):107–114.

71. Cohen SB, Towers JD, Zoga A, et al. Hamstring injuries in professional football players: magnetic resonance imaging correlation with return to play. *Sports Health.* 2011;3(5):423–430.

72. Drezner JA. Practical management: hamstring muscle injuries. *Clin J Sport Med.* 2003;13(1):48–52.

73. Çarli AB, Turgut H, Bozkurt Y. Choosing the right imaging method in muscle hernias: musculoskeletal ultrasonography. *J Sports Sci.* 2015;33(18):1919–1921.

74. Sokunbi G, Fowler JR, Ilyas AM, Moyer RA. A case report of myositis ossificans traumatica in the adductor magnus. *Clin J Sport Med.* 2010;20(6):495–496.

75. Alonso A, Hekeik P, Adams R. Predicting a recovery time from the initial assessment of a quadriceps contusion injury. *Aust J Physiother.* 2000;46(3):167–177.

76. Goyal K, Pettis CR, Bancroft AE, Wasyliw CW, Scherer KF. Myositis ossificans in the thigh of a lacrosse player. *Orthopedics.* 2015;38(8):468, 515–518.

CHAPTER 20

Knee

Michael C. Bond, MD

INTRODUCTION

The knee is a complex joint that is commonly injured. The accurate diagnosis of knee injuries requires a rather detailed knowledge of anatomy.

The knee is composed of three articulations: the medial and lateral condylar joints and the patellofemoral joint. The knee is capable of a wide range of motion, including flexion, extension, internal and external rotation, abduction, and adduction. In full extension, no rotary motion is permitted as the ligamentous structures are taut. This tightening with extension is referred to as "the screwing home mechanism." Beyond 20-degree flexion, the supporting ligaments are relaxed and axial rotation is permitted. At 90-degree flexion, there is a maximum of laxity allowing up to 40 degrees of rotation.

Examination

The surface anatomy, including the major muscles surrounding the knee, can be easily visualized and palpated. With the knee extended, the large, dominant vastus medialis and the smaller vastus lateralis can be visualized and palpated (Fig. 20–1A). The larger medialis pulls the patella medially during extension, thus preventing lateral subluxation or dislocation. The sartorius, gracilis, and semitendinosus muscles are palpable medially along their common insertion on the tibia, referred to as the pes anserinus (Fig. 20–1B). Laterally, the iliotibial tract and the tendon of the biceps femoris can be palpated.

The bony anatomy of the knee can also be palpated. The patella and patellar tendon are palpated along the anterior surface of the knee. Medially, the medial tibial plateau and medial femoral condyle are noted. The adductor tubercle extends posteriorly from the medial femoral condyle and can be palpated. The joint line can be readily located by noting the natural depression just medial and lateral to the patellar tendon with the knee in flexion. These indentations overlie the articular surfaces.

The patellar tendon inserts on the anterior tibial tubercle, which is easily palpable. The lateral tibial plateau is located just lateral to the tubercle. Posterior and lateral to the plateau is the fibular head, palpable just inferior to the lateral femoral condyle.

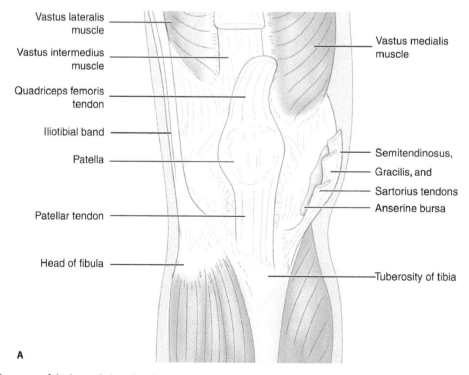

A

Figure 20–1. Anatomy of the knee. **A.** Anterior view.

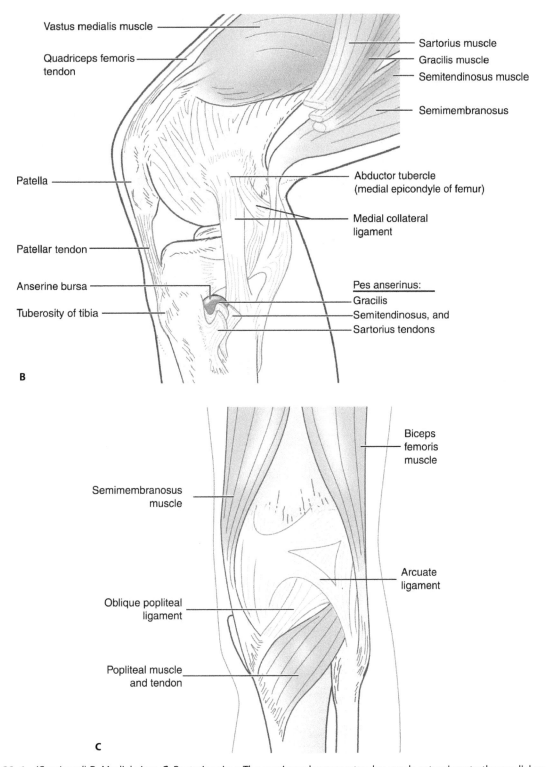

Figure 20–1. *(Continued) B.* Medial view. *C.* Posterior view. The semimembranosus tendon sends extensions to the medial meniscus and to the posterior aspect of the capsule. *(continued)*

The medial meniscus is palpable along the medial joint line as the knee is internally rotated and gently extended. The lateral meniscus is not palpable, although injury to this structure reliably produces joint line tenderness. The menisci of the knee migrate anteriorly with extension. The medial meniscus is less mobile because of its attachment to the medial collateral ligament (MCL). With flexion, there is posterior migration of both menisci, secondary to the pull of the (medial) semimembranosus and the (lateral) popliteus.

The supporting structures surrounding the knee can be divided into two groups: static (ligaments) stabilizers and dynamic (muscles) stabilizers. The static stabilizers can be further divided into medial, lateral, and posterior compartments.

The medial compartment static stabilizer is the MCL (Fig. 20-1B). This capsular structure, also known as the tibial collateral ligament, is the primary medial stabilizer against a valgus or rotary stress. It inserts on the medial femoral and tibial condyles. A deep portion of the ligament inserts on the medial meniscus. The MCL can also be divided into anterior, middle, and posterior components. The posterior component merges with the oblique popliteal ligament. The semimembranosus tendon inserts on the oblique popliteal ligament, adding stability and posterior mobility to the ligament as well as the medial meniscus during flexion (Fig. 20-1C).

The MCL is the most commonly injured ligament of the knee. This ligament normally glides anteriorly during extension and posteriorly during flexion and is taut only in extension. The ligament's normal function is to limit forward glide of the tibia on the femur and to limit rotation and abduction. The collaterals are twice as effective at inhibiting rotational laxity when compared with the cruciate ligaments.

The lateral compartment static stabilizer is the lateral collateral ligament (LCL) (Fig. 20-1D). This band-shaped ligament extends from the lateral femoral epicondyle to the fibular head. The ligament is extracapsular and does not insert on the lateral meniscus. This ligament offers little stability and is uncommonly injured. The LCL can be palpated laterally with the patient sitting cross-legged and the knee in 90-degree flexion.

The posterior compartment static stabilizer is the posterior capsule, which in reality is a continuation of the medial capsular ligament. The posterior capsular ligament is taut in extension and is the first line of defense against anteromedial or anterolateral rotary instability.

There are two noncapsular static stabilizers of the knee: the anterior and posterior cruciate ligaments. The cruciate ligaments extend from the area of the intercondylar fossa of the femur to the tibial intercondylar eminence. The ligaments cross over each other forming an "X" on lateral inspection (Fig. 20-2). The ligaments are named on the basis of their tibial attachment.

The anterior cruciate ligament (ACL) prevents anterior displacement of the tibia and excessive lateral mobility in flexion and extension, as well as controls tibial rotation. Some authors believe the ligament serves to prevent hyperextension and acts as a rotational guide in the screwing home (extension) mechanism. ACL injuries are rarely isolated and are typically associated with medial collateral tears. The ACL has a plentiful vascular supply and with appropriate treatment usually heals well after an injury. When it ruptures, a hemarthrosis is almost always present.

The posterior cruciate ligament (PCL) is regarded as the primary static knee stabilizer in preventing rotation. If ruptured, true anteroposterior (AP) and mediolateral instability can occur. Posterior cruciate injuries are rarely isolated and are typically associated with severe knee injuries.

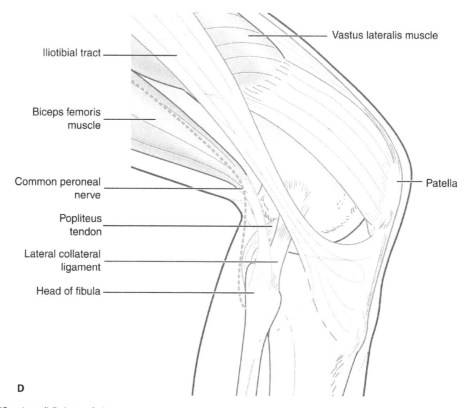

Iliotibial tract

Vastus lateralis muscle

Biceps femoris muscle

Common peroneal nerve

Popliteus tendon

Lateral collateral ligament

Head of fibula

Patella

D

Figure 20–1. *(Continued)* **D.** Lateral view.

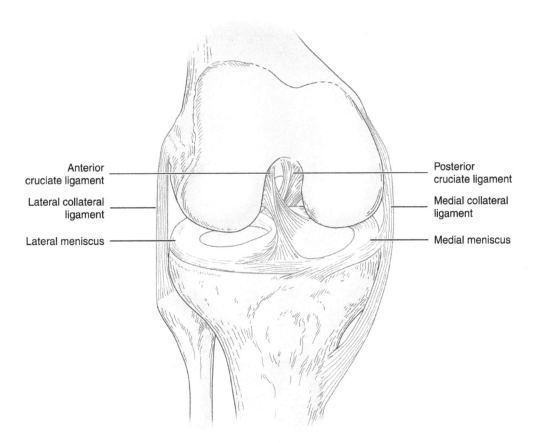

Anterior
cruciate ligament

Lateral collateral
ligament

Lateral meniscus

Posterior
cruciate ligament

Medial collateral
ligament

Medial meniscus

Figure 20–2. The ligamentous and meniscal structures of the knee.

The quadriceps tendon, a dynamic stabilizer, is a combination of the tendons of the vastus medialis, lateralis, and intermedius, along with the rectus femoris (Fig. 20–1A). The tendon encircles the patella and continues distally as the patellar tendon, inserting on the tibial tubercle. The quadriceps tendon is considered the primary dynamic stabilizer of the knee.

The pes anserinus, a dynamic stabilizer, is a medial structure formed from the conjoined tendons of the gracilis, sartorius, and semitendinosus (Fig. 20–1B). This tendon stabilizes the knee against excessive rotary and valgus motion.

The semimembranosus, a dynamic stabilizer, has three extensions that aid in stabilizing the knee (Fig. 20–1B and C). The oblique popliteal ligament extends from the tendon of the semimembranosus to the posterior capsule (posterior oblique ligament) and tightens the capsule when stressed. This tendon also inserts on the posterior horn of the medial meniscus, pulling it posteriorly during flexion. A final extension of the tendon is the insertion on the medial tibial condyle serving to flex and internally rotate the knee.

On the lateral surface of the knee, there are three dynamic stabilizing structures: the iliotibial tract, the biceps femoris, and the popliteus muscle (Fig. 20–1D). The iliotibial tract inserts on the lateral tibial condyle and moves anteriorly with extension and posteriorly with flexion. The biceps tendon inserts on the fibular head, lateral to the insertion of the LCL. The biceps

afford lateral stability as well as assisting the knee in flexion and external rotation. The popliteus is a posterior muscle inserting with a Y-shaped tendon called the arcuate ligament. One limb of the ligament inserts on the lateral femoral condyle and the other on the fibular head. Another limb inserts on the posterior portion of the lateral meniscus, providing for posterior mobility of the meniscus during flexion.

The posterolateral corner (PLC) of the knee has become increasingly recognized as an area responsible for stability in the varus and rotatory planes. This area was initially described in 1982; however, many providers are still not familiar with the importance of injuries to this area.[4] The PLC consists of static and dynamic restraints. The static restraints are the LCL, the arcuate ligament, the fabellofibular ligament, the popliteofibular ligament, the coronary ligament, and the joint capsule. The dynamic restraints are the biceps femoris and the popliteus muscle tendon. PLC injuries account for 5% to 9% of all injuries to the knee and are often associated with injuries to the ACL and the PCL.[5]

Similar to the PLC, the posteromedial corner (PMC) is also becoming recognized as an important anatomic structure of the knee that is often overlooked. The PMC lies between the posterior margin of the longitudinal fibers of the MCL and the medial border of the PCL.[6] It consists of five major components: (1) the semimembranous tendon, (2) the oblique popliteal ligament, (3) the posterior oblique ligament, (4) the posteromedial joint capsule, and (5) the posterior horn of the medial meniscus. Recognizing injuries to the PMC are important because they often result in anteromedial rotational instability (AMRI) and can lead to PCL and ACL graft failure if not corrected. The ACL and PCL are often injured along with the PMC as isolated injuries of the PMC are rare.

Imaging

Standard radiographs of the knee include an AP and lateral views (Fig. 20-3A and B). Oblique views are obtained to better evaluate the tibial plateau and spines (Fig. 20-3C). Other views include the skyline patellar and tunnel views. The skyline (or sunrise) patellar view is taken in the supine patient with the knees slightly flexed and the beam

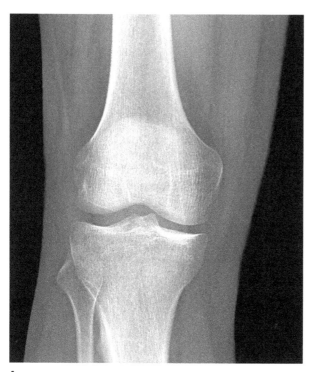

A

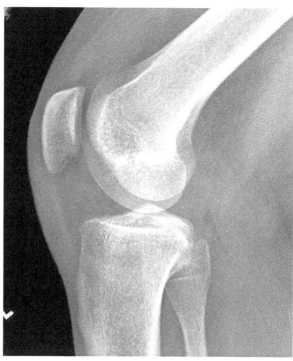

B

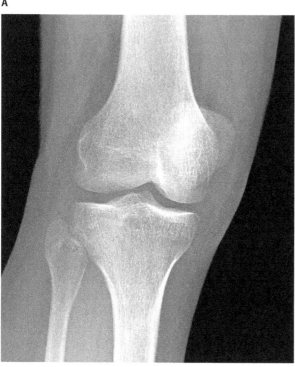

C

Figure 20-3. Normal knee radiographs. **A**. AP. **B**. Lateral. **C**. Oblique.

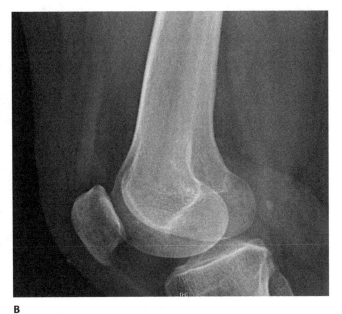

A   B

Figure 20–4. **A.** Knee effusion seen on the lateral radiograph as fluid density in the suprapatellar pouch (*white lines*). **B.** Normal lateral radiograph without distension of the normal fat in the suprapatellar area.

projected down toward the feet. It is useful to appreciate the relationship between the patella and the femoral condyles. The tunnel view is obtained with the patient lying prone and the knee flexed 40 degrees. The beam is directed down toward the feet, 40 degrees from vertical. This radiograph best demonstrates the intercondylar notch.

Identifying a fracture on knee radiographs can be both straightforward and difficult, depending on the circumstances. Occult fractures, especially of the tibial plateau, are not uncommon. An effusion of the knee is best appreciated on the lateral radiograph in the suprapatellar pouch because the normal hypodense fat is displaced by fluid (Fig. 20–4). This is sometimes confusing as it is the opposite appearance of the "fat pads" of an elbow effusion. To determine if the effusion represents the mixture of blood and fat seen in an intra-articular knee fracture, a cross-table lateral radiograph

may demonstrate lipohemarthrosis as a layering of the fat on top of the more dense blood on the bottom (Fig. 20–5). If there is still a question, an arthrocentesis of the knee will demonstrate the lipohemarthrosis as fat globules floating on the top of the blood (Fig. 20–6).

The decision to obtain a radiograph of the knee is based on many factors. In the emergency department (ED), in the setting of acute (<7 days) trauma, detection of a fracture is the most common reason. More than 1 million

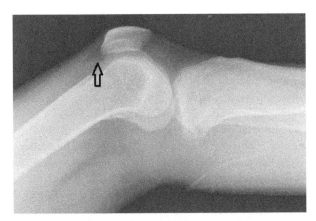

Figure 20–5. The cross-table lateral knee radiograph demonstrating lipohemarthrosis, the layering of fat and blood in an intra-articular fracture (*arrow*).

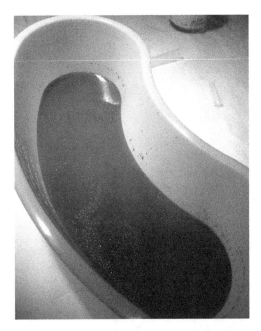

Figure 20–6. Lipohemarthrosis following knee arthrocentesis. Note the fat floating on top of the blood. This confirms an intra-articular fracture.

A knee x-ray series is only required for
knee injury patients with any of these findings:

1. Age 55 or older

2. Isolated tenderness of patella*

3. Tenderness at head of fibula

4. Inability to flex to 90 degree

5. Inability to bear weight both immediately
   and in the emergency department (four steps**)

*No bone tenderness of knee other than patella
**Unable to transfer weight twice onto each lower
limb regardless of limping.

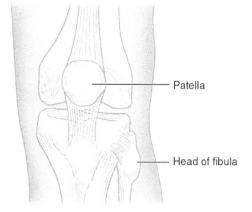

Patella

Head of fibula

Figure 20–7. Ottawa Knee Rules.

people present to EDs in the United States annually with acute knee trauma. Although the incidence of fractures in this population is between 6% and 12%, more than 90% receive a knee radiograph.

In an attempt to limit unnecessary radiographs and continue to diagnose clinically relevant fractures, the Ottawa knee rules were developed, validated, and tested (Fig. 20–7). Using five criteria, the clinician can exclude a clinically significant fracture with a pooled sensitivity of 98.5% and specificity of 48.6%. The reduction in the amount of knee radiographs obtained is between 25% and 50%. The rules apply to patients older than 18 years but have been tested in children older than 5 years with variable results. A recent meta-analysis by Vijayasankar et al demonstrated that the Ottawa knee rules had a pooled sensitivity of 99% and specificity of 46% in children older than 5 years, and they noted a reduction in radiographs between 30% and 40%. The Ottawa knee rules can be applied by triage nurses and have been shown to reduce

department length of stays and save money. The Pittsburgh knee rules are similar (Table 20–1) but have been tested in fewer patients. A recent study demonstrated that the Pittsburgh knee rules were more specific, with equal sensitivity in patients older than 18 years. Regardless of which rule is used, they both have demonstrated the ability to reduce radiographs without missing significant fractures or dislocations.

▶ **TABLE 20–1. PITTSBURGH KNEE RULES**

A knee x-ray series is only required for knee injury patients
  that answer "yes" to any one of the following:
  • Was the mechanism of injury blunt trauma or fall?
  • Is patient younger than 12 years?
  • Is the patient older than 50 years?
  • Is the patient unable to bear weight in the ED
    (for 4 steps, limping is allowed)?

KNEE FRACTURES

The bony anatomy of the knee includes the distal femur and the proximal tibia. The distal femur has a supracondylar portion and two condyles. The superior portion of the proximal tibia is the tibial plateau. The tibial spine is the site of attachment of ligamentous structures (Fig. 20–8).

DISTAL FEMUR FRACTURES

The classification system divides distal femur fractures into three types: (1) extra-articular (supracondylar), (2) partial articular (condylar), and (3) complete articular (bicondylar) (Fig. 20–9). The prognosis of the fracture progressively worsens with each type of fracture. A greater degree of comminution within these fracture subtypes worsens prognosis.

Supracondylar fractures involve the area between the femoral condyles and the junction of the metaphysis with the femoral shaft. These fractures are extra-articular and therefore not associated with knee joint distention. The remaining fracture types are intra-articular.

The musculature surrounding the distal femur is often responsible for fragment displacement after a distal femur fracture. The quadriceps extends along the anterior surface of the femur and inserts on the anterosuperior tibia. After a distal femur fracture, this muscle tends to pull the tibia and the attached proximal fragment in an anterosuperior direction. The hamstrings insert on the posterosuperior tibia. This muscle group tends to displace the tibia and the distal fragment in a posterosuperior direction. The gastrocnemius and the soleus insert on the posterior distal femur

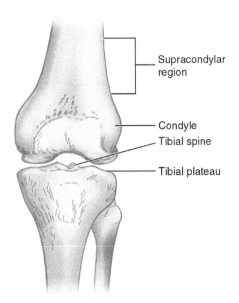

Figure 20–8. The anterior view of the knee. Note the supracondylar and condylar regions.

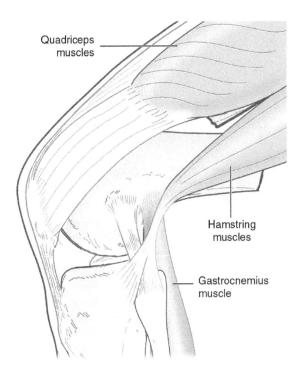

Figure 20–10. Note the typical fracture displacement in fractures of the supracondylar region of the distal femur. This displacement is caused by the traction of the hamstrings and quadriceps muscles in one direction and the traction of the gastrocnemius muscle on the distal fragment, producing posterior angulation and displacement.

and provide for inferior displacement after a fracture. The typical combined effect of these muscles is posterosuperior displacement (Fig. 20–10).

It is important to recall the close proximity of the distal femur to the popliteal artery and vein, along with the tibial and common peroneal nerves.

Distal femoral epiphyseal fractures are uncommon but serious injuries, which occur typically in children older than 10 years.[26] In children, 65% of the longitudinal growth of the lower extremity occurs around the knee, primarily the distal femoral epiphysis.[26] Leg shortening despite the maintenance of an anatomic reduction is common after these injuries, occurring in 25% of Salter type II injuries.[27] A Salter type II injury is the most common type of distal femoral epiphyseal fracture, and the poor prognosis is

in contradistinction to the generally favorable prognosis associated with Salter type I and II injuries in most other joints.[27-29]

Mechanism of Injury

Most of these fractures are secondary to direct trauma or have a component of direct force. Typical mechanisms include high-energy automobile collisions and falls. In

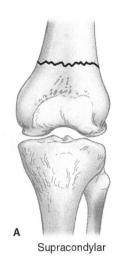

A Supracondylar

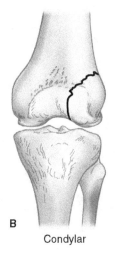

B Condylar

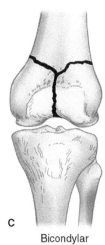

C Bicondylar

Figure 20–9. Distal femur fractures.

elderly patients, the force of injury may be much less. Condylar fractures are typically secondary to a combination of hyperabduction or adduction with direct trauma. Epiphyseal fractures are usually secondary to a medial or lateral blow resulting in fracture of the weaker epiphysis rather than the metaphysis. Another common mechanism involves hyperextension and torsion of the knee.

Examination

The patient with a distal femur fracture will present with pain, swelling, and deformity of the involved extremity. Palpable crepitus or bone fragments within the popliteal space may be present. Displaced supracondylar fractures typically present with leg shortening and external rotation of the femoral shaft. It is essential that the neurovascular status of the involved extremity be documented early in the patient assessment. Neurovascular injuries are uncommon, but they may be devastating if uncorrected. The web space between the first and second toe is innervated by the deep peroneal nerve and should be examined. Distal pulses should be documented. Distal capillary filling may persist despite an arterial injury secondary to an abundant collateral supply. Examine the popliteal space carefully for a pulsatile hematoma indicating an arterial injury.

Imaging

AP and lateral views are usually adequate in demonstrating the fracture (Fig. 20–11). Radiographs of the entire femur and hip should be obtained. Oblique and comparison views may be necessary to accurately diagnose a small condylar fracture. Comparison views should be obtained in all children younger than 10 years.

CT angiography may be indicated when physical examination suggests a vascular injury.

Associated Injuries

Distal femur fractures may be associated with the following:

* Ipsilateral acetabular or proximal femur fracture or dislocation
* Knee ligamentous injury (20% of patients)
* Vascular injury
* Peroneal nerve injury
* Damage to the quadriceps apparatus

Treatment

The ED management of these fractures includes immobilization in a long-leg posterior splint (Appendix A–17), analgesics, and emergent referral. The definitive treatment of distal femur fractures is open reduction with internal fixation. Operative fixation results in better functional results with a lower incidence of complications than closed techniques (i.e., skeletal traction).

Closed treatment can be successfully employed for nondisplaced or impacted supracondylar fractures that are extra-articular. In these patients, early use of a cast brace (hinged cast) with frequent radiographic reassessments may be definitive.

Today, skeletal traction is used only as a temporizing measure in patients awaiting operative repair or in patients with contraindications to surgery (i.e., frail elderly or those with associated medical conditions). In these patients, skeletal traction for 6 to 8 weeks is followed for an additional 6 to 8 weeks with a cast brace.

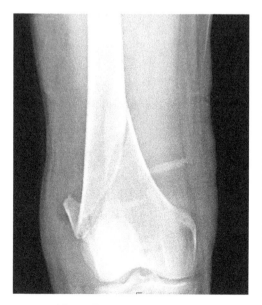 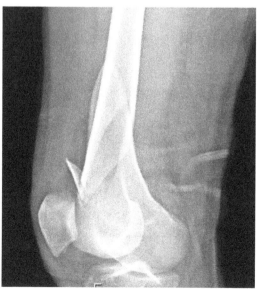

Figure 20–11. Distal femur fracture—an extra-articular (supracondylar) fracture. This displacement is caused by the traction of the hamstrings and quadriceps muscles in one direction and the traction of the gastrocnemius muscle on the distal fragment, producing posterior angulation and displacement.

In children with epiphyseal fractures, an anatomic reduction is very important. Associated physeal fractures (Salter type II) may be managed with the judicious use of internal fixation screws in order to maintain an anatomic reduction.[34]

Complications

Distal femoral fractures are associated with several significant complications:

* Venous thrombosis
* Delayed union or malunion may occur if reduction is incomplete or not maintained
* Intra-articular fractures may develop quadriceps adhesions or valgus/varus angulation deformities
* Intra-articular fractures may be complicated by the development of arthritis
* Femoral epiphyseal fractures are often followed by a growth disturbance in the involved extremity

PROXIMAL TIBIA FRACTURES

Proximal tibia fractures include those fractures above the tibial tuberosity. These fractures can be divided on the basis of their involvement of the articular surface. Articular fractures include the condylar (tibial plateau) fractures, whereas extra-articular injuries involve the tibial spine, tubercle, and subcondylar regions.

Essential Anatomy

The medial and lateral tibial condyles form a plateau that transmits the weight of the body from the femoral condyles to the tibial shaft. The intercondylar eminence includes the tibial spines, which provide the attachment site for the cruciate

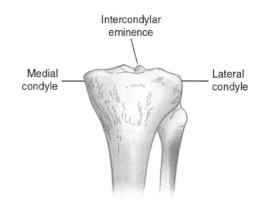

Figure 20–12. The tibial plateau.

ligaments and the menisci (Fig. 20–12). Condylar fractures are typically associated with some degree of depression secondary to the axillary transmission of the body's weight.

Classification

Proximal tibia fractures may be divided into five categories on the basis of anatomy:

* Tibial plateau fractures
* Spine fractures
* Tuberosity fractures
* Subcondylar fractures
* Epiphyseal fractures

Tibial Plateau Fractures

Many systems have been developed to classify these fractures. Schatzker developed the system most commonly used in North America. It groups fractures into six types (Fig. 20–13).[35,36] In discussing tibial plateau fractures, depression indicates more than 4 mm of inferior displacement.

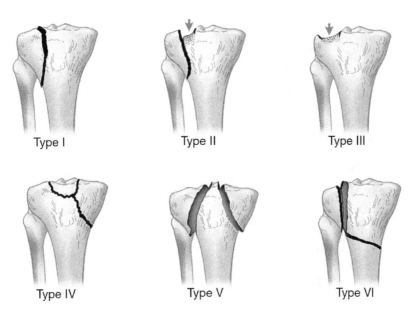

Figure 20–13. Classification of tibial plateau (condylar) fractures.

Types I to III are the result of low-energy trauma, whereas types IV to VI are generally due to high-energy trauma.

A type I fracture is of the lateral condyle. This fracture is referred to as a split fracture because the lateral portion of the condyle has sheared away from the remainder of the plateau. The articular surface is not depressed. These fractures are more common in young patients with strong cancellous bone that works to resist depression. Displacement of the lateral condylar fragment suggests a concomitant lateral meniscal injury.

Type II fractures are also lateral condylar fractures; they are differentiated from type I fractures in that the articular surface medially is depressed. These fractures are sometimes referred to as split-depression fractures because part of the lateral condyle is split, and the remaining portion is depressed. Type II fractures occur in patients older than 30 years because the subchondral bone is weaker.

Type III fractures result when there is isolated depression of the lateral condyle. The depression is usually central but can involve any part of the condyle. If the depression is located laterally, it is more likely to result in joint instability.

Type IV fractures involve the medial condyle. The force necessary to fracture the medial condyle is much higher than the lateral condyle. As a result, these fractures are much less common than the lateral condyle and are associated with a high incidence of associated injuries to the cruciate ligaments and popliteal artery. A type IV fracture may also be associated with a fracture of the intercondylar eminence.

Type V fractures are bicondylar and possess varying degrees of articular depression and displacement. The medial condyle is usually a split fracture, whereas the most common lateral condylar injury is either a split fracture or a depression fracture. These fractures are also associated with similar injuries as the type IV fractures.

Type VI fractures are similar to type V fractures with the addition of a disruption between the diaphysis and metaphysis of the tibia. These fractures are the result of the highest energy mechanism of injury and are usually associated with significant bony comminution, displacement, and depression.

Mechanism of Injury

The forces that normally act on the tibial plateau include axial compression and rotation. Fractures result when these forces exceed the strength of the bone.

A direct mechanism, such as a fall from a height, is responsible for approximately 20% of condylar fractures. Automobile–pedestrian collisions, where the car bumper strikes the patient over the proximal tibia, are responsible for approximately 50% of these fractures. The remainder of the fractures result from a combination of axial compression and rotational strain. Fractures of the lateral tibial plateau usually result from an abduction force on the leg. Medial plateau fractures typically result from adduction forces on the distal leg. If the knee is extended at the time of injury, the fracture tends to be anterior. Posterior condylar fractures usually follow injuries in which the knee was flexed at the time of impact.

Examination

The patient will usually present with a chief complaint of pain and swelling with the knee slightly flexed. There is frequently an abrasion indicating the point of impact, along with an effusion and reduced range of motion secondary to pain. Because these fractures are not always visualized on plain radiographs, tenderness over the tibial plateau (especially with an effusion) should alert the clinician to a possible fracture.

Imaging

AP, lateral, and oblique views are often adequate for demonstrating these fractures (Fig. 20–14). Although not

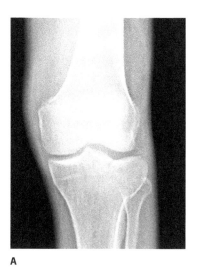
A

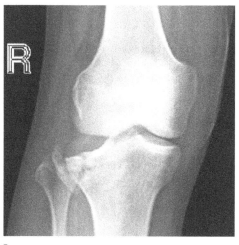
B

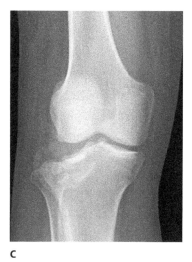
C

Figure 20–14. Tibial plateau fractures. **A.** Type I lateral condylar split fracture. **B.** Type II split-depression tibial plateau fracture. **C.** Type III lateral condyle compression.

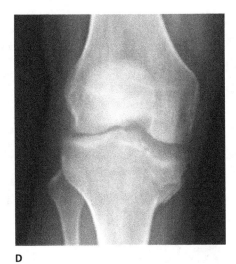
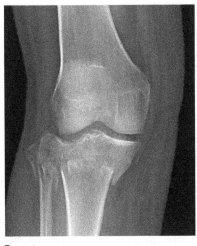

D   **E**

Figure 20–14. *(Continued)* **D.** Type IV medial plateau fracture. **E.** Type VI bicondylar fracture with diaphyseal disruption.

commonly performed, a tibial plateau view may be helpful in assessing the amount of depression in a tibial plateau fracture (Fig. 20–15).[38] Anatomically, the tibial plateau slopes down from anterior to posterior. Routine AP views do not detect this slope and may mask some depression fractures. The tibial plateau view compensates for this slope and allows a more accurate estimation of depressed tibial plateau fractures.

Because occult tibial plateau fractures are not uncommon, the clinician should look carefully at the radiographs, searching for an effusion or lipohemarthrosis as described previously. Depression fractures are seen as an abnormal increase in the density of the bone (Fig. 20–16). In cases in which a fracture is suspected clinically, but not seen on radiographs, treat the patient for a fracture or obtain further imaging studies (i.e., computed tomography [CT] scan).

CT scanning or magnetic resonance imaging (MRI), or both, are frequently used to determine the full extent of the injury.[39] In the ED, CT is much more readily obtained and will frequently be requested by the consulting orthopedist (Fig. 20–17). In one study, the addition of a CT to the plain radiographs changed the treatment plan in 26% of patients.[40] MRI is more valuable for delineating the extent of soft-tissue injuries, which are common following these fractures. Meniscal injuries occur in 55% of patients, whereas ligamentous injuries occur in 68%.[41]

Associated Injuries

Tibial condylar fractures are frequently associated with several significant knee injuries:

- Ligamentous injuries or meniscal injuries, or both, frequently accompany these fractures. With a lateral condylar fracture, MCL, anterior cruciate, and lateral meniscal injuries should be suspected. With a medial condylar fracture, LCL, cruciate, and medial meniscal injuries should be suspected.
- Vascular injuries, either acute or delayed in presentation, may be seen after these fractures, especially type IV through VI fractures.
- Compartment syndrome may occur but is rare.[42]

Treatment

The ED management of tibial plateau fractures includes immobilization in a long-leg posterior mold (Appendix A–17), ice, elevation, and analgesics. The patient should be instructed to use crutches and should not bear weight until evaluated by an orthopedic surgeon. Early consultation is strongly recommended. If surgery is indicated, a delay of 24 to 48 hours will not compromise treatment.

Definitive management is divided into operative versus closed treatment. The goals of definitive management are to restore the articular surface to normal, begin early knee

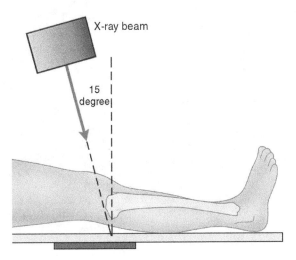

Figure 20–15. Tibial plateau view.

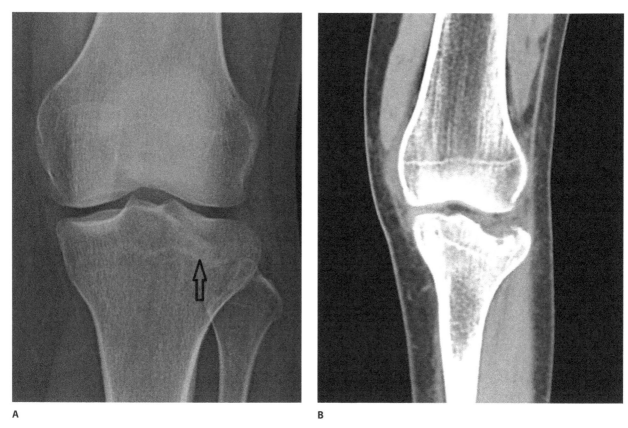

A

B

Figure 20–16. **A.** Increased density of the lateral tibial plateau is suggestive of a depression fracture. **B.** CT confirmed the suspicion.

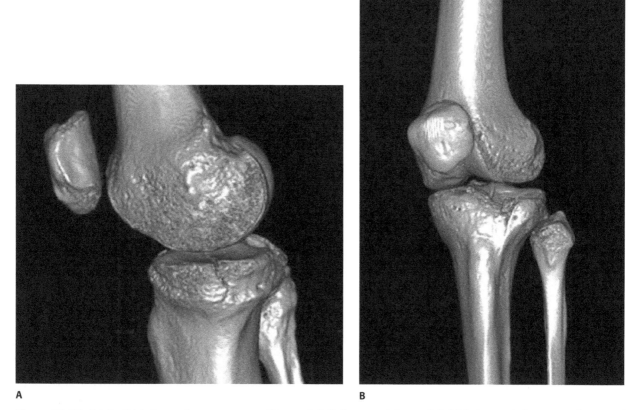

A

B

Figure 20–17. Subtle tibial plateau fractures seen on CT scan. **A.** Split fracture of the medial tibial plateau. **B.** Depression fracture of the lateral tibial plateau.

Type I
Incomplete avulsion
without displacement

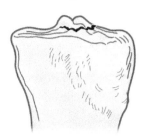

Type II
Displaced
incomplete avulsion

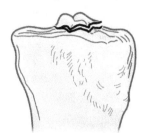

Type III
Complete

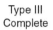
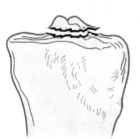

Figure 20–18. Tibial spine fractures.

motion to prevent stiffness, and delay weight bearing until healing is complete.[42]

The therapeutic modality selected depends on the type of fracture, the stability of the knee, the orthopedic surgeon's experience, and the age and comorbidities of the patient. Any articular fracture that results in instability of the knee joint requires operative fixation. In addition, the more anatomic the reduction is, the more likely the articular cartilage will regenerate. For these reasons, operative fixation is frequently the therapeutic modality of choice.

Nondisplaced, stable fractures without depression can be treated nonoperatively with protected mobilization. However, due to the high rate of complications with even minimally displaced fractures, it is important to provide orthopedic referral. Stability is difficult to determine in the ED unless the knee is examined following adequate anesthesia. Aspiration of the hemarthrosis followed by injection of 20 to 30 mL of local anesthetic may allow for testing knee joint stability, although general anesthesia is sometimes necessary (Video 20–1). Stability is defined as less than 10 degrees of movement with varus and valgus stresses at any point in the arc of movement from full extension to 90-degree flexion.[42]

Complications

Tibial plateau fractures may be followed by the development of several significant complications:

- Loss of full knee motion may follow prolonged immobilization.
- Degenerative arthritis may develop despite optimum therapy.
- Angular deformity of the knee may develop in the first several weeks, even with initially nondisplaced fractures.
- Knee instability or persistent subluxation may develop secondary to ligamentous damage.
- Infection may complicate the course of open fractures or those treated surgically.
- Neurovascular injuries and compartment syndromes may occur.

Tibial Spine Fractures

Isolated tibial spine fractures are uncommon injuries that typically occur in adolescents between the ages of 8 and 14. These fractures are analogous to an ACL injury in a skeletally mature patient. The anterior intercondylar eminence is 10 times more likely to be fractured than the posterior intercondylar eminence. The classification of these fractures is based on the system developed by Meyers and McKeever[43] (Fig. 20–18 and Table 20–2).

Mechanisms of Injury

Tibial spine fractures are the result of indirect trauma such as with an anterior or posterior force directed against the flexed proximal tibia. This mechanism results in cruciate ligament tension and avulsion of the spine. Hyperextension or violent abduction, adduction, or rotational forces may also result in fractures.

Examination

The patient will usually present with a suggestive history and a painful swollen knee. On examination, there will be an effusion. Following incomplete avulsions without displacement, knee extension is near normal unless an effusion is present. After displaced or complete fractures, a block to full extension is present. A positive drawer sign is present in most patients, but surrounding muscle spasm may prevent an accurate assessment. The remaining ligaments surrounding the knee should be examined carefully to exclude associated injuries.

▶ **TABLE 20–2. CLASSIFICATION OF TIBIAL SPINE FRACTURES**

Type	Description
I	Incomplete avulsion without displacement
II	Displaced incomplete avulsion of the tibial spine
III	Complete avulsion of the tibial spine

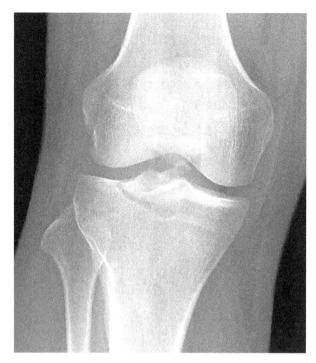

Figure 20–19. Tibial spine fracture.

Imaging

Routine radiographs, including a tunnel view (posteroanterior view with knee flexed to 40–50 degrees), are usually adequate in defining the fracture (Fig. 20–19). CT or MRI, or both, can be used to determine the full extent of the injury.

Associated Injuries

Collateral and cruciate ligamentous injuries are commonly associated with these fractures.

Treatment

The therapeutic objectives include joint stability and early restoration of motion. Early orthopedic consultation is recommended.

Type I—Incomplete Avulsion without Displacement. These fractures should be immobilized in a long-leg posterior splint (Appendix A-17) followed by cast immobilization with 5 degrees of flexion for 4 to 6 weeks. When there is associated ligamentous injury, operative repair is generally required.

Type II—Incomplete Avulsion with Displacement. These fractures are reduced with closed manipulation under general anesthesia. This is followed by cast immobilization in 5 degrees of flexion for 4 to 6 weeks. If closed treatment is not successful or there are associated ligamentous injuries, operative repair is required.

Type III—Complete. Operative therapy is indicated for these fractures. Reduction can be accomplished by either arthroscopy or limited arthrotomy. After reduction, a long-leg cast is applied in 5 degrees of flexion for 6 to 8 weeks.

Complications

The most frequent complication after this fracture is persistent pain and instability of the knee.

Tibial Tuberosity Fractures

These are uncommon fractures most often seen in adolescent patients (Fig. 20-20). The tibial tubercle is the insertion point of the quadriceps mechanism and accurate

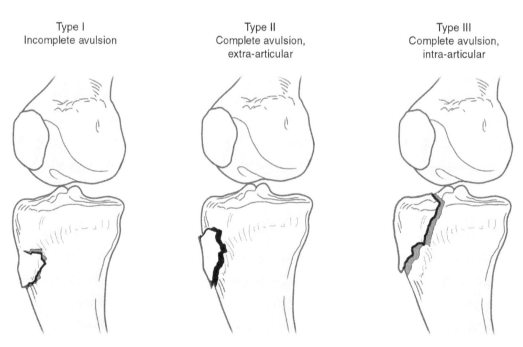

Figure 20–20. Tibial tuberosity fractures.

▶ TABLE 20–3. **CLASSIFICATION OF TIBIAL TUBEROSITY FRACTURES**

Type	Description
I	Incomplete avulsion
II	Complete avulsion without intra-articular extension
III	Complete avulsion with intra-articular extension

reduction is essential for proper function. These fractures may be classified into three types (Table 20–3).[45]

Mechanism of Injury
The mechanism of injury is indirect. With the knee in flexion and the quadriceps tightly contracted, a sudden flexion force is applied to the joint. The tightly contracted quadriceps resist this force and avulse the tibial tubercle.

Examination
The patient will present with pain that is exacerbated with attempted extension. Patients with incomplete or complete fractures may retain some degree of active extension because the patellar retinaculum usually remains intact.

Imaging
Routine radiographs are usually adequate in demonstrating the fracture. The lateral view best demonstrates the fracture (Fig. 20–21). In young patients, comparison views may be necessary when an incomplete avulsion injury is suspected.

Associated Injuries
A tear of the patellar retinaculum, including avulsion of the patellar ligament, may be associated with these fractures.[46]

Treatment
The emergency management of these fractures includes ice, immobilization (Appendix A–17), and emergent orthopedic consultation. Incomplete avulsions can be treated with cast immobilization if they are nondisplaced. However, even incomplete avulsions may become displaced during treatment, so close follow-up is required. Complete avulsion fractures require operative repair.

Complications
Most of these fractures heal without complications. Secondary postoperative displacement may follow inadequate immobilization or surgical fixation.

Subcondylar Tibial Fractures
This fracture involves the proximal tibial metaphysis and is typically transverse or oblique (Fig. 20–22). The fracture line may extend into the knee joint.

Mechanism of Injury
The fracture mechanism involves a rotational or angular stress accompanied by vertical compression.

Examination
The patient will present with tenderness and swelling over the involved area. A hemarthrosis indicates extension of the fracture line into the joint.

Imaging
Routine AP and lateral views are usually adequate in demonstrating this fracture.

Associated Injuries
Tibial condylar fractures are frequently associated with these injuries.

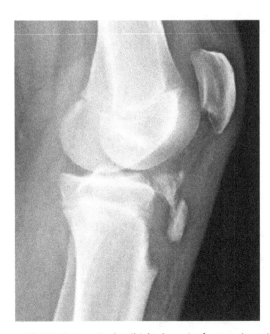

Figure 20–21. Intra-articular tibial tuberosity fracture (type III).

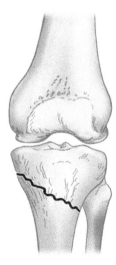

Figure 20–22. Proximal tibia fractures—subcondylar fractures.

Treatment

The emergency management of these fractures includes ice, immobilization in a long-leg posterior splint (Appendix A–17), and orthopedic consultation. Stable extra-articular, nondisplaced, nonangulated transverse fractures can be treated nonoperatively with a long-leg cast for 8 to 12 weeks. Operative management includes locked intramedullary nailing or a periarticular locking plate. Comminuted fractures or those associated with a condylar component require open reduction and internal fixation.

Complications

Subcondylar fractures are frequently associated with tibial plateau injuries and are thus subject to similar complications. Refer to the section on tibial plateau fractures for a review of these complications.

Epiphyseal Fractures

Epiphyseal fractures of the proximal tibia are uncommon injuries and are seen less frequently than are distal femoral or tibial tubercle epiphyseal fractures.

Mechanism of Injury

These injuries usually result from a severe valgus or varus strain on the knee.

Examination

The patient will present with pain and deformity of the knee. On examination, angulation is usually evident. Knee effusions are usually not seen with this fracture.

Imaging

Most of these fractures are Salter type II injuries and require comparison views for an accurate diagnosis.

Associated Injuries

These fractures are only infrequently associated with ligamentous or meniscal injuries.

Treatment

The emergency management of these fractures includes ice, immobilization in a long-leg posterior splint (Appendix A–17), and early orthopedic consultation for reduction. After reduction, most patients are immobilized in a long-leg cast for 8 weeks.

Complications

Growth abnormalities may follow proximal tibial epiphyseal fractures.

PROXIMAL FIBULA FRACTURES

Isolated proximal fibular fractures are relatively unimportant because the fibula does not support any weight. The most common fracture is of the fibular neck, although avulsion and comminuted fractures may also occur (Fig. 20–23). These fractures are significant in that they are frequently associated with other more serious knee injuries.

Axiom: *Proximal fibular fractures should be considered indicative of a significant knee injury until proven otherwise.*

Mechanism of Injury

Two mechanisms result in fractures of the proximal fibula. A direct blow over the fibular head may result in a comminuted fracture. An indirect varus stress to the knee may result in an avulsion fracture of the fibular head. A valgus strain on the knee may result in a lateral tibial condylar fracture associated with a proximal fibular fracture.

Examination

The patient will present with pain and tenderness over the fracture site. It is essential that the knee, distal leg, and foot be thoroughly examined to exclude associated neurovascular or ligamentous injuries.

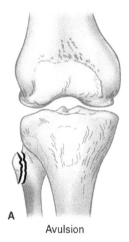 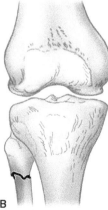

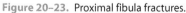
A   Avulsion

B   Fibula neck

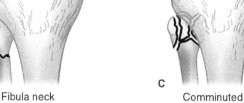
C   Comminuted

Figure 20–23. Proximal fibula fractures.

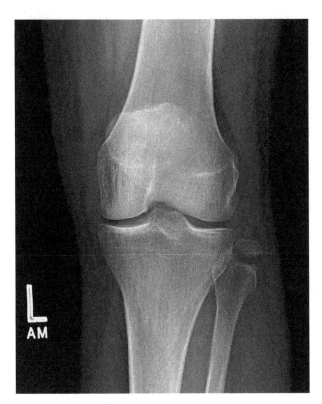

Figure 20–24. Avulsion fracture of the proximal fibula.

Imaging

AP and lateral views of the knee will demonstrate this fracture (Fig. 20–24).

Associated Injuries

As mentioned previously, proximal fibular fractures may be associated with a lateral condylar fracture or ligamentous injury to the ankle (see Chapter 22). Several serious neurovascular or ligamentous injuries are also associated with these fractures:

- The common peroneal nerve may be contused or lacerated. Most orthopedic surgeons will follow these injuries and repair them later if function does not return.
- The LCL may be ruptured or strained.
- Anterior tibial arterial injury with thrombosis (rare).

Treatment

The emergency management of these fractures includes ice, analgesics, and thorough evaluation and exclusion of serious associated injuries. Isolated fibular fractures are treated symptomatically.

Complications

Injuries associated with proximal fibular fractures are responsible for the majority of complications.

PATELLA FRACTURES

Patella fractures represent 1% of skeletal body injuries. These fractures are most common in patients between 20 and 50 years of age.[36] Patella fractures are classified into four types (Fig. 20–25). A transverse fracture is the most common patella fracture and represents more than half of all cases. Transverse fractures may occur in the middle of the patella or at the proximal or distal pole. Comminuted (stellate) fractures are the second most common type occurring in about one-third of patella fractures. Vertical fractures represent 10% to 20% of patella fractures.[47] Osteochondral fractures to the inferior patellar surface may also occur.

Mechanism of Injury

Two mechanisms result in fractures of the patella. A direct blow to the patella may result in transverse, comminuted, vertical, or osteochondral fractures. Secondary quadriceps pull may result in displacement of the fragments. Direct injuries are the most common mechanism and can occur from a fall or motor vehicle collision. The indirect mechanism occurs when an intense quadriceps contraction creates a force that exceeds the strength of the patella and results in an avulsion fracture. This injury may occur after a near fall and is more likely to result in a displaced transverse fracture.

Examination

The patient will present with tenderness and swelling of the knee. The undersurface of the patella must be palpated if an osteochondral fracture is suspected. This can be done by laterally and then medially, displacing the patella while using your other hand to feel the undersurface of the patella. The knee should be examined for active extension. If extension is absent, the quadriceps mechanism is disrupted. A palpable defect along the inferior pole of the patella indicates a disruption of the distal extensor mechanism.

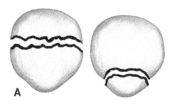
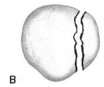
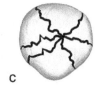
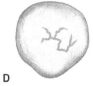

A   Transverse   B   Vertical   C   Comminuted   D   Osteochondral

Figure 20–25. Patella fractures.

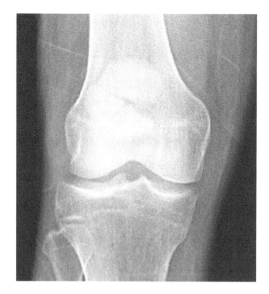

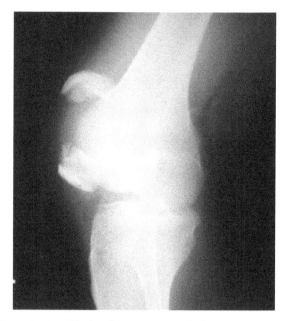

Figure 20–27. Displaced transverse patella fracture.

Associated Injuries

Direct patella fractures may be associated with other fractures and ligamentous injuries about the knee, as well as traumatic chondromalacia.

Treatment

The emergency management of these fractures includes aspiration of a tense hemarthrosis when present and immobilization in full extension. Immobilization can be accomplished with a long-leg posterior splint (Appendix A–17) or a knee immobilizer (Appendix A–16). The patient should then be referred for follow-up and the institution of quadriceps exercises within the first several days.

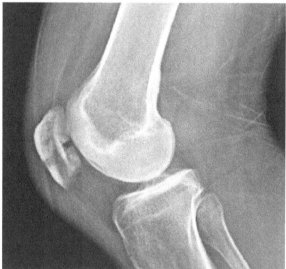

Figure 20–26. Comminuted patella fracture.

Imaging

AP, lateral, and sunrise (tangential view of flexed knee) views are usually adequate in defining these fractures (Figs. 20–26 and 20–27).

A bipartite patella may at times be difficult to differentiate from a fracture. A bipartite patella has smooth surfaces and is present in 2% to 8% of the population. The position of a bipartite patella is superolateral in 75% of cases, lateral in 20%, and interior in 5% (Fig. 20–28). Comparison views may be helpful in distinguishing these two entities because 50% are bilateral.

Osteochondral fractures are usually not detected on plain radiographs, although a small defect on the undersurface of the patella may be seen. MRI may be useful in delineating the full extent of the osseous and soft-tissue injuries. Ultrasound can also be used to evaluate the patella and femoral tendons for a visible defect that would suggest a disruption of the extensor mechanism.

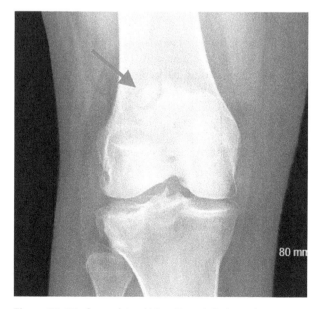

Figure 20–28. Superolateral bipartite patella (*arrow*).

Nonoperative management is appropriate for transverse, comminuted, and vertical patella fractures when displacement is less than or equal to 2 mm, the articular surface is intact, and the extensor mechanism is functional. Nonoperative therapy consists of a long-leg cylinder cast extending from the groin to the malleoli. The cast should be well molded around the patella, and the knee must be in full extension. A hinged knee brace locked in full extension may be used to permit early controlled motion. Vertical (regardless of displacement) and nondisplaced pole fractures can be managed with controlled range-of-motion exercises and modified activities for 3 to 6 weeks.[36]

Operative management is indicated for transverse and comminuted patella fractures if displacement is greater than or equal to 3 mm, the articular surface is disrupted more than 2 mm, or the extensor mechanism is functionally absent. Depending on the type of fracture and clinical situation, this can be accomplished with tension banding, cerclage, or screws. Osteochondral fractures require loose body repair or removal.

Severely comminuted fractures are usually treated with patellectomy because they are associated with a high incidence of degenerative arthritis. Partial patellectomy in comminuted fractures of the patella have produced satisfactory results if at least three-fifths of the patella could be preserved. Total excision of the patella is sometimes unavoidable.[48]

Complications

Patella fractures may be followed by the development of several significant complications:

- Degenerative arthritis is common, especially after osteochondral or comminuted fractures.
- Postoperative displacement of the fragments secondary to inadequate fixation or immobilization.
- The blood supply to the patella enters by way of central and distal polar vessels. Transverse or polar fractures may interrupt the blood supply, resulting in the development of avascular necrosis.

KNEE SOFT-TISSUE INJURY AND DISLOCATION

PATELLAR TENDINOPATHY (JUMPER'S KNEE)

Rapid repetitive acceleration, deceleration, jumping, and landing result in microtears of the extensor tendon matrix at three distinct locations: (1) the quadriceps tendon as it inserts into the patella, (2) the patellar tendon at the inferior aspect of the patella, and (3) the patellar tendon as it inserts into the tibial tubercle.[49]

The most common location for injury is the patellar tendon at the insertion of the inferior patella, termed "jumper's knee" or patellar tendinopathy.[50] Two-thirds of patients have been found to have structural tendon changes.[51] This condition can be disabling, with one-third of athletes unable to return to sports within 6 months and one-half of patients refraining from their sport due to the condition at 15 years of age.[52,53] Colosimo and Bassett classify jumper's knee into four stages (Table 20-4).[54]

▶ **TABLE 20-4. COLOSIMO AND BASSETT CLASSIFICATION FOR JUMPER'S KNEE**

Stage	Description
I	Pain after activity
II	Pain at the beginning of activity, disappearing after warm-up and reappearing after completion of activity
III	Pain remains during activity, precludes participation in sports
IV	Tendon rupture

Examination

During examination, the knee should be held at full extension. If the quadriceps tendon is involved, tenderness will be present over the insertion of the quadriceps tendon or the upper pole of the patella. Patients with patellar tendinopathy will have tenderness at the lower pole of the patella and the proximal portion of the patellar tendon.[49]

Imaging

Plain radiographs are usually normal. Occasionally, the patella will have an elongated or fragmented tip. Ultrasonography will reveal an enlarged and hypoechoic tendon and is used to confirm the diagnosis.[54] MRI will also be diagnostic.

Treatment

Treatment of jumper's knee includes avoiding the inciting activity and resting the affected extremity. The extent of treatment depends on the stage. Stages I and II are treated with adequate warm-up and ice packs or ice massage after the activity. Anti-inflammatory medications are administered for 10 to 14 days followed by physiotherapy. Eccentric training and shock wave therapy have proven to produce good results and should be used prior to surgical intervention.[55-58] Elastic knee support is recommended. Patients with stage III disease should undergo a prolonged period of rest, in addition to ice and anti-inflammatory medications. If this is not curative, the patient should consider either giving up sports or having surgery to excise abnormal tissue. Surgery is required for patients with stage IV disease (rupture). Arthroscopic treatment of this condition in

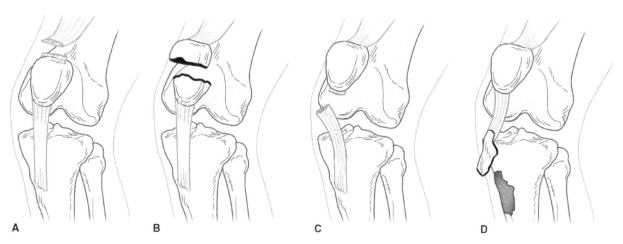

Figure 20–29. *A.* Rupture of quadriceps tendon. *B.* Fracture of the patella. *C.* Rupture of the patella tendon. *D.* Avulsion of the tibial tuberosity.

those that do not respond to conservative therapy produces good results.

Steroid injection is controversial. Some authors support its use, whereas others feel that it could lead to further damage and eventual rupture as it allows the athlete to continue to overload the weak tendon. Researchers are also evaluating the effectiveness of platelet-rich plasma injections, hyalyronan with and without botulinus toxin, and focused extracorporeal shock wave therapy, although these therapies are too new to recommend routinely.

EXTENSOR MECHANISM DISRUPTION

The extensor mechanism of the knee may be disrupted at four locations: (1) quadriceps tendon, (2) patella, (3) patellar tendon, and (4) tibial tubercle (Fig. 20–29). Patella and tibial tuberosity fractures are covered in the section on fractures. For this discussion, we focus on quadriceps and patellar tendon rupture.

The initial examiner misdiagnoses these injuries in 38% of patients. This fact is important because when treatment is delayed, functional results are poor. The clinical picture of an extensor mechanism disruption typically includes a history of a sudden buckling of the knee with extreme pain. After the acute injury, the pain is reduced.

Rupture of the quadriceps tendon is often seen in patients older than 40 years. The most common site of rupture is just proximal to the patellar insertion through an area of degenerated tendon. Patellar tendon ruptures are less common than quadriceps tendon ruptures and are typically seen in those younger than 40 years. Most patellar tendon ruptures occur at the site of insertion into the patella. Steroid injections are believed to predispose to rupture. Other factors predisposing to tendon rupture include tendon calcifications, arthritis, collagen disorders, fatty tendon degeneration, and metabolic disorders.

Mechanism of Injury

The injury may be either direct or indirect. The direct mechanism is less common and is the result of a violent impact against a taut quadriceps tendon. The more common indirect mechanism results from forced flexion when the quadriceps is contracted. This mechanism is commonly seen in patients who stumble while descending a staircase or stepping off a curb.

Examination

On examination, the position of the patella should be assessed. Inferior displacement of the patella with proximal ecchymosis and swelling indicates a quadriceps rupture. Superior displacement of the patella along with inferior pole tenderness and swelling indicates a patellar tendon rupture (Fig. 20–30). In both instances, the patient may have

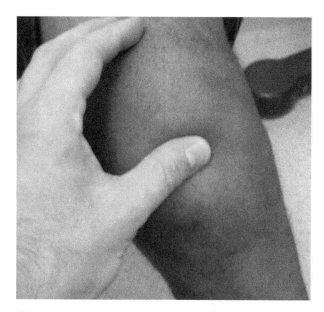

Figure 20–30. On examination, the patella is notably absent from the anterior knee and can be palpated superiorly.

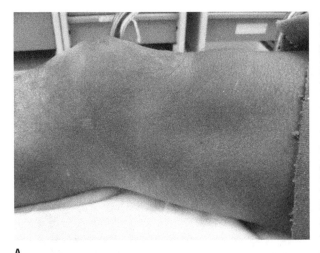

A

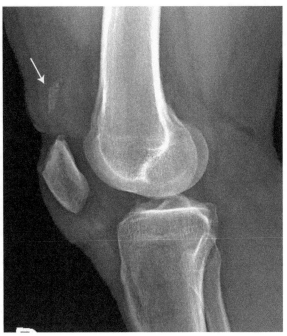

B

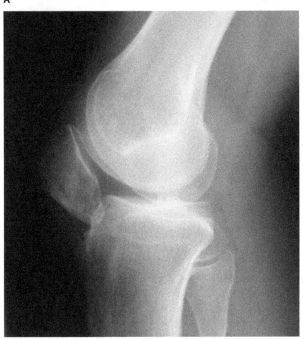

C

Figure 20–31. Quadriceps tendon rupture. **A.** The suprapatellar gap sign refers to the palpable depression superior to the patella. **B.** A superior pole patella avulsion fracture suggests a quadriceps tendon rupture (*arrow*). **C.** Patella baja refers to the inferiorly positioned patella on the lateral radiograph.

intact, "active" extension, but it will be very weak when compared with the uninjured extremity (Video 20–2). A quadriceps tendon rupture results in a suprapatellar gap just superior to the patella with swelling to the tissues above (Fig. 20–31A).[68] The most significant finding on clinical examination with extensor mechanism rupture is that the patient has loss of active extension of the knee or inability to maintain the passively extended knee against gravity. With partial ruptures, the patient may have active extension as previously indicated; however, it will be markedly weakened.

Imaging
The AP and lateral knee radiographs are often highly suggestive of these injuries. In the normal AP knee radiograph, the inferior aspect of the patella should lie within 2 cm of the distal femoral condyles. On the lateral view at 90-degree flexion, the patella should remain inferior to a line drawn along the anterior aspect of the femoral shaft. Inferior patellar displacement (patella baja) or a superior pole avulsion fragment suggests a quadriceps tendon rupture (Fig. 20–31B and C).[69] Superior displacement (patella alta) is diagnostic of a patellar tendon rupture (Fig. 20–32). An inferior bony avulsion fragment may also be present (Fig. 20–33). Comparison views may be helpful in diagnosing subtle patellar displacements.

Because treatment is altered depending on whether the injury is partial or complete, MRI or ultrasound is used to distinguish between cases that remain unclear after the initial assessment.

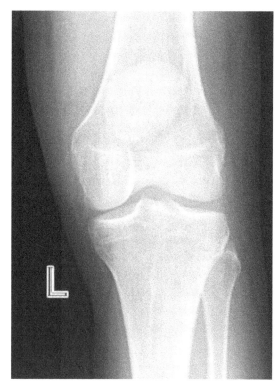
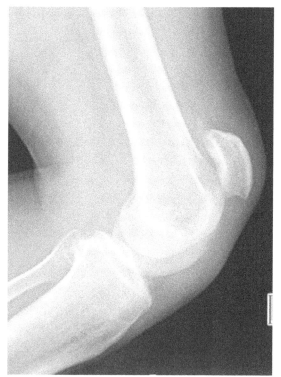

Figure 20–32. Patellar tendon rupture. On the AP view, the inferior aspect of the patella is more than 2 cm above a line drawn between the distal femoral condyles. Similarly, on the lateral view at 90-degree flexion, the patella is above a line drawn along the anterior femoral shaft.

Treatment

The initial treatment of partial and complete quadriceps and patellar tendon injuries is the same. Ice and a compression dressing are applied to reduce swelling. The knee is held in extension with a knee immobilizer (Appendix A–16).

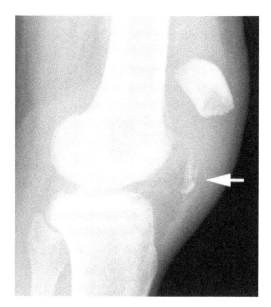

Figure 20–33. Patellar tendon rupture. Patella alta is seen on the lateral radiograph. An inferior body avulsion fragment is present (*arrow*).

In complete or severe injuries, the patient should not bear weight initially.

The definitive treatment of these injuries is different if the injury is partial or complete. A partial quadriceps or patellar tendon rupture requires early referral for the placement of a long-leg cylinder cast with the knee held in extension for 6 weeks. A complete quadriceps or patellar tendon tear is best treated with early surgical repair. Ideally, surgery is performed within 2 weeks of the injury. When performed after 6 weeks, results are inferior.

MUSCLE STRAIN AND TENDONITIS

The gracilis, the sartorius, and the semitendinosus insert on the medial tibia via the pes anserinus. Patients with tendonitis of the pes anserinus present with pain and tenderness 5 to 6 cm below the medial joint line. Other symptoms include pain on standing from a sitting position, pain at night, and "giving way" of the knee. It is most common in runners. Ultrasound will show an increase in the size of the tendon with heterogeneous echogenicity. Differentiating this condition from anserine bursitis is difficult clinically, but the conditions are treated the same. Tendonitis is less common and the response to treatment is less dramatic.

The semimembranosus inserts both medially and posteriorly along the knee. Semimembranosus tendonitis causes pain in the posteromedial aspect of the knee, immediately below the joint line.[73] The pain is worse after activity. This injury is often confused with a medial meniscus injury.

The biceps tendon inserts on the fibular head and the LCL. Sudden contraction against resistance as in running or jumping may strain or rupture the tendon and muscle. Pain and tenderness is present over the posterolateral portion of the knee.

The treatment of these injuries requires rest to allow healing and prevent further injury. Moderate strains consist of partial fiber tears with pain and bleeding. These injuries require 3 to 4 weeks of rest along with analgesics and ice. Heat is applied 48 hours after an acute injury. Complete ruptures are rare injuries that are best treated surgically.[74]

ILIOTIBIAL BAND SYNDROME

The iliotibial band originates from the fascia of the gluteus muscles and tensor fascia lata. It passes along the lateral portion of the thigh and inserts into a tubercle on the lateral tibial condyle. With the knee in extension, the iliotibial band lies anterior to the lateral femoral epicondyle. With flexion, the band slides posteriorly over the epicondyle (Fig. 20–34). Repetitive flexion and extension, as occurs with running or cycling, results in irritation of the iliotibial band and its bursa as it slides over the epicondyle.[75,76]

The patient presents with pain on the lateral side of the knee during activity that may radiate proximally or distally. Climbing stairs or walking up an incline will exacerbate the pain. On examination, there will be a focal area of tenderness over the lateral femoral epicondyle approximately 3 cm proximal to the joint. Full range of motion is typical, and the pain will be exacerbated with weight bearing on the flexed knee. Nobel's compression test will reproduce pain. To perform this test, the leg of the supine patient is elevated above the examination table. The examiner holds the ankle with one hand, while the thumb of the other hand compresses the lateral epicondyle of the femur. Active flexion and extension reproduce the pain.[77]

The recommended treatment includes a reduction in activity with the avoidance of hills or banked tracks. A lateral wedged orthotic, ice, anti-inflammatory medications, iliotibial band stretching, and local steroid injections are also useful.[78,79] Surgery is indicated in refractory cases.[75] This includes splitting the posterior 2 cm of the iliotibial band transversely at the area of the lateral condyle so this portion of the band is not taut.

FABELLA SYNDROME

The fabella is a sesamoid bone embedded in the tendon of the gastrocnemius muscle that articulates with the posterior portion of the lateral femoral condyle (Fig. 20–35). It serves as the site of attachment for fibers of the popliteus, arcuate complex, and fibular–fabellar ligament. The fabella is present in 11% to 13% of normal knees and is bilateral in 50% of these patients.

Fabella syndrome occurs when the fabella undergoes a degenerative or inflammatory process secondary to irritation. The condition is most common in adolescents but may also occur in adults. The clinical picture typically includes intermittent posterolateral knee pain exacerbated with extension.[80] Tenderness to palpation is localized over the fabella and is exacerbated with compression against the condylar surface.[71]

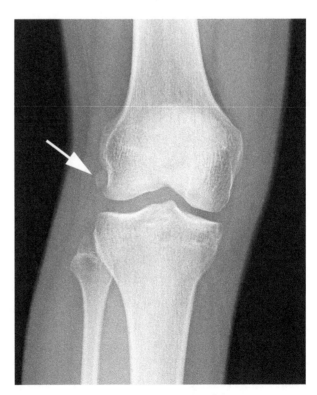

Figure 20–35. The fabella is a sesamoid bone embedded in the tendon of the gastrocnemius muscle (*arrow*).

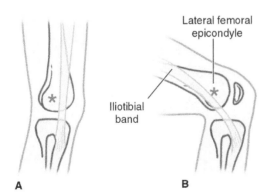

Figure 20–34. *A.* The iliotibial band lies anterior to the lateral femoral epicondyle when the knee is in extension and passes posterior to it with flexion. ***B.*** The coursing back and forth over this bony prominence is the cause of a symptom complex referred to as the *iliotibial band syndrome*.

Radiographs may not reveal evidence of a fabella if it has not ossified. The differential diagnosis should include injury to the posterior horn of the lateral meniscus, or tendonitis of the lateral head of the gastrocnemius, biceps femoris, or popliteus. The recommended treatment includes rest, analgesics, local anesthetic–steroid injection, and referral as surgical resection may be necessary when pain persists for more than 6 months. However, a recent study showed successful resolution of symptoms at 2 months in four patients using extracorporeal shock wave therapy. Larger studies are needed before this can become routine care, but this could be an interesting alternative treatment option.

BURSITIS

The normal function of a bursa is to permit friction-free movement between two structures. Because of the number of muscles and ligaments that come into contact with bony structures, the knee has many bursae, several of which can become injured or inflamed (Fig. 20–36).

Several knee bursae communicate with the joint space. The suprapatellar and popliteal bursae always communicate with the joint, whereas the semimembranosus only does some of the time. This communication is important for understanding Baker cysts, as well as evaluating for intra-articular involvement of foreign bodies or lacerations (Fig. 20–37). The suprapatellar bursa extends a full three fingerbreadths above the patella, and a laceration in this location that involves the bursa may result in septic arthritis.

Acute trauma or chronic occupational stresses cause bursitis around the knee. Other less common etiologies include infection or metabolic disorders such as gout or chronic arthritis. Clinically important bursae and their related conditions are discussed later. The treatment of bursitis surrounding the knee is similar and is discussed at the end of this section.

Prepatellar Bursitis. This bursa is located superficial to the patella and usually becomes inflamed 1 to 2 weeks after a direct traumatic injury such as a fall on the knee. Direct

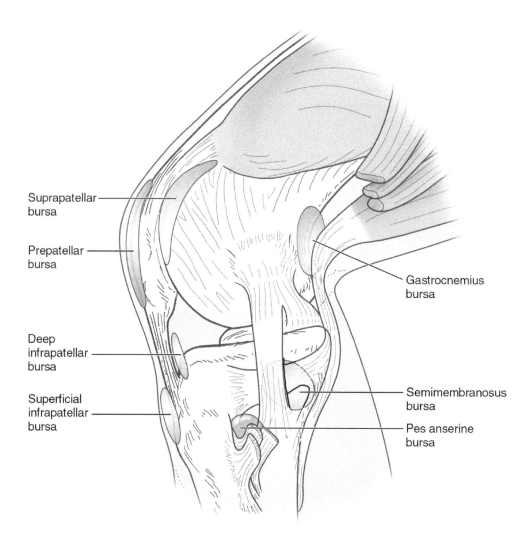

Figure 20–36. The bursa about the knee.

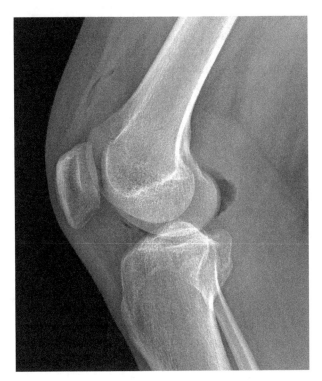

Figure 20–37. This patient sustained a laceration to the anterior knee just above the patella. He stated that he felt a crunching sound on bending the knee. Radiographs demonstrated air within the suprapatellar bursa and the joint space.

repeated trauma may also cause this condition, and this is why it is also referred to as "housemaid's knee."

The clinical presentation is typically one of pain with erythema, swelling, and increased warmth of the skin overlying the bursa (Fig. 20–38A). With palpation, the examiner will be able to identify the superficial bursal sac. Crepitation of the walls of the bursa may be noted. Knee motion is painless up to the point of skin tension, at which time pain is noted. Repeated trauma results in less pronounced symptoms and a palpably thickened bursal wall.

Like olecranon bursitis of the elbow, many cases of prepatellar bursitis are infectious. If infection is a consideration, aspiration of the fluid for diagnostic testing and antibiotics are indicated as outlined for olecranon bursitis in Chapter 14. Typically, the white blood cell (WBC) count is higher than 5000 WBC/mm³. Gram stain is positive in more than half of the cases. Treatment of noninfectious prepatellar bursitis is discussed at the end of this section.

Infrapatellar Bursitis. The superficial infrapatellar bursa is located just beneath the skin and superficial to the tibial tubercle. Superficial infrapatellar bursitis is also referred to as "clergyman's knee" because of its association with kneeling in a more erect position than would cause prepatellar bursitis. When inflamed, there will be swelling and tenderness inferior to the patella and over the tibial tubercle (Fig. 20–38B). In an adolescent, it may be difficult to differentiate this condition from Osgood–Schlatter disease.

The deep infrapatellar bursa is located beneath the patellar tendon, separating it from the underlying fat pad and tibia. The clinical picture includes pain-free passive extension and flexion. Pain will be elicited with active complete flexion and extension and with palpation of the margins of the patellar tendon. It may be difficult to differentiate fat pad syndrome from this disorder, although complete passive extension is usually painful with fat pad syndrome.

Anserine Bursitis. The anserine bursa lies under the pes anserine tendon. This is a conjoined tendon composed of the sartorius, gracilis, and semitendinosus muscles. This condition is more common in middle-age women and obese patients. Symptoms include knee pain, often nocturnal, particularly on walking upstairs or rising from a sitting position. Morning stiffness may last up to 1 hour. The

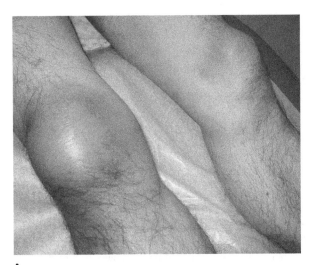

A

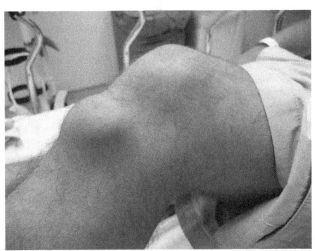

B

Figure 20–38. **A.** Infected prepatellar bursitis. **B.** Noninfected infrapatellar bursitis.

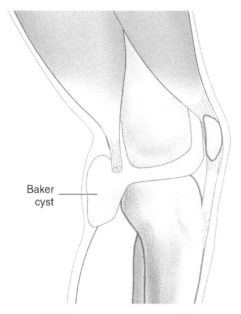

Figure 20–39. A Baker cyst (an extension of the semimembranosus bursa).

findings on physical examination are marked tenderness over the pes anserine, which is 5 to 6 cm below the medial joint line. Often, coexisting osteoarthritis is present. An ultrasound may show an enlarged anserine bursa.[84]

Baker Cyst. This entity, seen in the popliteal fossa behind the knee, is a benign outpouching of the semimembranosus bursa (Fig. 20–39). The incidence of Baker cysts is higher in patients with rheumatoid arthritis or osteoarthritis. A Baker cyst becomes enlarged when synovitis, arthritis, or any internal derangement of the knee results in the flow of excess synovial fluid into this bursa. At that point, the bursa expands posteriorly into the popliteal fossa.

The clinical picture usually includes a history of intermittent swelling behind the knee. On examination, a tense and sometimes painful fluid-filled sac is palpated within the popliteal fossa. A change in pressure in a Baker cyst with extension and flexion of the knee (Foucher sign) suggests the diagnosis. Additional complaints include chronic pain or a giving way of the knee. A Baker cyst should never be aspirated or injected.

Rupture of a Baker cyst presents with diffuse swelling in the leg as the synovial fluid dissects inferiorly. This entity may be clinically indistinguishable from a deep vein thrombosis. Nonruptured cysts must be differentiated from popliteal artery aneurysms, neoplasms, and true synovial hernias. The diagnosis can be confirmed by ultrasonography, CT, or MRI.[85]

Lateral Knee Bursitis. The popliteal bursa lies proximal to the joint line between the LCL and the popliteus tendon. The patient with popliteal bursitis presents with lateral joint line tenderness and swelling.

The fibular head is surrounded by a large bicipital bursa lying under the biceps femoris tendon, a bursa under the LCL, and a bursa under the lateral head of the origin of the gastrocnemius. Inflammation of these bursae creates a clinical picture that includes pain and tenderness around the fibular head, the LCL, or the biceps insertion. It may at times be difficult to differentiate bursitis from injuries to the LCL, the bicipital tendon, or the lateral meniscus.

Treatment of Bursitis

The treatment of acute traumatic or chronic occupational bursitis includes local heat, rest, and anti-inflammatory agents with protection from recurrent irritation. Patients with prepatellar and anserine bursitis respond well to the injection of a triamcinolone–bupivacaine mixture followed by a compression dressing. Ultrasonic treatment causes dramatic improvement in patients with anserine bursitis.

In some studies, steroid injection reduced the size of the cyst and led to increased comfort.[86,87] Ultrasound-guided aspiration, fenestration, and injection of 40 mg of triamcinolone and 2 mL of 0.5% bupivacaine has shown good clinical outcomes.[88] Those cases resistant to treatment may require surgical excision of the bursa. The treatment of a Baker cyst must be directed at the etiology, and early referral is recommended for diagnostic tests and possible closure of the synovial defect.

TRAUMATIC PREPATELLAR NEURALGIA

This is a well-recognized but uncommonly diagnosed syndrome following a direct blow to the front of the knee. The patient typically presents with a chief complaint of a persistent, dull ache deep to the patella that makes bending or climbing stairs difficult. Patients often complain of pain behind the knee on one or both sides. The disorder occurs secondary to contusion of the superficial prepatellar neurovascular bundle. Repeated trauma may cause secondary fibrosis of the neurovascular bundle.

On examination, the patient will complain of focal tenderness over the middle of the lateral border of the patella with no discomfort over the remainder of the patella.[89] Most patients respond to an injection of a lidocaine–steroid mixture. Unfortunately, the pain returns after a few weeks. Refractory cases require prepatellar neurectomy.[89]

FAT PAD SYNDROME

This syndrome is also known as Hoffa disease, infrapatellar fat pad syndrome, and synovial lipomatosis.[90] The fat pad, located beneath the patellar tendon, may become hypertrophied and inflamed in athletes secondary to repetitive trauma to the knee. The end result is pain on forced extension, catching, and anterior knee discomfort when sitting for long periods.

On examination, point tenderness is noted over the anteromedial or anterolateral joint line. The knee appears tender and puffy, and the fat pad bulges out on either side of the patellar tendon. Pain is reproduced when the slightly flexed knee is allowed to passively extend (bounce test). The provider must not confuse these symptoms with patellar tendinopathy or superficial or deep infrapatellar bursitis.

Treatment of this condition consists of rest, ice, and non-steroidal anti-inflammatory medications. Local anesthetic–steroid injection into the fat pad will also offer relief and aid in confirming the diagnosis. Heel lifts may reduce knee hyperextension and reduce pain. Operative resection is rarely necessary.

LIGAMENTOUS INJURIES

The stability of the knee is dependent on its surrounding ligaments and muscles. The knee is most stable in extension, yet the predominance of everyday activities is performed in some degree of flexion. The knee is thus predisposed to injury. The ligaments surrounding the knee function to guide motion and protect the knee from nonphysiologic movement.

These ligaments are innervated by myelin-free nerve fibers. It is characteristic of ligamentous injuries that a partial tear is typically more painful than a complete rupture.

Mechanism of Injury

The following discussion centers around six common mechanisms resulting in ligamentous injuries: (1) valgus, (2) varus, (3) hyperextension, (4) rotational, (5) anterior, and (6) posterior stresses.[58] It is important to determine if the knee was weight bearing or if a rotational force was present at the time of injury because these factors will increase the likelihood of an associated meniscal injury. In addition, the position of the knee (flexion or extension) at the time the force was applied will impact the structures involved.

Because the force of injury is more commonly a combination of stresses, it is difficult to predict the ligamentous injury pattern from the mechanism of injury alone. The following discussion should serve as a general guide to the types of injuries that are frequently the result of a particular mechanism. This is a controversial area, and the following tables include the predominant theories.

The most common mechanism of injury resulting in ligamentous damage is a valgus (*an abducting force that opens up the medial side*) stress with an external rotary component on the flexed knee. This is a common football or skiing injury where the patient typically complains of being clipped from the blind side or of catching a ski tip in the snow. The MCL is the first structure injured, making this ligament the most commonly injured ligament in the knee.[90] With increasing force, the ACL ruptures, followed by the medial meniscus or PCL. Injury to the MCL,

▶ **TABLE 20-5. PROGRESSIVE LIGAMENTOUS INJURY AFTER A VALGUS STRESS TO THE KNEE BASED ON THE POSITION OF THE KNEE AT THE TIME OF INJURY**

Flexion with External Rotation	Extension
MCL	MCL
↓	↓
ACL	ACL and medial portion of posterior capsule
↓	
	↓
Medial meniscus	Deep medial capsular ligament
↓	↓
PCL	PCL

MCL, medial collateral ligament; ACL, anterior cruciate ligament; PCL, posterior cruciate ligament.

ACL, and medial meniscus is referred to as the "unhappy triad" because of the common association of these structures following a valgus stress to the knee. Table 20–5 lists the sequence of events because an increasing valgus force is applied to the knee in flexion and extension.[75,79]

Varus (*an adducting force that opens the lateral side of the knee*) stress is believed to be the second most common mechanism resulting in ligamentous knee injuries. A varus stress may or may not be accompanied by an internal rotary force. The LCL is the first to be injured when this mechanism occurs in isolation, but the ACL, and finally the PCL, can also rupture when a combined varus and internal rotational force is applied.

A hyperextension stress usually results in injury to the cruciate ligaments. The ACL ruptures first, followed by the posterior capsule and PCL. The cruciate ligaments may rupture at their midpoint or at their femoral attachment.[91-93] An additional rotational stress may result in damage to the collateral ligaments.

There are two types of rotational stresses: internal and external. Internal rotational stresses result in ACL injury, followed by an LCL injury, whereas external rotational stresses may cause ACL, LCL, PCL, or meniscal injuries, depending on whether the knee was flexed, extended, or weight bearing at the time of injury.

Anterior and posterior stresses of the tibia on the femur may result in injuries to the cruciate ligaments. An anterior stress will rupture the ACL followed by the MCL. A posterior stress results in a PCL injury.

History

In addition to the mechanism of injury as described here, the emergency provider should inquire about other historic features. Pertinent questions in subacute and chronic cases include the location of the swelling and what activities reliably induce swelling. The usual duration of symptoms as well as the response to rest should be assessed.

The exact location of the pain after an injury and those factors that exacerbate the symptoms give important clues in the specific localization of a ligamentous injury. Partial ligament ruptures typically produce more pain than do complete tears. In one study, 76% of patients with a complete rupture of a ligament in the knee walked without assistance.

Several studies have indicated that during an injury an audible pop or snap is a reliable indicator of an anterior cruciate rupture. Some authors have stated that patients with this history have a 90% incidence of anterior cruciate rupture at surgery. Sixty-five percent of patients with a torn anterior cruciate, however, did not hear a pop or snap at the time of injury. Rupture of the anterior cruciate is usually followed by the rapid onset of a bloody effusion. In fact, the most common etiology for a traumatic hemarthrosis within 2 hours of injury is a rupture of the anterior cruciate.

> **Axiom:** *A history that includes a pop or snap at the time of injury suggests a rupture of the ACL until proven otherwise, especially when associated with the rapid development of a knee effusion.*

Examination

How Much Time Has Elapsed Since the Injury? The time between the injury and the examination is important in deciphering the physical findings. Immediately after an injury, there will be no effusion or spasm, and ligamentous injuries will be easily demonstrated. By the time the patient presents to the ED an hour later, these same injuries will be difficult to detect secondary to the surrounding muscular spasm. If spasm is present, ligamentous laxity may not be demonstrable. This patient must be reexamined after 24 hours when the spasm has been relieved.

Is There a Joint Effusion? The acutely injured knee should be examined methodically, and any swelling noted. When seen early, up to 64% of patients have localized edema at the site corresponding to the acute ligamentous tear. Complete ligamentous ruptures or capsule disruption may not exhibit swelling because the fluid extravasates through the torn capsule.

An effusion seen within 2 hours of an injury is suggestive of torn tissues, whereas those presenting 12 to 24 hours post injury are typically reactive synovial effusions. A tense and painful effusion that severely limits the range of motion can be relieved with aspiration in the ED.

A hemarthrosis that develops within the first 12 hours after injury most commonly suggests an ACL tear. After athletic injuries, 67% of patients with an acute hemarthrosis and no fracture on radiographs were found to have a partial or complete tear to the ACL. Other injuries included osteochondral fractures (13%) and meniscal tears (16%). Fat globules found in the bloody aspirate suggest an osteochondral fracture.

Is There Localized Tenderness? Next, the provider should gently palpate the knee in an attempt to localize tenderness. In one series, 76% of patients had their surgically confirmed injury initially localized on the basis of focal tenderness. Joint line tenderness suggests an injury to the capsule, ligaments, or menisci. At this point, the provider should perform a gentle examination to document the range of motion.

Are There Any Abnormalities with Stress Testing? Ligamentous injuries should be classified on the basis of involved ligaments as well as the degree of involvement (Table 20–6). Grade I (mild) sprains imply a stretching of the fibers without a tear. Grade II (moderate) sprains imply a tear in the ligament fibers without a complete rupture. Grade III (complete) sprains indicate a complete rupture of the ligament.

The use and interpretation of various tests to examine the acutely injured knee is controversial. After an acute injury, these tests are difficult to perform for the examiner and patient. The following discussion is based on published data and personal experience.

Stress testing for ligamentous injuries should be employed only after radiographs have ruled out the possibility of a fracture. It is important to document the feel of the joint at maximum stress (firm or "mushy"), along with the amount of joint opening. On stress testing, grade I and II injuries have a firm endpoint that does not exist for grade III injuries. Measuring the degree of joint opening on stress testing is an objective classification that requires examiner experience and a comparison to the opposite knee. Joints that open 0 to 5 mm suggest a mild (grade I) ligament tear, whereas joints that open 5 to 10 mm suggest a moderate (grade II) tear and more than 10 mm is consistent with a complete (grade III) tear.

▶ TABLE 20–6. **CLASSIFICATION OF LIGAMENT INJURY**

Grade I (Small Incomplete Tear)
- Local tenderness
- Minimal swelling
- No stress test instability with firm endpoint
- Little pain with stress testing

Grade II (Moderate Incomplete Tear)
- Local tenderness
- Moderate swelling
- 1+ stress instability with firm endpoint when compared with normal knee
- Moderately disabling

Grade III (Complete Rupture)
- Local tenderness but pain not proportional to degree of injury
- Swelling may be minimal or marked
- 2 to 3+ stress instability with mushy endpoint
- Severe disability may present

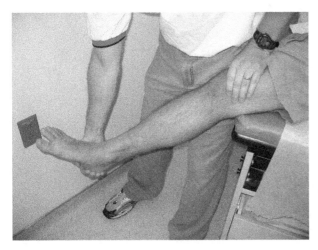

Figure 20–40. Valgus stress test of the medial collateral ligament.

The valgus stress test is performed with the hip in slight extension to relax the hamstrings (Fig. 20–40). This can be accomplished by hanging the thigh and the leg over the side of the table with the knee in 30-degree flexion and the patient supine. The examiner places his/her thigh against the lateral side of the patient's thigh to stabilize the femur. The examiner then places the fingers of one hand on the medial aspect of the joint line to feel for joint opening. The other hand grasps the foot and a gentle abduction stress, with external rotation of the foot, is applied. The slight external rotary stress tightens the medial capsular ligaments. It is essential that the stress examination of the injured extremity be compared with that of the uninjured extremity.

This test is a reliable indicator of injury to the MCL. In our experience and that of others, a torn anterior cruciate will result in a much greater degree of valgus instability. With extreme opening, the PCL may also be ruptured, and the knee should be treated as a reduced dislocation with potential for popliteal artery injuries.[99,100]

The valgus stress test in extension is performed after the flexion examination using the same technique but with the knee extended. The interpretation of this test is similar to the valgus stress test at 30-degree flexion, except that joint opening in extension suggests a greater degree of ligamentous injury. Remember, the knee joint is most stable in extension and when the ACL is taut. Joint laxity while in extension is therefore indicative of an anterior cruciate and a posterior capsular rupture, in addition to an MCL tear. When one suspects posterolateral instability, a careful valgus stress test in 0 and 30 degrees of knee flexion will often demonstrate the instability.[101]

The varus stress test is applied with the knee in 30-degree flexion with the foot and the leg internally rotated (Fig. 20–41).[102] The patient's thigh must be more abducted than during the valgus stress test because the applied force will be toward the examination table. The examiner starts

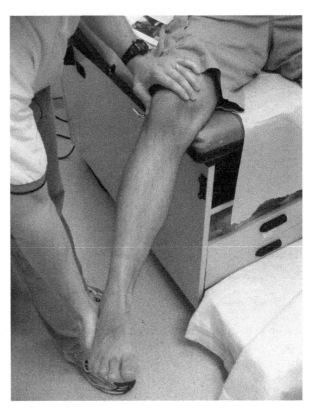

Figure 20–41. Varus stress test for the lateral collateral ligament.

by locating the lateral joint line. The thumb of the hand is placed on the lateral joint line with the rest of the hand stabilizing the medial aspect of the joint. The other hand is placed on the patient's foot, and a varus stress is applied. Joint opening is indicative of a rupture of the LCL. Wide opening suggests possible injury to the structures of the posterolateral knee complex (arcuate ligament, popliteus muscle, lateral head of the gastrocnemius, and iliotibial band) and ACL. Injury to the posterolateral knee complex is rare, reported in more than 2% of all acute ligamentous knee injuries.[103]

The varus stress test performed with the knee in extension with internal rotation of the leg can also be performed. Significant joint opening during this test is more likely to suggest injury to the LCL, posterolateral knee complex, or ACL than the varus stress test in flexion. A particularly wide opening may indicate a posterior cruciate rupture.[104]

The anterior drawer test assesses the integrity of the ACL. However, following an acute injury, this test is difficult to perform and lacks sensitivity. When performing the anterior drawer test, the patient must be in a supine, relaxed position. The hip should be in 45-degree flexion, with the knee in 80- to 90-degree flexion and the foot immobilized. The examiner should then place the hands on the upper tibia with the fingers in the popliteal fossa and ensure the hamstring muscles are relaxed. At this point, laxity is assessed by attempting to push and pull the tibia in an anterior–posterior direction. It is important to perform the

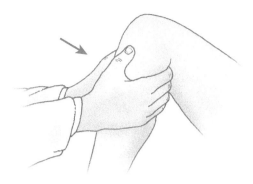

Figure 20–44. Posterior drawer sign of the knee. The arrow indicates the direction of force applied to the leg.

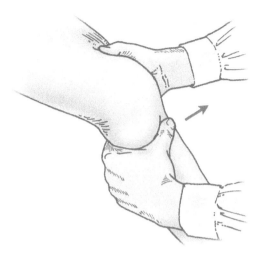

Figure 20–42. Lachman test.

test on both the injured and uninjured knee. The anterior drawer test is positive in up to 77% of patients with an ACL rupture. Unfortunately, this number overestimates the sensitivity of this test in patients with acute knee injuries.

The Lachman test is more sensitive for an acute ACL injury than the anterior drawer test. To perform the Lachman test, begin with the knee in full extension. Cup the distal femur in one hand and elevate it, allowing the knee to flex proximally (Fig. 20-42). Place the other hand on the proximal tibia at approximately the level of the tibial tuberosity and attempt to displace the tibia anteriorly on the femur. Anterior displacement as compared with the opposite side indicates a positive test. In one study, the Lachman test was positive in 99% of patients with rupture of the ACL. This test is more easily performed than the anterior drawer sign in the patient who has a markedly swollen knee. Palpable hamstring spasm when performing

the Lachman maneuver or the anterior drawer has been shown to interfere with the interpretation of this test in the awake patient.

The pivot shift test has also been described for the diagnosis of ACL tears. To perform this test, the examiner internally rotates the leg with one hand, while the other hand rests laterally at approximately the level of the fibular head (Fig. 20-43). A mild valgus stress is applied with slight traction on the fully extended knee. The knee is gradually flexed. With a positive test, the lateral femoral–tibial articulation, which starts out subluxed, is felt to "pop" back to a reduced state at approximately 30-degree flexion.

The posterior drawer test is performed in a similar manner to the anterior drawer test, except that a posterior force is applied to the anterior tibia (Fig. 20-44). A positive posterior drawer test indicates a rupture of the PCL. A negative test, however, does not exclude this injury. PCL injuries are more common than was once recognized. These injuries account for 1% to 20% of ligament injuries and occur most commonly after sports and motor vehicle collisions.

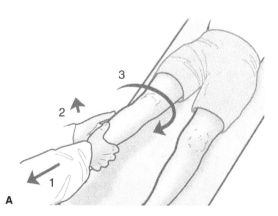
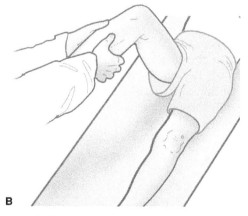

Figure 20–43. The pivot shift test for detection of an anterior cruciate ligament (ACL) tear. **A.** The examiner applies slight traction (1), valgus stress (2), and internal rotation (3) on the extended knee. **B.** The knee is gradually flexed until a "pop" is felt, indicating a positive test.

Is There Muscle Weakness? After a negative examination for ligamentous instability, the muscle strength of the involved extremity should be assessed and compared with the normal extremity. Loss of muscular strength may be seen after rupture of a musculotendinous unit.[112]

Imaging

Plain radiographs of the knee are usually necessary to rule out an associated fracture. A Segond fracture is a subtle avulsion fracture of the lateral tibial condyle that suggests a high likelihood of an ACL tear or menisci injury (Fig. 20–45). A "reverse Segond" fracture has also been described that was initially believed to suggest a high likelihood of a PCL tear or medial menisci injury.[113] However, more recent studies have showed that while a reverse Segond fracture is rare, it is not specifically associated with PCL or medial meniscus injury (these may actually remain intact) but is a marker of a ligamentous injury (i.e., ACL and MCL injuries).[114,115] A reverse Segond fracture is a subtle avulsion fracture of the medial tibial condyle that represents an avulsion of the deep portion of the MCL (Fig. 20–46). These films should precede an in-depth physical examination. If the radiographs are normal, diagnostic manipulation and stress testing can be undertaken.

It is likely that plain radiographs will be all that the emergency provider has at their disposal. The valgus stress test performed while taking a plain film is useful when uncertain of the degree of opening.[116] However, it should be understood that with the advent of MRI, the delineation of soft-tissue injuries has been revolutionized. The accuracy in diagnosing ligamentous injuries based on confirmation by arthroscopic findings may be as high as 99%.[117–123]

Initial Treatment

The initial management of ligamentous injuries of the knee should include ice, elevation, and a Jones compression dressing extending from the midcalf to the midthigh (Appendix A–15). Alternately, a knee immobilizer (Appendix A–16) or long-leg posterior splint (Appendix A–17) may be used.

Stable knee injuries refer to grade I or II injuries of a single ligament after an adequate examination can be performed. The treatment protocol for stable knee injuries is outlined in Table 20–7. The involvement of multiple ligaments or a single ligament with a grade III injury is considered unstable, requiring immobilization, nonweight bearing, and orthopedic referral.[124]

Frequently, an accurate initial examination will be impossible secondary to swelling and muscular spasm. When significant joint instability exists on stress testing, operative treatment is indicated. In the presence of significant spasm and a negative initial examination, the injured extremity should be reexamined 24 hours later for confirmation of the previous findings, and the patient should be kept nonweight bearing. Intravenous analgesics, intra-articular lidocaine, and even general anesthesia may be necessary to gain a reliable physical examination even after 1 to 2 days. Reexamination is indicated in a stable knee when any of the criteria listed in Table 20–8 are present.

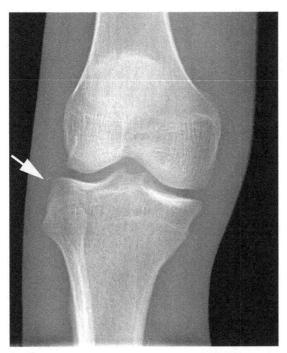

Figure 20–45. Segond fracture (*arrow*). This subtle avulsion fracture of the lateral tibial condyle is highly associated with an ACL tear or meniscal injury.

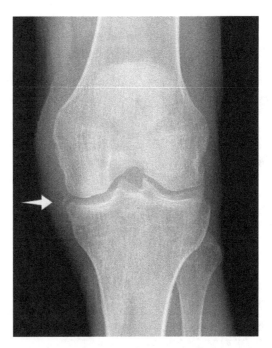

Figure 20–46. Reverse Segond fracture (*arrow*). This subtle avulsion fracture of the medial tibial condyle is highly associated with a PCL tear or medial meniscal injury. (*Used with permission from Michael C. Bond, MD.*)

▶ **TABLE 20-7. TREATMENT OF INCOMPLETE LIGAMENT INJURIES OF THE KNEE**

Mild Sprain
1. Ice and elevation
2. Jones compression dressing (Appendix A–15)
3. Ambulation with quadriceps exercises as soon as tolerated

Partial Tear
1. Ice and elevation
2. Posterior splint, immobilizer, or compression dressing (Appendix A–15 to A–17)
3. Nonweight bearing with crutches for 3 d
4. Knee immobilizer for 2 to 4 wk with gradual weight bearing as tolerated
5. Isometric quadriceps exercises
6. Early orthopedic follow-up; consider reevaluation in 24 h if examination is limited

Definitive Treatment

Collateral Ligaments. Nonoperative therapy for complete tears of the MCL with only mild-to-moderate joint instability is advocated. The treatment has been divided into three phases. In phase A, the leg is placed in an orthosis in approximately 30-degree flexion with partial weight bearing with crutches. Isometric quadriceps exercises and hip strengthening exercises are started in the second week. In phase B, which lasts for an additional 4 weeks, the orthosis is adjusted to allow 30 to 90 degrees of motion, and both isotonic and isokinetic exercises are performed. In phase C, which occurs 6 weeks after diagnosis, the orthosis is removed, and exercises are continued with a mild running program. When significant joint instability exists on stress testing, operative treatment is indicated.

It is important to rule out concomitant cruciate ligament ruptures or meniscus injury. When MCL and ACL injuries coexist, the majority of orthopedic surgeons treat the MCL injury first with conservative management, followed by delayed ACL reconstruction.

Isolated LCL injuries are also treated nonoperatively. When there is associated genu varum or injury to the posterolateral ligamentous complex or the PCL, surgery is indicated.

Cruciate Ligaments. Isolated ACL tears are common and can be treated with partial weight bearing with crutches.

▶ **TABLE 20-8. CRITERIA FOR REEVALUATING A "STABLE" KNEE**

High-energy mechanism of injury
History of a snap or pop at the time of injury
Hemarthrosis
Significant muscular spasm
Severe pain

Immobilization is not needed unless there are other ligamentous injuries and joint instability. The Management of ACL Injuries: Clinical Practice Guideline from the AAOS (American Association of Orthopaedic Surgeons) recommends against functional knee bracing for isolated ACL injuries because there is no demonstrated efficacy. Strengthening exercises are started after range of motion has returned. These injuries are managed operatively or nonoperatively. The decision to reconstruct the ligament depends on the patient's age, activity level, patient preferences, and presence of additional injuries. Operative repair is performed via arthroscopy in most cases. The ACL is reconstructed using autografts from the middle third of the patella tendon or a semitendinosus or gracilis graft.

In contrast to ACL injuries, isolated PCL tears are uncommon. When they do occur, they are usually treated nonoperatively. Isolated acute PCL injuries should be managed by splinting the knee in extension until the pain subsides and then allowing early motion. It is essential that the rehabilitation of this ligament emphasizes quadriceps strengthening.

Surgical reconstruction is reserved for symptomatic chronic PCL injuries and acute combined injuries (ACL, MCL, or posterolateral complex). In patients where a PCL injury is accompanied by a bony avulsion, operative treatment is recommended.

Complications

A small percentage of sprains become more painful during the healing phase. As the pain becomes severe, flexion may be limited. After 3 to 4 weeks, the plain film will show calcification in the area of the injured ligament. This condition is commonly referred to as posttraumatic periarticular ossification or Pellegrini–Stieda disease. Pathologically, calcium is deposited in the hematoma surrounding the partially torn ligament. This calcified mass may be connected to the underlying bone by way of a pedicle. In the early stages of development, massage or manipulation may worsen the symptoms. The recommended treatment includes a compression dressing and multiple punctures to enhance resorption of the calcium.

MENISCAL INJURIES

The medial meniscus is a "C"-shaped structure that is divided into an anterior and posterior horn. It is attached to the knee in three locations—on each end (intercondylar eminences) and at its midpoint (deep medial capsular ligament). The lateral meniscus also has an anterior and posterior horn. The lateral meniscus has more of an "O" shape and is attached medially to the intercondylar eminence (Fig. 20–47). The menisci move posteriorly with flexion and in an anterior direction with extension. Because of its single medial attachment, the lateral meniscus is more mobile than the medial meniscus.

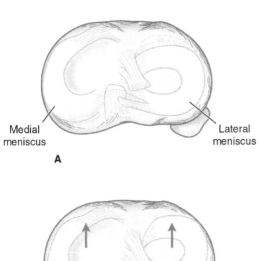

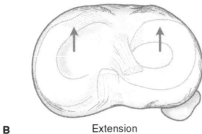

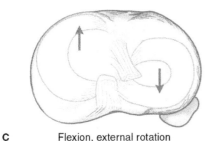

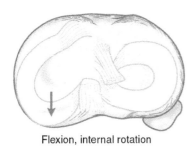

Figure 20–47. **A.** Articular surface of the tibia is shown with the menisci (as seen previously). Note the "O" shape of the lateral meniscus and the "C" shape of the medial meniscus. **B.** The position of the menisci with the knee in extension. **C.** Note the position of the menisci when the knee is flexed and in external rotation. The lateral meniscus is displaced posteriorly, and the anterior border of the medial meniscus protrudes forward. **D.** The position of the menisci with the knee in flexion and internal rotation of the tibia. Note that the medial meniscus retracts posteriorly.

Meniscal degenerative changes typically begin in the second decade of life and progress more rapidly under conditions of undue stress.[130] Several factors increase the propensity for meniscal injuries, including a congenitally discoid

meniscus, weakness of the surrounding musculature, and ligamentous laxity. Once an injury has occurred, healing is limited because the menisci are relatively avascular with a capillary supply limited to the peripheral one-fourth.

One-half to two-thirds of meniscal tears are longitudinal, extending from the anterior to the posterior horn (Fig. 20–48A and B). These injuries are referred to as "bucket handle tears" and can result in migration of the torn meniscus into the interior of the knee joint (Fig. 20–48C). The fragment may become uplifted, resulting in locking of the knee joint (Fig. 20–48D). The medial meniscus is more commonly affected because of its more secure attachments. Transverse tears are uncommon and may be seen in both the medial and lateral menisci (Fig. 20–48E). Transverse tears or spontaneous detachments are usually seen after a degenerative process with repeated exposure to minor stress.

Mechanism of Injury

Meniscal injuries occur frequently in patients with sudden rotary or extension–flexion motions. In older patients with degenerative disease of the menisci, a simple twist or squatting motion may result in a tear. With knee flexion, the femur rotates internally on the fixed tibia and displaces the medial meniscus toward the center of the joint. With a rapid forceful extension, the meniscus may be trapped centrally, resulting in peripheral segment stretching or tearing. With knee flexion, the lateral meniscus is also displaced centrally and a sudden forceful extension may result in a transverse tear at the junction of the anterior and middle thirds.

Examination

The sensitivity of detecting a meniscal lesion by any one clinical test is low.[129,130] The combined use of history and physical examination improves the ability of the experienced clinician to detect these injuries. The emergency provider should have a high index of suspicion for these injuries and refer patients to their primary care provider or an orthopedist when questions arise.

The menisci have no sensory nerve fibers, and the pain that results after these injuries is from irritation of the ligaments near the joint line. Several symptoms suggest the presence of a meniscal tear: (1) joint line pain, (2) joint effusion, (3) locking, and (4) giving way of the knee.

Joint Line Pain. Joint pain or tenderness on palpation of the joint line is seen in three-fourths of patients after a meniscal injury.[116] Bragard sign (indicating medial meniscus injury) refers to point tenderness along the anterior medial joint line that is increased with internal rotation and extension of the tibia. With internal rotation and extension, the torn medial meniscus is forced against the palpating finger of the examiner. To confirm a meniscal tear, Steinmann sign may be useful (Fig. 20–49). This sign is considered positive for a meniscal tear when flexion of the knee displaces the point of maximal tenderness posteriorly. This test is useful to distinguish meniscal from ligamentous

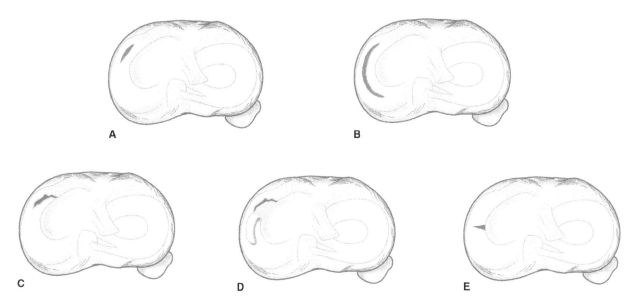

Figure 20–48. Medial meniscal tears. **A.** A partial longitudinal tear of the medial meniscus. **B.** A tear extending across the length of the meniscus is called a "bucket handle tear." The inner fragment can displace into the interior of the knee joint. **C.** A tear of the anterior horn. **D.** If the fragment becomes uplifted, it can produce locking of the knee. **E.** A transverse tear of the medial meniscus. This type of tear is more common in the lateral meniscus.

injuries because when the ligaments are the source of pain, the location of maximal tenderness will not change.

Joint Effusion. A joint effusion immediately after an injury suggests a ligamentous injury or an osteochondral fracture. Effusions developing 6 to 12 hours after an injury typically follow minor ligamentous sprains or meniscal tears. An acute tear in a degenerated meniscus may produce no effusion.

Locking. Knee locking may be of two types—true or pseudo. Pseudo locking is usually secondary to an effusion that causes pain and muscle spasm. True locking occurs spontaneously with some degree of flexion to the knee. A torn meniscus, loose body, rupture of the cruciate ligament, or an osteochondral fracture can all cause true locking. Childhood locking is rare; however, it may indicate a congenital discoid meniscus.

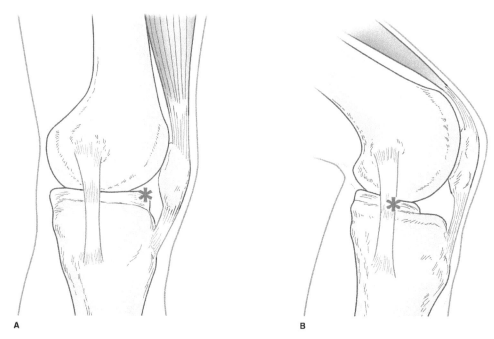

Figure 20–49. Steinmann sign. **A.** When the knee joint is extended, the meniscus lies anteriorly. **B.** Flexion of the knee displaces the point of tenderness from the anterior joint line back toward the collateral ligament. This indicates a meniscal problem rather than a ligamentous problem as the latter does not displace the point of maximal tenderness.

Only 30% of patients with meniscal injuries have true locking. Classically, the patient will complain of a sudden inability to fully extend the knee. Extension can be completed by rotating and passively extending the knee. True locking due to a meniscal tear is never complete because some extension against a rubbery resistance will be present. In addition, meniscal injuries rarely lock in full extension. An inability to fully extend the knee after trauma is usually secondary to muscular splinting, a loose body, or an effusion.

Knee Giving Way. Giving way of the injured knee is a common complaint of patients with meniscal tears.[131] It occurs when the knee cannot support weight on it irrespective of pain. When a patient reports that the knee gives way, the provider should ascertain the frequency, as well as any previous injuries to the knee. Other causes of this complaint include quadriceps weakness, patellar disorders, and ACL injuries.

There are several clinical signs that suggest the presence of a meniscal tear or help to differentiate it from a ligamentous tear:

- Payr sign involves placing the patient in a cross-legged position and pushing down on the thigh (Fig. 20–50). When this causes posterior knee pain, it suggests a tear of the posterior horn of the medial meniscus.
- Internal rotation of the flexed knee will result in pain in the anterolateral joint line in patients with a lesion of the lateral meniscus.
- Anteromedial joint line pain with external rotation of the flexed knee is indicative of a medial meniscus tear.

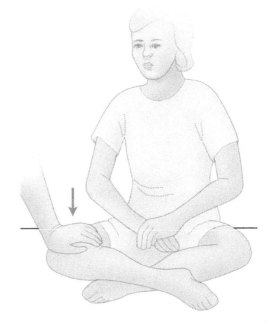

Figure 20–50. Payr sign. This produces pain with a lesion of the posterior horn of the medial meniscus.

- Apley test is performed on a prone patient with the knee flexed (Fig. 20–51). The examiner gradually extends the leg while it is externally rotated. This maneuver is repeated first while providing distraction and then compression. If the pain is worse with compression, the test is positive, indicating the possibility of a medial meniscus tear.

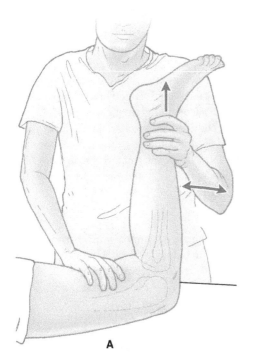

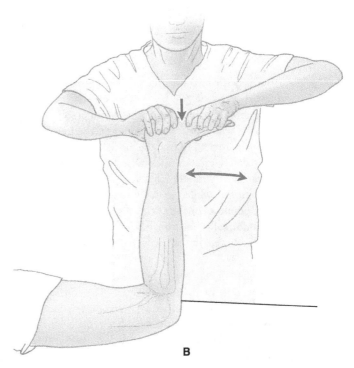

A   B

Figure 20–51. Apley test for medial meniscal tears. ***A.*** The leg is externally rotated and then extended while providing traction. ***B.*** The test is repeated, this time with compression.

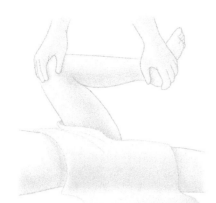

A

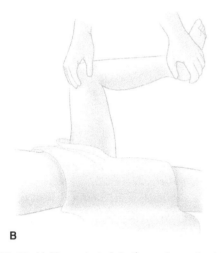

B

Figure 20–52. McMurray test. **A.** In the supine patient, flex the hip and knee. **B.** The knee and hip are then extended in either internal rotation (lateral meniscus) or external rotation (medial meniscus).

- McMurray test is performed with the patient supine and the hip and knee flexed (Fig. 20–52). To check the medial meniscus, the examiner palpates the posteromedial joint line with one hand while the other hand grasps the foot. The leg is externally rotated to trap the medial meniscus, and the knee is slowly extended. Conversely, the lateral meniscus is examined with the clinician palpating the posterolateral joint line while internally rotating the leg. A painful click, popping, or thud felt in early extension is considered abnormal. Unfortunately, McMurray test has been found to have a limited sensitivity in detecting meniscal lesions.

- Originally described in 2005, the Thessaly test is a newer test for the detection of meniscal tears. The Thessaly test is performed with the patient standing on the affected leg only while the examiner holds the patient's hands (Fig. 20–53). The patient flexes his/her knee to 5 degrees and then rotates his/her knee and body, internally and externally, three times, keeping the knee flexed. The test is repeated at 20 degrees of knee flexion. This

maneuver causes a dynamic reproduction of load transmission in the knee joint that subjects the meniscus to an excessive load and often reproduces the pain the patient reported. This test is considered positive if the patient experiences medial or lateral joint line discomfort or has the sense of locking or catching. The sensitivity and specificity of detecting injuries of the medial meniscus were 66% and 96%, respectively, at 5 degrees of flexion, and 89% and 97%, respectively, at 20 degrees of flexion. For the lateral meniscus, the sensitivity and specificity at 5 degrees of flexion were 81% and 91%, respectively, and at 20 degrees of flexion, 92% and 96%. Overall, accuracy for detecting a meniscal injury at 20 degrees of flexion was 94% for the medical meniscus and 96% for the lateral meniscus. A more recent study questioned the reproducibility of the sensitivity and specificity of the Thessaly test and found that it was no better than the other physical exam tests to identify a meniscal injury; therefore, it should not be used as a substitute for MRI.

Imaging

Plain films, although usually negative, should be obtained. MRI is useful in detecting meniscal injuries but is expensive and cannot be readily obtained from the ED. Many authors believe that the accuracy of the clinical evaluation is comparable with MRI and that this imaging modality should thus be used sparingly in cases where the diagnosis remains unclear. Other studies have shown that the physical exam can only identify about 60% of meniscal injuries.

The accuracy of MRI was initially reported between 80% and 90% for meniscal injuries; however, with improved technology and experience reading these films, accuracy has improved to 90% to 95%. However, relying blindly on MRI to determine surgical intervention would result in inappropriate treatment. In one study using MRI in asymptomatic patients, 13% of patients younger than 45 years and 36% of patients older than 45 years were diagnosed with a meniscal tear. In elderly patients, meniscal tears are found in 65% of asymptomatic patients.

Arthroscopy is considered the gold standard for making the diagnosis and is also valuable because it can provide definitive treatment. The accuracy of arthroscopy is as high as 98%, depending on the skill and the experience of the arthroscopist.

Associated Injuries

Meniscal injuries frequently accompany ligamentous knee injuries, particularly injuries to the MCL and ACL. One-third of all meniscal tears are associated with an ACL injury. Meniscal injuries are also frequently associated with tibial plateau fractures, occurring in up to 47% of patients.

Treatment

Patients presenting with an acute meniscal tear without ligamentous injuries should have a bulky compression dressing (Appendix A–15), knee immobilizer (Appendix A–16),

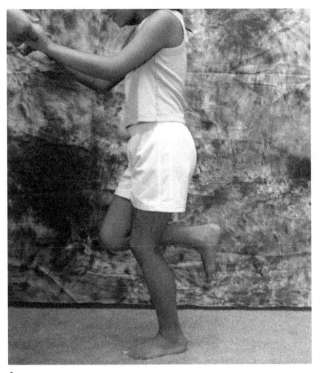

A

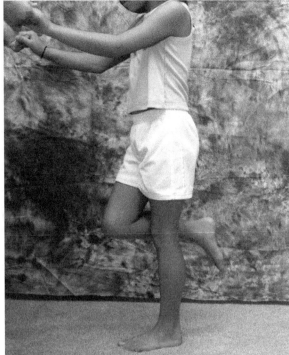

B

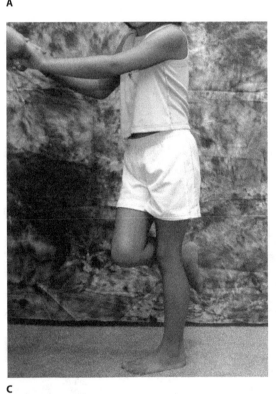

C

Figure 20–53. Thessaly test. **A.** Lateral view with the leg in 20-degree flexion with the examiner holding the patient's hands. **B.** Lateral view with the knee flexed to 5 degrees. **C.** Oblique view with the patient doing the twisting motion. *(Used with permission from Michael C. Bond, MD.)*

or a long-leg posterior splint applied (Appendix A–17). Twenty-four hours after the initial injury and treatment, the patient should be reexamined to exclude an occult ligamentous injury.[141] Those patients with meniscal tears without associated ligamentous injuries should be kept nonweight bearing if the pain is severe. It is important that immobilization does not persist for more than 2 to 4 days and that quadriceps-strengthening exercises are begun as early as possible. Referral to a primary care provider is appropriate for minor injuries, whereas orthopedic referral is needed whenever a significant effusion or instability of the joint is present. In patients with chronic symptoms, orthopedic referral should be provided whenever the patient reports locking, giving way, or catching.[140]

Nonoperative management is more likely to succeed in patients who are able to bear weight, who have developed swelling 24 to 48 hours after injury, who have minimal swelling, and who possess a full range of motion. Peripheral meniscal injuries also do better with nonoperative management because of improved vascularity to the peripheral portion of the meniscus. Limited improvement in symptoms after 3 weeks of conservative therapy suggests that surgery will likely be required.

The indications for arthroscopy include (1) persistent symptoms that affect daily activities, (2) positive physical findings of meniscal injury, (3) failure to respond to conservative management, and (4) absence of other causes of knee pain. Depending on the size, direction, and location of the tear, the surgeon may repair, remove, or leave the lesion to heal on its own.

Meniscal repair is preferable to maintain its important role in shock absorption within the knee. Meniscal tears that can be repaired have the following characteristics in common: (1) a tear is located no more than 3 mm from the meniscocapsular junction, (2) minimal damage has occurred to the body of the meniscus, (3) a tear that can be displaced with probing, and (4) a complete vertical longitudinal tear greater than 10 mm. When repair is not feasible, partial meniscectomy is advocated. In some instances, the meniscal lesion will heal spontaneously. Stable vertical longitudinal tears heal spontaneously without treatment in 65% of cases.

A locked knee secondary to a meniscal tear should be reduced within 24 hours after the injury. The knee can be reduced by positioning the patient with the extremity hanging off the edge of the table and the knee in 90-degree flexion. Gravity will distract the tibia from the femur. Intra-articular injection of 5 to 10 mL of local anesthetic will aid in unlocking the knee by reducing pain. The knee may unlock on its own after a period of rest (30 minutes) in this position. If it does not, mild rotation of the tibia with careful traction along the axis of the leg will usually result in reduction. If unsuccessful after a gentle attempt, a posterior splint should be applied. Manipulation of the acutely locked knee may further damage the involved meniscus, and therefore, consultation before further attempts at reduction is strongly recommended.

OSTEOCHONDRITIS DISSECANS

Osteochondritis dissecans, a condition of focal subchondral bone necrosis leading to articular cartilage disruption and displacement of a bony fragment into the joint space, is common in the knee joint, accounting for 75% of all cases. It occurs most frequently in the medial femoral condyle, but the lateral femoral condyle and patella are also affected. The remaining 25% of cases of osteochondritis dissecans occur in the elbow and ankle.

There are several proposed theories as to the etiology of osteochondritis dissecans, including localized ischemia and repetitive trauma. The surface of the joint becomes irregular, predisposing toward the development of osteoarthritis. In some instances, a sequestrum of bone or cartilage may become free in the joint and locking occurs.

Clinical Presentation

Frequently, this diagnosis is made in an asymptomatic patient on the basis of radiographic findings alone. Symptoms can include a persistent ache at rest, which is exacerbated with exercise. Some patients complain of a stiff sensation that is relieved by kicking. Recurrent knee effusions may be associated with this disorder. Percussion of the patella with the knee in flexion typically exacerbates the pain.

Imaging

The plain film will be negative in early cases. Later, a cavity surrounded by dense bone may be seen (Figs. 20–54 and 20–55).

Lesions are radiographically occult in up to 57% patients with chronic knee pain. Radionuclide bone scans, CT, and MRI are much more sensitive than plain films in identifying these lesions. MRI is of particular value in determining the need for operative intervention.

Treatment

The treatment of this condition is different in adults versus children. Children tend to heal well with conservative treatment, whereas adults frequently require surgery. Immobilization in a cast with nonweight bearing for 6 to 12 months frequently results in resolution of a newly acquired lesion

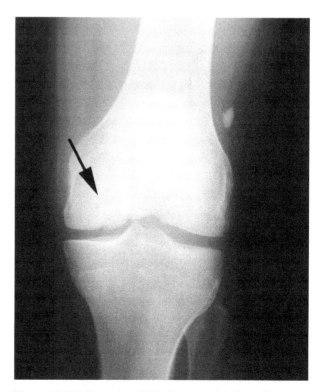

Figure 20–54. Osteochondritis dissecans of the knee (*arrow*).

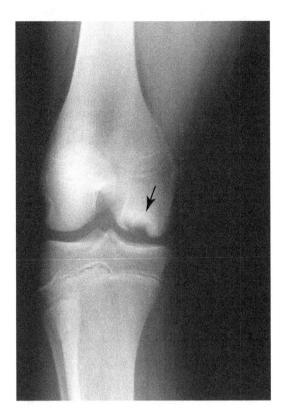

Figure 20–55. Osteochondritis dissecans. Note the development of fibrous tissue (*arrow*). *(Used with permission from John Fitzpatrick, MD.)*

in a child. Surgery is recommended in adults to prevent the development of premature degenerative arthritis. When a loose body is present in the joint space, surgical removal is indicated in both children and adults. Controversy exists as to the best surgical method to employ.[151–153] Arthroscopic surgery has yielded excellent results in this condition.[154–156]

OSTEOCHONDRAL INJURY

These injuries typically present with persistent pain after an injury without radiographic abnormalities. Chondral fractures involve only cartilage, whereas osteochondral fractures involve the cartilage as well as the subchondral bone. The most common mechanism is a direct impact over the involved area.

Examination

These injuries should be suspected if the patient's complaints are significant in the absence of physical findings. Acutely localized tenderness, joint locking, and hemarthrosis are frequently associated with this injury. These injuries are often confused with a meniscal tear, although arthroscopy will definitely exclude this problem.

Treatment

Arthroscopy is indicated in almost all cases. Degenerative arthritis with chronic pain, locking, and effusions develops if these injuries are left untreated.

▶ TABLE 20–9. **RISK FACTORS FOR PATELLOFEMORAL ARTHRITIS**

Increasing age
Obesity
Chronic overuse
Prior injuries (fractures, patellar dislocation, ACL tears)
Systemic inflammatory conditions

ACL, anterior cruciate ligament.

PATELLOFEMORAL DYSFUNCTION (CHONDROMALACIA PATELLAE)

Osteoarthritis of the knee is discussed in Chapter 3. Because the patellofemoral joint is unique, it is covered separately. Patellofemoral arthritis is the result of erosion and degeneration of the patellar cartilage. Risk factors for patellofemoral arthritis are listed in Table 20–9.[157] The terms *chondromalacia patellae* and *patellar malalignment syndrome* are used to describe premature patellar cartilage erosion occurring commonly in young adults, particularly women, due to patellar malalignment.

The patella acts to improve the function of the quadriceps mechanism and decreases the forces applied to the patellar tendon. The angle at which this force acts is believed to alter the patellofemoral mechanics and predispose to injury. When the angle is normal, pressure is distributed evenly across the patella. When the angle is increased, however, the lateral facet of the patella assumes a greater load and is injured.[157]

Patellar malalignment is determined clinically by measuring the Q angle (Fig. 20–56). Two lines intersecting

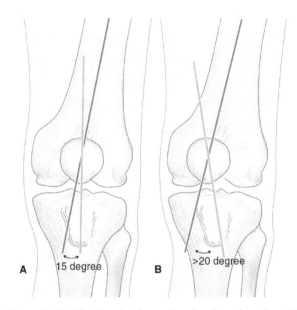

Figure 20–56. The Q angle is formed by a line drawn from the midpoint of the patella through the midpoint of the femoral shaft and a second line drawn from the midpoint of the patella through the tibial tuberosity. **A.** The normal Q angle is approximately 15 degrees. **B.** A Q angle of greater than 20 degrees is considered to be abnormal.

through the center of the patella form this angle. The first line is drawn from the middle of the femur through the center of the patella. The second line is drawn from the center of the patella through the tibial tubercle. The normal Q angle is 15 degrees, whereas measurements greater than 20 degrees are considered abnormal.

Clinical Presentation

When due to patellar malalignment, symptoms begin in the adolescent age group or the young adult. The patient will complain of a deep aching in the knees without a history of recent trauma. Strenuous athletic activities or prolonged sitting may exacerbate the pain hours later. Eventually, as the disorder progresses, slight exertion, as with climbing steps, will exacerbate the pain. The pain is usually localized to the anterior or medial portion of the knee. Acute trauma to the knee as during a fall may result in retropatellar pain and, in some instances, the development of chondromalacia patellae over a period of several weeks.

During the physical examination, the knee should be in slight flexion, thus drawing the patella into the femoral groove. Palpation and compression in this position will avoid synovial entrapment. Firm compression of the patella into the medial femoral groove will elicit pain, which is virtually pathognomonic. Anterior knee pain is present when the knee is maximally flexed. In addition, palpation of the undersurface of the medially displaced patella will typically yield tenderness and crepitus (Fig. 20–57). Knee extension against resistance is also painful through the terminal 30 to 40 degrees.

The patellar inhibition test is performed with the knee extended. The examiner pushes the patella inferiorly into the femoral groove. The patient is then asked to contract the quadriceps muscle while the patella is held firmly against the femoral condyles (Fig. 20–58). Pain, tenderness, and crepitus are diagnostic of patellofemoral joint arthropathy.

In addition to the Q angle, the examiner should note the course of the patella through flexion and extension of the knee. Normally with extension, the patella moves vertically with a slight medial shift as full extension is approached. A hypermobile or wandering patellae (patellar malalignment)

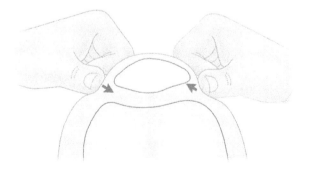

Figure 20–57. Palpation of the undersurface of the patella will elicit tenderness in chondromalacia of the patella.

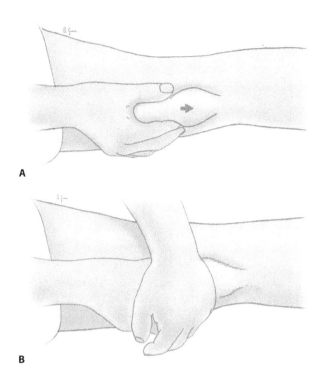

A

B

Figure 20–58. The patellar inhibition test is shown. **A.** With the quadriceps muscle relaxed push the patella inferiorly. **B.** Compress the patella into the femoral groove and ask the patient to tighten the quadriceps muscle. This will elicit pain and tenderness as the patella courses proximally.

with knee extension predispose to the development of chondromalacia patellae.

Patellofemoral arthritis may be confused with several other causes of anterior knee pain, including a torn medial meniscus, prepatellar bursitis, pes anserinus bursitis, fat pad syndrome, and osteochondritis dissecans.

Imaging

Radiographs are typically of little diagnostic value in a patient with this condition. Chronic changes such as sclerosis or osteophyte development, however, may occasionally be seen.

Treatment

Conservative treatment includes rest, nonsteroidal anti-inflammatory medications, and isometric quadriceps strengthening exercises. Isometric quadriceps exercises are performed with the patient lying down and the lower extremity held horizontal to the ground. The patient is instructed to lift the leg with the knee in full extension and hold this position for 5 seconds. This is repeated for three sets of 20 daily. The same technique is used with the knee held in 30-degree flexion. It is of critical importance to stress to the patient that the straight-leg exercises with the knee held at 30-degree flexion are key to resolution of the symptoms.

Steroid use is not recommended as it may increase the rate of cartilage degradation. The avoidance of activities such as squatting, running, kneeling, and climbing of steps is strongly recommended during the initial management phase. Immobilization is contraindicated because it leads to quadriceps atrophy that may exaggerate patellar malalignment.

KNEE DISLOCATIONS

Dislocations of the knee are considered orthopedic emergencies because an associated popliteal artery injury is present in one-third of these cases.[161] The incidence of knee dislocation has been estimated to be less than 0.02%, but this figure underestimates the true incidence because it does not take into account dislocations that have spontaneously reduced.[162] Therefore, the diagnosis can only be made if the examining provider retains a high index of suspicion.

Dislocations are classified as anterior (40%), posterior (33%), lateral (18%), medial (4%), or rotary (uncommon) on the basis of the direction of the tibia in relation to the femur (Fig. 20–59). Combinations of these dislocations also occur. The most common combination is the posterolateral dislocation.[163]

Bicruciate ligament injury without radiographic confirmation of dislocation is also considered a knee dislocation because these injuries are associated with the same high rate of associated neurovascular injury. In one series, more than half of the popliteal artery injuries occurred in patients with spontaneously reduced bicruciate ligament injuries.[164]

Mechanism of Injury

Knee dislocations are due to high-energy (motor vehicle collision, fall from height) and low-energy (minor fall, athletic activity) trauma. Motor vehicle collisions account for two-thirds of cases.[90,165] Low-energy mechanisms account for up to 20% of cases and are especially common in patients with a high body mass index after simple falls. Open dislocations are present in 16% of cases and are usually due to a high-energy mechanism.[164]

Anterior dislocations typically result from hyperextension. Hyperextension results in a tear of the posterior capsule followed by a rupture of the anterior cruciate and a partial tear of the posterior cruciate. Posterior dislocations usually result from a direct force applied to the anterior tibia with the knee flexed slightly. There is posterior displacement of the tibia with rupture of the posterior capsule and cruciates. A violent adduction force on the tibia against

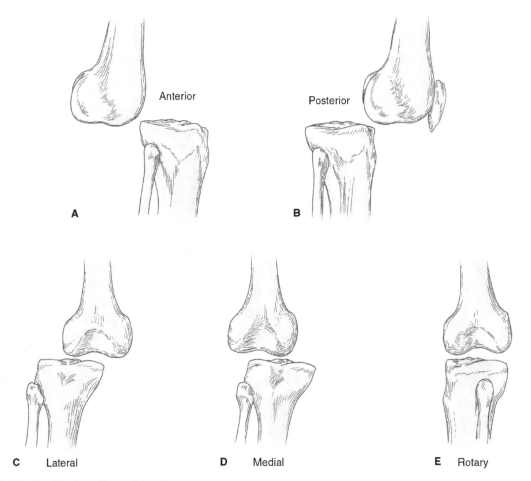

Figure 20–59. Classification of knee dislocations.

the femur may result in a medial dislocation. Rotary posterolateral dislocations are seen when an anteromedial force acts on the anterior tibia, resulting in a posterior dislocation with rotation. A posteromedial dislocation is the result of anterolateral force acting on the anterior tibia.

Examination

An accurate diagnosis of a knee dislocation is imperative and is based on a high index of suspicion. Spontaneous reduction prior to ED presentation is not uncommon and does not mean that the patient is not at risk for associated vascular injuries. A review of 63 knee dislocations noted that two-thirds were found in a reduced position at presentation.

> **Axiom:** *A grossly unstable knee after a traumatic injury should be considered a reduced dislocation.*

The initial assessment of a potentially dislocated knee is limited to inspection, palpation, and a distal neurovascular examination. Gross deformity may not be present due to significant adipose tissue or reduction prior to arrival in the ED (Fig. 20–60). There may or may not be an effusion because tears in the joint capsule will allow blood to dissect into the surrounding tissues.

The distal neurovascular status must be assessed early and completely in all patients. Diminished or absent distal pulses, distal ischemia, an ankle-brachial index (ABI) less than 0.9, or an expanding or pulsatile hematoma are hard evidence of a vascular injury and necessitate surgical exploration.

Nevertheless, a serious arterial injury may be present despite a warm foot or the presence of a distal pulse. Pulse examination is only 80% sensitive for detecting popliteal artery injury.

The ligamentous structures are examined, but this is difficult secondary to pain. A Lachman test and a posterior drawer test are used to assess the ACL and PCL, respectively. The collateral ligaments are stressed at 30-degree flexion. Hyperextension should be avoided because it places unnecessary traction on the peroneal nerve and popliteal artery.

Peroneal nerve injury is assessed by noting hypoesthesia in the first web space or loss of dorsiflexion of the foot. If significant swelling is present in a tense leg, compartment syndrome should be suspected.

Imaging

AP and lateral views demonstrate the knee dislocation (unless it has spontaneously reduced) and usually any associated fractures (Fig. 20–61).

Arteriography has been considered the gold standard for diagnosing popliteal artery injuries, including the difficult-to-detect intimal injury. However, CT angiography has surpassed arteriography because it is more readily available and has fewer complications when compared to traditional arteriography (Fig. 20–62).

CT is also playing a larger role in the evaluation of knee dislocations due to its higher sensitivity for fractures and associated proximal tibiofibular dislocations.

In patients without hard signs of vascular injury, duplex Doppler ultrasonography may be beneficial. The reported sensitivity is 95%, with a specificity of 99%. Ultrasound

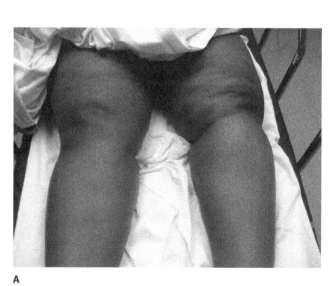 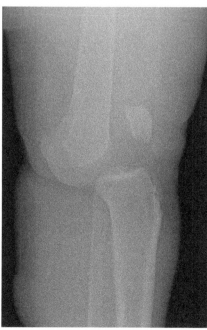

A   **B**

Figure 20–60. Dislocation of the left knee without significant deformity due to a large amount of adipose tissue. This injury occurred after a fall in the bathroom. **A.** Clinical photo. **B.** Lateral radiograph.

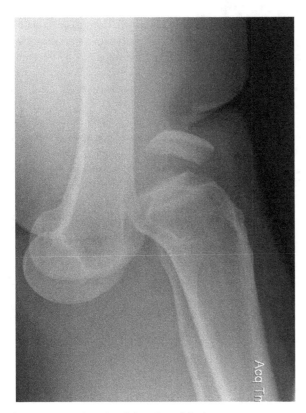

Figure 20–61. Anterior dislocation of the knee.

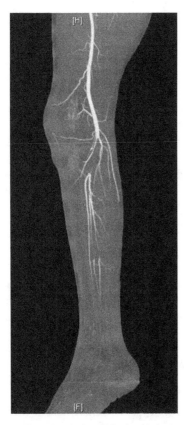

Figure 20–62. CT angiography of the leg demonstrating popliteal artery injury.

can miss intimal tears, however, so the gold standard remains arteriography or CT angiography.

Associated Injuries

Knee dislocations are associated with several significant injuries that are divided into three categories—vascular, ligamentous, and peripheral nerve injuries. In addition to the direct injuries that occur to the vessels and nerves following a knee dislocation, compartment syndrome may also occur due to significant soft-tissue swelling and hemorrhage. Concomitant fractures and other injuries are especially common when the dislocation is due to a high-energy mechanism.

Vascular Injury. Anatomically, the popliteal artery is firmly anchored proximally by the adductor magnus muscle and distally by the gastrocnemius and soleus muscles. These attachments make the artery susceptible to injury and account for the 30% to 40% incidence of vascular injury after a knee dislocation. A recent study reports that popliteal arteries are injured in 18% of cases, with hyperextension being the most common mechanism.[170] However, a large insurance database review of 8058 patients with knee dislocations showed that only 267 had an associated vascular injury for an overall frequency of 3.3%.[171] Vascular injury is more common after anterior and posterior dislocations, as well as following a high-energy mechanism.[172] When injured, emergent repair is indicated because, if delayed more than 8 hours, up to 86% of patients will require an amputation.[173]

Ligamentous Injury. Rupture of the ACL and PCL is present in all cases of knee dislocations with rare exception. The medial collateral is the next most common ligamentous injury, occurring in 50% of cases, whereas the posterolateral complex is injured in 28%.[164] The direction of the dislocation does not correlate with ligamentous injury. Muscle injury (gastrocnemii), meniscal damage, and chondral fractures may also be present.

Nerve Injury. Nerve injury associated with knee dislocations is present in 16% to 40% of cases.[162] The tibial and common peroneal nerves are not anchored as securely as the popliteal artery; therefore, they are injured less frequently. It is estimated that the common peroneal nerve is injured in 20% of cases.[170] These injuries range from simple neurapraxia to complete disruption of the neural elements, which is rare. The mechanism of neural damage is usually a traction injury. Traction injuries to the peroneal and tibial nerves are frequently seen after anterior dislocations. The treatment of these injuries is controversial and left to the consultant.

Treatment

The emergency management of these injuries includes reduction, immobilization, assessment of vascular injuries, and emergent referral. Reduction should be performed with adequate analgesia and procedural sedation as outlined in Chapter 2.

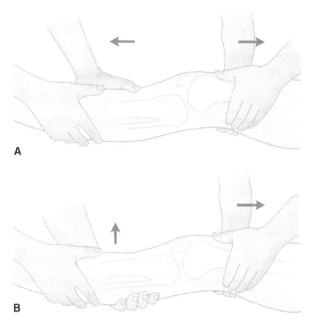

A

B

Figure 20–63. Reduction of a posterior dislocation. **A.** Distraction is the critical maneuver. **B.** Anterior pressure over the posterior tibia.

A posterior dislocation is reduced by having an assistant exert longitudinal traction while the proximal tibia is lifted anteriorly and reduced (Fig. 20–63). It should be noted that the distraction force should be gentle because excessive force may exacerbate arterial injury. An anterior dislocation is reduced in a similar manner, except the femur is lifted anteriorly into a reduced position (Video 20–3). Pressure over the popliteal space should be avoided. A posterolateral dislocation may be irreducible because the medial femoral condyle traps the medial capsule within the joint.

After reduction, the knee should be immobilized in a long-leg posterior splint (Appendix A–17) in 15-degree flexion to avoid tension on the popliteal artery.

Expeditious treatment of a vascular injury is critical to a good outcome. In approximately 10% of cases, normal pulses are restored after reduction of the knee. If signs of ischemia are present, emergent operative exploration is indicated with or without an intraoperative angiogram.

One study found that 4% of patients with a normal pulse examination who suffered a knee dislocation had a popliteal artery injury. If the pulses and perfusion are normal and there is no other evidence of vascular injury (i.e., expanding hematoma), the ABI is measured. The ABI is determined by dividing the systolic blood pressure (obtained by Doppler) of the affected leg by the same measurement in an unaffected upper extremity. The ABI has been found to be a helpful adjunct in detecting occult vascular injury when the rest of the vascular examination is normal. An ABI less than 0.9 is concerning in a patient with a knee dislocation and should warrant consultation and an arteriogram. However, ABIs will miss intimal flaps and false aneurysms as these injuries do not affect the flow of arterial blood. In patients with a normal vascular examination with an ABI measurement of greater than 0.9, diagnostic options include an arteriogram, CT angiography, or admission for serial examinations (Fig. 20–64). The option chosen may depend on the hospital setting or the preference of the consultant.

Once the possibility of vascular insufficiency has been resolved and the acute swelling has diminished, the patient will generally require operative ligamentous repair to achieve the best functional recovery possible. This procedure is generally performed 10 to 14 days following the injury, but it should not be delayed more than 3 weeks because excessive scarring makes the procedure more complicated. Surgical repair has good outcomes, with one study of 36 patients demonstrating that the mean time to surgery was 12 days (1–21 days), and after a mean follow-up of 10.1 years (7–19 years), patients had nearly normal knee function.

Complications

Knee dislocations are often complicated by the development of significant problems:

* Progressive distal ischemia resulting in amputation
* Degenerative joint disease with arthritis
* Persistent joint instability secondary to extensive ligamentous injuries

PROXIMAL TIBIOFIBULAR DISLOCATION

Pain along the lateral aspect of the knee must be carefully evaluated because the anatomy and the biomechanics of this region are very complex. Proximal tibiofibular dislocation occurs after trauma, whereas subluxation may be chronic and atraumatic. This injury is often confused with a torn lateral meniscus. Proximal tibiofibular dislocations can be anterior, posterior, or superior (Fig. 20–65). Anterior dislocations are most common. Superior dislocations are always accompanied by superior displacement of the lateral malleolus.

Subluxation of the proximal tibiofibular joint occurs when there is symptomatic hypermobility (Fig. 20–66).

Mechanism of Injury

Anterior dislocations typically result from a fall where the leg is flexed and adducted. Posterior dislocations are usually secondary to direct trauma to the flexed knee. A secondary mechanism involves a violent twisting motion as seen in athletics. In addition, violent twisting may rupture the ligaments and result in dislocation.

Examination

The location of the pain is generally along the lateral aspect of the knee. It radiates proximally into the region of the iliotibial band and medially into the patellofemoral joint. In

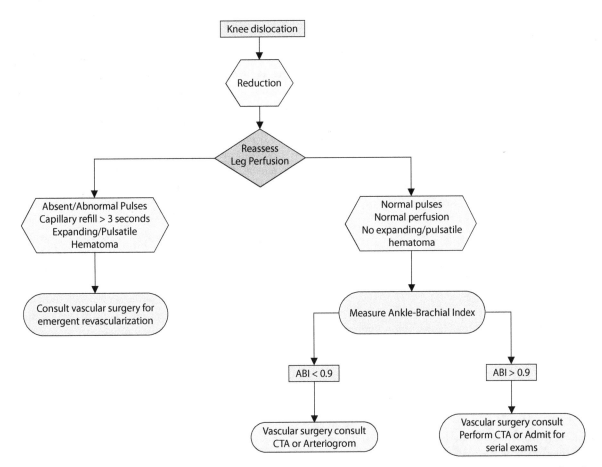

Figure 20–64. Algorithm for treating patients with knee dislocations or an unstable knee (presumed to be a spontaneously reduced dislocation). (CTA, computed tomography angiography).

cases of chronic subluxation, the patient will note a "clicking" or "popping" sensation in the front of the knee.[185,186]

On examination, there will be a localized exacerbation of pain with inversion or eversion of the ankle. Inspection of

the knee will reveal a prominent fibular head in an anterior lateral subluxation or dislocation. The pain will increase with palpation over the fibular head.[186] With an anterior dislocation, the fibular head will be more prominent when

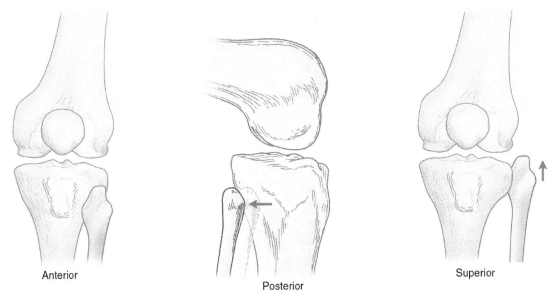

Figure 20–65. Proximal tibiofibular dislocations.

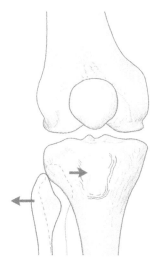

Figure 20–66. Proximal tibiofibular joint subluxation.

the knee is flexed. In addition, dorsiflexion and eversion will exacerbate the pain. Superior dislocations present with proximal displacement of the lateral malleolus.

Imaging

If this injury is suspected, comparison views are recommended. AP and lateral views are usually adequate in defining this injury. If plain films are not diagnostic, a CT is the most accurate imaging modality to detect this injury.

Associated Injuries

It is important to recall that the peroneal nerve passes inferior to the fibular head and encircles the neck of the fibula. Posterior dislocations are associated frequently with peroneal nerve injuries. Superior dislocations are always associated with interosseous membrane damage.

Treatment

Acute dislocations should be reduced by direct manipulation with the knee in flexion. An audible click is often heard as the fibula snaps back into position. Posterior dislocations with interposed soft tissues require operative reduction. After reduction, the patient should be on crutches and nonweight bearing for 2 weeks followed by progressive weight bearing over the next 6 weeks.

Treatment of chronic proximal tibiofibular subluxation involves modifying the patient's activities and the use of a supportive strap along with lower-leg strengthening exercises. For patients with chronic pain or instability, surgical correction is considered.

Complications

Peroneal nerve injury occurs in 5% of these dislocations and may present as a complication during the recuperation period. Posterior dislocations have a tendency to remain unstable and to develop recurrent subluxation. Degenerative joint disease with arthritis may develop after any of these dislocations.

PATELLAR DISLOCATION

Anatomically, the patella is an oval-shaped bone with two facets divided by a vertical ridge. The patella normally articulates in the groove between the femoral condyles. The vastus medialis, medial retinaculum, medial and lateral patellofemoral ligaments, and patellotibial ligaments prevent dislocation of the patella.

The most common location of patellar dislocations is lateral. Other dislocations that have been described include medial, superior, horizontal, and intercondylar (Fig. 20–67). Patellar dislocation with vertical axis rotation has also been described.

Patellar dislocations are typically seen in patients with chronic patellofemoral anatomic abnormalities. Dislocations and subluxations tend to be recurrent with redislocation rates ranging from 17% to 44%. Patellar subluxation is a common condition that usually occurs laterally and is associated with a tear of the retinaculum along the vastus medialis. Severe trauma is necessary for a dislocation to occur with a normal patellofemoral relationship. Patellar dislocations are associated with several conditions as shown in Table 20–10.

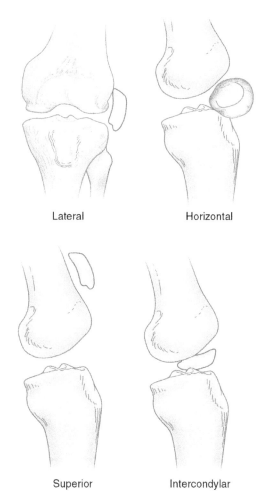

Lateral   Horizontal

Superior   Intercondylar

Figure 20–67. Patellar dislocations.

▶ **TABLE 20–10. CONDITIONS ASSOCIATED WITH PATELLAR DISLOCATIONS**

Genu valgum
Genu recurvatum
Excessive femoral neck anteversion or internal femoral torsion
External tibial torsion
Lateral insertion of patellar ligament on tibia
Contracture of lateral patellar retinaculum
Relaxation or attenuation of medial patellar retinaculum
Hypoplasia or dysplasia of patella
Hypoplasia or flattening of trochlear groove
Patella alta or high-riding patella
Atrophy of vastus medialis muscle
Pes planus
Generalized joint laxity

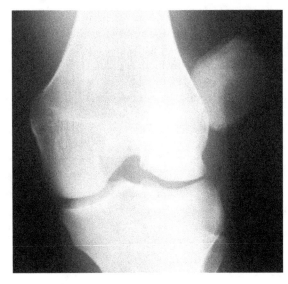

Figure 20–69. AP radiograph of a lateral patellar dislocation.

Mechanism of Injury

Two mechanisms result in patellar dislocations. A powerful contraction of the quadriceps in combination with sudden flexion and external rotation of the tibia on the femur is the most common cause of a lateral patellar dislocation.[187] Direct trauma to the patella with the knee in flexion may result in a dislocation, although this is uncommon. Horizontal dislocations are secondary to a direct blow on the superior pole of the patella followed by rotation.

Examination

The patient will relate a history of feeling the knee "go out" and will note a deformity followed by swelling (Fig. 20–68). Frequently, the patella will relocate prior to presentation. If the patella is still dislocated at presentation, deformity and hemarthrosis will be present and the knee will be flexed.

If spontaneous reduction has occurred, there is generally tenderness along the undersurface of the patella and the patellar apprehension test is positive. To perform this test, the knee is flexed to 30 degrees and the patella is pushed laterally; if the sensation of impending redislocation occurs, the test is considered positive.

Imaging

AP and lateral views are usually adequate in assessing this injury (Fig. 20–69). Radiographs should be obtained

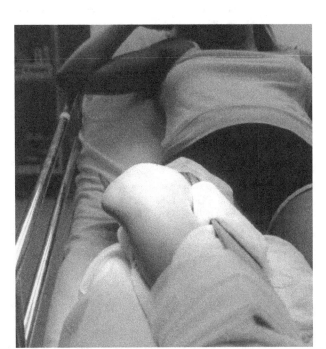

A

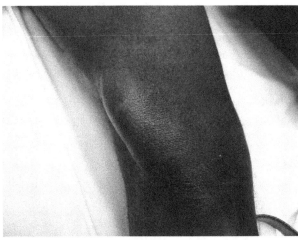

B

Figure 20–68. A. Lateral patella dislocation in a young woman. **B.** Patella dislocation with vertical-axis rotation. (**B,** Reproduced with permission from Sherman SC, Yu A: Patellar dislocation with vertical axis rotation, *J Emerg Med.* 2004 Feb;26(2):219–220.)

to exclude a fracture. The presence of a fat–fluid level is indicative of a bony or osteochondral fracture. Note that an abnormal patellofemoral angle is not a reliable radiologic sign of patellar instability in acute dislocation.[189]

Ultrasound and MRI do not need to be performed in the ED; however, one study showed that they have equal efficacy in detecting medial patellofemoral ligament tears after acute lateral patellar dislocation.[190]

Associated Injuries

The most common associated injury is an intra-articular loose body or osteochondral fracture of the medial facet of the patella or the lateral femoral condyle. Osteochondral injuries are present in 40% of cases.[160] These injuries are often difficult to see on plain radiographs.

Treatment

To reduce a lateral patella dislocation, flex the hip initially. Then, while extending the knee, apply a gentle pressure over the patella in a medial direction (Video 20–4). Intra-articular and horizontal dislocations are sometimes reduced by closed manipulation, although most require open reduction. Superior dislocations and lateral dislocations with vertical axis rotation usually require operative reduction.

After reduction, radiographs documenting the position of the patella should be obtained. The leg should be placed in a knee immobilizer (Appendix A–16) in full extension for 3 to 7 weeks. Ice is also recommended for the first 24 hours. Referral to an orthopedic surgeon is recommended. Some orthopedic surgeons believe that all first-time dislocations should be surgically repaired initially, whereas others elect for a more conservative approach. Recurrent patellar dislocations should be treated surgically; however, we do not advocate surgical treatment for first-time injuries.[191,192] Dislocations associated with an osteochondral fracture are best treated surgically.[193,194]

Patellar subluxation is managed conservatively; isometric exercises are initially undertaken to strengthen the quadriceps. Stretching exercises for the hamstrings are also advocated. In cases where tenderness is severe and one notices substantial laxity, the use of a patellar restraining brace is used. Operative therapy is reserved for patients who have failed conservative treatment after 6 to 12 months.

Complications

Patellar dislocations are subject to degenerative arthritis and recurrent dislocation and subluxation.

REFERENCES

1. Kennedy JC, Fowler PJ. Medial and anterior instability of the knee. An anatomical and clinical study using stress machines. *J Bone Joint Surg Am.* 1971;53(7):1257–1270.
2. Fetto JF, Marshall JL. Medial collateral ligament injuries of the knee: a rationale for treatment. *Clin Orthop.* 1978;(132):206–218.
3. Hughston JC, Andrews JR, Cross MJ, Moschi A. Classification of knee ligament instabilities. Part I. The medial compartment and cruciate ligaments. *J Bone Joint Surg Am.* 1976;58(2):159–172.
4. Seebacher JR, Inglis AE, Marshall JL, Warren RF. The structure of the posterolateral aspect of the knee. *J Bone Joint Surg Am.* 1982;64(4):536–541.
5. Pacheco RJ, Ayre CA, Bollen SR. Posterolateral corner injuries of the knee: a serious injury commonly missed. *J Bone Joint Surg Br.* 2011;93(2):194–197.
6. Lundquist RB, Matcuk GR, Schein AJ, Patel D. Posteromedial corner of the knee: the neglected corner. *Radiographics.* 2015;35(4):1123–1137.
7. Sanville P, Nicholson DA, Driscoll PA. ABC of emergency radiology. The knee. *BMJ.* 1994;308(6921):121–126.
8. Nichol G, Stiell IG, Wells GA, Juergensen LS, Laupacis A. An economic analysis of the Ottawa knee rule. *Ann Emerg Med.* 1999;34(4 pt 1):438–447.
9. Seaberg DC, Yealy DM, Lukens T, Auble T, Mathias S. Multicenter comparison of two clinical decision rules for the use of radiography in acute, high-risk knee injuries. *Ann Emerg Med.* 1998;32(1):8–13.
10. Stiell IG, Greenberg GH, Wells GA, et al. Prospective validation of a decision rule for the use of radiography in acute knee injuries. *JAMA.* 1996;275(8):611–615.
11. Stiell IG, Wells GA, Hoag RH, et al. Implementation of the Ottawa Knee Rule for the use of radiography in acute knee injuries. *JAMA.* 1997;278(23):2075–2079.
12. Emparanza JI, Aginaga JR, Estudio Multicéntro en Urgencias de Osakidetza: Reglas de Ottawa (EMUORO) Group. Validation of the Ottawa Knee Rules. *Ann Emerg Med.* 2001;38(4):364–368.
13. Stiell IG, Greenberg GH, Wells GA, et al. Derivation of a decision rule for the use of radiography in acute knee injuries. *Ann Emerg Med.* 1995;26(4):405–413.
14. Stiell IG, Wells GA, McDowell I, et al. Use of radiography in acute knee injuries: need for clinical decision rules. *Acad Emerg Med.* 1995;2(11):966–973.
15. Bachmann LM, Haberzeth S, Steurer J, ter Riet G. The accuracy of the Ottawa knee rule to rule out knee fractures: a systematic review. *Ann Intern Med.* 2004;140(2):121–124.
16. Bulloch B, Neto G, Plint A, et al. Validation of the Ottawa Knee Rule in children: a multicenter study. *Ann Emerg Med.* 2003;42(1):48–55.
17. Khine H, Dorfman DH, Avner JR. Applicability of Ottawa knee rule for knee injury in children. *Pediatr Emerg Care.* 2001;17(6):401–404.
18. Cohen DM, Jasser JW, Kean JR, Smith GA. Clinical criteria for using radiography for children with acute knee injuries. *Pediatr Emerg Care.* 1998;14(3):185–187.
19. Vijayasankar D, Boyle AA, Atkinson P. Can the Ottawa knee rule be applied to children? A systematic review and meta-analysis of observational studies. *Emerg Med J.* 2009;26(4):250–253.
20. Kec RM, Richman PB, Szucs PA, Mandell M, Eskin B. Can emergency department triage nurses appropriately utilize the Ottawa Knee Rules to order radiographs? An implementation trial. *Acad Emerg Med.* 2003;10(2):146–150.
21. Matteucci MJ, Roos JA. Ottawa Knee Rule: a comparison of physician and triage-nurse utilization of a decision rule for knee injury radiography. *J Emerg Med.* 2003;24(2):147–150.

22. Szucs PA, Richman PB, Mandell M. Triage nurse application of the Ottawa knee rule. *Acad Emerg Med.* 2001;8(2):112–116.

23. Jackson JL, O'Malley PG, Kroenke K. Evaluation of acute knee pain in primary care. *Ann Intern Med.* 2003;139(7):575–588.

24. Cheung TC, Tank Y, Breederveld RS, Tuinebreijer WE, de Lange-de Klerk ES, Derksen RJ. Diagnostic accuracy and reproducibility of the Ottawa Knee Rule vs the Pittsburgh Decision Rule. *Am J Emerg Med.* 2013;31(4):641–645.

25. Schatzker J. Fractures of the distal femur revisited. *Clin Orthop.* 1998;(347):43–56.

26. Crawford AH. Fractures about the knee in children. *Orthop Clin North Am.* 1976;7(3):639–656.

27. Stephens DC, Louis E, Louis DS. Traumatic separation of the distal femoral epiphyseal cartilage plate. *J Bone Joint Surg Am.* 1974;56(7):1383–1390.

28. Ehrlich MG, Strain RE Jr. Epiphyseal injuries about the knee. *Orthop Clin North Am.* 1979;10(1):91–103.

29. Lombardo SJ, Harvey JP Jr. Fractures of the distal femoral epiphyses. Factors influencing prognosis: a review of thirty-four cases. *J Bone Joint Surg Am.* 1977;59(6):742–751.

30. Walling AK, Seradge H, Spiegel PG. Injuries to the knee ligaments with fractures of the femur. *J Bone Joint Surg Am.* 1982;64(9):1324–1327.

31. Albert MJ. Supracondylar fractures of the femur. *JAAOS.* 1997;5(3):163–171.

32. Healy WL, Brooker AF Jr. Distal femoral fractures. Comparison of open and closed methods of treatment. *Clin Orthop.* 1983;(174):166–171.

33. Marks DS, Isbister ES, Porter KM. Zickel supracondylar nailing for supracondylar femoral fractures in elderly or infirm patients. A review of 33 cases. *J Bone Joint Surg Br.* 1994;76(4):596–601.

34. Graham JM, Gross RH. Distal femoral physeal problem fractures. *Clin Orthop.* 1990;(255):51–53.

35. Schatzker J, McBroom R, Bruce D. The tibial plateau fracture. The Toronto experience 1968–1975. *Clin Orthop.* 1979;(138):94–104.

36. Rockwood CA, Green DP, Bucholz RW. *Rockwood and Green's Fractures in Adults.* 7th ed. Philadelphia, PA: Wolters Kluwer Health/Lippincott Williams & Wilkins; 2010.

37. Apley AG. Fractures of the tibial plateau. *Orthop Clin North Am.* 1979;10(1):61–74.

38. Moore TM, Harvey JP Jr. Roentgenographic measurement of tibial-plateau depression due to fracture. *J Bone Joint Surg Am.* 1974;56(1):155–160.

39. Walker CW, Moore TE. Imaging of skeletal and soft tissue injuries in and around the knee. *Radiol Clin North Am.* 1997;35(3):631–653.

40. Chan PS, Klimkiewicz JJ, Luchetti WT, et al. Impact of CT scan on treatment plan and fracture classification of tibial plateau fractures. *J Orthop Trauma.* 1997;11(7):484–489.

41. Kode L, Lieberman JM, Motta AO, Wilber JH, Vasen A, Yagan R. Evaluation of tibial plateau fractures: efficacy of MR imaging compared with CT. *AJR Am J Roentgenol.* 1994;163(1):141–147.

42. Koval KJ, Helfet DL. Tibial plateau fractures: evaluation and treatment. *JAAOS.* 1995;3(2):86–94.

43. Meyers MH, McKeever FM. Fracture of the intercondylar eminence of the tibia. *J Bone Joint Surg Am.* 1970;52(8):1677–1684.

44. Wiley JJ, Baxter MP. Tibial spine fractures in children. *Clin Orthop.* 1990(255):54–60.

45. Hand WL, Hand CR, Dunn AW. Avulsion fractures of the tibial tubercle. *J Bone Joint Surg Am.* 1971;53(8):1579–1583.

46. Frankl U, Wasilewski SA, Healy WL. Avulsion fracture of the tibial tubercle with avulsion of the patellar ligament. Report of two cases. *J Bone Joint Surg Am.* 1990;72(9):1411–1413.

47. Bostman O, Kiviluoto O, Nirhamo J. Comminuted displaced fractures of the patella. *Injury.* 1981;13(3):196–202.

48. Bostrom A. Fracture of the patella. A study of 422 patellar fractures. *Acta Orthop Scand Suppl.* 1972;143:1–80.

49. Peers KH, Lysens RJ. Patellar tendinopathy in athletes: current diagnostic and therapeutic recommendations. *Sports Med.* 2005;35(1):71–87.

50. James SL. Running injuries to the knee. *JAAOS.* 1995;3(6):309–318.

51. Hoksrud A, Ohberg L, Alfredson H, Bahr R. Color Doppler ultrasound findings in patellar tendinopathy (jumper's knee). *Am J Sports Med.* 2008;36(9):1813–1820.

52. Cook JL, Khan KM, Harcourt PR, Grant M, Young DA, Bonar SF. A cross sectional study of 100 athletes with jumper's knee managed conservatively and surgically. The Victorian Institute of Sport Tendon Study Group. *Br J Sports Med.* 1997;31(4):332–336.

53. Kettunen JA, Kvist M, Alanen E, Kujala UM. Long-term prognosis for jumper's knee in male athletes. A prospective follow-up study. *Am J Sports Med.* 2002;30(5):689–692.

54. Colosimo AJ, Bassett FH III. Jumper's knee. Diagnosis and treatment. *Orthop Rev.* 1990;19(2):139–149.

55. Bahr R, Fossan B, Loken S, Engebretsen L. Surgical treatment compared with eccentric training for patellar tendinopathy (jumper's knee). A randomized, controlled trial. *J Bone Joint Surg Am.* 2006;88(8):1689–1698.

56. Jonsson P, Alfredson H. Superior results with eccentric compared to concentric quadriceps training in patients with jumper's knee: a prospective randomised study. *Br J Sports Med.* 2005;39(11):847–850.

57. Visnes H, Bahr R. The evolution of eccentric training as treatment for patellar tendinopathy (jumper's knee): a critical review of exercise programmes. *Br J Sports Med.* 2007;41(4):217–223.

58. Vulpiani MC, Vetrano M, Savoia V, Di Pangrazio E, Trischitta D, Ferretti A. Jumper's knee treatment with extracorporeal shock wave therapy: a long-term follow-up observational study. *J Sports Med Phys Fitness.* 2007;47(3):323–328.

59. Hyman GS. Jumper's knee in volleyball athletes: advancements in diagnosis and treatment. *Current Sports Med Rep.* 2008;7(5):296–302.

60. Fredberg U, Bolvig L. Jumper's knee. Review of the literature. *Scand J Med Sci Sports.* 1999;9(2):66–73.

61. Duthon VB, Borloz S, Ziltener JL. [Treatment options for patellar tendinopathy]. *Rev Med Suisse Romande.* 2012;8(349):1486–1489.

62. Vetrano M, Castorina A, Vulpiani MC, Baldini R, Pavan A, Ferretti A. Platelet-rich plasma versus focused shock waves in the treatment of jumper's knee in athletes. *Am J Sports Med.* 2013;41(4):795–803.

63. Petrella RJ, Wakeford C. Pain relief and improved physical function in knee osteoarthritis patients receiving ongoing hylan G-F 20, a high-molecular-weight hyaluronan, versus other treatment options: data from a large real-world longitudinal cohort in Canada. *Drug Des Devel Ther.* 2015;9: 5633–5640.

64. Siwek CW, Rao JP. Ruptures of the extensor mechanism of the knee joint. *J Bone Joint Surg Am.* 1981;63(6):932–937.

65. Perryman JR, Hershman EB. The acute management of soft tissue injuries of the knee. *Orthop Clin North Am.* 2002; 33(3):575–585.

66. Kuo RS, Sonnabend DH. Simultaneous rupture of the patellar tendons bilaterally: case report and review of the literature. *J Trauma.* 1993;34(3):458–460.

67. Schwartzberg RS, Csencsitz TA. Bilateral spontaneous patellar tendon rupture. *Am J Orthop.* 1996;25(5):369–372.

68. Adams SB Jr, Radkowski CA, Zura RD, Moorman CT III. Complete quadriceps tendon rupture with concomitant tears of the anterior cruciate ligament and lateral meniscus. *Orthopedics.* 2008;31(1):88.

69. Manaster BJ, Andrews CL. Fractures and dislocations of the knee and proximal tibia and fibula. *Semin Roentgenol.* 1994;29(2):113–133.

70. Haas SB, Callaway H. Disruptions of the extensor mechanism. *Orthop Clin North Am.* 1992;23(4):687–695.

71. Hamer AJ. Pain in the hip and knee. *BMJ.* 2004;328 (7447):1067–1069.

72. Valley VT, Shermer CD. Use of musculoskeletal ultrasonography in the diagnosis of pes anserine tendinitis: a case report. *J Emerg Med.* 2001;20(1):43–45.

73. Safran MR, Fu FH. Uncommon causes of knee pain in the athlete. *Orthop Clin North Am.* 1995;26(3):547–559.

74. Cohen S, Bradley J. Acute proximal hamstring rupture. *JAAOS.* 2007;15(6):350–355.

75. Barber FA, Sutker AN. Iliotibial band syndrome. *Sports Med.* 1992;14(2):144–148.

76. Hamill J, Miller R, Noehren B, Davis I. A prospective study of iliotibial band strain in runners. *Clin Biomech.* 2008; 23(8):1018–1025.

77. Rosenthal MD. Clinical testing for extra-articular lateral knee pain. A modification and combination of traditional tests. *N Am J Sports Phys Ther.* 2008;3(2):107–109.

78. Ellis R, Hing W, Reid D. Iliotibial band friction syndrome—a systematic review. *Manual Ther.* 2007;12(3):200–208.

79. Fredericson M, Weir A. Practical management of iliotibial band friction syndrome in runners. *Clin J Sports Med.* 2006; 16(3):261–268.

80. Zipple JT, Hammer RL, Loubert PV. Treatment of fabella syndrome with manual therapy: a case report. *J Orthop Sports Phys Ther.* 2003;33(1):33–39.

81. Dannawi Z, Khanduja V, Vemulapalli KK, Zammit J, El-Zebdeh M. Arthroscopic excision of the fabella. *J Knee Surg.* 2007;20(4):299–301.

82. Seol PH, Ha KW, Kim YH, Kwak HJ, Park SW, Ryu BJ. Effect of radial extracorporeal shock wave therapy in patients with fabella syndrome. *Ann Rehabil Med.* 2016;40(6): 1124–1128.

83. Rennie WJ, Saifuddin A. Pes anserine bursitis: incidence in symptomatic knees and clinical presentation. *Skeletal Radiol.* 2005;34(7):395–398.

84. Clapp A, Trecek J, Joyce M, Sundaram M. Radiologic case study. Pes anserine bursitis. *Orthopedics.* 2008;31(4):306, 407–408.

85. Treadwell EL. Synovial cysts and ganglia: the value of magnetic resonance imaging. *Semin Arthritis Rheum.* 1994; 24(1):61–70.

86. Acebes JC, Sanchez-Pernaute O, Diaz-Oca A, Herrero-Beaumont G. Ultrasonographic assessment of Baker's cysts after intra-articular corticosteroid injection in knee osteoarthritis. *J Clin Ultrasound.* 2006;34(3):113–117.

87. Labropoulos N, Shifrin DA, Paxinos O. New insights into the development of popliteal cysts. *Br J Surg.* 2004; 91(10):1313–1318.

88. Smith MK, Lesniak B, Baraga MG, Kaplan L, Jose J. Treatment of popliteal (Baker) cysts with ultrasound-guided aspiration, fenestration, and injection: long-term follow-up. *Sports Health.* 2015;7(5):409–414.

89. Ikpeme JO, Gray C. Traumatic prepatellar neuralgia. *Injury.* 1995;26(4):225–229.

90. Roberts DM, Stallard TC. Emergency department evaluation and treatment of knee and leg injuries. *Emerg Med Clin North Am.* 2000;18(1):67–84, v–vi.

91. McCarroll JR, Shelbourne KD, Patel DV. Anterior cruciate ligament injuries in young athletes. Recommendations for treatment and rehabilitation. *Sports Med.* 1995;20(2): 117–127.

92. Merrill KD. Knee dislocations with vascular injuries. *Orthop Clin North Am.* 1994;25(4):707–713.

93. Moyer RA, Marchetto PA. Injuries of the posterior cruciate ligament. *Clin Sports Med.* 1993;12(2):307–315.

94. Ginsburg JH, Ellsasser JC. Problem areas in the diagnosis and treatment of ligament injuries of the knee. *Clin Orthop.* 1978;(132):201–205.

95. Warren RF, Marshall JL. Injuries of the anterior cruciate and medial collateral ligaments of the knee. A retrospective analysis of clinical records—part I. *Clin Orthop.* 1978; (136):191–197.

96. Marshall JR, Warren R, Fleiss DJ. Ligamentous injuries of the knee in skiing. *Clin Orthop.* 1975;(108):196–199.

97. Maffulli N, Binfield PM, King JB, Good CJ. Acute haemarthrosis of the knee in athletes. A prospective study of 106 cases. *J Bone Joint Surg Br.* 1993;75(6):945–949.

98. Hough AJ Jr, Webber RJ. Pathology of the meniscus. *Clin Orthop.* 1990;(252):32–40.

99. Emerson RJ. Basketball knee injuries and the anterior cruciate ligament. *Clin Sports Med.* 1993;12(2):317–328.

100. Fanelli GC, Giannotti BF, Edson CJ. The posterior cruciate ligament arthroscopic evaluation and treatment. *Arthroscopy.* 1994;10(6):673–688.

101. Pritsch T, Blumberg N, Haim A, Dekel S, Arbel R. The importance of the valgus stress test in the diagnosis of posterolateral instability of the knee. *Injury.* 2006;37(10):1011–1014.

102. Fowler PJ. Bone injuries associated with anterior cruciate ligament disruption. *Arthroscopy.* 1994;10(4):453–460.

103. Medvecky MJ, Noyes FR. Surgical approaches to the posteromedial and posterolateral aspects of the knee. *JAAOS.* 2005;13(2):121–128.

104. Irrgang JJ. Modern trends in anterior cruciate ligament rehabilitation: nonoperative and postoperative management. *Clin Sports Med.* 1993;12(4):797–813.

105. Gibbs N. Common rugby league injuries. Recommendations for treatment and preventative measures. *Sports Med.* 1994;18(6):438–450.

106. Girgis FG, Marshall JL, Monajem A. The cruciate ligaments of the knee joint. Anatomical, functional and experimental analysis. *Clin Orthop.* 1975;(106):216–231.

107. Strand T, Engesaeter LB, Molster AO. Meniscus repair in knee ligament injuries. *Acta Orthop Scand.* 1985;56(2):130–132.

108. Donaldson WF III, Warren RF, Wickiewicz T. A comparison of acute anterior cruciate ligament examinations. Initial versus examination under anesthesia. *Am J Sports Med.* 1985;13(1):5–10.

109. Frank CB, Gravel JC. Hamstring spasm in anterior cruciate ligament injuries. *Arthroscopy.* 1995;11(4):444–448.

110. Cosgarea AJ, Jay PR. Posterior cruciate ligament injuries: evaluation and management. *JAAOS.* 2001;9(5):297–307.

111. Miller MD, Johnson DL, Harner CD, Fu FH. Posterior cruciate ligament injuries. *Orthop Rev.* 1993;22(11):1201–1210.

112. Covey DC, Sapega AA. Anatomy and function of the posterior cruciate ligament. *Clin Sports Med.* 1994;13(3):509–518.

113. Escobedo EM, Mills WJ, Hunter JC. The "reverse Segond" fracture: association with a tear of the posterior cruciate ligament and medial meniscus. *AJR Am J Roentgenol.* 2002;178(4):979–983.

114. Peltola EK, Lindahl J, Koskinen SK. The reverse Segond fracture: not associated with knee dislocation and rarely with posterior cruciate ligament tear. *Emerg Radiol.* 2014;21:245–249.

115. Kose O, Ozyurek S, Turan A, Guler F. Reverse Segond fracture and associated knee injuries: a case report and review of 13 published cases. *Acta Orthop Traumatol Turc.* 2016;50:587–591.

116. Sawant M, Narasimha Murty A, Ireland J. Valgus knee injuries: evaluation and documentation using a simple technique of stress radiography. *Knee.* 2004;11(1):25–28.

117. Behairy NH, Dorgham MA, Khaled SA. Accuracy of routine magnetic resonance imaging in meniscal and ligamentous injuries of the knee: comparison with arthroscopy. *Int Orthop.* 2009;33(4):961–967.

118. Kocabey Y, Tetik O, Isbell WM, Atay OA, Johnson DL. The value of clinical examination versus magnetic resonance imaging in the diagnosis of meniscal tears and anterior cruciate ligament rupture. *Arthroscopy.* 2004;20(7):696–700.

119. Rayan F, Bhonsle S, Shukla DD. Clinical, MRI, and arthroscopic correlation in meniscal and anterior cruciate ligament injuries. *Int Orthop.* 2009;33(1):129–132.

120. Andrews JR, Edwards JC, Satterwhite YE. Isolated posterior cruciate ligament injuries. History, mechanism of injury, physical findings, and ancillary tests. *Clin Sports Med.* 1994;13(3):519–530.

121. Khanda GE, Akhtar W, Ahsan H, Ahmad N. Assessment of menisci and ligamentous injuries of the knee on magnetic resonance imaging: correlation with arthroscopy. *J Pak Med Assoc.* 2008;58(10):537–540.

122. Tham SC, Tsou IY, Chee TS. Knee and ankle ligaments: magnetic resonance imaging findings of normal anatomy and at injury. *Ann Acad Med Singapore.* 2008;37(4):324–329.

123. Vaz CE, Camargo OP, Santana PJ, Valezi AC. Accuracy of magnetic resonance in identifying traumatic intraarticular knee lesions. *Clinics.* 2005;60(6):445–450.

124. Schulte KR, Chu ET, Fu FH. Arthroscopic posterior cruciate ligament reconstruction. *Clin Sports Med.* 1997;16(1):145–156.

125. Indelicato PA, Hermansdorfer J, Huegel M. Nonoperative management of complete tears of the medial collateral ligament of the knee in intercollegiate football players. *Clin Orthop.* 1990(256):174–177.

126. Cameron JC, Saha S. Management of medial collateral ligament laxity. *Orthop Clin North Am.* 1994;25(3):527–532.

127. Carey JL, Shea KG. AAOS Clinical Practice Guideline: Management of Anterior Cruciate Ligament Injuries: Evidence-Based Guideline. *J Am Acad Orthop Surg.* 2015;23(5):e6–e8. doi:10.5435/JAAOS-D-15-00095. Epub 2015 Mar 20.

128. Dye SF. The future of anterior cruciate ligament restoration. *Clin Orthop.* 1996;(325):130–139.

129. Greis PE, Bardana DD, Holmstrom MC, Burks RT. Meniscal injury: I. Basic science and evaluation. *JAAOS.* 2002;10(3):168–176.

130. Bessette GC. The meniscus. *Orthopedics.* 1992;15(1):35–42.

131. Steadman JR, Sterett WI. The surgical treatment of knee injuries in skiers. *Med Sci Sports Exerc.* 1995;27(3):328–333.

132. Evans PJ, Bell GD, Frank C. Prospective evaluation of the McMurray test. *Am J Sports Med.* 1993;21(4):604–608.

133. Solomon DH, Simel DL, Bates DW, Katz JN, Schaffer JL. The rational clinical examination. Does this patient have a torn meniscus or ligament of the knee? Value of the physical examination. *JAMA.* 2001;286(13):1610–1620.

134. Karachalios T, Hantes M, Zibis AH, Zachos V, Karantanas AH, Malizos KN. Diagnostic accuracy of a new clinical test (the Thessaly test) for early detection of meniscal tears. *J Bone Joint Surg Am.* 2005;87(5):955–962.

135. Blyth M, Anthony I, Francq B, et al. Diagnostic accuracy of the Thessaly test, standardised clinical history and other clinical examination tests (Apley's, McMurray's and joint line tenderness) for meniscal tears in comparison with magnetic resonance imaging diagnosis. *Health Technol Assess.* 2015;19(62):1–62. doi:10.3310/hta19620.

136. Stanitski CL. Correlation of arthroscopic and clinical examinations with magnetic resonance imaging findings of injured knees in children and adolescents. *Am J Sports Med.* 1998;26(1):2–6.

137. Gelb HJ, Glasgow SG, Sapega AA, Torg JS. Magnetic resonance imaging of knee disorders. Clinical value and cost-effectiveness in a sports medicine practice. *Am J Sports Med.* 1996;24(1):99–103.

138. Boden SD, Davis DO, Dina TS, et al. A prospective and blinded investigation of magnetic resonance imaging of the knee. Abnormal findings in asymptomatic subjects. *Clin Orthop.* 1992(282):177–185.

139. Bhattacharyya T, Gale D, Dewire P, et al. The clinical importance of meniscal tears demonstrated by magnetic resonance imaging in osteoarthritis of the knee. *J Bone Joint Surg Am.* 2003;85-A(1):4–9.

140. Jackson RW. The painful knee: arthroscopy or MR imaging? *JAAOS.* 1996;4(2):93–99.

141. Ott JW, Clancy WG Jr. Functional knee braces. *Orthopedics.* 1993;16(2):171–175; discussion 175–176.

142. Swenson TM, Harner CD. Knee ligament and meniscal injuries. Current concepts. *Orthop Clin North Am.* 1995;26(3):529–546.

143. Diment MT, DeHaven KE, Sebastianelli WJ. Current concepts in meniscal repair. *Orthopedics.* 1993;16(9):973–977.

144. Poulsen KA, Borris LC, Lassen MR. Thromboembolic complications after arthroscopy of the knee. *Arthroscopy.* 1993; 9(5):570–573.

145. Belzer JP, Cannon WD Jr. Meniscus tears: treatment in the stable and unstable knee. *JAAOS.* 1993;1(1):41–47.

146. Greis PE, Holmstrom MC, Bardana DD, Burks RT. Meniscal injury: II. Management. *JAAOS.* 2002;10(3):177–187.

147. Kollias SL, Fox JM. Meniscal repair. Where do we go from here? *Clin Sports Med.* 1996;15(3):621–630.

148. Schenck RC Jr, Goodnight JM. Osteochondritis dissecans. *J Bone Joint Surg Am.* 1996;78(3):439–456.

149. Tuite MJ, DeSmet AA. MRI of selected sports injuries: muscle tears, groin pain, and osteochondritis dissecans. *Semin Ultrasound CT MR.* 1994;15(5):318–340.

150. Kijowski R, Blankenbaker DG, Shinki K, Fine JP, Graf BK, De Smet AA. Juvenile versus adult osteochondritis dissecans of the knee: appropriate MR imaging criteria for instability. *Radiology.* 2008;248(2):571–578.

151. Cepero S, Ullot R, Sastre S. Osteochondritis of the femoral condyles in children and adolescents: our experience over the last 28 years. *J Pediatr Orthop B.* 2005;14(1):24–29.

152. Uematsu K, Habata T, Hasegawa Y, et al. Osteochondritis dissecans of the knee: long-term results of excision of the osteochondral fragment. *Knee.* 2005;12(3):205–208.

153. Wright RW, McLean M, Matava MJ, Shively RA. Osteochondritis dissecans of the knee: long-term results of excision of the fragment. *Clin Orthop.* 2004(424):239–243.

154. Detterline AJ, Goldstein JL, Rue JP, Bach BR Jr. Evaluation and treatment of osteochondritis dissecans lesions of the knee. *J Knee Surg.* 2008;21(2):106–115.

155. Kocher MS, Tucker R, Ganley TJ, Flynn JM. Management of osteochondritis dissecans of the knee: current concepts review. *Am J Sports Med.* 2006;34(7):1181–1191.

156. Murray JR, Chitnavis J, Dixon P, et al. Osteochondritis dissecans of the knee: long-term clinical outcome following arthroscopic debridement. *Knee.* 2007;14(2):94–98.

157. Boden BP, Pearsall AW, Garrett WE Jr, Feagin JA Jr. Patellofemoral instability: evaluation and management. *JAAOS.* 1997;5(1):47–57.

158. Davidson K. Patellofemoral pain syndrome. *Am Fam Physician.* 1993;48(7):1254–1262.

159. LaBrier K, O'Neill DB. Patellofemoral stress syndrome. Current concepts. *Sports Med.* 1993;16(6):449–459.

160. Crossley KM, Vicenzino B, Pandy MG, Schache AG, Hinman RS. Targeted physiotherapy for patellofemoral joint osteoarthritis: a protocol for a randomised, single-blind controlled trial. *BMC Musculoskelet Disord.* 2008;9:122.

161. Barnes CJ, Pietrobon R, Higgins LD. Does the pulse examination in patients with traumatic knee dislocation predict a surgical arterial injury? A meta-analysis. *J Trauma.* 2002; 53(6):1109–1114.

162. Rihn JA, Groff YJ, Harner CD, Cha PS. The acutely dislocated knee: evaluation and management. *JAAOS.* 2004; 12(5):334–346.

163. Good L, Johnson RJ. The dislocated knee. *JAAOS.* 1995; 3(5):284–292.

164. Wascher DC, Dvirnak PC, DeCoster TA. Knee dislocation: initial assessment and implications for treatment. *J Orthop Trauma.* 1997;11(7):525–529.

165. Perron AD, Brady WJ, Sing RF. Orthopedic pitfalls in the ED: vascular injury associated with knee dislocation. *Am J Emerg Med.* 2001;19(7):583–588.

166. Twaddle BC, Bidwell TA, Chapman JR. Knee dislocations: where are the lesions? A prospective evaluation of surgical findings in 63 cases. *J Orthop Trauma.* 2003;17(3):198–202.

167. Kremchek TE, Welling RE, Kremchek EJ. Traumatic dislocation of the knee. *Orthop Rev.* 1989;18(10):1051–1057.

168. Ahmad F, Turner SA, Torrie P, Gibson M. Iatrogenic femoral artery pseudoaneurysms—a review of current methods of diagnosis and treatment. *Clin Radiol.* 2008;63(12): 1310–1316.

169. Redmond JM, Levy BA, Dajani KA, Cass JR, Cole PA. Detecting vascular injury in lower-extremity orthopedic trauma: the role of CT angiography. *Orthopedics.* 2008; 31(8):761–767.

170. Keating JF. *Acute Knee Ligament Injuries and Knee Dislocation.* Berlin, Heidelberg: Springer Berlin Heidelberg; 2014:2949–2971.

171. Natsuhara KM, Yeranosian MG, Cohen JR, Wang JC, McAllister DR, Petrigliano FA. What is the frequency of vascular injury after knee dislocation? *Clin Orthop.* 2014;472(9):2615–2620.

172. Wascher DC. High-velocity knee dislocation with vascular injury. Treatment principles. *Clin Sports Med.* 2000; 19(3):457–477.

173. Green NE, Allen BL. Vascular injuries associated with dislocation of the knee. *J Bone Joint Surg Am.* 1977;59(2): 236–239.

174. Treiman GS, Yellin AE, Weaver FA, et al. Examination of the patient with a knee dislocation. The case for selective arteriography. *Arch Surg.* 1992;127(9):1056–1062; discussion 1062–1063.

175. Johansen K, Lynch K, Paun M, Copass M. Non-invasive vascular tests reliably exclude occult arterial trauma in injured extremities. *J Trauma.* 1991;31(4):515–519; discussion 519–522.

176. Hollis JD, Daley BJ. 10-year review of knee dislocations: is arteriography always necessary? *J Trauma.* 2005;59(3): 672–675; discussion 675–676.

177. Klineberg EO, Crites BM, Flinn WR, Archibald JD, Moorman CT III. The role of arteriography in assessing popliteal artery injury in knee dislocations. *J Trauma.* 2004; 56(4):786–790.

178. Mills WJ, Barei DP, McNair P. The value of the ankle-brachial index for diagnosing arterial injury after knee dislocation: a prospective study. *J Trauma.* 2004;56(6):1261–1265.

179. Almekinders LC, Dedmond BT. Outcomes of the operatively treated knee dislocation. *Clin Sports Med.* 2000; 19(3):503–518.

180. Brautigan B, Johnson DL. The epidemiology of knee dislocations. *Clin Sports Med.* 2000;19(3):387–397.

181. Dedmond BT, Almekinders LC. Operative versus nonoperative treatment of knee dislocations: a meta-analysis. *Am J Knee Surg.* 2001;14(1):33–38.

182. Shelbourne KD, Klootwyk TE. Low-velocity knee dislocation with sports injuries. Treatment principles. *Clin Sports Med.* 2000;19(3):443–456.

183. Khakha RS, Day AC, Gibbs J, et al. Acute surgical management of traumatic knee dislocations—average follow-up of 10 years. *Knee.* 2016;23(2):267–275.

184. Sekiya JK, Kuhn JE. Instability of the proximal tibiofibular joint. *JAAOS.* 2003;11(2):120–128.

185. Fatovich DM, Song S. Images in emergency medicine. Isolated proximal tibiofibular dislocation. *Ann Emerg Med.* 2006;48(6):759, 765.

186. Van Seymortier P, Ryckaert A, Verdonk P, Almqvist KF, Verdonk R. Traumatic proximal tibiofibular dislocation. *Am J Sports Med.* 2008;36(4):793–798.

187. Sherman SC, Yu A. Patellar dislocation with vertical axis rotation. *J Emerg Med.* 2004;26(2):219–220.

188. Iobst CA, Stanitski CL. Acute knee injuries. *Clin Sports Med.* 2000;19(4):621–635, vi.

189. Vainionpaa S, Laasonen E, Silvennoinen T, Vasenius J, Rokkanen P. Acute dislocation of the patella. A prospective review of operative treatment. *J Bone Joint Surg Br.* 1990;72(3):366–369.

190. Zhang G-Y, Zheng L, Ding H-Y, Li E-M, Sun B-S, Shi H. Evaluation of medial patellofemoral ligament tears after acute lateral patellar dislocation: comparison of high-frequency ultrasound and MR. *Eur Radiol.* 2014;25: 274–281.

191. Lim AK, Chang HC, Hui JH. Recurrent patellar dislocation: reappraising our approach to surgery. *Ann Acad Med Singapore.* 2008;37(4):320–323.

192. Shen HC, Chao KH, Huang GS, Pan RY, Lee CH. Combined proximal and distal realignment procedures to treat the habitual dislocation of the patella in adults. *Am J Sports Med.* 2007;35(12):2101–2108.

193. Joo SY, Park KB, Kim BR, Park HW, Kim HW. The "four-in-one" procedure for habitual dislocation of the patella in children: early results in patients with severe generalised ligamentous laxity and aplasis of the trochlear groove. *J Bone Joint Surg Br.* 2007;89(12):1645–1649.

194. Woods GW, Elkousy HA, O'Connor DP. Arthroscopic release of the vastus lateralis tendon for recurrent patellar dislocation. *Am J Sports Med.* 2006;34(5):824–831.

CHAPTER 21

Leg

Adriana Segura Olson, MD, George T. Chiampas, DO, and Jacob Stelter, MD

INTRODUCTION

The tibia is the only weight-bearing bone in the leg. The fibula is bound to the tibia by the interosseous membrane, which divides into a "Y" both proximally and distally. The proximal arm of the "Y" is composed of the anterosuperior tibiofibular ligament and the posterosuperior tibiofibular ligament. A similar division occurs distally with an antero-inferior tibiofibular ligament and a posteroinferior tibiofibular ligament. The upper portion of the fibula is of little importance and can be excised with little consequence. The lower portion cannot because of its importance in forming the ankle mortise.

The muscles of the leg are enclosed in four fascial compartments: anterior, peroneal, deep posterior, and superficial posterior compartments. The anterior compartment includes the ankle and the foot dorsiflexors, and the posterior compartments (superficial and deep) contain the plantar flexors. The peroneal compartment houses the foot evertors.

LEG FRACTURES

TIBIAL SHAFT FRACTURES

Tibial shaft fractures are the most common long bone fractures in the body. Because of the superficial location in the leg, the tibia is also the most common bone involved in open fractures.

Because the tibia and fibula run parallel to each other and are tightly bound together by ligaments, a displaced fracture of one bone is frequently associated with a fracture of the other bone.

Tibial shaft fractures are classified on the basis of principles established by Nicoll. Three factors determine the outcome of tibial shaft fractures:

- Initial displacement
- Comminution
- Soft-tissue injury

Fractures are divided based on displacement into three groups: (1) <50% displacement, (2) >50% displacement, and (3) complete displacement or severely comminuted (Fig. 21–1). Tibial shaft fractures with <50% displacement have a 90% chance of union, whereas fractures with complete displacement have only a 70% chance of union.

The degree of associated soft-tissue injury is an often unrecognized factor affecting prognosis and treatment of the fracture. Fractures associated with significant contusion of the overlying skin or muscles are associated with higher infection rates and poorer healing.

The average healing time for uncomplicated, non-displaced fractures is 3 months. For displaced, open, or comminuted fractures, the average healing time is 4 to 6 months.

Mechanism of Injury

Multiple mechanisms may result in fractures of the tibia and fibula shafts. Direct trauma is a common cause of injury and usually results in associated soft-tissue injury. These fractures are frequently secondary to automobile collisions and typically result in transverse or comminuted fractures.

Indirect trauma associated with rotary and compressive forces, as from skiing or falling, usually results in a spiral or

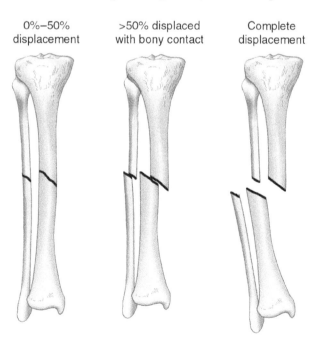

0%–50% displacement	>50% displaced with bony contact	Complete displacement

Figure 21–1. Fractures of the tibia and fibula shaft. Tibia shaft fractures can occur alone but are treated similarly to combined fractures.

oblique fracture. Rotary forces occur when the leg and body rotate around a planted foot and are most likely to cause a spiral fracture. Bending forces may also result in a fracture that is oblique or transverse. A tibial plafond fracture is typically secondary to a fall from a height that drives the talus up into the tibia. These fractures are intra-articular and are covered in Chapter 22.

Examination

Tibial shaft fractures usually present with pain, swelling, and deformity. Although neurovascular damage is not commonly seen after these injuries, documentation of pulses and peroneal nerve function (dorsiflexion and plantar flexion of the toes) is imperative. The dorsalis pedis pulse should be palpated and compared with the uninjured extremity. Other findings consistent with compartment syndrome should be sought, and the pertinent negative findings documented on the chart (see the Associated Injuries section).

Imaging

Anteroposterior and lateral views are generally adequate in defining the position of the fracture fragments (Figs. 21–2 to 21–4). When describing these fractures, it is important to assess the following:

- **Location:** proximal, middle, or distal third
- **Type:** transverse, oblique, spiral, or comminuted
- **Displacement:** percentage of fracture surface contact
- **Angulation:** valgus or varus of the distal fragment

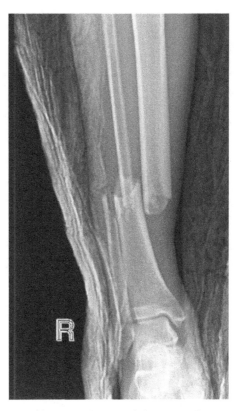

Figure 21–2. Tibia and fibula shaft fracture with 100% lateral displacement.

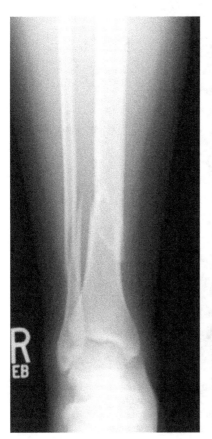
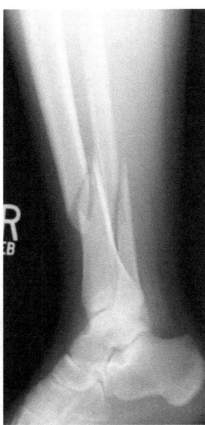

Figure 21–3. Spiral fractures of the distal third of the tibia and fibula shafts. There is <50% displacement and only slight angulation.

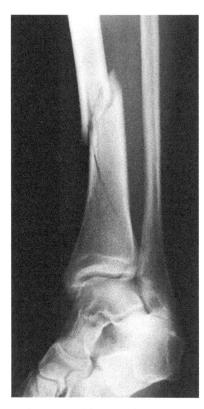

Figure 21–4. Comminuted fracture of the distal tibia with minimal displacement.

Associated Injuries

Compartment syndrome is a frequently associated finding after a tibia fracture, and the clinical evaluation and documentation should reflect that the clinician considered this diagnosis. Tibia fractures are the most common cause of compartment syndrome, accounting for 36% of all cases. The incidence of compartment syndrome after tibial shaft fractures is 4.3%. It is three times more common in individuals younger than 35 years.

Evidence of a compartment syndrome is usually present within the first 24 to 48 hours following the injury. The muscle compartments should be palpated for tenderness or tenseness. Pain with passive stretch should be noted as well as the sensation between the first and second toes as an indicator of peroneal nerve function. If a compartment syndrome is suspected, emergent orthopedic consultation is recommended. The determination of compartment pressures, in addition to a thorough clinical examination, will determine the subsequent management plan.

As mentioned previously, neurovascular damage at the time of injury is uncommon, although severe injuries may present with incomplete or complete disruption of the neurovascular structures.

Axiom: *Any patient with a tibia fracture and increasing pain 24 to 48 hours after casting should be suspected of having compartment syndrome.*

Treatment

The emergency department (ED) management of tibial shaft fractures includes immobilization in a long-leg splint with the knee in 10 to 15 degrees of flexion and the ankle flexed at 90 degrees. The splint should extend from the midthigh to the metatarsal heads. An emergent reduction of a closed fracture is indicated when there is a limb-threatening vascular compromise.

Open fractures may be gently cleaned and dressed (Fig. 21–5). Tetanus prophylaxis (when indicated) and parenteral antibiotics should be initiated. Emergency operative debridement with external or internal fixation is recommended.

Emergent orthopedic consultation is advised for patients with tibial shaft fractures because of the high incidence of compartment syndrome, which may evolve later. For this reason, patients with tibial shaft fractures and significant soft-tissue swelling should be hospitalized with elevation of the extremity and close observation for the development of a compartment syndrome.

Definitive treatment options include cast or brace immobilization, external fixation, and intramedullary nailing. Plating is occasionally used today, but the operation may cause additional soft-tissue injury. The degree of fracture displacement and comminution, mechanism of injury (high energy vs. low energy), and associated soft-tissue injury all play an important role in the surgeon's selection of therapy.

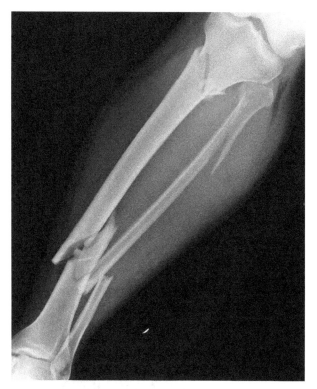

Figure 21–5. Open fracture of the tibia and fibula. (Used with permission from the Department of Emergency Medicine, Feinberg School of Medicine, Northwestern University. http://www.feinberg.northwestern.edu/emergencymed/)

Closed treatment with a long-leg, nonweight-bearing cast is reserved for patients with nondisplaced fractures with minimal soft-tissue injury. A displaced fracture that undergoes closed reduction can also be treated closed as long as it is stable. Tibial shaft fractures managed nonoperatively must be monitored with frequent radiographs to ensure the fracture does not displace during treatment. The cast can usually be removed within 6 to 8 weeks, after callus formation has occurred. Problems with cast immobilization include knee stiffness and difficulty ambulating following treatment.

When there is displacement, comminution, or instability, intramedullary nailing is the treatment of choice of most orthopedic surgeons.[3,10-13] The prevalence of nonunion and malunion is greatly decreased compared with the other methods of treatment. In addition, patients had less time off work with a more predictable and rapid return to full function.[12] In patients with severe open tibial shaft fractures, external fixation with delayed intramedullary nailing is preferred.[2,3]

Complications

Shaft fractures of the tibia and fibula have several significant complications:

- Nonunion or delayed union
- Compartment syndrome
- Chronic joint pain or stiffness

Pediatric Considerations

In patients younger than 18 years, tibial shaft fractures make up about 15% of long bone fractures.[14] Tibial fractures in children are the second most frequent fracture associated with nonaccidental trauma.[16] Hence, when evaluating children with these fractures, it is important to maintain clinical suspicion and evaluate for possible abuse. In addition, an important consideration in the evaluation of tibial injuries in children is the toddler's fracture. This fracture refers to a distal tibial shaft fracture in patients age 3 or younger that is not present on initial x-ray in the ED.[15] As a result, it is recommended that patients in this age range who have a mechanism of injury, point tenderness over the tibia, and inability to ambulate be treated for a presumed fracture with splinting, orthopedics follow-up, and repeat radiograph.[15] One particular study showed that in 39 children treated for a presumed toddler's fracture, 41% had a fracture noted on follow-up x-ray.[15] Management of tibial fractures present on initial x-ray in the ED should generally follow routine fracture care, including assessment of neurovascular status and evaluation of any signs of compartment syndrome followed by appropriate immobilization and follow-up care.

FIBULAR SHAFT FRACTURE

Isolated fibular shaft fractures are uncommon injuries usually associated with a tibia fracture (Fig. 21–6). They are often due to direct trauma over the lateral aspect of the leg or after a gunshot wound (Fig. 21–7).[4]

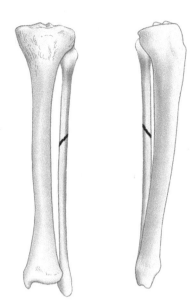

Figure 21–6. Fibula shaft fractures.

Fibular shaft fractures present with pain that is exacerbated with walking and a discrete area of tenderness over the fracture site. Examination should include a thorough assessment of the ankle. One must exclude a Maisonneuve fracture in which deltoid ligament rupture or a medial malleolus fracture accompanies a proximal fibula fracture.

Fibular shaft fractures without associated fracture of the tibia are treated symptomatically and usually heal without

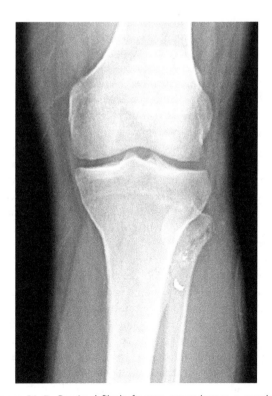

Figure 21–7. Proximal fibula fracture secondary to a gunshot wound.

complications. Splinting the leg can be used for pain relief. Some patients have little pain and tolerate initial crutch walking without immobilization.

TIBIAL STRESS FRACTURE

Stress fractures are common in the leg and are frequently misdiagnosed as contusions, strains, periostitis, exertional compartment syndrome, or nerve entrapment. The tibia is especially prone, accounting for almost one-half of cases. They occur in young athletes, dancers, or military recruits early in their training period. The most common location of a tibial stress fracture is the posteromedial cortex of the diaphysis. Anterior cortical stress fractures also occur and are more problematic because of decreased vascularity and the tension in this area.

Clinical Presentation

The patient complains of an insidious onset of soreness or a dull ache in the leg, which is increased with activity. Eventually, if untreated, the ache becomes continuous even at rest and at night. There may be localized tenderness with some soft-tissue swelling over the fracture site, which is usually at the upper third of the leg.

Imaging

Radiographs obtained early are negative, and the condition may be misdiagnosed. However, 2 weeks to 3 months later, a fine, transverse line with periosteal reactivity along one or both cortices will be present. Other diagnostic tests include bone scan and magnetic resonance imaging (MRI). Bone scan is very sensitive and reveals a focal area of uptake in all three phases. MRI is more specific than bone scan but is more expensive.

Treatment

Tibial stress fractures are most often treated nonsurgically. Rest and orthotics are usually required. Nonsteroidal anti-inflammatory agents (NSAIDs) should be avoided because of their inhibitory effects on bone healing. Gradual resumption of activity over the next 1 to 2 months is required for healing to take place, and the development of pain during that time necessitates a decrease in activity level.

Anterior cortical tibial stress fractures are treated with casting or surgical fixation. If there is suspicion of an anterior cortical stress fracture, the patient should be splinted and given crutches while awaiting definitive testing and referral to an orthopedic surgeon.

LEG SOFT-TISSUE INJURY

ACUTE COMPARTMENT SYNDROME

Compartment syndromes are among the most potentially devastating problems presenting to the ED. Volkmann ischemic contractures are the end result of muscle and nerve ischemia when the condition is not treated. Early diagnosis and the recognition of the early signs of this process are crucial to the emergency physician.

The leg is the most common location to develop a compartment syndrome, with the anterior compartment being most commonly involved. Other compartments in the leg include the superficial and deep posterior compartments and the peroneal (lateral) compartment (Fig. 21–8). The contents of each compartment are listed in Table 21–1.

Compartment syndromes of the leg can be caused by a number of conditions. A tibia fracture is the most common precipitant, but other conditions that may result in compartment syndrome include constrictive dressings or casts, crush injuries, and arterial injuries. Thus, an increase in compartmental pressure can be caused by (1) compression of the compartment (e.g., cast) or (2) volume increase within the compartment (e.g., hematoma). For an extensive list of the causes of compartment syndrome, refer to Chapter 4.

Clinical Presentation

Clinical evaluation begins with a high degree of suspicion. The earliest and most reliable sign of a compartment syndrome is *severe pain*, typically out of proportion to the

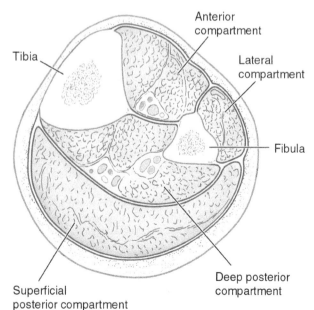

Figure 21–8. The compartments of the leg.

▶ TABLE 21–1. **RELATED ANATOMY OF TISSUE COMPARTMENTS OF THE LEG**

Compartment	Muscles	Vessels	Nerves	Pain
Anterior	Anterior tibialis, extensor hallucis longus, extensor digitorum longus, peroneus tertius	Anterior tibial artery	Deep peroneal • Weakness: Ankle dorsiflexion, toe extension • Paresthesia: Web space of first and second toes	Ankle plantar flexion, toe flexion
Lateral	Peroneus longus and brevis	None	Superficial peroneal • Weakness: Ankle dorsiflexion, foot eversion • Paresthesia: Dorsum of foot	Ankle plantar flexion, foot inversion
Deep posterior	Posterior tibialis, flexor digitorum longus, flexor hallucis longus	Peroneal artery, posterior tibial artery	Posterior tibialis • Weakness: Ankle plantar flexion, foot inversion, toe flexion • Paresthesia: Plantar aspect of foot	Ankle dorsiflexion, foot eversion, toe extension
Superficial posterior	Gastrocnemius, soleus, plantaris	None	Sural • Weakness: Ankle plantar flexion • Paresthesia: Lateral foot	Ankle dorsiflexion

apparent severity of the injury. The pain is not well localized, is progressive, and increases in intensity. In addition, palpation of the involved compartment will reveal that it is tense. *Pain with passive stretch* is an early sign but can be confused when there is a contusion. One must remember that paresis and paresthesias are not reliable and occur late, as do diminished pulses.

Because the anterior and deep posterior compartments of the leg are most commonly involved, a detailed description of those two presentations is outlined subsequently.[20]

> **Axiom:** *Increasing pain while an injured extremity is at rest should make the emergency physician suspect the diagnosis of compartment syndrome.*

Anterior Compartment Syndrome

This syndrome is characterized by anterior tibia pain, weakness of dorsiflexion of the ankle and the toes, and variable degree of sensory loss over the distribution of the deep peroneal nerve (web space between the first and second toes).

The emergency physician must not wait for the development of foot drop or paresthesias, as these are late findings. With the onset of severe pain over the anterior compartment, there is loss of function such that it becomes almost impossible to contract the muscles within the compartment. Passive stretching of the muscles causes significant pain. The skin over the compartment becomes erythematous and shiny and is warm and tender to palpation with what is described as a "woody" feeling.

Anterior compartment syndrome may be misdiagnosed as muscle spasms, shin splints, or contusions. However, if the examiner is aware that the previously mentioned conditions can result in a compartment syndrome, he/she will not miss the diagnosis.

> **Axiom:** *Any time a patient complains of intractable pain in the front of the leg with some loss of dorsiflexion of the toes and the foot, an anterior compartment syndrome should be suspected.*

Deep Posterior Compartment Syndrome

The deep posterior compartment encloses the flexor digitorum longus, the tibialis posterior, and the flexor hallucis longus, as well as the posterior tibial artery and nerve. The transverse crucial septum forms the posterior wall of the compartment, whereas the interosseous membrane forms the anterior wall.

The clinical picture of this syndrome is usually complicated by the involvement of other surrounding compartments. However, there is increased pain on passive extension of the toes, weakness of flexion, and hypesthesia over the distribution of the posterior tibial nerve along the sole. The patient also has tenseness and tenderness along the medial distal part of the leg. All of these signs may become evident within 2 hours to as long as 6 days from the injury.

Treatment

If one suspects this diagnosis, the compartment pressures must be measured in the ED. Compartment pressure can be quickly and easily measured using a commercially available battery-powered monitor (Stryker STIC monitor). A description of this technique is available in Chapter 4.

The normal compartment pressure is <10 mm Hg.[21] Pressures >20 mm Hg should prompt admission and surgical consultation. A pressure of 30 to 40 mm Hg is generally considered grounds for an emergent fasciotomy in the operating room.[22]

The fasciotomy is accomplished by making a longitudinal skin incision over the compartment. The underlying fascia is split along the length of the compartment, allowing the contained muscle to expand. Fasciotomy performed early, that is, <12 hours after the onset of symptoms, results in the return to normal function in 68% of patients, whereas only 8% of those with fasciotomies done after 12 hours had completely normal function. A complication rate of 54% is seen with delayed fasciotomy, compared to only 4.5% with early fasciotomy.   Traditionally, when all four compartments are involved in the syndrome, double incision fasciotomy or fibulectomy has been advocated.   However, more recently, it has been proposed that a single incision fasciotomy for the four compartments is also a safe alternative.

CHRONIC EXERTIONAL COMPARTMENT SYNDROME

Chronic exertional compartment syndrome (CECS) occurs after exercise when intramuscular pressure increases.   Swelling after strenuous activity results in up to a 20% increase in muscle volume.   The majority of cases occur after chronic overuse in an athlete, although acute cases have been described.   CECS is missed in 14% of cases after repeated consultations because of minimal findings on physical examination, and in some studies, misdiagnosis is much higher. CECS most commonly occurs in the lower leg.

Clinical Presentation
The clinical history of CECS of the lower leg is typically that of an athlete who describes recurrent pain in the area of the affected compartment during activity. The pain is usually depicted as an ache or tightness and can be localized over the involved compartment. The pain may not develop until 24 to 48 hours after the precipitating event.   After a period of rest, the pain characteristically subsides, only to recur again with the onset of the same exercise. In some patients, paresthesias may develop over an involved nerve. The condition is bilateral in more than 80% of patients. The majority of cases involve the anterior or posterior compartments.

Examination
The patient has a scarcity of definitive findings on examination.   In some cases, a sense of soft-tissue fullness, swelling, and thickening is present. Sensory loss on the plantar aspect of the foot is associated with CECS of the deep posterior compartment, whereas paresthesias on the dorsum of the foot may be present with anterior compartment involvement.

Diagnosis
When this syndrome is suspected on clinical grounds, a bone scan should be ordered to rule out a stress fracture or periostitis (shin splints).   MRI may reveal an increase in signal intensity between the resting and postexercise scans. The definitive diagnosis is established by intracompartmental pressure measurements, which reveal a preexercise compartment pressure of >15 mm Hg or a postexercise compartment pressure of >30 mm Hg 1 minute after exercise or >20 mm Hg 5 minutes after exercise.

Treatment
This condition is not as urgent as an acute compartment syndrome. The patient should be referred for compartment pressure measurements. Various treatment modalities such as physical therapy, orthotics, rest, and alternate activity have minimal or no effect.   Once the diagnosis of CECS is established, fasciotomy of the involved compartment is recommended.   Fasciotomy in CECS leads to sustained relief of leg pain and improved patient satisfaction.

SHIN SPLINTS

The term *shin splints* refers to the syndrome of pain in the leg from running and should exclude stress fractures, fascial hernias, or ischemic disorders.   This condition is also referred to as soleus syndrome and medial tibial stress syndrome (MTSS). MTSS is currently the preferred terminology. Hyperpronation of the foot, overuse, a sudden increase in exercise intensity, or a change in training surface may precipitate MTSS. The end result is a muscle-induced traction periostitis on the posteromedial border of the tibia.

Clinical Presentation
MTSS usually occurs early in the training period of athletes when running on hard surfaces. The pain of MTSS is a dull ache. The most common site of pain is the posteromedial surface of the distal two-thirds of the leg.

Examination
On examination, the hindfoot is in a valgus position and the forefoot may be hyperpronated. Palpable tenderness is elicited over the posteromedial border of the distal tibia. Percussion over this area of the tibia will cause pain, whereas passive or active ranges of motion of the ankle are not painful.

Diagnosis
Diagnosis is most frequently made by bone scan, which reveals diffuse, linear uptake. However, both plain films and bone scan may be normal. MRI will help differentiate MTSS from stress fractures.

Treatment
Many forms of treatment for shin splints have been advocated, but generally the pain does not subside until the patient stops running. The basic treatment is rest, ice, and analgesics. NSAIDs should be avoided if there is suspicion of a stress fracture.

MUSCLE INJURY

Contusion
Contusions are extremely common in the lower extremity because direct blows are frequent in this area. Four types of contusions are seen: (1) anterior leg producing severe pain caused by increased anterior compartment pressure; (2) subcutaneous

portion of the tibia, which, because of the superficial location of the tibia, often results in a *traumatic periostitis*; (3) posterior compartment, which is less common and not nearly as painful as contusions of the anterior compartment; and (4) lateral, where the peroneal nerve winds around the proximal fibula. Contusions laterally over the proximal fibula may produce a painful neuritis or even transient paralysis of the peroneal nerve with a secondary foot drop.

A hematoma may form at the site of the contusion, and if this occurs in the anterior compartment, the patient may present as a surgical emergency requiring fasciotomy to prevent ischemia and subsequent muscle necrosis.

The treatment of these injuries is contingent on the extent of damage and the structures involved. If there is a fresh, palpable hematoma, one may aspirate it by using an aseptic technique followed by a pressure bandage and cold compresses for the next 12 hours. If the contusion is limited to diffuse muscle involvement, the initial treatment should include ice packs and rest of the extremity with elevation for the first 48 hours.

In contusions involving the peroneal nerve, the patient will have local swelling and pain. The patient will complain of paresthesias, with pain shooting to the lateral side of the leg and extending into the foot. Tingling and numbness will remain after the pain is gone. Patients with severe contusions to the common peroneal nerve will have the initial symptoms followed by a pressure sensation over the nerve and functional loss. Sensory hypesthesia and weakness of the dorsiflexors are present. This period of functional loss is followed by a period when nerve function returns, initially sensation, followed by motor function. The return of nerve function may be complete or partial.

The treatment for a nerve contusion is initially nonspecific with ice packs followed in 48 hours by heat applications. If paresis is noted, the muscles must be protected by supporting the ankle and foot in a brace. The foot is held in a neutral position. In patients in whom the contusion is followed by a quiescent period and then rapid paralysis, surgical exploration is justified. When paralysis is immediate, a more conservative approach is usually taken. Referral is indicated in all patients with nerve involvement.

Strains

Muscle strains are common in the calf due to chronic overuse or forcible contraction. The treatment is symptomatic with a period of rest, local heat, and gradual return to activity. Athletes should be cautioned that early return to activity before complete healing may entail a risk for further and more severe injury of the muscle. NSAIDs are of some benefit early during treatment for pain control and functional improvement; however, long-term use of these agents beyond 2 to 3 days is detrimental to the repair process.

A common question relates to the usefulness of stretching to prevent muscle strains. Clinical studies have demonstrated that stretching appears to be beneficial, but forces in excess of 70% of the muscle's contractile force make the muscle more likely to be injured. Thus, when using stretching before running or other activities, one should use minimal force. Viscoelasticity is known to be temperature dependent, and warm-up is considered to protect against muscle strain.

Rupture

Gastrocnemius and Soleus

Rupture of the gastrocnemius or soleus can occur anywhere from the attachment on the femur to their attachment on the calcaneus, which is the most common site of rupture (along the musculotendinous junction). For more information regarding Achilles tendon rupture, the reader is referred to Chapter 22.

The patient notes pain and swelling with diffuse tenderness over the calf. Both active contraction and passive stretching cause pain along the muscle. The muscle may bunch up on any attempt at contraction. Surgical repair is indicated for complete ruptures. In patients with partial ruptures, an equinus cast is used until healing is complete. To detect a complete rupture, the physician should place the patient in a prone position with the feet hanging over the end of the table. Squeeze the upper calf and look for spontaneously occurring plantar flexion. If this does not occur, suspect a complete rupture.

Plantaris

This is a pencil-sized muscle that originates at the lateral condyle of the femur and passes beneath the soleus to attach on the Achilles tendon. In patients with plantaris rupture, pain is noted deep in the calf, which may be disabling. The patient may complain of a sudden sharp snap in the posterior part of the leg followed by a dull deep ache. Repair is not needed here; only symptomatic treatment is indicated.

Fascial Hernia

Fascial hernias are uncommon. The usual site is at the attachment of the anterior fascia along the anterior border of the tibia. The patient complains of an ache here that may initially be diagnosed as a contusion or periostitis. Later, a well-localized mass appears lateral to the tibial crest, which may be tender. The mass bulges when the muscle is flexed, and the examiner may feel a defect on palpation. These patients usually are asymptomatic; however, if symptoms are noted, surgical repair is indicated.

REFERENCES

1. Nicoll EA. Fractures of the tibial shaft. A survey of 705 cases. *J Bone Joint Surg Br.* 1964;46:373–387.
2. Tull F, Borrelli J Jr. Soft-tissue injury associated with closed fractures: evaluation and management. *J Am Acad Orthop Surg.* 2003;11(6):431–438.
3. French B, Tornetta P III. High-energy tibial shaft fractures. *Orthop Clin North Am.* 2002;33(1):211–230, ix.
4. Roberts DM, Stallard TC. Emergency department evaluation and treatment of knee and leg injuries. *Emerg Med Clin North Am.* 2000;18(1):67–84, v–vi.

5. McQueen MM, Gaston P, Court-Brown CM. Acute compartment syndrome. Who is at risk? *J Bone Joint Surg Br.* 2000; 82(2):200–203.

6. McQueen M, Duckworth A, Aitken S, Court-Brown CM. The estimated sensitivity and specificity of compartment pressure monitoring for acute compartment syndrome. *J Bone Joint Surg Am.* 2013;95(8):673–677.

7. Halvorson JJ, Anz A, Langfitt M, et al. Vascular injury associated with extremity trauma: initial diagnosis and management. *J Am Acad Orthop Surg.* 2011;19(8):495–504.

8. Griffin M, Malahias M, Khan W, Hindocha S. Update on the management of open lower limb fractures. *Open Orthop J.* 2012;6(suppl 3: M13):571–577.

9. Giannoudis PV, Papakostidis C, Kouvidis G, Kanakaris NK. The role of plating in the operative treatment of severe open tibial fractures: a systematic review. *Int Orthop.* 2009; 33(1):19–26.

10. Hooper GJ, Keddell RG, Penny ID. Conservative management or closed nailing for tibial shaft fractures. a randomised prospective trial. *J Bone Joint Surg Br.* 1991;73(1):83–85.

11. Rockwood CA, Green DP, Heckman JD, et al. *Rockwood and Green's Fractures in Adults.* 5th ed. Philadelphia, PA: Lippincott Williams & Wilkins; 2001.

12. Busse JW, Morton E, Lacchetti C, Guyatt GH, Bhandari M. Current management of tibial shaft fractures: a survey of 450 Canadian orthopedic trauma surgeons. *Acta Orthop.* 2008; 79(5):689–694.

13. Lefaivre KA, Guy P, Chan H, Blachut PA. Long-term follow-up of tibial shaft fractures treated with intramedullary nailing. *J Orthop Trauma.* 2008;22(8):525–529.

14. Mashru RP, Herman MJ, Pizzutillo PD. Tibial shaft fractures in children and adolescents. *J Am Acad Orthop Surg.* 2005; 13:345.

15. Halsey MF, Finzel KC, Carrion WV, Haralabatos SS, Gruber MA, Meinhard BP. Toddler's fracture: presumptive diagnosis and treatment. *J Pediatr Orthop.* 2001;21: 152–156.

16. Boden BP, Osbahr DC. High-risk stress fractures: evaluation and treatment. *J Am Acad Orthop Surg.* 2000;8(6):344–353.

17. Pell RF, Khanuja HS, Cooley GR. Leg pain in the running athlete. *J Am Acad Orthop Surg.* 2004;12(6):396–404.

18. Stovitz SD, Arendt EA. NSAIDs should not be used in treatment of stress fractures. *Am Fam Physician.* 2004;70(8):1452–1454.

19. Reuben A, Clouting E. Compartment syndrome after thrombolysis for acute myocardial infarction. *Emerg Med J.* 2005;22(1):77.

20. Whitesides TE, Heckman MM. Acute compartment syndrome: update on diagnosis and treatment. *J Am Acad Orthop Surg.* 1996;4(4):209–218.

21. Perron AD, Brady WJ, Keats TE. Orthopedic pitfalls in the ED: acute compartment syndrome. *Am J Emerg Med.* 2001;19(5):413–416.

22. Pearse MF, Harry L, Nanchahal J. Acute compartment syndrome of the leg. *BMJ.* 2002;325(7364):557–558.

23. Sheridan GW, Matsen FA III. Fasciotomy in the treatment of the acute compartment syndrome. *J Bone Joint Surg Am.* 1976;58(1):112–115.

24. Mubarak SJ, Owen CA. Double-incision fasciotomy of the leg for decompression in compartment syndromes. *J Bone Joint Surg Am.* 1977;59(2):184–187.

25. Maheshwari R, Taitsman LA, Barei D. Single-incision fasciotomy for compartmental syndrome of the leg in patients with diaphyseal tibial fractures. *J Orthop Trauma.* 2008;22(10):723–728.

26. Paik R, Pepples D, Hutchinson MR. Chronic exertional compartment syndrome. *BMJ.* 2013;346:f33.

27. Fraipont MJ, Adamson GJ. Chronic exertional compartment syndrome. *J Am Acad Orthop Surg.* 2003;11(4):268–276.

28. Green JE, Crowley B. Acute exertional compartment syndrome in an athlete. *Br J Plast Surg.* 2001;54(3):265–267.

29. Bong MR, Polatsch DB, Jazrawi LM, Rokito AS. Chronic exertional compartment syndrome: diagnosis and management. *Bull Hosp Jt Dis.* 2005;62(3–4):77–84.

30. Verleisdonk EJ, Schmitz RF, Van der WC. Long-term results of fasciotomy of the anterior compartment in patients with exercise-induced pain in the lower leg. *Int J Sports Med.* 2004;25(3):224–229.

31. Edmundsson D, Toolanen G, Sojka P. Chronic compartment syndrome also affects nonathletic subjects: a prospective study of 63 cases with exercise-induced lower leg pain. *Acta Orthop.* 2007;78(1):136–142.

32. Hislop M, Tierney P. Anatomical variations within the deep posterior compartment of the leg and important clinical consequences. *J Sci Med Sport.* 2004;7(3):392–399.

33. Farr D, Selesnick H. Chronic exertional compartment syndrome in a collegiate soccer player: a case report and literature review. *Am J Orthop.* 2008;37(7):374–377.

34. Pham TT, Kapur R, Harwood MI. Exertional leg pain: teasing out arterial entrapments. *Curr Sports Med Rep.* 2007; 6(6):371–375.

35. Edmundsson D, Svensson O, Toolanen G. Intermittent claudication in diabetes mellitus due to chronic exertional compartment syndrome of the leg: an observational study of 17 patients. *Acta Orthop.* 2008;79(4):534–539.

36. Shadgan B, Menon M, O'Brien PJ, Reid WD. Diagnostic techniques in acute compartment syndrome of the leg. *J Orthop Trauma.* 2008;22(8):581–587.

37. Tzortziou V, Maffulli N, Padhiar N. Diagnosis and management of chronic exertional compartment syndrome (CECS) in the United Kingdom. *Clin J Sport Med.* 2006;16(3):209–213.

38. Lohrer H, Nauck T. Endoscopically assisted release for exertional compartment syndromes of the lower leg. *Arch Orthop Trauma Surg.* 2007;127(9):827–834.

39. Stein DA, Sennett BJ. One-portal endoscopically assisted fasciotomy for exertional compartment syndrome. *Arthroscopy.* 2005;21(1):108–112.

40. Mouhsine E, Garofalo R, Moretti B, Gremion G, Akiki A. Two minimal incision fasciotomy for chronic exertional compartment syndrome of the lower leg. *Knee Surg Sports Traumatol Arthrosc.* 2006;14(2):193–197.

41. Orlin JR, Oen J, Andersen JR. Changes in leg pain after bilateral fasciotomy to treat chronic compartment syndrome: a case series study. *J Orthop Surg Res.* 2013;8(1):6–12.

42. Moen MH, Holtslag L, Bakker E, et al. The treatment of medial tibial stress syndrome in athletes: a randomized clinical trial. *Sports Med Arthrosc Rehabil Ther Technol.* 2012; 30(4):12.

43. Aoki Y, Yasuda K, Tohyama H, Ito H, Minami A. Magnetic resonance imaging in stress fractures and shin splints. *Clin Orthop.* 2004;(421):260–267.

CHAPTER 22

Ankle

Moira Davenport, MD and Madison M. Galasso, MD

INTRODUCTION

Ankle injuries are common and account for 30% of all sports injuries.[1] In the emergency department (ED), ankle injuries represent 12% of traumatic injuries with an overall incidence of more than 20%, fluctuating with season and physical activity.[2-4] Ligamentous injuries are more common than fractures by a ratio of 5:1.[5] A thorough understanding of the functional anatomy, fracture patterns, and soft-tissue injuries is important to the emergency physician.

Anatomy

The ankle is composed of the distal ends of the tibia and the fibula that form a mortise into which the talus fits. The ankle has been described in the past as a hinge joint, but it more accurately resembles a saddle joint.[6] The talar dome or saddle is wider anteriorly than it is posteriorly (Fig. 22–1). With dorsiflexion, the talar dome fits snugly into the ankle mortise, yielding greater stability when compared with plantar flexion (Fig. 22–2). With this in mind, it is easy to see why most ankle injuries occur when the ankle and the foot are in plantar flexion.

The only "pure" motion occurring at the ankle joint is plantar and dorsiflexion. Inversion and eversion take place at the subtalar joint formed by the talus and calcaneus. The subtalar joint is very strong, with firm ligamentous support, and the talus should always be thought of as moving with and in the same direction as the calcaneus. Because of the strength of the calcaneotalar joint, most inversion–eversion stresses injure the ankle joint rather than the subtalar joint.

To understand the disorders that occur around this crucial joint, the emergency physician must have good knowledge of the fundamental soft-tissue structures that surround it. These structures are best divided into three "layers" surrounding the joint. The deepest layer is the capsule, which contains the ligaments of the ankle; the middle layer includes the tendons, which traverse the joint to reach the foot; and the most superficial layer is made up of the fibrous bands (retinaculi), which hold the tendons in place as they act on the foot.

Capsular Layer

The capsule surrounds the ankle joint. It is weaker anteriorly and posteriorly but is strengthened laterally and medially by ligaments. The anterior ligament is thin, connects from the anterior tibia to the neck of the talus, and is commonly involved in extensive tears of the lateral ligaments. The posterior ligament is shorter than its anterior counterpart and extends from the posterior tibia to the posterior talus.

The lateral ligaments are the most commonly injured ligaments of the body. They are divided into three important components. Extending from the lateral malleolus to the neck of the talus is the anterior talofibular ligament (ATFL), the most commonly injured ligament in the ankle. From the lateral malleolus to the posterior tubercle of the talus is the posterior talofibular ligament (PTFL), and from the

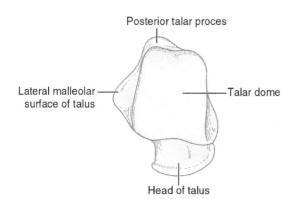

Figure 22–1. Note that the talar dome is wider anteriorly than it is posteriorly.

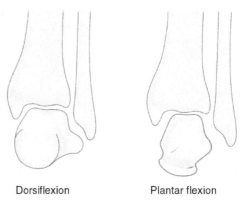

Dorsiflexion   Plantar flexion

Figure 22–2. In dorsiflexion, the wider anterior portion of the talar dome engages the ankle mortise and little motion is permitted. With the ankle in plantar flexion, the narrow posterior part of the talar dome lies within the mortise, permitting a significant degree of inversion–eversion "play" to occur in the joint.

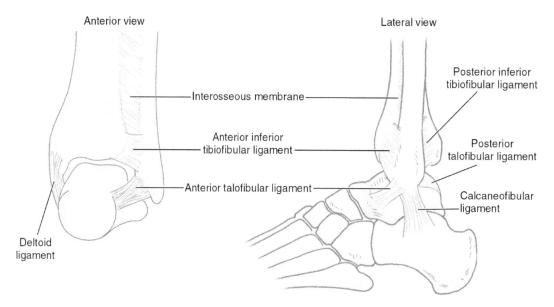

Figure 22–3. The essential ligaments of the anterior and lateral aspects of the ankle and the tibiofibular syndesmosis.

lateral malleolus to the calcaneus extends the calcaneofibular ligament (CFL) (Fig. 22–3).

Proximal to the lateral ligaments, the fibula is connected to the tibia by a series of tough fibrous structures together forming what is called the tibiofibular syndesmosis. This syndesmosis is composed of the interosseous ligament that connects the tibia and the fibula throughout their entire lengths. This ligament is strengthened inferiorly by two thickened fibrous bands: the anterior inferior tibiofibular ligament and the posterior inferior tibiofibular ligament.

The medial ligament is called the deltoid ligament and is a quadrangular structure that has the distinction of being the only ligament in the ankle to contain elastic tissue, giving it the ability to stretch rather than tear. The deltoid ligament is composed of four bands intermingled with each other and extending from the medial malleolus to the navicular, talus, and calcaneus. Two bands of the deltoid extend to the talus: one called the anterior tibiotalar ligament inserting to the neck of the talus, and the other called the posterior tibiotalar ligament, which is the deepest of the four structures. The portion of the deltoid that connects from the medial malleolus to the calcaneus is called the tibiocalcaneal ligament and attaches to the sustentaculum tali (Fig. 22–4).

A ligament of importance that is not included in the capsule of the ankle but is involved in injuries of the ankle and the middle part of the foot is the spring ligament. This ligament extends from the sustentaculum tali to the navicular and bridges the gap between the calcaneus and the navicular bones. It functions to give added support to the head of the talus against the weight of the body and is composed of dense fibrous tissue, portions of which resemble articular cartilage.

Tendon Layer

Superficial to the capsule of the ankle are a series of tendons, none of which attach to the ankle per se, but all of which traverse this joint and are important in considering associated injuries to the ankle. These tendons are subdivided into two groups: the extensors and the flexors of the foot. The extensors pass anteriorly to the ankle joint and the flexors pass posteriorly to the medial malleolus. A third group consists of the peroneal tendons, which pass posteriorly to the lateral malleolus (Fig. 22–5A). Synovial sheaths, some up to 8-cm long, surround these tendons.

Retinacular Layer

Superficial to the tendons are three divisions of thick fibrous bands that hold the tendons in place. These divisions follow the same categorization as the tendons and are similarly termed the extensor retinaculum, the flexor retinaculum, and the peroneal retinaculum. The extensor retinaculum is divided into the superior extensor retinaculum and the inferior extensor retinaculum. The flexor retinaculum consists of one fibrous band that courses posteriorly to the medial malleolus. The peroneal retinaculum has two divisions, the

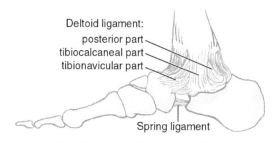

Figure 22–4. The ligaments of the medial ankle.

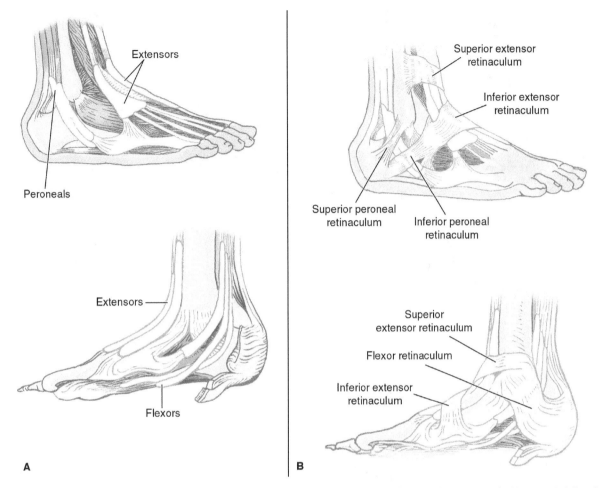

Figure 22–5. **A.** The tendons that traverse the ankle joint lie superficial to the capsular layer and are surrounded by synovial sheaths. **B.** The tendons are held in place by fibrous bands.

superior peroneal retinaculum and the inferior peroneal retinaculum (Fig. 22–5B).

Examination

The motions of the ankle and the foot are described by a number of interchangeable terms (Fig. 22–6).

- *Eversion*: External rotation
- *Inversion*: Internal rotation
- *Dorsiflexion*: Ankle flexion
- *Plantar flexion*: Ankle extension
- *Abduction*: Lateral deviation of the forepart of the foot on a longitudinal axis through the tibia
- *Adduction*: Medial deviation of the forepart of the foot on a longitudinal axis through the tibia
- *Supination*: Adduction and inversion
- *Pronation*: Abduction and eversion

These motions must be understood before any further discussion of fractures occurring at this joint. We use these terms in discussing ankle injuries throughout this chapter. In ankle injuries, inversion and eversion forces are common and are directed perpendicularly to plantar or dorsiflexion of the ankle.

Imaging

Routine ankle radiographs include an anteroposterior (AP), mortise, and lateral views (Fig. 22–7). On the AP view, there is overlap of the tibia and fibula. The mortise view is obtained with the ankle internally rotated 15 to 20 degrees. It represents the true AP projection of the ankle as the tibia and fibula are moved into a plain perpendicular to the x-ray beam. In the mortise view, the tibia and fibula do not overlap and the talar dome is visualized best. This is also the best view to detect a Tillaux (Salter–Harris III fracture of the distal tibial physis due to asymmetric closure of the physis) fracture in adolescents because the lateral aspect of the tibia is not obscured by the fibula. The lateral view provides the best visualization of the posterior aspects of the tibia, fibula, calcaneus, and talus.

Ankle radiographs account for 10% to 15% of all traumatic radiographs.[5,7,8] The Ottawa ankle rules were developed to predict fractures and reduce the number of

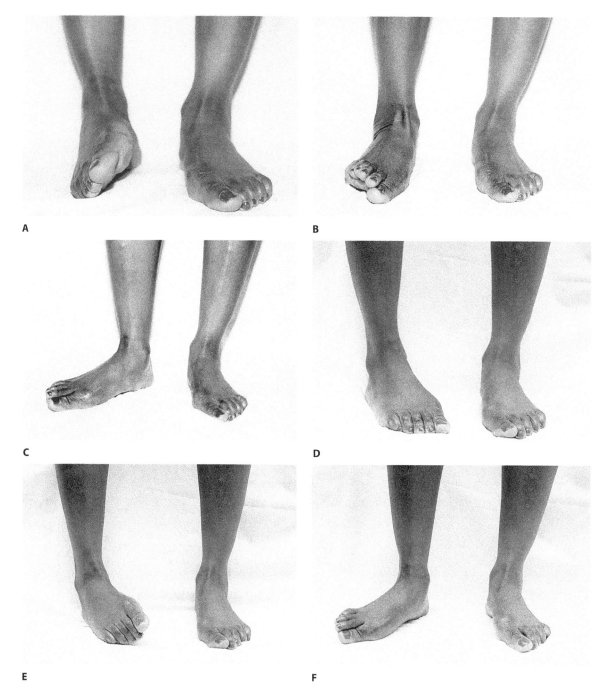

Figure 22–6. *A.* Inversion. *B.* Eversion. *C.* Abduction. *D.* Adduction. *E.* Supination. *F.* Pronation.

radiographs obtained (Fig. 22–8). By using physical examination, the authors detected 100% of all significant malleolar fractures and reduced ankle radiographs by 36%.

Since inception, this instrument has been validated in multiple clinical settings around the world and can be used by both physicians and nurses. A meta-analysis of 32 studies reported a sensitivity approaching 100%, with a reduction in the number of radiographs by 30% to 40%. The Ottawa ankle rules have been validated in children older than 5 years. However, the clinician should proceed

cautiously in preschool-age children, and the rules should not be employed in patients who are unable to communicate or have limited sensation.

Although the Ottawa ankle rules are very sensitive, they lack specificity, and thus, overestimate the need for radiographs. There have been several attempts at modification of these rules to increase specificity, including the Buffalo modification, tuning fork test, and Bernese ankle rules, none of which have been broadly adopted to date. Studies show that ultrasound can now be used as both a sensitive

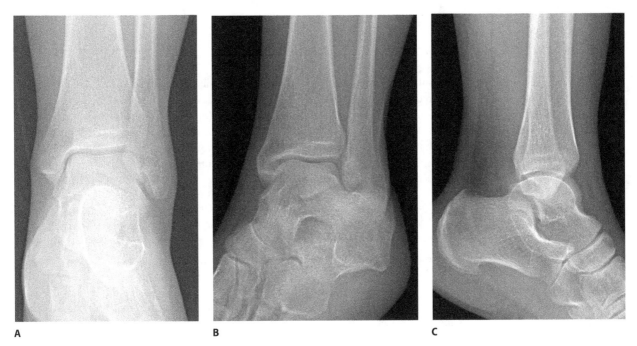

Figure 22–7. *A.* Normal anteroposterior. *B.* Mortise. *C.* Lateral views of the ankle.

and specific method to detect foot and/or ankle fractures, particularly fifth metatarsal, lateral, and medial malleolus fractures. The use of ultrasound in addition to the Ottawa ankle rules can significantly reduce the number of x-rays ordered, costs, and ED length of stay.[30–34]

When a fracture is suspected clinically but is not present on plain radiographs, the clinician should consider computed tomography (CT). Plain radiographs were only 85% sensitive to detect fractures about the ankle compared with multidetector CT.[35]

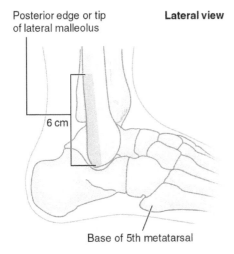

Posterior edge or tip of lateral malleolus

Lateral view

6 cm

Base of 5th metatarsal

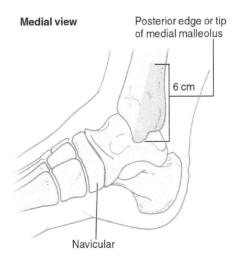

Medial view

Posterior edge or tip of medial malleolus

6 cm

Navicular

A foot x-ray series is only required if there is pain in the midfoot and any of these findings:
1. 5th metatarsal base tenderness
2. Navicular tenderness
3. Inability to bear weight both immediately and in ED

An ankle x-ray series is only required if there is pain in the ankle and any of these findings:
1. Lateral malleolus (posterior aspect) tenderness
2. Medial malleolus (posterior aspect) tenderness
3. Inability to bear weight both immediately and in ED

Figure 22–8. The Ottawa ankle rules.

ANKLE FRACTURES

The ankle bears more weight per unit area than any other joint in the body. It is essential for the physician to realize that ankle fractures and ligamentous injuries frequently coexist, and any treatment plan must include both types of injuries.

Ankle fractures are divided broadly into those due to rotational forces (i.e., malleolar fractures) and those secondary to axial loading forces (i.e., pilon fractures).

Malleolar Fractures

Many classification systems exist to describe ankle fractures due to rotational forces. The three most common include the Lauge-Hansen, Weber, and the Neer closed ring classification systems.

The *Lauge-Hansen classification system* was developed in 1949 by Niels Lauge-Hansen. This system took into consideration the position of the foot and the ankle at the time of injury. The first word refers to the position of the foot at the time the injuring force is applied—supination or pronation—and the second word pertains to the direction of the injuring force—external rotation (eversion), abduction, or adduction. Through cadaveric studies, the author found that the sequence of injured structures was similar and reproducible as the force of injury increased.

With the foot supinated, the lateral ankle structures are stressed. An external rotation or adduction force placed on the ankle results initially in a fracture of the distal fibula. If an external rotation force is applied, the fibula fracture is oblique and distal (Fig. 22-9). Adduction forces result in

a distal transverse fibula fracture (Fig. 22-10). Increasing amounts of force cause a posterior malleolus and a medial malleolus fracture (or deltoid ligament rupture). Fracture of the posterior malleolus is the result of avulsion from the posterior–inferior tibiofibular ligament. Supination-external rotation is the most common mechanism of an ankle fracture, accounting for 85% of cases.

In pronation, the medial structures of the ankle are now under stress. External rotation or abduction forces applied to the pronated ankle result initially in a medial malleolus fracture (or deltoid ligament rupture), and ultimately, as the force increases, a proximal transverse fibula fracture (Figs. 22-11 and 22-12). The pronation-external rotation (PER) fracture of the fibula is above the level of the tibial fibular syndesmosis and results in complete or partial rupture of the syndesmotic ligaments. The fibula fracture in PER injuries may be very proximal at the level of the fibular neck.

The *Weber classification system* categorizes ankle fractures by the level of the fibula fracture (Fig. 22-13). Class A fractures are distal to the level of the distal tibial fibular syndesmosis. Class B fractures are at the level of the syndesmosis, and class C fractures are proximal to the syndesmosis. Class A fractures were considered stable, not requiring surgical repair, whereas class B fractures were treated by fibular stabilization, and class C fractures required fibular stabilization and syndesmotic repair. This classification system was attractive because of its simplicity and because it was initially believed to guide therapy.

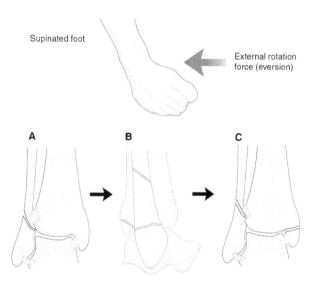

Figure 22–9. Schematic representing the progression of injury following forced eversion of the supinated foot. ***A.*** Distal oblique fibula fracture. ***B.*** With increasing force, the posterior malleolus avulses. ***C.*** Finally, the medial malleolus fractures, creating a trimalleolar fracture.

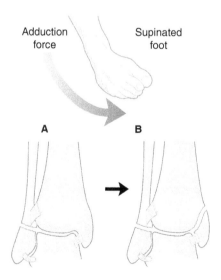

Figure 22–10. Schematic representing the progression of injury following forced adduction of the supinated foot. ***A.*** Distal transverse fibula fracture. ***B.*** With increasing force, the medial malleolus fractures, creating a bimalleolar fracture.

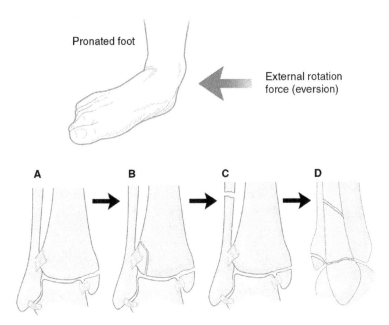

Figure 22–11. Schematic representing the progression of injury following forced eversion of the pronated foot. **A.** Isolated medial malleolus fracture. **B.** With increasing force, the anterior tibiofibular ligament avulses a portion of the distal tibia. **C.** High fibula fracture. **D.** Posterior malleolus fracture.

Unfortunately, the Weber classification ignores the medial injury, which is now believed to be of greater importance. Class B fractures, which are most common, only require surgical repair if the medial structures are injured.[36] In addition, the level of the fibula fracture did not always predict the need for syndesmotic repair. For these reasons, the Weber classification is rarely used.

The *closed ring classification system* is easy to understand and apply. In the closed ring classification system, the ankle is thought of as a ring of bone and ligaments surrounding the talus (Fig. 22–14). The ring in this conceptualization is composed of the tibia, tibiofibular ligament, fibula, lateral ligaments of the ankle, calcaneus, and deltoid ligament. A single disruption of the ring, whether osseous or ligamentous, results

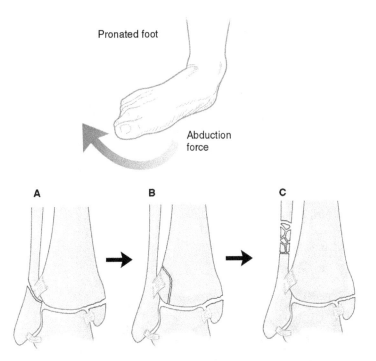

Figure 22–12. Schematic representing the progression of injury following forced abduction of the pronated foot. **A.** Isolated medial malleolus fracture. **B.** With increasing force, the anterior tibiofibular ligament avulses a portion of the distal tibia. **C.** Finally, a transverse or comminuted fibula fracture occurs.

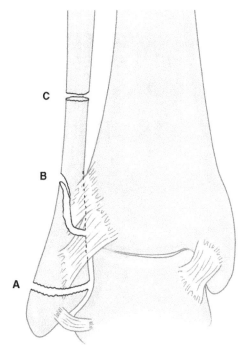

Figure 22–13. Weber classification system of ankle fractures. This system is based on the level of the distal fibula fracture in relation to the syndesmotic ligament.

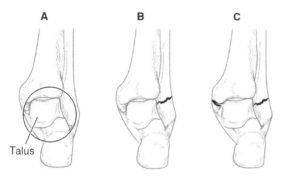

Figure 22–14. Closed ring classification system. **A.** The ankle is conceptualized as a closed ring surrounding the talus. **B.** A stable fracture is a single fracture without displacement. **C.** An unstable fracture involves a single fracture with a ligamentous disruption or two fractures in the ring.

in a stable injury. If the ring is disrupted in two places, an unstable injury is present. Unstable injuries can involve two bones (e.g., bimalleolar fracture) or a ligament and bone (e.g., lateral malleolus and deltoid ligament rupture). When fracture displacement is present, the clinician should suspect occult ligamentous disruption if it is not apparent initially.

Examination

The examination should begin with an assessment of the neurovascular status. Pulses, capillary refill, and sensation are tested. Gross deformity of the ankle is noted. The degree of ankle swelling and the presence of blisters or lacerations may affect patient management (Fig. 22-15).

The foot and knee are examined for evidence of associated injuries. The entire length of the fibula is palpated, searching for evidence of a more proximal fibula fracture consistent with a Maisonneuve injury, which can be easily missed without proper physical examination.

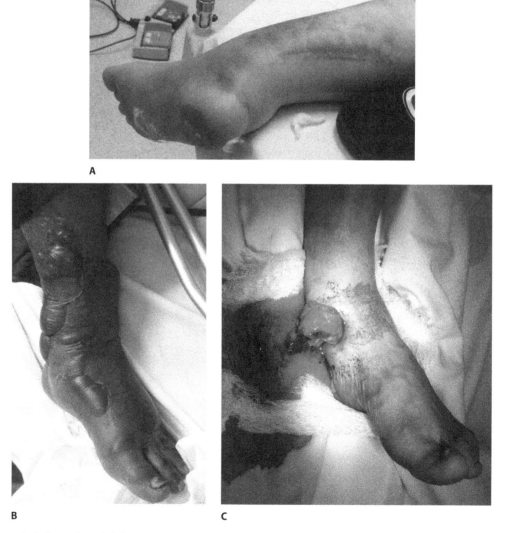

Figure 22–15. A. Ecchymosis and deformity suggesting an ankle fracture–dislocation. **B.** Significant fracture blisters from extensive soft-tissue swelling following an ankle fracture. **C.** An open fracture–dislocation of the ankle.

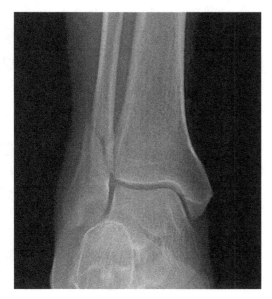

Figure 22–16. Isolated fibula fracture—stable.

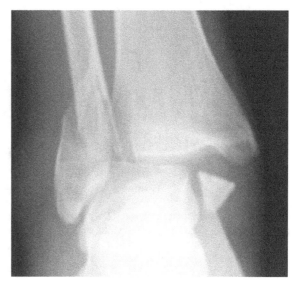

Figure 22–17. Two-part (bimalleolar) fracture—unstable.

The ankle is palpated for tenderness. The emergency physician should direct attention to the medial malleolus following rotational ankle injuries. Tenderness, swelling, or ecchymosis in this area suggests the possibility of injury to the medial structures (medial malleolus fracture or deltoid ligament rupture). If any of these findings are present, the emergency physician must pay special attention to these structures on the plain radiographs. The absence of medial tenderness rules out an acute deltoid ligament tear or medial malleolus fracture.[36]

Imaging

Routine views including AP, lateral, and mortise views are usually adequate. The mortise view is an AP view with 20 degrees of internal rotation. This view is useful for assessing the joint space and will detect ligamentous injury if widened.

Stable ankle fractures include an isolated distal fibula fracture (Fig. 22–16). Examples of unstable ankle injuries are bimalleolar (Fig. 22–17), trimalleolar (Fig. 22–18), and Maisonneuve fractures (Fig. 22–19). A lateral and medial malleolus fracture is referred to as a two-part ankle fracture

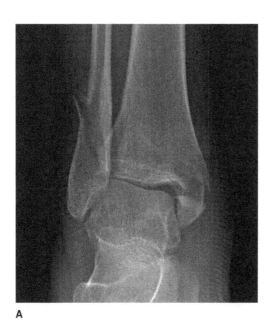

A

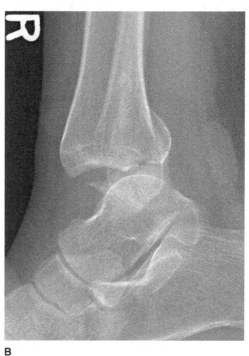

B

Figure 22–18. Three-part (trimalleolar) fracture of the ankle. **A.** AP view. **B.** Lateral view. Note the posterior dislocation of the talus.

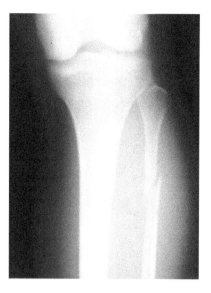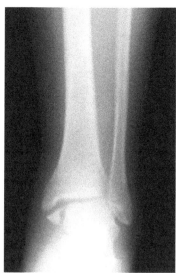

Figure 22–19. Maisonneuve fracture. This unstable fracture reflects injury to the interosseous ligament and stresses the importance of a thorough physical examination, including the proximal fibula.

(previously referred to as a bimalleolar fracture). When the posterior malleolus is also involved, the injury is called a three-part ankle fracture (previously called a trimalleolar fracture). A Maisonneuve fracture occurs when the fibula is fractured proximally in combination with a medial malleolus fracture (or deltoid ligament rupture) and disruption of the tibiofibular syndesmosis.

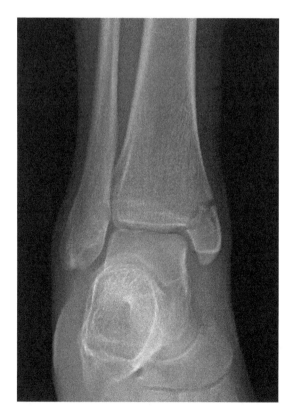

Figure 22–20. An isolated medial malleolus fracture. This injury pattern is less common and occurs after a pronated foot is externally rotated or abducted.

When physical examination findings suggest a medial injury, this portion of the plain radiograph should be scrutinized. A medial malleolus fracture is usually very apparent and may occur as an isolated injury (Fig. 22–20). Difficulty arises in determining the presence of deltoid ligament rupture. The best criterion for assessing deltoid ligament rupture is the presence of lateral talar shift on the AP or mortise views of the ankle. Lateral talar shift is present when the space between the medial malleolus and talus is greater than the space between the talar dome and tibial plafond (Fig. 22–21). This injury is referred to as a two-part equivalent fracture. A three-part equivalent injury pattern may also be seen (Fig. 22–22).

If radiographs are negative and medial malleolus tenderness is present, the injury should be presumptively treated as unstable or additional radiographs should be taken. A gravity stress view can help make the diagnosis. This AP radiograph is obtained with the leg horizontal to the floor with the medial side up and the ankle suspended over the edge of a pillow (Fig. 22–23). In cadaveric studies, an increase in the talar tilt >15 degrees or talar shift >2 mm occurs when the deltoid ligament is disrupted. Stress x-rays can cause a significant amount of patient discomfort. Advanced imaging (CT or MRI) should be considered to further evaluate the deltoid ligament.

An isolated posterior malleolar fracture has a low incidence and may be difficult to detect on plain radiographs, making this injury a potential diagnostic challenge (Fig. 22–24). If this injury is suspected, and because the lateral view may underestimate the size of the fragment, a CT scan may be required. Surgery is indicated when more than 25% of the articular surface is involved, there is more than 2 mm of displacement, or there is posterior subluxation of the talus.

Treatment

The ankle is considered stable when the talus moves in a normal pattern during range of motion. If talar movement

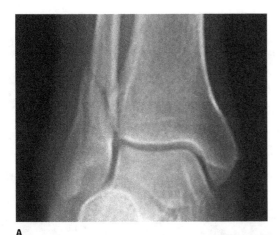

A

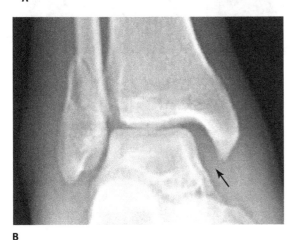

B

Figure 22–21. An oblique fibula fracture is noted in both radiographs. **A.** The distance between the talar dome and the tibial plafond is equal to the distance between the medial malleolus and the talus, indicating a stable fracture. **B.** Lateral talar shift is present, representing disruption of the deltoid ligament and an unstable fracture (*arrow*). This injury is also referred to as a bimalleolar equivalent fracture.

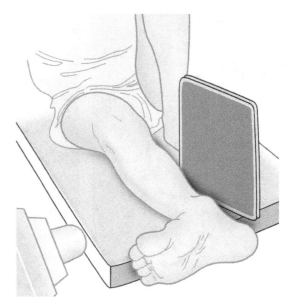

Figure 22–23. Gravity stress radiograph.

is abnormal, articular cartilage is damaged, degenerates, and leads to premature arthritis. For this reason, the determination of ankle stability is the most important factor to consider when treating ankle injuries. Stable injuries are treated nonsurgically, whereas unstable injuries require operative fixation.

It has been determined that the primary stabilizer of the ankle is not the lateral elements, as proposed by Weber, but the medial structures (medial malleolus, deltoid ligament).[36,42,43] A fracture of the fibula does not result in abnormal talar movement as long as the medial structures are intact.[44-46] Multiple studies have corroborated this fact by demonstrating successful long-term outcomes of isolated fibula fractures managed by closed methods.[47-50]

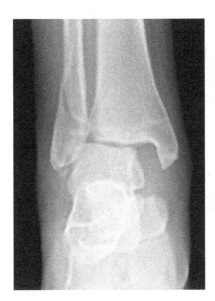
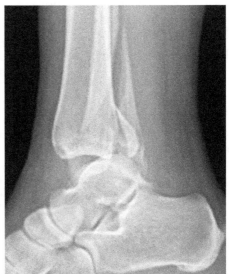

Figure 22–22. Trimalleolar equivalent fracture. Note the fractures of the distal fibula and posterior malleolus as well as the lateral talar shift.

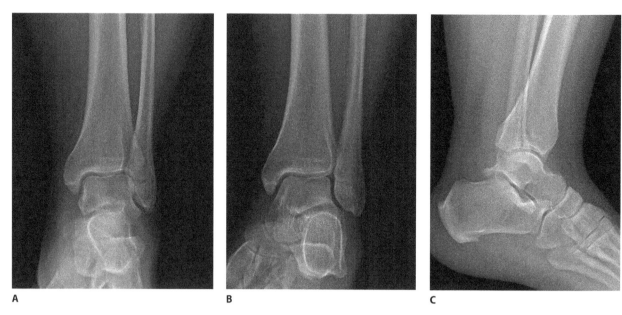

Figure 22–24. An isolated posterior malleolar fracture. **A.** AP. **B.** Mortise. **C.** Lateral radiographs.

On the contrary, when the medial malleolus is involved (as in a two-part ankle fracture), satisfactory results are obtained in only 65% of patients managed by closed means versus 90% treated operatively. Determining stability requires a review of the plain radiographs as well as a thorough physical examination.

Stable. Stable injuries require no reduction and have an excellent prognosis. Examples of stable ankle fractures include isolated distal fibula fractures (common) and some isolated distal medial malleolus fractures. Initially, these injuries are treated with a posterior splint (Appendix A–14), crutches, elevation, and ice until the swelling goes down. Definitive management of isolated distal fibula fractures includes a short-leg walking cast or cast boot for 4 to 6 weeks. The goal of therapy is protection from further injury, and the results are similar, even when a high-top tennis shoe is used for immobilization.

Although most medial malleolus fractures are treated operatively, a small avulsion can be treated nonoperatively if it is distal and minimally displaced.

Unstable. Unstable fractures that are displaced should undergo closed reduction and splinting in the ED. The definitive management of an unstable ankle fracture is surgery, but an accurate reduction in the ED is important because it prevents further injury to the articular cartilage, allows swelling to resolve more rapidly, and prevents ischemia to the skin.

Analgesia is necessary to perform the reduction. The ankle is usually easily reduced by applying gentle traction in line with the deformity, followed by gradual motion to return the talus into a reduced position. The ankle is splinted immediately to ensure the reduction is maintained. A posterior mold and a "U"-shaped splint on either side for added support and stability should be used (Video 22–1 and Appendix A–14). Postreduction films to confirm the reduction are obtained. If the reduction cannot be performed (soft-tissue interposition or impacted fragments) or maintained (large posterior malleolus fracture), urgent operative intervention is necessary. Orthopedic consultation should be obtained. More information about ankle fracture–dislocations is provided in the next section.

Although these injuries were traditionally treated surgically on an inpatient basis, a period of outpatient management before operative fixation is becoming common. Indications for admission include patient noncompliance, lack of social support, inability to manage crutches, or significant associated injuries.

The timing of surgery is dependent on several factors, including the type of fracture, condition of the soft tissue, and associated injuries. Even when severe soft-tissue swelling, fracture blisters, or abrasions delay surgery, no adverse outcomes are noted.

ANKLE FRACTURE–DISLOCATIONS

Dislocation of the ankle most commonly occurs in association with an unstable ankle and multiple fractures. These are open injuries in one-fourth of cases. Fracture–dislocations have three times the rate of major complications compared with simple fractures.

Early reduction of these injuries is encouraged to reduce the incidence of postoperative complications. Fracture–dislocations that are not anatomically reduced may result in osteochondral injury of the talar dome and pressure

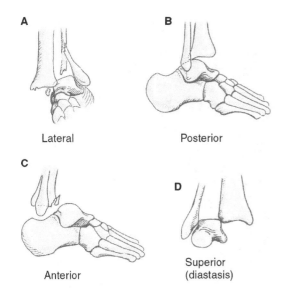

Figure 22–25. Ankle fracture–dislocations.

the fixed foot or forcible dorsiflexion of the foot such as occurs during a fall on the heel with the foot dorsiflexed.

Examination

Clinically, there is usually obvious deformity of the foot and ankle. In lateral dislocations, the foot is displaced laterally, and the skin on the medial aspect of the ankle joint is very taut (Figs. 22–26 and 22–27A). In patients with a posterior ankle dislocation, the foot is plantar-flexed and has a shortened appearance (Fig. 22–27B). Patient with an anterior dislocation presents with the foot in dorsiflexion and elongated. On examination, the supporting ligaments and capsule are disrupted. Anterior dislocations are associated with loss of a palpable dorsalis pedis pulse due to impingement by the talus.

Imaging

Whenever an ankle fracture–dislocation is suspected, assess the vascular integrity before obtaining radiographs to exclude compromise. If there is adequate perfusion to

necrosis of the overlying skin.⁴¹ This section addresses the relevant part of the examination and treatment of associated dislocations.

Fracture–dislocations of the ankle can be lateral, posterior, anterior, or superior (Fig. 22–25), with lateral ankle dislocation being the most common form seen in ED. These injuries are usually not open and are associated with either a fracture of the medial malleolus or, less commonly, rupture of the deltoid ligament. Posterior and posterolateral dislocations are also common. The mechanism causing posterior dislocations is a strong forward thrust of the posterior tibia, usually secondary to a blow. The patient is usually in plantar flexion when this occurs. Anterior dislocations are less common than posterior dislocations and are almost always associated with a fracture of the anterior lip of the tibia. The mechanism causing this type of dislocation is a force that causes posterior displacement of the tibia on

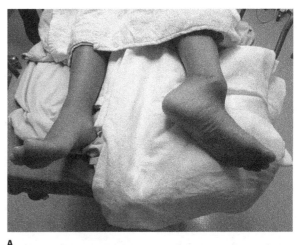

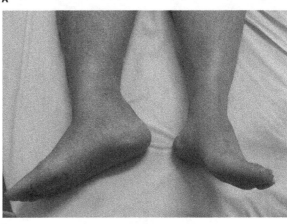

Figure 22–27. **A.** Posterolateral ankle fracture–dislocation of the left ankle. Note the taut appearance of the skin medially. **B.** Posterior ankle fracture–dislocation. The right foot is plantar-flexed and shortened.

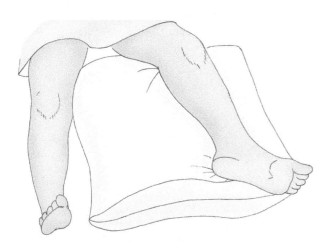

Figure 22–26. Lateral ankle dislocation—classic position.

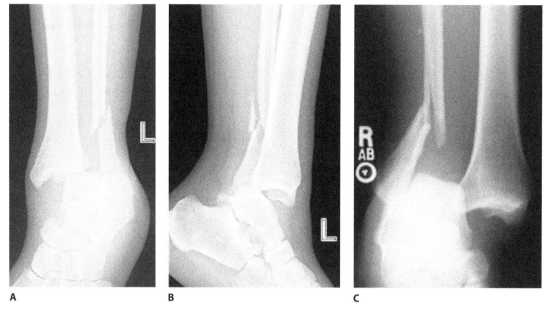

A   **B**   **C**

Figure 22–28. Ankle fracture–dislocations. **A.** Lateral dislocation of the ankle with associated fibula fracture and deltoid ligament rupture. **B.** Posterior dislocation. **C.** Superior dislocation. *(Used with permission from Kris Norland, MD.)*

the foot, an expedited radiograph can be obtained before reduction (Fig. 22–28). There is some evidence to suggest that CT scanning may further aid in operative planning and should be considered in the ED.

Treatment

As stated previously, early reduction is preferred following closed injuries. Open fracture–dislocations are reduced in the ED only if they are associated with vascular compromise. Anesthesia is administered using procedural sedation with the guidelines outlined in Chapter 2. Intra-articular

injection of local anesthetic into the ankle joint may provide enough pain relief to perform the reduction with a small amount of intravenous analgesics and without procedural sedation.

Hip and knee flexion to 90 degrees is recommended in all cases of ankle fracture–dislocations to relax the gastrocnemius–soleus complex and allow for an easier reduction. This is best achieved with an assistant who will hold the patient's lower extremity at the knee and provide countertraction during the reduction attempt (Fig. 22–29).

Lateral fracture–dislocation reductions involve axial traction with one hand on the heel and the other hand on the dorsum of the foot, while an assistant applies countertraction. Next, simple manipulation medially brings the ankle back into its normal position (Fig. 22–30 and Video 22–2).

Alternatively, the foot and leg can be suspended to allow gravity and the position of the ankle (plantar flexion and inversion) to aid in the reduction. This can be achieved with finger traps or Kerlix wrapped around the first and second

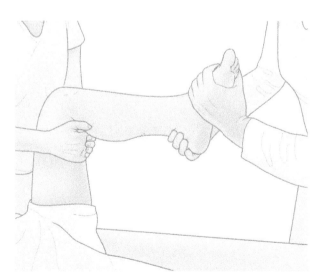

Figure 22–29. Reduction of an ankle fracture–dislocation should occur with the hip and knee flexed to 90 degrees. This position relaxes the gastrocnemius–soleus muscles and allows for an easier reduction.

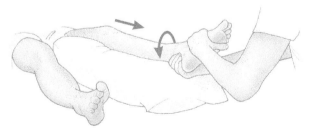

Figure 22–30. Lateral ankle fracture–dislocation. Distal traction to the plantar-flexed foot is applied initially followed by rotation of the foot to its proper anatomic position. This maneuver usually produces a palpable "thud."

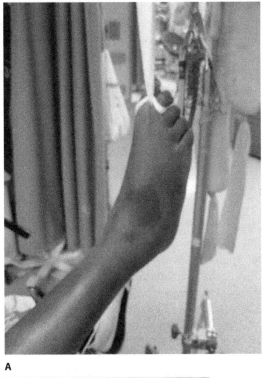

A

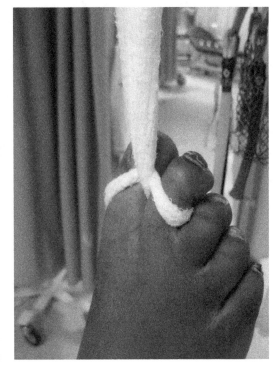

B

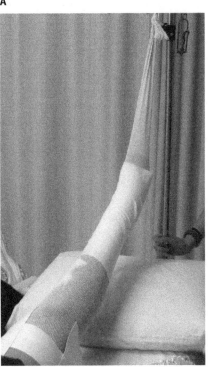

C

Figure 22–31. Methods to hang a fracture–dislocation of the ankle to allow the weight of the leg to help reduce the fracture. **A, B.** Hanging the toes with Kerlix (Quigley traction). **C.** The use of stockinette to hang the leg.

toes. A separate weighted IV pole or the pole attached to the stretcher should be used to avoid tipping the pole over. Another technique involves suspending the foot by a piece of stockinette on the leg that is taped to the thigh and runs distal to the toes. Both of these methods also aid in applying the splint following reduction (Fig. 22–31 and Video 22–3).

Posterior fracture–dislocations are reduced by grasping the heel with one hand and the forefoot with the other hand. First, plantar flex the foot while providing additional axial traction with the other hand. Next, the foot is dorsiflexed, and the heel is pushed forward while the tibia is pushed posteriorly (Fig. 22–32).

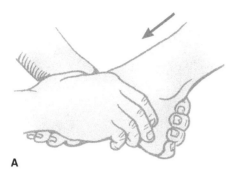

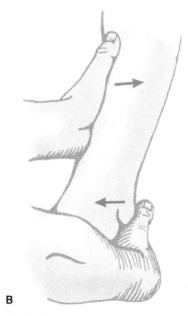

Figure 22–32. Reduction technique for a posterior ankle dislocation. **A.** Plantarflex the foot while providing additional axial traction with the other hand. **B.** Dorsiflex the foot and push the heel anteriorly while the tibia is pushed posteriorly.

Anterior fracture–dislocations are reduced by dorsiflexing the foot slightly to disengage the talus. Next, axial traction is applied. The foot is then pushed posteriorly back into its normal position, while an anterior force is applied to the distal tibia.

Superior fracture–dislocations (diastasis) are uncommon injuries often associated with articular damage. These cases should be splinted and emergent consultation obtained.

The Bosworth injury is the rare ankle fracture–dislocation that cannot be reduced. This injury results when a fibular fragment is lodged posterior to the tibia.[58,59] The external oblique x-ray view is most useful in differentiating this fracture from other bimalleolar fractures that are reducible.[60]

Following reduction, the neurovascular function of the extremity should be reassessed. A posterior splint with a U-shaped stirrup along the sides of the ankle is applied with the ankle at 90 degrees (Appendix A–14). Anterior dislocations are immobilized in slight plantar flexion. Because these fractures are usually unstable, care should be taken to avoid redislocation or displacement while the splint is being

applied. Gentle molding of the splint while it dries can be used to "fine tune" the reduction. Plaster splint material is preferred to commercially available fiberglass splints. Fluoroscopy is frequently used to confirm the adequacy of the reduction before the patient goes for a formal postreduction radiograph. For lateral dislocations, the joint space at the mortise should be no more than 3 mm.

The patient will require surgical repair, which is almost always indicated following these unstable ankle injuries. Many surgeons prefer early operative treatment, so consultation with an orthopedist before disposition is appropriate.

TIBIAL PLAFOND FRACTURES

Intra-articular fractures of the distal tibia are referred to as plafond (French for ceiling) fractures.[??] These fractures may be due to rotational force but are more common when the ankle undergoes an axial load. An axial load fracture of the tibial plafond is referred to as a pilon (French for pestle) fracture.[??] Intra-articular plafond fractures represent 1% to 10% of all lower-extremity fractures.

Mechanism of Injury
High-energy axial compression is the common mechanism for the majority of these fractures.[61-64] In this mechanism, the tibia is driven down into the talus and results in a comminuted intra-articular fracture of the distal tibia. Low-energy plafond fractures also occur and are associated with fewer complications because of a lesser degree of comminution and soft-tissue injury.[??] Low-energy fractures of the plafond may be due to rotational forces.[??]

The position of the ankle at the time of axial impact will create different fracture patterns (Fig. 22–33). If the ankle is dorsiflexed, the fracture pattern may be comminuted or an intra-articular anterior marginal fracture may be apparent. Alternatively, a plantar-flexed ankle will result in a posterior marginal fracture pattern.

Examination
The patient will present with pain and swelling that is initially localized but may later involve the ankle diffusely. The examiner should attempt to elicit an exact mechanism of injury and carefully examine the ankle for focal tenderness or swelling. Approximately 20% of these fractures are open.[61-64] The dorsalis pedis and posterior tibial pulses should be palpated and compared with the uninvolved extremity. Swelling or ecchymosis surrounding the Achilles tendon may indicate a posterior malleolar fracture.

Imaging
Routine views, including AP, lateral, and mortise views, are usually adequate (Figs. 22–34 and 22–35). Pilon fractures often require a CT scan to fully delineate the extent of injury. CT scan of the ankle is routinely obtained preoperatively and changes the surgeon's operative plan 64% of the time.[65,66]

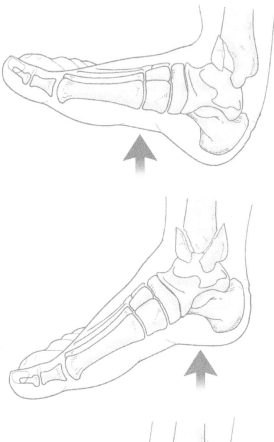

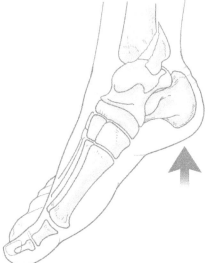

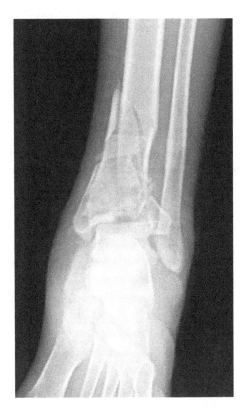

Figure 22–34. Tibial plafond fracture (pilon fracture) due to an axial compression force.

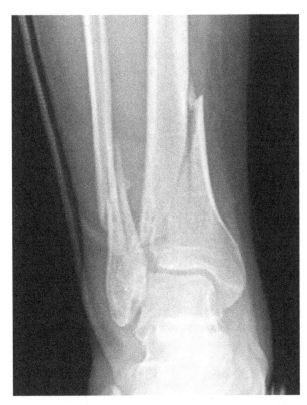

Figure 22–33. The position of the foot at the time of injury predicts that the portion of the tibial plafond will be fractured.

Associated Injuries

After an axial compression injury, calcaneal and spinal compression fractures may be seen. Compartment syndrome of the leg is also seen after these high-energy injuries.[61]

Treatment

The emergency management of plafond fractures should include ice, elevation, immobilization in a well-padded splint (Appendix A–14), and emergent referral.[63]

Figure 22–35. Plafond fracture due to a low-energy rotational mechanism. These fractures are associated with less soft-tissue injury and have a better functional outcome.

The definitive management of these injuries varies from casting to open reduction with internal fixation (ORIF) and, more recently, external fixation. Non-surgical treatment is rarely employed and is reserved for low-energy injuries without articular displacement. ORIF can be performed when the fracture is not associated with excessive soft-tissue damage (usually a low-energy mechanism). ORIF following high-energy injuries with extensive soft-tissue injury is associated with a high rate of complications, making external fixation the treatment of choice.

Complications

Ankle fractures may develop several significant complications. The incidence of severe complications following ORIF of the tibial plafond ranges from 10% to 55%. Complications include the following:

- Traumatic arthritis of the talar mortise (20%–40%). Comminuted tibial plafond fractures or those involving elderly patients are particularly predisposed to develop arthritis.
- Skin necrosis or wound breakdown following open reduction of high-energy tibial plafond fractures.
- Malunion or nonunion.
- Wound infection may be seen after open fractures or following operative repair due to extensive soft-tissue injury.
- Complex regional pain syndrome.
- Ossification of the interosseous membrane.
- Osteochondral fractures of the talar dome.

ANKLE SOFT-TISSUE INJURY AND DISLOCATION

ANKLE SPRAINS

Sprain is the most common ankle injury presenting to the ED, and perhaps the most commonly mistreated injury confronting the emergency physician. Many physicians have a limited understanding of the "simple sprain," yet this disorder confronts them more commonly than any other single entity involving the extremities. Inappropriate management of this common injury can result in chronic ankle instability in 30% of patients, further increasing the likelihood of traumatic osteoarthritis.

Sprains account for 75% of all injuries to the ankle. Females are at greater risk for ankle sprain than males, and children are at greater risk compared with adolescents and adults. Ankle sprains occur most often in athletes between 15 and 35 years of age involved in basketball, football, and running. Sprains of the lateral ligaments account for the vast majority, followed by the tibiofibular syndesmotic and medial ligaments. Given the high prevalence of lateral ankle sprain, one of the most common musculoskeletal injuries, and the associated chronic sequelae, this is a problem concerning more than just the young athlete.

Mechanism of Injury

Sprains are due to forced inversion or eversion of the ankle, usually while the ankle is plantar-flexed.

Inversion stresses account for 85% of all ankle sprains and result in lateral ligamentous injury. As force increases, a predictable sequence of structures is injured (Table 22–1). The lateral joint capsule and the anterior–inferior tibiofibular ligament (ATFL) are the first structures to be injured following an inversion stress. Isolated injury to the ATFL is present in 60% to 70% of all ankle sprains. With greater forces, a tear of the CFL occurs, and finally, the PTFL is injured. Injury to all three structures is seen in up to 9% of cases.

Eversion injuries to the ankle are much less likely to result in ankle sprains. In addition to the structures listed in Table 22–1, a lateral malleolus fracture is seen much more commonly following an eversion injury (Fig. 22–9). When the medial structures are injured, avulsion of the medial malleolus occurs more frequently than rupture of the strong and elastic deltoid ligament. As the force increases, the anterior–inferior tibiofibular ligament and the interosseous (syndesmotic) ligament will tear (Table 22–1). Medial ankle sprains account for approximately 5% to 10% of all ankle sprains.

Eversion of the ankle, internal rotation of the tibia, and excessive dorsiflexion may result in a tibiofibular syndesmotic ligament injury. This injury is termed the "high ankle sprain." In a series of ankle ligament ruptures, in 3% of cases, an isolated syndesmosis rupture was identified. Shoe design has no impact on the rate of ankle sprains.

Clinical Presentation

Ankle sprains were previously categorized as first-, second-, or third-degree injuries according to the clinical

▶ TABLE 22–1. **SEQUENCE OF STRUCTURES INJURED WITH INVERSION AND EVERSION ANKLE SPRAINS**

Inversion Stress	Eversion Stress
Anterior talofibular ligament	Medial malleolus avulses (deltoid ligament rupture)
↓	↓
Calcaneofibular ligament	Anterior–inferior tibiofibular ligament
↓	↓
Posterior talofibular ligament	Interosseous (syndesmotic) ligament

▶ TABLE 22–2. **CLASSIFICATION OF SPRAINS**

Grade	Signs and Symptoms
First-degree ligament injury without tear	Minimal functional loss (patient ambulates with minimal pain) Minimal swelling Mildly tender over involved ligament No abnormal motion or pain on stress testing
Second-degree incomplete tear of a ligament	Moderate functional loss (patient has pain with weight bearing and ambulation) Moderate swelling, ecchymosis, and tenderness Pain on normal motion Mild instability and moderate-to-severe pain on stress testing
Third-degree complete tear of a ligament	Significant functional loss (patient is unable to bear weight or ambulate) Egg-shaped swelling within 2 hours of injury May be painless with complete rupture Positive stress test

presentation and the instability demonstrated by stress testing (Table 22–2). However, these terms are no longer recommended as they do not specify the ligament or ligaments involved. Minor, moderate, and severe are now the preferred way to describe ankle sprains. Minor injuries are easy to diagnose, whereas difficulty exists in distinguishing between moderate and severe injuries.

In a minor ankle sprain, there is stretching of the fibers of the ligament without tear. The patient presents with no functional loss in the ankle and many of these patients often do not seek care, usually treating themselves at home. Patients with minor sprains demonstrate little or no swelling of the ankle, no pain on normal motion of the ankle, and only mild pain on stressing the joint in the direction of the insulting force, usually inversion.

Patients with a moderate ankle sprain are more difficult to diagnose because moderate sprains mean that the ligament is partially torn. This can run the gamut of anything from just a few fibers being torn to tears involving almost the entire ligament with only a few fibers remaining intact. The patient presents with moderate swelling and complains of immediate pain upon injuring the ankle. This is in contrast to patients with a first-degree injury who may not know they had a sprain until the next day or after a period of rest. The second-degree sprain is fraught with complications, including the possibility of ligamentous laxity and recurrent sprains due to instability.

A severe ankle sprain exists when there is a complete tear of the ligament. An "egg-shaped" swelling over the lateral ligaments of the ankle occurring within 2 hours of injury,

in most cases, indicates a severe injury of the ankle. It is often difficult to differentiate a moderate sprain from a severe injury without adequate stress testing or advanced imaging.[77] Because the ligaments are completely torn, there may be little or no pain, but there is usually swelling and tenderness of the ankle.

Examination

Careful examination of the ankle will give the emergency physician better insight into the ligamentous structures injured following an ankle sprain. If the swelling about the lateral malleolus increases the ankle circumference by 4 cm, then the probability of ligament rupture within the ankle is 70%. Tenderness over the CFL suggests rupture of this ligament in 72% of cases. Likewise, tenderness over the ATFL means that in 52% of cases, the ligament is ruptured. If all three symptoms are present, then there is a 91% chance of major ligament damage.[78]

Stress testing aids in differentiating moderate and severe ankle sprains. Frequently, pain and swelling secondary to the acute injury do not allow stress testing. In these cases, the ankle should be immobilized and the patient kept from weight bearing. Referral for serial examinations improves diagnostic accuracy.[79]

Injection of the ankle may allow performance of stress tests of the acutely injured ankle. This is done by injecting the joint opposite to the side of the injury (usually, medially) and infiltrating 5 to 10 mL of lidocaine. However, diagnostic accuracy is diminished following injection. The inversion stress test, for example, is only 68% accurate with anesthesia compared with 92% without anesthesia.[80]

The anterior drawer test is the first test to be performed because it examines for rupture of the ATFL. If this test is negative, then there is no need to go to the inversion stress test because it requires both the anterior talofibular and the CFL to be ruptured to be positive.

The anterior drawer test of the ankle can be done with the patient either sitting or supine (Fig. 22–36). The muscles surrounding the ankle should be relaxed. The knee should be flexed to relax the gastrocnemius muscle, and the

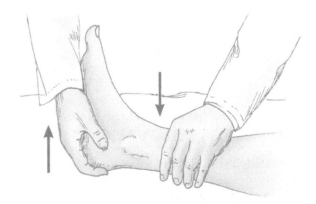

Figure 22–36. Technique for performing anterior drawer stress test of the ankle.

ankle should be held in a neutral position. If the ankle is plantar-flexed, a positive anterior drawer test will be impossible to demonstrate, even if the ligaments are completely disrupted. The examiner places the base of the hand over the anterior aspect of the tibia and applies a posteriorly directed force. At the same time, the other hand cups the heel and displaces the foot anteriorly. Rupture of ATFL is indicated by mild anterior displacement of the talus. Increasing laxity indicates additional injury to the calcaneofibular and PTFL. The degree of laxity should always be compared with the normal side.

Within the first 48 hours after injury, the anterior drawer test was found to have a sensitivity of 71%, with a specificity of 33%. Five days post injury, the sensitivity improved to 96% with a specificity of 84%.

An inversion stress test (talar tilt test) can be performed to identify rupture of the CFL. We do not recommend performing this test, however, because it can be quite painful and is not necessary in the acute setting. The inversion stress test measures the angle produced by the tibial plafond and the dome of the talus in response to forced inversion. To perform this test, the ankle is kept in a neutral position, and the examiner grasps the anterior tibia with one hand and the heel with the opposite hand. The ankle is inverted. A difference of 5% to 10% or 23-degree tilt indicates tears to the ATFL and the CFL. This examination technique is the same as that required to perform stress x-rays. Pain associated with this technique and the availability of advanced imaging have led to recommendations against stress x-rays in the acute setting. Eversion, in the manner described previously, detects injury to the deltoid ligaments.

Examination for the detection of a syndesmotic ligament sprain should include the *squeeze test*. To perform this test, the tibia and fibula are "squeezed" together at the midcalf. Pain in the ankle and lower leg on compression (in the absence of a fibula fracture) indicates injury to the syndesmotic ligaments. This injury should also be suspected when tenderness is present at the distal tibiofibular joint or pain is produced upon forced external rotation of the ankle.

Imaging

Radiographs of the ankle should be taken in most cases. The Ottawa ankle rules, as described previously, will aid the clinician in avoiding unnecessary ankle radiographs. In some patients with a moderate sprain, one may note a small flake of bone off of the lateral malleolus. This indicates an incomplete tear and is usually associated with a moderate injury to the lateral ligaments. Widening of the tibiofibular clear space to >6 mm suggests a syndesmotic ligament sprain. If syndesmotic ligament injury is suspected, MRI is still considered the imaging modality of choice. However, recently developed CT scan parameters to evaluate the anterior syndesmotic interval at the anterolateral tibial tubercle have been found to identify subtle syndesmotic disruptions. The ready availability of CT scanning in the

ED may increase diagnostic capability and better tailor patient therapy.

Ultrasound is another modality to be used in the evaluation of the ankle sprain patient. The superficial location of the ATFL lends itself very nicely to ultrasound evaluation.

Arthrography may be used to define the extent of ligamentous rupture. The benefit of this technique is controversial, and it is rarely used in the ED. To perform an arthrogram, the ankle is thoroughly prepped and a 22-gauge needle, attached to a 10-mL syringe, is inserted into the side opposite the injury and about 6 mL of contrast material is injected. A 1:1 mixture of Hypaque (50% diatrizoate meglumine and diatrizoate sodium) and sterile water is used. Radiographs of the ankle are then obtained. When ligamentous rupture is present, extravasation will be seen laterally outside the ankle joint along the lateral malleolus.

Associated Injuries

Osteochondral lesions of the talar dome occur in 6% to 22% of ankle sprains and are easily missed on the initial assessment. This lesion should be suspected when tenderness is present along the anterior joint line with the ankle plantar-flexed. Magnetic resonance imaging (MRI) or CT scan of the ankle will detect these injuries and should be considered in patients with sprains that remain symptomatic for 6 weeks after injury.

Treatment

The initial care of most lateral ankle sprains treated in the ED is similar, but important differences exist.

Mild Ankle Sprain. For the mild sprain, ice packs, elevation, and a functional bandage with early mobilization is the most appropriate treatment. Semi-rigid braces have been found to lead to better functional outcomes than taping or elastic bandages. Nonsteroidal anti-inflammatory medications provide analgesia and possibly improve outcomes.

Ice should be crushed, placed in a plastic bag, and covered with a thin protective cloth to avoid cold-induced injury to the skin. Ice application is recommended for 20 minutes four to six times a day for the first 2 days. The elastic bandage should extend just proximal to the toes to the level of the midcalf. Elevation of the injured extremity 15 to 25 cm above the level of the heart will facilitate venous and lymphatic drainage.

Weight bearing is encouraged as tolerated. Functional rehabilitation is begun immediately (Fig. 22-31). Return to full activity is usually achievable within a week, and patients should be referred to their primary physician.

Moderate Ankle Sprain. In moderate sprains, the initial treatment is similar to first-degree sprain, except the patient is kept from weight bearing for 48 to 72 hours. After that period, touchdown weight bearing with crutches should progress to crutch walking as soon as possible. An ankle support, which provides much more stability than an elastic

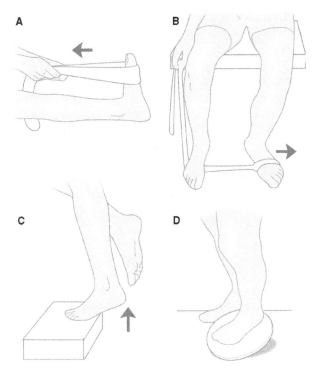

Figure 22-37. Functional rehabilitation following an ankle sprain consists of restoring range of motion, muscle strengthening exercises, proprioceptive training, and, finally, gradual return to activity. **A.** Achilles tendon stretching exercises should begin within 48 hours of injury. Other range-of-motion exercises include knee bends with the heel on the floor (five repetitions five times a day) and alphabet exercises, in which the patient "draws" the letters of the alphabet with the toes. **B, C.** Strengthening exercises begin once swelling and pain are controlled. Isometric exercises (plantar flexion, dorsiflexion, inversion, and eversion) against a wall are followed by isotonic exercises. **D.** Proprioceptive exercises begin once full weight bearing without pain has been achieved. A "wobble board" is used for 5 to 10 minutes two times a day, first while seated and then while standing. The patient rotates the board clockwise and counterclockwise.

bandage, is applied until healing is complete. These supports include lace-up braces, semirigid bimalleolar orthotics, and air splints (Appendix A–18).[85] Kinesio Tape has shown some promise as an additional modality of treatment as the patient progresses through physical therapy.[86] However, larger studies are needed to further evaluate this therapy.

Prolonged immobilization is a common error in the treatment of these injuries. Because second-degree sprains are stable injuries, rehabilitation should be started with range-of-motion exercises on day one. Functional rehabilitation stimulates healing by promoting collagen replacement. Lack of an appropriate rehabilitation program may delay return to activity by months.[87] Home-based physical therapy programs can be equally effective when compared to patients sent to a physical therapist.[88,89] Rehabilitation of the ankle includes strengthening of the elevators and the dorsiflexors.[90] Follow-up care with an orthopedist or sports medicine specialist is recommended.

Severe Ankle Sprain. These patients are treated initially with immobilization in a splint for 72 hours with ice, elevation, and referral.[91] When applying a splint, it is vital to keep the ankle out of equinus and in the neutral position.

Physical examination is notoriously difficult immediately following an injury due to pain and swelling. Patients in whom the differentiation between a moderate or severe sprain cannot be certain, it is recommended that the injury be treated as a severe sprain with reexamination after the swelling and pain has subsided. Delayed physical examination 5 days post injury has been shown to be more accurate than when performed in the first 2 days.[79,92]

The definitive treatment of patients with severe injury remains controversial. When significant talar instability is present, surgical repair is recommended by some authors, particularly in the young athletic patient, whereas others recommend early mobilization and physical therapy.[93] Orthopedic consultation for these injuries, as with any serious injury fraught with complications, is recommended.

Complications

The "simple sprain" can be associated with a high degree of morbidity. Although most patients return to normal activity within 4 to 8 weeks, as many as 20% to 40% of patients after third-degree sprains will have pain that limits their activity for years after the injury.[75]

The most common complication, lateral talar instability, will develop in as many as 40% of patients after an ankle sprain.[94] These patients complain of chronic instability of the ankle and "giving way." Many of these patients develop early onset posttraumatic osteoarthritis as well. If not treated correctly, these injuries pose a significant health care burden, given the long-term morbidity and high prevalence.[73] A majority of patients can be successfully treated with a rehabilitative exercise program and bracing to improve stability. However, in about 40% of ankle ligament injuries in athletes and in other severe or refractory cases, surgical intervention using a tendon graft to stabilize the joint is warranted.[94,95]

Peroneal nerve injury is another common complication following ankle sprains. In one series, 17% of patients with moderate sprains had mild peroneal nerve injuries, and 86% of patients with severe sprains injured either the peroneal or the posterior tibial nerve. Thus, impaired ability to walk 5 to 6 weeks after a sprain may be due to peroneal nerve injury. This injury is probably caused by mild nerve traction or a hematoma in the epineural sheath.

Peroneal tendon dislocation or subluxation, syndesmotic injuries, tibiofibular exostosis, sinus tarsi syndrome (subtalar sprain), talar dome osteochondral injuries, and complex regional pain syndrome are infrequent complications of lateral ligament sprains. These entities are all covered in the following sections with the exception of complex regional pain syndrome, which is described in Chapter 4.

SINUS TARSI SYNDROME

The sinus tarsi are spaces on the lateral aspect of the foot between the inferior neck of the talus and the superior aspect of the distal calcaneus. At the depth of this space is the interosseous talocalcaneal ligaments.   When these ligaments are injured after an inversion ankle injury, chronic pain and instability may result. This is termed the sinus tarsi syndrome. A feeling of hindfoot instability and pain while walking on uneven ground is characteristically relieved when at rest. It is difficult to differentiate this condition from a sprain of the ATFL.

This syndrome is a common complication of ankle sprains that was not recognized in the past.   The findings include tenderness at the lateral side of the foot over the opening of the sinus tarsi. This space is palpated inferior to the ATFL. Pain will also occur during walking and supination and adduction of the foot. The diagnosis is confirmed when injection of a local anesthetic into the sinus tarsi relieves symptoms (Fig. 22–38).

Even with stress radiographs, routine radiographic examination of the ankle and subtalar joint typically do not reveal any pathology.

The treatment of this condition includes anti-inflammatory agents, and the patient is fitted with an orthotic. Injection of a local anesthetic and steroid into the sinus tarsi can also be performed and may need to be repeated. When conservative treatment is unable to relieve the pain, surgical treatment of sinus tarsi syndrome can be performed. Subtalar arthrodesis is used if more conservative treatments are not successful.

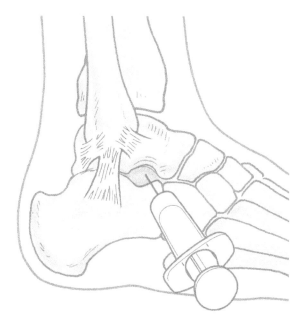

Figure 22–38. Injection of local anesthetic at the site of the sinus tarsi will relieve symptoms in patients with injury to the interosseous talocalcaneal ligament.

TALAR DOME OSTEOCHONDRAL INJURY

"Ankle sprain followed by traumatic arthritis" and "non-healing ankle sprain" are two common situations that should make the emergency physician consider the possibility of an osteochondral lesion.   There are two locations where the cartilage and bone of the talar dome of the ankle can be injured—the superolateral and superomedial margins. If the fragment dislodges, it grinds into the joint, resulting in irreversible chronic arthritis. Other less common sites for osteochondral injuries are the fibular edge and the posterior articular surface of the navicular.

Mechanism of Injury

An osteochondral lesion of the superolateral margin occurs secondary to dorsiflexion and inversion. The lateral ligaments may or may not rupture. This injury is seen more commonly in children due to a greater elasticity of the ligamentous tissue. Superomedial osteochondral fractures occur with plantar flexion, where the narrow talus engages the mortise with a "direct blow." This injury commonly occurs when a jumper comes down hard on the toes with the foot inverted.

Clinical Presentation

Patients complain of a painful ankle, resistant to treatment, with symptoms persisting longer than a sprain. There is usually no tenderness at the malleoli or over the ligaments during palpation. Patients' symptoms are aggravated by activity and completely relieved with rest, although there may be slight swelling with a dull ache after excessive walking. The entire examination may be negative except when the examiner palpates the talar dome with the ankle plantar-flexed. Point tenderness is elicited in this area. A synovitis may occur in the ankle joint with recurrent swelling. The most common site of injury in trauma is the posteromedial aspect of the talar dome.   Local anesthetic injection of the joint relieves the pain.

Imaging

Radiographs of the ankle may show a crater or a particle of bone that appears opaque, surrounded by radiolucency (Fig. 22–39). The best view to demonstrate a lateral lesion is an AP view with dorsiflexion of the ankle and 10 degrees of internal rotation. For medial lesions, the AP view is obtained in plantar flexion. Small lesions are not detectable with plain radiographs. Increased sensitivity is obtained using bone scanning, CT scan, or MRI.

Treatment

The patient should be referred for orthopedic consultation because traumatic arthritis is the sequel to delayed care. If this diagnosis is made in the ED, the patient should be placed in a posterior leg splint and be nonweight bearing. When treatment is delayed for more than 1 year, outcome is poor in most cases. Arthroscopy with debridement and removal of loose fragments offers the best opportunity for a good functional outcome.

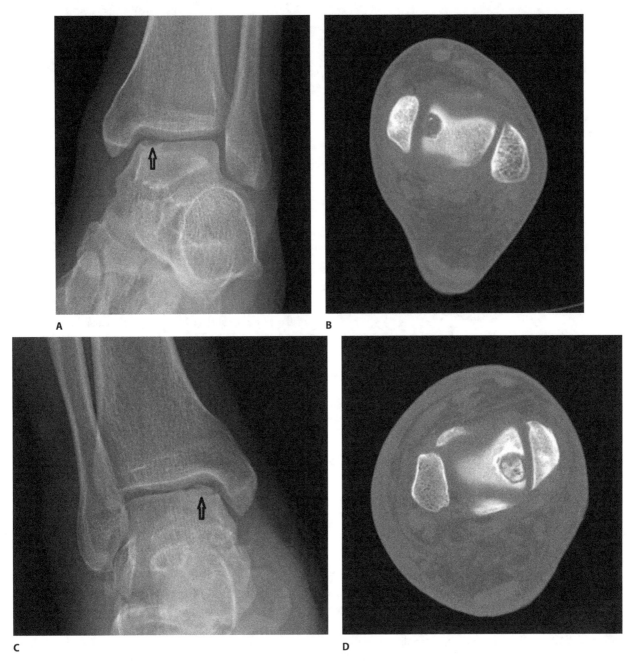

Figure 22–39. Osteochondral lesion of the talar dome. *A, B.* Plain film and CT demonstrating a defect of the talar dome (*arrow*). *C, D.* Another patient with a bony fragment of the talar dome visualized (*arrow*).

TALOTIBIAL EXOSTOSIS

Exostosis is the formation of a bony growth at the site of an irritative lesion or in response to direct trauma. Exostosis occurs in the anterior ankle due to repetitive trauma, usually in athletes.

In the normal ankle, the distal anterior aspect of the tibia is round, and there is a sulcus at the neck of the talus. As the ankle dorsiflexes, the anterior border of the tibia comes in contact with the sulcus (Fig. 22–40). After repetitive trauma, exostosis at the talar sulcus and anterior–inferior margin of the tibia may form. A third less common site is

at the medial and lateral malleolus because of direct trauma from the talus following sprains.

A large number of patients have exostosis that is asymptomatic. In others, pain is present at the anterior aspect of the ankle after activity, and the only finding is exostosis. In most patients, the primary complaint is a decreased activity level, and pain is present only on extreme dorsiflexion of the ankle. On examination, the physician will note some swelling of the anterior aspect of the joint with tenderness to palpation and increasing pain on hyperextension of the foot.

One must differentiate this condition from osteophytes that are a response to degenerative processes in the joint. In

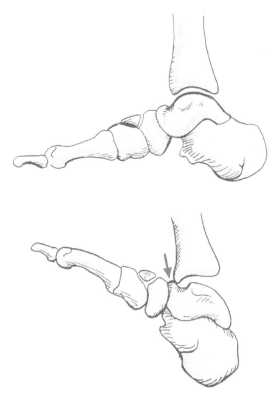

Figure 22–40. The mechanism by which a talotibial exostosis forms.

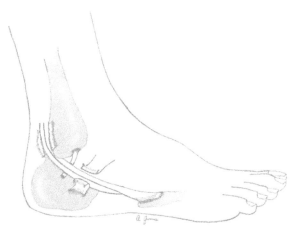

Figure 22–41. Dislocation of the peroneal tendon caused by rupture of the retinaculum is shown.

exostosis, there is no degeneration of the joint or chronic changes noted.

Treatment is usually conservative. Rest, activity modification, and physical therapy are attempted first. If symptoms continue, arthroscopic debridement is frequently curative.

PERONEAL TENDON DISLOCATION

The tendons of the peroneus longus and brevis muscles course down the posterior aspect of the fibula and attach to the base of the first and fifth metatarsals, respectively. These muscles act to evert and plantar flex the foot. The tendons are held in place behind the fibula by the superior and inferior peroneal retinaculum. Subluxation or dislocation occurs after injuries that disrupt the peroneal retinaculum (Fig. 22–41).

This condition may be due to laxity of the retinaculum or a congenitally absent retinaculum, but most cases occur after a sudden and forceful contraction of the peroneal muscles in association with forced plantar flexion and inversion of the foot and ankle. During injury, the peroneal muscles contract reflexively and overcome their fibroosseous sheath, causing the tendons to pass anteriorly.

This condition is sometimes confused with an ankle sprain; however, physical examination clearly distinguishes the two, based on tenderness behind the lateral malleolus following peroneal tendon injuries. Some factors may contribute to the frequency of dislocation, such as a convex or flat posterior surface of the distal fibula and a bifid peroneus brevis muscle. The condition may be acute or chronic in its presentation.

Clinical Presentation

The patient with acute subluxation will give a history of having sustained a blow to the back of the lateral malleolus, while the foot was taut in dorsiflexion and eversion. A snap may be heard or felt associated with severe pain initially that quickly improves. On examination, there is tenderness directly over the peroneal tendons. Tenosynovitis of the peroneal tendons will result in tenderness in the same location, but the history should help distinguish from peroneal retinaculum injury. Point-of-care ultrasound can also be used to quickly and accurately identify signs of peroneal tendon tenosynovitis, including synovial thickening, hyperemia, and effusion. A complete rupture of the retinaculum is distinguished from an incomplete rupture by noting the tendon ride up over the malleolus when the patient actively everts the ankle.

In patients with chronic subluxation, there is a history of slipping of the tendon with eversion of the foot. There is less pain than in the acute form, and the patient usually complains of a dull ache and the sensation of the tendon subluxating as it slips out of its normal position.

Treatment

The patient should be placed in a posterior splint (Appendix A–14) with a compression dressing over the lateral malleolus to stabilize the peroneal tendons in their functional position. They should remain nonweight bearing with crutches and receive orthopedic referral.

The definitive management is controversial. Most physicians recommend surgical treatment over conservative treatment in a cast for 6 weeks. In one large study, 74% of patients treated conservatively had to return for surgical correction at a later date.

TENOSYNOVITIS

The most common tendons involved in tenosynovitis around the ankle are the (1) posterior tibial, (2) peroneus longus, (3) anterior tibial, and (4) flexor hallucis longus. The Achilles tendon is also commonly involved and is covered in Chapter 23. There are two types of tenosynovitis: stenosing and rheumatoid. Stenosing tenosynovitis is common at the inferior retinaculum of the peroneal tendon with thickening of the sheath noted on examination. Rheumatoid tenosynovitis more commonly presents medially, involving the posterior tibial and flexor hallucis longus tendons.

Clinical Presentation

Dysfunction can be acute or chronic.[108] Most commonly, an acute tenosynovitis is present secondary to overuse. Chronic tenosynovitis, which is usually found in nonathletic patients, is associated with tendinosis and structural changes.[109] Localized swelling and tenderness is usually present over the involved tendon.[107] With continued use, partial or complete tears of the tendon may result.

Patients who have tenosynovitis of the tibialis posterior tendon report pain along the posteromedial aspect of the foot and ankle. Pain can occasionally extend into the arch of the plantar surface of the foot. The patient may develop structural abnormalities of the arch, particularly a flat foot. Approximately 80% of acquired flat foot deformities are due to posterior tibial tendon dysfunction.[110] This condition is frequently unilateral, providing a readily available point of comparison. A patient who has tibialis posterior tendon dysfunction may have an increased valgus posture of the calcaneus and a fullness that is seen just distal to the medial malleolus. Lack of heel inversion usually indicates dysfunction or weakness of the tibialis posterior tendon.[111] Frequently, patients with this condition are unable to stand on their tiptoes because of pain.

On examination, patients with stenosing tenosynovitis will have a thickened sheath palpated along its course. These patients are usually older than 40 years and have some predisposing occupational trauma. The tendon is tender to palpation and motion increases the pain with either form. Spontaneous rupture can occur, particularly in patients with rheumatoid arthritis or those with some unusual activity.

Treatment

Acute tenosynovitis, when it is mild, can be treated with a decrease in the level of activity. However, if the symptoms are moderate, the foot and ankle is put at rest and anti-inflammatory medication and ice are used. In some cases, immobilization (Appendix A–14) followed by a weight-bearing, below-the-knee cast for 4 weeks may be necessary. Rarely, if symptoms fail to respond after this initial treatment, surgical treatment is necessary in acute tenosynovitis.[109]

ANKLE DISLOCATION WITHOUT FRACTURE

Isolated dislocation without fracture is considered a rare injury but has been reported extensively.[112–116] The force required to produce a pure dislocation of the ankle without fracture is generally considered to be high energy, and often these dislocations are open. Predisposing factors include ligamentous laxity, weakness of peroneal musculature, medial malleolus hypoplasia, and previous ankle sprains.[113] Dislocations may be posterior (most frequent), anterior, medial, or lateral. Rotatory dislocation of the talus laterally from the tibiofibular joint without fracture has also been reported[117] (Fig. 22–42).

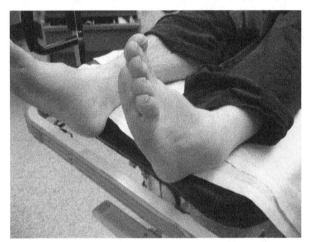

A

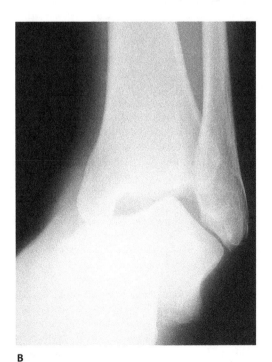

B

Figure 22–42. Isolated left ankle dislocation without fracture. **A.** Clinical photograph. **B.** Radiograph.

PEDIATRIC CONSIDERATIONS

Care must be taken when evaluating the pediatric patient. The presence of open physes necessitates a conservative approach to diagnosis and management of ankle injuries. Initial x-rays often do not fully evaluate the physes. Advanced imaging (MRI more so than CT) should be considered in this population. Children with suspected Salter–Harris injuries should be discharged fully nonweight bearing until definitive imaging and orthopedic follow-up is obtained.

REFERENCES

1. Wolfe MW, Uhl TL, Mattacola CG, McCluskey LC. Management of ankle sprains. *Am Fam Physician.* 2001;63(1):93–104.
2. Morris N, Lovell ME. Demographics of 3929 ankle injuries, seasonal variation in diagnosis and more fractures are diagnosed in winter. *Injury.* 2013;44(7):998–1001.
3. Darrow CJ, Collins CL, Yard EE, et al. Epidemiology of severe injuries among United States high school athletes: 2005–2007. *Am J Sports Med.* 2009;37(9):1798–1805. doi:10.1177/0363546509333015. Epub 2009 Jun 16.
4. Lucchesi GM, Jackson RE, Peacock WF, et al. Sensitivity of the Ottawa rules. *Ann Emerg Med.* 1995;26(1):1–5.
5. Birrer RB, Fani-Salek MH, Totten VY, Herman LM, Politi V. Managing ankle injuries in the emergency department. *J Emerg Med.* 1999;17(4):651–660.
6. Kleiger B. Mechanisms of ankle injury. *Orthop Clin North Am.* 1974;5(1):127–146.
7. Auletta AG, Conway WF, Hayes CW, Guisto DF, Gervin AS. Indications for radiography in patients with acute ankle injuries: role of the physical examination. *AJR Am J Roentgenol.* 1991;157(4):789–791.
8. Wedmore IS, Charette J. Emergency department evaluation and treatment of ankle and foot injuries. *Emerg Med Clin North Am.* 2000;18(1):85–113, vi.
9. Stiell IG, Greenberg GH, McKnight RD, Nair RC, McDowell I, Worthington JR. A study to develop clinical decision rules for the use of radiography in acute ankle injuries. *Ann Emerg Med.* 1992;21(4):384–390.
10. Stiell IG, Greenberg GH, McKnight RD, et al. Decision rules for the use of radiography in acute ankle injuries. Refinement and prospective validation. *JAMA.* 1993;269(9):1127–1132.
11. Papacostas E, Malliaropoulos N, Papadopoulos A, Liouliakis C. Validation of Ottawa ankle rules protocol in Greek athletes: study in the emergency departments of a district general hospital and a sports injuries clinic. *Br J Sports Med.* 2001;35(6):445–447.
12. Pijnenburg AC, Glas AS, De Roos MA, et al. Radiography in acute ankle injuries: the Ottawa ankle rules versus local diagnostic decision rules. *Ann Emerg Med.* 2002;39(6):599–604.
13. Markert RJ, Walley ME, Guttman TG, Mehta R. A pooled analysis of the Ottawa ankle rules used on adults in the ED. *Am J Emerg Med.* 1998;16(6):564–567.
14. Pigman EC, Klug RK, Sanford S, Jolly BT. Evaluation of the Ottawa clinical decision rules for the use of radiography in acute ankle and midfoot injuries in the emergency department: an independent site assessment. *Ann Emerg Med.* 1994;24(1):41–45.
15. Lucchesi GM, Jackson RE, Peacock WF, Cerasani C, Swor RA. Sensitivity of the Ottawa rules. *Ann Emerg Med.* 1995;26(1):1–5.
16. McBride KL. Validation of the Ottawa ankle rules. Experience at a community hospital. *Can Fam Physician.* 1997;43:459–465.
17. Auleley GR, Ravaud P, Giraudeau B, et al. Implementation of the Ottawa ankle rules in France. A multicenter randomized controlled trial. *JAMA.* 1997;277(24):1935–1939.
18. Salt P, Clancy M. Implementation of the Ottawa ankle rules by nurses working in an accident and emergency department. *J Accid Emerg Med.* 1997;14(6):363–365.
19. Auleley GR, Kerboull L, Durieux P, Cosquer M, Courpied JP, Ravaud P. Validation of the Ottawa ankle rules in France: a study in the surgical emergency department of a teaching hospital. *Ann Emerg Med.* 1998;32(1):14–18.
20. Mann CJ, Grant I, Guly H, Hughes P. Use of the Ottawa ankle rules by nurse practitioners. *J Accid Emerg Med.* 1998;15(5):315–316.
21. Perry S, Raby N, Grant PT. Prospective survey to verify the Ottawa ankle rules. *J Accid Emerg Med.* 1999;16(4):258–260.
22. Tay SY, Thoo FL, Sitoh YY, Seow E, Wong HP. The Ottawa ankle rules in Asia: validating a clinical decision rule for requesting x-rays in twisting ankle and foot injuries. *J Emerg Med.* 1999;17(6):945–947.
23. Springer BA, Arciero RA, Tenuta JJ, Taylor DC. A prospective study of modified Ottawa ankle rules in a military population. *Am J Sports Med.* 2000;28(6):864–868.
24. Yuen MC, Sim SW, Lam HS, Tung WK. Validation of the Ottawa ankle rules in a Hong Kong ED. *Am J Emerg Med.* 2001;19(5):429–432.
25. Broomhead A, Stuart P. Validation of the Ottawa ankle rules in Australia. *Emerg Med (Fremantle).* 2003;15(2):126–132.
26. Fiesseler F, Szucs P, Kec R, Richman PB. Can nurses appropriately interpret the Ottawa ankle rule? *Am J Emerg Med.* 2004;22(3):145–148.
27. Bachmann LM, Kolb E, Koller MT, Steurer J, ter Riet G. Accuracy of Ottawa ankle rules to exclude fractures of the ankle and mid-foot: systematic review. *BMJ.* 2003;326(7386):417.
28. Dowling S, Spooner CH, Liang Y, et al. Accuracy of Ottawa Ankle Rules to exclude fractures of the ankle and midfoot in children: a meta-analysis. *Acad Emerg Med.* 2009;16(4):277–287. doi:10.1111/j.1553–2712.2008.00333.x. Epub 2009 Feb 2.
29. Coll AP. Ottawa rules, OK? Rules are different in diabetes. *BMJ.* 2009;339:b3507. doi:10.1136/bmj.b3507.
30. Tollefson B, Nichols J, Fromang S, Summers RL. Validation of the Sonographic Ottawa Foot and Ankle Rules (SOFAR) study in a large urban trauma center. *J Miss State Med Assoc.* 2016;57(2):35–38.
31. Hedelin H, Goksör LÅ, Karlsson J, Stjernström S. Ultrasound-assisted triage of ankle trauma can decrease the need for radiographic imaging. *Am J Emerg Med.* 2013;31(12):1686–1689. doi:10.1016/j.ajem.2013.09.005. Epub 2013 Oct 21.

32. Atilla OD, Yesilaras M, Kilic TY, et al. The accuracy of bedside ultrasonography as a diagnostic tool for fractures in the ankle and foot. *Acad Emerg Med*. 2014;21(9):1058–1061. doi:10.1111/acem.12467.

33. Ekinci S, Polat O, Günalp M, et al. The accuracy of ultrasound evaluation in foot and ankle trauma. *Am J Emerg Med*. 2013;31(11):1551–1555.

34. David S, Gray K, Russell JA, et al. Validation of the Ottawa Ankle Rules for Acute Foot and Ankle Injuries. *J Sport Rehabil*. 2016;25(1):48–51.

35. Haapamaki VV, Kiuru MJ, Koskinen SK. Ankle and foot injuries: analysis of MDCT findings. *AJR Am J Roentgenol*. 2004;183(3):615–622.

36. Michelson JD. Ankle fractures resulting from rotational injuries. *J Am Acad Orthop Surg*. 2003;11(6):403–412.

37. Ostrum RF, Litsky AS. Tension band fixation of medial malleolus fractures. *J Orthop Trauma*. 1992;6(4):464–468.

38. Toolan BC, Koval KJ, Kummer FJ, Sanders R, Zuckerman JD. Vertical shear fractures of the medial malleolus: a biomechanical study of five internal fixation techniques. *Foot Ankle Int*. 1994;15(9):483–489.

39. Taweel NR, Raikin SM, Karanjia HN, Ahmad J. The proximal fibula should be examined in all patients with ankle injury: a case series of missed Maisonneuve fractures. *J Emerg Med*. 2013;44(2):e251–e255.

40. Michelson JD, Varner KE, Checcone M. Diagnosing deltoid injury in ankle fractures: the gravity stress view. *Clin Orthop*. 2001;(387):178–182.

41. Earll M, Wayne J, Brodrick C, Vokshoor A, Adelaar R. Contribution of the deltoid ligament to ankle joint contact characteristics: a cadaver study. *Foot Ankle Int*. 1996;17(6):317–324.

42. Miller JM, Svoboda SJ, Gerber JP. Diagnosis of an isolated posterior malleolar fracture in a young female military cadet: a resident case report. *Int J Sports Phys Ther*. 2012;7:167–172.

43. Michelsen JD, Ahn UM, Helgemo SL. Motion of the ankle in a simulated supination-external rotation fracture model. *J Bone Joint Surg Am*. 1996;78(7):1024–1031.

44. Clarke HJ, Michelson JD, Cox QG, Jinnah RH. Tibiotalar stability in bimalleolar ankle fractures: a dynamic in vitro contact area study. *Foot Ankle*. 1991;11(4):222–227.

45. Burns WC, Prakash K, Adelaar R, Beaudoin A, Krause W. Tibiotalar joint dynamics: indications for the syndesmotic screw—a cadaver study. *Foot Ankle*. 1993;14(3):153–158.

46. Brown TD, Hurlbut PT, Hale JE, et al. Effects of imposed hindfoot constraint on ankle contact mechanics for displaced lateral malleolar fractures. *J Orthop Trauma*. 1994;8(6):511–519.

47. Kristensen KD, Hansen T. Closed treatment of ankle fractures. stage II supination-eversion fractures followed for 20 years. *Acta Orthop Scand*. 1985;56(2):107–109.

48. Yde J, Kristensen KD. Ankle fractures: supination-eversion fractures of stage IV. Primary and late results of operative and non-operative treatment. *Acta Orthop Scand*. 1980;51(6):981–990.

49. Bauer M, Jonsson K, Nilsson B. Thirty-year follow-up of ankle fractures. *Acta Orthop Scand*. 1985;56(2):103–106.

50. Michelson JD, Ahn U, Magid D. Economic analysis of roentgenogram use in the closed treatment of stable ankle fractures. *J Trauma*. 1995;39(6):1119–1122.

51. Michelson JD. Fractures about the ankle. *J Bone Joint Surg Am*. 1995;77(1):142–152.

52. Konrath G, Karges D, Watson JT, Moed BR, Cramer K. Early versus delayed treatment of severe ankle fractures: a comparison of results. *J Orthop Trauma*. 1995;9(5):377–380.

53. Carragee EJ, Csongradi JJ, Bleck EE. Early complications in the operative treatment of ankle fractures. Influence of delay before operation. *J Bone Joint Surg Br*. 1991;73(1):79–82.

54. Watson JA, Hollingdale JP. Early management of displaced ankle fractures. *Injury*. 1992;23(2):87–88.

55. Black EM, Antoci V, Lee JT, et al. Role of preoperative computed tomography scans in operative planning for malleolar ankle fractures. *Foot Ankle Int*. 2013;34:697–704.

56. Gibb S, Abraham A. A reliable technique for early reduction of ankle fracture dislocations. *Ann R Coll Surg Engl*. 2005;87(3):208–209.

57. Abraham A. Emergency treatment of ankle fracture dislocations—a reliable technique for early reduction. *Ann R Coll Surg Engl*. 2003;85(6):427.

58. Schepers T, Hagenaars T, Den HD. An irreducible ankle fracture dislocation: the Bosworth injury. *J Foot Ankle Surg*. 2012;51:501–503.

59. Ellanti P, Hammad Y, Grieve PP. Acutely irreducible ankle fracture dislocation: a report of a Bosworth fracture and its management. *J Emerg Med*. 2013;44:e349–e352.

60. Yang KH, Won Y, Lim JR, et al. Assessment of Bosworth-type fracture by external oblique radiographs. *Am J Emerg Med*. 2014;32(11):1387–1390.

61. Bonar SK, Marsh JL. Tibial plafond fractures: changing principles of treatment. *J Am Acad Orthop Surg*. 1994;2(6):297–305.

62. Germann CA, Perron AD, Sweeney TW, Miller MD, Brady WJ. Orthopedic pitfalls in the ED: tibial plafond fractures. *Am J Emerg Med*. 2005;23(3):357–362.

63. Sirkin M, Sanders R. The treatment of pilon fractures. *Orthop Clin North Am*. 2001;32(1):91–102.

64. Helfet DL, Koval K, Pappas J, Sanders RW, DiPasquale T. Intraarticular "pilon" fracture of the tibia. *Clin Orthop*. 1994;(298):221–228.

65. Borrelli J Jr, Catalano L. Open reduction and internal fixation of pilon fractures. *J Orthop Trauma*. 1999;13(8):573–582.

66. Tornetta P III, Gorup J. Axial computed tomography of pilon fractures. *Clin Orthop*. 1996;(323):273–276.

67. Brumback RJ, McGarvey WC. Fractures of the tibial plafond. Evolving treatment concepts for the pilon fracture. *Orthop Clin North Am*. 1995;26(2):273–285.

68. Karas EH, Weiner LS. Displaced pilon fractures. An update. *Orthop Clin North Am*. 1994;25(4):651–663.

69. Borrelli J Jr, Ellis E. Pilon fractures: assessment and treatment. *Orthop Clin North Am*. 2002;33(1):231–245, x.

70. Thordarson DB. Complications after treatment of tibial pilon fractures: prevention and management strategies. *J Am Acad Orthop Surg*. 2000;8(4):253–265.

71. Wikstrom EA, Hubbard-Turner T, McKeon PO. Understanding and treating lateral ankle sprains and their consequences: a constraints-based approach. *Sports Med*. 2013;43:385–393.

72. Doherty C, Delahunt E, Caulfield B, et al. The incidence and prevalence of ankle sprain injury: a systematic review

and meta-analysis of prospective epidemiological studies. *Sports Med.* 2014;44(1):123–140.

73. Gribble PA, Bleakley CM, Caulfield BM, et al. 2016 consensus statement of the International Ankle Consortium: prevalence, impact and long-term consequences of lateral ankle sprains. *Br J Sports Med.* 2016;50:1493–1495.

74. Johnson KA, Teasdall RD. Sprained ankles as they relate to the basketball player. *Clin Sports Med.* 1993;12(2):363–371.

75. Renstrom PA. Persistently painful sprained ankle. *J Am Acad Orthop Surg.* 1994;2(5):270–280.

76. Curtis CK, Laudner KG, McLoda TA, McCaw ST. The role of shoe design in ankle sprain rates among collegiate basketball players. *J Athl Train.* 2008;43(3):230–233.

77. Lamy C, Stienstra JJ. Complications in ankle arthroscopy. *Clin Podiatr Med Surg.* 1994;11(3):523–539.

78. Boruta PM, Bishop JO, Braly WG, Tullos HS. Acute lateral ankle ligament injuries: a literature review. *Foot Ankle.* 1990;11(2):107–113.

79. van Dijk CN, Lim LS, Bossuyt PM, Marti RK. Physical examination is sufficient for the diagnosis of sprained ankles. *J Bone Joint Surg Br.* 1996;78(6):958–962.

80. Lassiter TE Jr, Malone TR, Garrett WE Jr. Injury to the lateral ligaments of the ankle. *Orthop Clin North Am.* 1989; 20(4):629–640.

81. Beumer A, Swierstra BA, Mulder PG. Clinical diagnosis of syndesmotic ankle instability: evaluation of stress tests behind the curtains. *Acta Orthop Scand.* 2002;73(6): 667–669.

82. Linklater JM, Hayter CL, Vu D. Imaging of acute capsuloligamentous sports injuries in the ankle and foot: sports imaging series. *Radiology.* 2017;283(3):644–662.

83. Croy T, Saliba SA, Saliba E, Anderson MW, Hertel J. Differences in lateral ankle laxity measured via stress ultrasonography in individuals with chronic ankle instability, ankle sprain copers, and healthy individuals. *J Orthop Sports Phys Ther.* 2012;42:593–600.

84. Lardenoye S, Theunissen E, Cleffken B, Brink PR, de Bie RA, Poeze M. The effect of taping versus semi-rigid bracing on patient outcome and satisfaction in ankle sprains: a prospective, randomized controlled trial. *BMC Musculoskelet Disord.* 2012;13:81.

85. Sitler MR, Horodyski M. Effectiveness of prophylactic ankle stabilisers for prevention of ankle injuries. *Sports Med.* 1995;20(1):53–57.

86. Bicici S, Karatas N, Baltaci G. Effect of athletic taping and Kinesiotaping® on measurements of functional performance in basketball players with chronic inversion ankle sprains. *Int J Sports Phys Ther.* 2012;7:154–166.

87. Kerkhoffs GM, Rowe BH, Assendelft WJ, Kelly KD, Struijs PA, van Dijk CN. Immobilisation for acute ankle sprain. A systematic review. *Arch Orthop Trauma Surg.* 2001;121(8): 462–471.

88. Bassett SF, Prapavessis H. Home-based physical therapy intervention with adherence-enhancing strategies versus clinic-based management for patients with ankle sprains. *Phys Ther.* 2007;87(9):1132–1143.

89. van Rijn RM, van Os AG, Kleinrensink GJ, et al. Supervised exercises for adults with acute lateral ankle sprain: a randomised controlled trial. *Br J Gen Pract.* 2007;57(543): 793–800.

90. Mitchell A, Dyson R, Hale T, Abraham C. Biomechanics of ankle instability. Part 1: reaction time to simulated ankle sprain. *Med Sci Sports Exerc.* 2008;40(8):1515–1521.

91. Lamb SE, Marsh JL, Hutton JL, Nakash R, Cooke MW; Collaborative Ankle Support Trial (CAST Group). Mechanical supports for acute, severe ankle sprain: a pragmatic, multicentre, randomised controlled trial. *Lancet.* 2009; 373(9663):575–581.

92. van Dijk CN. Management of the sprained ankle. *Br J Sports Med.* 2002;36(2):83–84.

93. Martin RL, Stewart GW, Conti SF. Posttraumatic ankle arthritis: an update on conservative and surgical management. *J Orthop Sports Phys Ther.* 2007;37(5):253–259.

94. Knupp M, Lang TH, Zwicky L, Lötscher P, Hintermann B. Chronic ankle instability (medial and lateral). *Clin Sports Med.* 2015;34(4):679–688. doi:10.1016/j. csm.2015.06.004. Epub 2015 Jul 23.

95. Colville MR. Surgical treatment of the unstable ankle. *J Am Acad Orthop Surg.* 1998;6(6):368–377.

96. Jotoku T, Kinoshita M, Okuda R, Abe M. Anatomy of ligamentous structures in the tarsal sinus and canal. *Foot Ankle Int.* 2006;27(7):533–538.

97. Lektrakul N, Chung CB, Lai Y, et al. Tarsal sinus: arthrographic, MR imaging, MR arthrographic, and pathologic findings in cadavers and retrospective study data in patients with sinus tarsi syndrome. *Radiology.* 2001;219(3):802–810.

98. Swain RA, Holt WS Jr. Ankle injuries. Tips from sports medicine physicians. *Postgrad Med.* 1993;93(3):91–100.

99. Dellon AL, Barrett SL. Sinus tarsi denervation: clinical results. *J Am Podiatr Med Assoc.* 2005;95(2):108–113.

100. Lee KB, Bai LB, Song EK, Jung ST, Kong IK. Subtalar arthroscopy for sinus Tarsi syndrome: arthroscopic findings and clinical outcomes of 33 consecutive cases. *Arthroscopy.* 2008;24(10):1130–1134. doi:10.1016/j.arthro.2008.05.007. Epub 2008 Jun 16.

101. Finger A, Sheskier SC. Osteochondral lesions of the talar dome. *Bull Hosp Jt Dis.* 2003;61(3–4):155–159.

102. Mintz DN, Tashjian GS, Connell DA, Deland JT, O'Malley M, Potter HG. Osteochondral lesions of the talus: a new magnetic resonance grading system with arthroscopic correlation. *Arthroscopy.* 2003;19(4):353–359.

103. Naran KN, Zoga AC. Osteochondral lesions about the ankle. *Radiol Clin North Am.* 2008;46:995–1002, v.

104. Butler BW, Lanthier J, Wertheimer SJ. Subluxing peroneals: a review of the literature and case report. *J Foot Ankle Surg.* 1993;32(2):134–139.

105. Brage ME, Hansen ST Jr. Traumatic subluxation/dislocation of the peroneal tendons. *Foot Ankle.* 1992;13(7):423–431.

106. Shewmaker DM, Guderjahn O, Kummer T. Identification of peroneal tenosynovitis by point-of-care ultrasonography. *J Emerg Med.* 2016;50(2):e79–e81.

107. Jones DC. Tendon disorders of the foot and ankle. *J Am Acad Orthop Surg.* 1993;1(2):87–94.

108. Garrett WE Jr. Muscle strain injuries. *Am J Sports Med.* 1996;24(6 suppl):S2–S8.

109. Teitz CC, Garrett WE Jr, Miniaci A, Lee MH, Mann RA. Tendon problems in athletic individuals. *Instr Course Lect.* 1997;46:569–582.

110. Crevoisier X, Assal M, Stanekova K. Hallux valgus, ankle osteoarthrosis and adult acquired flatfoot deformity: a review of

three common foot and ankle pathologies and their treatments. *EFORT Open Rev.* 2016;1(3):58–64. doi:10.1302/2058-5241.1.000015. Epub 2016 Mar 22.

111. Gerow G, Matthews B, Jahn W, Gerow R. Compartment syndrome and shin splints of the lower leg. *J Manipulative Physiol Ther.* 1993;16(4):245–252.

112. Gogi N, Khan SA, Anwar R. Anterior dislocation of the tibio-talar joint without diastasis or fracture—a case report. *Foot Ankle Surg.* 2008;14(1):47–49.

113. Rivera F, Bertone C, De Martino M, Pietrobono D, Ghisellini F. Pure dislocation of the ankle: three case reports and literature review. *Clin Orthop.* 2001;(382):179–184.

114. Frankel MR, Tucker DJ. Ankle dislocation without fracture in a young athlete. *J Foot Ankle Surg.* 1998;37(6):548.

115. Wehner J, Lorenz M. Lateral ankle dislocation without fracture. *J Orthop Trauma.* 1990;4(3):362–365.

116. Wroble RR, Nepola JV, Malvitz TA. Ankle dislocation without fracture. *Foot Ankle.* 1988;9(2):64–74.

117. Wilson AB, Toriello EA. Lateral rotatory dislocation of the ankle without fracture. *J Orthop Trauma.* 1991;5(1):93–95.

118. Endele D, Jung C, Bauer G, Mauch F. Value of MRI in diagnosing injuries after ankle sprains in children. *Foot Ankle Int.* 2012;33:1063–1068.

CHAPTER 23

Foot

Dennis Hanlon, MD and Christopher Morris, DO

INTRODUCTION

The foot has a wide range of normal motion, including flexion, extension, inversion, and eversion. In addition, supination and pronation are part of the normal range of foot motion. The foot contains two arches: a longitudinal arch (midfoot) and a transverse arch (forefoot). Weight is normally distributed equally on the forefoot and the heel. Weight is not equally distributed on the metatarsal heads because the first bears twice as much weight as the remaining four. The maximum weight applied to the foot occurs during the push-off phase of walking and running.

The foot contains 28 bones and 57 articulations (Figs. 23–1 and 23–2). Conceptually, the foot can be divided into three regions: the hindfoot (talus and calcaneus), the midfoot (navicular, cuneiforms, and cuboid), and the forefoot (metatarsals and phalanges).

Foot fractures are common and account for 10% of all fractures. They are generally the result of one of three basic mechanisms of injury—direct trauma, indirect trauma, and overuse.

Imaging

The Ottawa foot rules recommend a radiographic series of the foot if there is bony tenderness at the base of the fifth metatarsal or over the tarsal navicular and if the patient is unable to take four steps both immediately and in the emergency department (ED). These rules apply to just the midfoot. Routine radiographs of the foot include the antero-posterior (AP), oblique, and lateral views (Fig. 23–3). These radiographs can be difficult to interpret because bones overlap in all projections. The AP radiograph is used to best assess the medial two tarsometatarsal joints, whereas the oblique image provides the best view of the lateral three tarsometatarsal joints. This alignment is important and will be altered in patients with Lisfranc fracture–dislocations. The lateral radiograph is best for detecting calcaneus fractures. Advanced imaging will be required with certain injuries and conditions.

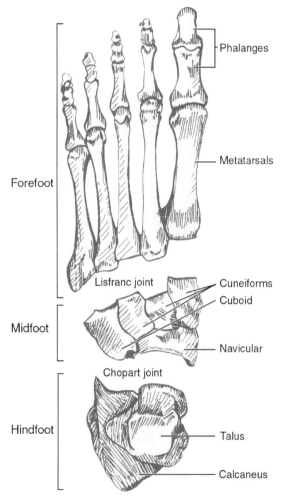

Figure 23–1. The foot is divided into a hindfoot, a midfoot, and a forefoot. Chopart joint separates the hindfoot from the mid-foot, and Lisfranc joint separates the midfoot from the forefoot.

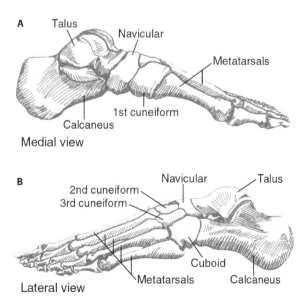

Figure 23–2. A. Medial. **B.** Lateral views of the foot.

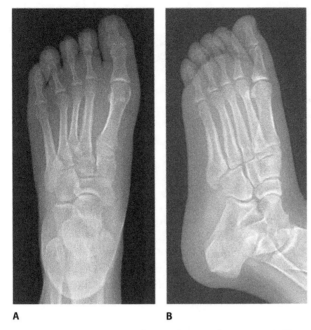

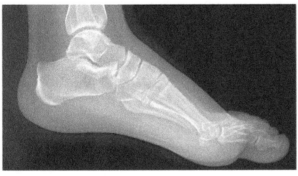

Figure 23–3. Normal radiographs of the foot. **A.** Anteroposterior (AP). **B.** Oblique. **C.** Lateral images.

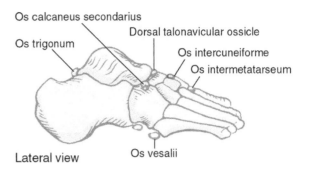

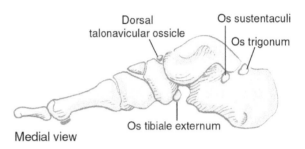

Figure 23–4. The sesamoids of the foot. These bones are commonly confused for fractures.

There is conflicting evidence of the overall effectiveness of bedside ultrasonography in the evaluation of potential foot and ankle fractures.

The radiologic diagnosis of foot fractures is frequently complicated by the secondary ossification centers and sesamoids (Fig. 23–4). Commonly seen sesamoids include the os trigonum, os tibiale externum, os peroneum, and os vesalianum. Sesamoids can be distinguished from fractures by their smooth sclerotic bony margins.

FOOT FRACTURES

CALCANEUS FRACTURES

The calcaneus is the largest and most frequently fractured tarsal bone, representing 60% of all tarsal fractures and 2% of all fractures in general.

The anterior portion of the calcaneus is the body. Fractures of the body may be intra-articular or extra-articular. The posterior portion of the calcaneus is the tuberosity. At the base of the tuberosity are the medial and lateral processes that serve as points of insertion for the planter fascia. The Achilles tendon inserts on the posterior portion of the tuberosity. The principal articulation of the calcaneus is with the talus, forming the subtalar joint. Three articular surfaces exist—an anterior, middle, and posterior articular facet. The sustentaculum talus is a medial extension of the calcaneus that supports the anterior and middle articular

facets. The peroneal tubercle is on the lateral surface and provides a groove for the peroneal tendons and a site of attachment for the inferior peroneal retinaculum.

Fractures may occur at any of these sites. Excluding avulsion fractures, 75% of calcaneal fractures are intra-articular (involving the subtalar joint) and 75% of these are depressed. Extra-articular fractures account for 25% of calcaneus fractures and include fractures of the anterior process, sustentaculum tali, lateral calcaneal process and peroneal tubercle, medial calcaneal process, and tuberosity.

Calcaneal Body Fractures

Intra-articular calcaneal body fractures are not only the most common, but also most likely to result in long-term disability (Fig. 23–5).

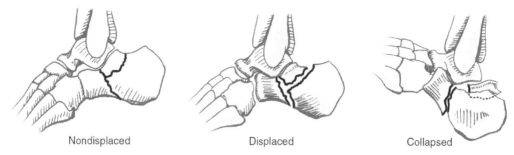

Nondisplaced   Displaced   Collapsed

Figure 23–5. Calcaneal body fractures—intra-articular.

It is uncommon that a calcaneal body fracture does not involve the subtalar joint. Although patients with extra-articular fractures have a better prognosis than patients with intra-articular fractures, they may still change the articular configuration of the calcaneus and result in long-term problems.

Mechanism of Injury

The most common mechanism is a fall from a significant height where the weight of the body is absorbed by the heel. In most individuals, a height of 8 feet or higher is needed to produce such a fracture, but in older, osteoporotic patients, falls from shorter distances can produce these injuries.

Examination

The patient will present with pain, swelling, and plantar ecchymosis (Mondor sign) with loss of the normal depressions along both sides of the Achilles tendon. Fracture blisters usually develop within the first 24 to 48 hours and may be clear or blood-filled. If these blisters are extensive, surgery may be delayed to avoid higher rates of postoperative infections. Despite these findings, the diagnosis can be missed because significant associated injuries distract the patient and clinician. Occasionally, the patient may not complain of significant heel pain and may be able to bear weight, although this is usually quite painful.

Imaging

Routine radiographic views are generally adequate in diagnosing this fracture. Depressed fractures are more challenging to detect but are diagnosed by noting an increased density of the bone and loss of the normal bony trabecular pattern (Fig. 23–6). The AP view is used to assess involvement of the calcaneocuboid joint. The lateral view demonstrates intra-articular involvement and allows for an assessment of Bohler angle. Bohler angle should be calculated to help identify subtle fractures and measure the degree of fracture depression. This angle is calculated by measuring the intersection of two lines: (1) from the superior margin of the posterior tuberosity of the calcaneus through the superior tip of the posterior facet and (2) from the superior tip of the anterior facet to the superior tip of the posterior facet (Figs. 23–7 and 23–8).

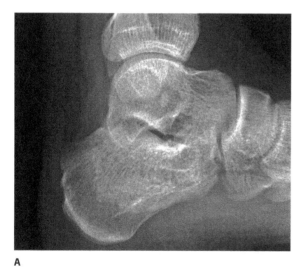

A

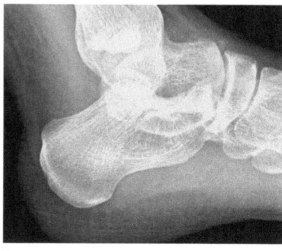

B

Figure 23–6. **A.** Depression fracture of the body of the calcaneus. Note the increased density of the compressed bone and loss of trabecular pattern. **B.** Normal lateral radiograph for comparison.

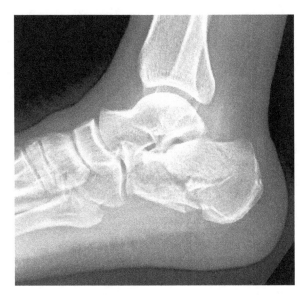

Figure 23–7. Calcaneus fracture. This fracture is comminuted, intra-articular, and depressed. Bohler angle is 0 degrees.

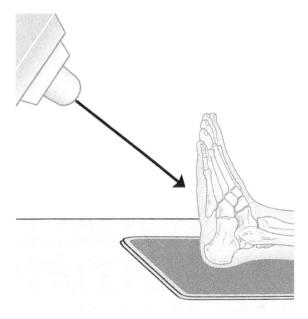

Figure 23–9. The technique for obtaining a Harris view. This view is helpful in defining the extent of intra-articular involvement and degree of depression of the fracture fragments.

Normally, Bohler angle measures 20 to 40 degrees. If the angle is less than 20 degrees, a depressed fracture is present even if it is not directly visualized on the plain radiographs. It should be noted that Bohler angle can be normal despite the presence of a severely comminuted fracture; therefore, this angle cannot be used to exclude a calcaneus fracture.[10] The most important function of Bohler angle is its significant prognostic ability. Fractures with a diminished Bohler angle have worse outcomes, regardless of intervention.[11]

The Harris view is helpful in defining the extent of intra-articular involvement and degree of depression of the fracture fragments. It is taken with the ankle dorsiflexed and the x-ray beam angled obliquely across the plantar aspect of the heel (Fig. 23–9). This view has become less important with the more liberal use of computed tomography (CT).

CT has become routine to fully delineate the extent of fractures and the degree of subtalar joint involvement (Fig. 23–10).[5,6] CT is especially useful to the surgeon

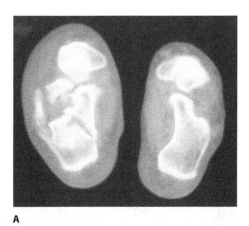

A

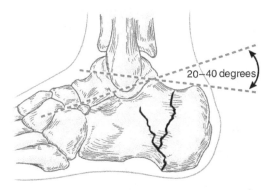

Figure 23–8. Bohler angle is calculated whenever a calcaneus fracture is diagnosed. If the angle measures <20 degrees, a depressed fracture is diagnosed.

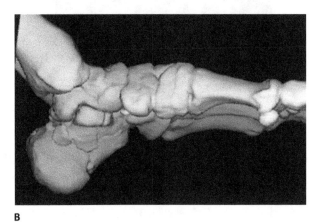

B

Figure 23–10. Calcaneal body fractures **A.** Coronal CT image demonstrating a normal calcaneus in the patient's left foot and a comminuted fracture of the right calcaneus. **B.** 3D reconstruction CT scan.

planning operative intervention. Plain radiographs alone fail to identify the degree of fracture extension in almost half of the cases.

Associated Injuries

The majority of calcaneus fractures are associated with additional injuries. Thirty percent of calcaneus fractures are associated with another fracture to the lower extremities. Calcaneus fractures are bilateral in 7% of cases. Compression fractures of the thoracolumbar spine are associated with 10% to 15% of calcaneus fractures. Compartment syndrome develops in up to 10% of patients, with many of these patients going on to develop significant foot deformities.

Treatment

Intra-Articular Calcaneal Body Fractures. The emergency management of these fractures includes ice, elevation, and immobilization in a bulky compressive dressing with a posterior splint (Appendix A–14). The patient should be kept nonweight bearing and given crutches. Ice and a bulky dressing are important to prevent soft-tissue injuries such as fracture blisters and skin sloughing, which ultimately delay surgery or make it more difficult. The presence of an intra-articular fracture necessitates consultation with the orthopedics service for definitive management. Patients with significant swelling and the possibility of developing compartment syndrome should be admitted.

In addition to compartment syndrome, the clinician should also identify and note the significance of a "tongue-type" calcaneus fracture. This intra-articular fracture is unique in that it is longitudinal and exits the tuberosity posteriorly distal to the Achilles tendon insertion. The fracture fragment is pulled superiorly and very close to the skin by the Achilles tendon (Fig. 23–11A). Early operative intervention is recommended to avoid skin necrosis in these patients (Fig. 23–11B). Splint the ankle in plantar flexion. Consult an orthopedist from the ED for these fractures.

Definitive management of an intra-articular calcaneal body fracture depends on the degree of displacement. Nondisplaced fractures may be treated with nonweight-bearing status for 6 to 8 weeks and hydrotherapy, followed by a gradual increase in activity. The treatment of displaced fractures is controversial and varies from a conservative approach to surgical repair. For this reason, early consultation and referral are strongly recommended in the management of these injuries. When indicated, surgery is not emergent (unless a fasciotomy is required for compartment syndrome) and generally occurs 5 to 10 days after injury; however, surgery can take place up to several weeks post injury if swelling is significant. Bilateral calcaneal fractures do not routinely require surgery, and the decision to operate should be made on the basis of each individual fracture. Pediatric calcaneal fractures tend to be caused by lower

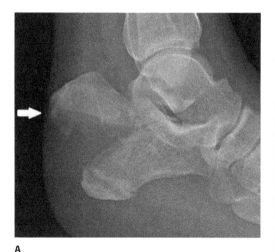

A

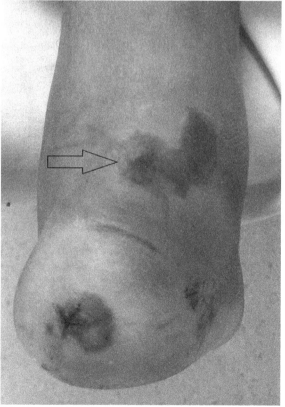

B

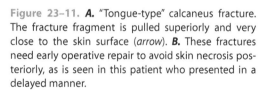

Figure 23–11. A. "Tongue-type" calcaneus fracture. The fracture fragment is pulled superiorly and very close to the skin surface (*arrow*). **B.** These fractures need early operative repair to avoid skin necrosis posteriorly, as is seen in this patient who presented in a delayed manner.

impact trauma and have favorable outcomes with conservative treatment.[17]

In patients with comminuted, displaced, or depressed intra-articular fractures, a good outcome requires the reestablishment of joint congruity and the elevation of depressed fragments. Open reduction with internal fixation is recommended in these patients.[18,19]

Extra-Articular Calcaneal Body Fractures.

The emergency management of these fractures includes ice, elevation, and immobilization in a bulky dressing, crutches, and early referral.

Nondisplaced fractures are treated with nonweight bearing, hydrotherapy, and ambulation after a minimum of 4 to 6 weeks. Displaced fractures are managed similarly to displaced intra-articular calcaneal body fractures. Early ice and elevation are important in preventing the formation of skin blisters. Operative management is preferred.

Complications

Calcaneus fractures are associated with up to 10% incidence of compartment syndrome of the foot.[13] Highly comminuted intra-articular fractures are at the highest risk of compartment syndrome.[20] Symptoms such as tense swelling and severe pain may be associated with a wide spectrum of long-term problems, including clawing of the toes, stiffness, chronic pain, weakness, sensory changes, atrophy, and forefoot deformities. The diagnosis can be made in the acute phase using pressure measurements within the involved compartment. Fasciotomy is the recommended treatment. Open calcaneal fractures have up to a 10% risk of below-the-knee amputation.[21]

The long-term consequences of these fractures are disabling. Posttraumatic arthritis with stiffness and chronic pain is the most frequent complication. Spur formation with chronic pain or nerve entrapment may complicate the management of these fractures. Intra-articular calcaneus fractures have a very poor prognosis with the incidence of long-term problems approaching 50% despite optimal treatment.[6]

Extra-articular calcaneal body fractures may be associated with sural nerve entrapment in addition to the other complications of intra-articular calcaneal body fractures.

Extra-Articular Calcaneus Fractures

Extra-articular calcaneus fractures are those fractures that do not involve the posterior articular surface (Fig. 23-12). These fractures account for 25% of all calcaneus fractures

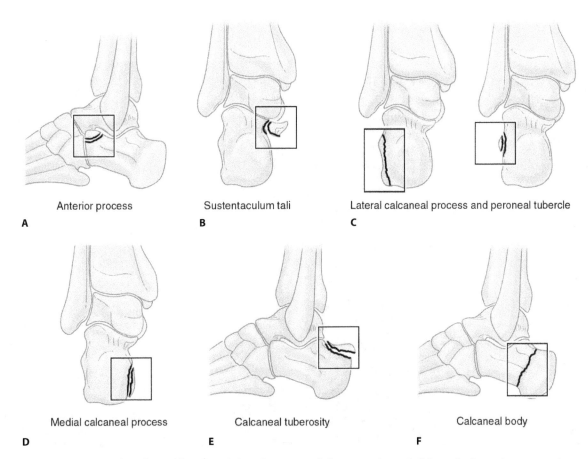

Anterior process

A

Sustentaculum tali

B

Lateral calcaneal process and peroneal tubercle

C

Medial calcaneal process

D

Calcaneal tuberosity

E

Calcaneal body

F

Figure 23–12. Extra-articular calcaneal fractures. **A.** Anterior process. **B.** Sustentaculum tali. **C.** Lateral calcaneal process and peroneal tubercle. **D.** Medial calcaneal process. **E.** Calcaneal tuberosity. **F.** Calcaneal body.

and include fractures of the anterior process, sustentaculum tali, lateral calcaneal process and peroneal tubercle, medial calcaneal process, and tuberosity. Extra-articular calcaneus body fractures are considered in the previous section.

Mechanism of Injury

These fractures occur as a result of minor falls and twisting injuries or can be due to avulsions from strong muscular contractions. The force required to sustain an extra-articular calcaneus fracture is generally less than intra-articular fractures.

Examination

Pain may be localized to the specific region in question. Diffuse pain may be present on attempts at weight bearing.

Imaging

Routine views are usually adequate for defining the fracture fragments (Fig. 23–13). The lateral projection of the hindfoot is especially helpful in visualizing subtle fractures. CT analysis is used to more accurately delineate the anatomy of injuries (Fig. 23–14). Stress fractures of the calcaneus are typically posterior and may be difficult to see on plain films despite months of symptoms.

Associated Injuries

Extra-articular calcaneus fractures are associated with fewer injuries than intra-articular fractures.

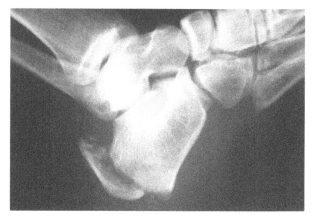

Figure 23–13. Calcaneal tuberosity fracture secondary to avulsion by the Achilles tendon mechanism.

Treatment

Anterior Process Fracture. These fractures, which account for 15% of all calcaneus fractures, are avulsion fractures secondary to abduction with the foot in plantar flexion. This position stresses the bifurcate ligament, which inserts on the calcaneus as well as both the cuboid and the navicular. Severe stress results in ligamentous rupture or an avulsion fracture of the calcaneus. The patient will usually present with a history of "twisting" the foot and complain of pain, swelling, and tenderness just distal to the lateral malleolus.

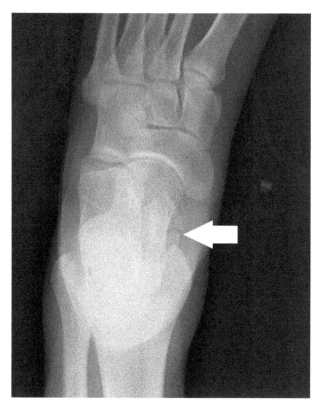

A

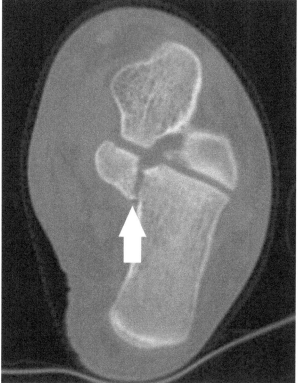

B

Figure 23–14. Sustentaculum tali fracture. ***A.*** AP view of the foot. ***B.*** CT image shows an obvious fracture.

The recommended management of these injuries includes ice, elevation, and weight bearing as tolerated. A removable fracture boot is applied for 4 to 6 weeks. Open reduction with internal fixation is considered for large or displaced fragments. Orthopedic referral for follow-up is recommended.

Sustentaculum Tali Fracture. This is uncommon as an isolated injury. The most common mechanism of injury is axial compression on the heel with marked inversion of the foot. The patient will present with pain, tenderness, and swelling just distal to the medial malleolus and over the medial heel. The pain will be exacerbated by inversion of the foot or hyperextension of the great toe, as this will pull on the flexor hallucis longus, which passes beneath the sustentaculum tali.

The management of these fractures includes ice, elevation, and immobilization in a compression dressing for 24 to 36 hours. Nondisplaced fractures should then be cast and remain nonweight bearing for 8 weeks. Orthopedic referral is mandatory because many of these fractures are followed by chronic pain. Displaced fractures require emergent orthopedic consultation for consideration of open reduction. The flexor hallucis longus tendon may be interposed. Accurate analysis of fragment position by CT is recommended. Surgery is performed within 3 weeks (optimally, 10 days or less) after foot and ankle swelling has reduced.[19]

Lateral Calcaneal Process and Peroneal Tubercle Fractures. These are uncommon injuries that result from plantar flexion and inversion or direct trauma. Localized tenderness and swelling is present in the lateral heel. Treatment is symptomatic with weight bearing allowed with a soft ankle support for 4 to 6 weeks.

Medial Calcaneal Process Fractures. The mechanism of injury of this structure is a direct blow. Pain and swelling is localized to the medial heel. Treatment includes a compressive soft-tissue dressing and a posterior splint (Appendix A–14). Weight bearing is allowed as tolerated after the initial swelling has decreased. Some authors primarily recommend open reduction with internal fixation; thus, early consultation is recommended.[19]

Calcaneal Tuberosity Fractures. The most common mechanism of injury for this fracture is avulsion by the insertion of the Achilles tendon, as may occur during a fall or a jump landing on the dorsiflexed foot with the knee extended. The patient will present with pain, swelling, and tenderness over the fracture; inability to walk; and weak plantar flexion of the foot.

Nondisplaced fractures are treated in a nonweight-bearing cast with the foot in slight plantar flexion for 6 to 8 weeks. Early referral is strongly recommended. Displaced fractures require orthopedic consultation for consideration of open reduction. If the fracture fragment is placing tension on the overlying skin, surgical intervention is performed earlier to minimize the risk of soft-tissue injury.

TALUS FRACTURES

The talus, or astragalus, is the second largest and second most frequently fractured tarsal bone.[22] Despite this, talus fractures are still uncommon and account for less than 1% of all fractures.[23] Added to their uncommon frequency is the difficultly visualizing talus fractures on plain radiographs. Therefore, without some knowledge of these fractures, they may remain occult with the patient frequently receiving a misdiagnosis of ankle sprain.[24,25]

The talus is divided anatomically into three segments—the head, the neck, and the body. It is held in place by ligaments and has no sites of muscle insertion. In addition, 60% of its surface is covered by articular cartilage.[22] The vascular supply to the bone does not penetrate the articular cartilage but enters by way of the deltoid ligament, the talocalcaneal ligament, the anterior capsule, and the sinus tarsi. The blood supply is, therefore, somewhat tenuous, and avascular necrosis (AVN) is not uncommon after displaced fractures. The rate of osteonecrosis is estimated to be 20% to 50% with higher rates in comminuted or open fractures.[23] Proximal talar fractures are particularly predisposed to develop AVN of the proximal fragment.

Talus fractures are divided into major and minor categories. Major talus fractures involve the head, neck, or central portion of the body. Minor talus fractures are fractures of the body of the talus that do not traverse the central portion of the bone. Minor talus fractures include lateral process, posterior process, and osteochondral talar dome fractures.

The most common fractures of the talus are to the neck.[23] Osteochondral fractures are the most common fracture of the talar body. Osteochondral fractures of the talar dome are discussed in more detail in Chapter 22. Fractures of the lateral and posterior processes of the body are less common, whereas fractures of the main portion of the talar body and the head are uncommon.

Major Talus Fractures

Major talus fractures are those that involve the head, neck, or central portion of the body (Fig. 23–15). Talar neck fractures are most common, representing 50% of all major talus fractures.

Talar neck fractures have been classified by Hawkins.[23,24] Type I fractures are nondisplaced. Type II fractures result in displacement with subluxation or displacement of the subtalar joint. Type III fractures possess displacement with dislocation of the talus from the subtalar and ankle joints. Type IV fractures are displaced from the subtalar joint with the talar head dislocated. This classification correlates with the risk of AVN, with the majority of Hawkins type III and IV fractures developing AVN.[23,24]

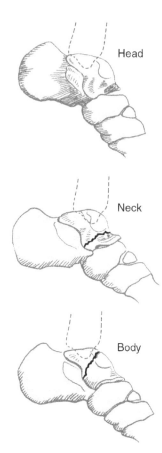

Figure 23–15. Talus fractures—major.

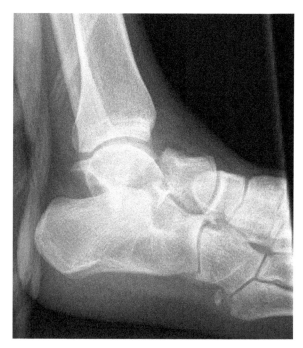

Figure 23–16. Lateral view demonstrates talar neck fracture with displacement. An avulsion fracture of the base of the fifth metatarsal is also present.

Mechanism of Injury

Talar head fractures are usually the result of direct impact, such as falling on the fully extended foot. The force is transmitted from the forefoot to the talus, which impacts the anterior edge of the tibia.

Talar neck fractures typically follow acute dorsiflexion of the ankle and are frequently seen after automobile collisions or falls from heights. This fracture is also referred to as "*aviator's astragalus*" because it occurred in World War II pilots after the rudder from their plane forcibly dorsiflexed the ankle while crash landing their planes on return from bombing missions. With dorsiflexion, the neck of the talus impacts the anterior edge of the tibia. Continuation of the force may result in ligamentous tearing, fragment displacement, or subtalar and talar body dislocation. Fracture–dislocations require a more severe force.

Nondisplaced talar body fractures are the result of an acute hyperextension injury. Comminuted or displaced fractures are typically the result of axial compression with hyperextension.

Examination

The patient will usually present with pain, swelling, ecchymosis, and tenderness. With talar head fractures, the tenderness is concentrated over the talar head and the talonavicular joint. Ankle motion will be normal, although inversion of the foot will exacerbate the pain over the talonavicular joint. Patients with neck fractures and associated dislocation will present with the foot locked into a hyperextended position. When the body is fractured, intense, diffuse ankle pain, tenderness, and swelling are present.

Imaging

Routine views often do not adequately demonstrate these fractures. Talar neck fractures are best visualized on the routine lateral view (Fig. 23–16). The oblique view may be helpful in the presence of subtle subluxation or dislocation. If a talus fracture is strongly suspected, a CT scan will be required in most cases.

Treatment

The emergency management of a major talus fracture should include ice, elevation, immobilization (Appendix A–14), crutches, and early consultation.

Definitive treatment of talar head fractures is a nonweight-bearing cast for 6 to 8 weeks. Open reduction with internal fixation is recommended if the fragment causes instability of the talonavicular joint, is displaced resulting in an articular step-off, or is larger than 50% of the articular surface.

Nondisplaced talar neck fractures are treated with a short-leg nonwalking cast for 6 weeks, followed by 3 weeks of partial weight bearing. Displaced fractures or those associated with dislocations require a neurovascular assessment followed by an emergent orthopedic consultation for an operative anatomic reduction to avoid the high incidence of

AVN.[22–24] Hawkin type II, III, and IV fractures will need prompt ORIF because of the difficulty to obtain anatomic reduction by a closed means.[24] Delayed reductions are associated with an increased incidence of skin necrosis and AVN.

Definitive treatment of nondisplaced talar body fractures is with a short-leg nonwalking cast for 6 to 8 weeks. The prognosis for these injuries is very good. Displaced or comminuted fractures require an anatomic reduction, and early consultation and referral is strongly recommended.

Complications

Talar head fractures may be complicated by the development of talonavicular osteoarthritis or chondromalacia. Talar neck fractures may be complicated by the development of peroneal tendon dislocations, AVN of the talus, or delayed union. Fracture–dislocations are particularly predisposed to the development of AVN. Displaced or comminuted body fractures are often complicated by the development of AVN.

Minor Talus Fractures

These fractures are not necessarily as "minor" as the name implies, frequently requiring careful consideration to make the diagnosis and initiate the appropriate treatment plan. This category includes fractures of the body of the talus that do not involve the central portion of the bone. They include fractures of the lateral process, posterior process, and osteochondral talar dome (Fig. 23–17). Osteochondral fractures are discussed in Chapter 22.

Mechanism of Injury

The lateral process of the talus is fractured with axial loading, dorsiflexion, eversion, and external rotation. This combination of forces can result from falls or automobile collisions but has been noted to be a commonly associated injury during snowboarding.[28–32] Because of this association, lateral process fractures are frequently referred to as "*snowboarder's ankle.*" This fracture has also been reported in a kayaker with her feet dorsiflexed and planted in the foot peg.[31] A posterior process fracture is often the result of

extreme plantar flexion with impingement of the posterior process against the posterior tibia and calcaneus. Inversion may produce an avulsion fracture.

Examination

The patient with a lateral process talus fracture will have pain and swelling over the lateral malleolus and localized tenderness just anterior and inferior to the tip of the lateral malleolus. Because this presentation is so similar to a lateral ankle sprain, the fracture is missed in up to 40% of cases on initial presentation.[25]

Posterior process fractures typically present with posterior lateral pain, tenderness, and swelling. The pain is exacerbated by activities that require plantar flexion. The tenderness is present with deep palpation anterior to the Achilles tendon over the posterior talus. Occasionally, dorsiflexion of the great toe will exacerbate the pain because of movement of the flexor hallucis longus tendon as it passes along the bone.

Imaging

Minor talus fractures typically present with only minimal radiographic findings. The abnormalities may be limited to a tiny avulsion fragment of bone over the involved area. The best radiograph to see a lateral process fracture is the mortise view, whereas the lateral view is the best opportunity to diagnose a posterior process fracture. The smoothly round sesamoid, os trigonum, may be confused with a posterior process fracture, but knowledge of its typical location and shape will aid in avoiding this confusion. Special oblique views or CT are often necessary to adequately evaluate these fractures. If there is lateral tenderness with a dorsiflexion injury, a CT should be strongly considered.[31]

Treatment

Lateral process fractures are treated with ice, elevation, and immobilization in a short-leg splint (Appendix A–14). The ankle is kept in a neutral position, and the patient is given crutches and an orthopedic referral. Definitive treatment depends on the size of the fracture and the amount of displacement. Nonoperative treatment is reserved for nondisplaced (<2 mm) fragments. Large fragments that are displaced will require open reduction and internal fixation, whereas small fragments and comminuted fractures will undergo debridement.[29]

Posterior process fractures are treated as previously discussed, except the foot is splinted in 15 degrees of plantar flexion. Nondisplaced fractures can be treated definitively with cast immobilization, whereas larger and more displaced fractures may require operative treatment.[25]

Complications

Lateral process fractures may be complicated by malunion and nonunion. Because the lateral process articulates with the calcaneus, forming the lateral portion of the subtalar joint, degenerative changes in this joint may occur.

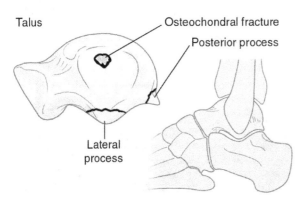

Figure 23–17. Talus fractures—minor.

Posterior process fractures are generally not complicated by any long-term disorders. If the fragments are large, nonunion with migration may result in joint locking, and eventually, traumatic arthritis. Also, if the posterior process fracture is missed and the diagnosis is delayed, the patient will most likely need excision of the nonunited fragment.

MIDFOOT FRACTURES

The midfoot is the least mobile portion of the foot and includes the *navicular, cuboid,* and three *cuneiforms.* These fractures are rare but, when present, typically involve multiple fractures or fracture–dislocations. The detection of these fractures on plain radiographs is limited. The sensitivity of radiographs is 25% to 33% when compared with multidetector CT.

Midfoot fractures are classified on the basis of anatomy:

- Navicular fractures
  - Dorsal avulsion fractures
  - Tuberosity fractures
  - Body fractures
  - Compression fractures
- Cuboid and cuneiform fractures
  - Cuboid fractures
  - Cuneiform fractures

Navicular Fractures

The most common midfoot fracture is the navicular fracture (Fig. 23–18). Of navicular fractures, the dorsal avulsion fracture is the most frequent. Tuberosity fractures are second in frequency and are followed by navicular body fractures, which may be transverse or horizontal. Body fractures and compression fractures of the navicular are rare injuries. Stress fractures of the navicular may also occur.

Mechanism of Injury
Dorsal avulsion fractures are usually the result of acute flexion with inversion of the foot. The talonavicular joint capsule is stressed and avulses the proximal dorsal aspect of the navicular. Tuberosity fractures are also avulsion fractures and typically follow an acute eversion force on the foot. Eversion of the foot results in increased tension on the tibialis posterior tendon, which avulses a portion of the navicular tuberosity. Previously reported mechanisms of injury include acute hyperextension with compression, direct trauma, or extreme flexion with rotation.

Examination
The patient will present with pain, swelling, and tenderness over the involved area. For dorsal avulsion fractures, the dorsal and medial aspect of the midfoot will be tender. Tuberosity fractures present with pain localized distally and anteriorly to the medial malleolus, which is exacerbated with eversion of the foot.

Imaging
AP, lateral, and oblique views may demonstrate these injuries (Fig. 23–19). Subtle, nondisplaced fractures may be difficult to diagnose and require comparison views, follow-up films, or CT scan for adequate visualization. Navicular body fractures should have a CT scan to determine displacement, which is inadequately demonstrated on plain radiographs. An accessory bone, the os tibiale externum, is often confused with an avulsion fracture of the navicular (Fig. 23–20). Stress fractures of the navicular may require a bone scan, CT, or magnetic resonance imaging (MRI).

Associated Injuries
Dorsal avulsion fractures are often associated with lateral malleolar ligament injuries. Tuberosity fractures are often accompanied by cuboid fractures. With all navicular fractures, injury to adjacent structures is common and should be sought.

Treatment
Dorsal Avulsion Fracture. Small chip fractures are treated symptomatically with ice, elevation, and a compressive

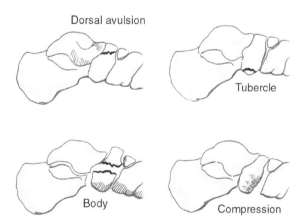

Figure 23–18. Navicular fractures.

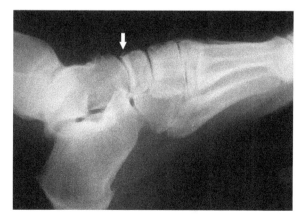

Figure 23–19. Dorsal chip fracture of the navicular.

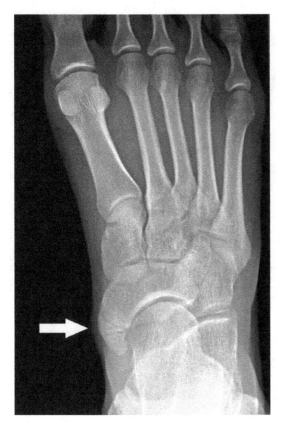

Figure 23–20. The os tibiale externum is frequently confused with a navicular tuberosity fracture (*arrow*).

swelling, a well-molded short-leg cast with the foot in inversion should be used for 6 weeks. This position reduces the pull of the posterior tibial tendon. Significant displacement of the avulsed fragment will require emergent orthopedic referral for consideration of surgical reattachment.[34,35]

Body Fractures. The emergency management of these fractures includes ice, elevation, and a posterior splint (Appendix A–14). Definitive management of nondisplaced body fractures includes a well-molded, below-the-knee walking cast for 6 to 8 weeks. After this, longitudinal arch support should be employed. Displaced navicular body fractures require open reduction with internal fixation in the active ambulatory patient. Nonambulatory patients may be treated symptomatically with a compressive dressing. Navicular fracture–dislocations require open reduction with internal fixation.

Compression Fractures. These fractures are treated similarly to dorsal avulsion fractures with ice, elevation, and a compressive dressing.

Complications

Navicular tuberosity fractures are often complicated by nonunion. Body fractures may develop aseptic necrosis or traumatic arthritis.

dressing. The patient may bear weight with the aid of crutches for 2 weeks or until the pain subsides. The compressive dressing should be applied from the midtarsal region to above the ankle joint, including the heel. Definitive management of large avulsion fragments >25% of the articular surface includes reduction and fixation with Kirschner wires.[32]

Tuberosity Fracture. Small, nondisplaced avulsion fractures can be treated with a compression dressing and a short-leg splint (Appendix A–14). With the reduction in

Cuboid and Cuneiform Fractures

Cuboid and cuneiform fractures usually occur in combination (Fig. 23–21). Isolated injuries are uncommon, and the clinician should consider the possibility of injury to the Lisfranc joint in any patient with these injuries.

Mechanism of Injury

Cuboid and cuneiform fractures are often the result of direct crush injuries to the foot. Cuboid fractures can also occur with extreme plantar flexion of the forefoot, which compresses the cuboid between the bases of the fourth and

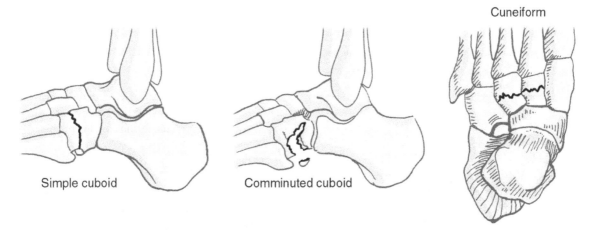

Cuneiform

Simple cuboid　　Comminuted cuboid

Figure 23–21. Cuboid and cuneiform fractures.

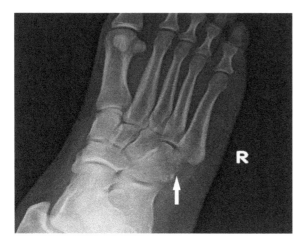

Figure 23–22. An oblique radiograph demonstrating an isolated cuboid fracture (*arrow*).

fifth metatarsals and calcaneus like a nutcracker. Cuboid and cuneiform dislocations are rare injuries and are secondary to acute inversion or eversion of the foot.

Examination

The patient will present with severe pain, tenderness, and swelling over the involved area. Midfoot motion will exacerbate the pain. Dislocations present with a palpable deformity and severe pain.

Imaging

AP, lateral, and oblique views may visualize these fractures (Figs. 23–22 and 23–23). CT scan can evaluate the articular surface and bony comminution and identify associated fractures if present (Fig. 23–24).

Associated Injuries

Cuboid and cuneiform fractures are associated with significant soft-tissue injuries. Cuboid fractures are associated with calcaneus fractures. Cuboid and cuneiform fractures may be seen with metatarsal fractures or tarsometatarsal fracture–dislocations.

> **Axiom:** *Distal cuboid or cuneiform fractures are associated with a tarsometatarsal dislocation that may have spontaneously reduced. This injury should be assumed to be present until proven otherwise.*

Treatment

Fractures of the cuboid and cuneiform are treated with ice, elevation, and a splint (Appendix A–14) with crutches.

Definitive management of nondisplaced cuboid or cuneiform fractures consists of a well-molded, short-leg cast (nonweight bearing) for 6 to 8 weeks. After cast removal, a longitudinal arch support is used for 5 to 6 months. Displaced fractures require operative fixation. Comminuted

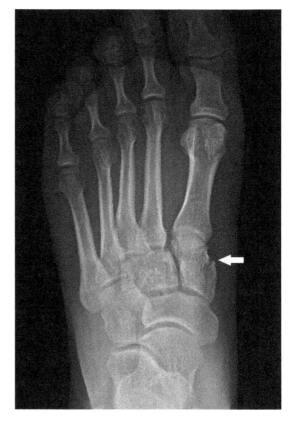

Figure 23–23. Medial cuneiform fracture (*arrow*).

cuboid fractures frequently require an external fixator as definitive treatment.

Dislocations or fracture–dislocations of the cuboid or cuneiforms are frequently unstable after reduction and, thus, early consultation is strongly recommended. In fact, some authorities recommend open reduction of dislocated cuneiforms due to potential interposed ligaments or tendons.

LISFRANC FRACTURE–DISLOCATION

Injuries to the Lisfranc (tarsometatarsal) joint involve a spectrum of injury from the subtle sprain to the complex and unstable fracture–dislocation. *Lisfranc fracture–dislocations* are rare, accounting for 0.2% of all fractures. They are associated with a high incidence of chronic pain and functional disability. This fact, combined with studies that report a 20% rate of misdiagnosis, make this injury one of the most common reasons for malpractice lawsuits against emergency physicians.

Anatomy

The Lisfranc joint is defined by the articulation of the midfoot and metatarsals. The base of the first three metatarsals aligns with the cuneiforms, whereas the fourth and fifth metatarsals articulate with the cuboid bone.

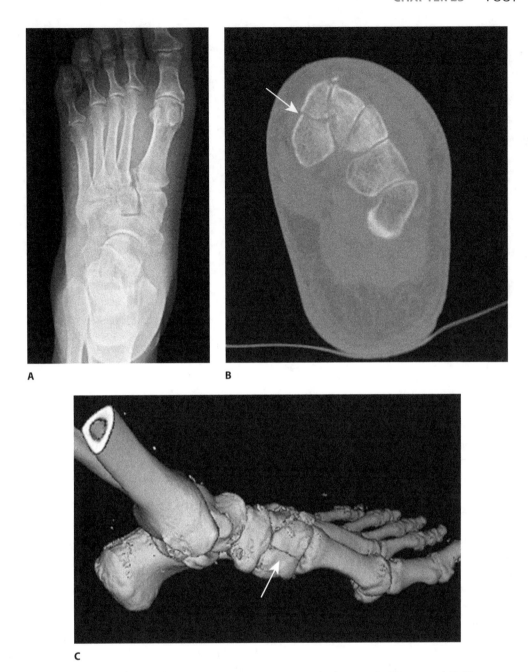

Figure 23–24. Medial cuneiform fracture. **A.** Plain images did not detect the fracture. **B.** CT scan and **C.** 3D reconstruction were performed because of significant pain and swelling and demonstrated a transverse fracture of the medial cuneiform (*arrows*).

Ligaments are essential in the stability of the tarsometatarsal joint. A tarsometatarsal ligament binds each of the metatarsal bones to a bone of the midfoot. In addition, the proximal aspects of the second through the fifth metatarsals are bound by a strong, transverse intermetatarsal ligament. These ligaments have a stronger plantar component than dorsal. No ligament connects the bases of the first and second metatarsals (Fig. 23–25).[42]

The second metatarsal is firmly bound in place by its tarsometatarsal ligament, intermetatarsal ligament, and strong Lisfranc ligament, which extends obliquely to the medial cuneiform. This strong, recessed articulation of the second metatarsal bone acts as the primary stabilizing force of the tarsometatarsal complex and makes a proximal second metatarsal fracture more likely than dislocation. Therefore, fracture at the base of the second metatarsal suggests a high likelihood of injury to the remaining ligamentous structures of the Lisfranc joint.

> **Axiom:** *A fracture of the base of the second metatarsal suggests a Lisfranc fracture–dislocation until proven otherwise.*

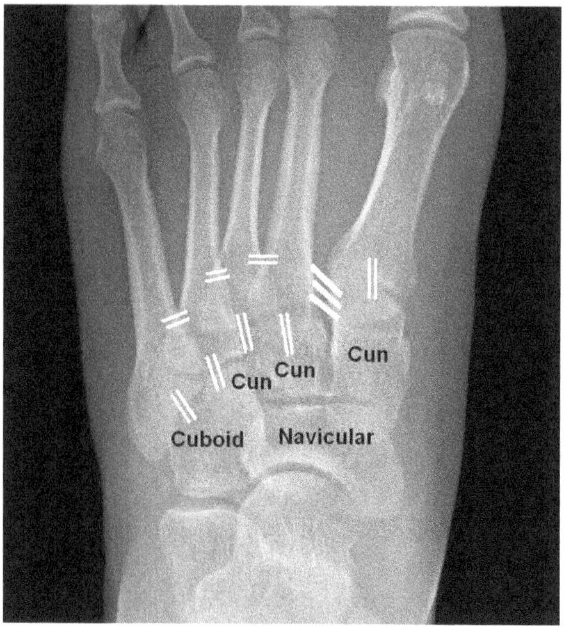

Figure 23–25. Ligamentous anatomy of the Lisfranc joint with tarsometatarsal, intermetatarsal, and the strong Lisfranc ligament (three oblique lines).

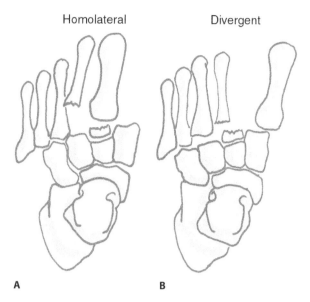

Figure 23–26. *A.* Lisfranc fracture–dislocation with total lateral incongruity of the entire joint (homolateral). ***B.*** Divergent Lisfranc fracture–dislocation.

Classification

Lisfranc fracture–dislocations exist in several variations. They are classified based on whether all Lisfranc joints are disrupted, termed total or partial incongruity. In addition, the direction of displacement is noted: medial, lateral, dorsal, or plantar. Homolateral dislocations are common and refer to lateral displacement of four or all five metatarsals in the same direction. If displacement is in opposing directions, then the fracture–dislocation is referred to as divergent (Fig. 23–26). Divergent dislocations usually occur between the first and second metatarsals because this is where the ligamentous attachments are the weakest. Unfortunately, no classification system is helpful in determining management or prognosis.

Mechanisms of Injury

Lisfranc fracture–dislocations generally occur after a high-energy trauma such as a fall from a great height or motor vehicle collision. Motor vehicle collisions account for 45% of these injuries. A more subtle injury after a lower-energy mechanism can also occur and accounts for up to 30% of the cases.

The mechanism of injury is either direct or indirect. Direct injuries involve a high-energy blunt trauma, usually to the dorsum of the foot. The direct mechanism is associated with significant soft-tissue injury and the development of compartment syndrome. Indirect trauma is more common and usually involves axial loading of the plantar-flexed foot. A twisting force across the Lisfranc joint with the foot planted can disrupt the ligaments as well.

Homolateral dislocations may follow a fall with the foot landing in plantar flexion. Compressive forces, such as those that occur during an automobile collision or rotational stress, may also produce this type of dislocation. Divergent dislocations typically follow a compressive force that splits the groove between the first and second metatarsals.

Examination

A patient with a mild sprain will exhibit tenderness at the Lisfranc joint, minimal swelling, and no instability. The patient with a fracture–dislocation will present with extreme midfoot pain and swelling. This swelling may mask any deformity. The patient may be able to ambulate despite a significant injury, so this feature cannot be used to exclude the diagnosis. There may be a prominence of the base of the first metatarsal or an apparent shortening of the forefoot. The forefoot may also appear widened or flat. Ecchymosis may be present on the plantar aspect of the foot (Fig. 23–27). Pain on passive abduction and pronation of the forefoot is suggestive of injury. Severe pain on passive dorsiflexion of the toes suggests a concomitant compartment syndrome. The neurovascular status of the foot should be carefully examined and documented, although vascular injury is rare.

Imaging

AP, oblique, and lateral radiographs are obtained and the relationship between the tarsal and metatarsal bones is scrutinized (Figs. 23–28 and 23–29). The AP view allows for better visualization of the first and second metatarsal, whereas the oblique view allows for better visualization of the bases of the fourth and fifth metatarsals.

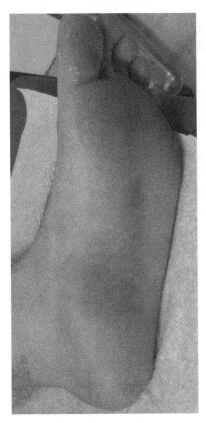

Figure 23-27. An ecchymosis on the plantar aspect of the foot should alert the clinician to a possible Lisfranc injury. This finding may also be present in patients with calcaneus fractures.

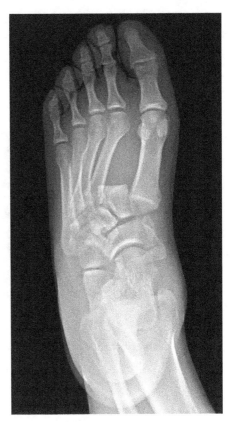

Figure 23-28. A divergent-type Lisfranc fracture–dislocation with first metatarsal dislocated medially while the remainder of the metatarsals are dislocated laterally. *(Used with permission from Eric Brader, MD.)*

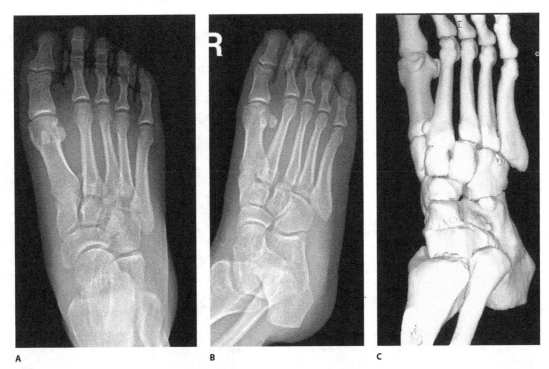

A   B   C

Figure 23-29. Another example of a Lisfranc fracture–dislocation. **A.** AP image demonstrated normal alignment of the first and second metatarsals with the medial and middle cuneiforms, respectively. **B.** The oblique view demonstrated loss of alignment of the third metatarsal and lateral cuneiform that was not readily apparent on the AP view. **C.** CT 3D reconstruction with the same malalignment. *(continued)*

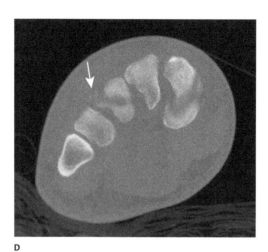

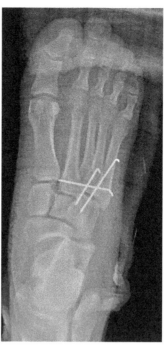

D

E

Figure 23–29. *(Continued)* **D.** CT also demonstrated avulsion fractures of the third and fourth metatarsals *(arrow)*. **E.** Surgical stabilization of the injury with Kirschner wires.

AP View. Evaluate the normal alignment of the first and second metatarsal with their respective cuneiforms:

- The medial borders of the second metatarsal and middle cuneiform are aligned.
- The first metatarsal aligns with the borders of the medial cuneiform.
- The distance between the bases of the first and second metatarsals should be less than 3 mm.

Oblique View. Evaluate the normal alignment of the third and fourth metatarsal with the cuboid and lateral cuneiform.

- The medial borders of the fourth metatarsal and cuboid are aligned.
- The lateral borders of the third metatarsal and lateral cuneiform are aligned.

Lateral View. This view is used to evaluate dorsal or plantar dislocation of the metatarsals. In the normal foot, a line drawn along the dorsal surface of the foot at the level of the tarsometatarsal joint will not be disrupted. A metatarsal should never be more dorsal than its respective tarsal bone.

> **Axiom:** *The medial aspect of the middle cuneiform and second metatarsal align. Any disruption of this alignment is indicative of a dislocation, which may have spontaneously reduced.*

Another radiographic sign of a spontaneously reduced Lisfranc fracture–dislocation is the *fleck sign* (Fig. 23–30). This sign is present in 90% of cases and occurs due to an avulsion of bone from the second metatarsal or medial cuneiform.

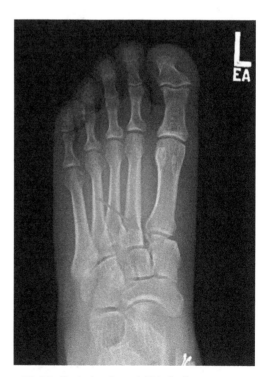

Figure 23–30. Fleck sign *(arrow)*. This finding suggests a spontaneously reduced Lisfranc fracture–dislocation.

Weight-bearing views may be required to detect subtle injuries. Some authors have suggested that up to 10% of Lisfranc injuries cannot be detected without weight-bearing views.[33] The radiographic findings are the same as nonweight-bearing views. Weight-bearing views are often difficult to obtain due to patient discomfort.

A CT scan should be obtained if there is a high clinical suspicion and the patient cannot tolerate stress views. CT scanning is more sensitive and has proven to be a valuable diagnostic tool for delineating occult injuries.[50] Displacement of up to 2 mm may not be visible on plain films but is seen on CT. In one study, plain films missed one-fourth of all cases.[26] MRI has been shown to correlate very well with intraoperative findings.[39] These advanced imaging studies can be performed in early, outpatient follow-up.

Associated Injuries

Tarsometatarsal dislocations are associated with the following injuries:

- Fracture of the base of the second metatarsal
- Avulsion fractures of adjacent tarsals or metatarsals
- Cuboid, cuneiform, or navicular fractures
- Compartment syndrome

Treatment

The ED management of these injuries includes analgesics, ice, elevation, and immobilization (Appendix A–14). Even a mild sprain of the joint with normal radiographs should be kept nonweight bearing until further evaluation due to the potential for disability with these injuries.[41,45] Fracture–dislocations almost always require orthopedic consultation and operative repair. If developing compartment syndrome is suspected, emergent orthopedic consultation and admission are indicated.

The orthopedic surgeon may consider nonoperative management of Lisfranc joint sprains (normal weight-bearing radiographs) with nonweight bearing and a short-leg cast for 6 weeks.[42,45] For fracture–dislocations, closed reduction with casting will usually result in reduction but is not sufficient to produce a stable anatomic reduction. Percutaneous reduction and fixation provide an excellent outcome, with less soft tissue disruption in low-energy Lisfranc injuries.[46] With high-impact Lisfranc injuries, open reduction and internal fixation with pins or screws are necessary. After surgical reduction, a short-leg cast is applied for 6 to 12 weeks. A custom arch support is used for the following 12 months. Proper management yields a good clinical result in 90% of cases.

Complications

Tarsometatarsal dislocations are frequently complicated by the development of degenerative arthritis, chronic pain, and chronic instability.

METATARSAL FRACTURES

Metatarsal fractures are classified on the basis of anatomy and therapy:

- First metatarsal
- Central (second, third, and fourth) metatarsals
- Fifth metatarsal (proximal)
  - Tuberosity avulsion fracture
  - Jones fracture
  - Diaphyseal stress fracture

First Metatarsal Fractures

Significant forces act on this bone during ambulation, making it essential that it remains anatomically intact in relation to the other bones of the foot. Unlike the second through fourth metatarsals, the first metatarsal does not have interconnecting ligaments, allowing it to move independently.

Mechanism of Injury

The majority of metatarsal fractures are the result of a direct crush injury, as when a heavy object is dropped on the foot. An indirect twisting mechanism can also cause these fractures.

Examination

First metatarsal fractures usually present with pain, swelling, and tenderness localized over the dorsal and medial part of the foot. Axial compression along the first metatarsal will exacerbate the pain. The strength and quality of the dorsalis pedis pulse should be documented in all patients.

Imaging

AP, lateral, and oblique views are usually adequate in demonstrating this fracture.

Associated Injuries

First metatarsal fractures may be accompanied by phalanx, second through fourth metatarsal, or tarsal fractures. In addition, compartment syndrome may develop when soft-tissue swelling is significant.

Treatment

First metatarsal fractures require ice, elevation, analgesics, and immobilization (Appendix A–14). Special care should be taken to ensure the metatarsophalangeal (MTP) joints are kept in a neutral position. The patient should be given crutches and instructed to avoid weight bearing. Definitive management of stable, nondisplaced fractures includes a cast for 4 to 6 weeks. Stability is not definite until the fracture is noted not to displace while weight bearing (stress radiographs). Displaced neck fractures require early referral for open reduction and fixation. Severely comminuted fractures require external fixation.

Complications

Nonunion and malunion may occur after these fractures. Degenerative arthritis is also a complication of intra-articular fractures.

Central Metatarsal Fractures

The second, third, and fourth metatarsals are bound by several ligamentous attachments that provide inherent stability to these bones. Fractures of the central metatarsals are much more common than the first metatarsal. Fractures can occur in the shaft, head, neck, or base. When diagnosing fractures of the base, however, the emergency physician should consider the possibility of instability within the Lisfranc joint.

Mechanism of Injury

The majority of these fractures are the result of a direct crush injury, as when a heavy object is dropped on the foot. An indirect twisting mechanism can also cause these fractures. Stress fractures, common in the second and third metatarsals, are seen after repetitive trauma to the forefoot.

Examination

Central metatarsal fractures usually present with pain, swelling, and tenderness localized over the dorsal middle part of the foot. Axial compression along the involved metatarsal will exacerbate the pain.

Imaging

AP, lateral, and oblique views are usually adequate in demonstrating these fractures (Fig. 23–31). The flexor tendons frequently force the distal fragment in a plantar and proximal direction.

Associated Injuries

Central metatarsal fractures are frequently accompanied by phalanx fractures. The alignment of the bones of the Lisfranc joint should be assessed, especially when fractures are seen proximally.

Treatment

The ED management of these fractures includes elevation, ice, and analgesics. Isolated metatarsal fractures are usually nondisplaced because of the stabilizing effect of the adjacent metatarsals. Nondisplaced fractures generally heal well and may be treated with a hard-sole shoe. The hard-sole shoe functions to keep weight distributed evenly and prohibit motion at the MTP joints. Weight bearing can progress as tolerated.

Displaced (>3 mm) or angulated (>10 degree) metatarsal fractures involving the second through the fifth metatarsals require closed reduction. Allowing displacement or angulation to persist will disrupt normal weight bearing across the forefoot. After adequate analgesia, the toes are hung with finger traps and countertraction applied to the distal tibia by a sling with weights. Postreduction

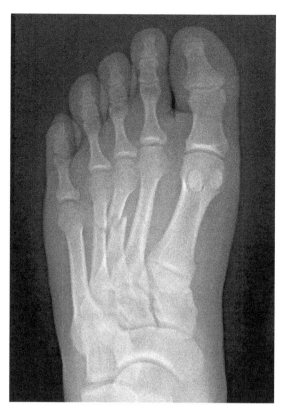

Figure 23–31. Metatarsal shaft fractures of the second, third, and fourth metatarsals.

radiographs are recommended. Following reduction, the patient is splinted (Appendix A–14) and kept nonweight bearing. Surgery may be required for unstable fractures and those fractures resistant to closed attempts. Open reduction is more common when multiple metatarsals are fractured because the stabilizing effect of the adjacent metatarsals is lost.

Fractures of the middle and distal fifth metatarsal are treated in a similar manner to corresponding fractures of the central metatarsals.

Complications

Nonunion and malunion may occur after these fractures. Degenerative arthritis is also a complication of intra-articular fractures.

Proximal Fifth Metatarsal Fractures

The most common site of midfoot fractures is the proximal fifth metatarsal. Three types of fractures that differ in their etiology and treatment occur at the proximal portion of the fifth metatarsal. These fractures can be distinguished by both the history and the zone of injury demonstrated on radiographic images. Proximal fifth metatarsal fractures consist of (A) tuberosity avulsion fractures, (B) Jones fractures, and (C) diaphyseal stress fractures (Fig. 23–32).

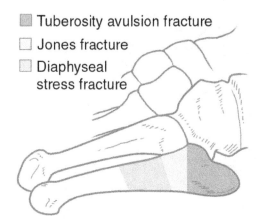

Figure 23–32. Proximal fifth metatarsal fractures.

Tuberosity avulsion fractures, also called "pseudo-Jones fractures," are the most common type and account for approximately 90% of fractures at the base of the fifth metatarsal.[55] These fractures are defined as occurring proximal to the articulation between the fourth and fifth metatarsals. These fractures are transverse or oblique and usually extra-articular, although they may extend into the intra-articular space between the cuboid and fifth metatarsal.[56]

The Jones fracture—an acute fracture at the junction of the diaphysis and metaphysis—is named after Sir Robert Jones, who described these fractures in 1902. These fractures involve the articular facet between the fourth and fifth metatarsal.[57] Jones fractures are important to distinguish from the tuberosity fracture because of concern that they may disrupt the blood supply to the distal portion of the proximal fragment and therefore heal poorly.

A third fracture type begins just distal to the ligamentous attachments of the bone and extends 1.5 cm into the diaphysis. This zone is the most common location for stress fractures of the fifth metatarsal.

Mechanism of Injury

Tuberosity avulsion fractures occur after forced inversion with the foot and ankle in plantar flexion. This mechanism avulses the tuberosity by tension from the peroneus brevis tendon and the lateral cord of the plantar aponeurosis (Fig. 23–33). Both structures attach to the tuberosity. Recent studies suggest it is more likely the lateral band of the plantar fascia that produces the avulsion.[58]

A Jones fracture occurs most often after a laterally directed force on the forefoot disrupts the plantar-flexed foot. This injury is commonly reported in basketball or football.

Stress fractures can be distinguished because they are often symptomatic for several days before presentation, unlike the Jones and avulsion fractures, which are acutely injured. These injuries occur in individuals engaged in strenuous physical activities.

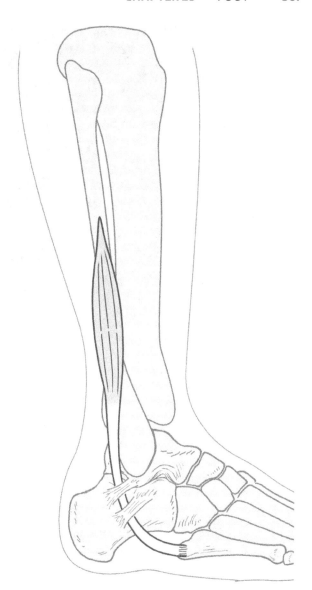

Figure 23–33. Avulsion of the base of the fifth metatarsal by the peroneus brevis tendon. Traditional proposed mechanism.

Examination

Proximal fifth metatarsal fractures usually present with tenderness localized to the involved area and only minimal swelling. Ecchymosis is present following acute injuries. Horizontal compression of the metatarsal heads produces pain at the base of the fifth metatarsal.

Imaging

AP, lateral, and oblique views are usually adequate in demonstrating these fractures (Fig. 23–34). The presence of the *os vesalianum* (a secondary center of ossification) at the base of the fifth metatarsal may be confused with a fracture (Fig. 23–4). Secondary ossification centers are typically smooth, rounded, bilateral, and often have sclerotic margins. These apophyses are parallel to the bone rather than oblique or transverse. Ultrasound is

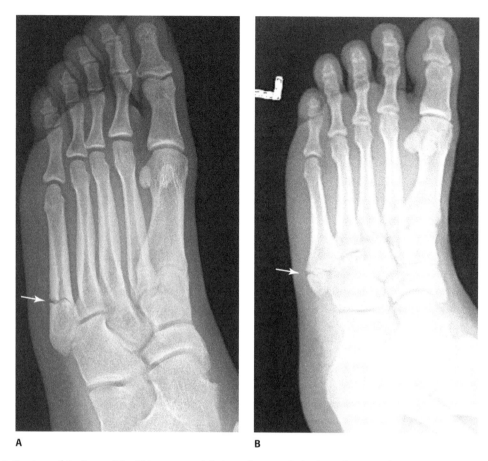

A   **B**

Figure 23–34. Fracture of the base of the fifth metatarsal. **A.** Jones fracture. **B.** Avulsion fracture of the tuberosity.

being used to image fractures at the bedside (Fig. 23-35). Recent studies have suggested that ultrasound is at least equivocal to plain films for diagnosing fractures of the fifth metatarsal.

Associated Injuries
Metatarsal fractures are frequently accompanied by phalanx fractures.

Treatment
Tuberosity Avulsion Fracture. The emergency management of these fractures includes ice; elevation; and a compression dressing, hard-soled or cast shoe, and weight bearing as tolerated. Elastic bandages have been shown to be equally as effective as a walking cast.

Healing occurs within 4 to 6 weeks and is excellent in most cases. In one study from Scotland, patients with these fractures were not provided with any follow-up appointment and told to call the fracture clinic only if the pain persisted after several months.

Because some surgeons treat displaced avulsion fractures with a nonweight-bearing period, it may be prudent to use a posterior splint with crutches in this scenario, at least until the patient has seen the specialist.

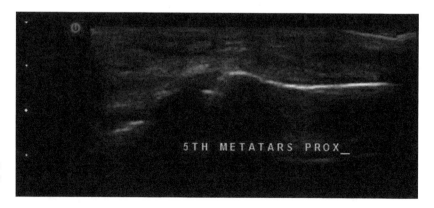

Figure 23–35. Bedside ultrasound of a Jones fracture. *(Used with permission from Eric Brader, MD.)*

Operative intervention is rarely necessary, occurring in only 1% of patients in one study.[62] It may be considered for comminuted fractures or when intra-articular involvement between the metatarsal and cuboid is >30% with significant step-off. Either finding should prompt placement of a posterior splint with crutches and referral to an orthopedic surgeon.[51,61]

Jones Fracture.   The emergency management of these fractures includes ice, elevation, immobilization (Appendix A–14), and crutches. These patient should be nonweight bearing initially and requires referral to a surgeon.

Definitive management is controversial and should be individualized to the patient and, ultimately, determined by the specialist. Options include early surgery with screw fixation and casting with crutches/nonweight bearing for 6 to 8 weeks, and more recent evidence suggests that these fractures might heal well with functional treatment in a similar manner to the tuberosity avulsion fracture.[57,64,65]

Early surgical intervention with screw fixation results in a high rate of primary union.[57,66] This technique is frequently employed in young, active patients (e.g., athletes) to decrease union time and promote an earlier return to activity.[57,61,66,67] Patients with displaced fractures are also more likely to undergo operative fixation.[57,61] If nonoperative treatment is initially chosen, some evidence suggests that up to one-half of fractures later required surgery because of nonunion or refracture.[68,69]

Diaphyseal Stress Fracture.   The emergency management of these fractures includes ice, elevation, immobilization (Appendix A–14), and crutches. These patient should be nonweight bearing and require referral to a surgeon.

Acute diaphyseal stress fractures are frequently managed with screw fixation or bone grafting.[57] These fractures have a high rate of nonunion. If a nonoperative route is chosen, the patient will be immobilized and nonweight bearing for 6 to 10 weeks.[51,66] Up to 20 weeks of immobilization is required in some cases, and nonunions can still occur.

Complications

The most common complication is nonunion, which is most frequent after diaphyseal stress fractures.

TOE FRACTURES

Phalanx fractures are the most common forefoot fracture (Fig. 23–36). The proximal phalanx of the great toe is most frequently injured, followed by proximal phalangeal fractures of the fifth toe.[70]

Mechanism of Injury

The majority of phalanx fractures are the result of a direct blow, such as when a heavy object is dropped on the foot. An axial force caused by "stubbing the toe" may also result in these fractures. An abrupt abduction force commonly

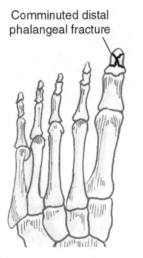
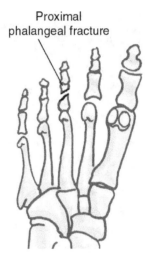

Figure 23–36. Toe fractures.

produces a fracture of the lesser toes. This injury is referred to as a "night walker's" fracture. Less commonly, hyperextension of the toe, an indirect mechanism, may result in a spiral or avulsion fracture.

Examination

Phalanx fractures present with pain, swelling, and ecchymosis. Point tenderness is present on examination, and there may be visible deformity of the toe. Subungual hematomas may develop within the first 12 hours.

Imaging

Phalanx fractures are usually best seen on AP and oblique views (Figs. 23–37 and 23–38). Lateral views are difficult to interpret due to overlying bone shadows. With the exception of the great toe, many toe fractures can be diagnosed clinically and may not require x-rays.

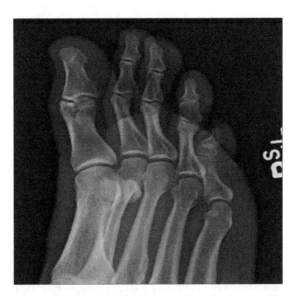

Figure 23–37. Intra-articular fracture of the distal aspect of the first proximal phalanx.

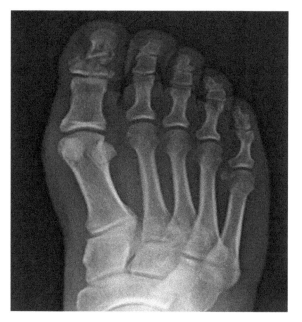

Figure 23–38. Comminuted first distal phalanx fracture.

Treatment

Most toe fractures are nondisplaced or minimally displaced. Nondisplaced phalanx fractures involving the second through the fifth digits are treated with dynamic splinting and a hard-soled open shoe to prevent movement. Dynamic splinting involves the use of cotton padding between the affected toe and its neighbor. The injured toe is then securely taped to the adjacent uninjured toe (Fig. 23–39). The splint should be changed every few days and used for a period of 2 to 3 weeks. These minimally displaced phalanx fractures involving the second through fifth digits do not require orthopedic follow-up. Significant subungual hematomas can be drained using electrocautery or an 18-gauge needle.

Because of the great toe's importance in weight bearing and balance, these fractures require referral more often than other lesser toe fractures. If the fracture involves more than 25% of the joint space, then referral is recommended. Nondisplaced fractures of the great toe phalanx can be treated with buddy tape and a hard-soled shoe, although if pain is significant, a posterior splint is preferred. Comminuted fractures of the great toe require a walking cast because dynamic splinting offers insufficient immobilization.

Displaced phalanx fractures can be reduced by the emergency physician (Fig. 23–40). The toe is anesthetized with a digital block, and traction is applied to manipulate the toe into proper position. Alignment of the nails is used to detect subtle rotational abnormalities. A near anatomic alignment is most important when reducing great toe fractures. Postreduction films are indicated, and, if stable, these fractures are treated with buddy tape and a hard-soled open shoe.

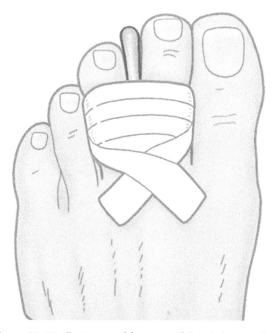

Figure 23–39. Treatment of fractures of the phalanges of the toes. A piece of cotton padding is placed between the toes, and the fractured toe is taped to the adjacent toe. Taping can extend all the way to the nails for additional support.

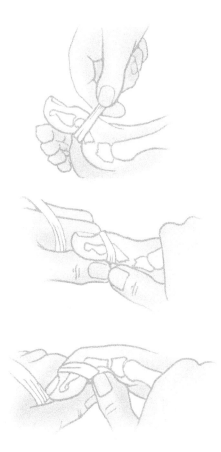

Figure 23–40. Closed reduction of the displaced phalanx fracture.

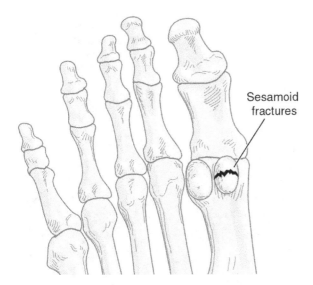

Figure 23–41. Sesamoid fractures.

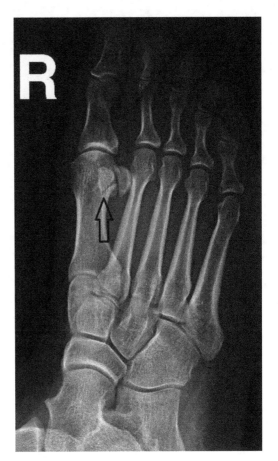

Figure 23–42. Bipartite medial sesamoid.

SESAMOID FRACTURES

Two sesamoids are commonly found within the tendon of the flexor hallucis brevis and are only infrequently fractured (Fig. 23–41). Sesamoid fractures are usually the result of acute or chronic direct trauma. Medial sesamoid fractures are more common than lateral. Sesamoid fractures present with localized pain to palpation over the plantar aspect of the first metatarsal head. Extension of the first phalanx results in an exacerbation of pain referred to the plantar aspect of the metacarpal joint. Sesamoid fractures require oblique tangential views for adequate visualization. Bipartite sesamoids are smooth, rounded structures not frequently confused with acute fractures (Fig. 23–42).

Treatment of sesamoid fractures is conservative, with orthotic inserts and a hard-soled shoe to take weight off the painful area. However, if the symptoms are severe, a short-leg walking cast is indicated. Excision can be performed when conservative treatment fails.

FOOT SOFT-TISSUE INJURY AND DISLOCATIONS

SUBTALAR DISLOCATION

Subtalar dislocations are a rare entity accounting for only 1% to 2% of all dislocations. This injury, also termed a *peritalar dislocation*, describes dislocation of the talus from both the calcaneus and navicular bones (Fig. 23–43). Subtalar dislocations may be classified as medial or lateral depending on the position of the foot relative to the distal tibia. The more common medial type represents 80% to 85% of all subtalar dislocations.[73–74] Medial subtalar dislocations are known as "basketball foot" or acquired clubfoot.[74] Lateral subtalar dislocations are less common. Lateral subtalar dislocations have been called "acquired flatfoot."[74] Anterior and posterior subtalar dislocation may also occur but are unusual.

Dislocation of the talus above the ankle mortise and below the calcaneus and navicular bones is termed a *total talar dislocation* and is extremely rare.[75] With total talar dislocations, the talus is completely dislocated out of the ankle mortise and rotated such that the inferior articular surface points posteriorly and the talar head points medially.

Mechanism of Injury
Subtalar dislocations can occur after both low-energy (e.g., stepping off a curb) and high-energy (e.g., fall from a height) trauma.[73–76] A medial subtalar dislocation typically follows an inversion and plantar flexion injury. The talocalcaneal and talonavicular ligaments rupture as the bones of the foot are displaced medially.

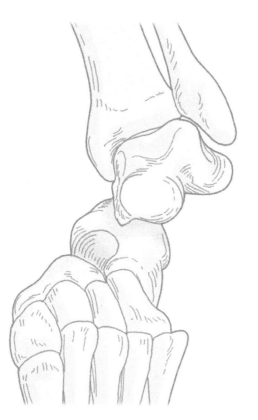

Figure 23–43. Subtalar dislocation (medial).

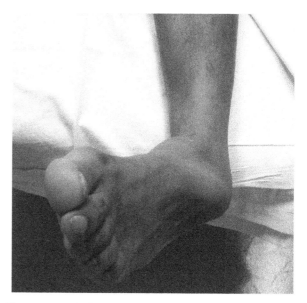

Figure 23–44. Subtalar dislocation (medial).

In lateral dislocations, there is a forcible eversion of the foot. The talar head is forced through the capsule of the talonavicular joint and the calcaneus. The remainder of the forefoot displaces laterally from the talus.

Examination

The patient will present with a relatively obvious deformity of the foot (Fig. 23–44). There is generally marked pain,

swelling, and tenderness. With medial dislocations, the foot will be displaced medially and the talus palpable laterally. The skin is taut over the lateral surface of the foot, and the vascular supply is often compromised. Open dislocations may also occur and should be suspected whenever there is disruption of the skin laterally.

Imaging

Routine views including AP, lateral, and oblique are usually adequate in demonstrating a subtalar dislocation (Fig. 23–45). Fractures are associated in approximately two-thirds of cases. Malleolar, talar neck, and osteochondral fractures are the most common. Postreduction films are required for documentation as well as to exclude the presence of occult fractures. Postreduction CT identifies

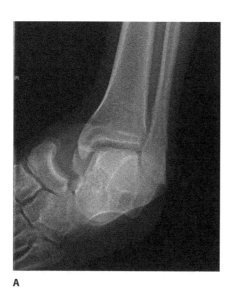

A

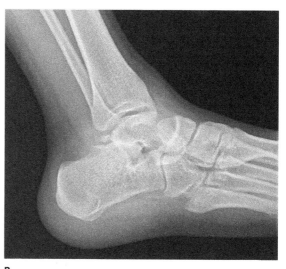

B

Figure 23–45. Radiographs of a subtalar dislocation (medial). *A.* AP. *B.* Lateral.

additional fractures and changes the management in nearly half of the cases.[77]

Associated Injuries

Subtalar dislocations are associated with fractures (tarsal, malleolar, talar neck, and osteochondral) and ligamentous injury.

Treatment

The emergency management of closed injuries includes analgesics and prompt reduction to avoid the complication of skin necrosis (Video 23–1). If prompt consultation is not available, an attempt at closed reduction should be made.[78,79]

The knee is held in flexion to relax the gastrocnemius and allow for an easier reduction. To reduce a medial dislocation, traction is applied to the foot and heel in line with the deformity. Counter traction is applied to the leg. This is followed by pressure over the talar head with an abduction force concomitantly applied to the forefoot. Lateral dislocations are reduced by firm traction followed by adduction over the forefoot. Subtalar dislocations are irreducible in almost one-third of cases.[80] Medial subtalar dislocations have a higher rate of successful reduction than lateral dislocations, which require open reduction in half of the cases.[80,81]

Complications

Subtalar dislocations may be complicated by the development of several significant disorders[82]:

- AVN of the talus (rare)
- Subtalar osteoarthritis (main long-term complication)
- Ischemic skin loss secondary to underlying talar pressure

TOE DISLOCATION

MTP dislocations are a rare injury and usually occur in a dorsal direction. Dislocations of the great toe MTP are more common than the lesser toes.[51] MTP dislocations are classified as simple or complex based on the presence of interposed soft tissues or sesamoid bones (Fig. 23–46). The interphalangeal (IP) joint can be dislocated in a dorsal or volar direction. IP dislocations, like MTP dislocations, are rare.[51]

Mechanism of Injury

Dislocations of the MTP joint are secondary to axial load with extreme dorsiflexion of the proximal phalanx. Classically, this injury occurs in football players competing on artificial turf.[83] If the force generated does not result in a dislocation, a sprain is diagnosed, commonly referred to as "turf toe." With greater forces (e.g., motor vehicle collisions), the plantar capsule avulses, and a dorsal dislocation of the proximal phalanx on the metatarsal occurs. Medial or

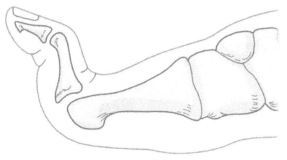

Simple dislocation

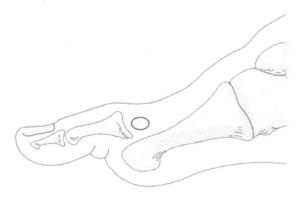

Complex dislocation

Figure 23–46. Metatarsophalangeal dislocations.

lateral MTP dislocations are the result of injury forces that abduct or adduct the toe.

Examination

Patients with dislocation of the MTP joint present with pain, swelling, inability to walk, and visible deformity. Typically, the toe is hyperextended, resting on the dorsum of the metatarsal. The sesamoid may be palpable on the dorsal aspect if the dislocation is complex. Patients with IP dislocations will present with similar findings. If swelling is significant, the deformity might not be as obvious (Fig. 23–47A).

Imaging

MTP dislocations may be diagnosed on the AP view because there is generally an overlap between the distal metatarsal and proximal phalanx. IP dislocations are best seen on the AP and oblique views (Fig. 23–47B and C). With a complex MTP dislocation, the volar plate of the great toe, along with the sesamoid, entraps the phalanx on the dorsal surface of the metatarsal.

Associated Injury

IP dislocations are frequently associated with fractures.

Treatment

IP dislocations may be treated with closed reduction followed by dynamic splinting. Unstable reductions require

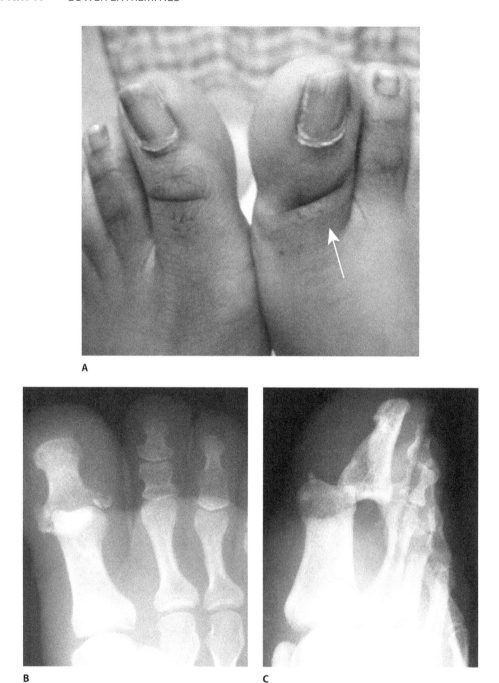

Figure 23–47. Dorsal dislocation of the right great toe interphalangeal joint. **A.** Patient photograph (*arrow*). **B.** AP radiograph. **C.** Oblique radiograph.

early referral for internal fixation. Dorsal MTP dislocations are reduced using hyperextension with distal traction (Fig. 23–48 and Video 23–2). Stable reductions require a hard-soled shoe and dynamic splinting. Dislocations resistant to reduction have interposed soft tissues and usually require open reduction, although successful percutaneous reduction has been reported. Unstable reductions or crepitus after reduction, suggesting an intra-articular loose body, are also indications for operative repair.

FOOT COMPARTMENT SYNDROME

For a full discussion of compartment syndrome, refer to Chapter 4. This section addresses unique aspects of compartment syndrome of the foot. The foot is the most challenging location in the body to diagnose compartment syndrome because the presentation is subtle. The emergency physician should have a high index of suspicion for this diagnosis to avoid the chronic sequelae of a missed diagnosis.

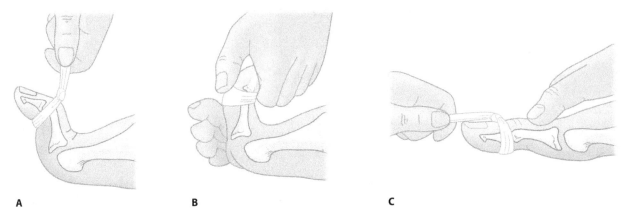

A   **B**   **C**

Figure 23–48. Reduction of the metatarsophalangeal joint. **A.** Traction is applied in the line of deformity. **B.** Hyperextension is used to reproduce the injuring force. **C.** With traction maintained, reduction is accomplished.

The foot contains a total of nine separate compartments. Three compartments—the medial, lateral, and central (superficial)—run along the entire plantar surface of the foot (Fig. 23–49). The medial compartment is located inferior and medial to the first metatarsal and contains the abductor hallucis and flexor hallucis brevis muscles. The lateral compartment is found inferior and lateral to the fifth metatarsal. This compartment contains the abductor digiti minimi and flexor digiti minimi brevis. The central (superficial) compartment contains the flexor digitorum longus and brevis muscles.

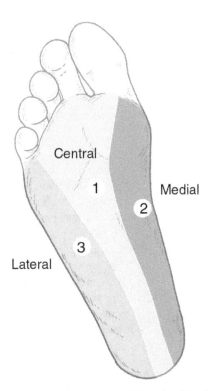

Figure 23–49. The compartments of the sole of the foot. *(Used with permission from Eric Brader, MD)*

The remaining six compartments do not run along the entire length of the foot (Fig. 23–50). These compartments include the four interosseous compartments and the calcaneus and adductor compartments. The four interosseous compartments exist dorsally between the metatarsals. These compartments contain the interosseous muscles. The calcaneus compartment is deep to the central compartment within the heel of the foot. This compartment contains the quadratus plantae muscle and communicates with the deep posterior compartment of the leg through the flexor retinaculum. The adductor compartment is within the deep plantar aspect of the forefoot and contains the adductor hallucis muscle.

Similar to compartment syndromes in other parts of the body, fractures are a major cause of foot compartment syndrome, along with significant crush injuries, infection, and iatrogenic causes.[85] The fractures most likely to produce a compartment syndrome in the foot include multiple metatarsal fractures, Lisfranc fracture–dislocations, and intra-articular calcaneal fractures.[85] Foot compartment syndrome occurs after 10% of intra-articular calcaneal fractures.[13,85] Of these, one-half develop a claw toe deformity due to contracture of the quadratus plantae muscle within the calcaneal compartment. In one study, foot compartment syndrome was due to calcaneal fractures in 42%, multiple metatarsal fractures in 25%, and Lisfranc fracture–dislocation in 17%. The remaining 17% of patients did not have injury to the foot, but suffered from foot swelling due to more proximal orthopedic injuries (tibia plafond, open femur, tibial plateau).[86] Delayed presentations of up to 36 hours have been reported in patients who sustained less severe mechanisms of trauma (kicked in the foot during a soccer game).[87]

As with all compartment syndromes, the degree of pain is out of proportion to the injury, but it is generally more vague and ill defined. The pain is not relieved by immobilization or with pain medication. The pain caused by compartment syndrome in the foot may be *exacerbated* by elevation.

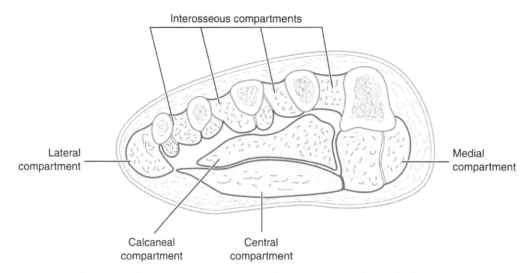

Figure 23–50. Cross-section schematic of the compartments of the foot at the level of the proximal metatarsal head.

The affected compartment will be tense on examination. Pain with passive stretching of the involved muscles is an important sign, but it is difficult to isolate the muscles of the foot. After several hours, signs of neurologic compromise may appear, including numbness, burning, and paresthesias. Again, these findings are less dramatic in the foot when compared with other locations of the body. Also, the vascular exam is not helpful because the palpable pulses in the foot are located extra-compartmentally.

The emergency physician must have a high index of suspicion for this condition in patients with significant bony or soft-tissue injuries or in patients who present after minor trauma with pain that appears out of proportion to what is expected. Orthopedic consultation should be obtained, and compartmental pressure readings are measured. Treatment involves decompression with an emergent fasciotomy.

PLANTAR PUNCTURE WOUNDS

Puncture wounds to the plantar aspect of the foot are associated with a higher rate of infection than similar wounds elsewhere on the body. The penetrating agents include needles, nails, glass, wood splinters, thorns, and toothpicks. Retained foreign bodies are present in 3% of cases and include pieces of clothing, rust, gravel, or dirt. The presence of a foreign body is associated with soft-tissue infection and osteomyelitis.

Ten percent of patients experience late infection. In a study by Fitzgerald and Cowan,[89] 132 of 774 children examined with puncture wounds experienced cellulitis and 16 had osteomyelitis. The most common bacterial pathogens causing soft-tissue infections are staphylococci, including methicillin-resistant *Staphylococcus aureus* (MRSA) and streptococci, whereas pseudomonas causes 90% of the cases

of osteomyelitis. Other organisms that cause osteomyelitis include *Escherichia coli*, *S aureus*, and mixed flora.

Classification
Puncture wounds of the foot can be separated into five types depending on the degree of penetration and infection and the presence of the foreign body. Type I involves superficial cutaneous penetration into the epidermis or the dermis with no signs or symptoms of infection. Type II puncture wounds are subcutaneous or involve a joint without signs or symptoms of infection. This is the most common type of puncture wound. Type III puncture wounds are divided into those that involve soft-tissue infection, including septic arthritis and a retained foreign body (type IIIA), and those with penetration of the foreign body into the bone (type IIIB). Type IV puncture wounds are associated with osteomyelitis.

Examination
Findings on physical examination are usually minimal immediately following injury and include a small laceration or puncture wound (Fig. 23–51A). If the injury is several days old, the original wound may be partially healing. In these cases, the patient is usually presenting because of erythema, discharge, warmth, and pain associated with an infection (Fig. 23–52). If the presence of a foreign body is unclear, use a cotton-tipped applicator to palpate around the puncture site and ask the patient if there is any area of significant tenderness. If the wound is *tender*, the likelihood of a retained foreign body is greater, and the area of tenderness is likely its location.

Imaging
Plain radiographs should be taken when a patient presents with a puncture wound and the examiner is uncertain if a retained foreign body is present. Glass and metal are usually

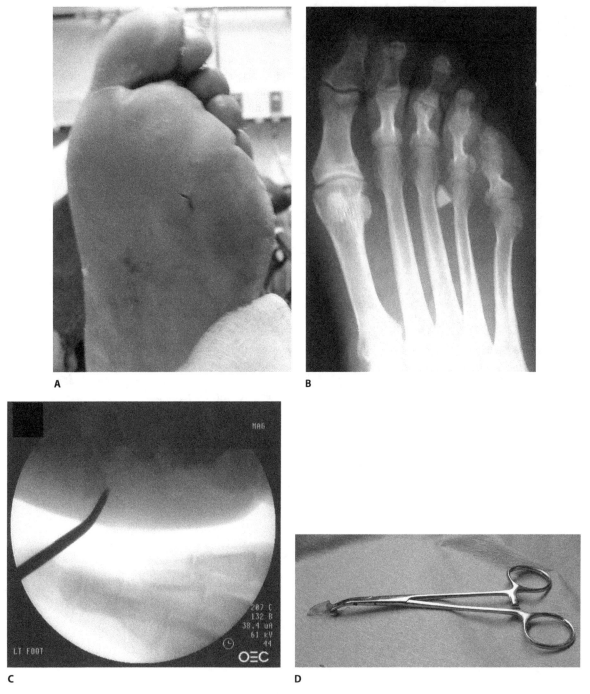

Figure 23–51. Plantar foreign body removal. **A.** Plantar puncture wound. **B.** Radiograph demonstrates a triangular glass foreign body. **C.** Fluoroscopy is used to locate the glass. **D.** The glass is grasped and removed.

easily seen on radiographs (Fig. 23–51B). To localize a metal foreign body, ultrasonography or fluoroscopy is useful. These modalities are especially useful because real-time images can be obtained that will also aid in the removal of larger foreign bodies. For radiopaque foreign materials, removal is aided because the clinician can visualize both the instrument and the foreign body (Fig. 23–51C and D). Ultrasonography and CT better demonstrate plastic or wood foreign bodies.

Treatment

Because of the high rate of infection, these wounds require special attention. The treatment of superficial, noninfected puncture wounds (type I) includes tetanus and local wound care. The patient is instructed to clean the area twice daily and wear a protective covering. If there is discomfort when walking, nonweight-bearing activities are recommended. When the depth of the wound cannot be determined, the penetration should be assumed to be deep and the wound treated as such.

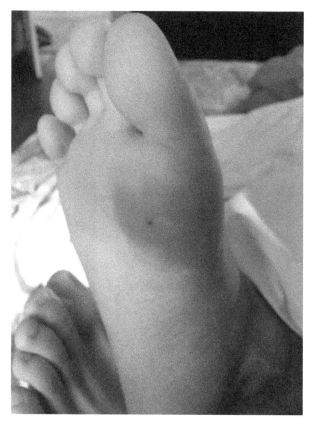

Figure 23–52. Infection complicating a plantar puncture wound. *(Used with permission from Elizabeth Palomaki Lazowski.)*

Deeper wounds (type II) usually require exploration. A local anesthetic or a regional nerve block (ankle block of sural and posterior tibial nerves) should be administered. Multiple options for exploration exist, and the best method is unknown. Blunt probing with splinter forceps may simply force objects deeper. Excision of a block of tissue around the puncture will aid in foreign body removal and assist in irrigation (Fig. 23–53). Extending the uninfected wound is recommended to remove wood or other contaminated objects or when a nail puncture occurs through a shoe. These injuries are especially likely to become infected. To prevent the inoculation of healthy tissues, the wound should not be closed. It must be noted, however, that it is not necessary to remove a foreign body if it is inert, asymptomatic, not a threat to function, and not within a joint. Unfortunately, prophylactic antibiotics have not been shown to reduce the infection rate.

Puncture wounds that are infected and have a foreign body (type IIIA) require antibiotics and surgical intervention. When penetration of foreign material is into bone (type IIIB), the foreign body must be surgically removed with curettage of the osseous defect, debridement of soft tissue, copious lavage, and open packing. Empiric intravenous antimicrobial agents are administered, pending intraoperative cultures results.

Puncture wounds of the foot that result in osteomyelitis (type IV) are unusual. The condition does occur, and wider recognition of the entity will help in prevention and early

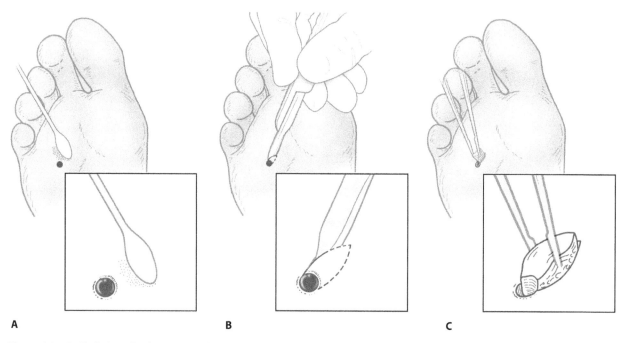

A   **B**   **C**

Figure 23–53. Technique for detecting and removing a foreign body within a plantar puncture wound. ***A.*** Palpate around the wound with a cotton-tipped applicator. The site of greatest tenderness is the location of the foreign body. ***B.*** A small 2- to 3-mm elliptical incision is made toward the presumed location of the foreign body. ***C.*** The tissue is removed with forceps. The foreign body may be located within the tissue.

diagnosis. Once infection develops in a puncture wound. Antibiotic coverage should include gram-positive and *Pseudomonas* coverage.[92] Wound care must be aggressive, including surgical exploration of the wound, debridement, and removal of all foreign material.[90,93]

ACHILLES TENDON RUPTURE

Rupture of the Achilles tendon is relatively common, occurring in 18 per 100,000 persons.[94] This condition is misdiagnosed in 20% to 30% of cases because of insignificant pain or an incomplete examination. The diagnosis is delayed more commonly in those patients injured while not participating in sports and patients with a high BMI. This delay is due to a lower index of suspicion and a technically difficult examination.[95] This injury is more common in men between the ages of 30 and 50 years who participate in recreational sports (weekend warrior). This condition also occurs in serious athletes.[80] Chronic oral corticosteroid administration and fluoroquinolone usage predispose to rupture.[94-97] Rupture of the Achilles tendon occurs most commonly at the narrowest portion of the tendon, approximately 2 to 6 inches above its point of attachment to the calcaneus.[98]

Mechanism of Injury

The mechanisms of injury include an extra stretch applied to a taut tendon, forceful dorsiflexion with the ankle in a relaxed state, or direct trauma to a taut tendon. Only one-third of patients will have symptoms prior to rupture. Patients report a sudden onset of pain and the sensation that they were struck or kicked in the back of the leg. An audible snap may be heard.

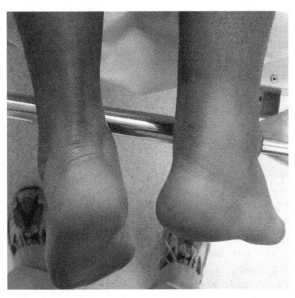

Figure 23–54. Achilles tendon rupture of the right foot. Note the edema in the heel and loss of plantar flexion when compared with the uninjured side.

Examination

The patient complains of acute pain in the lower calf that makes walking almost impossible. A partial tear may be difficult to diagnose and is often misdiagnosed as a strained muscle; however, most Achilles tears are complete.

On examination, diffuse swelling and bruising is present, and there may be loss of plantar flexion (Fig. 23–54). A palpable defect may be present, unless swelling is severe. The patient will have some ability to plantar flex the ankle because of the action of the posterior tibial muscle, but weakness will be noted.

Several clinical tests are described to aid in the diagnosis. The *calf-squeeze test* is performed while the patient lies prone on the examination table with the feet hanging off the edge. The calves are squeezed bilaterally, and the foot is observed for plantar flexion. If a complete rupture is present, little or no foot movement will occur (Fig. 23–55 and Video 23–3). The description of this test is commonly credited to Thompson; however, it was described 5 years earlier by Simmonds.[99-101]

Other tests include the *knee flexion test* and *sphygmomanometer test*. To perform the knee flexion test, the supine patient is asked to flex the knee to 90 degrees. The foot is

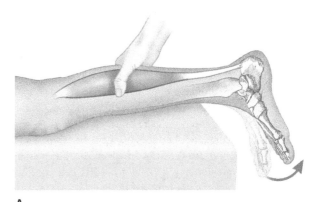

A

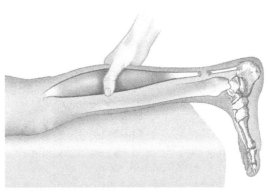

B

Figure 23–55. Thompson test. **A.** When the Achilles mechanism is intact, squeezing the calf will cause plantar flexion of the foot. **B.** In patients with a ruptured Achilles tendon, there is no plantar flexion. *(Used with permission from Melissa Leber, MD.)*

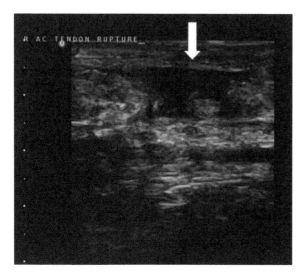

Figure 23–56. Ultrasound of an Achilles tendon rupture. *(Used with permission from Eric Brader, MD.)*

observed during this movement and will fall into neutral or dorsiflexion when a tendon tear is present. The sphygmomanometer test is performed by inflating the cuff to 100 mm Hg while wrapped around the midcalf. The foot is dorsiflexed, and the manometer pressure is noted. When the tendon is intact, the pressure should rise to approximately 140 mm Hg.

Imaging
Radiographs are usually not necessary to make the diagnosis. A lateral radiograph of the ankle may reveal loss of the regular configuration between the superior aspect of the calcaneus and the posterior aspect of the tibia (Kager triangle). When rupture is present, this space becomes smaller. Bedside ultrasound can confirm the diagnosis, but it is an operator-dependent test (Fig. 23–56). MRI can confirm the diagnosis, but it is not required in the ED.

Treatment
Achilles tendon rupture should be treated with ice, analgesics, and immobilization in the "gravity equinus position" with the ankle plantar flexed to a comfortable position. Crutches should be given and the patient instructed not to bear weight. Referral to an orthopedic surgeon should be made within 2 days.

There continues to be controversy regarding the most appropriate treatment for Achilles tendon rupture. There is a suggested ultrasound-based criteria for choosing nonoperative treatment. In ruptures with a gap of greater than 10 mm that were managed nonsurgically, there was a significantly higher rate of re-rupture than nonsurgically treated gaps of less than 10 mm. It was also noted that nonsurgical management of ruptures with a gap of greater than 5 mm led to inferior outcomes for heel-rise height and heel-rise work compared with surgical management. Nonsurgical treatment consists of splint immobilization in 20

degrees of plantar flexion for 2 weeks to allow hematoma consolidation. Following this period, the lower extremity is immobilized in a short-leg cast or removable boot with an elevated heel for 6 to 8 weeks. After immobilization is complete, gradual range of motion is initiated and a 2-cm heel lift is weaned over the next 2 months. Disadvantages of this method include decreased muscle strength due to lengthening of the healed tendon and a higher rate of recurrent rupture (8%–39%).

Surgical treatment is frequently preferred in younger or more athletic patients. Range-of-motion exercises can be initiated 3 to 7 days after surgery, but a walking boot must be worn for 6 weeks. Outcomes after surgery reveal improved strength when compared with nonoperative management. Risk of recurrent rupture is significantly decreased (approximately 5%). Disadvantages of this treatment method include higher costs and postsurgical complications (infection, skin sloughing, nerve injury). In patients whom the diagnosis is delayed for less than 1 week, surgical treatment is generally preferred. If managed nonoperatively, these patients exhibit tendon lengthening upon healing that inhibits muscle strength.

ACHILLES TENDINOPATHY

The Achilles tendon constitutes the distal insertion of the gastrocnemius and soleus muscles into the calcaneus. Achilles tendinopathy is a painful condition due to inflammation of the Achilles tendon. This condition is also referred to as Achilles tendonitis, tenosynovitis, peritendinitis, paratenonitis (acute disease), tendinosis (chronic disease), and achillodynia.

Mechanism of Injury
The acute phase of Achilles tendinopathy is secondary to acute overexertion, blunt trauma, or chronic overuse and muscle fatigue. Achilles tendinopathy is the third most common problem in distance runners and the most frequent injury in ballet dancers. The annual incidence in elite runners is 7% to 9%. Improper muscle flexibility, increased foot pronation, and leg-length discrepancy are other predisposing factors for this condition. It is the most common tendinopathy associated with fluoroquinolone use.

Examination
Patients present with swelling and tenderness around the tendon. Fine crepitus is perceived on motion of the foot due to the presence of fibrin exudate within the tendon. In most cases, the tender region is well localized, and the patient holds the foot plantar flexed to relieve the discomfort. Passive dorsiflexion will aggravate the pain. There is often a palpable nodular thickening over the tendon or peritendinous tissues as previously described. Morning stiffness is common, but pain is typically increased with activity and relieved by rest.

Imaging

The diagnosis is made on clinical grounds. Ultrasonography and MRI are confirmatory but are not necessary.

Treatment

Conservative management includes decreasing activity and elevating the heel inside the shoe with a small felt pad. The runner should be encouraged to perform sustained stretching exercises of the Achilles complex. Oral anti-inflammatory agents may be used, whereas steroid injections should be avoided as they may lead to rupture. Eccentric loading exercises are recommended. Ice is used after activity. If the pain is acute and other measures have not helped, then a short-leg walking cast can be used for 10 days. Injectible therapies such as platelet-rich plasma have had variable results.[111] Operative treatment to release the thickened tenosynovium is recommended in patients who do not respond to a 6-month trial of conservative treatment.[102]

PLANTAR FASCIITIS

This condition is the most common cause of heel pain and represents up to 15% of foot problems.[113,114] The typical patient is 40 to 60 years old, but the condition occurs at an earlier age in runners, where the incidence is as high as 10%.[115] The patient presents with pain on the undersurface of the heel on standing or walking and relief with rest. Frequently, patients note pain after a period of bed rest that lessens after some activity but then becomes severe again after an increased duration of weight bearing.

Mechanism of Injury

Plantar fasciitis develops as an inflammatory and degenerative condition at the site of origin of the plantar fascia (medial tuberosity of the calcaneus). Irritation of the periosteum results in secondary subperiosteal ossification and the development of a bone spur.

The condition is most commonly secondary to overuse. Several risk factors have been identified, including occupations that involve excessive walking or standing, poorly cushioned footwear, obesity, and running. Patients who are excessive pronators (pes planus) or have reduced ankle dorsiflexion are also at a higher risk of developing plantar fasciitis.[113]

Examination

Local tenderness is noted to palpation at the anteromedial surface of the calcaneus where the plantar fascia attaches (Fig. 23–57). Passive dorsiflexion of the toes accentuates the pain. The pain and tenderness are always anterior to the heel with radiation to the sole being a frequent accompaniment.

Associated Injuries

The condition is bilateral in up to one-third of cases. When plantar fasciitis is bilateral, it is associated with rheumatologic conditions such as rheumatoid arthritis, systemic lupus erythematosus, and gout.

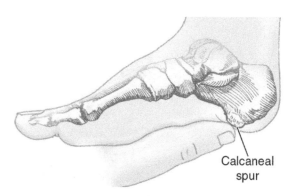

Figure 23–57. Palpation in this area is painful in patients with plantar fasciitis. A calcaneal spur is shown, which is commonly associated with this condition. *(Used with permission from Melissa Leber, MD.)*

Imaging

The diagnosis of plantar fasciitis is a clinical one in most cases. Radiographs or bone scan may be useful to rule out other diagnoses, such as a calcaneal stress fracture.

Radiographs demonstrate a calcaneal bone spur in 50% of cases. Heel spurs occur on the plantar aspect of the calcaneus at the attachment of the plantar aponeurosis, where a bony prominence develops and extends across the plantar surface of the bone. Many patients with a calcaneus spur are asymptomatic, however, and 15% to 25% of the general population have these spurs.[116]

Treatment

Several therapies exist to treat plantar fasciitis, including rest, physical therapy, stretching, change in footwear, arch supports, orthotics, night splints, anti-inflammatory agents, and surgery. With proper treatment, 80% of patients will see a resolution of their symptoms within 12 months. Early treatment within 6 weeks of the development of symptoms is believed to hasten recovery.[113,117]

The ED treatment should include rest, ice, and nonsteroidal anti-inflammatory drugs (NSAIDs). The patient should be instructed to use a heel pad (one-half inch), arch support to reduce the stretch of the plantar fascia, or taping (Fig. 23–58A–C).[116,118] In addition, the patient should be advised not to walk barefoot and to replace worn-out footwear.

Stretching exercises of the Achilles tendon should also be prescribed (Fig. 23–58D). The best method for performing these stretches is to lean against a wall with the forefoot while keeping the heel on the ground and knees straight. The patient should be instructed to stand approximately 1 foot away from the wall with the opposite foot and gradually lean the hips forward until the Achilles is felt to stretch. This position is held for 10 seconds and then repeated three times. The stretch should initially be performed frequently during the day (up to five times) and then continued at a rate of a few a day to prevent recurrence.

Another method that can be employed in the ED is strapping the plantar aspect of the foot. Using a roll of

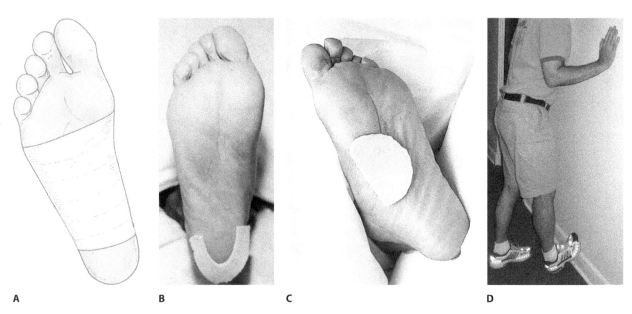

A **B** **C** **D**

Figure 23–58. **A.** Planter fascia taping technique. **B.** Heel pad for treating plantar fasciitis. **C.** Plantar fascia arch support padding. **D.** Stretches for plantar fasciitis.

2-inch tape, several pieces are measured out that extend along the plantar aspect of the foot from the head of the fifth metatarsal to the head of the first metatarsal. The strips are applied so they overlap by one-fourth to one-half inch. The tape should be bow strung in the arch area.

Local steroid–anesthetic injection along the medial aspect of the heel often provides relief but may be associated with fat pad atrophy and is recommended in resistant cases. Steroid injections can be done using ultrasound to guide needle placement.[119,120] Steroid injections may predispose to rupture.[11] In a recent study, the injection of botulinum toxin A in the calf muscles produced faster and more sustained results than intralesional steroids.[121] More recently, a study demonstrated that the injection of botulin toxin directly into the affected foot was significantly better than placebo.[122] Plantar fascial release, including the first layer of intrinsic muscles, has been shown to be effective in recalcitrant cases.[11] Endoscopic plantar fasciotomy is a reasonable option where conservative therapy has failed.[119,123]

HEEL PAD ATROPHY

The calcaneal fat pad is composed of multiple fibroelastic tissue compartments composed of adipose cells. A painful heel pad is due to atrophy of the subcalcaneal fat pad and repetitive heel loading during walking. This condition is common, especially in the elderly. Obesity and prolonged ambulatory activity, particularly on hard floors, aggravates the condition. Furthermore, acute stress on the pad may rupture or strain the compartments, causing temporary loss of compressibility.

On examination, pain is generalized over the whole heel. Pain is especially prominent on standing, and rest gains relief. Radiographs may demonstrate a smooth undersurface of the

calcaneus in some patients; otherwise, they are normal. Conservative treatment includes rest, NSAIDs, and a dispersion pad (U pad). A flexible heel protector is a tight-fitting plastic that cups the heel and squeezes all fat under the calcaneus, providing more cushioning. Over-the-counter, silicone-based heel cushions are also available. To prevent recurrence, shoe modification with heel dispersion padding or a foot orthotic is used, and the patient is referred to an appropriate clinician.

CALCANEAL BURSITIS

Two bursae are involved in inflammatory processes around the heel. The *retrocalcaneal bursa* is located between the calcaneus and the Achilles tendon. The *posterior calcaneal bursa* is located more superficially between the Achilles tendon and the skin (Fig. 23–59).[116]

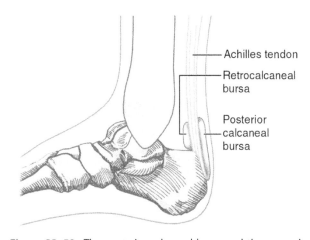

Achilles tendon

Retrocalcaneal bursa

Posterior calcaneal bursa

Figure 23–59. The posterior calcaneal bursa and the retrocalcaneal bursa.

Posterior calcaneal bursitis is usually secondary to friction from ill-fitting shoes and is especially common in women who wear high heels.[124] The bursa is usually distended with fluid and visibly inflamed. In chronic cases, the bursa and overlying skin is thickened with tenderness and swelling noted in the back of the heel. In retrocalcaneal bursitis, the patient complains of pain on motion, and localized tenderness is noted to palpation just anterior to the Achilles tendon.

The treatment of calcaneal bursitis is rest, heat, NSAIDs, and elevation. In patients with posterior calcaneal bursitis, proper fitting shoes with low heels are essential. The back of the shoe may have to be cut out in acute cases. Local anesthetic–steroid injection provides prompt relief of symptoms.

CALCANEAL BONE CYST

A simple bone cyst is a relatively common bone tumor and accounts for about 3% of all bone tumors. Males are more commonly affected in their first and second decades of life. A simple bone cyst can be asymptomatic or it may produce localized pain and swelling. The radiograph demonstrates a cystic structure in the bone. Steroid injection therapy has been shown to be successful and is preferable to surgical curettage.[125]

FOOT STRAIN

Bones and ligaments maintain the normal resting position of the foot. The muscles act to protect the bones and ligaments from excessive stress. Foot pain on standing, therefore, is not muscular in etiology but mechanical, osseous, or ligamentous. Pain on walking, however, may be muscular or from other soft tissues.

The foot has two arches: a *longitudinal arch* and a *transverse arch*. The longitudinal arch extends from the calcaneus to the metatarsal heads. The transverse arch runs across the metatarsals. The arches are maintained by skeletal components held in place by ligaments. The longitudinal arch is maintained by the relationship of the talus and the calcaneus, the interosseous ligaments, the long and short plantars, and the spring ligament. The function of this arch is to provide a springboard for weight bearing and forward motion. When the ligaments are stretched by excessive weight, pressure, or poor muscle tone, the foot is strained. Foot strain can be acute, subacute, or chronic. Acute foot strain is seen most commonly after recent overuse, such as occurs with prolonged standing. Chronic foot strain is secondary to excessive stresses on normal structures or to normal stresses on abnormal structures.

Clinical Presentation

As mentioned, most patients with these injuries have recently increased activity levels. In other cases, excessive weight and exercise or incorrectly fitting shoes may be the causative factors. The patient complains of pain over the inner border of the foot with standing or walking and relief with rest. The patient has tenderness over the strained ligament that is often well localized under the navicular and anterior and posterior arches. Passive dorsiflexion of the foot intensifies the pain, and plantar flexion is usually painless. The patient may have such significant strain that he or she may be unable to bear weight and complains of pain radiating to the calf.

Treatment

The treatment of the acute form of foot strain that is most commonly seen in the ED is rest and hot soaks. Support for the longitudinal arch can be provided with a sponge rubber pad fitted into the shoe. Acute foot strain subsides with simple rest and gradual return to activity. All these patients should be referred for podiatric consultation to avoid complications such as ligamentous elongation, joint inflammation, degeneration, and arthrosis.

METATARSALGIA

Metatarsalgia is characterized by pain and tenderness of the plantar heads of the metatarsals. It occurs when the transverse arch becomes depressed and the middle metatarsal heads bear a disproportionate amount of the weight. It is seen in patients with cavus deformity of the foot and in patients who wear high-heeled shoes.

In normal weight bearing, the first metatarsal head and the two sesamoids bear one-third of the body's weight. In the flattened foot, the second, third, and fourth metatarsal heads bear greater weight. There are many common factors that cause the syndrome of metatarsalgia. These include ligamentous stretching that permits the transverse arch to become more relaxed and subject to strain, muscle weakness of the intrinsics, and traumatic factors. Metatarsalgia is a symptom, not a disease, and refers only to pain around the metatarsal heads.

Clinical Presentation

The patient presents with pain and decreased willingness to bear weight in the forefoot. The dorsum of the foot may be edematous. Tenderness is noted at the middle of the shafts with flexion or extension of the toes. Pain subsides with rest and nonweight bearing but recurs with any exertion. The site of initial tenderness is over the metatarsal heads.

Treatment

The treatment must be directed at the causative factor and is symptomatic initially, which may include anti-inflammatory agents. The patient must be instructed to use low-heeled shoes only. Ultrasound has been used to treat this condition, and metatarsal pads fitted to the patient's foot have yielded good results.[126] Referral to a podiatrist is indicated on a nonurgent basis.

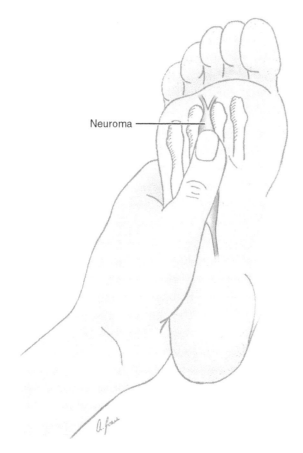

Figure 23–60. Morton neuroma.

MORTON NEUROMA

Morton neuroma is an entrapment neuropathy of the interdigital nerve (Fig. 23–60). This condition most commonly affects middle-age women and is usually unilateral. Morton neuroma is a type of metatarsalgia characterized by sudden attacks of sharp pain that radiate to the toes. The cutaneous branches of the digital nerves divide on the plantar aspect of the transverse metatarsal ligament and supply the nerves to the sides of the toes.

Pathologically, the neuroma is a fusiform swelling occurring proximal to the bifurcation of the nerve that consists primarily of proliferative connective tissue and an amorphous eosinophilic material, which may be the result of a nonspecific inflammatory neuritis or some type of localized arteritis. The deposition of these materials is followed by slow degeneration of the nerve fiber.

Clinical Presentation
The patient usually complains of a *burning pain* localized to the plantar aspect of the metatarsal heads, which *radiates* to the toes and may be accompanied by paresthesias and numbness. The most common site is between the second and third metatarsals. The pain is usually described as a lancinating, sharp pain that feels "like walking on a stone."

Initially, the pain occurs only with walking or standing but later persists even at rest. The patient obtains relief by removing the shoe and massaging the foot. This relieves the pressure between the metatarsal heads.

After these sudden attacks, the tenderness may persist for days. The foot appears normal; however, on firm palpation, one finds a small area of exquisite tenderness located in the web space. In late stages, one may elicit crepitation and palpate a small tumor in the web space. This condition can be differentiated from other causes of metatarsalgia because pressure between the metatarsal heads reproduces the pain.

If the toes are hyperextended at the MTP joint, a throbbing type of pain occurs in the involved toes. The most useful clinical test for the diagnosis of Morton neuroma is to perform a web space compression test. Severe pain is produced by squeezing the metatarsal heads together with one hand and simultaneously compressing the involved web space with the thumb and the index finger of the opposite hand. This compression test can also produce a painful and palpable click known as a Mulder sign.

The clinical assessment was as accurate as ultrasound in the diagnosis of Morton neuroma. The differential diagnosis includes a foreign body, an epithelial cyst, and a traumatic bursitis.

Treatment
There are several important components of the treatment of Morton neuroma. First, the patient's footwear must be examined to make sure that the forefoot and the toe box are large enough. Steroid injection within the affected area followed by ultrasound, forefoot mobilization, and a temporary metatarsal pad will also decrease symptoms. If these conservative measures fail, the patient is referred for surgical treatment, which consists of division of the transverse ligament with or without the excision of the neuroma. Alcohol injections under ultrasound guidance have also been used, which may obviate the need for surgery.

NAVICULAR STRESS FRACTURE

Navicular stress fracture is a relatively uncommon injury most often seen in elite-level athletes with repetitive push-off activities such as sprinters and gymnasts. The navicular most commonly succumbs to stress in the central third. Because this bone is relatively avascular, similar to its counterpart in the wrist, it is prone to developing delayed union or nonunion if not diagnosed and treated properly. The patient will complain of pain that is insidious in onset. Palpation of the proximal dorsal portion of the navicular will elicit tenderness and is the key to making the diagnosis. Like stress fractures in the rest of the body, plain radiography is not sensitive, and the clinician will need to rely on bone scan, CT, or MRI. Treatment includes nonweight-bearing immobilization for 6 weeks followed by a gradual return to activity.[132] Screw fixation is required for those patients that develop nonunion or do not respond to conservative treatment.[131] Some authors have advocated operative fixation to promote an earlier return to sports participation, but this has not been clearly demonstrated.[131,132]

METATARSAL STRESS FRACTURE

No discussion of painful disorders of the forefoot would be complete without including stress fractures of the metatarsals called *March fractures.* The patient usually gives a history of an increase in physical activity with no clear history of preceding trauma.

On examination, there is tenderness at the middle of the shaft of the third metatarsal, which is the one most commonly involved. The pain is worse with ambulation and flexion or extension of the toes and subsides with rest. Initial radiographs are negative, but within 2 weeks, a callus is seen in the midshaft of the metatarsal (Fig. 23–61). MRI has replaced bone scan as the test of choice in patients with negative x-rays but suspected stress fracture.[133]

When the fracture involves the first, third, fourth, and distal aspect of the second metatarsals, the treatment is

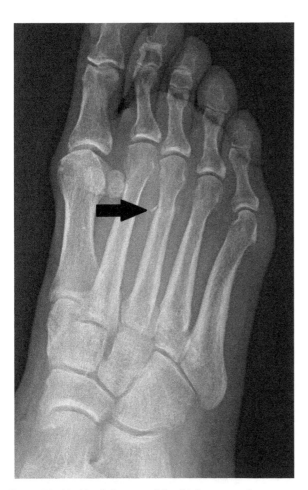

Figure 23–61. March fracture of the third metatarsal.

symptomatic with relative rest. Patients may benefit from a walking boot or crutches if the pain is severe. Once tenderness to palpation and pain with ambulation has resolved, the patient may gradually commence activity. Cardiovascular fitness can be maintained with pool running, or cycling.

Stress fractures at the base of the second metatarsal should be treated with weight-bearing rest for a period of 6 weeks. CT or MRI may be needed to rule out a subtle Lisfranc fracture in this location.[134] Diaphyseal fractures of the fifth metatarsal are prone to nonunion, and these patients should be nonweight bearing for 6 to 10 weeks.[134]

FOREFOOT BURSITIS

Most of the bursae in this area are "adventitial bursa." They are found in the joints of the foot that are exposed to pressure, often from a shoe. The most common sites are as follows:

- Dorsal IP joints of the toes
- Navicular tuberosity
- Medial first MTP joint
- Lateral fifth MTP joint

In acute bursitis, the patient presents with tenderness to palpation of the involved site along with erythema and edema. The treatment includes elimination of the inciting cause. One must protect the area from further irritation using ice therapy, NSAIDs, and steroid injection therapy to relieve swelling and acute pain.

SESAMOIDITIS

The first metatarsal sesamoids can become inflamed following trauma or increased ambulation. Examination demonstrates point tenderness beneath the metatarsal head that increases with dorsiflexion of the MTP joint. Low-heeled shoes and a metatarsal bar proximal to the metatarsal heads are usually satisfactory to alleviate the symptoms. Taping of the great toe, slight plantar flexion, and anti-inflammatory drugs are also useful. If persistent, sesamoid stress fracture needs to be ruled out.

NAVICULAR OSTEOCHONDROSIS

The navicular is the last tarsal bone to ossify and is subject to AVN, which usually occurs between the ages of 4 and 6 years and is often bilateral.[135] The etiology of this disorder is unclear, but the condition is usually self-limited and tends toward spontaneous recovery.

On examination, the patient is most often a boy between the ages of 4 and 10 years who complains of pain over the region of the navicular, usually accompanied by a limp. Palpation elicits tenderness over the navicular, and there is usually no history of trauma.

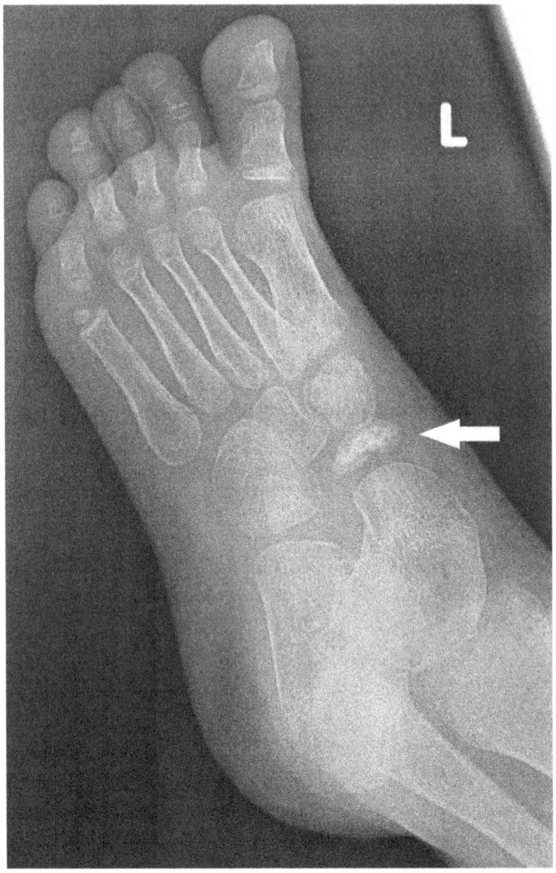

Figure 23–62. Radiograph of a 5-year-old demonstrates increased density and irregular appearance of the tarsal navicular consistent with AVN (*arrow*). *(Used with permission from Melissa Leber, MD.)*

Radiographs of the foot should be obtained with comparison views that demonstrate an increased density and loss of the trabecular pattern of the navicular, which is irregular in outline and often has a crushed appearance (Fig. 23–62).

The treatment consists of protecting the bone in the acute stage with restricted activity and casting for 6 to 8 weeks in more severe cases. Complete ossification occurs in 2 to 3 years, and no permanent disability is expected.

FREIBERG DISEASE

Initially described by Dr. Alfred Freiberg, this entity is an AVN of a metatarsal head, most commonly the second metatarsal. Freiberg disease is five times more common in females than males. There is no consensus on the cause, whether the etiology is repetitive trauma, vascular, or multifactorial.

Clinical Presentation
Most commonly, an adolescent or a female in her early twenties presents with forefoot pain that increases with activity. Stiffness, limp, and vague pain are the primary complaints. Tenderness and decreased range of motion will be noted.

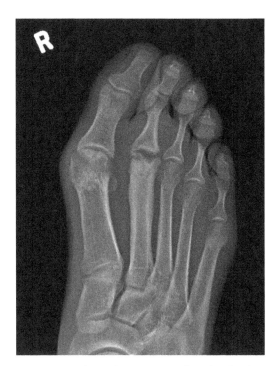

Figure 23–63. Frieberg disease is noted in the distal second metatarsal.

Imaging
Radiographs will demonstrate sclerosis and flattening of the metatarsal head, which may show collapse in more advanced cases (Figs. 23–63 and 23–64).

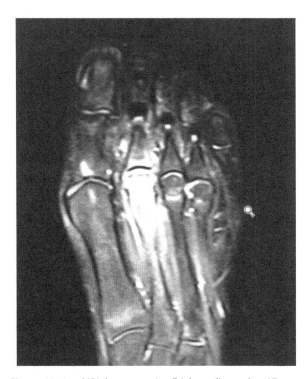

Figure 23–64. MRI demonstrating Frieberg disease in a 17-year-old female. *(Used with permission from Melissa Leber, MD.)*

Treatment

Initial therapy includes anti-inflammatory medications, immobilization, limited weight bearing, and orthopedic follow-up. Further treatments may include physical therapy, orthotics, and steroid injections. Surgery is reserved for refractory cases.[136,138]

SYNOVIAL GANGLION

Synovial herniation occurs after a chronic sprain that is accompanied by weakness of the capsules of one of the many joints of the foot. A frequent site is near the peroneal tendon insertion distal to the lateral malleolus, where it may be quite large. Another site is at the dorsum of the foot. In this case, the ganglion arises along the long extensor tendon sheath or the tarsal joints. The treatment is surgical removal; however, in some cases, aspiration followed by a pressure dressing may yield good results.

ENTRAPMENT NEUROPATHIES

Tarsal Tunnel Syndrome

The tarsal tunnel is located on the medial aspect of the foot posterior to the medial malleolus. It is formed by the flexor retinaculum, which makes up the roof of the tunnel. Tarsal tunnel syndrome results from compression of the posterior tibial nerve within the fibro-osseous tunnel (Fig. 23–65).[139]

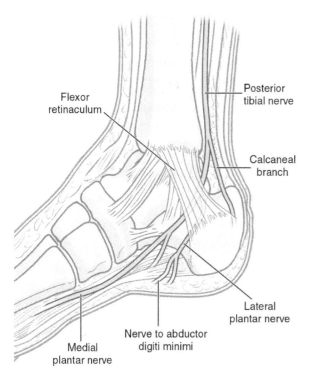

Figure 23–65. Medial view of the ankle demonstrating the course of the posterior tibial nerve within the tarsal tunnel.

Pes planus is a common cause of this condition because increased abduction of the forefoot and valgus deviation of the hindfoot increase tension on the nerve.[124] Tarsal tunnel syndrome is commonly seen in athletes involved in strenuous sporting activities that place a great deal of stress on the tibiotalar joint.[140]

Patients complain of an insidious onset of pain described as burning in nature. It originates at the medial malleolus and radiates to the sole and heel. The pain is increased with activity and decreased with rest. Paresthesia, dysesthesia, and hypesthesia may be present within the same distribution. However, the presentation varies, with some patients complaining of pain only in the metatarsal area and others noting pain along the lateral aspect of the foot. About one-half of patients state that the pain radiates superiorly along the medial side of the calf. Rubbing of the foot seems to offer temporary relief.

The feature that clinches the diagnosis is a *positive Tinel sign*, with pain radiating down the medial or lateral plantar nerve distribution on percussion of the nerve within the canal.[141] Pain is also reproduced by dorsiflexion and eversion of the foot. The diagnosis can be confirmed by nerve conduction studies.

Orthotics, stretching, rest, and NSAIDs are prescribed. Steroid and local anesthetic injection of the tunnel at the point where percussion tenderness is maximal will also be effective in relieving symptoms.[142] Surgical release of the flexor retinaculum is the treatment of choice for this condition, and patients should be appropriately referred when the diagnosis is suspected.[139]

Lateral Plantar and Calcaneal Nerve Entrapment

The posterior tibial nerve gives rise to the medial and lateral plantar nerves and the calcaneal nerve. The lateral plantar and calcaneal nerves can become entrapped between the deep fascia of the abductor hallucis muscle and the medial caudal margin of the quadratus plantar muscle. The result is pain within the nerves' distribution—the heel.

Approximately 10% to 15% of athletes with chronic unresolved heel pain have entrapment of these nerves. The patient presents with chronic heel pain that is dull, aching, or sharp in character. The pain may radiate into the ankle and is intensified by walking or running. Point tenderness over the first branch of the lateral plantar nerve deep to the abductor hallucis muscle is present. Variable success rates have been shown with orthotics. Frequently, these patients require surgical neurolysis.

Medial Plantar Nerve Entrapment

This condition is most commonly known as jogger's foot. Entrapment of the medial calcaneal branch of the posterior tibial nerve causes acute irritation and inflammation and chronic fibrosis and neuroma formation. The patient complains of aching pain along the medial border of the heel that is more severe on weight bearing but does not radiate further into the foot. If the foot is in hyperpronation, this tends to aggravate the condition further. Anti-inflammatory agents and a custom molded orthotic are useful. If the patient does not respond after several months, referral for operative neurolysis is indicated.

Sural Nerve Entrapment

Sural nerve entrapment occurs secondary to recurrent ankle sprains and running. The patient presents with a shooting pain and paresthesias, typically extending to the lateral foot border, which is confirmed by local tenderness, a positive Tinel sign, and occasionally an area of hyperesthesia. A trial of NSAIDs is useful; however, injection therapy should be tried, and orthotics may be necessary. If conservative therapy fails, surgical release usually is definitive.

Ski Boot Compression Syndrome

In this condition, pain is felt on the dorsum of the foot when the *deep peroneal nerve* is injured (Fig. 23-66). The nerve is superficial, and a contusion to the dorsum of the foot or compression by the "tongue" of a ski boot will cause nerve injury and pain. The deep peroneal nerve can

also be entrapped, most commonly under the inferior extensor retinaculum. The superficial peroneal nerve can be entrapped at its exit from the deep fascia. Recurrent ankle sprains or repetitive trauma from running causes both of these entrapment neuropathies.

This nerve supplies sensation to the area between the first and second toes, and the patient has pain radiating to this region. When entrapment is the cause, the pain is reproduced with either dorsiflexion or plantar flexion. Superficial neuropathy is suggested by pain; paresthesias; or numbness over the outer border of the distal calf, dorsum of the foot, and ankle, but sparing the first web space.

On examination, light palpation evokes severe pain over the dorsum of the foot. When entrapment is the cause, there may be point tenderness where the nerve emerges from the deep fascia. Sensation in the web space between the first and second toes is almost absent, and the sensation over the remainder of the dorsum of the foot is decreased.

For ski boot compression syndrome, the treatment includes elevation of the extremity, ice packs, and mild analgesics, with resolution usually occurring in 36 hours; however, sensation may not return to normal for up to 4 weeks. In refractory cases, injection of steroids is recommended. Entrapment neuropathies are also treated with conservative modalities such as NSAIDs, orthotics, or injection therapy. Neurolysis is reserved for cases of intractable pain or atrophy.

DIABETIC FOOT ULCERS AND INFECTION

Diabetic foot ulcers are common conditions seen in the ED. They develop in 15% of diabetics. In diabetics that require foot amputation, 85% had ulceration initially. Foot ulcers occur in diabetics with and without neuropathy. The annual incidence of foot ulcers is 2% in diabetics but increases to 7.5% in diabetics with peripheral neuropathy. Peripheral neuropathy results in a loss of protective mechanisms because the patient can no longer sense when an injury has occurred. Other predisposing factors in the development of a diabetic foot ulcer include calluses, peripheral vascular disease, and deformity. Trauma is a common precipitant, which may be as minor as improperly fitted shoes.

The evaluation of a patient with foot ulceration should include a thorough sensory examination and palpation of the peripheral pulses. If foot pulses are present, neuropathy is the major cause of the ulcer. Ischemic ulcers should be recognized by clinical examination and evaluated for the possible need of revascularization. Neuropathic ulcers are subdivided into mild, moderate, or severe, depending on the depth of the ulcer and the presence or absence of bone involvement.

Infection is a common complication (Fig. 23-67A). The ulcer provides an easy entry for bacteria in a patient with a diminished resistance to infection. Infection is defined as the presence of local signs and symptoms (erythema,

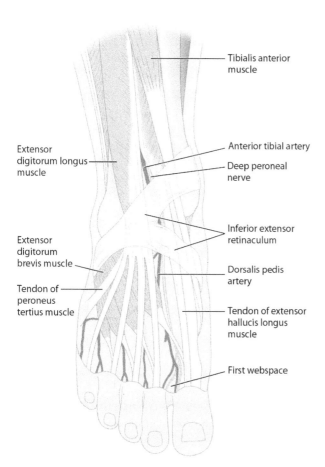

Tibialis anterior muscle

Extensor digitorum longus muscle

Anterior tibial artery

Deep peroneal nerve

Inferior extensor retinaculum

Extensor digitorum brevis muscle

Dorsalis pedis artery

Tendon of peroneus tertius muscle

Tendon of extensor hallucis longus muscle

First webspace

Figure 23–66. Anterior view of the foot demonstrating the deep peroneal nerve.

warmth, induration, and pain) combined with either systemic symptoms or purulent discharge. Infections are typically polymicrobial with aerobic gram-positive, gram-negative, and anaerobic organisms present. Osteomyelitis is present in up to two-thirds of diabetic foot ulcers.[146] The ability to touch bone with a blunt sterile instrument had a positive predictive value for osteomyelitis of 89% in one study.[147] A radiograph should be obtained to look for evidence of osteomyelitis (bone destruction or periosteal reaction) or gas in the surrounding soft tissues (Fig. 23–67B). When infection is present, a deep-tissue culture should be obtained and is superior to superficial swab specimens for identifying the causative organism.[148]

Treatment

The treatment of neuropathic ulcers includes the avoidance of pressure to the ulcer (i.e., nonweight bearing with crutches or a walking cast/shoe). Debridement of necrotic tissue, callus, and infected foreign material is crucial and best performed with a scalpel.[145] Soaking of the wound macerates the tissue but does not debride the necrotic tissue and should be avoided. Enzymatic chemical debridement and whirlpool soaks are not useful. Surgical treatment is indicated for severe claudication, intractable rest pain, necrosis, or nonresponding ulcers.[149]

The choice of dressing is important. A sterile nonadherent gauze dressing is preferred to either plain gauze or occlusive/semiocclusive dressing. Newer dressings contain cellulose or collagen–protease modulating materials or hyaluronan and are designed to promote healing.[145]

Clinical signs of infection are treated with antibiotics. Empiric choices for mild foot infections include clindamycin, levofloxacin, trimethoprim–sulfamethoxazole, or amoxicillin–clavulanic acid for outpatient therapy. Intravenous antibiotics for inpatient care include imipenem, piperacillin–tazobactam, or broad-spectrum cephalosporins. Vancomycin should also be considered to cover resistant gram-positive organisms. Soft-tissue infections usually require 1 to 2 weeks of therapy, whereas patients with osteomyelitis require 6 weeks or more of treatment. Surgical debridement of infected bone is also important in eradicating osteomyelitis.

One of the most important aspects in treating patients with diabetic foot ulcers is to make certain that they are referred to an appropriate clinic where preventive care at 2- to 3-month intervals can be performed. Blood sugar control, pressure reduction, debridement, and antibiotics when necessary are critical measures. Preventive care includes nail care and removal of any calluses as well as fitting the patient with appropriate shoes.

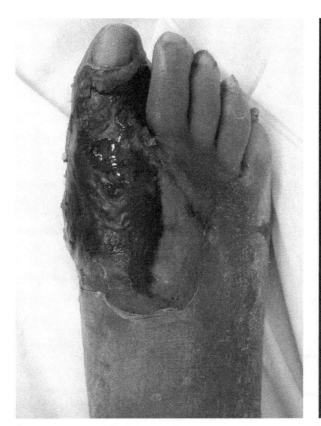
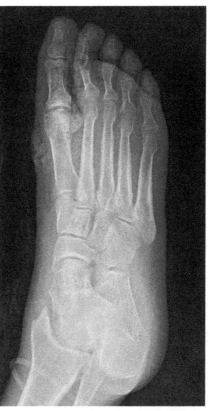

A   B

Figure 23–67. A. A necrotic diabetic foot infection. **B.** Radiograph of the same patient demonstrating gas in the tissues.

PLANTAR WARTS

Verruca vulgaris are common and occur on the plantar surface of the feet. Plantar warts cause significant pain with standing and walking. These lesions appear as a firm white growth, which is flat or raised. Warts can be differentiated from calluses and corns by superficial sharp debridement of the lesions, which reveals punctate black dots that are thrombosed capillary vessels in patients with warts. Spontaneous regression is quite common in children, with almost 50% of warts disappearing within 6 months. Unfortunately, warts are more persistent in adults. Mosaic warts can occur when small warts coalesce.

Treatments can be categorized as topical, intralesional, oral, and destructive. Large plantar warts are treated conservatively with weekly paring and the application of a keratolytic agent such as salicylic acid. Painful lesions are treated with more invasive techniques, including cryotherapy with liquid nitrogen, local curettage, laser therapy, and electrosurgery. These patients should be referred for therapy.

Although surgical removal has been shown to be effective, complications include pain and wound healing. Topical treatments use salicyclic acid preparations, podophyllotoxin, retinoids, silver nitrate, and topical immunotherapeutic agents. The early success of intralesional immunomodulators is a promising treatment that requires further study.

INGROWN TOENAIL

The ingrown toenail, or onychocryptosis, is a commonly occurring problem that is easily treated in the ED (Fig. 23–68). This condition must be distinguished from subungual exostosis, which is a benign condition that can look like an ingrown nail. An ingrown toenail occurs when the lateral margins of the nail dig into the surrounding nail fold and cause discomfort that may lead to a paronychial infection. The causes of this condition include excessive external pressure (i.e., poorly fitted shoes), improperly trimmed nails, or hyperhidrosis. The condition is most common in 20- to 30-year-old individuals, and most often involves the great toe.

The treatment depends on the stage at which the condition is seen. In the early stages, the examiner will notice only erythema and some swelling of the nail fold where the nail is penetrating the skin. At this stage, treatment should consist of warm soaks and elevation of the leading corner of the nail with a cotton pledget soaked in an antiseptic solution. The patient should be advised on how to trim the nails properly and cautioned against wearing shoes that are narrow or have a high heel.

In the later stages, when the nail fold is acutely inflamed or there is a paronychial infection, excision of the lateral nail plate is accompanied by lateral matricectomy. To perform this procedure, the great toe is prepped with povidone–iodine solution and blocked with a local anesthetic (Video 23–4). A fine pair of scissors or hemostat is used to carefully lift the lateral nail plate. A scissors is then used to cut the nail plate and the nail is removed. The nail matrix is now exposed and the tissue can be ablated with a cotton-tipped applicator soaked with phenol or electrocautery (Fig. 23–69 and Video 23–5). It is important that the nail matrix is ablated beneath the nail fold or a portion of the nail will grow back.

SUBUNGUAL EXOSTOSIS

This is an uncommon benign bony tumor that manifests as a painful, firm hyperkeratotic nodule at the free edge of the nail plate. Subungual exostosis forms over the distal portion of the distal phalanx and is most common in the great toe. The patient presents with complaints of pain and swelling along with increased sensitivity of the toe over the exostosis. The toe deviates laterally, causing difficulty with walking. Subungual exostosis more commonly affects women than men by a ratio of 2:1. Most lesions occur in children and young adults. The treatment for the condition is surgical removal.

HALLUX VALGUS

Hallux valgus (bunion) is a deformity in which the large toe deviates laterally and a bony prominence develops over the medial aspect of the first metatarsal head and neck. The medial portion of the first metatarsal head enlarges, and a bursa forms over the medial MTP joint that may become inflamed and thickened. It is this bursitis that may

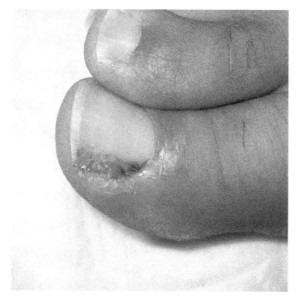

Figure 23–68. Ingrown toenail.

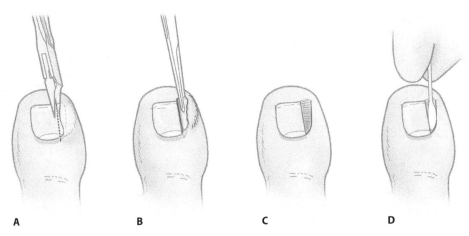

Figure 23–69. Ingrown toenail removal. **A.** After a hemostat is used to elevate the ingrown toenail, cut the nail plate with scissors. **B.** The lateral portion of the nail plate is removed. **C.** The nail matrix is now exposed. **D.** A cotton-tipped applicator soaked in phenol is used to destroy the nail bed matrix of the toe so this portion of the toenail does not grow back.

bring the patient to the ED. Treatment is the application of warm moist soaks to the region. A pad is placed over the medial aspect of the toe for comfort. A large number of different surgical procedures have been described for this common condition. These patients should be referred to a podiatrist for definitive care.

REFERENCES

1. Bachman LM, Kolb E, Koller MT, Steurer J, ter Reit G. Accuracy of Ottawa ankle rules to exclude fractures of the ankle and mid-foot: systemic review. *BMJ.* 2003;326:417–420.
2. Pearse EO, Klass B, Bendall SP. The "ABC" of examining foot radiographs. *Ann R Coll Surg Engl.* 2005;87(6):449–451.
3. Ekinci S, Polat O, Gunalp M, et al. The accuracy of ultrasound evaluation in foot and ankle trauma. *Am J Emerg Med.* 2013;31:1551–1555.
4. Atilla OD, Yesilaras M, Kilic TY, et al. The accuracy of bedside ultrasound as a diagnostic tool for fractures in the ankle and foot. *Acad Emerg Med.* 2014;21:1058–1061.
5. Hanlon DP. Leg, ankle, and foot injuries. *Emerg Med Clin North Am.* 2010;28(4):885–905.
6. Germann CA, Perron AD, Miller MD, Powell SM, Brady WJ. Orthopedic pitfalls in the ED: calcaneal fractures. *Am J Emerg Med.* 2004;22(7):607–611.
7. Perron AD, Brady WJ. Evaluation and management of the high-risk orthopedic emergency. *Emerg Med Clin North Am.* 2003;21(1):159–204.
8. Richman JD, Barre PS. The plantar ecchymosis sign in fractures of the calcaneus. *Clin Orthop.* 1986;207:122–125.
9. Lim EV, Leung JP. Complications of intraarticular calcaneal fractures. *Clin Orthop.* 2001;(391):7–16.
10. Newton EJ, Love J. Emergency department management of selected orthopedic injuries. *Emerg Med Clin North Am.* 2007;25(3):763–776.
11. Loucks C, Buckley R. Bohler's angle: correlation with outcome in displaced intra-articular calcaneal fractures. *J Orthop Trauma.* 1999;13(8):554–558.
12. Miric A, Patterson BM. Pathoanatomy of intra-articular fractures of the calcaneus. *J Bone Joint Surg Am.* 1998;80(2):207–212.
13. Kalsi R, Dempsey A, Benney EB. Compartment syndrome of the foot after calcaneal fracture. *J Emerg Med.* 2012;43(2):e101–e106.
14. Macey LR, Benirschke SK, Sangeorzan BJ, Hansen ST. Acute calcaneal fractures: treatment options and results. *J Am Acad Orthop Surg.* 1994;2(1):36–43.
15. Barei DP, Bellabarba C, Sangeorzan BJ, Benirschke SK. Fractures of the calcaneus. *Orthop Clin North Am.* 2002;33(1):263–285.
16. Dooley P, Buckley R, Tough S, et al. Bilateral calcaneal fractures: operative versus nonoperative treatment. *Foot Ankle Int.* 2004;25(2):47–52.
17. Mora S, Thordarson DP, Zionts LE, et al. Pediatric calcaneal fractures. *Foot Ankle Int.* 2001;22(6):471–477.
18. Thermann H, Krettek C, Hufner T, Schratt HE, Albrecht K, Tscherne H. Management of calcaneal fractures in adults. Conservative versus operative treatment. *Clin Orthop.* 1998;353:107–124.
19. Sanders R. Intra-articular fractures of the calcaneus: present state of the art. *J Orthop Trauma.* 1992;6(2):252–265.
20. Rosenthal R, Tenenbaum S, Thein R, et al. Sequelae of undiagnosed foot compartment syndrome after calcaneal fractures. *J Foot Ankle Surg.* 2013;52:158–161.
21. Worsham JR, Elliott MR, Harris AM. Open calcaneal fractures and associated injuries. *J Foot Ankle Surg.* 2016;55:68–71.
22. Archdeacon M, Wilber R. Fractures of the talar neck. *Orthop Clin North Am.* 2002;33(1):247–262.
23. Lin S, Hak DJ. Management of talar neck fractures. *Orthopedics.* 2011;34(9):715–721.
24. Vallier HA, Nork SE, Barei DP, et al. Talar neck fractures: results and outcomes. *J Bone Joint Surg Am.* 2004;86A(8):1616–1624.
25. Judd DB, Kim DH. Foot fractures frequently misdiagnosed as ankle sprains. *Am Fam Physician.* 2002;66(5):785–794.
26. Haapamaki VV, Kiuru MJ, Koskinen SK. Ankle and foot injuries: analysis of MDCT findings. *AJR Am J Roentgenol.* 2004;183(3):615–622.

27. Adelaar RS. The treatment of complex fractures of the talus. *Orthop Clin North Am.* 1989;20(4):691–707.

28. Funk JR, Srinivasan SC, Crandall JR. Snowboarder's talus fractures experimentally produced by eversion and dorsiflexion. *Am J Sports Med.* 2003;31(6):921–928.

29. Valderrabano V, Perren T, Ryf C, Hintermann B. Snowboarder's talus fracture: treatment outcome of 20 cases after 3.5 years. *Am J Sports Med.* 2005;33(6):871–880.

30. Boon AJ, Smith J, Zobitz ME, Amrami KM. Snowboarder's talus fracture. Mechanism of injury. *Am J Sports Med.* 2001; 29(3):333–338.

31. Yan AY, Mesfin M, Schon LC. Lateral process talus fracture in a kayaking injury. *Orthopedics.* 2011;34(4):296–299.

32. Miller CM, Winter WG, Bucknell AL, Jonassen EA. Injuries to the midtarsal joint and lesser tarsal bones. *J Am Acad Orthop Surg.* 1998;6(4):249–258.

33. Rockett MS, Brage ME. Navicular body fractures: computerized tomography findings and mechanism of injury. *J Foot Ankle Surg.* 1997;36(3):185–191.

34. Valkosky GJ, Pachuda NM, Brown W. Midfoot fractures. *Clin Podiatr Med Surg.* 1995;12(4):773–789.

35. Davis CA, Lubowitz J, Thordarson DB. Midtarsal fracture-subluxation. Case report and review of the literature. *Clin Orthop.* 1993;(292):264–268.

36. Hsu J-C, Chang J-H, Wang S-J, Wu S-S. The nutcracker fracture of the cuboid in children: a case report. *Foot Ankle Int.* 2004;25(6):423–425.

37. van Raaij TM, Duffy PJ, Buckley RE. Displaced isolated cuboid fractures: results of four cases with operative treatment. *Foot Ankle Int.* 2010;31(3):242–246.

38. Mehlhorn AT, Schmal H, Legrand MA, et al. Classification and outcome of fracture-dislocation of the cuneiform bones. *J Foot Ankle Surg.* 2016;55:1249–1255.

39. Rosenbaum A, Dellenbaugh S, DiPreta J, Uhl R. Subtle injuries to the Lisfranc joint. *Orthopedics.* 2011;34(11): 882–887.

40. Saab M. Lisfranc fracture-dislocation: an easily overlooked injury in the emergency department. *Eur J Emerg Med.* 2005; 12(3):143–146.

41. Perron AD, Brady WJ, Keats TE. Orthopedic pitfalls in the ED: Lisfranc fracture-dislocation. *Am J Emerg Med.* 2001; 19(1):71–75.

42. Philbin T, Rosenberg G, Sferra JJ. Complications of missed or untreated Lisfranc injuries. *Foot Ankle Clin.* 2003;8(1): 61–71.

43. Gupta RT, Wadhwa RP, Learch TJ, Herwick SM. Lisfranc injury: imaging findings for this important but often-missed diagnosis. *Curr Probl Diagn Radiol.* 2008;37(3):115–126.

44. Thompson MC, Mormino MA. Injury to the tarsometatarsal joint complex. *J Am Acad Orthop Surg.* 2003;11(4):260–267.

45. Latterman C, Goldstein JL, Wukich DK, Bach BR Jr. Practical management of Lisfranc injuries in athletes. *Clin J Sport Med.* 2007;17:311–315.

46. Vosbikian M, O'Neill JT, Piper C, Huang R, Raikin SM. Outcomes after percutaneous reduction and fixation of low-energy Lisfranc injuries. *Foot Ankle Int.* 2017;38(7):710–715. doi:10.1177/1071100717706154. Epub 2017 May 8.

47. Raikin SM, Elias I, Dheer S, Besser MP, Morrison WB, Zoga AC. Prediction of midfoot instability in the subtle Lisfranc injury. *J Bone Joint Surg Am.* 2009;91:892–899.

48. Englanoff G, Anglin D, Hutson HR. Lisfranc fracture-dislocation: a frequently missed diagnosis in the emergency department. *Ann Emerg Med.* 1995;26(2):229–233.

49. Ross G, Cronin R, Hauzenblas J, Juliano P. Plantar ecchymosis sign: a clinical aid to diagnosis of occult Lisfranc tarsometatarsal injuries. *J Orthop Trauma.* 1996;10(2):119–122.

50. Zgonis T, Roukis TS, Polyzois VD. Lisfranc fracture-dislocations: current treatment and new surgical approaches. *Clin Podiatr Med Surg.* 2006;23(2):303–322.

51. Armagan OE, Shereff MJ. Injuries to the toes and metatarsals. *Orthop Clin North Am.* 2001;32(1):1–10.

52. Schenck RC Jr, Heckman JD. Fractures and dislocations of the forefoot: operative and nonoperative treatment. *J Am Acad Orthop Surg.* 1995;3(2):70–78.

53. Fetzer GB, Wright RW. Metatarsal shaft fractures and fractures of the proximal fifth metatarsal. *Clin Sports Med.* 2006; 25:139–150.

54. Shuen WM, Boulton C, Batt ME, Moran C. Metatarsal fractures and sports. *Surgeon.* 2009;7:86–88.

55. Den Hartog BD. Fracture of the proximal fifth metatarsal. *J Am Acad Orthop Surg.* 2009;17(7):458–464.

56. Nunley JA. Fractures of the base of the fifth metatarsal: the Jones fracture. *Orthop Clin North Am.* 2001;32(1):171–180.

57. Rosenberg GA, Sferra JJ. Treatment strategies for acute fractures and nonunions of the proximal fifth metatarsal. *J Am Acad Orthop Surg.* 2000;8(5):332–338.

58. DeVries JG, Taefi E, Bussewitz BW, et al. The fifth metatarsal base: anatomic evaluation regarding fracture mechanism and treatment algorithms. *J Foot Ankle Surg.* 2015; 54:94–98.

59. Jones SL, Phillips M. Early identification of foot and lower limb stress fractures using diagnostic ultrasonography: a review of 3 cases. *Foot Ankle Online J.* 2010;3(4):3. doi:10.3827/faoj.2010.0304.0003.

60. Akimau PI, Cawthron KL, Dakin WM, Chadwick C, Blundell CM, Davies MB. Symptomatic treatment or cast immobilisation for avulsion fractures of the base of the fifth metatarsal: a prospective, randomised, single-blinded non-inferiority controlled trial. *Bone Joint J.* 2016;98-B(6):806–811. doi:10.1302/0301-620X.98B6.36329.

61. Hatch RL, Alsobrook JA, Clugston JR. Diagnosis and management of metatarsal fractures. *Am Fam Physician.* 2007; 76:817–826.

62. Ferguson KB, McGlynn J, Jenkins P, et al. Fifth metatarsal fractures—is routing follow-up necessary? *Injury.* 2015;46(8):1664–16648.

63. Parekh S, Baravarian B, Pedowitz D, et al. Treatment of fifth metatarsal fractures in adults. *Foot Ankle Spec.* 2016; 9(1):48–51.

64. Polzer H, Polzer S, Mutschler W, et al. Acute fractures to the proximal fifth metatarsal bone: development of classification and treatment recommendations based on the current evidence. *Injury.* 2012;43(10):1626–1632.

65. Marecek GS, Earhart JS, Croom WP, et al. Treatment of acute Jones fractures without weightbearing restriction. *J Foot Ankle Surg.* 2016;55(5):961–964.

66. Carreira DS, Sandilands SM. Radiographic factors and effect of fifth metatarsal Jones and diaphyseal stress fractures on participation in the NFL. *Foot Ankle Int.* 2013;34(4): 518–522.

67. Japjec M, Staresinic M, Starjacki M, et al. Treatment of proximal fifth metatarsal bone fractures in athletes. *Injury*. 2015; 46(suppl 6):S134–S136.

68. Portland G, Kelikian A, Kodros S. Acute surgical management of Jones' fractures. *Foot Ankle Int*. 2003;24(11): 829–833.

69. Mologne TS, Lundeen JM, Clapper MF, O'Brien TJ. Early screw fixation versus casting in the treatment of acute Jones fractures. *Am J Sports Med*. 2005;33:970–975.

70. Van Vliet-Koppert ST, Cakir H, Van Lieshout EM, De Vries MR, Van Der Elst M, Schepers T. Demographics and functional outcome of toe fractures. *J Foot Ankle Surg*. 2011;50(3):307–310. doi:10.1053/j.jfas.2011.02.003. Epub 2011 Mar 25.

71. Hatch RL, Hacking S. Evaluation and management of toe fractures. *Am Fam Physician*. 2003;68(12):2413–2418.

72. Eves TB, Oddy MJ. Do broken toes need follow-up in the fracture clinic? *J Foot Ankle Surg*. 2016;55:488–491.

73. Bryant J, Levis JT. Subtalar dislocation. *West J Emerg Med*. 2009;10(2):92.

74. Pesce D, Wethern J, Patel P. Rare case of medial subtalar dislocation from a low-velocity mechanism. *J Emerg Med*. 2011; 41(6):e121–e124.

75. Sharda P, DuFosse J. Lateral subtalar dislocation. *Orthopedics*. 2008;31(7):718.

76. Love JN, Dhindsa HS, Hayden DK. Subtalar dislocation: evaluation and management in the emergency department. *J Emerg Med*. 1995;13(6):787–793.

77. Bibbo C, Lin SS, Abidi N, et al. Missed and associated injuries after subtalar dislocation: the role of CT. *Foot Ankle Int*. 2001;22(4):324–328.

78. de Palma L, Santucci A, Marinelli M, Borgogno E, Catalani A. Clinical outcome of closed isolated subtalar dislocations. *Arch Orthop Trauma Surg*. 2008;128(6):593–598.

79. Jerome JT. Antero-lateral subtalar dislocation. *J Foot Ankle Surg*. 2008;14(1):36–39.

80. Bibbo C, Anderson RB, Davis WH. Injury characteristics and the clinical outcome of subtalar dislocations: a clinical and radiographic analysis of 25 cases. *Foot Ankle Int*. 2003; 24(2):158–163.

81. Barg A, Tochigi Y, Amendola A, Phisitkul P, Hintermann B, Saltzman CL. Subtalar instability: diagnosis and treatment. *Foot Ankle Int*. 2012;33(2):151–160.

82. Ruhlmann FR, Poujardieu C, Vernois J, Gayet LE. Isolated acute traumatic subtalar dislocations: review of 13 cases at a mean follow-up of 6 years and literature review. *J Foot Ankle Surg*. 2017;56(1):201–207. doi:10.1053/j.jfas.2016.01.044. Epub 2016 Mar 2.

83. McCormick JJ, Anderson RB. Rehabilitation following turf toe injury and plantar plate repair. *Clin Sports Med*. 2010; 29:313–323.

84. Woon CY. Dislocation of the interphalangeal joint of the great toe: is percutaneous reduction of an incarcerated sesamoid an option? *J Bone Joint Surg Am*. 2010;92:1257–1260.

85. Towater LJ, Heron S. Foot compartment syndrome: a rare presentation to the emergency department. *J Emerg Med*. 2013;44(2):e235–e238.

86. Manoli A, Fakhouri AJ, Weber TG. Concurrent compartment syndromes of the foot and leg. *Foot Ankle*. 1993; 14(6):339.

87. Myerson MS, Berger BI. Isolated medial compartment syndrome of the foot: a case report. *Foot Ankle Int*. 1996;17(3): 183–185.

88. Towater LJ, Heron S. Foot compartment syndrome: a rare presentation to the emergency department. *J Emerg Med*. 2013;44(2):e235–e238.

89. Fitzgerald RH Jr, Cowan JD. Puncture wounds of the foot. *Orthop Clin North Am*. 1975;6(4):965–972.

90. Resnick CD, Fallat LM. Puncture wounds: therapeutic considerations and a new classification. *J Foot Surg*. 1990; 29(2):147–153.

91. Miron D, Raz R, Kaufman B, Fridus B. Infections following nail puncture wound of the foot: case reports and review of the literature. *Isr J Med Sci*. 1993;29(4):194–197.

92. Rubin G, Chezar A, Raz R, et al. Nail puncture wound through a rubber-soled shoe: a retrospective study of 96 adult patients. *J Foot Ankle Surg*. 2010;49:421–425.

93. Brook JW. Management of pedal puncture wounds. *J Foot Ankle Surg*. 1994;33(5):463–466.

94. Maffulli N. Rupture of the Achilles tendon. *J Bone Joint Surg Am*. 1999;81(7):1019–1036.

95. Raikin SM, Garras DN, Krapchev PV. Achilles tendon injuries in a United States population. *Foot Ankle Int*. 2013; 34(4):475–480.

96. Budny AM, Ley AN. Fluoroquinolone-mediated Achilles rupture: a case report and review of the literature. *J Foot Ankle Surg*. 2015;54:494–496.

97. Cetti R, Christensen SE, Ejsted R, Jensen NM, Jorgensen U. Operative versus nonoperative treatment of Achilles tendon rupture. A prospective randomized study and review of the literature. *Am J Sports Med*. 1993;21(6): 791–799.

98. Ufberg J, Harrigan RA, Cruz T, Perron AD. Orthopedic pitfalls in the ED: Achilles tendon rupture. *Am J Emerg Med*. 2004;22(7):596–600.

99. Simmonds FA. The diagnosis of the ruptured Achilles tendon. *Practitioner*. 1957;179(1069):56–58.

100. Thompson TC, Doherty JH. Spontaneous rupture of tendon of Achilles: a new clinical diagnostic test. *J Trauma*. 1962;2:126–129.

101. Thompson TC. A test for rupture of the tendon Achilles. *Acta Orthop Scand*. 1962;32:461–465.

102. Saltzman CL, Tearse DS. Achilles tendon injuries. *J Am Acad Orthop Surg*. 1998;6(5):316–325.

103. Mazzone MF, McCue T. Common conditions of the Achilles tendon. *Am Fam Physician*. 2002;65:1805–1810.

104. Deangelis JP, Wilson KM, Cox CL, Diamond AB, Thomson AB. Achilles tendon rupture in athletes. *J Surg Orthop Adv*. 2009;18:115–121.

105. Bhandari M, Guyatt GH, Siddiqui F, et al. Treatment of acute Achilles tendon ruptures: a systematic overview and metaanalysis. *Clin Orthop*. 2002;(400):190–200.

106. Westin O, Nilsson Helander K, Grävare Sibernagel K, Möller M, Kälebo P, Karlsson J. Acute ultrasonography investigation to predict reruptures and outcomes in patients with an Achilles tendon rupture. *Orthop J Sports Med*. 2016; 4(10):2325967116667920. eCollection 2016 Oct.

107. Paavola M, Kannus P, Jarvinen TA, et al. Achilles tendinopathy. *J Bone Joint Surg Am*. 2002;84-A(11):2062–2076.

108. Soma CA, Mandelbaum BR. Achilles tendon disorders. *Clin Sports Med.* 1994;13(4):811–823.

109. Fernandez-Palazzi F, Rivas S, Mujica P. Achilles tendinitis in ballet dancers. *Clin Orthop.* 1990;(257):257–261.

110. Lysholm J, Wiklander J. Injuries in runners. *Am J Sports Med.* 1987;15(2):168–171.

111. Gross CE, Hsu AR, Chahal J, Holmes GB. Injectable treatments for noninsertional Achilles tendinosis: a systematic review. *Foot Ankle Int.* 2013;34(5):619–628.

112. Skjong CC, Meininger AK, Ho SSW. Tendinopathy treatment: where is the evidence? *Clin Sports Med.* 2012;31:329–350.

113. Buchbinder R. Clinical practice. Plantar fasciitis. *N Engl J Med.* 2004;350(21):2159–2166.

114. Elizondo-Rodriguez J, Araujo-Lopez Y, Moreno-Gonzalez JA, Cardenas-Estrada E, Mendoza-Lemus O, Acosta-Olivo C. A comparison of botulinum toxin A and intralesional steroids for the treatment of plantar fasciitis: a randomized, double-blinded study. *Foot Ankle Int.* 2013;34(1):8–14.

115. Ballas MT, Tytko J, Cookson D. Common overuse running injuries: diagnosis and management. *Am Fam Physician.* 1997;55(7):2473–2484.

116. Singh D, Angel J, Bentley G, Trevino SG. Fortnightly review. Plantar fasciitis. *BMJ.* 1997;315(7101):172–175.

117. Young CC, Rutherford DS, Niedfeldt MW. Treatment of plantar fasciitis. *Am Fam Physician.* 2001;63(3):467–468.

118. Saxena A, Fullem B. Plantar fascia ruptures in athletes. *Am J Sports Med.* 2004;32(3):662–665.

119. Urovitz EP, Birk-Urovitz A, Birk-Urovitz E. Endoscopic plantar fasciotomy in the treatment of chronic heel pain. *Can J Surg.* 2008;51(4):281–283.

120. Butcher JD, Salzman KL, Lillegard WA. Lower extremity bursitis. *Am Fam Physician.* 1996;53(7):2317–2324.

121. Ahmad J, Ahmad SH, Jones K. Treatment of plantar fasciitis with botulin toxin: a randomized, controlled study. *Foot Ankle Int.* 2017;38(1):1–7. doi:10.1177/1071100716666364. Epub 2016 Oct 1.

122. Karr SD. Subcalcaneal heel pain. *Orthop Clin North Am.* 1994;25(1):161–175.

123. Cottom JM, Maker JM, Richardson P, Baker JS. Endoscopic debridement for treatment of plantar fasciitis: an innovative technique and prospective study of 46 consecutive patients. *J Foot Ankle Surg.* 2016;55(4):748–752. doi:10.1053/j.jfas.2016.02.005. Epub 2016 Apr 5.

124. Aldridge T. Diagnosing heel pain in adults. *Am Fam Physician.* 2004;70(2):332–338.

125. Smith SB, Shane HS. Simple bone cyst of the calcaneus. A case report and literature review. *J Am Podiatr Med Assoc.* 1994;84(3):127–130.

126. DiDomenico LA, Masternick EB. Anterior tarsal tunnel syndrome. *Clin Podiatr Med Surg.* 2006;23(3):611–620.

127. Brantingham JW, Snyder WR, Michaud T. Morton's neuroma. *J Manipulative Physiol Ther.* 1991;14(5):317–322.

128. Wu KK. Morton's interdigital neuroma: a clinical review of its etiology, treatment, and results. *J Foot Ankle Surg.* 1996;35(2):112–119.

129. Mahadevan D, Venkatesan M, Bhatt R, et al. Diagnostic accuracy of clinical tests for Morton's neuroma with ultrasonography. *J Foot Ankle Surg.* 2015;54:549–553.

130. Hughes RJ, Ali K, Jones H, Connell DA. Treatment of Morton's neuroma with alcohol injection under sonographic guidance: follow-up of 101 cases. *AJR Am J Roentgenol.* 2007;188(6):1535–1539.

131. McCormack JJ, Bray CC, Davis WH, Cohen BE, Jones CP III, Anderson RB. Clinical and computed tomography evaluation of surgical outcomes in tarsal navicular stress fractures. *Am J Sports Med.* 2011;39(8):1741–1748.

132. Torg JS, Moyer J, Gaughan JP, Boden BP. Management of tarsal navicular stress fractures. *Am J Sports Med.* 2010;38(5):1048–1053.

133. McCormack F, Nwachukwu BU, Provencher MT. Stress fractures in runners. *Clin Sports Med.* 2012;31:291–306.

134. Goulart M, O'Malley MJ, Hodgkins CW, Charlton TP. Foot and ankle fractures in dancers. *Clin Sports Med.* 2008;27:295–304.

135. Manusov EG, Lillegard WA, Raspa RF, Epperly TD. Evaluation of pediatric foot problems: part II. The hindfoot and the ankle. *Am Fam Physician.* 1996;54(3):1012–1026, 1031.

136. Love JN, O'Mara S. Freiberg's disease in the emergency department. *J Emerg Med.* 2010;38(4):e23–e25.

137. Carmont MR, Rees RJ, Blundell CM. Current concepts review: Frieberg's disease. *Foot Ankle Int.* 2009;30(2):167–176.

138. Cerrato RA. Frieberg's disease. *Foot Ankle Clin.* 2011;16(4):647–658.

139. Hirose CB, McGarvey WC. Peripheral nerve entrapments. *Foot Ankle Clin.* 2004;9(2):255–269.

140. Kinoshita M, Okuda R, Yasuda T, Abe M. Tarsal tunnel syndrome in athletes. *Am J Sports Med.* 2006;34(8):1307–1312.

141. Barry NN, McGuire JL. Acute injuries and specific problems in adult athletes. *Rheum Dis Clin North Am.* 1996;22(3):531–549.

142. Tallia AF, Cardone DA. Diagnostic and therapeutic injection of the ankle and foot. *Am Fam Physician.* 2003;68(7):1356–1362.

143. Jeffcoate W. The causes of the Charcot syndrome. *Clin Podiatr Med Surg.* 2008;25(1):29–42.

144. Murray HJ, Boulton AJ. The pathophysiology of diabetic foot ulceration. *Clin Podiatr Med Surg.* 1995;12(1):1–17.

145. Boulton AJ, Kirsner RS, Vileikyte L. Clinical practice. Neuropathic diabetic foot ulcers. *N Engl J Med.* 2004;351(1):48–55.

146. Newman LG, Waller J, Palestro CJ, et al. Unsuspected osteomyelitis in diabetic foot ulcers. Diagnosis and monitoring by leukocyte scanning with indium in 111 oxyquinoline. *JAMA.* 1991;266(9):1246–1251.

147. Grayson ML, Gibbons GW, Balogh K, Levin E, Karchmer AW. Probing to bone in infected pedal ulcers. A clinical sign of underlying osteomyelitis in diabetic patients. *JAMA.* 1995;273(9):721–723.

148. Pellizzer G, Strazzabosco M, Presi S, et al. Deep tissue biopsy vs. superficial swab culture monitoring in the microbiological assessment of limb-threatening diabetic foot infection. *Diabet Med.* 2001;18(10):822–827.

149. Giurini JM, Rosenblum BI. The role of foot surgery in patients with diabetes. *Clin Podiatr Med Surg.* 1995;12(1):119–127.

150. Hsu AR, Hsu JW. Topical review: skin infections in the foot and ankle patient. *Foot Ankle Int.* 2012;33(7):612–619.

151. Sinha S, Relhan V, Garg VK. Immunomodulators in warts: unexplored or ineffective? *Indian J Derm*. 2015;60(2):118–129.

152. Esterowitz D, Greer KE, Cooper PH, Edlich RF. Plantar warts in the athlete. *Am J Emerg Med*. 1995;13(4):441–443.

153. Aggarwal K, Gupta S, Jain VK, Mital A, Gupta S. Subungual exostosis. *Indian J Dermatol Venereol Leprol*. 2008;74(2):173–174.

154. Lee SK, Jung MS, Lee YH, Gong HS, Kim JK, Baek GH. Two distinctive subungual pathologies: subungual exostosis and subungual osteochondroma. *Foot Ankle Int*. 2007;28(5):595–601.

155. Zuber TJ. Ingrown toenail removal. *Am Fam Physician*. 2002;65(12):2547–2552, 2554.

156. Noel B. Surgical treatment of ingrown toenail without matricectomy. *Dermatol Surg*. 2008;34(1):79–83.

PART V

Appendix

APPENDIX

Splints, Casts, and Other Techniques

UPPER EXTREMITY

A-1 DISTAL PHALANX SPLINTS

Dorsal Distal Phalanx Splints

Dorsal and volar splints are very useful in treating avulsion fractures of the distal phalanx as discussed in the text. Our preference is the dorsal splint, which provides more support because there is less "padding" on the dorsal aspect of the finger. The splint is in closer contact with the bone. When using these splints, do not hyperextend the distal interphalangeal joint as was previously recommended in older texts. Full extension is the position of choice when applying the splint.

Hairpin Splint

This splint is made from a thin metal strip. It provides protection for distal phalangeal fractures resulting from external injury. This splint provides no structural support.

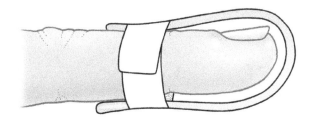

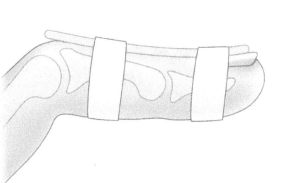

A–2 FINGER SPLINTS

Dorsal and Volar Finger Splints

These splints are fashioned from commercially available metallic splints that have sponge rubber padding on one side. The splint is cut to the proper size and shaped as desired.

The splints should be applied with the metacarpophalangeal joint at 50 degrees of flexion and the interphalangeal joints flexed approximately 15 to 20 degrees.

Dynamic Finger Splinting

The injured finger is splinted to the adjacent normal finger. This provides support of the injured digit while permitting motion of the metacarpophalangeal joint and some motion at the interphalangeal joint. This type of splinting is used commonly in sprains of the collateral ligaments of the interphalangeal joints and other injuries discussed in the text. A piece of cast padding cut to proper size is inserted between the fingers and the two digits are taped together.

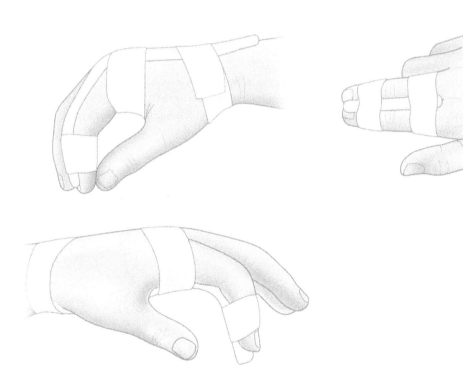

A-3 GUTTER SPLINTS

Ulnar Gutter Splint

Gutter splints are used for the treatment of phalanx and metacarpal fractures. Fractures of the ring and little finger are immobilized in an ulnar gutter splint. The MCP joint should be flexed 50 to 90 degrees, and the PIP and DIP joints are extended. Remember to place a piece of padding between the fourth and fifth digits.

Radial Gutter Splint

Radial gutter splints are used to treat fractures of the index and long fingers. A hole is cut out so that the thumb is free to move normally. Padding is placed between the second and third digits. The position of immobilization of the digits is the same as the ulnar gutter splint (Video A–3A).

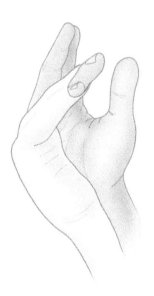

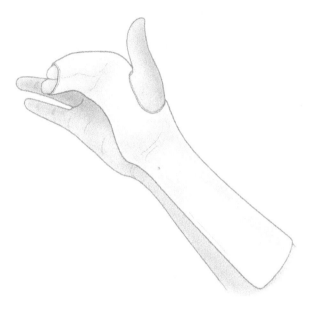

A-3 GUTTER SPLINTS (PLASTER APPLICATION)

The splint is made by using approximately 10 plaster sheets cut to the proper size (Video A-3B).

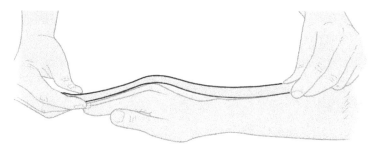

A. The measurement should be from the tip of the finger to a point two-thirds of the way down the forearm.

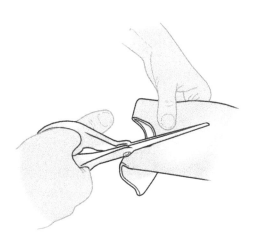

B. When applying a radial gutter splint, cut out a hole for the thumb.

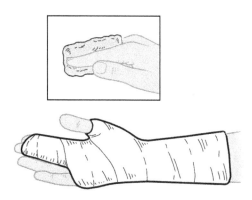

C. Next, apply Webril to the fingers, hand, and forearm, making sure to pad between the fingers.

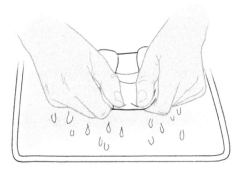

D. The plaster is soaked in warm water, and then the excess is squeezed out.

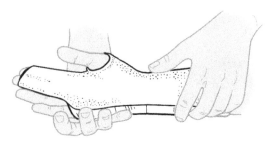

E. The wet plaster is then smoothed out and placed on the patient's extremity.

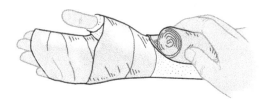

F. A piece of cotton roll (Webril) can be placed on the wet plaster before wrapping the extremity with the elastic bandage. The proper final position for the plaster splint is 50 to 90 degrees of flexion at the metacarpophalangeal joint, 15 degrees of extension at the wrist, and full extension at the interphalangeal joints.

A–4 DORSAL SPLINT WITH EXTENSION HOOD ("CLAM DIGGER") SPLINT

This splint is placed over the dorsum of the forearm and includes the second, third, fourth, and fifth digits. It covers the DIP joint. To decrease swelling and stretch the collateral ligaments during healing, the MCP joint should be flexed 60 to 90 degrees, the PIP and DIP joint are fully extended, and the wrist is extended approximately 15 degrees.

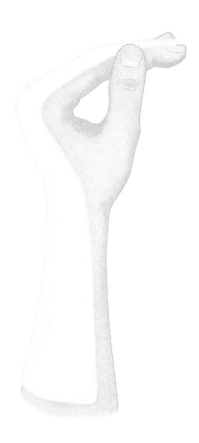

A-5 UNIVERSAL HAND DRESSING

The universal hand dressing is used when treating inflammatory conditions that affect the hand. This is a soft dressing that places the hand in a position that allows for maximal drainage.

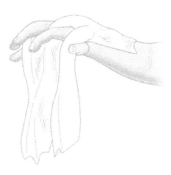

A. In applying this dressing, the fingers are separated by gauze (4 × 4) that is unfolded and layered in between the digits.

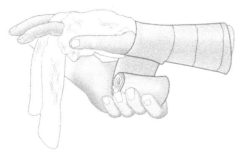

B. Once the gauze sufficiently pads between the fingers, an elastic bandage is applied around the forearm and onto the hand.

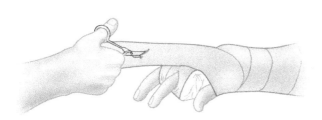

C. When encircling the fingers, the elastic bandage is cut to allow the fingers to go through the bandage.

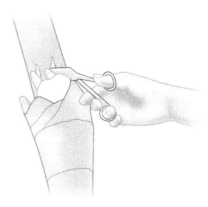

D. In the final stages of encircling the digits, the elastic bandage courses along the palmar aspect of the hand and holes are cut to incorporate the fingers.

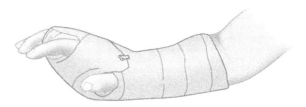

E. The hand is pulled back so the wrist is held in extension and the elastic bandage is secured.

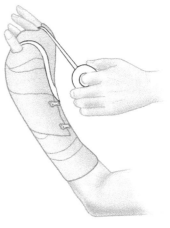

F. To assist in maintaining the wrist at 15 degrees of extension with the fingers separated, tape is used between the fingers, applied from the palmar aspect to the dorsum of the hand so as to pull back the wrist.

A-6 THUMB SPICA CAST

This cast is made by applying stockinette dressing to the arm extending from the hand to the midarm. This is followed by application of cotton bandage (Webril), which is then followed by plaster rolls. The method of applying the plaster rolls is discussed in Chapter 1. Before application of the final roll, the stockinette is folded back over the cast and the final plaster roll is applied.

Note the position of the thumb that must be maintained in applying this cast (abducted with the IP joint in extension as if holding a can of soda). The interphalangeal joint is incorporated in the cast in the figure below, although controversy exists as to whether this is necessary. The fingers are left free so there is full motion of the metacarpophalangeal joints. The position of the wrist shown here is the neutral position. In using this cast for fractures of the scaphoid, we advocate extending it to above the elbow, making it a long-arm cast.

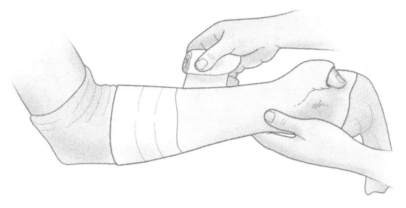

A. Following application of stockinette and cotton padding, wet plaster rolls are applied.

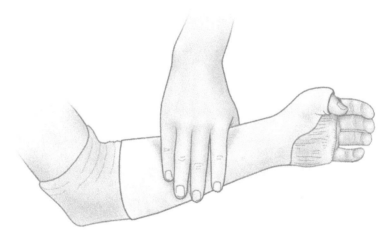

B. Stockinette is folded back before the final roll of plaster.

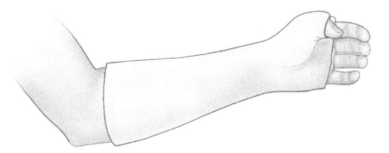

C. Proper positioning of the hand.

A-7 SHORT- AND LONG-ARM THUMB SPICA SPLINTS

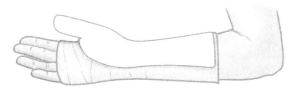

A. The short-arm thumb spica splint is made by applying a plaster slab from the tip of the thumb to approximately two-thirds of the way along the forearm.

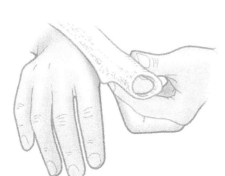

B. In applying the plaster, be certain that the width is enough so the two ends overlap at the distal tip of the thumb.

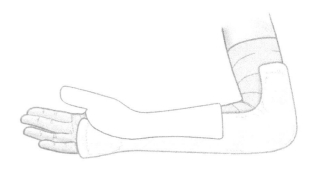

D. To create a long-arm thumb spica splint, add a volar splint to include the wrist and the elbow. If fiberglass is used, a single slap extending beyond the elbow is acceptable.

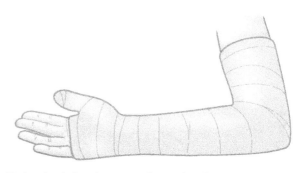

E. An elastic bandage is used over the plaster (Video A-7).

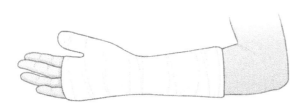

C. An elastic bandage is applied.

A–8 SHORT-ARM CAST

A short-arm cast is used for immobilizing a number of fractures of the forearm. A long-arm cast is produced in a similar fashion except that it is extended above the elbow to approximately the midarm.

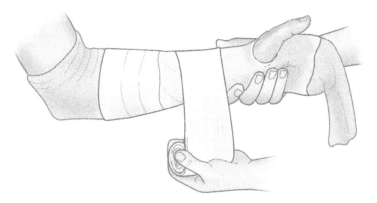

A. The cast is made by applying a stockinette from the fingers to above the elbow. Cotton bandage (Webril) is then applied over the stockinette with the thumb remaining free at the metacarpophalangeal joint and the fingers free at the same level.

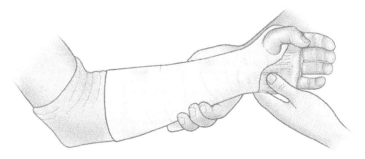

B. Plaster rolls are used while the hand is maintained in position.

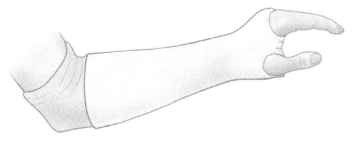

C. The stockinette is folded down over the cast and cut, and the final roll of plaster bandage is then applied. Note that the fingers and thumb are free and the patient is able to use the fingers without any impingement on normal motion.

A-9 LONG-ARM POSTERIOR SPLINT

A long-arm posterior splint is used to immobilize a number of injuries to the elbow and forearm. The splint is produced by wrapping a cotton bandage (Webril) around the forearm from the midpalmar region to the midarm. Next, a posterior plaster splint is applied to the arm held in a position of 90-degree flexion at the elbow and neutral position at the wrist. This is followed by an elastic bandage to hold the posterior slab in position. A sling should be applied after the splint is in position (Video A-9).

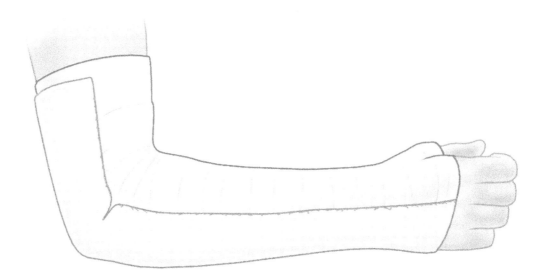

A-10 LONG-ARM ANTERIOR–POSTERIOR SPLINT

This splint is used for fractures of the distal humerus, combined fractures of the radius and ulna, and an unstable distal radius or proximal ulna fracture. Generally speaking, the arm, forearm, and wrist are placed in a position most comfortable for the patient. This position usually conforms to the most relaxed placement of the muscles.

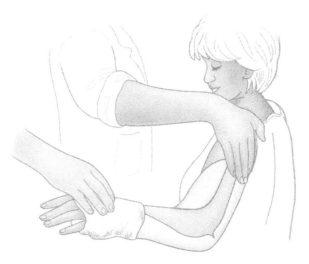

A. Apply a plaster slab over the volar and dorsal portion of the arm and forearm. The plaster slab should extend from the midarm to the dorsum of the hand, incorporating both the elbow and wrist joints. It is important that the volar (anterior) and dorsal (posterior) slabs do not meet to form a circumferential "cast." After measuring the slabs, place cotton roll on the undersurface and apply the plaster slab to the extremity. Use a small amount of gauze wrapping at the distal end of the splint to keep the slab in place during application. An assistant can hold the upper end.

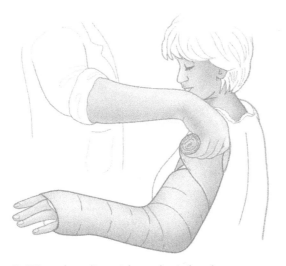

B. Wrap the splint with an elastic bandage.

A-11 SUGAR-TONG SPLINT

This splint is used in distal forearm fractures, especially fractures of the distal radius (Colles fracture). The forearm can be supinated or pronated during the application of the splint. A cotton bandage is first applied to the injured limb. Next, a single long plaster splint is applied by encircling the elbow.

The splint should extend from the metacarpophalangeal joint palmarly around the elbow to the dorsal aspect of the hand just proximal to the metacarpophalangeal joint. The excess plaster, created by encircling the elbow, is tucked. An elastic bandage holds the splints in position. The advantage of this splint is that it permits immobilization in a position of pronation or supination without a circumferential cast being applied to the extremity. A sling should be used with the splint (Video A-11).

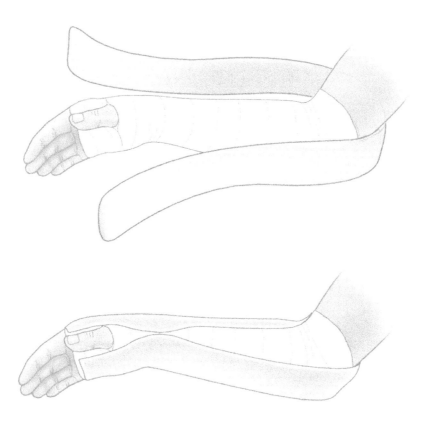

A-12 COAPTATION SPLINT

This splint is used for the acute management of humeral shaft fractures. Following the application of padding to protect the skin, the splint is applied to extend from the axilla, around the elbow, to above the shoulder. The arm is kept adducted, and the elbow is flexed 90 degrees. Elastic bandage is wrapped around the splint. The weight of this splint will aid in keeping the fracture aligned. For this reason, a collar and cuff is recommended over a traditional sling.

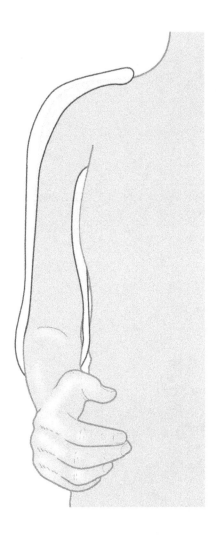

A-13 SLINGS

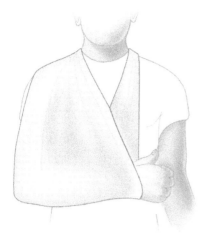

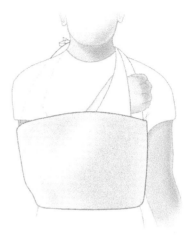

A. A commercial sling is used to support the arm for a number of injuries as discussed in the text.

C. A *stockinette Valpeau* and swathe (the component encircles the patient's waist) is used in situations where there is an unstable fracture of the proximal humerus, which has a tendency to displace due to contraction of the pectoralis major muscle. This position relaxes the pectoralis major.

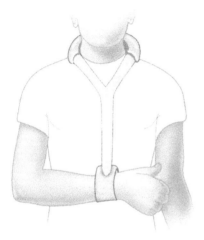

B. A *collar and cuff* is an alternate method used to support the forearm in patients with a humeral fracture treated with a coaptation splint.

LOWER EXTREMITY

A-14 POSTERIOR LEG SPLINT

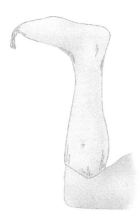

A. Stockinette is applied over the foot and ankle with the patient lying in the prone position.

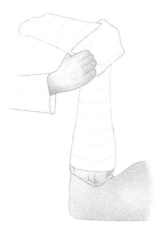

B. Next, cotton roll (Webril) is applied over the stockinette with extra padding applied over the malleoli and heel.

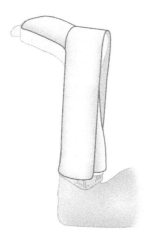

C. Premeasured plaster slab is applied from the base of the toes to just below the knee. For additional support, a U-shaped splint can be added.

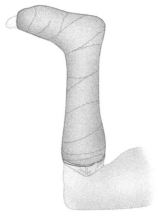

D. Finally, an elastic bandage is applied over the plaster splints. The ankle is held in a neutral position when treating ankle sprains or most fractures.

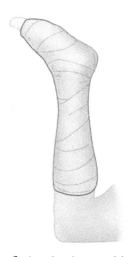

E. Ankle plantar flexion (equinus position) is used when treating Achilles tendon injuries (Video A–14).

A-15 JONES COMPRESSION DRESSING

A Jones compression dressing is used for soft-tissue injuries of the knee. This dressing provides immobilization of the limb while permitting some flexion and extension and provides a compressive force that limits swelling at the knee. The dressing is made by applying a layer of cotton bandage (Webril) extending from the groin to just above the malleoli of the ankle. After this, an elastic wrap is applied circumferentially. A second layer of cotton bandage is then applied followed by another elastic wrap. This additional layer provides added support that may or may not be necessary depending on the condition being treated (Video A-15).

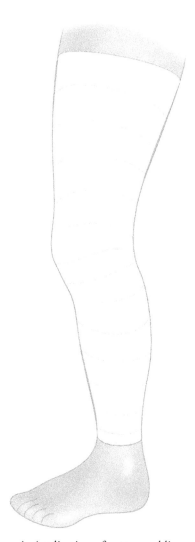

A. Application of cotton padding.

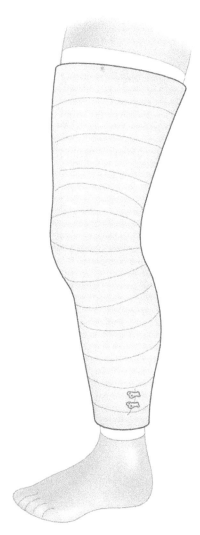

B. Elastic bandage.

A–16 KNEE IMMOBILIZER

This commercially available splint is used when ligamentous instability exists within the knee.

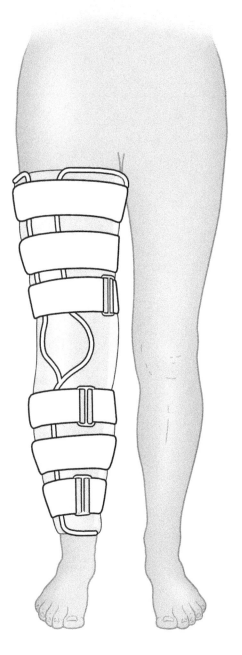

A–17 LONG-LEG POSTERIOR SPLINT

The long-leg posterior splint is used to immobilize fractures of the distal femur and tibia. The splint extends from the toes to the middle of the thigh. The ankle is kept at 90 degrees, and the knee is flexed 15 to 20 degrees.

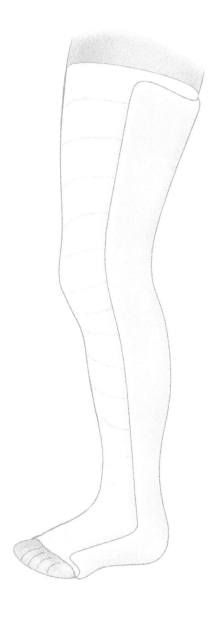

A-18 AIR STIRRUP ANKLE BRACE

This commercially available splint manufactured by Aircast (Summit, NJ) limits inversion and eversion of the ankle while allowing for normal ambulation. It is used for added support after the second- and third-degree ankle sprains.

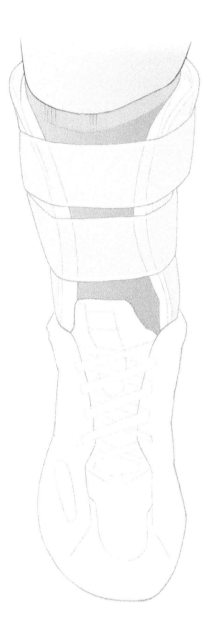

A–19 RADIOGRAPHIC VIEWS OF THE EXTREMITIES

Extremity	Standard Views	Additional Views
Hand	AP, lateral, oblique	
Wrist	AP, lateral, oblique (better visualization of the distal scaphoid and trapezium)	Scaphoid view (PA in ulnar deviation) Carpal tunnel view (axial view for hamate hook fractures) MDCT or MRI (occult carpal fractures, especially scaphoid)
Forearm	AP, lateral	
Elbow	AP, lateral, oblique (best view to see radial head/neck fractures)	
Arm	AP, lateral	
Shoulder	AP in external and internal rotation, scapular "Y" view	Axillary view (helpful for posterior shoulder dislocation)
Pelvis	AP	Judet views (oblique views for acetabular fractures) Inlet/outlet views (pelvic ring fractures) MDCT
Hip	AP, lateral (cross table; in the setting of possible fracture)	"Frog leg" lateral (if suspicion of slipped capital femoral epiphysis)
Thigh	AP, lateral	
Knee	AP, lateral, oblique (better visualization of tibial plateau and spine)	Axial sunrise or skyline view (slightly flexed knees with beam projected to foot; patella fractures) Tunnel view (best view of the intercondylar notch) MDCT (tibial plateau fractures)
Leg	AP, lateral	
Ankle	AP, lateral, mortise (15-degree internal rotation)	
Foot	AP, lateral, oblique	MDCT

AP, anteroposterior; MDCT, multi-detector computed tomography; MRI, magnetic resonance imaging; PA, posteroanterior.

A-20 IMMOBILIZATION OF VARIOUS EXTREMITY INJURIES

Injury	Immobilization
Distal phalanx fracture	Hairpin splint (A–1) or finger splint (A–2)
Mallet finger	Dorsal distal phalanx splint (extension) (A–1)
Jersey finger	Dorsal distal phalanx splint (flexion) (A–1)
Central slip rupture of extensor tendon	Dorsal splint of PIP joint in extension
Middle/proximal phalanx fracture	Finger splint (A–2) or gutter splint (A–3)
PIP or MCP dislocation	Finger splint or dynamic finger splint, if stable (A–2)
Hand infections	Universal hand dressing (A–5)
Ulnar collateral ligament (Gamekeeper's thumb)	Thumb spica splint (A–7)
Metacarpal fractures (4th/5th)	Ulnar gutter splint (A–3) or Dorsal splint with extension hood (A–4)
Metacarpal fractures (2nd/3rd)	Radial gutter splint (A–3) or Dorsal splint with extension hood (A–4)
Metacarpal fracture (1st)	Thumb spica splint (A–7)
Scaphoid fracture	Thumb spica splint (A–7)
Distal radius fracture	Sugar-tong splint (A–11)
Nightstick fracture	Long-arm posterior splint (A–9)
Radius/ulna fracture	Long-arm anterior–posterior splint (A–10)
Radial head/neck fracture	Long-arm posterior splint (A–9)
Elbow dislocation	Long-arm posterior splint (A–9)
Olecranon fracture	Long-arm posterior splint with 60-degree flexion (A–9)
Humeral shaft fracture	Coaptation splint (A–12)
Proximal humerus or clavicle fracture	Sling (A–13)
Shoulder dislocation	Sling and swathe (A–13) or shoulder immobilizer
Femoral neck/intertrochanteric fracture	Nonweight bearing and admit
Femur fracture	Long-leg posterior splint (A–17)
Patella fracture or dislocation	Knee immobilizer (A–16)
Ligamentous knee injury	Jones compression dressing (A–15)
Patella tendon or quadriceps rupture	Knee immobilizer (A–16)
Knee dislocation	Long-leg posterior splint (A–17)
Tibial plateau fracture	Long-leg posterior splint (A–17)
Tibia fracture	Long-leg posterior splint (A–17)
Ankle fracture	Posterior leg splint ± stirrup (A–14)
Achilles tendon rupture	Posterior leg splint with "gravity" plantar flexion (A–14)
Calcaneus fracture	Posterior leg splint (bulky dressing) (A–14)
Lisfranc fracture–dislocation	Posterior leg splint (A–14)
Metatarsal fractures	Posterior leg splint (A–14) with occasional use of hard-soled shoe (see text for details)
Ankle sprain	Elastic bandage or posterior leg splint (A–14)
Toe fracture	Hard-soled shoe with partner (buddy) tape

MCP, metacarpophalangeal; PIP, proximal interphalangeal.

A-21 SPLINT TREATMENT TABLE

Splint	Indications	Notes
Ulnar Gutter	4th/5th Metacarpal fractures (including boxer's fracture) 4th/5th phalangeal fractures	Padding between 4th and 5th digits MCP joints flexed 60–90 degrees
Radial Gutter	2nd/3rd Metacarpal fractures 2nd/3rd Phalangeal fractures	Must cut out hole for thumb MCP joints flexed 60–90 degrees
"Clam Digger"	Metacarpal and/or phalangeal fractures of 2nd–5th digits	Dorsal splint keeping MCP joints flexed to 90 degrees with wrist extended 20 degrees and PIP and DIP joints fully extended
Thumb Spica	Scaphoid fracture 1st Metacarpal or phalangeal fractures	Immobilizes IP of thumb, 1st MCP joint, wrist, and elbow Elbow immobilization takes away supination/pronation, which further immobilizes scaphoid Can use two slabs of fiberglass (pictured) or a single slab extending above elbow
Long Arm	Elbow fractures (most commonly supracondylar, olecranon, and radial head/neck)	Includes wrist and elbow
"Sugar Tong"	Distal radius fractures	Most commonly for Colles fractures (wrist in slight flexion and ulnar deviation) Elbow at 90 degrees
Coaptation	Humeral shaft fractures	Extends from axilla around to AC joint of the shoulder NOT the proper splint for proximal humerus fractures (sling)
Posterior Leg with "Stirrups"	Ankle fractures (distal fibula, bi- and trimalleolar fractures) Achilles tendon rupture	Simple posterior splint from toes to two-thirds of way up leg is sufficient for isolated distal fibula fractures (stable) If injury to both sides of ankle, add second "stirrup" slab from medial to lateral surfaces Ankle is immobilized at 90 degrees unless Achilles tendon rupture (slight plantar flexion)
Long Leg	Knee fractures (most commonly tibial plateau) Tibia fractures	Slight flexion of the knee Ankle at 90 degrees

AC, acromioclavicular; DIP, distal interphalangeal; IP, inter phalangeal; MCP, metacarpophalangeal; PIP, proximal interphalangeal.

INDEX

Note: Page numbers followed by t and f indicate tables and figures, respectively.

Printed in the USA
CPSIA information can be obtained
at www.ICGtesting.com
CBHW080753250624
10286CB00012B/55